Grainger & Allison's
Diagnostic Radiology
Essentials

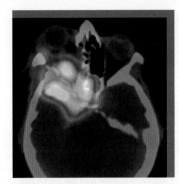

Second Edition

Grainger & Allison's
Diagnostic Radiology
Essentials

Lee Alexander Grant MBChB, BA(Oxon), MRCS, FRCR
Consultant Radiologist
The Royal Free NHS Foundation Trust
London, UK

Nyree Griffin MBChB(Hons), MD, MRCS, FRCR
Consultant Radiologist
Guy's and St Thomas' NHS Foundation Trust
London, UK

ELSEVIER

ELSEVIER

©2019 Elsevier Ltd. All rights reserved.
First edition 2013
Second edition 2019

ISBN: 978-0-7020-7311-3
E-ISBN: 978-0-323-56884-5

Printed in China
Last digit is the print number: 9 8 7 6 5 4 3 2 1

Content Strategist: Michael Houston
Content Development Specialist: Joanne Scott
Project Manager: Andrew Riley
Designer: Renee Duenow

Working together
to grow libraries in
developing countries

www.elsevier.com • www.bookaid.org

CONTENTS

CONTENTS

CONTENTS

PREFACE

This second edition of *Grainger & Allison's Diagnostic Radiology Essentials* is the culmination of one year's hard work on the part of the editors to update and extensively revise the original first edition. There are now new sections on functional imaging and interventional radiology as well as the latest 8th edition of TNM staging for cancers.

This book is based on the current sixth edition of *Grainger & Allison's Diagnostic Radiology*. Again, the overriding vision is to provide a unique single volume general radiology textbook, which attempts to encapsulate all the core information provided in its parent book, but presents it in an easy to read format. With this in mind, we have again made use of standardized headings throughout the book and have again directly linked images with the relevant text by placing them on the facing page. We have again made use of colour formatting throughout the book, to make it more accessible to the reader and facilitate quicker referencing. Inevitably due to limitations of space not every detail or as many figures could be included as we would have liked. However, we hope we have achieved, within space limitations, what we set out to do.

As with the first edition, the aim of this textbook is to provide as close as is possible a 'one-stop reference guide' for both trainees and practising consultants. Since the first edition was published we have continually received enthusiastic feedback from radiology trainees as to how this book has become an essential study aid in helping them successfully pass their FRCR part 2A examinations.

We are extremely grateful to Michael Houston for giving us the opportunity to build on the success of our first edition and the continuing support given to us by the editors of the *Grainger & Alison's Diagnostic Radiology* series. We would like to acknowledge the important groundwork that Joannah Duncan put in to creating the first edition, and single out Joanne Scott for special praise in working tirelessly with us in helping create this second updated and improved edition.

Lee Grant BA FRCR
Nyree Griffin MD FRCR
2018

ACKNOWLEDGEMENTS

Listed below are the sources for borrowed and adapted material. Due to space limitations within the book symbols have been used instead of full citations after figure and table legends. Below is a list of the symbols and their corresponding citations.

©1 Edey AJ, Hansell DM. Incidentally detected small pulmonary nodules on CT. Clinical Radiology 2009;64: 872–884

©2 Hansell DM, Lynch D, McAdams HP, Bankier AA. Imaging of diseases of the chest. Mosby, 2009

©10 O'Connor JH, Cohen J. Dating fractures. In: Kleinman PK (ed). Diagnostic imaging of child abuse. Williams & Wilkins, 1987, p.112

©11 Kleinman PK (ed). Diagnostic imaging of child abuse. Williams & Wilkins, 1998, p.179

©12 Chapman S, Nakielny R. Aids to radiological differential diagnosis, 4th edn. Saunders, 2003

©13 Abrams HL, Sprio R, Goldstein N. Metstases in carcinoma. Analysis of 1000 autopsied cases. Cancer 1950;3:74–85

©20 Gore RM, Levine MS. Textbook of gastrointestinal radiology. Saunders/Elsevier, 2007

©21 Lim JS, Yun MJ, Kim MJ, et al. CT and PET in stomach cancer: preoperative staging and monitoring of response therapy. RadioGraphics 2006;26(1): 143–156

©24 Slovis TL. Caffey's pediatric diagnostic imaging, 11th edn. Elsevier, 2008

©27 De Bruyn R. Paediatric ultrasound: how, why and when, 2nd edn. Elsevier/Churchill Livingstone, 2010

©28 Bates J. Abdominal ultrasound: how, why and when. Churchill Livingstone, 2011

©30 Turgut AT, Altin L, Topcu S, et al. Unusual imaging characteristics of complicated hydatid disease. European Journal of Radiology 2007;63(1):84–93

©31 Parizel PM, Makkat S, Van Miert E, et al. Intracranial hemorrhage: principles of CT and MRI interpretation. European Radiology 2001;11:1770–1783

©32 Eisenhauer EA, Therasse P, Bogaerts J, et al. New response evaluation criteria in solid tumours: revised RECIST guideline (version 1.1). European Journal of Cancer 2009;45(2);228–247

©33 Royal College of Radiologists; Standards for intravascular contrast agent administration to adult patients, 2nd edn. The Royal College of Radiologists, April 2010

©34 El-Khoury GY, Bennett DL, Stanley MD. Essentials of MSK imaging, 1st edn. Churchill Livingstone, 2002

©35 Pope T, Morrison WB, Bloem HL, et al. Imaging of the musculoskeletal system. Saunders, 2008

* Adam A, Dixon AK, Grainger RG, Allison DJ. Grainger & Allison's diagnostic radiology, 5th edn. Churchill Livingstone, 2007

** Adam A, Dixon AK, Gillard JH, Schaefer-Prokop CM. Grainger and Allison's Diagnostic Radiology 6th edition, Elsevier, 2015

† Sutton D. Textbook of radiology and imaging, 7th edn. Churchill Livingstone, 1998

‡ McLoud T. Thoracic radiology: The requisites. Mosby, 1998

¶ Middleton WD, Kurtz AB, Hertzberg BS. Ultrasound: The requisites. Mosby, 2004

¶¶ Kaufman J, Lee M. Vascular and interventional radiology: The requisites. Mosby, 2003

§ Blickman J, Parker B, Barnes P. Pediatric radiology: The requisites. Mosby, 2009

§§ Ziessman HA, O'Malley JP, Thrall JH. Nuclear medicine: The requisites. Mosby, 2006

∫ Zagoria R. Genitourinary radiology: The requisites. Mosby, 2004

∫∫ Weissleder R, Wittenberg J, Harisinghani M, Chen J. Primer of diagnostic imaging, 4th edn. Mosby, 2007

• Miller S. Cardiac imaging: The requisites. Mosby, 2004

•• Halpert R. Gastrointestinal imaging: The requisites, 3rd edn. Mosby, 2006

+ Grossman R, Yousem D. Neuroradiology: The requisites. Mosby, 2003

++ Soto J, Lucey B. Emergency radiology: The requisites. Mosby, 2009

■ Naidich T, Castillo M, Cha S, Raybaud C, Kollias S, Smirniotopoulos J. Imaging of the Spine. Saunders, 2011

SECTION 1

CHEST

1.1 CHEST WALL AND PLEURA

RIB LESIONS

Benign

Congenital abnormalities The upper ribs are commonly bifid, splayed, fused, or hypoplastic ▶ they are occasionally associated with syndromes (e.g. basal cell naevus syndrome) or other anomalies (e.g. Sprengel's deformity)
- *Cervical rib:* this arises from C7 (affecting 1–2% of the population) and consists of an initially downward sloping rib just lateral to the spine (cf. an initially upward sloping normal rib) ▶ it can cause a thoracic outlet syndrome and is often bilateral and asymmetrical

Callus Post fracture this can mimic an intrapulmonary opacity

Rib notching This is due to external pressure on a rib (e.g. coarctation of the aorta, neurofibromatosis type I (NF2))

Benign primary tumours These are infrequent ▶ they are most commonly cartilaginous tumours (e.g. a chondroma or osteochondroma) ▶ they are predominantly found in an anterior location and may show characteristic cartilaginous calcification

Other benign rib lesions Fibrous dysplasia ▶ histiocytosis X ▶ haemangioma ▶ aneurysmal bone cyst

Aggressive

Destructive rib lesions These are most commonly an osteomyelitis or a neoplastic disease
- *Malignant rib tumours:* these are commonly metastatic deposits or myeloma ▶ primary malignant tumours are rare (but usually a chondrosarcoma)
- *Osteomyelitis:* this is uncommon ▶ it may be due to haematogenous spread (e.g. staphylococcal or tuberculous), or it may be caused by direct spread from the lung or pleural space (e.g. actinomycosis)

Bronchial carcinoma (including pancoast's tumours) These can spread from the lung to a rib ▶ MRI can determine the extent of a Pancoast's tumour (and assess the relationship between the tumour and the plexus brachialis)

DIFFERENTIAL OF RIB NOTCHING

Inferior rib notching	**Arterial:** Coarctation of the aorta, aortic thrombosis, subclavian obstruction, any cause of pulmonary oligaemia **Venous:** Superior vena cava obstruction **Arteriovenous:** Pulmonary arteriovenous malformation, chest wall arterial malformation **Neurogenic:** Neurofibromatosis (ribbon ribs)
Superior rib notching	**Connective tissue diseases:** Rheumatoid arthritis, SLE, Sjögren's, scleroderma **Metabolic:** Hyperparathyroidism **Miscellaneous:** Neurofibromatosis, restrictive lung disease, poliomyelitis, Marfan's syndrome, osteogenesis imperfecta, progeria
©12	

CLAVICLES

Definition Together with the spine the medial clavicular heads can assess rotation ▶ the joints at both ends are synovial and may be eroded in any synovitis appearing more ill defined (e.g. rheumatoid arthritis, hyperparathyroidism)

Pearl Neoplasms of the clavicle are usually malignant (myeloma or metastatic)
- Other primary tumours/tumour-like conditions:
  - Osteosarcoma ▶ Ewing's sarcoma ▶ post radiation sarcoma ▶ aneurysmal bone cyst ▶ histiocytosis X ▶ intersternocostoclavicular hyperostosis

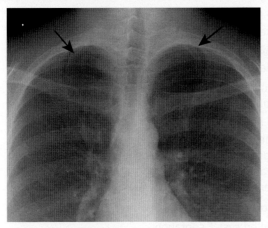

Cervical ribs. Bilateral downsloping cervical ribs (arrows).

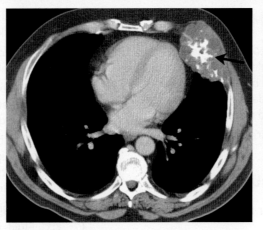

Axial CT. Chondrosarcoma of an anterior left rib demonstrating a large soft tissue component with internal punctuate calcification (arrow).

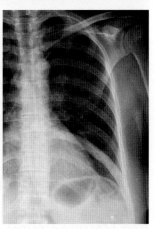

Fibrous dysplasia in a rib. CXR detail of the left lung. Compared with the other ribs the 9th rib shows an increase in density and is slightly broadened.*

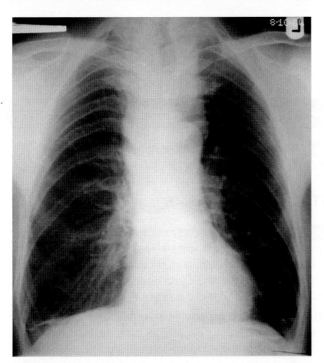

Chest radiograph in a patient with coarctation. There is rib notching and enlargement of the left subclavian artery, causing a '3' sign.

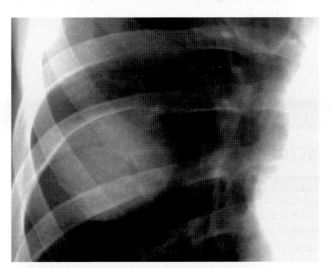

Neurofibromatosis type 1 (NF-1): skeletal findings. Pressure erosion of a rib due to a neurofibroma. (Most rib deformities in NF-1 are due to the skeletal dysplasia, not pressure erosion.)

SOFT TISSUE LESIONS

POLAND'S SYNDROME

Definition An autosomal condition where there is unilateral absence or hypoplasia of the pectoralis major muscle ▶ it is accompanied by ipsilateral hand and arm anomalies (particularly syndactyly), rib anomalies and hypoplasia of the breast and nipple

CXR Unilateral lung transradiancy and an abnormal anterior axillary fold

SOFT TISSUE TUMOURS

Benign (rib separation or notch-like remodelling from pressure erosion)

Lipoma The most common benign chest wall tumour

CT A low-density well-demarcated homogeneous mass (−90 to −150HU) ▶ soft tissue components suggest a liposarcoma

MRI T1WI: high SI ▶ T2WI: intermediate SI (and low SI with fat suppression)

Neurofibroma Rib splaying and pressure erosion ▶ widened intervertebral foramina

CT Lower density than muscle before and after IV contrast medium

MRI T1WI: low to intermediate SI ▶ T2WI: high SI ▶ T1WI + Gad: marked contrast enhancement

Haemangiomas An uncommon anterior mediastinal lesion (± phleboliths)

CT A smooth, sharp, lobulated mass with central heterogeneous enhancement ▶ there may be bone remodelling and hypertrophy

MRI The best investigation for delineating its extent ▶ there are signal inhomogeneities generated by vessels, soft tissue and haemorrhage
- T1WI: intermediate SI ▶ T2WI: high SI

Lymphangiomas

CT Fluid-filled cyst ± septation

MRI Features of a cyst with a low protein content

Malignant (bony destruction)
- Malignant primary chest wall tumours are rare ▶ the most common are lipo- or fibrosarcomas
- Secondary tumours of the chest wall are common, particularly if there is local tumour spread (e.g. carcinoma of the breast and lung)

STERNAL LESIONS

PECTUS EXCAVATUM

Definition A depressed sternum resulting in the anterior ribs projecting more anteriorly than the sternum (funnel chest) ▶ it may be an isolated abnormality or associated with other disorders such as Marfan's syndrome or congenital heart disease (particularly an ASD)

CXR The condition is best assessed on a lateral CXR ▶ PA CXR: leftward shift of the heart ▶ straightening of the left heart border with prominence of the main pulmonary artery segment ▶ an indistinct right heart border simulating middle lobe disease (the sternum replaces aerated lung at the right heart border) ▶ a steep inferior slope of the anterior ribs ▶ undue clarity of the lower dorsal spine seen through the heart

Pearl Pigeon chest (pectus carinatum): the reverse deformity, which may be congenital or acquired

STERNAL NEOPLASMS

Definition These are usually malignant: myeloma ▶ chondrosarcoma ▶ lymphoma ▶ metastatic carcinoma
- The most common benign tumour is a chondroma
- Relevant non-neoplastic processes: osteomyelitis ▶ histiocytosis X ▶ Paget's disease ▶ fibrous dysplasia

CT This is the recommended investigation: it eliminates any overlapping structures, detects bony destruction and allows imaging of the adjacent soft tissues

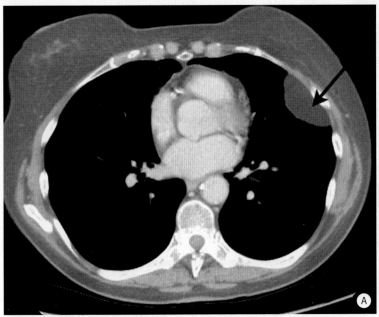
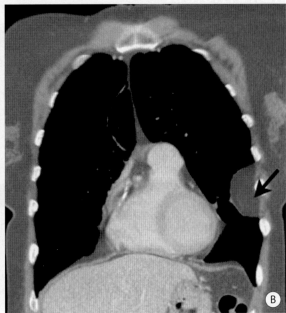

Axial (A) and coronal (B) CT images of a chest wall lipoma.

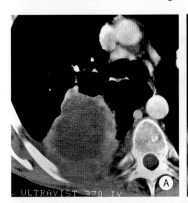
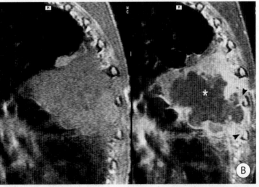

Invasive malignant T-cell lymphoma. (A) CECT. Enhancing peripheral tumour tissue is widely invading the posterior chest wall. (B) Sagittal T1WI (left) and T1WI + Gad (right) demonstrating the widespread invasion of the posterior chest wall by enhancing tumour tissue. There is invasion of 2 ribs, including cortical rib destruction (arrowheads). The central non-enhancement of the tumour is due to necrosis (asterisk).*

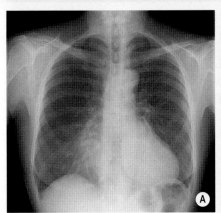
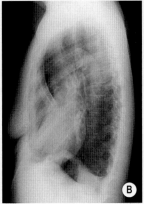
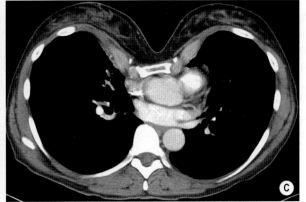

Depressed sternum. (A) PA CXR. The depressed sternum displaces the heart to the left and rotates it so that the left heart border adopts a straight configuration. The ill-defined right heart border simulates middle lobe collapse. Horizontal (posterior) and steeply oblique (anterior) ribs. (B) Lateral CXR demonstrates posterior sternal displacement. (C) Axial CT.*

PLEURAL THICKENING AND FIBROTHORAX

DEFINITION

- Pleural thickening usually represents an organized end stage of infective or non-infective inflammation
- If generalized and gross it is termed a fibrothorax and may cause significant ventilatory impairment
  - *Common causes:* empyema ▶ tuberculosis ▶ haemorrhagic effusions
  - Extensive calcification favours TB or empyema

RADIOLOGICAL FEATURES

XR Fixed shadowing (water density) located within the dependent parts of the pleural cavity ▶ costophrenic angle blunting is common

- *In profile:* it appears as band of soft tissue density (up to 10 mm thick) parallel to the chest wall and with a sharp lung interface
- *En face:* it appears as an ill-defined veil-like shadowing
- *Fibrothorax:* a smooth uninterrupted pleural density extending over at least $\frac{1}{4}$ of the chest wall

US A homogeneous echogenic layer just inside the chest wall ▶ US is only reliable if this is > 1 cm thick

CT The most sensitive modality ▶ pleural thickening is seen particularly on the medial rib aspect

- *Fibrothorax:* pleural thickening (> 3 mm) extending > 8 cm (craniocaudal) or > 5 cm (laterally)

MRI Low SI is a reliable indicator of benign pleural disease

PEARLS

- Extensive pleural calcification favours previous tuberculosis or empyema ▶ an asbestos-related fibrothorax is usually bilateral and rarely calcified

Apical pleural CAP Unilateral or bilateral fibrous pleural thickening is common in the apical pleural cupola (with an unknown aetiology but which may be secondary to TB or because the apices are relatively ischaemic areas of lung) ▶ it should be distinguished from a Pancoast's tumour (if in doubt perform a CT or MRI)

Asbestos exposure This can induce fibrous pleural thickening ▶ it can be diffuse but is more often multifocal

and often calcified ▶ it is most commonly found along the lower thorax and diaphragmatic pleura

CXR Calcified plaques may have a 'holly leaf' configuration when viewed *en face*

CT Circumscribed areas of pleural thickening separated from an underlying rib and extrapleural soft tissues by a thin layer of fat ▶ they may be calcified

LOCALIZED FIBROUS TUMOUR (LOCALIZED MESOTHELIOMA)

DEFINITION

- A localized fibrous tumour of the pleura ($\frac{2}{3}$ are benign) ▶ there is no relation to previous asbestos exposure

CLINICAL PRESENTATION

- It presents in middle age and 50% are asymptomatic
- Hypertrophic osteoarthropathy is a well-recognized complication (10–30%) ▶ it uncommonly produces hypoglycaemia

RADIOLOGICAL FEATURES

CXR A pleurally based, well-demarcated, slightly lobulated mass ▶ there can be marked positional variation with postural change (as it may be pedunculated) ▶ it can be massive (measuring up to 10-20 cm, with malignant tumours usually > 10 cm)

CT A heterogeneous mass (necrosis or haemorrhage) ▶ it frequently enhances but is rarely calcified

MRI T1WI / T2WI: low SI

PEARLS

- The visceral pleura is more commonly involved
- The invasive form only grows locally (cf. a malignant mesothelioma)
- Pleural fibromas usually make an obtuse angle with the chest wall (extra pulmonary origin)
- Rarely arise within a fissure

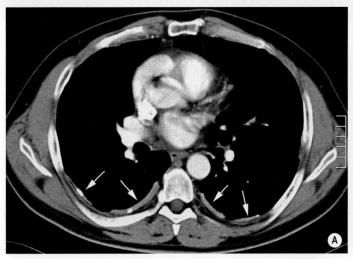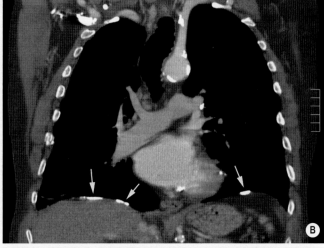

Pleural plaques caused by asbestos exposure. (A) Axial and (B) coronal CT. Pleural plaques are most commonly found along the lower thorax and on the diaphragmatic pleura (arrows). They can partially or completely calcify or ossify.*

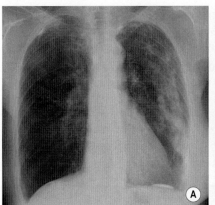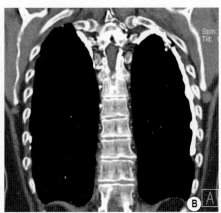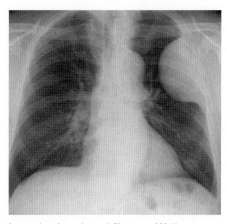

Pleural calcification. (A) On the CXR an extensive sheet-like calcification of the left pleura is seen together with focal calcifications of the diaphragmatic pleura. (B) CT demonstrates the extent and thickness of the pleural calcification.**

Large benign pleural fibroma. Well demarcated and homogeneneous mass making an obtuse angle with the chest wall. **

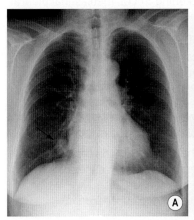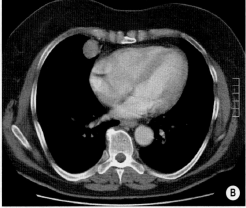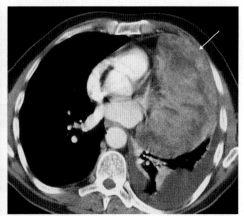

Benign pleural fibroma. (A) PA CXR demonstrating a small well-demarcated, homogeneous, slightly lobulated mass (arrow). (B) CT shows that the mass is pleurally based, sharply defined and slightly enhancing.*

Malignant fibrous tumour of pleura. Note the pleural effusion and the local invasion of the chest wall (arrow).

MALIGNANT MESOTHELIOMA

DEFINITION

- A rare primary pleural neoplasm strongly related to prior asbestos exposure (particularly crocidolite and amosite fibres)
- It predominantly involves the parietal pleura ▶ it can also involve the abdominal peritoneal lining

CLINICAL PRESENTATION

- Chest wall pain, dyspnoea and weight loss ▶ 4M:1F
- There is a latency period of 20–40 years post exposure ▶ it is associated with a poor prognosis

RADIOLOGICAL FEATURES

- It is radiographically indistinguishable from pleural metastases

XR Irregular nodular pleural thickening that is almost always associated with a pleural effusion (which is often haemorrhagic) ▶ it is usually confined to one hemithorax

CT Circumferential nodular pleural thickening (>1 cm) extending into the fissures or over the mediastinal surface, it can invade the chest wall ▶ there may be low attenuation necrotic areas present ▶ Metastatic mediastinal nodes in up to 50%

- *Lung encasement and volume loss:* there is a relative absence of any mediastinal shift even if there is a large effusion due to fixation of the mediastinum by tumour
- Previous evidence of asbestos exposure (e.g. calcified pleural plaques) is usually *absent*

MRI This is superior in assessing any mediastinal and chest wall involvement

- T1WI/T2WI: slightly greater SI than muscle

FDG PET Increased uptake (not tumour specific)

PEARLS

- **Diagnosis:** percutaneous needle biopsy (US or CT guidance)

PERICARDIAL MALIGNANT MESOTHELIOMA

- The most common primary pericardial malignancy (with a possible asbestos link) ▶ it presents with a haemorrhagic effusion (+/− cardiac tamponade)

CT/MRI A well-defined single mass, multiple nodules or diffuse plaques wrapping around the heart and great vessels

PLEURAL METASTASES

DEFINITION

- Malignant pleural disease due to haematogenous spread from primary tumour elsewhere ▶ occasionally it is from direct seeding (e.g. malignant thymoma)
- This is the most common pleural neoplasm (and is more common than a mesothelioma)
- It is usually an adenocarcinoma
- Primary tumour is often lung, breast, lymphoma, ovary, stomach

CLINICAL PRESENTATION

- Chest wall pain, dyspnoea

RADIOLOGICAL FEATURES

CT There are usually multiple foci but there can be diffuse tumoural pleural thickening extending into the fissures (mimicking a mesothelioma) ▶ it is often accompanied by a pleural effusion ▶ pleural thickening is often lobulated

- Signs suggesting malignancy: circumferential thickening, nodularity, parietal thickening >1 cm, mediastinal pleural involvement

MRI DWI and DCE MRI may aid differentiation

FDG PET Increased uptake in malignant disease, but it is not completely tumor specific with uptake in some benign inflammatory lesions.

PEARLS

- Metastatic disease to the pleura is the second most common cause of a pleural effusion in patients >50 years (after congestive heart failure)
- It is the commonest cause of a pleural exudate

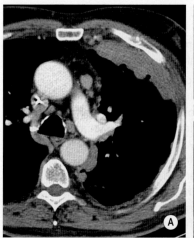

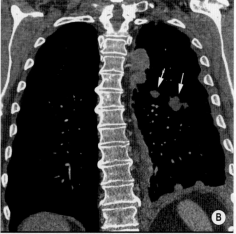

Malignant mesothelioma. (A, B: axial and coronal CT). Diffuse lobulated and nodular thickening of the pleura with tumour extension into the lobar fissure (arrows). Note the metastatic hilar and mediastinal adenopathy.*

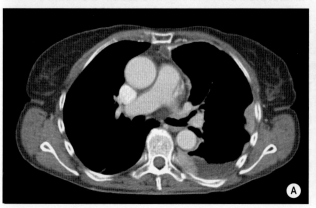

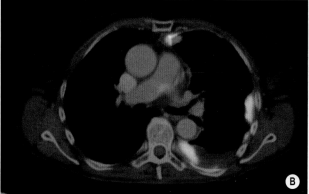

Malignant mesothelioma. CT and PET-CT fusion image showing tumour extent.**

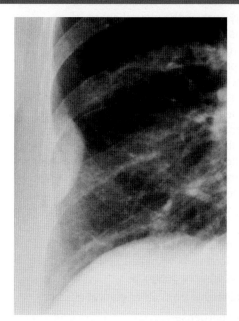

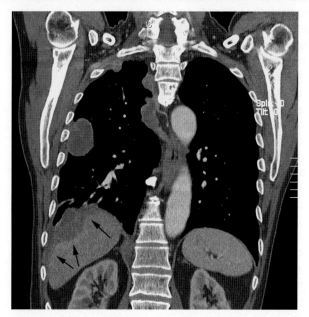

Pleural metastasis from carcinoma of uterus. This case is unusual in that the lesion is solitary and no pleural effusion is present.

Malignant pleural thickening caused by metastatic pleural disease. Note the compression on the right hemidiaphragm and the extension of the tumour into the liver (arrows).*

PLEURAL EFFUSION

Definition

- Accumulation of fluid within the pleural space
  - **Transudate:** the rate of pleural fluid accumulation exceeds resorption, leading to a plasma ultrafiltrate (with a low protein content)
    - *Causes:* cardiac failure ▶ lymphatic obstruction
  - **Exudate:** increased pleural permeability leads to the accumulation of proteinaceous pleural fluid
    - *Causes:* neoplasia (including metastases and mesothelioma) ▶ pleural inflammation ▶ infection (parapneumonic effusions) ▶ collagen vascular disease ▶ pulmonary embolism
  - **Additional causes of a pleural effusion:** cytotoxic drugs ▶ cirrhosis (with transdiaphragmatic passage of ascites + hypoalbuminaemia) ▶ renal disease (uraemia) ▶ immunocompromise ▶ a subphrenic abscess (which is often accompanied by basal atelectasis, consolidation and a subdiaphragmatic air-fluid level)

Radiological features

XR All types of simple pleural effusion are radiographically identical

- *Small effusions:*
  - Lateral decubitus CXR: this can detect as little as 10 ml of fluid
  - Lateral CXR: blunting of the posterior angles (approximately 50 ml)
  - PA CXR: blunting of the lateral costophrenic angles (200–500 ml)
- *Larger effusions:* homogeneous opacification of the lower chest with obliteration of the costophrenic angle and hemidiaphragm ▶ a superior meniscus (concave to the lung and higher laterally)
- *Massive effusions:* dense opacification of the hemithorax with contralateral mediastinal shift (unless there is associated obstructive collapse of the ipsilateral lung or extensive pleural malignancy) ▶ it may cause diaphragmatic inversion (particularly on the left as there is no liver support)
- *Localized subpulmonary effusion:* a 'high hemidiaphragm' with a contour that peaks more laterally than usual – the straight medial segment falls rapidly away to the costophrenic angle laterally ▶ separation of the gastric bubble from the diaphragm
- *Supine position:* generalized 'veil-like' haze with no meniscus present ▶ preserved lung vascular markings
- *Loculated effusion:* Fluid collecting between pleural layers ▶ a lenticular configuration with smooth margins ▶ usually there are additional clues indicating additional pleural disease

US Pleural fluid is usually echo-free with a highly echogenic line at the fluid–lung interface ▶ exudative and haemorrhagic effusions may be echogenic (homogeneous, complex or septated) and are often accompanied by pleural thickening

- Fluid bronchograms and vessels on Doppler examination will identify consolidation

CT A pleural effusion appears as a dependent sickle-shaped opacity of low attenuation ▶ CT characterizes the morphology of any pleural thickening that may accompany an effusion (nodular malignant or uniform benign) ▶ it identifies any causative underlying disease ▶ it can distinguish between free and loculated fluid (but cannot distinguish between a transudate or exudate)

- *Pleural lesions:* these make an obtuse angle with the chest wall (cf. intrapulmonary lesions which make an acute angle with the chest wall)
- *Parietal pleural thickening:* this usually indicates a pleural exudate
- *Liver interface:* this is indistinct with pleural fluid, but sharp with ascites

Pearls

- **Right-sided effusion:** this is associated with ascites, heart failure and liver abscesses
- **Left-sided effusion:** this is associated with pancreatitis (with a high pleural fluid amylase level), pericardial disease, oesophageal rupture and aortic dissection
- **Bilateral pleural effusions:** these tend to be transudates and are secondary to generalized changes affecting both pleural cavities (e.g. uraemia or the nephrotic syndrome)
- **Massive effusions:** these are often due to malignant disease (particularly lung or breast metastases) but can also occur with heart failure, cirrhosis, TB and trauma
- **Empyema:** a collection of pus within a naturally existing anatomical cavity such as the pleural space (cf. an abscess, which is a collection of pus in a newly formed cavity) ▶ this commonly follows a pneumonia and associated parapneumonic effusion
- **Bronchopleural fistula:** a communication with the pleural space via the proximal airways (cf. distal air spaces with a pneumothorax) ▶ this occurs following lung resection or a necrotizing infection
- **Chylothorax:** milky chylous effusions (containing triglycerides) following thoracic duct rupture or seepage from any collaterals ▶ high protein content prevents expected reduction in attenuation

  MRI T1WI: this may demonstrate high SI (due to a high protein content)

- **Haemothorax:** this demonstrates a tendency for loculation if the blood clots with pleural thickening and calcification as recognized sequelae

  CXR Indistinguishable from other pleural effusions

  CT It may be hyperdense

  MRI T1WI / T2WI: high SI (if subacute or chronic with a possible haemosiderin low SI rim)

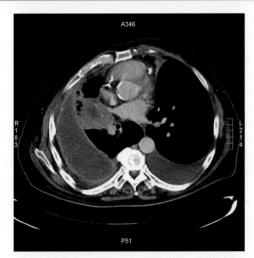

Empyema. CECT shows a thickened and enhanced smooth pleura in keeping with an empyema. Contrast this with the simple left pleural effusion.**

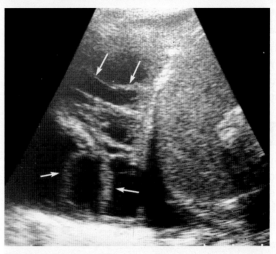

US of an empyema. The pleural fluid is separated by septa (arrows). Although the pleural fluid is echo-free in part, some areas return echoes owing to the turbid nature of the empyema fluid.*

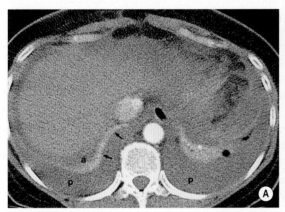

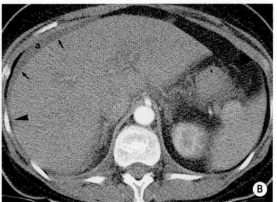

CT signs which may differentiate pleural effusion and ascites. Scans through lower thorax/upper abdomen in patient with bilateral pleural effusions and ascites. (A) *Displaced crus sign*: The right pleural effusion collects posterior to the right crus of the diaphragm (arrows) and displaces it anteriorly. *Diaphragm sign:* The pleural fluid (p) is over the outer surface of the dome of the diaphragm, whereas the ascitic fluid (a) is within the dome. (B) *Interface sign:* The interface (arrows) between the liver and ascites is usually sharper than between liver and pleural fluid. *Bare area sign:* Peritoneal reflections prevent ascitic fluid from extending over the entire posterior surface of the liver (arrowhead), in contrast to pleural fluid in the posterior costophrenic recess.†

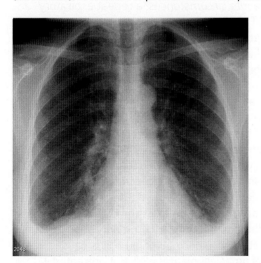

Bilateral pleural effusions. Erect CXR. The pleural effusion obscures the diaphragm and both costophrenic angles. It has a curvilinear upper margin concave to lung and is higher laterally than medially.*

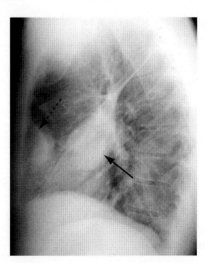

Encapsulated fluid on a lateral CXR. Pleural fluid is encapsulated in the major fissure (arrows) and against the anterior chest wall (dotted arrow). These encysted fluid collections can mimic a lung tumour.*

PNEUMOTHORAX

DEFINITION

- Air within the pleural space – if liquid is present the nomenclature depends on the relative volumes and liquid type: (hydro-, haemo-, pyo-, chylo-) pneumothorax

CLINICAL PRESENTATION

- Sudden dyspnoea ▶ chest pain
- Adhesions can limit collapse but may also account for continued air leakage from the lung surface, and can bleed if teared ▶ appear as straight band shadows extending from the lung to chest wall

Causes of a secondary adult pneumothorax*	
Airflow obstruction	Asthma Chronic obstructive pulmonary disease (COPD) Cystic fibrosis
Pulmonary infection	Cavitary pneumonia Tuberculosis Fungal disease AIDS Pneumatocele
Pulmonary infarction	
Neoplasm	Metastatic osteosarcoma
Diffuse lung disease	Histiocytosis X Lymphangioleiomyomatosis Fibrosing alveolitis Other diffuse fibroses
Hereditable disorders of fibrous connective tissue	Marfan's syndrome
Endometriosis	
Catamenial pneumothorax: pleural endometrial deposits leading to recurrent pneumothoraces associated with the menses	
Traumatic, noniatrogenic	
Ruptured oesophagus/trachea	
Closed chest trauma (± rib fractures)	
Penetrating chest trauma	
Traumatic, iatrogenic	
Thoracotomy/thoracocentesis	
Percutaneous biopsy	
Tracheostomy	
Central venous catheterization	

RADIOLOGICAL FEATURES

Typical CXR signs A separate visceral pleural line from the chest wall commonly seen at the lung apex (erect CXR) ▶ a transradiant zone devoid of vessels lateral to the pleural line ▶ it may be more evident on expiratory films (due to an increased relative size of the pleural space)

- Skin folds can cause diagnostic problems (particularly in neonates and the elderly)

Supine pneumothorax Pleural air rises and collects anteriorly (particularly medially and basally) with no obvious lung edge visible

  CXR Ipsilateral lung transradiancy ▶ a deep lateral finger-like costophrenic sulcus ▶ a transradiant band parallel to the diaphragm or mediastinum ▶ undue clarity of the mediastinal border ▶ diaphragmatic depression

- 'Double diaphragm' sign: visualization of the undersurface of the heart (visible anterior costophrenic recess)

Tension pneumothorax A life-threatening complication present when the intrapleural pressure is positive relative to the atmospheric pressure (air can enter but not leave the pleural space) ▶ the mediastinal displacement can have an adverse effect on gas exchange and cardiovascular performance with a rapid clinical deterioration

  CXR Absent lung markings on the affected side ▶ moderate or gross mediastinal displacement away from the side of the pneumothorax ▶ eversion of the diaphragm

- The diagnosis is made clinically and a CXR should not usually be performed

PEARLS

- A pneumothorax can be confirmed with a lateral decubitus view or a supine decubitus projection (immobile patients)
  - *Indeterminate circumstances:* a repeat expiratory CXR or CT
- A haemopneumothorax is a common complication of a traumatic pneumothorax
- Re-expansion oedema can follow rapid therapeutic lung expansion
- **Features that help identify artefacts and skin folds:**
  - Extension of the 'pneumothorax' line beyond the margin of the chest cavity ▶ laterally located vessels ▶ an orientation of a line that is inconsistent with the edge of a slightly collapsed lung ▶ a skin fold margin tends to be much wider than the normally thin visceral pleural line
- **Primary spontaneous pneumothorax (PSP):** the most common adult pneumothorax (commonly seen in young males with otherwise normal lungs) ▶ it is caused by rupture of an apical pleural bleb ▶ if untreated it commonly recurs on the same side

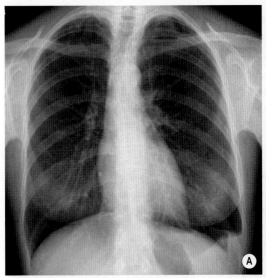

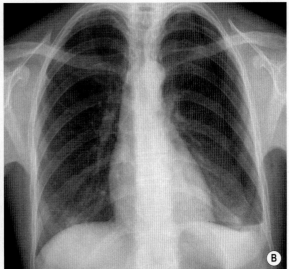

Left primary spontaneous pneumothorax. CXR (A) at deep inspiration and (B) deep expiration. The pneumothorax is accentuated on the CXR at suspended deep expiration (B).*

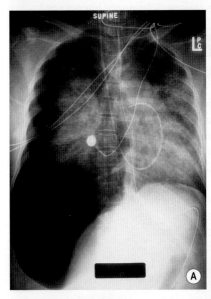

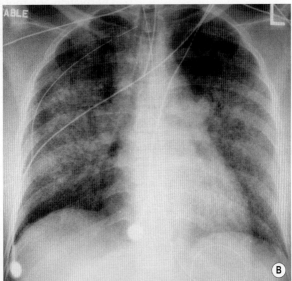

(A) Tension pneumothorax following a transbronchial lung biopsy. There is inversion of the right hemidiaphragm, and deviation of the mediastinum to the opposite side. (B) Following insertion of a right-sided chest drain the diaphragm and mediastinum have returned to a normal position. The diffuse bilateral infiltrate is due to pre-existing pulmonary haemorrhage.†

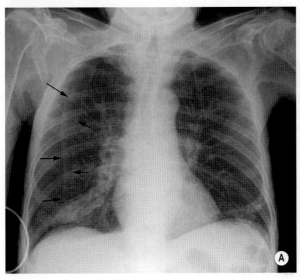

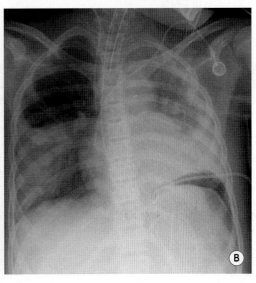

(A) Skin fold mimicking a right pneumothorax: laterally located blood vessels, margin of the lines, inconsistent orientation of the lines with the edge of a collapsed lung. (B) Supine pneumothorax. Increased transradiation at the left base and the costophrenic sulcus laterally is more pronounced ('sulcus' sign).**

DIAPHRAGMATIC HERNIA/EVENTRATION

DEFINITION

- **Hernia:** intrathoracic movement of the abdominal contents through a diaphragmatic defect
  - The diaphragm initially develops as an incomplete septum – the septum is derived from several separate elements which fuse between the 6th and 7th weeks of gestation to close the posterolateral diaphragmatic defects that are initially present
  - *Bochdalek hernia:* the most common type (70%) ▶ this occupies a posterolateral location through the pleuroperitoneal foramen
  - *Morgagni hernia:* anterior herniation through the formamen of Morgagni ▶ this usually presents later in childhood or adult life
- **Eventration:** part of the normal diaphragm is replaced by a thin layer of connective tissue and a few muscle fibres (the unbroken continuity differentiates this from a hernia) ▶ it also includes elevation as a result of acquired paralysis and associated muscular atrophy

CLINICAL PRESENTATION

- Asymptomatic in an adult ▶ respiratory distress in the newborn

RADIOLOGICAL FEATURES

Adults

Bochdalek (posterior) hernia A defect through the pleuroperitoneal foramen, the majority are left sided ▶ it usually contains retroperitoneal fat, kidney or spleen

CXR A well-defined, dome-shaped, soft tissue opacity midway between the spine and lateral chest wall (PA) ▶ a focal bulge 4–5 cm anterior to the posterior diaphragmatic insertion (lateral CXR)

CT/MRI A soft tissue mass protruding through the posteromedial aspect of either hemidiaphragm

Morgagni (anterior) hernia

CXR/CT An opacity at the right cardiophrenic angle frequently containing omentum or gut ▶ it demonstrates a smooth, well-defined margin and its soft tissue radiodensity allows differentiation from a fat pad collection (although it is more difficult to differentiate from a pericardial cyst)

Paediatric

Antenatal US This allows a diagnosis to be made

CXR An opaque hemithorax with mediastinal deviation away from the lesion ▶ once the GI tract begins to fill with air, radiolucencies will be seen within the affected hemithorax with progressive mediastinal deviation ▶ a NGT can determine the position of the stomach (an intrathoracic stomach is associated with earlier herniation and more severe pulmonary hypoplasia)

PEARLS

- **Total eventration:** this demonstrates a left-sided predominance
- **Localized eventration:** this predominantly affects the anteromedial right hemidiaphragm
- **Neonatal diaphragmatic hernia:** this can be compounded by severe respiratory difficulties secondary to any associated pulmonary hypoplasia, persistent fetal circulation and a degree of surfactant deficiency ▶ malrotation and small bowel malfixation are also associated problems
  - *Treatment:* surgical repair

Causes of bilateral symmetrical elevation of the diaphragm
Supine position
Poor inspiration
Obesity
Pregnancy
Abdominal distension (ascites, intestinal obstruction, abdominal mass)
Diffuse pulmonary fibrosis
Lymphangitis carcinomatosa
Disseminated lupus erythematosus
Bilateral basal pulmonary emboli
Painful conditions (after abdominal surgery)
Bilateral diaphragmatic paralysis

Causes of unilateral elevation of the diaphragm
Posture – lateral decubitus position (dependent side)
Gaseous distension of stomach or colon
Dorsal scoliosis
Pulmonary hypoplasia
Pulmonary collapse
Phrenic nerve palsy
Eventration
Pneumonia or pleurisy
Pulmonary thromboembolism
Rib fracture and other painful conditions
Subphrenic infection
Subphrenic mass

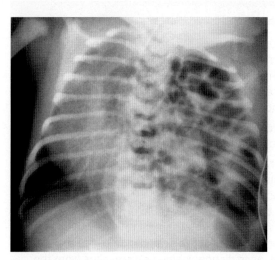

Congenital diaphragmatic hernia showing bowel extending from the abdomen in the left hemithorax and shift of the mediastinum to the right side.*

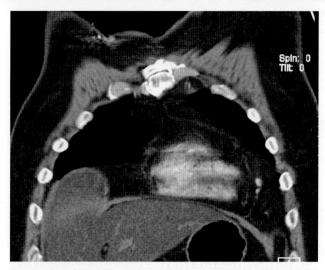

Focal eventration. CT shows the presence of liver under the elevated part of the diaphram.**

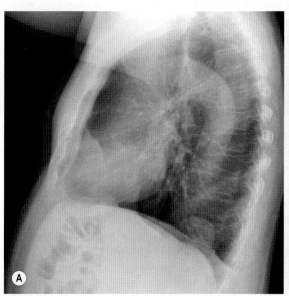

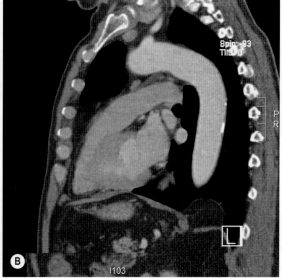

Bochdalek hernia. (A) Lateral CXR shows a focal bulge on the diaphragmatic contour just above the posterior costophrenic recess. (B) CT shows a fatty mass abutting the defect in the posteromedial aspect of the left hemidiaphragm.**

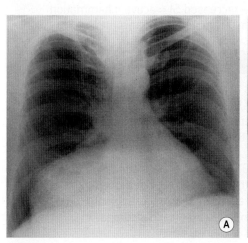

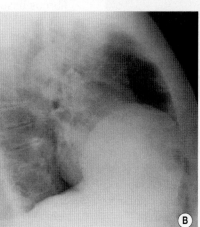

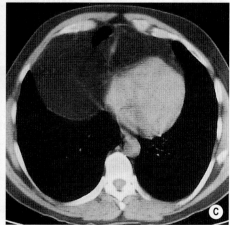

Morgagni's hernia. (A) PA and (B) lateral CXRs show a large mass in the right cardiophrenic angle. CT (C) confirms the presence of a Morgagni hernia.†

1.2 MEDIASTINUM

ACUTE MEDIASTINITIS

DEFINITION

- Acute infection of the mediastinum ▶ this is rare
- It is most commonly due to an oesophageal perforation (e.g. following endoscopy or from a swallowed object) – the alimentary contents serve as an infective source

Other causes

- Boerhaave's syndrome (forceful vomiting that tears the oesophagus) with the tear almost invariably just above the gastro-oesophageal junction ▶ leakage through a necrotic neoplasm ▶ post sternotomy ▶ infective extension from the neck, retroperitoneum or adjacent intrathoracic or chest wall structures

CLINICAL PRESENTATION

- Patients are often very ill with a high fever, tachycardia and chest pain
- 5–30% associated mortality with acute mediastinitis from oesophageal perforation even with treatment

RADIOLOGICAL FEATURES

CXR Widening and lack of clarity of the mediastinal outline ▶ streaks or round collections of air within the mediastinum ▶ mediastinal air-fluid levels ▶ pleural effusions are frequent (more commonly on the left) ▶ lower lobe pneumonia or atelectasis ▶ air within neck soft tissues

Barium swallow This may show the perforation site (a non-ionic contrast medium must be used)

CT Obliteration of the normal mediastinal fat planes ▶ gas bubbles within the mediastinum ▶ a walled-off discrete fluid or air-fluid collection (abscess) ▶ empyema, subphrenic or pericardial collection formation

- *Post sternotomy:* distinguishing a retrosternal haematoma from reactive granulation tissue or cellulitis is difficult, as is distinguishing osteomyelitis from the direct effects of the surgical incision
  - Substernal fluid collections and small amounts of air are normal in the first 20 postoperative days ▶ de novo postoperative or worsening gas collections should raise concern

FIBROSING MEDIASTINITIS (SCLEROSING MEDIASTINITIS/MEDIASTINAL FIBROSIS)

DEFINITION

- Proliferation of fibrous tissue and collagen within the mediastinum
- This is usually due to previous histoplasmosis or tuberculosis infection ▶ it is usually maximal within the upper mediastinum, but may extend to the lung roots
- *Other causes:* idiopathic (similar to retroperitoneal fibrosis or peri-aortitis) ▶ autoimmune disease ▶ radiation therapy ▶ drugs (particularly methysergide)

CLINICAL PRESENTATION

- SVC obstruction ▶ occasionally central pulmonary artery or venous obstruction

RADIOLOGICAL FEATURES

CXR Non-specific features ▶ CXR often underestimates the disease extent, but may show calcification of the mediastinal or hilar lymph nodes (if it is due to previous tuberculous or fungal infection)

CT An infiltrative (often extensively calcified) hilar and mediastinal process ▶ it is relatively focal if it is secondary to previous histoplasmosis or tuberculosis infection (a more diffuse appearance is seen with the idiopathic form) ▶ airway narrowing ▶ vascular encasement ± obstruction

MRI This provides similar information to CT ▶ however, MRI lacks sensitivity for detecting calcification (which is an important feature differentiating fibrosing mediastinitis from other infiltrative disorders of the mediastinum such as lymphoma or metastatic carcinoma) ▶ extensive regions of decreased signal intensity help differentiate fibrosing mediastinitis from other infiltrative mediastinal lesions

- T1WI: heterogeneous infiltrative mass of intermediate SI
- T2WI: more variable ▶ reduced SI = calcification or fibrous tissue, increased SI = active inflammation
- T1WI + Gad: heterogeneous enhancement

PEARL

- Two patterns of fibrosing mediastinitis:
  - Focal (80%): caused by histoplasmosis ▶ mass of soft tissue attenuation that is often calcified ▶ usually located in the right paratracheal, subcarinal or hilar regions
  - Diffuse (20%): not related to histoplasmosis ▶ often occurs in the setting of retroperitoneal fibrosis ▶ manifests as a diffusely infiltrating non-calcified mass affecting multiple mediastinal compartments

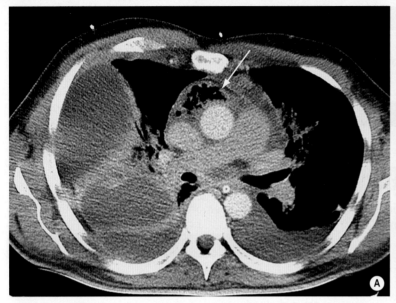
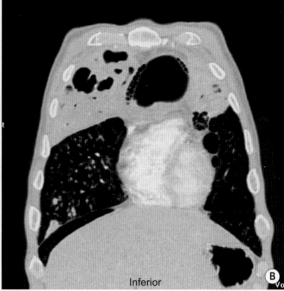

Abscess formation. (A) CT of an anterior mediastinal abscess (arrow). (B) Coronal CT (different patient) demonstrating a tuberculous mediastinal abscess and associated lung changes.*

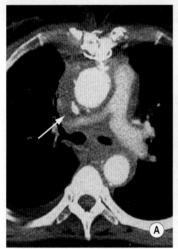
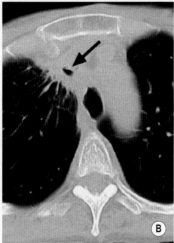
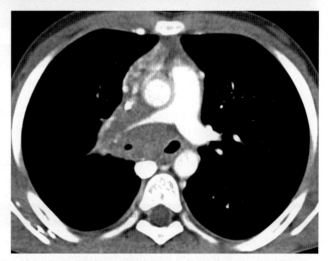

Mediastinitis. (A) Fibrosing mediastinitis. There is confluent soft tissue infiltration throughout the mediastinum without evidence of a discrete mass. Note the marked narrowing of the SVC (white arrow). (B) Tracheal narrowing from mediastinal fibrosis of unknown cause (different patient). The trachea (black arrow) is markedly narrowed and distorted and lies within the fibrotic scarring. The more posterior oesophagus is relatively dilated and gas filled.*

Fibrosing mediastinitis. CECT shows a partly calcified hilar mass secondary to histoplasmosis causing stenosis of the right pulmonary artery.**

THYROID MASSES

DEFINITION

- Most mediastinal thyroid masses are downward extensions of a multinodular colloid goitre (occasionally an adenoma or carcinoma)

CLINICAL PRESENTATION

- Usually an incidental CXR finding

RADIOLOGICAL FEATURES

XR A well-defined mass (spherical or lobular) within the superior aspect of the anterior or middle mediastinum ▶ tracheal displacement (± narrowing)

Scintigraphy ^{123}I or ^{131}I will demonstrate a thyroid mediastinal mass

CT This is almost as specific as scintigraphy but it will also demonstrate the shape and position of the mass ▶ the mass is invariably continuous with the thyroid gland in the neck ▶ it will demonstrate higher attenuation values than muscle pre and post IV contrast medium administration (due to its inherent iodine content) ▶ intense and prolonged enhancement ▶ areas of low attenuation are due to cystic degeneration ▶ retrotracheal masses will separate the trachea and oesophagus – this is virtually diagnostic of a thyroid mass

- *Benign disease:* this may demonstrate rounded or irregular well-defined areas of calcification
- *Carcinoma:* this occasionally demonstrates amorphous cloud-like calcification

MRI This identifies any cystic and solid components together with any haemorrhage (but not calcification)

PEARL

- It is not possible to determine any malignant potential on CT unless the tumour has clearly spread beyond the thyroid gland

PARATHYROID MASSES

DEFINITION

- Parathyroid tumours causing hyperparathyroidism are commonly located near the thyroid thymus
- *Causes of primary hyperparathyroidism:* single adenoma (80%) ▶ hyperplasia (15%) ▶ carcinoma (4%) ▶ multiple adenomas (1%)
  - Occasionally it can be due to hormone excretion from an ectopic bronchial carcinoma

RADIOLOGICAL FEATURES

- Small tumours are almost never visible on plain radiographs ▶ they are best detected using either US or ^{99m}Tc-MIBI

US An oval, well-defined anechoic or hypoechoic mass posterior to the thyroid gland (approximately 10 mm in size but can grow to 4–5 cm) ▶ larger tumours are more likely to be multilobulated and to contain echogenic areas, cysts and calcification ▶ retropharyngeal and mediastinal nodes are not very accessible ▶ a parathyroid gland can be mistaken for an ectopic thyroid nodule or a hyperplastic lymph node

CT This is useful for assessing sites inaccessible by US

MRI T1WI: isointense to muscle ▶ T2WI: high SI

Scintigraphy

- *Subtraction imaging:* a ^{99m}Tc or ^{123}I image (thyroid uptake only) is subtracted from a ^{201}Tl or ^{99m}Tc-MIBI image (uptake within both the thyroid and parathyroid glands)
- *Timed imaging:* ^{99m}Tc-MIBI (sestamibi)
  - *Early (15 min post injection):* thyroid and parathyroid uptake
  - *Delayed (90 min post injection):* there is significantly longer parathyroid tracer retention with thyroid 'washout'

PEARLS

- *Normal arrangement:* usually 4 glands are found adjacent to the thyroid lobes, thoracic inlet or mediastinum (up to 5 mm in long axis)
  - Ectopic glands can be found anywhere from behind the angle of the mandible down to the aortic root
- Selective arteriography, venous sampling and venography can be used for further assessment
- It is associated with the MEN I syndrome

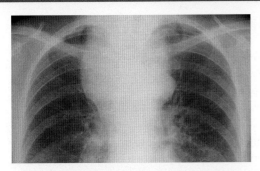

PA CXR of an intrathoracic thyroid mass.*

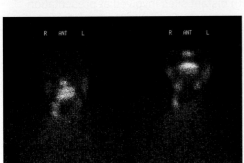

^{123}I radionuclide imaging of the face and neck demonstrates iodine uptake of the goitre.**

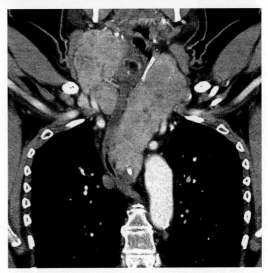

Coronal CT demonstrating thyroid intrathoracic extension. The thyroid demonstrates heterogeneous contrast medium enhancement and there are flecks of calcification in the gland.*

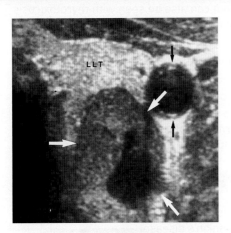

High-resolution US of the left lobe of the thyroid (LLT) anterior to a parathyroid adenoma (white arrows). There is a small area of cystic degeneration within the posterior aspect of the adenoma. Carotid artery (black arrows).*

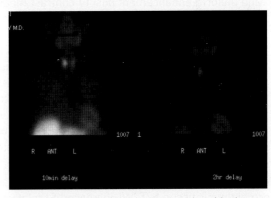

Role of scintigraphy in detecting parathyroid adenomas. A 66-year-old woman with hypercalcaemia. CT (not shown) did not reveal a parathyroid adenoma. ^{99m}Tc-sestamibi radionuclide imaging demonstrates uptake in both thyroid and parathyroid parenchyma in the 10-minute delayed image (left); however, at 2-hour delay, imaging (right) demonstrates persistent uptake in the right lobe of the thyroid gland, representing the parathyroid adenoma.**

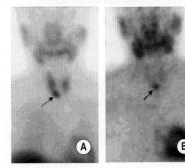 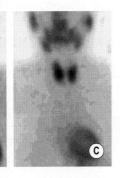

Parathyroid adenoma. ^{99m}Tc-MIBI images at 10 min (A) and 3 h (B) showing a persistent focus of activity inferior to the right lobe of the thyroid; ^{99m}TcO$_4$ image (C) shows normal thyroid uptake but the adenoma is not visualized.

THYMOMA

Definition

- A thymic epithelial neoplasm (usually low grade), which is the most common primary adult tumour of the anterior mediastinum
- An invasive thymoma (25%) demonstrates contiguous spread and is histologically indistinguishable from a benign tumour ▶ it is only identified by any extra-capsular spread

Clinical presentation

- It is rare under the age of 20 years – the average age at diagnosis is 50 years (but earlier in those with myasthenia gravis) ▶ M = F
- It is asymptomatic in up to 50% of patients – any symptoms are caused by compression or invasion of nearby mediastinal structures
- Up to 50% of patients have myasthenia gravis ▶ approximately 10–20% of patients with myasthenia gravis have a thymoma

Radiological features

CT This is the best imaging modality ▶ 90% arise within the upper anterior mediastinum (usually anterior to the ascending aorta and lying above the right ventricular outflow tract and pulmonary artery)

- A thymoma is spherical or oval in shape with lobulated borders (± cystic areas) ▶ there may be punctate or curvilinear calcification ▶ there is homogeneous density and uniform enhancement post IV contrast medium
  - Asymmetrical focal swelling (cf. generalized hyperplasia with myasthenia gravis)
- **Invasive thymoma:** a poorly marginated mass (which does not respect tissue planes) ▶ invasion of the mediastinal fat and pleura ▶ vascular encasement
  - *Pleural metastases:* via drop metastases once the pleural space has been breached
  - *Trans-diaphragmatic spread:* via the retrocrural space (30%) to involve the peritoneal surfaces and para-aortic regions

MRI T1WI: similar SI to that of muscle and adjacent normal thymic tissue ▶ T2WI: increased SI relative to adjacent mediastinal fat ▶ heterogeneity of SI can be caused by cystic change and haemorrhage

Pearls

- Thymoma can be difficult to diagnose in young patients as the normal gland is variable in size
- *Other syndromes associated with a thymoma:* hypogammaglobulinaemia ▶ red cell aplasia
- *Thymic cysts:* uncommon ▶ if congenital tend to be simple/unilocular ▶ acquired tend to be multilocular and are seen in association with thymic tumours, Langerhans cell histiocytosis or following irradiation

OTHER THYMIC TUMOURS

THYMIC CARCINOMA

Definition An aggressive and locally invasive malignancy (particularly invading the mediastinum, pericardium and pleura) with a poor prognosis

- It presents with chest pain and weight loss, usually in adults

CT A large heterogeneous mass with areas of necrosis and calcification ▶ it frequently metastasizes to the regional lymph nodes with distant sites involved at presentation

THYMOLIPOMA

Definition A rare benign encapsulated tumour composed of mature fat and normal thymic tissue ▶ it is associated with myasthenia gravis, aplastic anaemia, Graves' disease and hypogammaglobulinaemia

- Age range: 3–60 years ▶ it is usually asymptomatic although it can be large at presentation

CT/MRI It can grow to a large size before discovery and, being soft, moulds itself to the adjacent mediastinum ▶ the mass is fatty in nature ▶ occurs low in the anterior mediastinum (often the cardiophrenic angle)

THYMIC HYPERPLASIA

Definition This is most commonly associated with myasthenia gravis, but can also be seen with thyrotoxicosis and collagen vascular diseases

CT/MRI It rarely causes visible thymic enlargement ▶ if it is visible both the lobes are usually uniformly enlarged

Pearl The thymus may atrophy with stress or as a consequence of steroid or anti-neoplastic drug therapy – it usually returns to its original size on recovery but it may undergo rebound thymic hyperplasia making it difficult to distinguish from neoplastic involvement

THYMIC LYMPHOMA

Definition This is usually part of a generalized disease (most commonly Hodgkin's disease)

CT/MRI Imaging features are similar to thymoma

THYMIC CARCINOID

Definition An APUDoma which is histologically distinct from a thymoma (but with identical imaging features) ▶ it forms part of the MEN I syndrome ▶ aggressive tumour

Pearl It may secrete adrenocorticotrophic hormone in sufficient quantities to cause Cushing's syndrome (40%)

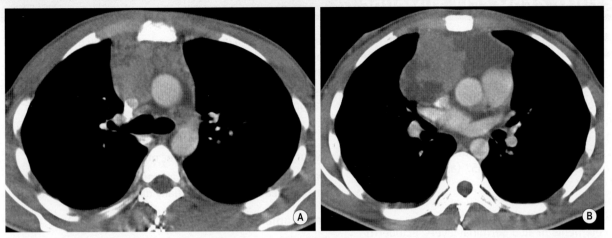

Thymic carcinoma. A 16-year-old man with history of weight loss and night sweats. Contrast medium-enhanced CT images show a heterogeneously enhancing anterior mediastinal mass arising from the right lobe of the thymus (A), with cystic (or necrotic) components. It extends inferiorly in the retrosternal space (B) and has no clear fat plane between it and the mediastinal structures (B). It was surgically excised and pathological examination revealed thymic carcinoma.**

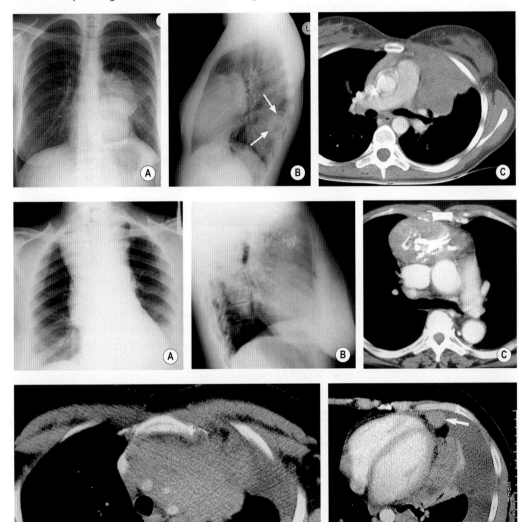

Malignant thymic mass. (A) PA and (B) lateral CXRs – the lateral view demonstrates pleural metastases posteriorly (arrows). (C) CT confirms the anterior position of the primary tumour suspected from the filling of the retrosternal window apparent on the lateral CXR.*

Thymoma. (A) CXR demonstrating a large anterior mediastinal mass (A) with coarse calcification visible on (B) the lateral view and (C) CECT.*

Invasive thymoma in a young man. (A) A lobular anterior mediastinal mass associated with a pleural effusion. (B) Image obtained through the lower chest demonstrates mixed soft tissue (arrows) and fluid attenuation owing to transpleural spread of tumour.*

MEDIASTINAL GERM CELL TUMOURS

DEFINITION

- Germ cell tumours of the mediastinum are derived from primitive germ cell elements left behind after embryonal cell migration ▶ the anterior mediastinum is the commonest extragonadal site (60%) ▶ malignant tumours are almost always seen in male patients ▶ almost all are in intimate contact with the thymus
- Anterior mediastinal masses: 10-15% (adults) ▶ 25% (children)
- **BENIGN** (70%)
  - MATURE (usually cystic) TERATOMAS
  - Contain elements of all 3 germinal layers: ectoderm (skin, teeth, hair) ▶ mesoderm (bone, cartilage, muscle) ▶ endoderm (bronchial / GI epithelium)
  - Usually benign but malignant tumours have a poor prognosis
- **MALIGNANT** (30%)
  - SEMINOMAS (majority)
    - Most common malignant mediastinal germ cell tumour
  - NON- SEMINOMATOUS GERM CELL TUMOURS (NSGCTs)
    - Include malignant teratoma, embryonal carcinoma, choriocarcinoma, endoderm sinus tumour and mixed cell types ▶ they are generally more aggressive and have an association with Klinefelter's syndrome and haematological malignancies (e.g. the acute leukaemias)

CLINICAL PRESENTATION

- Usually present during the 2nd to 4th decades
- TERATOMAS
  - They are usually asymptomatic and are diagnosed incidentally on CXR or CT ▶ can give symptoms if compress the bronchial tree or SVC ▶ haemorrhage or infection can lead to a rapid size increase ▶ they predominantly affect young adolescents ▶ women slightly outnumber men
- SEMINOMAS
  - Occur almost exclusively in men (2nd to 4th decade)
- NSGCTs
  - 90% are seen in young adult male patients ▶ more commonly symptomatic due to mass effect or invasion

RADIOLOGICAL FEATURES

Mature teratoma

A well defined, rounded or lobulated anterior mediastinal mass localized to the anterior mediastinum ▶ it can frequently be of a large size (and can occupy the entire haemothorax) ▶ haemorrhage or infection can lead to a rapid size increase ▶ it can occasionally rupture into the mediastinum or lung (mimicking the appearance of a malignant lesion)

CT A combination of fat, fluid and soft tissue components (± calcification which can occasionally represent a tooth) favour a mature teratoma over other causes

MRI This provides similar information but may not detect any calcification ▶ fat is virtually diagnostic of a teratoma

Seminoma

CT/MRI Well-defined solid masses ▶ possibly small areas of haemorrhage and necrosis ▶ homogenous attenuation and signal intensity

NSGCTs

These are often more lobular in outline ▶ they grow rapidly and metastasize readily to the liver, lungs, bones or pleura ▶ adjacent mediastinal fat planes may be obliterated

CT Lobular asymmetrical mass ▶ homogenous soft tissue density or multiple areas of contrast enhancement ▶ decreased attenuation can be due to necrosis and haemorrhage

- NSGCTs tend to be more heterogenous and demonstrate more contrast enhancement than seminomas

PEARLS

- Malignant tumours secrete human chorionic gonatotrophin and α-fetoprotein ▶ these can be used as tumour markers

Treatment

- *Teratomas:* benign course ▶ surgical resection treatment of choice due to low malignant potential
- *Seminomas:* radiotherapy (it is very radiosensitive) ± chemotherapy ± surgery
- *NSGCTs:* chemotherapy ± surgical resection of any residual tissue

Prognosis Teratomas and seminomas have a good prognosis (however, teratomas should be removed as 20% are malignant)

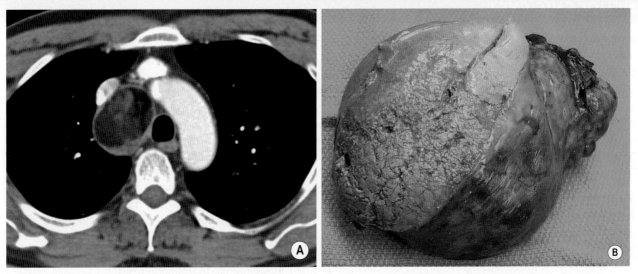

Cystic teratoma. (A) CT shows a heterogeneous mass with areas of fat attenuation. (B) Gross pathological specimen demonstrated sebaceous material and pieces of hair (not shown).**

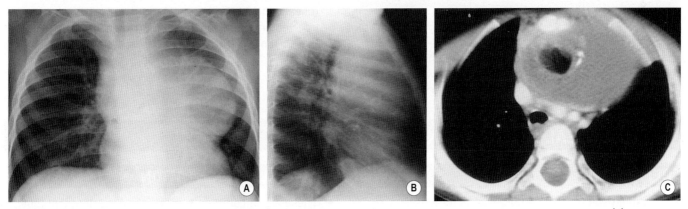

Benign teratoma. AP (A) and lateral (B) chest films demonstrate an oval anterior mediastinal mass overlying the left hilum. (C) CT demonstrates an oval mass of soft tissue density containing fat and calcification.†

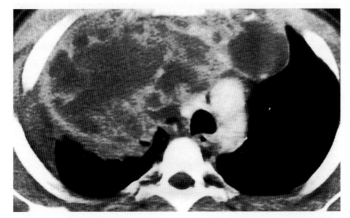

Malignant germ-cell tumour. CT shows a lobular asymmetrical mass with low attenuation areas corresponding to necrotic tumour intersected by neoplastic septation.*

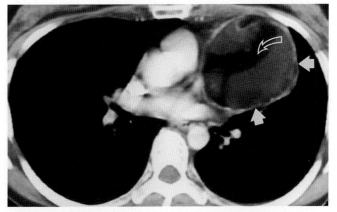

Teratoma. Contrast-enhanced CT reveals a heterogeneous anterior mediastinal mass with a calcified rim (short white arrows). There is also fat attenuation within the mass (curved open arrow).‡

BRONCHOGENIC CYST

DEFINITION

- A cyst derived from the embryological foregut
- Following abnormal budding of the developing tracheobronchial tree with separation of the buds from the normal airways
- It has a *thin*-walled fibrous capsule which is lined with respiratory epithelium, and usually contains thick mucoid material

CLINICAL PRESENTATION

- A solitary asymptomatic mediastinal mass presenting at any age
- Can grow very large without causing symptoms but can compress surrounding structures causing symptoms (particularly airways)

RADIOLOGICAL FEATURES

- Most are located adjacent to the trachea or main bronchi (commonly a subcarinal location)

CXR A spherical or oval mass with a smooth outline ▶ most are unilocular ▶ calcification of the cyst wall is rare ▶ a subcarinal cyst may resemble a large left atrium

CT A thin-walled mass demonstrating no contrast enhancement ▶ it is often in contact with the carina or main bronchus ▶ it can push the carina forward and the oesophagus backward (such displacement is almost never seen with other masses except for a thyroid mass or an aberrant left pulmonary artery) ▶ it frequently projects into the middle (± posterior) mediastinum

- *Cyst contents:* these are of usually uniform attenuation (close to water) ▶ they can have attenuation values similar to soft tissue and therefore tumour ▶ it may also show uniform high density due to high protein or calcium within the fluid, or as a liquid/calcium level due to milk of calcium (rare)

MRI T1WI: variable SI (protein, blood or mucous contents) ▶ T2WI: hyperintense (paralleling CSF)

PEARLS

- 25% are located within the pulmonary parenchyma (usually the medial lower lobe) ▶ rarely it may become infected or there may be haemorrhage into the cyst (which can be life-threatening)

OESOPHAGEAL DUPLICATION (ENTERIC) CYST

DEFINITION

- A cyst derived from the embryological foregut
- It has a *thick* wall (due to smooth muscle within its walls) ▶ it is lined with gastrointestinal epithelium (which is commonly gastric) ▶ it may become infected or the ectopic gastric mucosa may cause haemorrhage or perforation

	Bronchogenic cyst	Enteric cyst
Common location	Subcarinal	Intimately related to the oesophagus
Cyst wall	Thin	Thick
Symptoms	Asymptomatic (unless large)	Symptomatic (peptic ulceration)

CLINICAL PRESENTATION

- These are uncommon ▶ many are clinically silent (but usually present first in childhood) ▶ they may cause dysphagia, pain or symptoms due to the compression of adjacent structures

RADIOLOGICAL FEATURES

Barium swallow Extrinsic or intramural oesophageal compression

CT/MRI Imaging features are identical to those of a bronchogenic cyst (except that an oesophageal duplication cyst will have thicker walls, a more tubular shape and be in more intimate contact with the oesophagus)

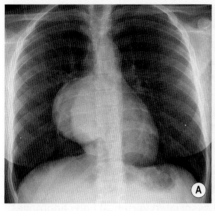 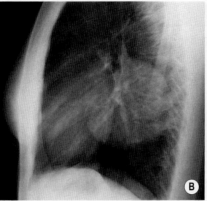 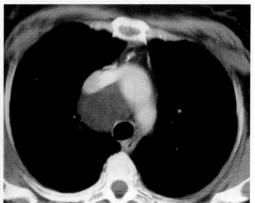

Bronchogenic cyst in a young woman with cough. (A) Frontal and (B) lateral chest radiographs show a large, smooth, well-marginated mass in the middle mediastinum – the most common location for a bronchogenic cyst.

Bronchogenic cyst. The CT attenuation was almost the same as that of the other soft tissue structures and it was not possible to predict the cystic nature of the mass. The cyst was surgically removed.*

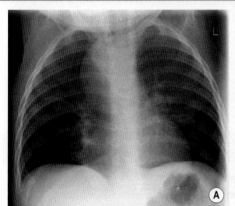 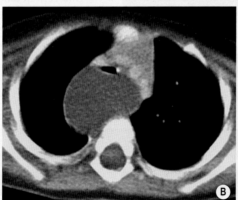 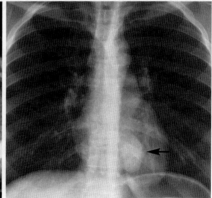

Oesophageal duplication cyst on (A) CXR and (B) CT. This case shows the typical features of a well-defined spherical mass projecting from the mediastinum.*

Oesophageal duplication cyst. Frontal chest radiograph shows a lobulated left retrocardiac mass (arrow).

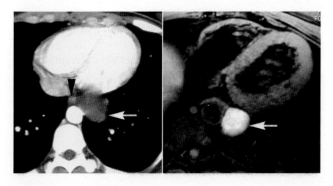

Oesophageal duplication cyst. Contrast-enhanced CT (left panel) shows a well-marginated water attenuation mass (arrow) that is closely associated with the distal oesophagus (arrowhead). Note that the lesion is homogeneous and of high signal intensity on T2WI MRI (right panel). **27**

NEURENTERIC CYSTS (SEE ALSO CONGENITAL SPINAL ANOMALIES)

DEFINITION

- This results from incomplete separation of the foregut from the notochord during early embryonic life ▶ the cyst wall contains both gastrointestinal and neural elements with an enteric epithelial lining
- There is usually a fibrous connection to the spine or an intraspinal component ▶ communication with the gastrointestinal tract may be present (but communication with the oesophageal lumen is rare)

CLINICAL PRESENTATION

- These frequently produce pain and are therefore seen early in life

RADIOLOGICAL FEATURES

- A well-defined, round, oval or lobulated mass within the middle and posterior mediastinum ▶ it is located between the oesophagus (which is usually displaced) and the spine

CT/MRI Appearances are similar to other foregut duplication cysts ▶ MRI is the investigation of choice for demonstrating the extent of any intraspinal involvement

PEARL

- Typically there are associated vertebral body anomalies (e.g. a butterfly or hemivertebra)

PERICARDIAL CYSTS

DEFINITION

- An outpouching of the parietal pericardium, representing the most common pericardial mass ▶ if it communicates with the pericardial cavity it is known as a pericardial diverticulum
- It is lined by mesothelial cells and usually contains clear fluid

CLINICAL PRESENTATION

- Asymptomatic

RADIOLOGICAL FEATURES

XR A well-defined oval mass within the cardiophrenic angle

CT/MRI A well-defined, oval fluid-filled cyst attached to the pericardium (and surrounded by normal pericardium)

PEARLS

- It is usually located at the anterior right cardiophrenic angle
- It can occur within the left cardiophrenic angle in up to $\frac{1}{3}$ of cases
- Differential diagnoses of a cardiophrenic angle mass: lipoma ▶ pericardial fat pad ▶ foramen of Morgangi hernia ▶ enlarged epicardial lymph nodes ▶ pleural tumour

PNEUMOMEDIASTINUM

DEFINITION

- A pneumomediastinum, in itself, is of little consequence ▶ however, the underlying cause may be of great significance
- **Intrathoracic causes:** asthma ▶ blunt trauma ▶ vomiting ▶ straining against a closed glottis
- **Extrathoracic causes:** dissection of air from the neck or retroperitoneum

RADIOLOGICAL FEATURES

Signs:
- *'Ring around the artery'*: air around the pulmonary artery
- *'Sail sign'*: elevation of the thymus
- 'Continuous diaphragm sign': air trapped posterior to the pericardium
- *'Extrapleural sign'*: air extending laterally between the parietal pleura and diaphragm
- *'Tubular artery sign'*: air adjacent to the major branches of the aorta
- *'Double bronchial wall sign'*: air adjacent to the bronchus

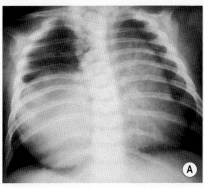
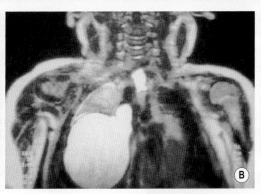
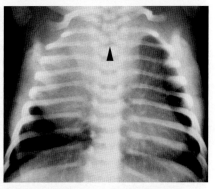

Neurenteric cyst. (A) CXR showing multiple segmentation anomalies affecting the cervicothoracic spine with a large soft tissue mass occupying the right hemithorax. (B) Coronal T2WI showing the high SI cystic mass originating from the cervicothoracic spine and causing compressive atelectasis of the right upper lobe.†

Neurenteric cyst in an infant. Frontal chest radiograph shows a large right-sided mediastinal mass. Note the butterfly vertebral body (arrowhead). (Courtesy of Helen Carty, Liverpool, UK.)

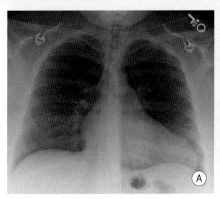
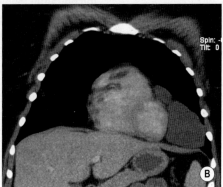
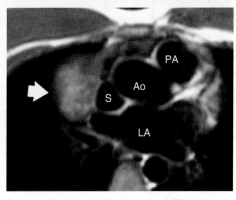

Pericardial cyst. (A) Frontal chest radiograph of a 33-year-old woman shows an abnormal mass-like contour of the left ventricle. (B) Coronal contrast medium-enhanced CT image demonstrates a mass of fluid attenuation without internal enhancement and no perceptible wall, located anterior and to the left of the heart.**

Pericardial cyst. Axial spin-echo MRI at the base of the heart. An intermediate signal intensity smooth mass extrinsic to the heart is identified (arrow). Ao = ascending aorta, LA = left atrium, PA = main pulmonary artery, S = superior vena cava.*

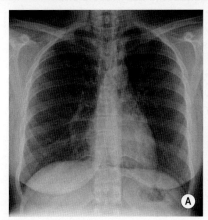
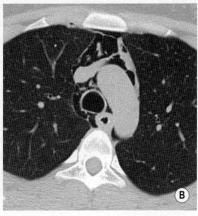
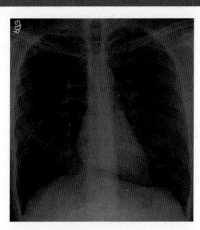

Pneumomediastinum. (A) CXR shows vertical lucent lines in the neck extending into the mediastinum. (B) CT demonstrating air tracking around the mediastinal structures.**

Continuous diaphragm sign in pneumomediastinum. Frontal chest radiograph shows an uninterrupted outline of the diaphragm indicative of a pneumomediastinum.**

MEDIASTINAL ADENOPATHY

DEFINITION

- Mediastinal nodes > 2 cm (short-axis diameter) are likely to represent metastatic carcinoma, malignant lymphoma, sarcoidosis, tuberculosis or fungal infection
  - *Smaller mediastinal nodes:* the differential also includes lymph node hyperplasia and pneumoconiosis
  - *Widespread moderate enlargement:* this is seen with chronic diffuse lung disease and bronchiectasis

RADIOLOGICAL FEATURES

CXR Right paratracheal nodes widen the right paratracheal stripe ▶ azygos nodes displace the azygos vein laterally ▶ nodes beneath the aortic arch obliterate the aortopulmonary window ▶ hilar lymph nodes enlarge the hilar shadows ▶ subcarinal nodes widen the carinal angle ▶ posterior mediastinal nodes displace the paraspinal or para-oesophageal lines

CECT This is a sensitive imaging modality ▶ short-axis lymph node measurements are the most representative (the long axis can vary according to the nodal orientation within a CT slice)

- Moderate nodal contrast enhancement is non-specific (it can be seen with inflammatory disorders) ▶ when striking it suggests a metastatic neoplasm from a hypervascular primary (e.g. melanoma, renal or thyroid carcinoma, carcinoid)
- Low-density centre with rim enhancement of an enlarged node is a useful pointer towards TB

Lymph node calcification This is seen with tuberculosis, fungal infections, sarcoidosis, silicosis and amyloidosis

- It is rare with metastatic neoplasms (although it may be seen with an osteosarcoma, chondrosarcoma or mucinous colorectal and ovarian tumours)
- It is virtually unknown with an untreated lymphoma ▶ it is occasionally seen with treated Hodgkin's disease
- The common patterns: course irregularly distributed clumps within the node ▶ homogeneous calcification of the whole node
- *'Eggshell' calcification:* a ring of calcification at the periphery of a node ▶ this is seen particularly with sarcoidosis and silicosis
- Pneumocystis jiroveci *infection (AIDS patients):* this leads to a strikingly foamy appearance

Low attenuation nodes (necrosis) Tuberculosis ▶ metastatic neoplasms (notably testicular) ▶ lymphoma ▶ attenuation values below that of water have been seen in Whipple's disease

PEARLS

Sarcoidosis *Symmetrical* hilar lymphadenopathy (in almost all cases) ▶ this is the most common cause of intrathoracic lymphadenopathy ▶ the anterior nodes occasionally increase in size (posterior nodal enlargement is very unusual) ▶ stippled or eggshell calcification

- *Garland's triad ('1-2-3' sign):* symmetrical hilar adenopathy + right paratracheal adenopathy

Malignant lymphoma *Asymmetrical* hilar lymphadenopathy involving multiple nodal groups ▶ nodal enlargement is seen in a higher proportion of Hodgkin's than non-Hodgkin's disease

- Anterior mediastinal and paratracheal nodes are the most frequently involved (subcarinal nodes are also often involved) ▶ contiguous retroperitoneal disease is likely
- The posterior mediastinal and paracardiac nodes are infrequently involved (the latter are important sites of recurrent disease as they may not be included in the initial radiotherapy field)
- Hilar nodal enlargement is rare without mediastinal nodal enlargement ▶ usually seen with mediastinal enlargement
- Hodgkin's disease (particularly the nodular sclerosing form) has a propensity to involve the anterior mediastinal and paratracheal nodes
- Nodal enlargement in lymphoma and leukaemia has the same pattern
- Can have rapid response with therapy

Tuberculosis and histoplasmosis These may affect any nodal group ▶ associated pulmonary consolidation may or may not be present ▶ involved nodes often return to a normal size with healing ▶ dense calcification is frequent ▶ rim enhancement with a low-density centre may be seen

Castleman's disease A benign lymph node hyperplasia of uncertain aetiology with substantial lymph node enlargement seen throughout the body (but is often localized to one area) ▶ it appears as a smooth lobulated hilar mass ▶ any involved nodes may calcify ▶ the nodal enlargement is very vascular (with strikingly uniform enhancement)

- *Thorax:* it is usually situated within the middle or posterior mediastinum ▶ affected in 70% of cases
- *Abdomen, pelvis or retroperitoneum:* affected in 10–15% of cases

Metastatic carcinoma As well as from bronchial carcinoma, metastases can also occur from any extrathoracic primary carcinoma (e.g. the GI tract, kidney, testis, head and neck tumours, breast)

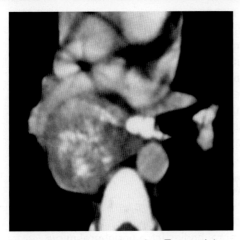

High-attenuation lymph nodes. Transaxial image of chest CT shows a calcified mediastinal lymphadenopathy. Such dystrophic calcification is common as a sequela of *Histoplasma capsulatum* infection ▶ however, it can also be seen with metastatic lymphadenopathy of mucinous adenocarcinomas.**

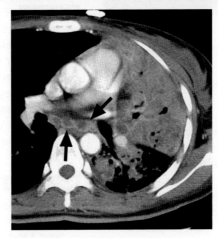

Tuberculous lymphadenopathy. Following contrast enhancement there is rim enhancement and central low attenuation due to caseation (arrows).*

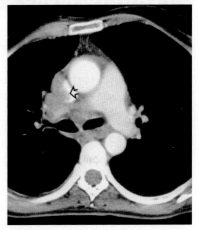

Metastatic malignant teratoma involving mediastinal nodes and directly invading the lumen of the SVC (arrow), where it is outlined by IV contrast medium.*

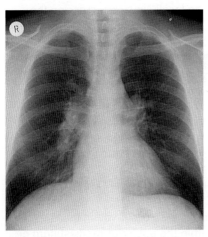

Sarcoidosis producing symmetrical bilateral hilar lymph node enlargement.*

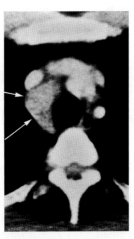

Right paratracheal lymph node enlargement (arrows) due to sarcoidosis.*

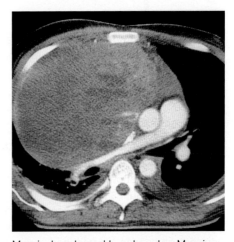

Massively enlarged lymph nodes. Massive anterior mediastinal nodal enlargement secondary to Hodgkin's disease. There is marked compression and distortion of the mediastinal structures and bilateral small pleural fluid reactions.*

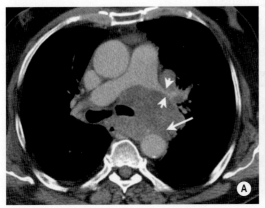

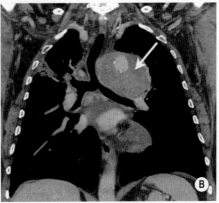

Non-small cell lung carcinoma. (A) Axial and (B) coronal CT demonstrating massive mediastinal adenopathy partially encasing the thoracic aorta (arrows) as well as compressing and nearly occluding the left main pulmonary artery (arrowheads). The trachea and left main bronchus are also displaced by the mass. The patient presented with a hoarse voice due to involvement of the recurrent laryngeal nerve by this mass.

PERIPHERAL NERVE SHEATH TUMOURS

Definition

- Most common posterior mediastinal tumour ▶ adults > children
- These originate from a paravertebral intercostal nerve within the posterior mediastinum
- **Benign:**
  - *Neurofibroma:* a non-encapsulated tumour with a central position within a nerve (containing all the nerve elements) ▶ it affects patients during the 2nd–4th decade
  - *Schwannoma (neurilemmoma):* an encapsulated tumour that is eccentrically placed within a nerve (arising from the nerve sheath) ▶ it affects patients during the 5th decade
- **Malignant:**
  - *Nerve sheath tumours (neurogenic sarcomas):* these are rare ▶ they affect patients during the 3rd–5th decades (with an earlier presentation in NF-1)

Clinical presentation

- Often asymptomatic (and an incidental CXR finding) ▶ mass effect or nerve entrapment ▶ pain should raise the possibility of a malignant lesion

Radiological features

Benign tumours

CXR A well-defined round or oval posterior mediastinal mass ▶ any pressure deformity causes a smooth, scalloped indentation on the adjacent ribs, vertebral bodies (dural ectasia causes posterior vertebral body scalloping), pedicles or transverse processes ▶ there is preservation of the scalloped cortex (which is often thickened) ▶ the adjacent rib spaces are widened

NECT A widened intervertebral foramina in 10% (with an associated dumb-bell-shaped mass extending through the foramina) ▶ homogeneous or heterogeneous appearance (± punctate foci of calcification) ▶ generally < 2 vertebral bodies long

CECT Heterogeneous enhancement

MRI T1WI: variable SI (similar to the spinal cord) ▶ T2WI: the 'target' sign: a characteristic high SI peripherally with low SI centrally ▶ T1WI + Gad: uniform enhancement

Malignant tumours

CT These are usually larger masses (>5 cm)

MRI This cannot reliably differentiate a malignant from a benign tumour ▶ heterogeneous SI (haemorrhage or necrosis) or infiltration of any adjacent structures are concerning as is a sudden size change ▶ haematogenous lung metastases have been reported

SYMPATHETIC GANGLION TUMOURS

Definition
Rare ▶ originate from nerve cells rather than nerve sheaths within sympathetic ganglia/adrenal glands

- **Ganglioneuroma:** a *benign* form ▶ this occurs in children or young adults
- **Ganglioneuroblastoma:** an *intermediate* form (with variable degrees of malignancy) ▶ this occurs in children
- **Neuroblastoma:** a *highly malignant* form ▶ this occurs in children younger than 5 years of age ▶ the posterior mediastinum is the most common extra-abdominal location

Radiological features

- A well-defined elliptical mass ▶ a vertical orientation along the course of the sympathetic chain and extends over 3 to 5 vertebral bodies (cf. a peripheral nerve tumour which is generally < 2 vertebral bodies long) ▶ calcification in 25% of cases

CT Variable appearances

MRI T1WI/T2WI: ganglioneuromas and ganglioneuroblastomas demonstrate homogeneous intermediate SI ▶ neuroblastomas are more heterogeneous (due to haemorrhage, necrosis and cystic degeneration) and may be locally invasive, crossing the midline

MEDIASTINAL PARAGANGLIOMAS

Definition

- Tumours arising from the paraganglion cells of the sympathetic system (benign or malignant)
  - *Chemodectoma:* almost all are close to the aortic arch (aortic body tumours) with other mediastinal chemodectomas rarely seen ▶ they are usually single tumours
  - *Phaeochromocytoma:* < 2% occur within the chest ▶ most are found within the posterior mediastinum or closely related to the heart (particularly the left atrial wall or interatrial septum)

Clinical presentation

- A third of mediastinal phaeochromocytomas are asymptomatic (non-functioning) ▶ the remainder present clinically with catecholamine overproduction

Radiological features

CXR/CT Rounded soft tissue masses which are very vascular and therefore enhance intensely

MRI T1WI: SI similar to muscle ▶ T2WI: high SI

Scintigraphy Radio-iodine MIBG or somatostatin receptor scintigraphy demonstrates increased activity ▶ this is useful for identifying extra-adrenal phaeochromocytomas

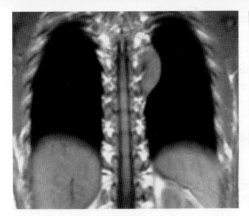

Neurofibroma in the left paravertebral region. Coronal T1WI demonstrates the tumour well and shows that it does not enter the spinal canal or encroach significantly on the adjacent foramina.*

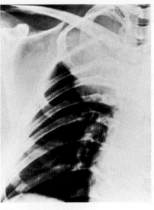

Neurofibrosarcoma showing widening and pressure deformity of adjacent ribs. A benign neurofibroma would have had identical features.*

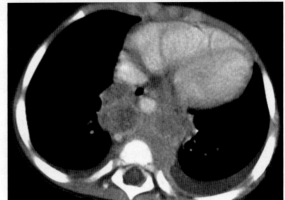

Neuroblastoma. Contrast-enhanced CT shows an infiltrative posterior mediastinal mass that encases the descending thoracic aorta. (Courtesy of Donald Frush, Durham, NC.)

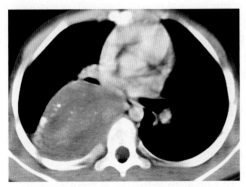

Ganglioneuroma in a 7-year-old girl with cough. Contrast-enhanced CT shows that the mass is heterogeneous and contains punctuate and chunk-like calcification.

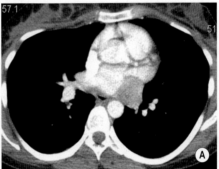

Paraganglioma. CT of the chest demonstrates an enhancing mediastinal mass arising in the middle mediastinum adjacent to the left atrium, and protruding into it (A). I-131 *meta*-iodobenzylguanidine (MIBG) scintigraphy shows increased uptake, revealing that it is a paraganglioma (B).**

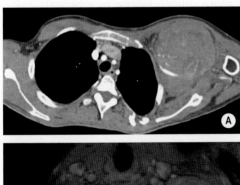

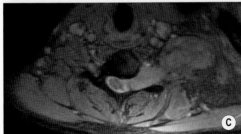

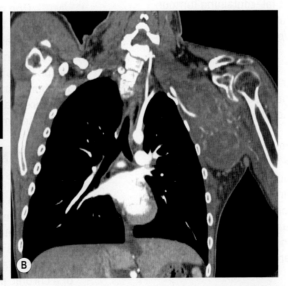

Malignant nerve sheath tumour. A 23-year-old patient with left axillary mass and left shoulder pain. (A) Axial and (B) coronal contrast medium-enhanced CT images show a large heterogeneously enhancing mass in the left axilla, which encases the left subclavian artery. Axial contrast medium-enhanced MRI demonstrates that this enhancing mass expands the neural foramen of the spine, with no erosion of the vertebral body, suggesting that this is a neurogenic tumour (C).**

LYMPHANGIOMAS (CYSTIC HYGROMAS)

Definition

- Focal mass-like congenital malformations of the lymphatic system composed of complex lymph channels or cystic spaces (containing clear or straw-coloured fluid)
- Classified as simple (capillary), cavernous or cystic (hygroma) depending on the size of the lymphatic channels ▶ cystic are the most common
- It is usually as part of an extension from a lymphangioma within the axilla or neck (but occasionally wholly confined to the mediastinum) ▶ it is most commonly seen within the anterior or superior mediastinum ▶ complete resection may be difficult due to their insinuating nature

Clinical presentation

- A neck mass presenting in early life ▶ purely mediastinal lymphangiomas present in older children and adults as an asymptomatic mediastinal mass

Radiological features

CT A cystic mass whose contents mirror the attenuation values of water ▶ envelops rather than displaces structures

MRI T1WI/T2WI: signal characteristics compatible with fluid contents ▶ septations can be seen

Pearl Complete resection may be difficult due to their insinuating nature

FATTY TUMOURS OF THE MEDIASTINUM

Definition

- *Lipoma*: a benign fatty tumour
- *Liposarcoma*: a malignant fat-containing tumour
- *Lipoblastoma*: a benign tumour of childhood
- *Angiolipoma and myelolipoma*: benign tumours

Radiological features

CT Regardless of whether they are benign or malignant, fatty tumours are well-defined round or oval mediastinal masses ▶ they are usually located within the anterior or middle mediastinum

- *Lipoma*: uniform fat attenuation (a few strands of soft tissue may be present) ▶ there is usually no mass effect (as it is a soft tumour that does not compress surrounding structures unless it is very large)
- *Liposarcoma*: heterogeneous fat attenuation ▶ large areas of soft tissue attenuation ▶ local invasion/infiltration
- *Lipoblastoma/angiolipoma/myelolipoma*: fat and soft tissue attenuation ▶ it can be indistinguishable from a liposarcoma

Pearls

Mediastinal lipomatosis Massive (usually symmetrical) collections of fat throughout the mediastinum (most prominent in upper mediastinum) ▶ it is seen especially in

Cushing's disease, steroid therapy and in obese subjects
- Relatively large fat collections are often 'normally' present within the cardiophrenic angles of obese patients

Abdominal fat herniation Herniation of omental and peri-gastric fat commonly herniates via the oesophagel hiatus or formamen (Morgagni / Bochdalek)

LATERAL THORACIC MENINGOCELE

Definition

- A rare lesion due to protrusion of redundant spinal meninges through an intervertebral foramen ▶ filled with CSF
- Asymptomatic
- It is commonly associated with neurofibromatosis (as are neurofibromas)

Radiological features

CXR A posterior mediastinal mass (often with pressure deformity on the adjacent bone) ▶ it is indistinguishable from a neurofibroma

CT/MRI A fluid-filled mass (rather than solid) ▶ intrathecal contrast medium (CT) demonstrates flow into the lesion

EXTRAMEDULLARY HAEMATOPOIESIS

Definition

- Compensatory expansion of the bone marrow seen with thalassaemia, hereditary spherocytosis and sickle cell anaemia ▶ this leads to extrusion of bone marrow through the cortex, with creation of a paravertebral mass
- Asymptomatic

Radiological features

CT/MRI One or more smooth, lobular or spherical masses within the paravertebral gutters (usually located within the lower thorax) ▶ these are usually bilateral and symmetrical and of homogeneous soft tissue attenuation (occasionally a fatty component is visible)
- The bones may appear normal or demonstrate an altered lace-like trabecular pattern (due to the associated marrow expansion)

MEDIASTINAL PANCREATIC PSEUDOCYST

Definition

- This follows extension of a pancreatic pseudocyst into the posterior mediastinum ▶ this occurs via the oesophageal or aortic hiatus and therefore lies adjacent to the oesophagus ▶ usually middle or posterior mediastinum
- Most cases are seen in adults with clinical features of a chronic pancreatitis (it can also occur in children following trauma)

Radiological features

CT A thin-walled cyst continuous with the pancreas ▶ left-sided or bilateral pleural effusions

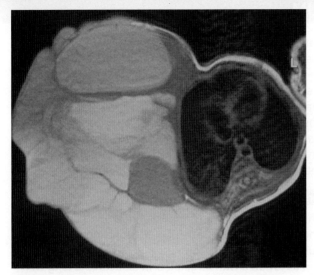

T2WI. Extrathoracic cystic hygroma (lymphangioma) in a neonate showing high SI due to the dilated lymphatic spaces.[†]

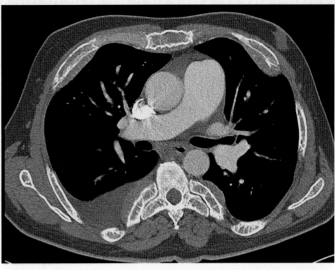

Extramedullary haematopoiesis showing smooth pleurally based masses and altered bone texture in this patient with thalassaemia. There is also a small right pleural effusion.*

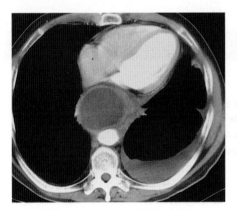

Pancreatic pseudocyst. CECT shows a round posterior mediastinal cystic mass located behind the heart and demonstrating enhancing walls. Note the associated left pleural effusion.[†]

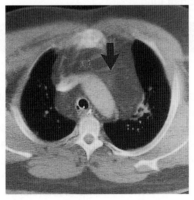

Mediastinal lipomatosis. CECT shows excess mediastinal fat deposition, particularly anteriorly (arrow).[†]

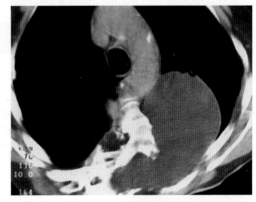

Lateral thoracic meningocele. Non-contrast CT shows a well-marginated water attenuation mass arising from the spinal canal. Note the marked widening of the neural foramen.

Summary of mediastinal masses

Anterior mediastinum	Middle mediastinum	Posterior mediastinum
Hernia (Morgagni)	Hernia (hiatus/aortic)	Hernia (Bochdalek)
Aortic aneurysm	Aortic aneurysm	Aortic aneurysm
Cystic hygroma	Lymph nodes (sarcoidosis/TB/lymphoma/metastases)	Myeloma/metastases
Diaphragmatic eventration	Foregut duplication cysts	Diaphragmatic eventration
Thymic tumours*	Neurenteric cyst	Sympathetic ganglion cell tumours
Retrosternal thyroid mass*	Mediastinal paragangliomas	Peripheral nerve tumours
Germ cell tumour*	Carcinoma of the bronchus	Lateral thoracic meningocoele
Lymph nodes (lymphoma)*	Fatty mediastinal tumours/mediastinal lipomatosis	Extramedullary haematopoiesis
Pericardial cyst		Paravertebral abscess
Pericardial fat pad		Pancreatic pseudocyst
Sternal masses		Neurenteric cyst

*Anterior mediastinal masses: '4 Ts' – **T**hymic, **T**hyroid, **T**eratoma or **T**errible lymphoma

CONGENITAL ABSENCE OF THE PERICARDIUM

Definition

- A congenital pericardial defect caused by vascular compromise to the pleuropericardial membrane during development
- This varies from a small defect to complete (bilateral) absence of the pericardium ▶ complete absence commonly affects the left pericardium (bilateral and isolated right-sided lesions are very rare)

Clinical presentation

- Complete absence is usually asymptomatic ▶ partial absence may be complicated by herniation or cardiac chamber entrapment (particularly affecting the left atrial appendage)

Radiological features

CXR/CT/MRI

- *Complete absence of the left pericardium:* cardiac displacement into the left chest ▶ interposition of lung between the aorta and pulmonary artery (also between the left hemidiaphragm and cardiac silhouette) ▶ an ill-defined right cardiac border (due to leftward cardiac displacement and rotation) ▶ medial/lateral borders of the main pulmonary artery may be more visible due to absence of anterior pericardial reflection
- *Partial pericardial defect:* varying degrees of pulmonary artery or left atrial appendage prominence ▶ the heart retains its normal position

Pearls

- This is associated with congenital heart and lung anomalies: ASD ▶ TOF ▶ PDA ▶ bronchogenic cysts ▶ pulmonary sequestration
- It is associated with large pleural defects (the lung can herniate and surround the intrapericardial vascular structures)

PERICARDITIS

Definition

- Pericardial inflammation caused by: myocardial infarction (Dressler syndrome) ▶ mediastinal irradiation ▶ infection (viral or bacterial) ▶ connective tissue diseases (rheumatoid arthritis or SLE) ▶ metabolic disorders (uraemia or hypothyroidism) ▶ neoplasia ▶ AIDS ▶ TB (immunocompromised) ▶ trauma

Clinical presentation

- Chest pain ▶ dyspnoea ▶ pericardial friction rub ▶ pulsus paradoxus

Radiological features

CXR Acute pericarditis commonly manifests as a pericardial effusion (which is usually diagnosed with echocardiography) ▶ >50 ml fluid ▶ CXR positive if >200 ml

- *Pericardial effusion:* a sudden increase in the cardiac silhouette without specific chamber enlargement ▶ filling in of the retrosternal space ▶ effacement of the normal cardiac borders ▶ a 'water bottle' cardiac configuration ▶ the bilateral 'hilar overlay' sign ▶ the 'epicardial fat pad' sign (with an anterior pericardial stripe > 2 mm on a lateral CXR)

CT Pericardial enhancement (increased attenuation suggests haemorrhage) ▶ increased pericardial thickness

MRI In the absence of haemorrhage, effusions are predominantly low SI ▶ haemorrhagic effusions are of variable SI (depending upon the blood product age)

- *Inflammatory conditions:* T2WI: thickened inflamed pericardium returns moderate to high SI ▶ T1WI + Gad: enhancement

Pearls

- **Causes of a transudative pericardial effusion:** cardiac surgery ▶ CCF ▶ uraemia ▶ myxoedema ▶ collagen vascular diseases
- **Causes of a haemopericardium:** trauma ▶ aortic dissection or rupture ▶ neoplasm
- **Constrictive pericarditis:** this represents a chronic phase of fibrous scarring, pericardial thickening and obliteration of the pericardial cavity ▶ it can result in restriction of diastolic cardiac filling
  - The aetiology is usually unknown (but is presumed secondary to an occult viral pericarditis) ▶ it can follow mediastinal irradiation or following cardiac surgery ▶ neoplastic infiltration can follow carcinoma of the lung or breast, lymphoproliferative malignancies and melanoma
  - **CT/MRI** Pericardial thickening ≥ 4 mm ▶ there is commonly pericardial calcification ▶ a reduced right ventricular volume ▶ a dilated right atrium, SVC and IVC ▶ hepatomegaly and ascites ▶ little enhancement
- **Pericardial neoplasms:** metastases are much more common than rare primary pericardial tumours ▶ metastases to consider: lung/lymphoma/breast/melanoma/colon ▶ most common primary malignancy is malignant mesothelioma (haemorrhagic effusion) ▶ pericardial effusion is the most common finding ± a mass

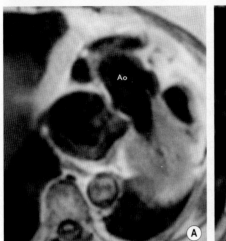
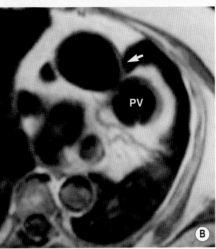
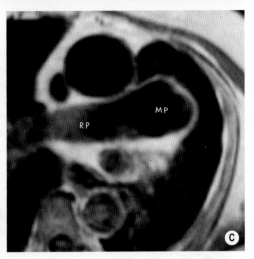

Partial absence of the pericardium. T1WI. (A) Image through the aortic valve and proximal ascending aorta (Ao). The heart is displaced into the left chest and rotated in a clockwise manner. (B) Image through the pulmonary valve (PV). A sliver of lung (arrow) invaginates to come into contact with the ascending aorta. (C) Image through the main (MP) and transverse right (RP) pulmonary arteries. The MP protrudes to the left and is in contact with the lung.*

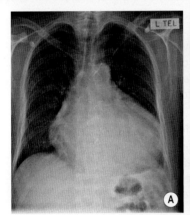
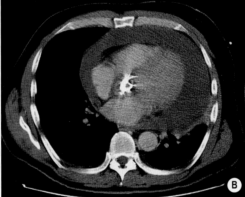
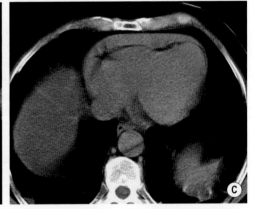

Pericardial effusion. (A) The heart had become rapidly enlarged in this patient who had previously undergone aortic valve replacement. (B) NECT through the level of the valve replacement demonstrates the large pericardial effusion. (C) A large haemopericardium complicating a type A aortic dissection (different patient). The haemopericardium is the same attenuation as soft tissue on this unenhanced image.*

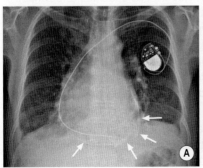
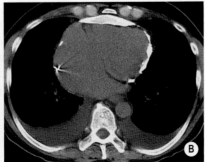

Dense pericardial calcification demonstrated on (A) CXR (arrows) and (B) CT. There are bilateral pleural effusions in this patient with constrictive calcific pericarditis (previous TB).*

1.3 PULMONARY INFECTION

LOBAR PNEUMONIA

Definition
- An infection developing within the distal airspaces (and adjacent to the visceral pleura) ▶ it spreads via collateral air drift (pores of Kohn), producing homogeneous opacification of partial or complete lung segments (and occasionally an entire lobe) ▶ any lung opacification is limited by the fissures and is usually unifocal
- As the airways are not primarily involved and remain patent there is little or no volume loss ▶ there is also associated air bronchogram formation
- On CT appears as lobar/sublobar sharply demarcated consolidation

Streptococcus pneumoniae (pneumococcal pneumonia)
- *The most common community-acquired adult bacterial pneumonia*
  - **Predisposing factors:** *chronic illness ▶ alcoholism ▶ sickle-cell disease ▶ splenectomy*

CXR/CT Homogeneous consolidation that crosses segmental boundaries but only involves one lobe (± air bronchograms or a parapneumonic effusion) ▶ it is commonly basal and solitary (but may be multifocal) ▶ the lobar volume is usually unchanged (and rarely increases) ▶ there is a fairly rapid XR resolution (total resolution usually occurs within 2–6 weeks)
- Empyema and cavitation formation are infrequent ▶ effusions are common
- **Round pneumonia:** a spherical pneumonia (with ill-defined margins) that is usually seen in children (due to the lack of collateral air drift) ▶ it can demonstrate a rapid change in size and shape ▶ it may simulate a lung mass
  - *Organisms: Haemophilus influenzae ▶ Streptococcus ▶ pneumococcus*
  - *Location:* it is always within the posterior (usually lower) lobes

Klebsiella

CXR/CT A homogeneous opacity similar to that seen with *S. pneumoniae* (or it may produce a bronchopneumonia pattern) ▶ there is rapid cavitation of any lobar consolidation ▶ early abscess formation ▶ ground-glass attenuation on CT
- It is often accompanied by bulging fissures (signifying a very exudative response)

Legionella (Legionnaires' disease)
- *This is acquired in a community, nosocomial, or an epidemic fashion and is associated with a contaminated water source ▶ there is rapid progression (with up to a 30% mortality rate)*
  - *Predisposing factors: post-transplantation (immuno-suppression) ▶ COPD ▶ heart failure ▶ renal disease*

CXR Solitary or multifocal, lobar pneumonia-like, homogeneous opacities simulating *S. pneumoniae* infection (with a tendency to a round and mass-like appearance) ▶ there is rapid spread of the initial consolidation to the other lobes ▶ cavitation can be seen in immunocompromised and post renal transplant patients ▶ pleural effusions are present in 10–35% of cases ▶ can mimic round pneumonia

Actinomycosis
- *An anaerobic, Gram-positive bacterium (Actinomyces israelii): this is a mouth commensal, causing infection when it accesses devitalized tissues (particularly within the cervicofacial region and abdomen) ▶ it generates a chronic inflammatory reaction, causing abscess and fistula formation (which contain tiny sulphur granules)*
  - *Lung involvement is seen in <25% of cases (due to aspiration or spread from other foci)*

CXR Homogeneous opacification (as a lobar-type pneumonia or as a mass) ▶ cavitation is common and can mimic the appearance of a bronchogenic carcinoma ▶ focal fibrosis (± contraction) may be severe ▶ there are associated pleural effusions, pleural thickening, empyema formation and disease extension into the contiguous soft tissues or bones (the resultant periostitis sets this apart from other infections)

CT Scattered peripheral areas of homogeneous consolidation with central low attenuation and adjacent pleural thickening

Nocardiosis
- *An aerobic, Gram-positive bacillus (Nocardia asteroides): most cases arise within North America in immunocompromised patients ▶ the initial pulmonary focus may disseminate to other organs (notably the brain)*

CXR There is usually unifocal or multifocal pulmonary consolidation ▶ there can be single or multiple pulmonary nodules (which can mimic a primary lung cancer or metastatic disease) ▶ there may be lymphadenopathy and chest wall involvement ▶ cavitation and pleural effusions are frequent

Chlamydial pneumonia
- **Chlamydia psittaci:** *this causes psittacosis (ornithosis) and is usually seen following direct bird contact*

CXR Small to large homogeneous opacities (± perihilar or basal reticular opacities) ▶ there are occasionally enlarged hilar nodes and small effusions ▶ any radiographic opacities clear slowly
- **Chlamydia pneumoniae:** *this causes an asymptomatic or mild adult respiratory infection – it is one of the commonest causes of a community-acquired pneumonia*

  CXR/CT
  - *Primary disease:* a unifocal homogeneous opacity (occasionally multifocal) ▶ bronchovascular thickening ▶ lymphadenopathy ▶ reticular or linear opacities ▶ airway dilatation
  - *Recurrent disease:* bilateral and more heterogenous changes ▶ small or moderate pleural effusions (up to 50%)

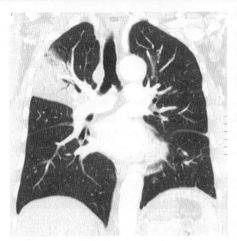

Lobar pneumonia. A 36-year-old man with *S. pneumoniae* pneumonia. Coronal reformatted CT image shows a homogeneous focal area of consolidation in the right upper lobe. Patent bronchi (air bronchograms) are seen within the area of consolidation.**

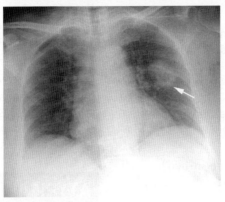

Round pneumonia. A previously healthy 64-year-old man with fever and productive cough. Chest radiograph shows a mass-like area of consolidation in the left upper lobe (arrow).**

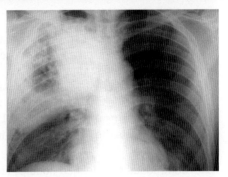

Legionnaires' disease. The PA CXR demonstrates homogeneous opacities in the right upper lobe. The medial one resembles a mass.*

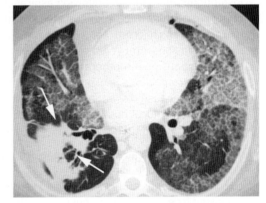

Alveolar proteinosis and *Nocardia* pneumonia. A 42-year-old man with alveolar proteinosis who presented with fever. CT at the level of the lower lobes shows bilateral areas of extensive ground-glass opacities with superimposed smooth septal lines and intralobular lines, resulting in a pattern known as 'crazy-paving'. Note a localised area of consolidation (arrows) and a right pleural effusion.**

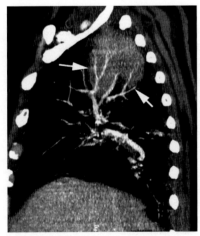

Segmental *Pneumoccocal pneumonia* pneumonia. 48-year-old man with fever and a right upper lobe pneumonia. Sagittal reformatted minimum intensity projection (MIP) image from dynamic contrast-enhanced MDCT shows a normal pattern of pulmonary vasculature within a homogeneous right upper lobe consolidation (CT angiogram sign) (arrows).**

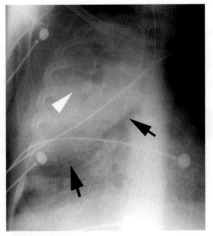

Klebsiella pneumonia. A 50-year-old man with fever and a severe right pneumonia. Posteroanterior chest radiograph shows dense consolidation of the right upper lobe with visible areas of abscessification (arrowhead). Note an inferior convexity of the major fissure ('bulging fissure' sign) (arrows) characteristic of lobar expansion.**

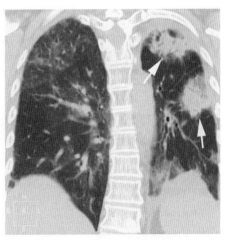

Chlamydia pneumoniae pneumonia. A 67-year-old woman with chest pain, fever and non-productive cough. Coronal reformatted CT shows multiple ill-defined, rounded areas of consolidation in the left upper lobe with visible air bronchogram and poorly defined margins (arrows).**

BRONCHOPNEUMONIA

Definition

- A multifocal infection centred within and along the course of the distal airways ▶ predominantly peribronchiolar inflammation
- Bronchial spread results initially in large heterogeneous scattered opacities
- Air bronchograms are usually absent as the disease primarily affects the bronchi (filling them with inflammatory fluid)

CT Centrilobular ill-defined nodules ('tree-in-bud')/branching linear opacities/airspace nodules/multifocal lobular consolidation

SPECIFIC INFECTIONS

Staphylococcus aureus

- This usually affects debilitated hospitalized or institutionalized patients (following aspiration from the upper respiratory tract) ▶ pneumatoceles may form (particularly in children)
- Pleural effusions, empyemas and cavitation are common ▶ spontaneous pneumothoraces can also occur
- *Septicaemic infections* (e.g. drug addicts, infective endocarditis): can cause disseminated, poorly marginated and peripheral multifocal nodules which can cavitate

Gram-negative pneumonias

- These are usually caused by hospital-acquired enterobacteria in debilitated patients (e.g. *Proteus, E. coli, Pseudomonas* and *Haemophilus*) ▶ the bacteria are aspirated from a colonized upper respiratory tract
- *E. coli*: multilobar bronchopneumonia (usually lower lobes)
- *Pseudomonas*: extensive confluent bronchopneumonia ▶ frequently cavitates ▶ predominantly upper lobe
- *Haemophilus influenzae*: multilobar, lobar or segmental consolidation ± effusions

ANAEROBIC PNEUMONIA

Definition

- This usually results following the aspiration of anaerobic bacteria ▶ it is associated with altered consciousness and mechanical ventilation

Radiological features

CXR Changes are usually delayed by 24–72 hours ▶ heterogeneous opacities are seen in the dependent lung segments (uni- or bilaterally) ▶ multiple cavities (reflecting severe lung necrosis) may be seen 1–3 weeks following aspiration

- Delayed presentation is associated with discrete thick irregular-walled lung abscesses (⅔ are within the upper lobe apico-posterior segments or lower lobe superior segments)

Pearls

Empyema A suppurative infection of the pleural space ▶ this is a common complication of anaerobic infections (and may occur without any XR evidence of pneumonia)

US Septations ± echogenic internal material (representing pus)

CT A 'split' enhancing thickened pleura ▶ displaced lung and vessels (± gas within the empyema collection)

- *Long-term sequelae:* fibrothorax ▶ sheet-like pleural calcification (especially following TB)

ATYPICAL PNEUMONIA

Mycoplasma pneumonia

Definition The major non-bacterial cause of a community-acquired pneumonias (20 and 40 years) ▶ it resembles a viral infection with spread from the upper to lower respiratory tract ▶ it is usually self-limiting

CXR There is most commonly a unilateral lower lobe process beginning as a heterogeneous, reticular, segmental or peribronchial region of opacification that may become lobar or homogeneous ▶ pleural effusions and nodal enlargement are uncommon

HRCT Ground-glass and homogeneous opacities ▶ bronchiolitis with centrilobular nodules ▶ bronchovascular thickening (80%)

Viral pneumonias

Definition These are common in children (and unusual in adults) ▶ they predispose to secondary bacterial infection

Influenza A and B

- A common cause of an adult pneumonia (particularly affecting the elderly) and immunocompromised

CXR Scattered homogeneous opacities that rapidly become bilateral, extensive and confluent ▶ pleural effusions are rare ▶ clinical relapse may be due to a secondary bacterial pneumonia

HRCT Ground-glass opacities ▶ nodules ▶ a 'tree-in-bud' appearance

Varicella

- This affects young adults more frequently than children ▶ there is an increased risk with lymphoma, pregnancy and steroid therapy ▶ pulmonary involvement follows a skin rash by 1–6 days

CXR/CT Widespread 5–10 mm poorly marginated nodules or acinar opacities (which may become confluent) ▶ the nodules usually resolve in 1–2 weeks but can persist for months ▶ numerous residual small irregular calcified nodules may remain

Herpes simplex virus type I (HSV-1)

- Immunocompromised or ventilated patients

CT Patchy consolidation ▶ ground-glass opacities ▶ 'tree-in-bud' appearance

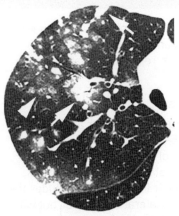

Mycoplasma pneumonia. A 35-year-old man presents with non-productive cough and fever. CT shows airspace nodules, focal areas of lobular consolidation (arrows) and patchy ground-glass opacities (arrowhead).**

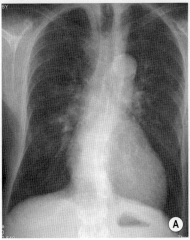
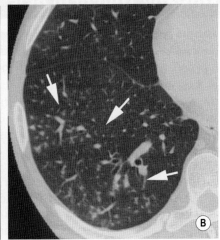

Cellular bronchiolitis. A 71-year-old man with fever of 48-h duration. (A) Posteroanterior chest radiograph is normal. (B) Complementary CT shows centrilobular branching nodular and linear opacities resulting in a 'tree-in-bud' appearance (arrows). *Mycoplasma* bronchiolitis was diagnosed.**

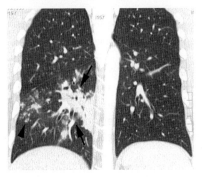

Bronchopneumonia caused by *H. influenzae*. A 48-year-old man with productive cough and fever. Coronal reformatted CT shows a focal area of consolidation in the right lower lobe with visible air bronchogram and poorly defined margins (arrows). Also evident are small nodular opacities and a few 'tree-in-bud' opacities (arrowhead).**

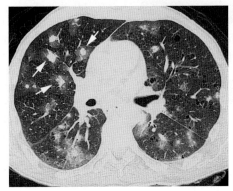

Herpesvirus pneumonia. A 34-year-old severely immunocompromised patient with fever. CT at the level of the bronchus intermedius in a patient with herpesvirus infection shows multiple, bilateral and randomly distributed pulmonary nodules surrounded by a 'halo' of ground-glass opacity (arrows).**

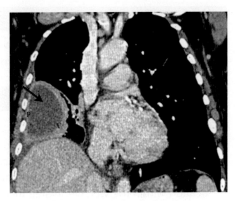

Coronal CT demonstrating a right lower lobe empyema (arrow). The central low attenuation collection of pus is surrounded by enhancing pleura. This demonstrates the 'split pleura' sign with separation of the visceral (v) from the parietal (p) pleural surfaces.

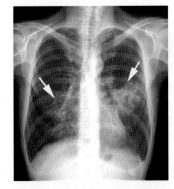

Haemophilus influenzae pneumonia. A 49-year-old man with fever. Posteroanterior chest radiograph shows bilateral areas of consolidation with ill-defined margins. A community-acquired *H. influenzae* pneumonia was diagnosed.**

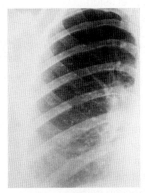

Multiple calcified varicella scars.†

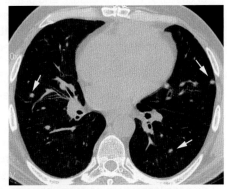

Varicella pneumonia. A 30-year-old man with lymphoma and new development of fever and skin rash. CT of the lower lobes shows multiple, bilateral and randomly distributed well-defined small pulmonary nodules (arrows).**

41

PULMONARY TUBERCULOSIS

DEFINITION

- Infection with *Mycobacterium tuberculosis* (95%) ▶ it is acquired via droplet inhalation
  - **Primary TB:** this is commonly seen in infants and children if previously unexposed to TB (hypersensitivity is absent) ▶ the patient is immunologically able to kill the organism and heals with fibrosis (± calcification)
  - **Post-primary TB:** if hypersensitivity is present (e.g. due to previous infection or BCG vaccination) a greater inflammatory reaction and caseous necrosis results ▶ this is usually due to reactivation of a quiescent lesion (and occasionally due to a new exogenous infection)
  - **Progressive primary TB:** direct transition from primary to post primary disease

CLINICAL PRESENTATION

- Loss of weight or appetite ▶ malaise ▶ fever ▶ night sweats ▶ cough (productive with haemoptysis)

RADIOLOGICAL FEATURES

Primary tuberculosis

- *Homogeneous pneumonia:* (mimicking a community-acquired pneumonia) ▶ any lobe may be involved to any size ▶ there is commonly a subpleural location within the well-ventilated lower lobes ▶ multifocal involvement and cavitation is unusual (cavitation suggests progressive primary disease) ▶ a pneumothorax can occur due to rupture into the pleural space
- *Nodal enlargement:* ipsilateral hilar ± mediastinal adenopathy ▶ this is the most common manifestation in children but is less commonly seen in adults (50% of cases) ▶ nodal pressure and bronchial erosion may cause segmental or lobar collapse (commonly the anterior segment of the RUL or ML) ▶ bronchial perforation and subsequent endobronchial spread can mimic a bronchopneumonia
- *Ghon lesion or focus:* in ⅓ of cases a residual well-defined rounded or irregular linear opacity remains (± calcification)
- *Ranke complex:* irregular and heterogeneous nodal calcification within the ipsilateral hilum or mediastinum which is seen in conjunction with a Ghon lesion
- *Miliary TB:* this is classically a manifestation of primary disease (representing overwhelming infection with haematogenous spread) – although it is now more commonly seen with post primary disease
  - Multiple small 1–2 mm discrete nodules (which are rarely calcified) are scattered evenly throughout both lungs

- *Pleural effusion:* this follows a subpleural infection ▶ it is often large, unilateral and isolated ▶ it is seen in children and young adults ▶ residual pleural change is unusual

Post-primary tuberculosis

- *Initial lesions:* Poorly marginated, nodular and linear opacities (approximately 5–10 mm) arising within the apico-posterior segments of an upper lobe or superior segment of a lower lobe (isolated involvement of the anterior segment of an upper lobe virtually excludes the diagnosis) ▶ they can be unilateral or bilateral, but with progression these opacities may coalesce
- *Cavitation:* this affects 40–80% of cases ▶ cavities may be single or multiple, large or small, or thin or thick walled (air-fluid levels are unusual)
  - *Rasmussen aneurysm:* a rare granulomatous weakening of a pulmonary arterial wall which can be life threatening
- *Pleural effusions:* these often progress to an empyema ▶ healing is complicated by pleural thickening and calcification
- *Healing:* the resultant fibrosis and scar formation results in well-defined upper lobe nodular or linear opacities ▶ there is associated volume loss, pleural thickening and occasional calcification (which is less common than with primary TB) ▶ bronchiectasis, cysts and bullae can develop
- *Miliary TB:* endobronchial spread can occur, appearing similar to that seen in primary TB
- *Tuberculoma:* this is due to repeated episodes of activation and healing which generates a growing nodule (10–15 mm in diameter) ▶ it is commonly solitary and well defined (calcification is common) ▶ there may be satellite lesions nearby ▶ it can also be seen with primary TB
- *Signs suggestive of active disease:* ill-defined coalesced nodules ▶ poorly marginated linear opacities ▶ cavitation ▶ unstable radiographic appearances

PEARLS

- Chemotherapy is successful and surgery is rarely required (including phrenic nerve ablation, plombage and thoracoplasty)
- **Non-tuberculous mycobacterial disease:** this is usually due to *M. kansasii* or *M. avium-intracellulare* complex (MAC)
  - *M. kansasii:* this resembles post-primary TB
  - *MAC:* this is an indolent process and does not resemble post-primary TB

  HRCT Small centrilobular nodules (with no lobar predilection) ▶ small airway ectasia (lingular and middle lobe bronchiectasis) ▶ 'tree in bud' opacities ▶ pleural effusions and lymphadenopathy are rare

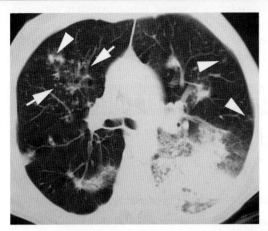

Endobronchial spread of tuberculosis. A 56-year-old man with post-primary tuberculosis. CT shows a non-cavitating consolidation in the left lung. Note typical images of 'tree-in-bud' opacities (arrows) and variable-sized bilateral nodular lesions (arrowheads).**

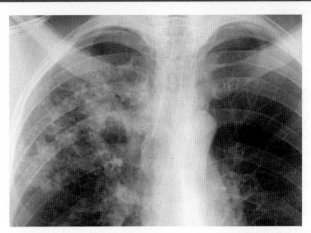

Post-primary tuberculosis. Magnified PA CXR demonstrates coalescence of poorly marginated reticular and nodular opacities in the right upper lobe with an irregularly margined moderately thick-walled cavity and small air–fluid level.*

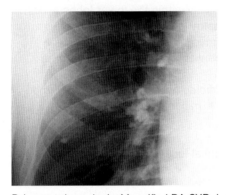

Primary tuberculosis. Magnified PA CXR demonstrates a right mid lung calcified nodule (Ghon focus) together with ipsilateral right hilar lymph node calcification (Ranke complex).*

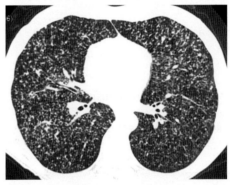

Miliary tuberculosis. A 26-year-old man with fever and shortness of breath. CT shows a random distribution of multiple, discrete 1–2 mm in diameter nodules.**

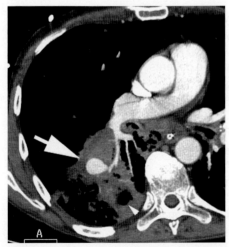

Rasmussen aneurysm. A 65-year-old man with chronic destructive pulmonary tuberculosis. Contrast-enhanced CT at the level of the right pulmonary artery shows a contrast-filling aneurysm (arrow) within parenchymal consolidation in a superior segment of the right lower lobe. Note an associated parenchymal cavity (arrowhead).**

	Primary TB	Post-primary TB
Consolidation	Can affect an entire lobe ▶ multifocal involvement is rare	Poorly marginated ▶ can be multifocal
Location	Lung bases	Upper lobes
Lymphadenopathy	Common	Rare
Pleural effusion	Common	More likely to be an empyema
Cavitation	Rare	Common (active disease)
Miliary TB	Yes	Yes

43

CRYPTOCOCCOSIS (TORULOSIS)

Definition

- This follows infection with *Cryptococcus neoformans* (an encapsulated yeast-like fungus found in soil and bird droppings)

Clinical presentation

- Many patients are asymptomatic
- 50% of symptomatic infections are associated with immunodeficiency
- It may spread to other organs, with the central nervous system being the most frequently affected site

Radiological features

CXR 3 patterns:
- *Pulmonary masses* (which can be very large, are usually single, have ill-defined edges and which may cavitate)
- *Homogeneous segmental or lobar opacification (± air bronchograms, cavitation and lymphadenopathy)*
- *Diffuse nodular (occasionally miliary) or reticulonodular opacities*

CT Similar findings: 'acinar' nodules – but there is no 'tree-in-bud' change

Pearls

- Cavitation, adenopathy and pleural effusion are all uncommon
- Meningoencephalitis is the most serious CNS complication

HISTOPLASMOSIS

Definition

- This follows infection with *Histoplasma capsulatum* (a fungus found in moist soil, bird or bat excreta)
- It is common in North America

Clinical presentation

- Most cases are asymptomatic

Radiological features

CXR/CT Multiple poorly defined nodules (5–10 mm) ▶ there is less commonly a segmental or lobar pneumonia
- *Chronic pulmonary histoplasmosis:* this resembles a post-primary tuberculosis:
  - The hilar and mediastinal nodes are frequently enlarged ▶ there are multiple calcified 3–4 mm sharply marginated round nodules ▶ calcified lymph nodes are seen within the hila and mediastinum

- *Histoplasmoma:* a solitary well-defined nodule ▶ the calcified centre forms a 'target' lesion (which is very specific sign)
- *Fibrosing mediastinitis:* this may occur with constriction of the SVC and pulmonary vessels

OTHER FUNGAL INFECTIONS

COCCIDIOIMYCOSIS

Definition

- This follows inhalation of *Coccidioides immitis* spores

Clinical presentation

- Usually asymptomatic

Radiological features

CXR
- Consolidation, especially within the lower lobes ▶ hilar/mediastinal adenopathy in 20% ▶ it usually resolves
- Chronic coccidioidomycosis occurs in 5% of cases ▶ solitary/multiple nodules, which cavitate to become thin-walled cavities
- Disseminated coccidioidomycosis is very rare ▶ small nodules (5–10 mm) ▶ miliary appearance

Pearl

- Reactivation of an initial focus can occur (e.g. with tuberculosis)

CANDIDIASIS

Definition

- This is caused by various organisms in the *Candida* group, especially *Candida albicans* (a commensal within the oral pharynx) ▶ infection occurs in immunocompromised patients

Clinical presentation

- It usually infects mucous membranes and skin
- Pulmonary infection is rare, due to aspiration

Radiological features

CXR Areas of consolidation – multiple, patchy and bilateral
- Cavitation and hilar adenopathy are very rare
- Pleural effusion occurs in 25%

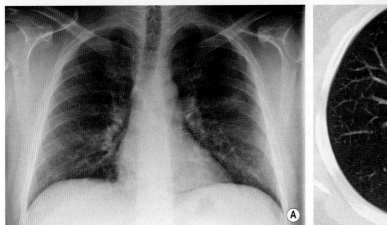
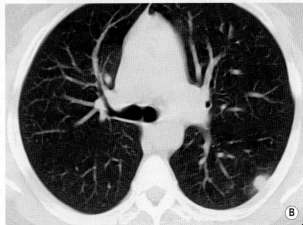

Cryptococcus. (A) PA CXR demonstrates a poorly marginated left mid lung nodular opacity. (B) CT demonstrates a solid left lower lobe nodule with minimal surrounding halo.*

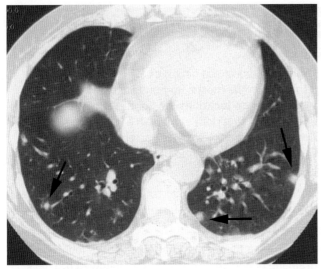

Candida pneumonia. A 52-year-old man who underwent bone marrow transplantation. CT shows multiple ill-defined bilateral nodules (arrows).**

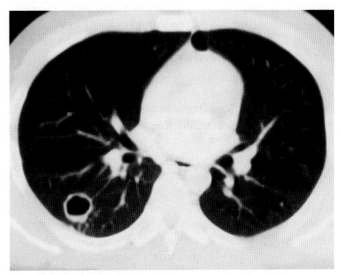

Coccidioidomycosis. CT demonstrates a relatively thin-walled cavity in the right lower lobe. The classic lesion of coccidioidomycosis has a paper-thin wall.

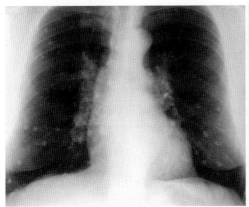

Chronic histoplasmosis. PA CXR demonstrates several well-defined uniform-sized calcified nodules in both lungs with bilateral hilar and mediastinal lymph node calcification.*

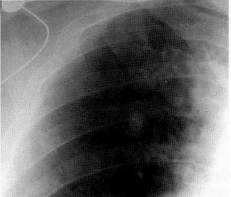

The right upper lobe demonstrates central target calcification with surrounding soft tissue opacity very suggestive of histoplasmoma.*

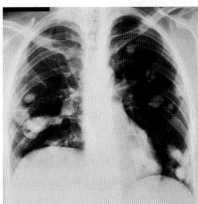

Multiple calcified histoplasmomas. The denser nodules are heavily calcified.

ASPERGILLUS INFECTION

Definition

- This is caused by infection with *Aspergillus fumigatus* ▶ the disease type depends on an individual's immune response

Radiological features

Aspergilloma *There is a normal immune status* ▶ there is colonization of a pre-existing lung cavity with little invasion of the surrounding lung – as most cavities are due to sarcoidosis or TB mycetomas these tend to be located within the upper lobes ▶ the majority are asymptomatic although haemoptysis is an important complication (which may warrant surgical lung resection or bronchial artery embolization)

CXR A fungal mass (mycetoma) within a cavity with thickened walls (± adjacent pleura) ▶ it may demonstrate a freely moving fungus ball on decubitus imaging ▶ there may be an 'air crescent' sign around the mycetoma ▶ calcification and fluid levels are infrequent

Allergic bronchopulmonary aspergillosis (ABPA) *This is due to a hypersensitivity reaction (type I) within the major airways leading to wall damage, bronchiectasis and fibrosis* ▶ there is an elevated serum IgE and a positive skin test ▶ it is common in asthma and cystic fibrosis

CXR/CT Consolidation (± a surrounding ground-glass 'halo') ranging from subsegmental to lobar involvement ▶ when the consolidation clears, any residual bronchiectasis creates a favourable environment for fungal recolonization ▶ atelectasis and occasionally cavitation are seen ▶ upper lobe predominance

- *Mucoid impaction:* this obstructs the airways (the lung parenchyma remains aerated by collateral drift, permitting visualization of an impacted airway)
  - *'Finger in glove' appearance:* bronchoceles appearing as branching thick tubular opacities pointing to the hilum
- *Bronchiectasis:* this is permanent and indicates irreversible lung damage ▶ it affects the proximal bronchi more commonly than other bronchiectatic diseases ▶ there can be air trapping
  - *'Tree in bud' appearance:* mucoid impaction within dilated bronchioles
- *Late disease:* there is upper lobe fibrotic volume loss (the overall lung volume is frequently increased due to lower lobe overinflation, small airway obstruction and upper lobe bullae and cavitation)

Chronic necrotizing (semi-invasive) aspergillosis *There is a normal or mildly impaired immune status* ▶ this demonstrates a more chronic disease course than seen with invasive aspergillosis ▶ there is local lung invasion (upper lobes) ▶ it affects debilitated patients or patients with pre-existing lung damage or chronic disease

CXR/CT Heterogeneous opacities (resembling TB) followed by enlarging thick-walled cavity (weeks later)

▶ adjacent pleural thickening ▶ occasionally mycetoma formation ▶ bilateral and multiple nodules have been reported

Invasive aspergillosis *This affects immunocompromised hosts* ▶ there is aggressive vascular invasion and parenchymal necrosis (with a high mortality) ▶ acute tracheobronchitis, bronchiolitis and bronchopneumonia

CXR/CT Rounded poorly marginated nodules (± air bronchograms) which may resemble a mass ▶ 50% cavitate forming an 'air crescent' (which indicates recovery) ▶ there are rarely miliary nodules

- *'Angioinvasive disease':* wedge-shaped peripheral opacities due to vascular invasion and lung infarction

HRCT Perinodular ground-glass haloes (due to associated haemorrhage) ▶ pleurally based wedge-shaped consolidation

COMPLICATIONS OF PNEUMONIA

Lung abscess

- **Definition:** Localised necrotic cavity containing pus
- Aspiration is the most common cause
- **Most common locations:** posterior segment of an upper lobe / superior segment of a lower lobe
- **Common causes:** anaerobic bacteria / *S. aureus* / *P aeruginosa* / *K. pneumonia*

Pulmonary gangrene

- **Definition:** fragments of necrotic lung within an abscess cavity (pulmonary sequestrum)

Pneumatocele

- **Definition:** a thin-walled, gas-filled space following drainage of a focus of necrotic lung followed by check valve obstruction of the subtending airway
- *Common causes: S. aureus* (infants) ▶ *P. jiroveci* (AIDS)

Septic emboli

- **Definition:** Septic foci can originate from cardiac valves (endocarditis) / peripheral veins (thrombophlebitis) / venous catheters
- *Imaging:* solid nodules ± cavitation ▶ 'feeding vessel' sign

Empyema

- **Definition:** a collection of pus within the lung
- *Common organisms: S. pneumonia / S. pyogenes / S. aureus*

Bronchoplueral fistula

- **Definition:** a sinus tract between the bronchus and pleural space
- *Causes:* necrotizing pneumonia / surgery / tumour / trauma
- *Imaging:* increased intrapleural air space / new or changes in an air-fluid level / tension pneumothorax

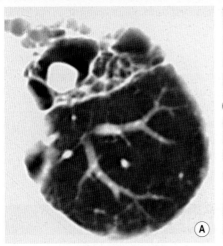
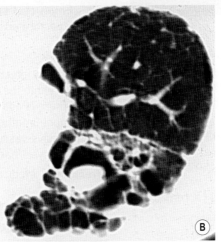

Aspergilloma. (A) Supine and (B) prone CT of the upper lobe demonstrate a fungus ball moving within the left upper lobe cavity.*

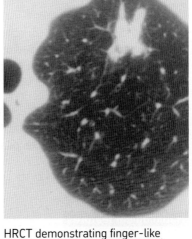

HRCT demonstrating finger-like opacities due to dilated mucous-filled bronchi.[†]

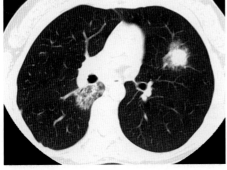

Invasive aspergillosis. CT demonstrating heterogeneous and ground-glass opacity in the azygo-oesophageal lung recess as well as a nodule within the lingular lobe consisting of an opaque centre and ground-glass halo.*

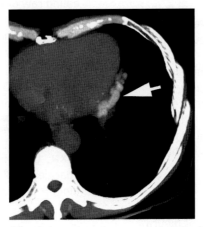

Allergic bronchopulmonary aspergillosis. A 43-year-old asthmatic man with cough. Non-enhanced CT section shows a tubular opacity in the lingula containing a hyperdense mucoid impaction.**

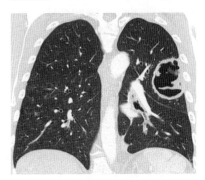

Lung abscess. A 35-year-old man with high fever and large purulent sputum production with positive culture for *P. aeruginosa*. Coronal reformatted CT shows a large cavity in the left upper lobe. Note intracavitary thick septa.**

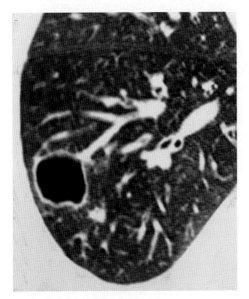

Pneumatocele. A 32-year-old woman with previous *S. aureus* pneumonia. CT shows thin-walled cystic lesion (pneumatocele) in the right lower lobe.**

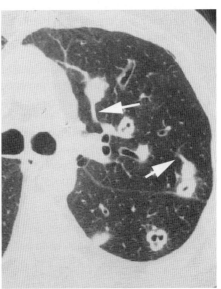

Septic embolism. A 40-year-old male, intravenous drug user with fever. CT shows multiple cavitated nodules in the left upper lobe. Different vessels (arrows) course into the nodules. Blood cultures were positive for *S. aureus*.**

HYDATID DISEASE

Definition

- Hydatid disease (echinococcosis) is a metazoal infestation caused by a tapeworm (usually *Echinococcus granulosus*) ▶ humans are accidental hosts – infection is acquired by ingesting ova (e.g. from contaminated water) and by direct contact with dogs
- Cysts develop within the lungs (less commonly within the mediastinum) and are usually solitary
  - 10% of cysts are multiple, bilateral, or associated with liver cysts
  - At presentation ⅔ of cysts are ruptured (⅓ remain intact)

Radiological features

Unruptured pulmonary cysts

- One or more homogeneous, roughly spherical or oval, sharply demarcated mass lesions (1–10 cm) ▶ these occur particularly within the mid or lower lobes ▶ they are of soft tissue density and almost never calcify (unlike their mediastinal counterparts)
- The cysts are easily deformed where they come up against any major bronchovascular structures:
  - This leads to lobulation or an eccentric contour, or flattening of their peripheral aspects where they come into contact with the chest wall or mediastinum
  - They can also demonstrate changes in shape with breathing

Ruptured pulmonary cysts

- These are usually associated with secondary infection and rupture may occur into the airways or pleural spaces ▶ this is associated with acute symptoms which often precipitates presentation
- Cyst wall layers:
  - *Pericyst:* adventitia formed of compressed host lung tissue
  - *Ectocyst:* middle layer of friable tissue
  - *Endocyst:* inner germinal layer from which are produced the scolices
- If the two inner layers remain intact then airway communication results in a ring opacity containing a rounded, homogeneous density resembling the air crescent of a mycetoma
- If there is disruption of the inner layers a complex cavitary lesion results which can demonstrate an air-fluid level or the following signs:
  - *'Double wall' sign:* ectocyst has separated from the pericyst
  - *'Water lily'/'camalote' sign:* a floating membrane
  - *'Rising sun'/'serpent' sign:* an essentially dry cyst with crumpled membranes lying at its bottom

- *'Empty cyst' sign:* a cyst with all its contents expectorated

Pearls

- Secondary infection may produce a lung abscess
- Rupture into the pleural space can cause an effusion or if there is additional airway communication a hydropneumothorax
- Aggressive vascular invasion may result in massive haemoptysis/haemorrhage

Treatment Medical (albendazole) ▶ surgical resection

PARAGONIMIASIS

Definition A metazoal infestation due to a fluke (*Paragonimus westermani*) that develops from a larval form in the lung and produces ova ▶ it is acquired from eating raw or incompletely cooked freshwater crabs and crayfish
- *Intermediate hosts:* water snails and crustaceans
- It is mostly found within the Far East, Southeast Asia and Africa

Diagnosis Ova within the sputum ▶ anti-*Paragonimus* antibody within the blood

Clinical presentation Chronic cough ▶ sputum ▶ haemoptysis

CXR Consolidation, nodules, band, tubular and ring opacities (5–30 mm) within any lobe (especially the mid lung) ▶ pleural effusions are seen in up to 50% of cases

CT As above, but in addition peripheral lineal opacities (representing worm migration tracks) may be seen

ENTAMOEBA HISTOLYTICA

Definition A protozoal infection – pleuropulmonary amoebiasis is usually secondary to liver involvement (developing in ⅕ of patients with liver disease) ▶ lung is the second most common site after the liver
- It characteristically affects young adults (M>F)

CXR Lung involvement usually occurs at the right lung base with hemidiaphragmatic elevation, and a pleural effusion (± thickening and plate-like atelectasis) ▶ if a liver abscess erodes through the diaphragm the basal homogeneous opacification can cavitate
- Haematogenous spread can occasionally give rise to similar appearances within other lung segments
- Haemoptysis can occur secondary to fistulation into a major bronchus, containing the 'anchovy paste' pus coming from the amoebic abscess

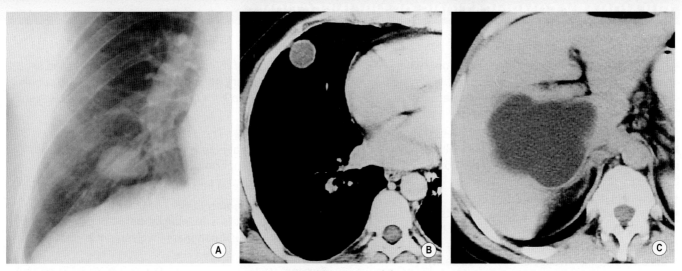

Pulmonary hydatid disease. (A) A well-defined right basal pulmonary mass. (B) The CT reveals a well-defined wall and cystic contents. (C) The patient also had a large hepatic hydatid cyst.[†]

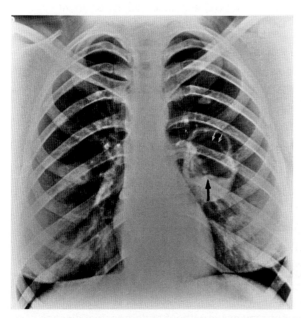

Hydatid cysts. There are multiple nodules in both lungs, some of which have cavitated. A meniscus or crescent can be identified (small arrows) in the large cyst in the left lung, which also displays an air-fluid level and 'water lily' sign (black arrows).[‡]

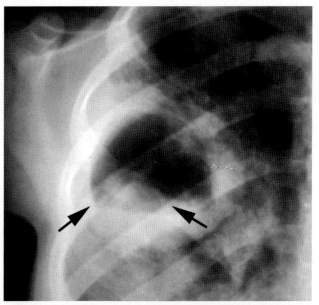

Ruptured hydatid cyst. A 65-year-old male shepherd with abrupt onset of expectoration and pruritus. Close-up view of the right upper lung shows a cystic lesion surrounded by a parenchymal consolidation due to a massive aspiration of intracystic content. Note a rounded opacity immediately above the fluid level ('water lily' sign (arrows).[**]

PULMONARY COMPLICATIONS OF HIV INFECTION

Pneumocystis jiroveci (formerly *carinii*)

Definition A fungal infection manifesting only when immunosuppressed (CD4 ≤ 100 cells/mm³) ▶ elevated serum lactase dehydrogenase (LDH) is a sensitive (but non-specific) indicator

CXR/CT 5–10% have a normal CXR at presentation ▶ classically diffuse bilateral interstitial infiltrates in a perihilar distribution ▶ usually there are no sequelae but pulmonary fibrosis can develop
- *Pleural fluid or adenopathy:* this is rare
- *Pneumatocele:* this affects 10% of patients ▶ they may rapidly increase or decrease in size and then gradually resolve ▶ they appear within a few days and can persist as a chronic thin-walled and air-filled cavity
- *Spontaneous pneumothorax* (5%): this is due to multiple upper lobe pneumatocoeles ▶ management is difficult as bronchopleural fistulas are common
- *Unusual presentations:* diffuse or focal miliary nodules ▶ homogeneous opacities ▶ solitary or multiple well-formed nodules ▶ moderate to thick-walled cavitary nodules
- Upper lobe involvement is common as aerosolized pentamidine may not reach the upper lobes (which can resemble reactivation TB)

Mycobacterium tuberculosis Clinical features depend on the stage of immunosuppression at infection (and which may be indistinguishable from 'ordinary' disease with early stage HIV) ▶ in late stage HIV there is often a negative tuberculin skin test with >50% of patients having extrapulmonary (especially lymph node) involvement
- *Primary TB:* lymphadenopathy ± consolidation ▶ residual Ghon focus / Ranke complex
- *Reactivation / Reinfection TB:* more frequent cavitation (active disease), upper lobe predilection ▶ military TB ▶ endobronchial spread ('tree-in-bud')

Pulmonary non-tuberculous Mycobacteria (NTMB) Due to *Mycobacterium avium* complex or *M. kansasii* ▶ disease status depends on any underlying lung disease / immunocompetence
- *Mycobacterium avium complex:* there are no distinctive features (diffuse bilateral opacities, focal consolidation, pleural fluid, adenopathy)
- *M. kansasii:* indistinguishable from reactivation / reinfection TB

Pyogenic organisms Community-acquired pneumonias (*S. pneumoniae* / *H. influenzae*) are common in HIV-infected patients ▶ the radiographic features are similar to those seen in non-immunosuppressed individuals

Candidiasis

CXR/CT multiple bilateral nodular opacities ± consolidation / ground-glass opacities ▶ less common: pleural effusion / bronchial wall thickening / cavitation

Mucormycosis

CXR/CT Lobar / multilobar consolidation and solid or multiple pulmonary nodules or masses with a surrounding ground-glass halo ▶ cavitation (up to 40%) ▶ 'air crescent' sign

Cytomegalovirus This is well documented in post transplantation patients ▶ its role in HIV pneumonia is unclear (due to superimposed infections)

CXR/CT A bilateral fine reticular pattern (similar to PCP)

Cryptococcus neoformans The usual disease process seen in HIV patients is meningitis, but ⅓ of patients will have simultaneous pulmonary involvement ▶ (CD4 ≤ 100 cells/mm³)

CXR/CT Pulmonary masses (5 mm ± can be very large) with a possible halo similar to *Aspergillus* ▶ homogenous segmental / lobar opacifications ▶ miliary, reticular interstitial pattern

Histoplasma capsulatum

CXR/CT Normal (50%) ▶ diffuse nodular or linear opacities (50%) ▶ pleural effusions (20%) ▶ adenopathy (10%)
- Coarse and nodular lung changes, or adenopathy, distinguishes this from PCP ▶ fibrosing mediastinitis can develop

Coccidioidomycosis

CXR/CT Diffuse, medium to coarse nodular opacities (similar to histoplasmosis or disseminated TB) ▶ can have a classic CT appearance of central soft tissue attenuation with a ground-glass halo ▶ cavitation and adenopathy is seen in 35% of cases ▶ miliary appearance in disseminated disease

Aspergillosis This is relatively infrequent in HIV patients

Kaposi's sarcoma

Definition This is caused by the human herpes virus 8 (in association with AIDS) ▶ it is rare in the lung in the absence of any cutaneous involvement ▶ parenchymal involvement may occur without endobronchial disease

CXR/CT Linear, rounded or reticulonodular shadowing predominantly in a perihilar distribution (reflecting the bronchocentric distribution of the disease) ▶ there is a tendency for the shadowing to coalesce (unlike lymphoma) ▶ lymphadenopathy and pleural effusions (tending to be bilateral and large) are common ▶ cavitation is rare
- Rapid progression to airspace consolidation usually represents lung haemorrhage
- Endobronchial disease may result in atelectasis or a postobstructive pneumonia

Pearls Focal segmental or lobar opacities are usually due to the tumour itself ▶ the pulmonary opacities seen with Kaposi's sarcoma do not tend to fluctuate in severity

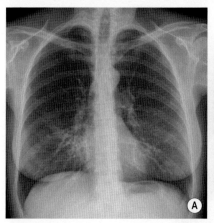
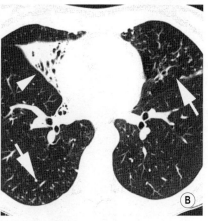

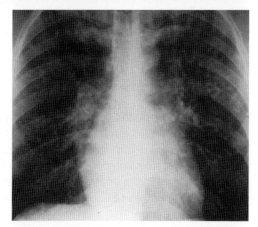

Mycobacterium avium–intracellulare complex. A 65-year-old woman with chronic cough. (A) Posteroanterior chest radiograph shows bilateral opacities in the right middle lobe and lingula. (B) CT at the level of the inferior pulmonary veins shows complete collapse of the middle lobe containing visible bronchiectasis (arrowhead). Note the presence of small nodular opacities and few tree-in-bud opacities in the lingula and in the superior segment of the right lower lobe (arrows).**

Tuberculosis. A PA CXR demonstrates a diffuse, bilateral coarse nodular pattern associated with right hilar adenopathy. This combination of findings should suggest the presence of fungal or mycobacterial disease.*

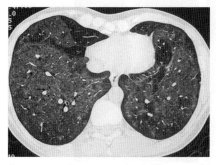
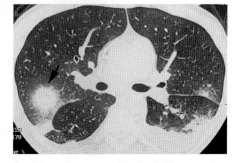
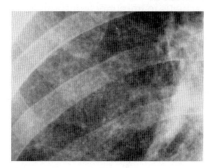

Pneumocystis pneumonia. A 45-year-old homosexual man with severe dyspnoea. CT shows extensive bilateral ground-glass opacities. Bronchoalveolar lavage showed *P. jiroveci*.**

Angioinvasive aspergillosis. A 65-year-old man with immunosuppression and severe neutropenia presents with fever. CT shows a nodule with surrounding ground-glass attenuation (CT halo sign) (arrow). Note also bilateral poorly marginated peripheral areas of consolidation.**

Cryptococcosis. A 24-year-old HIV-positive man with dyspnoea and fever. Close-up view of a posteroanterior chest radiograph shows diffuse small ill-defined nodules.**

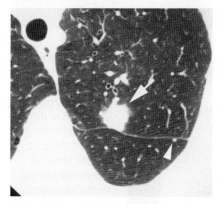
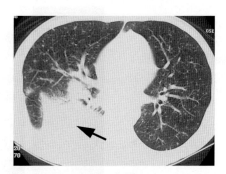
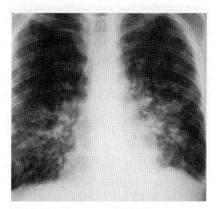

Histoplasmoma. A 62-year-old asymptomatic woman living in an area endemic for histoplasmosis. An incidental nodule was found on routine chest radiography. CT shows a rounded opacity in the left upper lobe (arrow). A 3-mm nodule (arrowhead) is also seen in the superior segment of the left lower lobe.**

Coccidioidomycosis. A 38-year-old man with vague chest pain and fever. CT shows a parenchymal consolidation in the superior segment of the right lower lobe (arrow). Note multiple miliary nodules randomly distributed through both lungs.**

Kaposi's sarcoma. A PA CXR demonstrates coarse linear opacities in the perihilar regions. Some nodular opacities are noted in the right upper lobe. Left pleural fluid is present. This constellation of findings is highly suggestive of Kaposi's sarcoma.*

1.4 LARGE AIRWAY DISEASE

POST-TRAUMATIC STRICTURES

Definition These are usually secondary to damage from external neck trauma or from a cuffed endotracheal or tracheostomy tube

CXR/CT A focus of circumferential or eccentric tracheal narrowing associated with a segment of increased soft tissue

- *Postintubation stenosis:* this extends for several cm ▶ it typically involves the trachea above the level of the thoracic inlet
- *Post-tracheostomy stenosis:* this typically begins 1–1.5 cm distal to the inferior margin of the tracheostomy stoma ▶ it involves 1.5–2.5 cm of tracheal wall

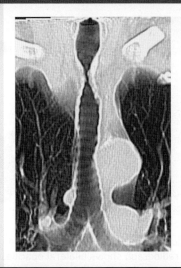

Post-intubation tracheal stenosis in severe COPD. Coronal oblique average image (21-mm-thick slab). Note the visibility of the tracheal cartilage.**

INFECTIOUS TRACHEOBRONCHITIS

Definition This is most commonly due to a bacterial tracheitis in immunocompromised patients ▶ it is also seen with TB, rhinoscleroma and necrotizing invasive aspergillosis

CT Irregular and circumferential tracheobronchial thickening ± mediastinitis

- *Active phase:* a narrowed and irregularly thickened trachea ± the main bronchi
- *Fibrotic/healed phase:* a narrowed trachea with a smooth wall of normal thickness

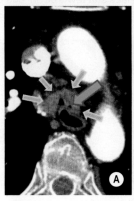
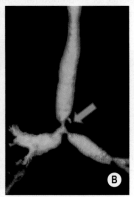

Infectious tracheobronchitis. (A) Severe stenosis of the distal trachea (orange arrows) and proximal main bronchi associated with a fistulous tract (blue arrow) connecting with a paratracheal submucosal abscess. (B) 3-D reconstruction.**

TRACHEOBRONCHIAL FISTULA AND DEHISCENCE

Bronchopleural fistula This is most commonly caused by a necrotizing pneumonia or secondary to trauma

Nodobronchial/nodobroncho-oesophageal fistula This is commonly caused by *Mycobacterium tuberculosis* ▶ it is characterized by gas within a cavitated hilar or mediastinal lymphadenopathy

Tracheo-oesophageal fistulas The most common cause is a malignant neoplasia (particularly oesophageal) ▶ infection and trauma are other causes

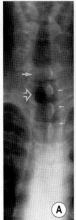
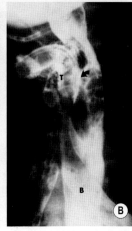

Tracheo-oesophageal fistula following prolonged intubation and an indwelling NGT. (A) PA XR of the trachea reveals a tracheal stenosis (arrow) proximal to a tracheostomy stoma (open arrow). The proximal oesophagus is distended with air (arrows) close to the fistula. (B) A contrast study demonstrates filling of the fistula (arrow) and aspiration of contrast medium from the oesophagus (O) into the trachea (T) and main bronchi (B).‡

TRACHEAL NEOPLASMS

Benign

Definition This is most commonly a hamartoma, leiomyoma, neurogenic tumour or lipoma

CT A well-demarcated and round lesion (< 2 cm) ▶ a smoothly marginated intraluminal polyp (hamartomas and lipomas may demonstrate fat attenuation)

Malignant

Definition These are uncommon – the vast majority are a squamous cell or adenoid cystic carcinoma

CT A soft tissue mass (usually involving the posterior and lateral walls) ▶ it is often sessile and eccentric resulting in asymmetrical luminal narrowing ▶ can be polypoid and mostly intraluminal (with mediastinal extension seen in 30–40%)

Secondary malignant neoplasms

Definition These can be due to a haematogenous metastasis (commonly renal cell carcinoma and melanoma) or following direct local invasion

CT Intraluminal soft tissue nodules and wall thickening

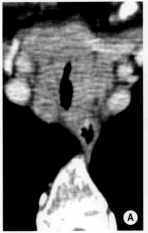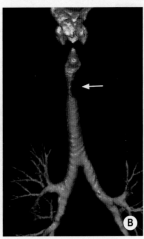

Adenoid cystic carcinoma of the trachea. (A) Axial CT at the level of the supra-aortic part of the mediastinum. Irregular stenosis of the tracheal lumen due to a soft tissue mass developing from the posterior and left lateral wall of the trachea. (B) Coronal 3D external volume rendering. The level, length and degree of the tracheal lumen involvement (arrow) is accurately assessed.*

TRACHEOBRONCHIAL PAPILLOMATOSIS

Definition This is caused by human papillomavirus infection (and usually acquired at birth from an infected mother) ▶ it usually involves the larynx – occasionally extension into the trachea and proximal bronchi is seen

CT Typically multiple small nodules projecting into the airway lumen or diffuse nodular thickening of the airway wall ▶ although benign it may undergo transformation to a squamous cell carcinoma

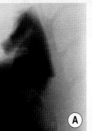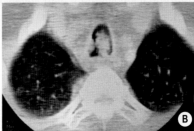

Diffuse tracheobronchial papillomatosis. (A) Lateral soft tissue view of the neck reveals nodular masses in the larynx and proximal trachea representing multiple papillomas. (B) CT reveals near obstruction of the tracheal lumen by irregular polypoid masses.‡

TRACHEOBRONCHOMALACIA

Definition This results from weakened tracheal cartilage rings ▶ It is seen in association with tracheobronchomegaly, COPD, relapsing polychondritis and following trauma

CT Luminal diameter narrowing > 70% on expiration compared with inspiration ▶ calibre changes >50% can be seen at expiration with normal tracheal compliance with high dynamic pressure gradients (e.g. COPD) ▶ a coronal tracheal diameter significantly larger than the sagittal diameter (producing a lunate configuration)

- Central tracheobronchial tree involvement may be either diffuse or focal

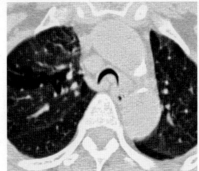

Tracheobronchomalacia. Axial CT acquired during a dynamic expiratory manoeuvre. The collapse of the tracheal lumen is almost complete. The tracheal lumen is crescentic in shape because of the bowing of the posterior membranous trachea.*

ANCA-ASSOCIATED GRANULOMATOUS VASCULITIS

Definition Large airway involvement is common (± subglottic or bronchial stenosis, ulceration and pseudotumour formation)

CT Thickening of the subglottic region and proximal trachea (smooth symmetrical or asymmetrical narrowing over a variable length) ▶ nodular or polypoid lesions may be seen on the inner airway contour ▶ luminal stenosis may affect any main, lobar or segmental bronchus

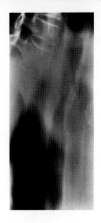

An oblique tracheal tomogram reveals an hourglass stenosis of the mid trachea, representing changes of Wegener's granulomatosis.[‡]

RELAPSING POLYCHONDRITIS

Definition A rare systemic autoimmune disease affecting the cartilage of the ears, nose, joints and tracheobronchial tree (inflammation is followed by fibrosis) ▶ usually there is a symmetrical subglottic stenosis – with disease progression the distal trachea and bronchi may become involved

CT Smooth airway wall thickening associated with diffuse narrowing ▶ early sparing of the posterior tracheal wall (circumferential involvement with advanced disease) ▶ the trachea may become flaccid with considerable collapse at expiration ▶ fibrotic cartilaginous ring destruction may cause stenosis

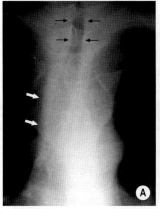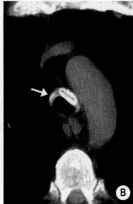

Relapsing polychondritis. (A) PA CXR demonstrating narrowing of the upper tracheal lumen (black arrows). The right paratracheal band is abnormally thickened (white arrows). (B) Axial CT showing abnormal thickening of the anterior and lateral walls of the trachea associated with calcium deposits (arrow). The posterior membranous wall of the trachea is unaffected.[*]

TRACHEOBRONCHIAL AMYLOIDOSIS

Definition This is seen in association with systemic amyloidosis or as an isolated manifestation – therefore it can form either multifocal or diffuse submucosal plaques or masses (with an intact overlying mucosa) ▶ dystrophic calcification or ossification is frequently present

CT Focal or diffuse airway wall thickening and luminal narrowing (proximal bronchial narrowing can lead to distal atelectasis, bronchiectasis or an obstructive pneumonia)

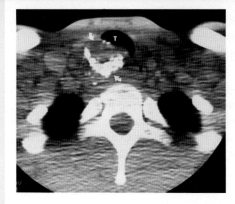

Tracheal amyloidosis. CT of the proximal trachea demonstrating pronounced tracheal narrowing (T) by a large calcified soft tissue mass arising from the right posterolateral tracheal wall (arrows).[‡]

SABRE-SHEATH TRACHEA

Definition

Diffuse narrowing involving the intrathoracic trachea (the pathogenesis is probably related to the abnormal pattern of intrathoracic pressures generated by the usually coexistent COPD)

CT The internal side-to-side diameter of the trachea is halved or less than the corresponding sagittal diameter ▶ the narrowing usually affects the whole intrathoracic trachea (with an abrupt return to a normal calibre at the thoracic inlet) ▶ frequently there is calcification of the tracheal cartilage rings

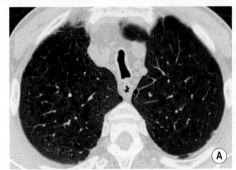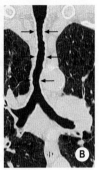

Sabre-sheath trachea in a patient with COPD. (A) Axial CT shows a significant reduction of the coronal diameter of the trachea. Bilateral centrilobular and paraseptal emphysematous areas are also present. (B) Coronal oblique reformat demonstrating a reduction of the coronal diameter of the tracheal lumen (arrows). The upper part of the trachea above the thoracic inlet has a normal appearance.*

TRACHEOBRONCHOMEGALY (MOUNIER–KUHN DISEASE)

Definition Marked dilatation of the trachea and mainstem bronchi (atrophy affects the elastic and muscular elements of the trachea)

- The immediate subglottic trachea has a normal diameter but expands as it passes to the carina (and continuing into the major bronchi) ▶ atrophic mucosa prolapses between the cartilage rings giving the trachea a corrugated outline (this may become exaggerated to form sacculations)
- It is often associated with tracheal diverticulosis, recurrent lower respiratory tract infections and bronchiectasis

Diagnostic criteria Tracheal diameter > 3 cm (measured 2 cm above the aortic arch) ▶ diameters > 2.4 and 2.3 cm for the right and left main bronchi, respectively

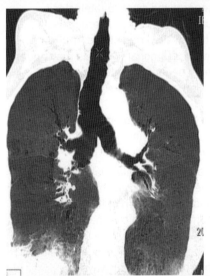

Tracheobronchomegaly. Coronal oblique MIP reformat with dilatation of the trachea into the proximal bronchi. There is a scalloped appearance of the airway due to mucosal protrusion between cartilaginous rings.**

TRACHEOBRONCHOPATHIA OSTEOCHONDROPLASTICA

Definition This is rare and characterized by multiple cartilaginous nodules and bony submucosal nodules on the inner surface of the trachea and proximal airways (with sparing of the posterior tracheal wall as this contains no cartilage) ▶ the nodules contain heterotopic bone, cartilage and calcified acellular protein matrix with normal overlying bronchial mucosa ▶ M>F (usually > 50 years old)

CT Thickened tracheal cartilage rings with irregular calcifications ▶ nodules may protrude from the anterior and lateral luminal walls into the lumen (usually with foci of calcification)

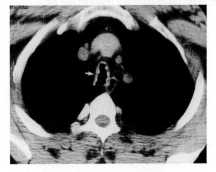

Tracheobronchopathia osteochondroplastica. CT of the trachea demonstrates nodularity of the anterior and lateral cartilaginous tracheal walls with a smooth normal-appearing posterior wall.‡

BRONCHIECTASIS

DEFINITION

- Local, irreversible dilatation of the bronchi which is usually associated with inflammation ▶ the mechanisms include:
  - *Bronchial obstruction and bronchial wall damage:* the common factor is a combination of mucous plugging and bacterial colonization leading to a vicious cycle of increasing airway damage
  - *Parenchymal fibrosis:* with bronchial dilatation secondary to external fibrotic retraction

CLINICAL PRESENTATION

- Cough ▶ sputum ▶ haemoptysis ▶ digital clubbing
- There is an increasing prevalence with age (except if secondary to cystic fibrosis)

RADIOLOGICAL FEATURES

CXR Dilated bronchi filled with mucus or pus resulting in tubular or ovoid opacities of varying sizes ▶ overinflation is often present with generalized disease (atelectasis can be seen with localized forms) ▶ cystic bronchiectasis manifests as multiple thin-walled ring shadows often containing air fluid levels ▶ pulmonary vessels may appear increased in size and may be indistinct due to adjacent peribronchial inflammation and fibrosis ▶ thickened bronchial walls:

- *'Tramlines':* single or parallel line opacities
- *'Ring shadows':* poorly defined ring or curvilinear opacities are seen when enface

HRCT Bronchial dilatation ± bronchial wall thickening ▶ lack of peripheral tapering of the bronchial lumen with visualization of the bronchi within 1 cm of the costal pleura or abutting the mediastinal pleura (a cardinal sign of bronchiectasis) ▶ subtle lower lobe volume loss in early disease with crowding of the dilated bronchi ▶ possible complete collapse with bronchiectatic airways

- *'Signet ring' sign:* the internal bronchial diameter is greater than that of the adjacent pulmonary artery
- *'Finger in glove' sign:* secretion and mucus accumulation within the bronchiectatic airways can lead to V- or Y-shaped densities ▶ if 'en face' can appear as nodular opacities running alongside adjacent pulmonary arteries

General distribution of bronchiectatic diseases

Bilateral upper lobes	Cystic fibrosis/ABPA
Unilateral upper lobe	TB
Lower lobes	Childhood viral infections

PEARLS

- **Causes include:**
  - **Congenital:** cystic fibrosis ▶ Kartagener's syndrome (abnormal mucociliary transport)
  - **Post infection** (bronchial wall damage): childhood pneumonia (pertussis and measles) is a common cause ▶ allergic bronchopulmonary aspergillosis (ABPA) ▶ chronic granulomatous infection
  - **Obstructive:** neoplasm ▶ lymphadenopathy ▶ aspiration ▶ foreign body
  - **External:** parenchymal fibrosis ('traction' bronchiectasis)
- It is classified into three subtypes (reflecting an increasing disease severity):
  - **Cylindrical:** relatively uniform airway dilatation
  - **Varicose:** non-uniform and somewhat serpiginous dilatation
    - *'String of pearls':* the bronchial lumen assumes a beaded configuration on HRCT
  - **Cystic:** saccular dilatation ▶ multiple thin-walled ring shadows often containing air-fluid levels
    - *'Cluster of grapes':* a string of cysts or clusters of cysts on HRCT
- **Bronchiolitis:** this is seen in about 70% of bronchiectatic patients (and may precede the development of bronchiectasis)

  HRCT Peripheral airway involvement leads to areas of decreased attenuation and vascularity – the resultant mosaic perfusion pattern and expiratory air trapping reflects the extent of any obliterative bronchiolitis
  - *'Tree-in-bud' appearance:* small centrilobular nodular or linear branching opacities which are seen with an inflammatory or infectious bronchiolitis

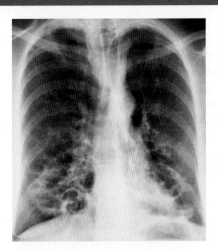

Bronchiectasis. Multiple ring shadows, many containing air-fluid levels, are present throughout the lower zones of this patient with cystic bronchiectasis.†

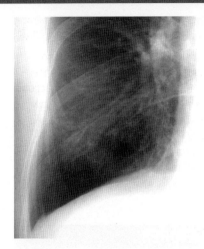

Bronchiectasis. Targeted image of a right lower lung base shows tramlines and ring opacities.*

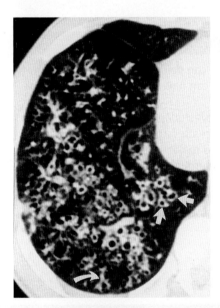

Bronchiectasis. CT demonstrating dilated subsegmental bronchi. The bronchi are larger than the accompanying vessels with some demonstrating the 'signet ring' sign (arrows). Plugging of peripheral smaller bronchi is also evident (curved arrow).†

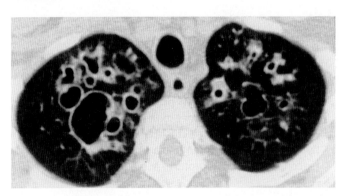

Cystic bronchiectasis. CT demonstrates multiple ring shadows due to irregularly dilated bronchi.†

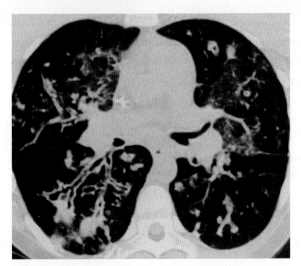

Cylindrical bronchiectasis. The bronchi fail to taper and have irregular thickened walls.†

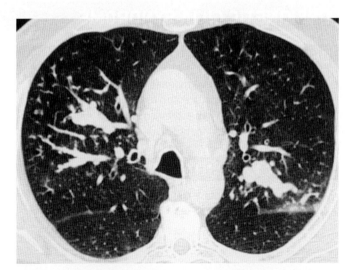

ABPA. HRCT demonstrating mucoid impactions within segmental and subsegmental dilated bronchi in the upper lobes. Small centrilobular linear branching opacities are seen in the periphery of the right upper lobe.*

CYSTIC FIBROSIS

DEFINITION

- An autosomal recessive genetic defect leading to an abnormal cystic fibrosis transmembrane conductance regulator protein and impaired chloride transport across epithelial membranes ▶ the resultant abnormally low water content of the airway mucus leads to decreased mucus clearance, airway mucous plugging and increased incidence of bacterial infections
- Associated bronchial wall inflammation, progressing to secondary bronchiectasis, is always present in long-standing disease

RADIOLOGICAL FEATURES

CXR

- **Early:** hyperinflation (small airway obstruction) ▶ linear opacities within the upper lungs (bronchial wall thickening)
- **Late:** the above findings together with the following: increased lung volumes ▶ proximal bronchiectasis and mucoid impaction ▶ upper lobe cystic bronchiectasis, cavities, bullae and atelectasis ▶ pulmonary hypertension or cor pulmonale ▶ pneumothoraces (secondary to bullae rupture) ▶ pleural effusions

CT

- **Early:** focal areas of decreased lung attenuation representing air trapping and mosaic perfusion (representing small airway obstruction)

  - *'Tree-in-bud' appearance:* centrilobular nodular and branching linear opacities representing mucous impaction within dilated bronchioles (± associated peribronchiolar inflammation)
- **Late:** peripheral (± central) bronchiectasis with an upper lobe predominance ▶ bronchial wall and peribronchial interstitial thickening ▶ mucous plugging within all lobes (25–50%) ▶ collapse or consolidation in up to 80% (commonly staphylococcal or pseudomonal infections) ▶ lobar volume loss ▶ pleural thickening

MRI

- **T2W1:** high bronchial wall signal with inflammation ▶ high T2 signal mucous plugs (without enhancement)
- **T1W1+C:** enhancement of thickened bronchial wall with inflammation

PEARLS

- Cystic bronchiectasis can be difficult to distinguish from a lung abscess (both can have air-fluid levels) or from upper lobe bullae
- *Non-pulmonary manifestations:* pancreatic insufficiency associated with pancreatic fatty replacement (presenting with steatorrhoea and malabsorption) ▶ liver cirrhosis ▶ sinusitis ▶ male infertility ▶ neonatal meconium ileus and intussusception

DYSKINETIC CILIA SYNDROME

DEFINITION

- An autosomal recessive disease characterized by abnormal ciliary structure and function ▶ the resultant reduced mucociliary clearance commonly leads to chronic airway infection, bronchiectasis and sinusitis

CLINICAL PRESENTATION

- Recurrent pneumonia ▶ sinusitis

RADIOLOGICAL FEATURES

CXR/CT Bilateral bronchiectasis with a basal (lower or middle lobe) predominance ▶ cylindrical bronchiectasis is the most common type ▶ a diffuse bronchiolitis may be present

PEARLS

- Situs inversus is seen in 50% (Kartagener's syndrome: bronchiectasis + sinusitis + situs inversus)
- There is an equal sex incidence (leading to infertility in men)

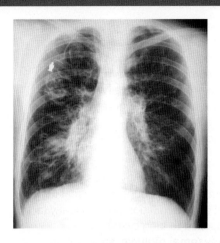

Cystic fibrosis. The PA CXR shows slight overinflation and the presence of multiple thin-walled ring shadows in the right lung and the upper part of the left lung, reflecting cystic bronchiectasis. Some ring shadows contain air-fluid levels.*

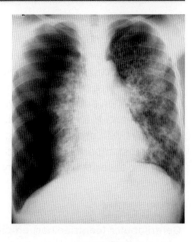

Cystic fibrosis. There are widespread bronchiectatic changes and a large right pneumothorax ▶ a small left apical pneumothorax is also present.*

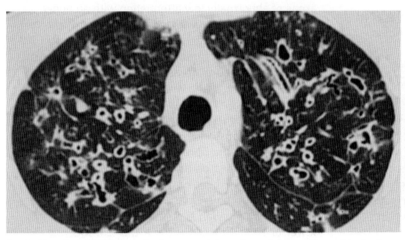

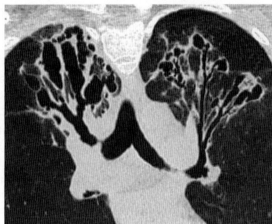

Cystic fibrosis. HRCT image in the upper lobes shows bilateral bronchiectasis and bronchial wall thickening.*

Cystic fibrosis. Coronal MIP image showing a combination of varicose and cystic bronchiectatic change.**

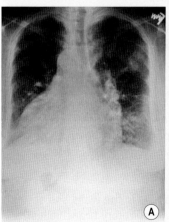

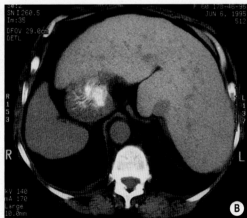

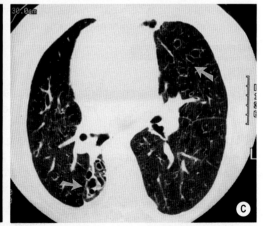

Kartagener's syndrome. (A) PA CXR demonstrates complete situs inversus (the gastric bubble is also in the right upper quadrant). Irregular parenchymal opacities represent bronchiectasis. An incidental left upper lobe carcinoma is also present. (B) CT showing the spleen and stomach in the right upper quadrant. (C) HRCT. Cystic bronchiectasis is present bilaterally.‡

EMPHYSEMA

Definition

- Permanent and abnormal airspace enlargement distal to the terminal bronchioles accompanied by wall destruction without fibrosis ▶ this is caused by elastic fibre destruction and the mechanical stresses of ventilation and coughing (with no obvious fibrotic component) ▶ the airways collapse as their elastic recoil declines with progressive lung destruction
- The most important aetiological factor is smoking
- Genetic associations: α_1-antitrypsin deficiency ▶ Marfan syndrome

Classification

Centrilobular (centriacinar) emphysema A selective process affecting mainly the proximal respiratory bronchioles (the alveoli within the central acinus are spared until later) ▶ there is an upper lung predominance ▶ it is strongly associated with cigarette smoking

Paraseptal emphysema This selectively involves the alveoli at the lobule margins, subpleurally and adjacent to the bronchovascular bundles ▶ the airspaces may become confluent, forming bullae (particularly within the upper zones)

Panlobular (panacinar) emphysema Involvement of the entire acinus and lobule (the most severe type) ▶ progressive destruction leaves residual thin strands of tissue surrounding the blood vessels ▶ seen throughout the lungs but with a basal predominance (bullae formation has no particular distribution) ▶ occurs in α_1-antitrypsin (protease inhibitor) deficiency

Irregular (paracicatricial) emphysema Irregular airspace enlargement in pulmonary fibrosis

Clinical presentation

- Asymptomatic or dyspnoea ▶ M>F smoking
- Panacinar emphysema is associated with air trapping and usually causes symptoms ▶ centriacinar and paraseptal emphysema are not associated with air trapping and are usually asymptomatic

Radiological features

CXR

- Bronchial wall thickening (tubular + ring shadows) ▶ 'dirty chest': a loss of clarity and accentuated linear lung markings
- **Lung overinflation:** height of the right lung > 29.9 cm ▶ the right hemidiaphragm at or below the anterior 7th rib ▶ hemidiaphragm flattening ▶ retrosternal space enlargement ▶ sternodiaphragmatic angle widening ▶ transverse cardiac diameter narrowing ▶ a 'barrel chest' appearance
- **Lung vessel alteration:** arterial depletion ▶ vessel absence or displacement by bullae ▶ widened branching angles (with side branch loss) ▶ central pulmonary arterial enlargement (pulmonary arterial hypertension) ▶ signs of cor pulmonale (left heart failure)

- **Bullae:** these may be small (1 cm) or occupy the whole hemithorax ▶ bullae may enlarge progressively over months or years or may disappear spontaneously
    - *Complications:* pneumothorax (commonly at the apices) ▶ infection or haemorrhage (which may develop an air-fluid level with a thickened wall and mimicking a lung abscess)
        - *Bullous emphysema:* emphysema + bullae

CT

- **Emphysema:** this is characterized by areas of abnormally low attenuation surrounding normal lung parenchyma ▶ focal low attenuation areas usually lack distinct walls (as opposed to lung cysts)
- **Centrilobular emphysema:** multiple, small round areas of abnormally low attenuation with an upper lobe predominance ▶ with increasing severity the centrilobular distribution becomes less apparent
- **Paraseptal emphysema:** areas of low attenuation within the subpleural areas, along the peripheral and mediastinal pleura, and within the fissures ▶ emphysematous spaces often have thin walls (the interlobular septa are thickened by associated fibrosis) ▶ predilection for anteroposterior upper lobes and posterior lower lobes ▶ may mimic fibrotic honeycombing, but the cysts are usually small, only a single layer and lack architectural distortion ▶ bullae may be large
- **Panlobular emphysema:** widespread areas of abnormally low attenuation ▶ pulmonary vessels appear fewer or smaller than normal ▶ this is frequently associated with bronchiectasis if it is secondary to α_1-antitrypsin deficiency (α_1-antitrypsin is a protease inhibitor)
- **Irregular (paracicatricial) emphysema:** irregular low attenuation areas associated with fibrosis ▶ it is seen adjacent to localized parenchymal scars, in diffuse pulmonary fibrosis and with pneumoconiosis (especially progressive massive fibrosis)
- **Bullae:** avascular low attenuation areas (> 1 cm in diameter) that can have a thin but perceptible wall ▶ inspiratory and expiratory CT images indicate if a bulla is ventilated

Pearls

- **COPD:** slowly progressive airway obstructive disorder following an exaggerated inflammatory response to pollutants leading to lung parenchyma destruction (emphysema) and irreversible airway calibre reduction (obstructive bronchiolitis)
- Small airway disease
    - *Initial:* inflammatory changes in the walls and around respiratory bronchioles (respiratory bronchiolitis)
    - *Intermediate:* obstruction of small airway lumen by plugs of inflammatory exudate and pus
    - *Advanced:* narrowing of terminal bronchiole lumen by peribronchiolar fibrosis (obstructuve bronchiolitis)
- **Large airway disease:** this includes inflammation and remodelling of the trachea and bronchi

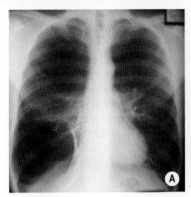
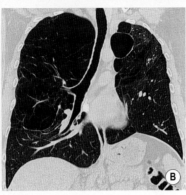
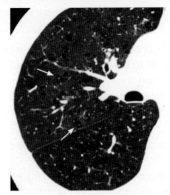

Giant bullous emphysema. (A) The PA CXR shows large avascular transradiant areas in the upper and lower parts of the right lung. The bullae are marginated with thin curvilinear opacities. (B) CT coronal reformat demonstrates large confluent bullae within the right lung associated with destruction of the right upper lobe. Presence of paraseptal emphysematous bullae within the left upper lobe along the mediastinum is also seen.*

Centrilobular emphysema. HRCT of the right lung shows multiple small round areas of low attenuation that are distributed through the lungs, mainly around the centrilobular arteries (arrows).*

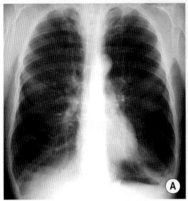
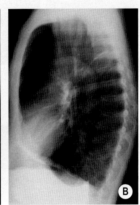

Severe diffuse emphysema. The diaphragm is displaced downwards and appears flattened. On the PA CXR (A) the transverse cardiac diameter is reduced. Note the depression of vessels in the periphery of the lungs. On the lateral CXR (B) there is a widening of the sternodiaphragm angle and an increase of dimensions of the retrosternal transradiant area.*

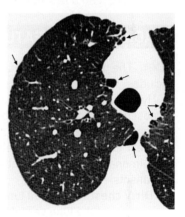

Paraseptal emphysema. HRCT of the right upper lobe shows multiple small areas of low attenuation distributed along the peripheral and mediastinal pleura (arrows).*

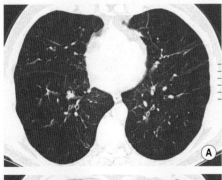

Panlobular emphysema in a patient with α_1-antitryspin deficiency. Axial CT at the levels of the mild (A) and lower parts (B) of the lung with diffuse lung attenuation and paucity of the pulmonary vessels. The presence of multiple thin lines, particularly throughout the lung bases, reflects a distortion of the anatomical structure of the lung parenchyma and thickening of the remaining interlobular septa by lung fibrosis.**

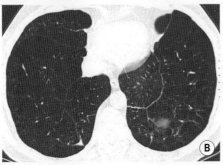

Advanced centrilobular emphysema in a smoker. Axial CT at the level of the upper lobes shows large and coalescent areas of low attenuation with lobular margins corresponding to advanced centrilobular emphysematous spaces predominantly distributed on the right side. The patient had a history of left upper lobectomy for bronchopulmonary carcinoma. Note the thickened bronchi related to associated airway remodelling (arrow).**

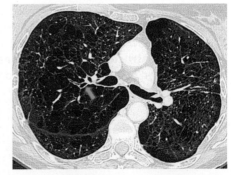

CHRONIC BRONCHITIS

DEFINITION

- Excessive mucus secretion by the bronchial tree ▶ this is usually related to cigarette smoking (but also air pollution and infection)
- *Pathology:* bronchial submucosal hyperplasia ▶ smooth muscle hypertrophy ▶ chronic inflammation and small airway obstruction
- Airflow obstruction is concentrated within the small bronchioles
  - *Reversible component:* mucous plugging ▶ inflammation ▶ smooth muscle hypertrophy
  - *Irreversible component:* fibrosis and stenosis

CLINICAL PRESENTATION

- A chronic or recurring productive cough on most days for more than 3 months of each of 2 successive years

RADIOLOGICAL FEATURES

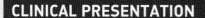 **CXR** The majority are normal, however, abnormalities include:

- Hyperinflation and oligaemia (which can occur in the absence of emphysema) ▶ bronchial wall thickening (leading to tubular and ring shadows) ▶ accentuation of linear lung markings ▶ a sabre-sheath trachea and cor pulmonale (which occurs almost exclusively in hypoxic patients)
- **'Dirty chest':** increased lung markings leading to a loss in clarity of the lung vessels

CT Bronchial wall thickening with air-filled outpouchings or diverticula (reflecting mucous gland enlargement and mucosal herniation between small muscle bundles) ▶ prominent airway lumen collapse with a maximum forced expiratory manoeuvre (due to a bronchial cartilage defect and occurring predominantly within the lower lobes)

PEARLS

- The extent of lung hypoattenuation at expiration probably reflects air trapping more than a reduction of the alveolar wall surface
- **Pulmonary function tests:** there is a normal total lung capacity and normal elastic recoil, but a reduced expiratory flow and elevated residual volumes
- **Chronic obstructive pulmonary disease (COPD):** this is composed of two components: chronic bronchitis + emphysema

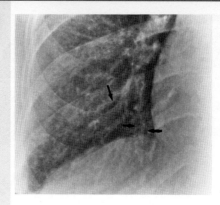

Chronic bronchitis. PA CXR demonstrates bronchial wall thickening in profile– 'tram tracking' (arrows). Bronchi are also seen more peripherally in the lungs than is normally the case.‡

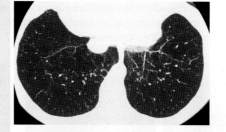

Chronic bronchitis. Small poorly defined opacities are present throughout both lungs, producing the 'dirty chest'.*

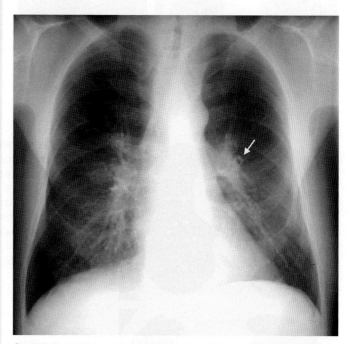

Chronic bronchitis and obstructive lung disease. PA CXR shows mild overinflation. A ring shadow is visible above the left hilum (arrow) reflecting bronchial wall thickening. There is also accentuation of linear markings in the right lung base.*

ASTHMA

DEFINITION

- A chronic inflammatory condition (IgE mediated) involving the airways and leading to a generalized increase in the existing bronchial hypersensitivity to a variety of stimuli
- Chronic inflammation can cause structural changes: new vessel formation ▶ airway smooth muscle thickening and fibrosis (which may result in irreversible airway narrowing)

CLINICAL PRESENTATION

- Recurrent episodes of wheezing, chest tightness, breathlessness and coughing ▶ it is usually associated with widespread but variable airflow obstruction
- It is often reversible either spontaneously or with treatment

RADIOLOGICAL FEATURES

CXR The majority are normal
- **Hyperinflation:** this is often transient but may be a permanent change
- **Bronchial wall thickening:** this appears as parallel or single line opacities (more frequently in children but usually irreversible when seen in adults)
- **Complications:** consolidation (commonly infective but may be related to ABPA) ▶ atelectasis due to mucoid impaction within the large airways or small airway mucous plugging (lobar to subsegmental collapse) ▶ pneumothorax ▶ pneumomediastinum

HRCT Bronchial dilatation and wall thickening ▶ mucoid impaction ▶ decreased lung attenuation ▶ air trapping (due to airway luminal obstruction) ▶ small centrilobular opacities
- **Bronchial wall thickening:** this increases with asthma severity and correlates with the degree of airflow obstruction (irreversibility suggests airway wall remodelling due to smooth muscle hyperplasia and hypertrophy)
- **Decreased lung attenuation:** with focal and diffuse areas (occurring in 20–30% and more conspicuous on expiratory CT) ▶ it results from a combination of air trapping and pulmonary oligaemia (due to hypoxic vasoconstriction)
  - A mosaic perfusion pattern is frequently seen in patients with moderate persistent asthma (in severe persistent asthma diffuse decreased lung attenuation and expiratory air trapping makes the pattern difficult to distinguish from obliterative bronchiolitis)

PEARL

- Emphysematous changes with chronic asthma are invariably related to cigarette smoking and not asthma per se

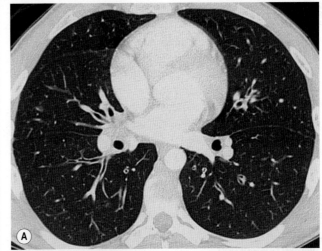

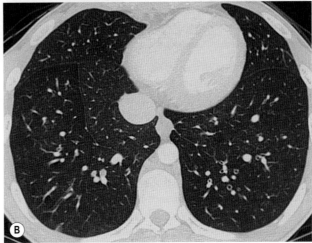

Moderate persistent asthmatic patient. Axial CT at the levels of mid (A) and lower (B) parts of the lungs. Diffuse bronchial wall thickening with mucoid impactions in the subsegmental and segmental bronchi in the basilar segments of the right lower lobe. Patchy areas of hypoattenuation in the anterior, lateral and posterobasal segments of the right lower lobe and the posterior segment of the left lower lobe, reflecting the presence of small airway remodelling.**

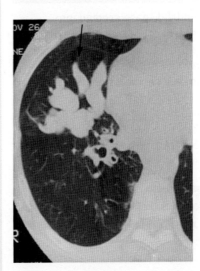

Mucoid impaction with ABPA in an asthmatic patient. Branching V-shaped, mucous-filled, dilated bronchi are identified (arrow).‡

OBLITERATIVE (CONSTRICTIVE) BRONCHIOLITIS

DEFINITION

- Characterized by irreversible, circumferential and submucosal bronchiolar or peribronchiolar inflammation and fibrosis ▶ it ultimately leads to luminal obliteration affecting the membranous and respiratory bronchioles
- The fibrosis impairs collateral ventilation and leads to airflow obstruction ▶ the accompanying artery can also be obliterated by fibrosis
- It is the result of a variety of causes but is rarely idiopathic (see table)

CLINICAL PRESENTATION

- Progressive shortness of breath ▶ functional evidence of airflow obstruction

RADIOLOGICAL FEATURES

CXR This is often normal ▶ occasionally there is mild hyperinflation, subtle peripheral attenuation of any vascular markings, widespread and conspicuous abnormalities in lung attenuation, or central bronchiectasis

HRCT Bronchial wall thickening and bronchiectasis (central and peripheral)

- **Mosaic perfusion**
  - Affected areas demonstrate decreased lung attenuation associated with *vessels of decreased calibre* on inspiratory imaging (the vessels are not distorted as in emphysema) ▶ unaffected areas demonstrate *compensatory vessel diameter enlargement* resulting in areas of normal lung demonstrating relatively increased attenuation
    - Involved areas are heterogeneously distributed throughout the lungs
- Areas of mosaic perfusion can be poorly defined or sharply demarcated giving a geographical outline ▶ any regional inhomogeneity is accentuated during expiratory imaging (the high attenuation areas increase in density as air is removed – the low attenuation areas remain unchanged as there is 'air trapping') ▶ the mosaic pattern can be lost with severe and widespread disease
- Mosaic attenuation due to an infiltrative lung disease with a patchy distribution will have vessels of the same calibre within both the high and normal attenuation areas (cf. vessels of decreased calibre within low attenuation areas with mosaic perfusion due to an obliterative bronchiolitis)

PEARLS

- **Swyer–James/MacLeod syndrome:** a variant form of postinfectious obliterative bronchiolitis affecting predominantly a single lung
- **Respiratory bronchiolitis-associated interstitial lung disease (RB-ILD):** this is seen in heavy smokers and is an inflammatory process affecting the respiratory bronchioles and alveoli
- **Panbronchiolitis (Japanese panbronchiolitis):** a diffuse panbronchiolitis commonly seen in Asia
- **Air trapping:** assessed by comparing a post-expiratory (forced expiration) with a matched inspiratory image – redistributed blood to normally ventilated areas increases attenuation which becomes more pronounced on expiratory imaging

BRONCHOLITHIASIS

DEFINITION

- Peribronchial calcified nodal disease eroding into or distorting an adjacent bronchus ▶ the underlying abnormality is usually a granulomatous lymphadenitis caused by *Mycobacterium tuberculosis* or fungi such as *Histoplasma capsulatum* ▶ it can occasionally be caused by silicosis
- Calcified material within a bronchial lumen (or bronchial distortion by peribronchial disease) can result in airway obstruction leading to collapse, obstructive pneumonitis, mucoid impaction or bronchiectasis

CLINICAL PRESENTATION

- Cough ▶ haemoptysis ▶ recurrent episodes of fever ▶ purulent sputum

RADIOLOGICAL FEATURES

CXR Calcified hilar or mediastinal nodes are a key feature ▶ three major types of changes may be seen:
- Disappearance of a previously identified calcified nidus
- Change in position of a calcified nidus
- Evidence of airway obstruction: segmental or lobar atelectasis ▶ mucoid impaction ▶ obstructive pneumonitis ▶ obstructive oligaemia with air trapping

PEARL

- It is more commonly seen on the right - obstructive changes particularly affect the middle lobe

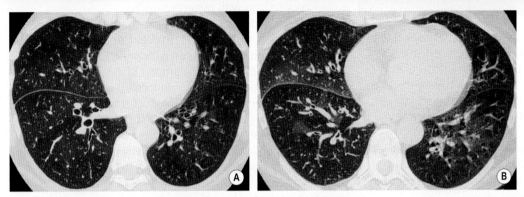

Obliterative bronchiolitis. HRCT acquired at (A) full inspiration and (B) full expiration. The mosaic perfusion appearance is very difficult to perceive on the inspiration image (A). The contrast in attenuation between normal and abnormal areas is accentuated at expiration. The areas that did not change in attenuation between inspiration and expiration represent areas of lung parenchyma containing obliterative lesions on the bronchioles. These low attenuation areas have failed to deflate due to 'air trapping'.*

Causes of and association with obliterative (constrictive) bronchiolitis	
Post infection	*Childhood viral infection:* adenovirus, respiratory syncytial virus, influenza, parainfluenza *Adulthood and childhood: Mycoplasma pneumoniae, Pneumocystis carinii* in AIDS patients, endobronchial spread of tuberculosis, bacterial bronchiolar infection
Post inhalation (toxic fumes and gases)	Nitrogen dioxide (silo filler's disease), sulphur dioxide, ammonia, chlorine, phosgene, hot gases
Gastric aspiration	Diffuse aspiration bronchiolitis (chronic occult aspiration in the elderly, patients with dysphagia)
Connective tissue disorders	Rheumatoid arthritis, Sjögren's syndrome
Allograft recipients	Bone marrow transplant, heart–lung or lung transplant
Drugs	Penicillamine, lomustine
Other conditions	Ulcerative colitis, bronchiectasis, chronic bronchitis, cystic fibrosis, hypersensitivity pneumonitis, sarcoidosis

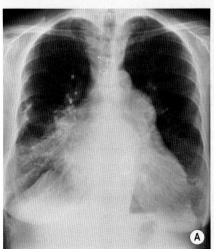
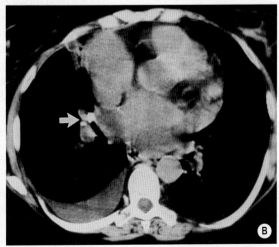

Broncholithiasis. (A) CXR – there is middle lobe collapse. (B) CT demonstrating the calcified broncholith (arrow) that is obstructing the middle lobe bronchus.‡

1.5 PULMONARY LOBAR COLLAPSE

MECHANISMS AND CAUSES OF LOBAR COLLAPSE

- **Lobar collapse:** this is divided into those causes due to an endobronchial obstruction (intrinsic or extrinsic) or those causes without obstruction
  - A segment of atelectatic lung pivots around the central hilum via its attaching bronchovascular structures – any fissures will also influence the direction of collapse
- **Common causes differ between adults and children:**
  - *Adults:* intrinsic obstruction is commonly due to a bronchogenic tumour (especially in middle-aged or elderly smokers) or mucous plugs
    - *Rarer causes:* foreign bodies ▶ broncholiths ▶ focal bronchostenosis due to inflammation or trauma
  - *Children:* intrinsic obstruction is commonly due to an inhaled foreign body or mucous plugs ▶ tumours are very rare
- **Subsegmental atelectasis (linear or plate atelectasis):** this describes atelectasis involving less than a whole segment ▶ it is usually a thin horizontal linear opacity abutting the pleura
  - It is commonly located within the mid or lower lung and can cross segmental boundaries

RADIOGRAPHIC CONSIDERATIONS

- **Increased opacity of the affected lobe:** this is due to retained secretions and a reduction in lobe aeration
- **Silhouette sign:** this describes loss of an air–soft tissue interface when a segment of collapsed lung abuts an adjacent soft tissue structure (e.g. a heart border)
- **Direct signs of volume loss:** fissure displacement ▶ displacement and crowding of the pulmonary vessels and bronchi
  - *Upper lobe collapse:* hilar elevation ▶ the ipsilateral main bronchus becomes more horizontally orientated
  - *Lower lobe collapse:* a 'small hilum' – the collapsed lower lobe obscures the lower lobe artery and therefore smaller vascular structures are seen at the expected hilar position ▶ the ipsilateral main bronchus becomes more vertically orientated
- **Indirect signs of volume loss:** compensatory shifts of adjacent structures (e.g. hyperinflation of the remaining lobes in proportion to the degree of volume loss) ▶ the contralateral lung may extend across the midline ▶ the anterior junctional line is displaced to the contralateral side ▶ displacement of the azygo-oesophageal or posterior junctional lines on a PA CXR ▶ rib crowding
  - *A juxtaphrenic diaphragmatic peak:* this describes a small triangular density at the highest point of the hemidiaphragm dome with upper lobe (± middle lobe) collapse – this is a useful ancillary sign

- *'Shifting granuloma' sign:* a change in position of a granuloma with hyperexpansion
- *Mediastinal shift:* this is greatest with a lower lobe collapse, and least with middle lobe collapse ▶ little mediastinal shift is seen with an acute upper lobe collapse but there is a greater shift with chronic fibrotic upper lobe volume loss
- *Luftsichel sign:* paramediastinal translucency secondary to an overinflated superior segment of the ipsilateral lower lobe occupying the space between the mediastinum and medial aspect of the collapsed upper lobe ▶ L > R ▶ typical of left upper lobe collapse
- An elevated hemidiaphragm (particularly with left upper lobe collapse) is of limited value
- **Ancillary features:** absence of air bronchograms within an affected lobe should raise the possibility of a central obstructing lesion
  - *'Golden's S' sign:* this describes the S shape (reverse S on the right) of a major fissure due to a combination of collapse and a central mass ▶ it is commonly seen in the right upper lobe (but can be seen in any lobe)
    - Focal central convexity: collapse around the central mass
    - Concave outline peripherally: peripheral collapse not occurring around a central mass

COMPUTED TOMOGRAPHY OF LOBAR COLLAPSE

- Accurate delineation of a tumour mass from surrounding collapsed lung can be difficult but collapsed lung will usually enhance more than a tumour (the maximal difference is seen between 40 s and 2 min post IV injection) ▶ increased uptake on PET-CT within tumour vs lung collapse
- **CT mucous bronchogram sign:** tubular, low attenuation branching airways that are dilated with inspissated secretions and seen within the enhancing collapsed lobe (post IV contrast administration) – this is highly suggestive of an obstructing lesion causing lobar collapse
  - However this can also be caused by excessive mucus production combined with decreased mucociliary function (e.g. ABPA, asthma, cystic fibrosis)
- **Potential pitfalls:** air bronchograms may be seen in peripheral collapsed lobes (due to collateral air drift or tumour necrosis) ▶ a proximal obstructing lesion may not cause complete lobar collapse (if a fissure is incomplete and allows collateral air drift) ▶ occasionally the parenchyma and airways can become fluid filled due to a central obstructing lesion with little or no volume loss giving rise to the appearance of a 'drowned lobe' ▶ false-positive diagnoses may be due to bronchial strictures, mucous plugs, or compression by a large pleural effusion

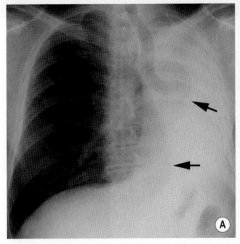
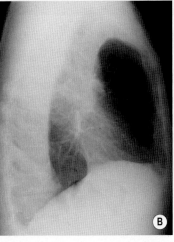

Total left lung collapse. (A) PA and (B) lateral CRXs. The cause of the collapse is a bronchogenic carcinoma ▶ the endobronchial component is visible as an abrupt cut-off of the left main bronchus. Note the marked displacement of the right lung anteriorly and posteriorly across the midline (arrows). Note the marked anterior hyperlucency of the thorax on the lateral view (B).*

Total right lung collapse in a neonate. The patient was ventilated for respiratory distress syndrome and the cause of the total lung collapse was a mucous plug.*

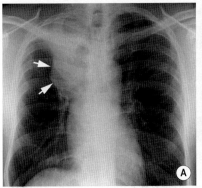
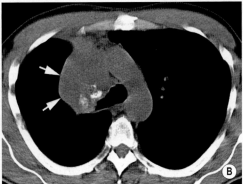
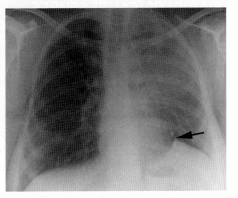

Golden's S sign. (A) PA CXR – a right upper lobe collapse demonstrating peripheral concavity and central convexity (arrows) due to an underlying bronchogenic carcinoma resulting in a reverse S shape. (B) CT demonstrating a convex border of the collapsed lobe (arrows) which is the CT equivalent of Golden's S sign.*

Juxtaphrenic peak sign. A small triangular density (arrow) is seen in a left upper lobe collapse. The sign is due to reorientation of an inferior accessory fissure.*

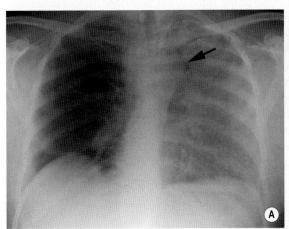
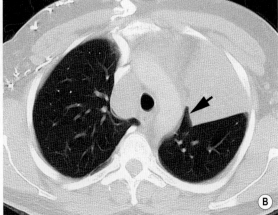

Luftsichel sign. (A) A left upper lobe collapse demonstrating paramediastinal lucency (arrow). (B) CT shows interposition of aerated lung between the collapse and the mediastinum (arrow). There is also a large right paratracheal node causing some distortion of the SVC.*

RIGHT UPPER LOBE COLLAPSE

RADIOLOGICAL FEATURES

PA CXR Increased density at the apex of the right hemithorax adjacent to the right mediastinum ▶ an elevated horizontal fissure with a concave inferior outline

Lateral CXR Approximation and superomedial displacement of both the horizontal and oblique fissures with the collapsed lobe forming a superior ill-defined wedge-shaped density ▶ in severe cases the horizontal fissure parallels the mediastinum and appearances may simulate an apical cap of pleural fluid

CT A triangular density with the base set anteriorly against the chest wall and the apex at the hilum
- Compensatory hyperinflation of the middle, left upper and both lower lobes (resulting in elevation and a more horizontal course of the lower lobe pulmonary artery and right main bronchus)

LEFT UPPER LOBE COLLAPSE

RADIOLOGICAL FEATURES

- There is rarely a left horizontal fissure, so the features of a left upper lobe collapse are different from a right upper lobe collapse (consequently the main direction of volume loss is anteriorly and medially rather than superiorly)

PA CXR A 'veil-like' increased density affecting the whole left hemithorax (the density is often greatest at the hilum and fading out laterally, superiorly and inferiorly without a clear inferior demarcation of the horizontal fissure as with a right upper lobe collapse) ▶ loss of the normal silhouette of the structures adjacent to the collapse (such as the left heart border, mediastinum and aortic arch) ▶ a more horizontal course of the left main bronchus
- In severe collapse the apical segment of the left lower lobe is hyperexpanded superiorly adjacent to the aortic arch (and therefore, paradoxically, the aortic knuckle is visible in severe cases)
- *Luftsichel sign:* a particular manifestation of hyperexpansion with an 'air crescent' between the aortic arch and the medial border of the collapse

CT Appearances are similar to a right upper lobe collapse (with a triangular soft tissue density with its apex at the origin of an upper lobe bronchus and its base against the anterior chest wall adjacent to the left mediastinal border) – however, the lingular segment is seen as a density closely opposed to the left heart border

- Rarely a left upper lobe collapse may mimic a right upper lobe collapse ▶ this is due to collapse of the apicoposterior and anterior segments of the left upper lobe with sparing of the lingular portion resulting in a concavity to the inferior border of the collapse ▶ an isolated lingular collapse appears similar to a middle lobe collapse (but on the left)

PEARL

- Combinations of lobar collapse:
  - *Obstructing lesion of the bronchus intermedius:* this can give rise to a middle and right lower lobe collapse ▶ the features are similar to a right lower lobe collapse although the opacity extends laterally to the costophrenic angle (PA CXR) and from the front to the back of the hemithorax (lateral CXR)
  - *Collapse of the right upper and right middle lobes:* this is more unusual as there is no common bronchial origin, which spares the lower lobe ▶ the cause is often a carcinoma obstructing one bronchus and causing extrinsic compression of the other (mass effect) ▶ the appearances are very similar to a left upper lobe collapse on both a PA and lateral CXR
  - *Bilateral lower lobe and upper lobe collapse:* this is exceedingly rare (and can be caused by metachronous bronchial neoplasms or mucous plugging)

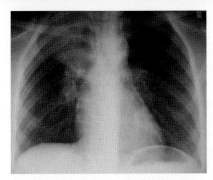

Right upper lobe collapse. Typical example of a collapsed right upper lobe demonstrating the slightly concave inferior border of the opacified lung due to the horizontal fissure.*

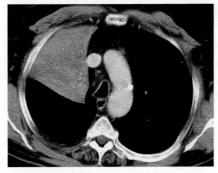

CT of right upper lobe collapse. The collapsed lobe forms a triangular wedge of soft tissue anteriorly in the right hemithorax.*

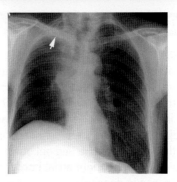

Right upper lobe collapse. An example of right upper lobe collapse mimicking an apical cap of fluid (arrow).**

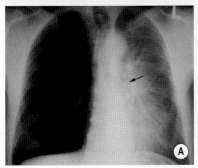
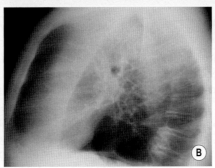
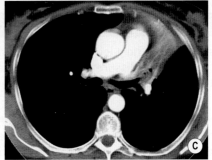

Left upper lobe collapse. (A) A typical example of left upper lobe collapse demonstrating increased angulation between the left main bronchus and the lower lobe bronchus (arrow) on the frontal view. The aortic knuckle is visible in this example due to compensatory hyperinflation of the left lower lobe. There is a 'veil-like' opacity overlying the left hemithorax with an indistinct left heart border. (B) The lateral view demonstrates anterior displacement of the oblique fissure. (C) CECT demonstrating an increased wedge-shaped density of the left upper lobe adjacent to the mediastinum. Note the displacement of the right lung across the midline anteriorly, resulting in retrosternal hyperlucency and increased clarity of the anterior ascending thoracic aorta on the lateral view (seen on the lateral CXR).*

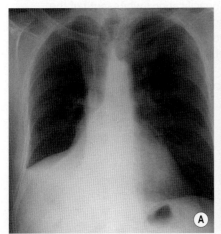
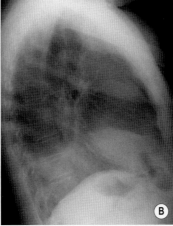
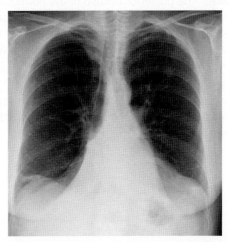

Combined right middle and right lower lobe collapse. (A) On the PA CXR the increased density extends to the right costophrenic angle. (B) On the lateral CXR the increased density also extends from the anterior to the posterior chest wall. The cause in this case was a bronchogenic carcinoma obstructing the bronchus intermedius.*

Bilateral lower lobe collapse. Bilateral triangular densities are seen with obscuration of the medial portions of the hemidiaphragms. The cause was mucous plugging.*

MIDDLE LOBE COLLAPSE

RADIOLOGICAL FEATURES

PA CXR The radiographic findings can be very subtle ▶ the collapsed lobe lies adjacent to the right heart border with variable loss of this structure's silhouette

- If the collapse is parallel to the XR beam or the patient is in a lordotic position, a triangular sail-shaped density adjacent to the right heart border may be seen
- If the collapsed lobe lies obliquely, the only sign may be an indistinct right atrial border (± a recognizable increase in density)

Lateral CXR A triangular density of collapsed middle lobe is easy to identify (approximation of the minor and inferior major fissures with a triangular apex at the hilum) ▶ in severe collapse the fissures can become almost parallel (with only a thin wedge of density separating them)

CT A triangular-shaped density adjacent to the right heart border

- *'Middle lobe syndrome':* a collapsed middle lobe with associated bronchiectasis – this is due to a focal bronchostenosis secondary to pulmonary TB (the middle lobe is the most commonly affected)

RIGHT AND LEFT LOWER LOBE COLLAPSE

RADIOLOGICAL FEATURES

- Features of left and right lower lobe collapse are very similar ▶ the oblique fissure is displaced posteriorly and medially ▶ the collapsed lobe lies in the posteromedial chest

PA CXR A triangular density behind the heart ▶ obscuration of the medial hemidiaphragm (as it is no longer outlined by aerated lung – but if the inferior pulmonary ligament is incomplete and does not attach to the diaphragm the medial hemidiaphragm may still be visualized) ▶ the lower lobe pulmonary artery is no longer visualized (as this is also no longer outlined by aerated lung) ▶ there is a more vertical orientation of the main bronchi

Lateral CXR The posterior portion of the hemidiaphragm may not be seen (it may reappear in severe collapse as it becomes outlined by a hyperexpanded upper lobe) ▶ there is a progressively dense inferior vertebral column (the converse is seen on a normal lateral view)

CT A triangle of soft tissue density is seen posteromedially within the thorax (adjacent to the spine) ▶ on the left the collapsed lobe is seen to drape over the descending aorta

- *'Superior triangle sign':* a triangular density seen adjacent to the right mediastinum with a right lower lobe collapse (caused by displacement of the anterior junctional structures)
- *'Flat waist sign':* this is seen with extensive left lower lobe collapse and describes flattening of the contours of the aortic knuckle and main pulmonary artery (due to cardiac rotation and leftward displacement)
- The outline of the superior aortic knuckle may be lost with severe left lower lobe collapse

PEARL

- Whole lung collapse:
  - This is usually due to an obstructing neoplasm in the left or right main bronchi
  - **CXR** Complete opacification ('white-out') of the affected hemithorax
  - There is marked volume loss with compensatory hyperinflation of the contralateral lung across the midline
  - **Lateral CXR** Accentuation of the retrosternal space

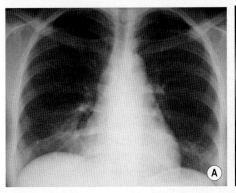

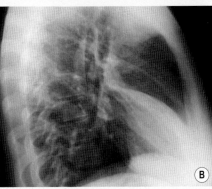

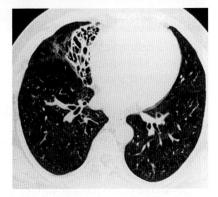

Middle lobe collapse. (A) PA CXR of a typical example showing loss of clarity of the right heart border. (B) The lateral view shows the wedge-shaped density extending anteriorly from the hilum.*

Middle lobe syndrome. High-resolution CT showing right middle lobe collapse and bronchiectasis due to previous tuberculous infection.*

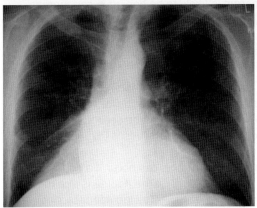

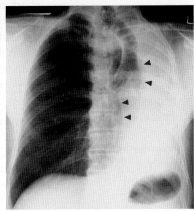

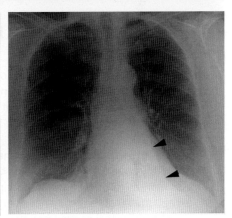

Right lower lobe collapse. PA CXR of right lower lobe collapse demonstrating a triangular density which does not obscure the right hemidiaphragm silhouette.*

Complete collapse of the left lung due to a left hilar tumour. Air–soft tissue interfaces due to hernation of the right lung (arrowheads).†

Left lower lobe collapse. A typical appearance with a triangular density behind the heart (arrowheads). The contour of the medial left hemidiaphragm is lost.*

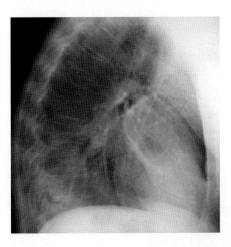

Right lower lobe collapse. The lateral CXR shows the typical features of increased density of the posterior costophrenic angle and loss of the silhouette of the right diaphragm posteriorly.*

Complete collapse of the left lung due to a left hilar tumour. CT demonstrates herniation of both the retrosternal lung and the azygo-oesophageal reflection. The oesophagus contains a small amount of air (arrow).†

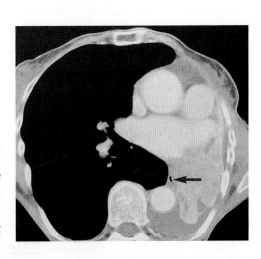

1.6 PULMONARY NEOPLASMS

EVALUATION OF THE SOLITARY PULMONARY NODULE

DEFINITION

- This is defined as a solitary circumscribed pulmonary opacity with no associated pulmonary, pleural, or mediastinal abnormality ▶ it measures < 3 cm in diameter
- Many are discovered incidentally (but up to 40% may be malignant)
- <10% are due to a solitary pulmonary metastasis
- **Benign intrapulmonary lymph nodes:** nodules <15 mm from the pleural surface ▶ ellipsoid in shape, usually connected to the pleural surface by a fine linear opacity
- **Ground-glass nodules:**
  - *Ground-glass density:* focal area of increased lung attenuation (well or poorly defined) through which normal structures can be seen
  - *Pure ground-glass nodule:* no soft tissue component
  - *Part solid ground-glass nodule:* a solid component obscuring lung architecture

DIFFERENTIATION BETWEEN BENIGN AND MALIGNANT MASSES

- The two primary criteria are the rate of growth (or stability over time) and the attenuation of the nodule ▶ the patient's age is also a significant distinguishing feature (a carcinoma is only seen in < 1% of patients < 35 years old)
  - **Rate of growth/stability over time:** benign lesions invariably have a doubling time of < 1 month or > 18 months (bronchoalveolar carcinomas are an exception in that they may have very slow growth rates) ▶ bronchial carcinomas usually have a doubling time of between 1 and 18 months

- **Attenuation/enhancement:** a dense central nidus or lamellated calcification indicates a granulomatous process (e.g. tuberculosis, histoplasmosis) ▶ irregular 'popcorn' calcification suggests a hamartoma ▶ fat is virtually diagnostic of a hamartoma ▶ a lack of enhancement (<15HU) following IV contrast medium is indicative of benignity
  - Granular calcification is seen on CT in up to 7% of carcinomas (and can represent either tumour calcification or a granuloma engulfed by tumour) ▶ eccentric or stippled calcification within soft tissue may indicate malignancy
  - A mixture of soft tissue and ground-glass attenuation nodules is more likely to be malignant than soft tissue nodules alone
- **Size:** this is of little diagnostic value ▶ most benign nodules are <2 cm ▶ round, flat or tubular nodules tend to be benign
- **Margins:** a well-defined mass with a smooth pencil sharp margin is likely to be benign ▶ carcinomas typically have ill-defined margins which are irregular, spiculated, or lobulated and may exhibit umbilication or a notch – unfortunately all these features can be seen with benign disease

FDG-PET This is useful for nodules >1 cm ▶ a positive result is 97% sensitive and 82% specific for malignancy
- **False-positive result:** this can be secondary to an infectious or inflammatory processes (e.g. TB, sarcoid or rheumatoid nodules)
- **False-negative result:** this can occur if a nodule is <1 cm ▶ it can also occur if the nodule is due to a carcinoid tumour or a slow-growing adenocarcinoma subtype

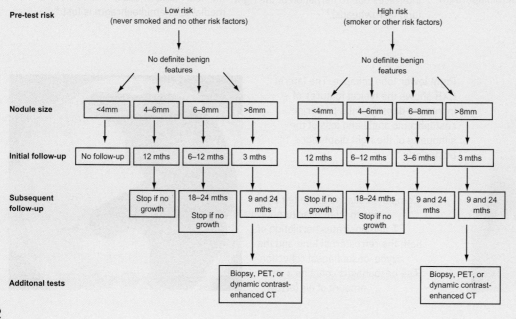

Pre-test risk	Low risk (never smoked and no other risk factors)				High risk (smoker or other risk factors)				
			No definite benign features				No definite benign features		
Nodule size	<4mm	4–6mm	6–8mm	>8mm	<4mm	4–6mm	6–8mm	>8mm	
Initial follow-up	No follow-up	12 mths	6–12 mths	3 mths	12 mths	6–12 mths	3–6 mths	3 mths	
Subsequent follow-up		Stop if no growth	18–24 mths Stop if no growth	9 and 24 mths	Stop if no growth	18–24 mths Stop if no growth	9 and 24 mths	9 and 24 mths	
Additonal tests				Biopsy, PET, or dynamic contrast-enhanced CT				Biopsy, PET, or dynamic contrast-enhanced CT	

The Fleischner Society guidelines: a strategy for follow-up and management of pulmonary nodules in patients over 35 years of age with no known malignancy.©1

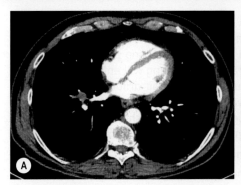 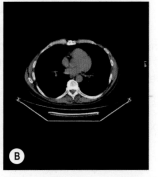 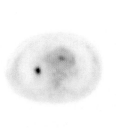 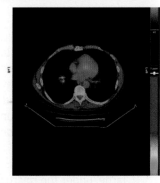

Axial image from a contrast enhanced CT and CT image, FDG PET image and fused image from a CT PET study, demonstrating a PET positive right lung nodule. (A) Lung nodule close to the right hilum with (B) increased uptake on PET/CT corresponding to lung cancer.**

Recommendations for the management of subsolid pulmonary nodules detected at CT: a statement from the Fleischner Society		
Nodule type	**Management recommendations**	**Additional remarks**
Solitary pure GGNs		
≤5 mm	No CT follow-up required	Obtain contiguous 1-mm-thick sections to confirm that nodule is truly a pure GGN
>5 mm	Initial follow-up CT at 3 months to confirm persistence then annual surveillance CT for a minimum of 3 years	FDG PET is of limited value, potentially misleading, and therefore not recommended
Solitary part-solid nodules	Initial follow-up CT at 3 months to confirm persistence. If persistent and solid component <5 mm, then yearly surveillance CT for a minimum of 3 years. If persistent and solid component ≥5 mm, then biopsy or surgical resection	Consider PET/CT for part-solid nodules >10 mm
Multiple subsolid nodules		
Pure GGNs ≤5 mm	Obtain follow-up CT at 2 and 4 years	Consider alternate causes for multiple GGNs ≤5 mm
Pure GGNs >5 mm without a dominant lesion(s)	Initial follow-up CT at 3 months to confirm persistence and then annual surveillance CT for a minimum of 3 years	FDG PET is of limited value, potentially misleading, and therefore not recommended
Dominant nodule(s) with part-solid or solid component	Initial follow-up CT at 3 months to confirm persistence. If persistent, biopsy or surgical resection is recommended, especially for lesions with >5 mm solid component	Consider lung-sparing surgery for patients with dominant lesion(s) suspicious for lung cancer

Note—These guidelines assume meticulous evaluation, optimally with contiguous thin sections (1 mm) reconstructed with narrow and/or mediastinal windows to evaluate the solid component and wide and/or lung windows to evaluate the nonsolid component of nodules, if indicated. When electronic calipers are used, bidimensional measurements of both the solid and ground-glass components of lesions should be obtained as necessary. The use of a consistent low-dose technique is recommended, especially in cases for which prolonged follow-up is recommended, particularly in younger patients. With serial scans, always compare with the original baseline study to detect subtle indolent growth.

LUNG CANCER: RADIOLOGICAL FEATURES

Definition

- **SCLC:** small (oat) cell carcinoma
  - This originates from submucosal neuroendocrine cells ▶ it rapidly spreads haematogenously and to the lymph nodes ▶ it behaves as a systemic disease and is usually disseminated at presentation
- **NSCLC:** non-small cell lung cancer
  - *Squamous cell carcinomas:* arises from the proximal airway epithelium
  - *Large cell carcinomas:* atypical cells that appear 'large' under the microscope
  - *Adenocarcinomas:* arising from the bronchial glands
- **Risks:** tobacco smoke (20- to 30-fold increased risk) – has the greatest association with squamous cell carcinomas and weakest association with bronchoalveolar carcinomas ▶ asbestos exposure, interstitial pulmonary fibrosis and radiotherapy are additional risks

Clinical presentation

- *Asymptomatic* (25%): asymptomatic peripheral tumours are more likely to be incidental findings and surgically resectable
- *Symptomatic:* recurrent pneumonia ▶ cough ▶ wheeze ▶ haemoptysis
- *Paraneoplastic syndromes:* inappropriate ADH secretion ▶ Cushing's syndrome (ACTH) ▶ carcinoid syndrome ▶ hypercalcaemia (PTH)
- *Poor prognostic features:* hoarseness ▶ chest pain ▶ brachial plexus neuropathy or Horner's syndrome (due to a Pancoast's tumour) ▶ SVC obstruction ▶ dysphagia

Radiological features

Peripheral tumours

- The majority are spherical or oval in shape ▶ lobulated masses can occur due to uneven growth rates ▶ there may be a 'corona radiata' due to numerous fine strands radiating into the lung ▶ a bronchocele or mucoid impaction can be seen distal to an obstructing carcinoma ▶ collapse and consolidation is less commonly seen than with central tumours
  - Cavitation with irregular thick walls (≥8 mm) ± fluid levels (particularly squamous tumours)
  - Calcification is rare (6–10%) and may represent engulfed granulomatous disease ▶ amorphous or cloud-like calcification can be seen with dystrophic tumour calcification (10%)
  - Air bronchograms are rare but can be seen with adenocarcinoma
  - Ground-glass attenuation is associated with a higher risk of malignancy (and commonly seen with lepidic or invasive mucinous adenocarcinoma)

Central tumours

- Collapse or consolidation can be seen peripheral to the tumour (due to bronchial narrowing ± hilar enlargement) ▶ any peripheral collapsed lung will enhance more than a central tumour ▶ collateral air drift may prevent some post-obstructive changes
  - *'Golden S' sign:* a fissure may show a central bulge due to collapse around a central tumour

Hilar enlargement (N1-N3)

- This is a common presenting feature and may reflect a proximal central tumour, lymphadenopathy or consolidated lung ▶ extensive hilar and mediastinal lymphadenopathy is typical of small cell tumours ▶ simple pneumonias rarely cause hilar adenopathy

Chest wall invasion (T3)

- This does not preclude surgical resection (although it adversely affects the prognosis)
- **CT:** assessment is unreliable (with local chest wall pain remaining the most specific indicator) ▶ contact with or a thickened pleura does not necessarily indicate invasion ▶ a clear extrapleural fat plane is helpful but not definitive ▶ reliable signs include clear-cut bone destruction or a large soft tissue mass
- **MRI:** this is better than CT in selected cases ▶ it is the optimal modality for demonstrating the extent of a superior sulcus tumour
- **Transthoracic ultrasound:** this is an accurate technique
- **^{99m}Tc radionuclide skeletal scintigraphy:** this is sensitive (and may detect bone invasion before plain radiography) ▶ PET-CT is now the technique of choice for distant spread

Mediastinal invasion (T4)

- **CT/MRI indicators:** visible tumour deep within the mediastinal fat (mediastinal contact alone is not enough to diagnose invasion) ▶ encasement of the mediastinal vessels, oesophagus, or proximal mainstem bronchi ▶ SVC obstruction ▶ an elevated hemidiaphragm (indicating phrenic nerve involvement)
- **Criteria for resectability:** < 3 cm of contact with the mediastinum ▶ < 90° of circumferential contact with the aorta ▶ a visible mediastinal fat plane between the mass and any vital mediastinal structure
- **Irresectability:** tumours obliterating fat planes or showing greater contact than that described above (although less certain)

Bone involvement (M1)

- Direct rib or spine invasion ▶ haematogenous osteolytic bone metastases ▶ hypertrophic osteoarthopathy

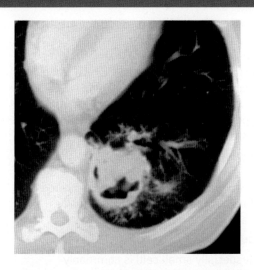

Cavitating squamous cell carcinoma. CT – the wall of the cavity is variable in thickness.*

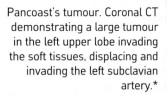

Pancoast's tumour. Coronal CT demonstrating a large tumour in the left upper lobe invading the soft tissues, displacing and invading the left subclavian artery.*

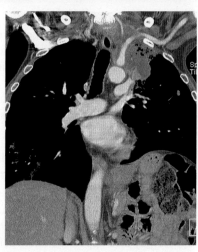

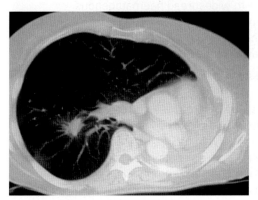

CT demonstrating a second primary bronchogenic carcinoma in the right lung in a patient who had undergone a previous left pneumonectomy. The new tumour has spiculated edges infiltrating into the adjacent lung (corona radiata).*

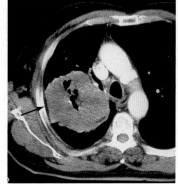

Cavitating bronchogenic carcinoma. There is preservation of the extrapleural fat plane at the point of contact with the chest wall (arrow). Although the pleura may be involved, the chest wall is likely to be otherwise spared.*

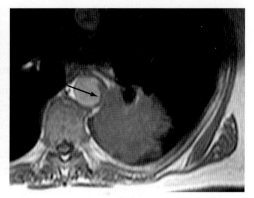

MRI of a left lower lobe tumour that has directly invaded the aortic wall, which has altered the signal adjacent to the tumour (arrow).*

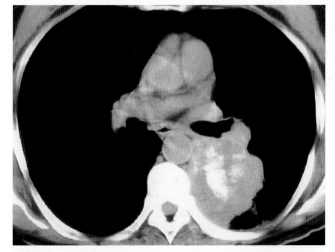

Tumour calcification. Large bronchial carcinoma within the left lower lobe showing extensive amorphous and cloud-like calcification.*

New classification for adenocarcinomas	
Premalignant	**Malignant**
Atypical adenomatous hyperplasia	*Minimally invasive adenocarcinoma*
Adenocarcinoma in situ	predominantly lepidic growth pattern
lepidic growth pattern (no solid components)	≤3 cm
pure ground-glass opacity on CT	invasive component <5 mm
	subsolid nodules on CT
	Lepidic predominant adenocarcinoma
	>5 mm invasion
	previously known as non-mucinous bronchoalveolar carcinoma
	Invasive mucinous adenocarcinoma
	previously known as mucinous bronchoalveolar carcinoma

LUNG CANCER: PEARLS

Pleural effusions (M1a)

- They may occur due to direct spread, lymphatic involvement, or tumour emboli (an adenocarcinoma may cause lobular pleural thickening indistinguishable from a malignant mesothelioma)
- A pleural effusion designates a tumour as M1a (unless clinically there is another cause and the pleural cytology is negative)

Lepidic predominant adenocarcinoma/invasive mucinous adenocarcinoma (formerly bronchoalveolar carcinoma)

- This can appear as a solitary lobulated or spiculated pulmonary mass with air bronchograms and cavitation ▶ it may also appear as an ill-defined opacity resembling a pneumonia, homogeneous consolidation, multiple ill-defined nodules throughout the lung, or a focal ground-glass opacity
  - They are often PET negative

Pancoast's tumour (superior sulcus tumour)

- A Pancoast's tumour is an apical lung tumour which can extend into the chest wall and may resemble apical pleural thickening (and is commonly a squamous carcinoma) ▶ it can invade the subclavian vessels, brachial plexus (with pain radiating into the arm) and cervical sympathetic chain (leading to Horner's syndrome)
- MRI is the optimal modality for assessment but CT is used for assessing bony involvement

Lymph Node Staging

- Lung cancers normally spread sequentially to the ipsilateral hilar nodes, ipsilateral mediastinal nodes and then the contralateral mediastinal and supraclavicular nodes
  - Skip metastases to the mediastinal nodes (in the absence of hilar nodes) can occur in $\frac{1}{3}$ of patients
- Other causes of enlarged nodes: previous tuberculosis ▶ histoplasmosis ▶ pneumoconiosis ▶ sarcoidosis ▶ reactive hyperplasia to the tumour or an associated pneumonia

CXR This is insensitive

CT/MRI Generally nodes with a short-axis diameter of > 10 mm are considered enlarged (normal subcarinal and lower mediastinal nodes can be up to 10 mm – upper paratracheal nodes rarely exceed 7 mm) ▶ increased signal on STIR imaging in abnormal nodes ▶ however microscopic tumour involvement can be present in normal-sized nodes

EUS This can assess nodal size and morphology, and guide fine needle aspiration of the aortopulmonary, subcarinal and posterior mediastinal nodes ▶ it has greater sensitivity and specificity than CT or PET in some series

FDG PET This assesses the lung mass (± any involved mediastinal nodes and any extrathoracic metastases) ▶ it has a greater sensitivity and specificity than CT but requires lesions to be > 1 cm in diameter ▶ fused PET–CT imaging is more accurate than PET or CT alone in staging NSCLC
- *False-positive results:* these can be due to inflammation or reactive hyperplasia (therefore positive PET findings still require histology)

Mediastinoscopy/mediastinotomy The most widely used techniques for mediastinal lymph node sampling ▶ they have a high sensitivity and specificity and are indicated prior to thoracotomy (biopsy confirmation is usually essential before a patient is denied surgery)

Extrathoracic Staging

- Lung cancer (especially small cell) is commonly associated with widespread haematogenous dissemination at presentation (to the adrenal glands, bones, brain, liver and distant lymph nodes)
- Metastatic disease precludes surgical resection

Features Suggesting a Pneumonia Is Secondary to a Neoplasm

- An altered shape of a collapsed or consolidated lobe (due to underlying tumour bulk) ▶ a visible mass or an irregular stenosis within a mainstem or lobar bronchus
- Pneumonia in an at-risk patient confined to one lobe (or more lobes if there is a common supplying bronchus) which persists unchanged for more than 2–3 weeks ▶ a pneumonia that recurs in the same lobe (particularly if there is volume loss and no air bronchograms)
- Mucous-filled dilated bronchi should prompt a search for a centrally obstructing tumour
  - Complete pneumonia resolution virtually excludes an obstructing neoplasm
  - A simple pneumonia rarely causes visible hilar adenopathy on CXR (although enlarged central nodes may be seen on CT)
- Drowned lobe: an opacified lobe appears larger than normal because of a build-up of secretions beyond the obstruction

Treatment

- **SCLC:** initially responsive to radiotherapy and chemotherapy but associated with early recurrence ± prophylactic cranial radiotherapy (as it is usually disseminated at presentation)
- **NSCLC:** surgical resection ± neoadjuvant chemotherapy to 'down-stage' a tumour ▶ surgery is not curative for N3 (contralateral mediastinal nodes) or symptomatic N2 (ipsilateral mediastinal nodes) disease ▶ T4 tumours are irresectable (the results for T3 tumours are worse than for T1 and T2 tumours)
  - Irresectable tumours: chemotherapy ± radical radiotherapy

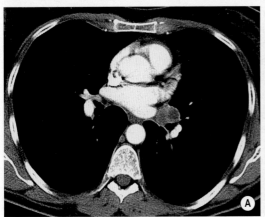 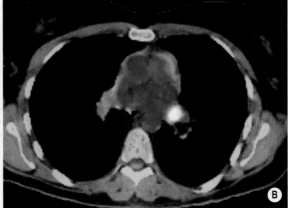

Recurrent malignant left hilar lymph nodes from a small peripheral non-small cell lung cancer. (A) CT demonstrates nodes at the left hilum. (B) The PET–CT image confirms high FDG uptake.*

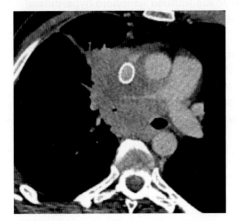 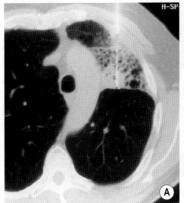 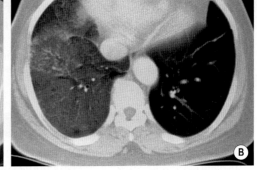

Mediastinal invasion. Tumour is obstructing the right main bronchus and encasing the stented SVC and the aorta.**

Lepidic predominant adenocarcinoma. (A) CT obtained during fine needle aspiration biopsy demonstrating lepidic growth in the left upper lobe. (B) Tumour presenting as diffuse consolidation and ground-glass shadowing on CT.*

Tumour	Incidence	Location	Pearl
Adenocarcinoma*	30–35% (and rising)	Peripheral (72%)	Cavitation is rare ▶ can arise within scar tissue ▶ smaller volume mediastinal and hilar adenopathy than with small cell tumours ▶ small (<4 cm) peripheral tumours ▶ pleural effusions
Squamous cell carcinoma	30–35% (and decreasing)	Central	Commonest tumour to cavitate (12%) ▶ slowest growth rate ▶ commonest tumour causing collapse and consolidation of the peripheral lung
Large cell carcinoma	10–15%	Peripheral (63%)	Early, significant mediastinal and hilar adenopathy ▶ large peripheral masses
Small cell carcinoma	20–30%	Central	Most aggressive tumour with the fastest growth rate (usually disseminated at diagnosis) ▶ early and often massive mediastinal and hilar adenopathy (78%) ▶ collapse and consolidation of the peripheral lung ▶ chemotherapy sensitive

*Includes lepidic predominant and invasive mucinous adenocarcinoma (whose relative incidence is decreasing)

LYMPHOCYTIC INTERSTITIAL PNEUMONIA/PSEUDOLYMPHOMA

DEFINITION

- A chronic antigenic stimulus generates a lymphoproliferative response – this can lead to a non-neoplastic disorder characterized by infiltration of the pulmonary parenchymal interstitium by lymphocytes and plasma cells
  - *Diffuse disease:* LIP
  - *Focal disease:* pseudolymphoma
  - *Disease centred on the small airways:* follicular bronchiolitis

CLINICAL PRESENTATION

- Cough ▶ dyspnoea ▶ it commonly affects females (at around 50 years of age)

RADIOLOGICAL FEATURES

- **Diffuse disease:** bilateral areas of ground-glass opacification, centrilobular nodules and thin-walled cysts (average 5 mm) ▶ it may rarely proceed to fibrosis with late honeycombing ▶ lymphadenopathy is rare ▶ pleural effusions may occur
- **Focal disease:** central airspace consolidation with air bronchograms or a mass ▶ the disease extends peripherally over time

PEARLS

- A histological differentiation between benign proliferation and a low-grade lymphoma can be difficult

- LIP may rarely occur as an isolated entity (it is included in the classification of the idiopathic interstitial pneumonias) ▶ however, it is more commonly seen in association with an underlying immunological abnormality (e.g. Sjögren's disease, rheumatoid arthritis or AIDS)

  Pseudolymphoma A rare condition demonstrating benign behaviour which arises from mucosa-associated lymphoid tissue (MALT) and which is considered a low-grade B-cell lymphoma

  CXR/CT Solitary or multiple areas of pulmonary consolidation ▶ air bronchograms and cavitation can be seen ▶ lymphadenopathy and pleural effusions are rare
- It is initially central in location with later growth out towards the periphery
- It rarely undergoes malignant transformation to a pulmonary lymphoma

  Follicular bronchiolitis (diffuse lymphoid hyperplasia) Hyperplasia of the bronchial MALT occurring in relation to the airways

  CXR/CT Reticular or reticular nodular shadowing with centrilobular nodules and ground-glass opacification ▶ occasionally bronchial wall thickening, bronchial dilatation, interlobular septal thickening and peribronchovascular airspace consolidation is demonstrated

LEUKAEMIA

DEFINITION

- Various acute or chronic neoplastic diseases of the bone marrow
- Pulmonary infiltration is seen in $\frac{2}{3}$ of patients at autopsy ▶ it is usually asymptomatic and rarely a cause of significant pulmonary opacities on imaging

CLINICAL PRESENTATION

- It is usually asymptomatic (however, dyspnoea can occur due to obliteration of small pulmonary blood vessels by leukaemic cells)
- Disease complications are the likely cause of any symptoms (pulmonary infection, oedema or haemorrhage)

RADIOLOGICAL FEATURES

CXR/MRI Diffuse bilateral reticulation and patterns resembling interstitial oedema ▶ lymphangitis carcinomatosa, small nodules, ground-glass opacification and consolidation can also be seen ▶ hilar and mediastinal lymph node enlargement closely resembling lymphoma (this can be massive with T-cell leukaemia with a rapid response to treatment) ▶ pleural effusions are common
- Granulocytic sarcoma or chloroma: rarely there can also be pleural thickening in myeloid leukaemia due to a mass of leukaemic cells

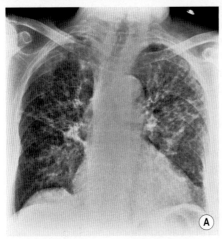
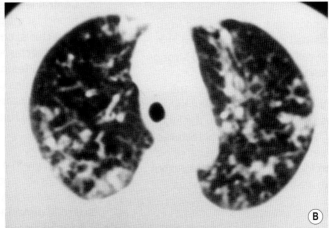

Lymphocytic interstitial pneumonitis. (A) PA CXR shows a coarse reticulonodular pattern diffusely throughout both lungs. (B) CT demonstrating a predominantly nodular pattern with a lymphatic distribution both along the bronchovascular bundles and in the subpleural zones.‡

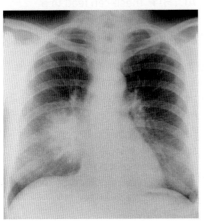
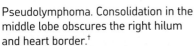
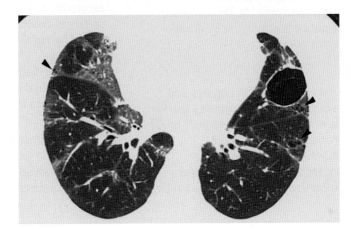

CT through the lower lobes shows scattered areas of ground-glass abnormality. The large cyst in the lingula and the scattered smaller cysts (arrowheads) are important clues to the diagnosis of LIP.

Pseudolymphoma. Consolidation in the middle lobe obscures the right hilum and heart border.†

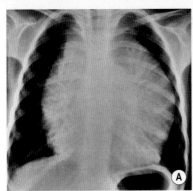
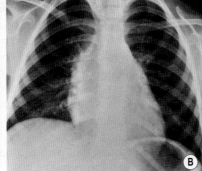
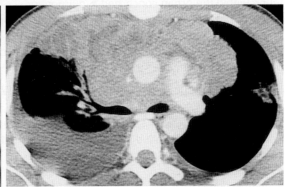

T-cell leukaemia/lymphoma in a 4-year-old girl. (A) Massive mediastinal adenopathy. (B) Following very rapid response to chemotherapy.

Leukaemia. CT demonstrating massive anterior mediastinal adenopathy with a large pleural effusion.†

BRONCHIAL CARCINOID

Definition

- An uncommon neuroendocrine tumour derived from bronchial APUD cells (small cell carcinomas are also derived from the same cell type) ▶ there is no strong association with smoking
  - **Typical** (90%): these commonly arise within the central airways ▶ they demonstrate benign behaviour
  - **Atypical** (10%): these usually arise within the lung periphery ▶ their histological and clinical features are intermediate between a typical bronchial carcinoid and a small cell carcinoma of the lung ▶ they often metastasize with an associated poor prognosis

Clinical presentation

- Cough ▶ wheeze ▶ post-obstructive pneumonia ▶ haemoptysis ▶ Cushing's syndrome (ACTH secretion)
- The peak age of presentation is during the 5th decade (2M:1F)

Radiological features

- **Bronchial lesions:** a mass with smooth borders and without necrosis or cavitation ▶ it demonstrates marked contrast enhancement ▶ calcification is seen in ⅓ on CT
  - *'Iceberg' lesion:* carcinoids arising within a central bronchus (80–90%) often have a larger mass component external to the bronchus – the extra-bronchial component may be visible as a hilar mass

- Central lesions usually produce partial or complete bronchial obstruction ▶ there may be associated atelectasis, pneumonia (± a lung abscess), distal bronchiectasis or a mucocele
- **Peripheral lesions** (10–20%): solitary spherical or lobular nodules (2–4 cm) with well-defined smooth edges ▶ they can resemble a bronchial carcinoma and are therefore frequently removed surgically

Pearls

- Although given a benign classification, carcinoids can invade locally and metastasize to the hilar or mediastinal lymph nodes as well as to the brain, liver and bone (with sclerotic metastases)
- Carcinoids may secrete various hormones (e.g. serotonin, histamine, ACTH) ▶ these can lead to a carcinoid syndrome – this is very rare if the disease is confined to the lung and usually indicates hepatic metastases
- Differential diagnosis for central lesions: adenoid cystic carcinoma and mucoepidermoid carcinoma (both are salivary gland malignancies that can develop in the main airways)

DIPNECH: diffuse idiopathic pulmonary neuroendocrine cell hyperplasia – preinvasive form ▶ multiple small nodules <5 mm seen in association with a mosaic attenuation pattern in the setting of a known carcinoid tumour

OTHER BENIGN PULMONARY NEOPLASMS

Pulmonary hamartoma

Definition A hamartoma is a tumour-like malformation composed of abnormal mature tissues that are normally found within the organ concerned ▶ pulmonary hamartomas consist predominantly of cartilage, bronchial epithelium and fat and demonstrate slow growth ▶ malignant transformation is extremely rare ▶ they can very occasionally be multiple

Clinical presentation An asymptomatic pulmonary nodule presenting between young adulthood and old age

CXR/CT A spherical or slightly lobulated well-defined nodule (<4 cm) surrounded by normal lung ▶ cavitation is rare

- A central fat density or 'popcorn' calcification (increasing with lesion size) is virtually diagnostic of a hamartoma

Pearl A hamartoma demonstrates an opposite distribution to a bronchial carcinoid: 90% are peripheral (as a solitary pulmonary nodule) and 10% arise within a major bronchus (which may also lead to major airway obstruction)

- *Carney's triad:* pulmonary chondroma(s) + gastric epithelioid leiomyosarcoma (leiomyoblastoma) + functioning extra-adrenal paragangliomas

Leiomyoma of the lung

Definition This may be a solitary lesion (multiple leiomyomas, which can present as multiple discrete lung nodules, are also known as benign metastasizing leiomyomas) ▶ they are radiographically indistinguishable from other benign connective tissue neoplasms ▶ they may represent a very slow-growing metastasis from a uterine leiomyoma

Plasma cell granuloma of the lung (inflammatory pseudotumour)

Definition This is presumed to be reactive inflammatory granulomatous tissue ▶ it affects a wide age range (including children) ▶ it presents as an asymptomatic solitary pulmonary nodule and can demonstrate occasional cavitation or calcification

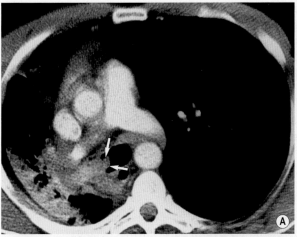

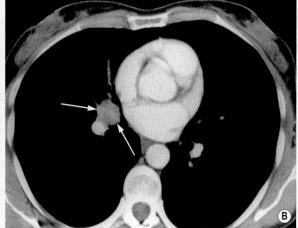

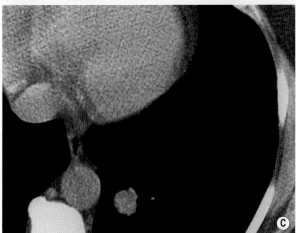

Carcinoid tumour. (A) A small tumour is completely occluding the right main bronchus and causing extensive collapse in the right lung. The endoluminal component is well seen (arrows), but there is poor differentiation of the tumour from adjacent collapsed lung. (B) A well-defined perihilar carcinoid tumour (arrows) is demonstrated anterior to the artery to the right lower lobe. (C) A small peripheral carcinoid tumour indistinguishable from a number of other causes of a solitary pulmonary nodule.*

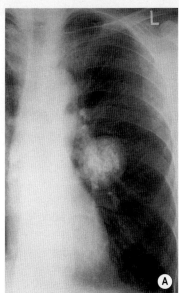

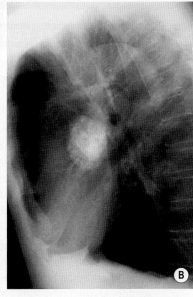

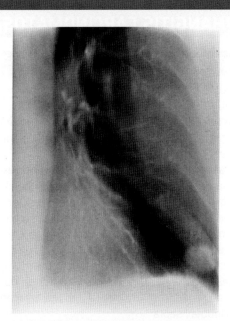

Hamartoma of the lung. (A,B) A round, completely smooth hamartoma. There is typical coarse popcorn calcification in this lesion, which is unusually large.*

Plasma cell granuloma. AP tomogram shows a smooth, well-defined peripheral lung nodule.‡

PULMONARY METASTASES

DEFINITION

- Adult pulmonary metastases are usually from the following primaries: breast, GI tract, kidney, testes, head and neck tumours or a variety of bone and soft tissue sarcomas
- There are 3 modes of spread: haematogenous (most common), lymphatic and endobronchial (rare)
- Their growth rates can be very variable, ranging from very slow (e.g. metastatic thyroid carcinoma) to very fast (e.g. metastatic choriocarcinoma or an osteosarcoma)

RADIOLOGICAL FEATURES

Haematogenous metastases

- These usually present as multiple discrete pulmonary nodules (75%) ▶ the nodules can measure up to a few cm in size and tend to be spherical with a well-defined margin
  - An irregular edge is commonly seen with metastatic adenocarcinoma
  - An ill-defined margin may signify haemorrhage (classically a choriocarcinoma)
  - Cavitation is most commonly seen with metastatic squamous carcinoma
  - Calcification is unusual but when seen is usually due to an osteosarcoma (rarely a chondrosarcoma or mucinous adenocarcinoma)
- Metastases are usually bilateral, and within the peripheral subpleural regions (where the tumour cells are trapped in the smallest vessels) ▶ there is also a basal predominance (the region of greatest gravitational perfusion)
- A pneumothorax may be seen with cavitation of subpleural metastases (especially with a sarcoma)

Endobronchial metastases

- These are rare ▶ melanoma, renal, colorectal and breast carcinomas are the most frequent
- A hilar mass ± airway obstruction (with atelectasis) may be seen

Miliary metastases

- These are rare ▶ they appear as multiple small (approximately 2 mm) parenchymal nodules representing 'millet' seeds
- They are commonly seen with thyroid and renal carcinomas

Tumour emboli

- Pulmonary arterial hypertension can rarely occur secondary to tumour emboli blocking small pulmonary arteries (HCC/breast/renal/stomach/prostate/choriocarcinoma)

PEARL

- Approximately 3% of asymptomatic pulmonary nodules are metastases – it may be the presenting feature in a patient without a known primary tumour

LYMPHANGITIS CARCINOMATOSA

DEFINITION

- This is due to the permeation of the pulmonary lymphatics (± the adjacent interstitial tissue) by neoplastic cells ▶ common causative tumours include carcinomas of the bronchus, breast, stomach and prostate
- **Bilateral symmetric pulmonary abnormalities:**
  - These are secondary to blood-borne emboli lodging within the smaller pulmonary arteries ▶ there can be subsequent spread into the perivascular interstitium or lymphatic vessels
- **Localized pulmonary abnormalities:**
  - Direct extension of tumour from the hilar lymph nodes into the peribronchovascular interstitium
  - Direct spread from the pleura into the adjacent interlobular septa
  - Direct spread from a lung primary carcinoma into the adjacent peribronchovascular interstitium

RADIOLOGICAL FEATURES

- Lymphangitis may involve all zones of both lungs or may be centrally or peripherally predominant ▶ it may be confined to a lobe or one lung (particularly if due to a bronchial carcinoma) ▶ hilar adenopathy is rarely seen

CXR Fine reticulonodular shadowing (± thickened septal lines) – this is due to a combination of dilated lymphatics, interstitial oedema, shadowing due to tumour cells and any associated desmoplastic response
- Subpleural oedema results from tumour lymphatic obstruction and can lead to fissure thickening and pleural effusions (30%)

CT Non-uniform (often nodular) thickening of the interlobular septa ▶ irregular thickening of the central bronchovascular bundles ▶ small peripherally located wedge-shaped densities can be seen ▶ there is often patchy airspace shadowing with nodular shadows scattered throughout the parenchyma

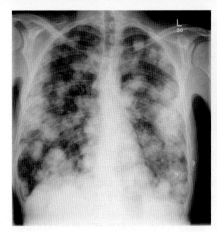

Typical pulmonary metastases. CXR showing multiple, well-defined spherical nodules in the lungs.

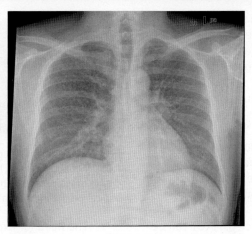

Miliary metastases. CXR showing multiple small nodules throughout both lungs from a thyroid carcinoma.

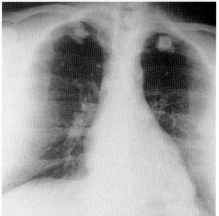

Pulmonary metastases from an osteosarcoma. Densely calcified masses are seen throughout both lungs.[†]

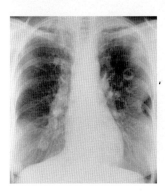

Pulmonary metastases from carcinoma of the cervix. Multiple cavitating masses are present in both lungs.[†]

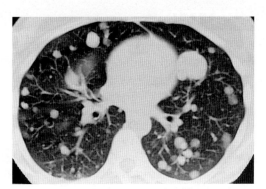

Pulmonary metastases. Soft tissue sarcoma. CT demonstrating the subpleural location of several of the metastases.[†]

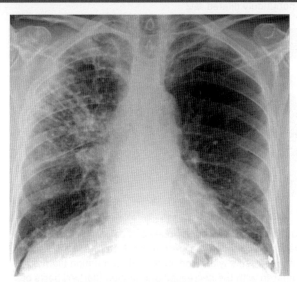

Unilateral lymphangitic carcinomatosis. Carcinoma of the bronchus, showing thickened septal lines and nodules confined to the right lung.**

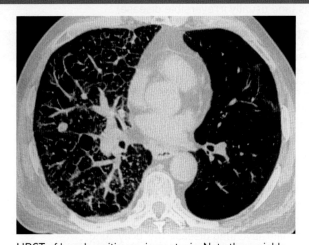

HRCT of lymphangitic carcinomatosis. Note the variable thickening of the interlobular septa and the enlargement of the bronchovascular bundle in the centre of the secondary pulmonary lobules. The polygonal shape of the walls (septa) of the secondary pulmonary lobules is particularly well shown anteriorly. The pulmonary nodule is due to a discrete metastasis, a relatively frequent finding in this condition.*

1.7 HIGH-RESOLUTION COMPUTED TOMOGRAPHY (HRCT)

HRCT TECHNIQUE

- Thin collimation (1-2 mm) with a high spatial frequency algorithm reconstruction ▶ interspaced versus volumetric acquisition (dose considerations)
- Reducing slice thickness < 1 mm will not increase spatial resolution but increase image noise
- A sharp reconstruction algorithm reduces images smoothing making structures visibly sharper (at the cost of increased image noise)
- IV contrast should be avoided if possible as it can spuriously increase parenchymal opacification
- Images usually acquired in the supine position from the apices to lung bases at full inspiration (at 1-2 cm intervals if non-volumetric)
  - If early interstitial fibrosis is suspected, HRCT can be performed in the prone position to distinguish from potential dependent change that can be seen in the posterobasal segments when supine

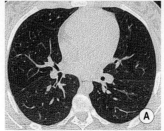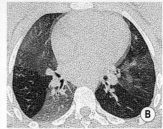

Mosaic attenuation in a patient with bronchiectasis in the lower lobes (not shown). HRCT image taken in inspiration (A) shows subtle mosaicism, emphasized in the section acquired at end-expiration (B), indicating small airways disease.**

  - The need for expiratory CT is controversial – although end-expiration images can reveal subtle areas of air trapping, if clinically significant this is usually evident on inspiratory images

GROUND-GLASS PATTERN

Definition A non-specific feature representing a generalized increase in lung parenchymal opacification that does not obscure the pulmonary vessels ▶ it represents a combination of partial airspace filling, interstitial thickening and displacement of air from the lung

- *Causes:* subacute hypersensitivity pneumonitis ▶ acute respiratory distress syndrome (ARDS) ▶ acute interstitial pneumonia (AIP) ▶ non-specific interstitial pneumonia (NSIP) ▶ diffuse pneumonias (particularly *Pneumocystis jiroveci (P. carinii)* pneumonia in AIDS patients)

HRCT Identification of dilated airways within areas of ground-glass opacification is usually an indication of fine fibrosis (and usually irreversible disease)

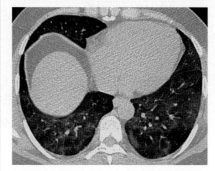

Widespread ground-glass opacification in a patient with desquamative interstitial pneumonia. The pulmonary vasculature is not obscured by this degree of opacification and the air-filled bronchi not unduly dilated. ©2

MOSAIC ATTENUATION PATTERN

Definition A non-specific sign representing regional lung parenchymal attenuation differences ▶ lung attenuation depends on the amount of blood, parenchymal tissue and air and is therefore a non-specific sign

- This is the dominant abnormality in small airways disease, occlusive vascular disease and infiltrative lung disease
  - In small airways and occlusive vascular disease the 'black' lung demonstrating decreased attenuation is abnormal
  - In infiltrative lung disease the 'grey' lung demonstrating normal or increased attenuation is abnormal

HRCT Bronchial abnormalities and the presence of air trapping on expiratory CT are the most useful discriminatory features in identifying small airways disease as the cause of mosaic attenuation

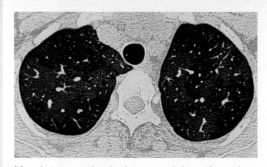

Mosaic attenuation in the upper lobes of a patient with sickle cell disease and pulmonary hypertension. Note the increased calibre of the vessels within the increased attenuation (lighter) lung compared with the decreased attenuation (darker) parts of the lung, suggesting a vascular cause of the mosaic attenuation pattern in this case. ©2

RETICULAR PATTERN

Definition This is caused by thickened interlobular or intralobular septa or honeycomb (fibrotic) destruction ▶ it almost always represents significant interstitial lung disease (ILD)

- Causes include infiltration by fibrosis (interstitial fibrosis), abnormal cells (lymphangitis carcinomatosa) or fluid (pulmonary oedema)
- *Smooth interlobular septal thickening:* pulmonary oedema or alveolar proteinosis
- *Irregular interlobular septal thickening:* lymphangitic spread of tumour or the nodular septal thickening seen in sarcoidosis

HRCT

- *A fine reticular pattern* (most commonly seen with idiopathic pulmonary fibrosis)
- *A coarse reticular pattern:* this occurs with severe fibrosis and is characterized by interlacing irregular linear opacities ▶ an end-stage fibrotic (honeycomb) lung is characterized by cystic airspaces surrounded by irregular walls
  - *Traction bronchiectasis/bronchiolectasis:* extensive fibrosis can distort the lung morphology resulting in irregular segmental or subsegmental airway dilatation
- *Ground-glass opacification* (if the septal thickening is very fine)

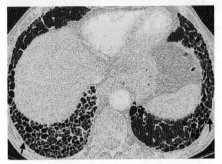

Reticular pattern: HRCT showing a coarse reticular pattern with extensive subpleural and basal honeycombing (arrows) in a patient with usual interstitial pneumonia.

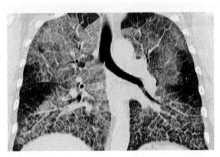

Widespread smooth thickening of the interlobular and intralobular septa in areas of ground-glass opacification in a patient with pulmonary alveolar proteinosis. ©2

NODULAR PATTERN

Definition This is a feature of both interstitial and airspace disease

Nodules within the lung interstitium This is seen within the interlobular septa and the subpleural and peribronchovascular regions (especially those related to lymphatic vessels) ▶ nodules can be < 5 mm from the pleural surface

- *Causes:* sarcoidosis ▶ lymphangitis carcinomatosa

Centrilobular nodules These are related to endobronchial and small airway disease ▶ most peripheral nodules are > 5 mm from the pleural surface ▶ a 'tree-in-bud' appearance suggests endobronchial disease

- *Causes:* subacute hypersensitivity pneumonitis ▶ respiratory bronchiolitis–interstitial lung disease (RB–ILD) ▶ diffuse panbronchiolitis ▶ endobronchial spread of TB ▶ cryptogenic organizing pneumonia

Random distribution The distribution is not related to the secondary pulmonary lobule and can involve the pleural surface

- *Causes:* haematogenous spread of TB ▶ pulmonary metastases ▶ pneumoconiosis ▶ sarcoidosis (rare)

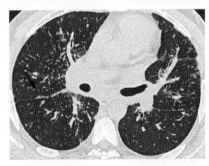

Nodular pattern: HRCT showing scattered nodules within the lung interstitium in a peribronchovascular distribution, with beading along the fissures (arrows) in a patient with pulmonary sarcoidosis.

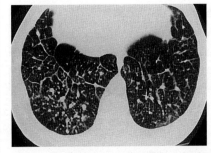

Marked thickening of the interlobular septa with randomly distributed small nodules in an individual with silicosis. ©2

IDIOPATHIC PULMONARY FIBROSIS (IPF)

DEFINITION

- Progressive fibrosis and end-stage lung destruction of unknown cause
- It is also known as cryptogenic fibrosing alveolitis (CFA) or usual interstitial pneumonia (UIP) ▶ UIP specifically refers to the *histopathological* pattern seen in patients with the clinical presentation of CFA or IPF

Clinical presentation Cough ▶ dyspnoea ▶ weight loss ▶ clubbing ▶ it commonly affects patients who are 40–70 years old (M>F)

RADIOLOGICAL FEATURES

CXR Bilateral asymmetric peripheral reticular opacities ▶ these are most profuse at the lung bases ▶ although there is associated volume loss, the lung volumes may be preserved or increased if there is coexisting emphysema

HRCT Ground-glass change is not predominant ▶ with disease progression the lung changes 'creep' around the lung periphery to involve the anterior aspects of the upper lobes (this is an important discriminator between UIP and other conditions with a similar clinical presentation) ▶ mediastinal adenopathy is frequently seen (up to 2 cm and unrelated to infection or malignancy) ▶ pleural effusions are uncommon ▶ pulmonary hypertension can be seen with severe disease

- *Early stage:* ground-glass change
- *Late stage:* a predominantly subpleural bibasal reticular pattern
- *End stage:* areas of honeycomb destruction (end stage) with associated traction bronchiectasis

PEARL

- Other causes of a UIP-type histological pattern: chronic hypersensitivity pneumonitis ▶ asbestosis ▶ connective tissue disease ▶ rarely drugs
- A confident HRCT diagnosis of UIP is difficult without honeycombing
- Extent of fibrosis is predictive of survival and mortality

NON-SPECIFIC INTERSTITIAL PNEUMONIA (NSIP)

DEFINITION

- Varying degrees of interstitial inflammation and fibrosis without any specific features to allow a diagnosis of UIP or DIP to be made

Clinical presentation As for UIP ▶ it commonly affects patients who are aged between 40 and 50 years (M = F)

RADIOLOGICAL FEATURES

HRCT A predominant pattern of ground-glass opacification (with a basal and subpleural distribution) ± associated airway distortion ▶ a reticular pattern is common ▶ there may be significant fibrosis (temporally uniform in comparison with UIP) but honeycombing is sparse ▶ abnormalities are usually peribronchovascular or peripheral, and occasionally spare the subpleural lung

- NSIP may be distinguished from UIP by more prominent ground-glass attenuation, a finer reticular pattern and an absence of honeycombing

PEARLS

- The heterogeneity of pathological processes encompassed by NSIP makes a confident CT diagnosis less likely than with UIP
- NSIP has a better prognosis than UIP

CRYPTOGENIC ORGANIZING PNEUMONIA (COP)

DEFINITION

- A clinicopathological entity of an isolated organizing pneumonia seen in patients without an identifiable associated disease (e.g. infection, malignancy or connective tissue disease)
- COP was previously known as bronchiolitis obliterans organizing pneumonia (BOOP)

Clinical presentation A non-productive cough ▶ dyspnoea ▶ malaise ▶ weight loss ▶ it commonly affects patients during the 6th decade (M = F)

RADIOLOGICAL FEATURES

CXR Areas of patchy consolidation which is often subpleural and basal (with a propensity to progress and change location over time) ▶ there is lung volume preservation

HRCT Consolidation corresponding with areas of organizing pneumonia is commonly seen within the lower zones with either a subpleural or a peribronchial distribution (the peribronchial distribution is typically seen in patients with polymyositis or dermatomyositis) ▶ ground-glass opacification, subpleural linear opacities and a distinctive perilobular pattern is commonly seen ▶ the lung architecture is generally well preserved with cavitation rarely seen

- 'Reverse halo' sign: multifocal areas of ground-glass opacification with a surrounding rim of consolidation

PEARL

- There is usually a complete response to a long (2–3 months) course of high-dose steroids

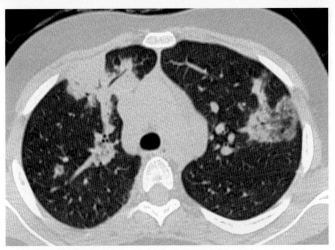

Cryptogenic-organizing pneumonia. HRCT through the upper lobes demonstrates areas of consolidation in a subpleural and peribronchial distribution in association with areas of ground-glass opacification (left upper lobe).*

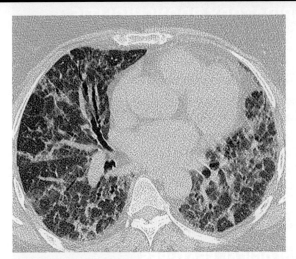

Biopsy-proven-organizing pneumonia. There are poorly defined arcade-like and polygonal opacities (the perilobular pattern) in the subpleural and posterior regions of both lungs. The opacities resemble ill-defined thickened interlobular septa.*

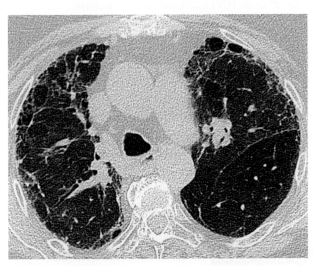

Usual interstitial pneumonia. In the upper lobes anteriorly there are peripheral irregular lines with areas of honeycombing.*

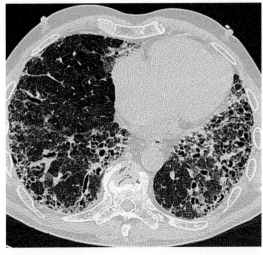

Usual interstitial pneumonia. HRCT abnormalities predominate in the posterior, and subpleural regions of the lower lobes and comprise honeycombing and traction bronchiectasis within the abnormal lung.*

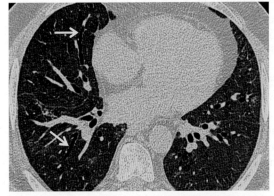

There is generalized ground-glass opacification and a few thickened interlobular septa. There is marked dilatation of the bronchi (arrows) reflecting the presence of fine interstitial fibrosis. Biopsy-proven non-specific interstitial pneumonia. ©2

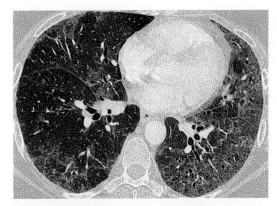

Non-specific interstitial pneumonia. The predominant abnormality is patchy, bilateral ground-glass opacification, mild reticulation and traction bronchiectasis. There is no frank honeycombing destruction.*

RESPIRATORY BRONCHIOLITIS–INTERSTITIAL LUNG DISEASE (RB–ILD) AND DESQUAMATIVE INTERSTITIAL PNEUMONIA (DIP)

DEFINITION

- This is characterized by alveolar space filling with macrophages and a strong association with cigarette smoking
- RB–ILD and DIP are part of the same disease spectrum, with DIP the more severe form

Clinical presentation Insidious dyspnoea ▶ cough

RADIOLOGICAL FEATURES

CXR This is relatively insensitive

HRCT

- **RB–ILD:** areas of patchy ground-glass opacification (due to macrophage accumulation within the alveolar spaces and ducts) ▶ poorly defined low attenuation centrilobular nodules ▶ upper lobe centrilobular emphysema and areas of air trapping (usually to a limited extent and reflecting the bronchiolitic element)
  - Thickening of the interlobular septa and features of interstitial fibrosis is unusual
- **DIP:** ground-glass opacification is the dominant feature ▶ this typically affects the peripheral lower zones and may be patchy ▶ occasionally there are features of established fibrosis (which is usually to a limited extent)

PEARLS

- It demonstrates a relatively stable clinical course
- Smoking cessation is an important part of the management
- Because of significant overlap, 'smoking-related interstitial lung disease' (SR-ILD) has been proposed to encompass DIP, RB-ILD, LCH and interstitial fibrosis

LYMPHOID INTERSTITIAL PNEUMONIA

DEFINITION

- This is due to a widespread interstitial lymphoid lung infiltrate ▶ it resembles lymphoma but its clinical course is more akin to a chronic interstitial pneumonia

Clinical presentation Progressive cough and dyspnoea (2F : 1M)

RADIOLOGICAL FEATURES

HRCT Nodules of varying sizes (which may be ill-defined) ▶ ground-glass opacification ▶ thickened bronchovascular bundles and interlobular septal thickening ▶ discrete thin-walled cysts lying deep within the lung parenchyma (measuring up to 3 cm)

- Airspace disease, large nodules and pleural effusions are rare

PEARLS

- Evolution to a frank lymphoproliferative disease is rare
- It occurs in association with autoimmune diseases (e.g. Sjögren's syndrome), dysproteinaemias, autologous bone marrow transplantation, infection (viral, mycobacterial, HIV) and Castleman's disease

ACUTE INTERSTITIAL PNEUMONIA/DIFFUSE ALVEOLAR DAMAGE (FORMERLY HAMMAN–RICH SYNDROME)

DEFINITION

- This can be regarded as an idiopathic form of adult respiratory distress syndrome (ARDS)
- It consists of diffuse alveolar damage – there is an acute exudative phase with subsequent organizing and fibrotic phases

Clinical presentation An acute onset with a similar presentation to ARDS (M = F)

RADIOLOGICAL FEATURES

CXR Bilateral patchy airspace opacification

HRCT Ground-glass opacification and consolidation (all phases) ▶ bronchial dilatation and architectural distortion (fibrotic phase)

PEARLS

- With resolution there is clearing of any ground-glass attenuation leaving residual fibrosis – fibrosis is more common than that seen in ARDS
- It has a poor prognosis

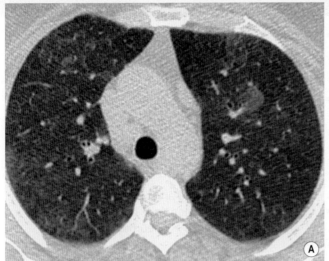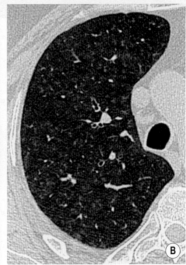

RB–ILD. HRCT shows (A) subtle areas of ground-glass opacification and (B) ill-defined centrilobular nodules.*

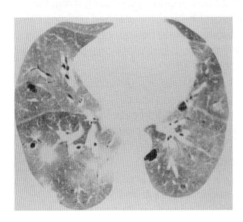

DIP. There is diffuse ground-glass opacification throughout the lungs due to inflammatory infiltrate.†

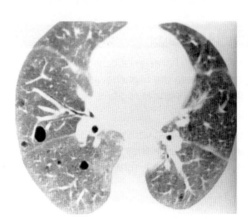

Lymphocytic interstitial pneumonitis. There is a background of ground-glass opacification and a few thin-walled cystic airspaces (the pathogenesis of these cysts is unclear).*

Clinico–radiological–pathological criteria	Histological pattern	HRCT features*
Idiopathic pulmonary fibrosis	Usual interstitial pneumonia	Peripheral (subpleural) and basal reticular opacities ▶ honeycombing ▶ areas of ground-glass opacity (associated with traction bronchiectasis)
Non-specific interstitial pneumonia	Non-specific interstitial pneumonia	Areas of ground-glass opacity ± traction bronchiectasis ▶ minimal honeycombing
Cryptogenic organizing pneumonia	Organizing pneumonia	Peripheral or peribronchial consolidation ▶ areas of ground-glass opacity ▶ a perilobular pattern is increasingly recognized
Acute interstitial pneumonia	Diffuse alveolar damage	Consolidation (within the dependent lung) ▶ areas of ground-glass opacity ▶ traction bronchiectasis (organizing phase)
Respiratory bronchiolitis–interstitial lung (RB–ILD)	RB–ILD	Poorly defined centrilobular nodules ▶ areas of ground-glass opacity ▶ bronchial wall thickening ▶ limited emphysema
Desquamative interstitial pneumonia (DIP)	DIP	Areas of ground-glass opacity ▶ features of interstitial fibrosis
Lymphoid interstitial pneumonia (LIP)	LIP	Areas of ground-glass opacity ▶ poorly defined centrilobular nodules ▶ thickened interlobular septa ▶ thin-walled discrete cysts ▶ air trapping

SARCOIDOSIS

DEFINITION

- A multisystem non-caseating granulomatous disorder of unknown aetiology
- The lungs, hilar and mediastinal nodes are the most commonly affected organ system
  - *Other affected organs:* skin > peripheral lymph nodes > eyes > spleen > CNS > parotid glands > bones

CLINICAL PRESENTATION

- Fatigue ▶ malaise ▶ weight loss ▶ fever and night sweats ▶ dyspnoea ▶ erythema nodosum ▶ arthralgia ▶ 30% of patients are asymptomatic
  - Respiratory symptoms are most commonly seen in the black female population
- Onset is usually during the 2nd to 4th decades (F>M)

RADIOLOGICAL FEATURES

- Lung granulomas have a characteristic distribution along the lymphatics within the bronchovascular sheath, interlobular septa and subpleural regions

CXR (lymphadenopathy)

- Lymph nodes appear lobulated with a well-demarcated outline (they can be massive) ▶ they can calcify in a characteristic 'eggshell' fashion ▶ airway or vascular compression is unusual
- *Garland's triad:* bilateral *symmetrical* hilar and paratracheal lymphadenopathy
  - The lymphadenopathy can occasionally (1–5%) be asymmetrical or unilateral – marked asymmetry should bring the diagnosis into question ▶ unilateral paratracheal lymphadenopathy is usually right-sided (left-sided lymphadenopathy causes enlargement of the aortopulmonary window nodes)
- 40% of patients with nodal enlargement will develop parenchymal opacities within 1 year – of these ⅓ ▶ will develop persistent fibrotic shadowing (± traction bronchiectasis)
  - Nodal enlargement does not develop after parenchymal opacification

CXR (parenchymal changes)

- Parenchymal changes appear as any nodal enlargement subsides (these tend to progress in unison in lymphoma)

Causes of eggshell nodal calcification*
Sarcoidosis
Silicosis
Histoplasmosis
Lymphoma (post-irradiation)
Blastomycosis
Amyloidosis

- *The most common pattern:* rounded or irregular moderately well-defined nodules (2–4 mm) ▶ very small aggregated opacities can give a ground-glass appearance
- *The second most common pattern:* peribronchovascular patchy airspace consolidation ▶ this usually demonstrates a nodular pattern but can also contain air bronchograms and have ill-defined margins ▶ a conglomerate opacity resembling progressive massive fibrosis can develop
  - Both types have a mid and upper zone predominance
- *Complications:* cor pulmonale ▶ bullous disease (± mycetoma formation) ▶ pneumothorax

HRCT

- Perilymphatic nodular opacities (1–5 mm) within the subpleural regions and along the bronchovascular bundles and interlobular septae (generating irregular and beaded interfaces) ▶ larger ill-defined nodules can develop – these rarely cavitate but can demonstrate air bronchograms ▶ patchy ground-glass opacification ▶ air trapping is commonly seen
  - Parenchymal consolidation and ground-glass opacification is usually reversible
  - Fibrosis occurs in advanced disease in one-third and is usually irreversible (affecting the mid to upper zones)

Other thoracic findings

- Pleural thickening and effusions are unusual (any effusion seen is usually unilateral and small)
- Intrinsic mural sarcoidosis can rarely cause airway narrowing (with single or multiple lesions seen down to a segmental level) ▶ there is a potential for significant airflow obstruction or atelectasis (particularly involving the middle lobe)

PEARLS

- Sarcoidosis is the most common cause of intrathoracic lymph node enlargement ▶ symmetry is the important diagnostic feature
  - The anterior mediastinal nodes are occasionally enlarged – posterior mediastinal nodal enlargement is unusual
- 67Gallium accumulation is a sensitive but non-specific indicator of active inflammation in sarcoidosis
- **Diagnosis:** transbronchial biopsy
- **Staging (CXR)**
  - *Stage 0:* normal CXR
  - *Stage I:* lymphadenopathy
  - *Stage II:* lymphadenopathy with parenchymal opacification
  - *Stage III:* parenchymal opacification only
  - *Stage IV:* pulmonary fibrosis

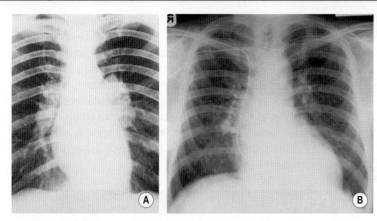

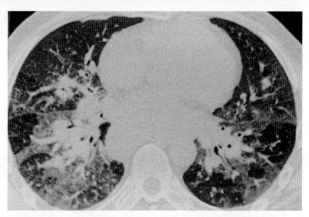

Sarcoidosis. (A) Bilateral hilar node enlargement. In a different patient (B) there is peripheral hilar node calcification ('eggshell' calcification). A pacing electrode is present for heart block, which is an occasional complication.†

Sarcoidosis. Expiratory HRCT. There is air trapping, as evidenced by parenchymal areas that remain low attenuation on expiration.†

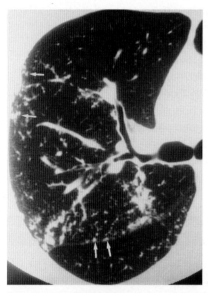

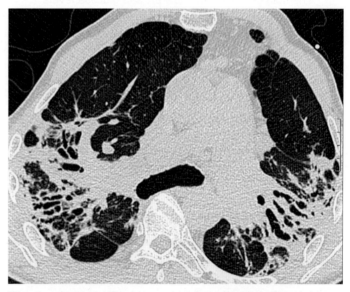

Sarcoidosis. HRCT shows nodularity of the bronchovascular bundles due to multiple sarcoid granulomas. Nodules are also evident in the subpleural regions adjacent to the chest wall and major fissure (arrows).†

Fibrotic sarcoidosis. There are areas of conglomerate fibrosis in a perihilar distribution with associated bronchial distortion and volume loss. The appearances superficially mimic progressive massive fibrosis seen in the pneumoconioses.*

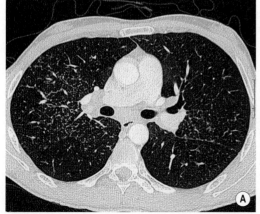

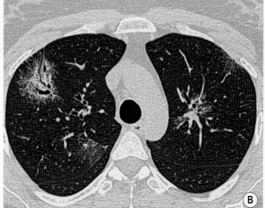

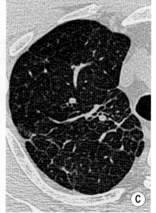

Sarcoidosis. Typical HRCT features are (A) nodular opacities which (B) may become confluent, and (C) interlobular septal thickening.*

RHEUMATOID DISEASE

DEFINITION

- Rheumatoid disease is associated with a broad spectrum of pleural and pulmonary manifestations ▶ most patients with pleuropulmonary disease have other clinical signs of RA ▶ pleuropulmonary involvement is not related to the severity of the arthritis
- The most common histopathological pattern is UIP

RADIOLOGICAL FEATURES

CXR Erosion of the lateral clavicles
- *Pleural effusions or thickening:* these are common ▶ effusions can be unilateral or bilateral and are usually small or moderate in size ▶ the majority resolve spontaneously
  - The fluid demonstrates low pH and glucose levels

HRCT The features are indistinguishable from idiopathic UIP cases (reticular opacities with honeycombing predominantly in the subpleural lung) ▶ it demonstrates a basal predominance (due to the higher blood flow)
- NSIP is also seen but is less prevalent than in other connective tissue diseases (e.g. systemic sclerosis)

Rheumatoid (necrobiotic) pulmonary nodules These are usually asymptomatic ▶ they are uncommonly seen and are usually associated with subcutaneous nodules (and like them they may wax and wane) ▶ they appear as well-circumscribed nodules (± cavitation) that can be single or multiple and which can vary in size (several mm to several cm) ▶ they may occur in association with pulmonary fibrosis and pleural changes ▶ there is an association with pneumothoraces ▶ FDG uptake on PET
- **Caplan's syndrome:** radiologically identical nodules can occur in RA patients exposed to silica (they appear rapidly and in crops) ▶ radiographic features of pneumoconiosis may also be present but are not prominent

PEARLS

- **Other pulmonary abnormalities:** bronchiectasis (up to 30%) ▶ obliterative bronchiolitis (leading to hyperinflation) ▶ methotrexate-induced pneumonitis ▶ cryptogenic-organizing pneumonia (COP)
- **Follicular bronchiolitis:** diffuse peribronchiolar proliferation of hyperplastic lymphoid follicles and alveolar interstitial inflammation ▶ it is usually associated with connective tissue diseases (e.g. RA, Sjögren's and scleroderma) and presents in young adults with an insidious dyspnoea

  HRCT Centrilobular nodules (1–12 mm) associated with peribronchial nodules and patchy areas of ground-glass opacity ▶ it is generally bilateral and diffuse

SJÖGREN'S SYNDROME

DEFINITION

- A chronic autoimmune inflammatory disease

CLINICAL PRESENTATION

- Dry mouth (xerostomia) ▶ dry eyes (keratoconjunctivitis sicca) ▶ arthritis ▶ F>M

RADIOLOGICAL FEATURES

- NSIP is the most common entity ▶ other pathologies include bronchiolitis, lymphoma, amyloidosis, atelectasis and LIP
- Most frequent interstitial pneumonia is SNIP and LIP
- Mild bronchiectasis is common
- Lymphoproliferative disease may occur on a background of LIP

PEARL

- It can occur alone (primary) or in association with other autoimmune diseases (secondary)

Intrathoracic manifestations of rheumatoid disease*
Pleural effusion or thickening
Interstitial fibrosis (most frequently usual interstitial pneumonia type)
Constrictive obliterative bronchiolitis
Bronchiectasis
Organizing pneumonia
Follicular bronchiolitis
Drug-induced lung disease (methotrexate)
Necrobiotic nodules/Caplan's syndrome

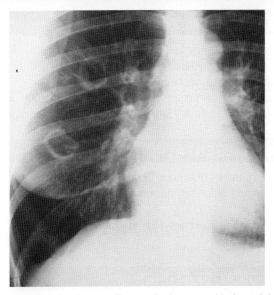

Rheumatoid disease. Two cavitating necrobiotic nodules are visible.†

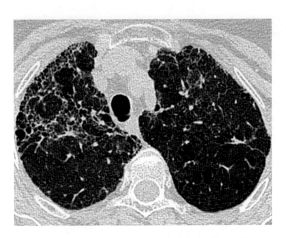

Rheumatoid arthritis with a UIP-type pattern. In this case the HRCT appearances of peripheral reticular abnormality and honeycombing are indistinguishable from that of UIP.*

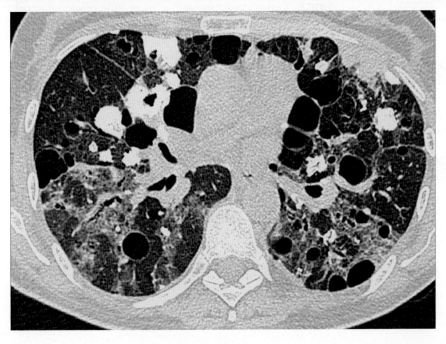

Sjögren's syndrome – LIP and amyloid. There are numerous thin-walled cysts in association with multiple irregular solid nodules, some of which are heavily calcified. Histopathological examination showed marked thickening of the interstitium with an infiltrate of small, mature lymphocytes and plasma cells. Multiple deposits of amyloid were seen throughout the specimen and there was no evidence of malignancy.*

PROGRESSIVE SYSTEMIC SCLEROSIS (SCLERODERMA)

DEFINITION

- A collagen vascular disease characterized by the deposition of excessive extracellular matrix with subsequent vascular occlusion
- It can involve several organs: the skin (scleroderma) ▶ peripheral vasculature ▶ kidneys ▶ oesophagus ▶ lungs

CLINICAL PRESENTATION

- Cutaneous features (Raynaud's phenomenon, skin thickening and tightening) dominate the clinical picture ▶ F>M
- The prognosis is determined by any heart, lung or kidney involvement

RADIOLOGICAL FEATURES

- ILD is common and causes considerable morbidity and mortality (the interstitium and pulmonary vasculature is predominantly affected)
- The interstitium and pulmonary vasculature are the predominant sites affected

- Scleroderma has the highest incidence of fibrosis amongst the connective tissue diseases

HRCT Peripheral reticular opacities, ground-glass attenuation, traction bronchiectasis and occasionally honeycomb destruction ▶ pleural disease is much less commonly seen than in the other connective tissue diseases ▶ enlarged mediastinal lymph nodes (due to reactive hyperplasia) is a frequent finding

- NSIP and OP are increasingly regarded as the prevalent histological patterns ▶ UIP patterns are thought to occur in 5–10%

PEARLS

- Oesophageal involvement (resulting in abnormal motility and a dilated oesophagus with an air-fluid level) may cause reflux and a subsequent aspiration pneumonia which predominantly affects the lung bases
- There is an increased lung cancer prevalence

POLYMYOSITIS/DERMATOMYOSITIS

DEFINITION

- **Polymyositis:** an idiopathic autoimmune inflammatory myopathy resulting in proximal muscle weakness
- **Dermatomyositis:** this is similar to polymyositis except that it is accompanied by a skin rash

CLINICAL PRESENTATION

- Initially a cough, dyspnoea and fever occurs prior to any arthralgia, myalgia or weakness (30% of patients) ▶ a simultaneous presentation can occur in 20% of patients

RADIOLOGICAL FEATURES

- Aspiration pneumonia (due to respiratory muscle weakness and a poor cough reflex) is the most important pulmonary disease – this is due to its high prevalence and the associated morbidity and mortality

- NSIP and OP are the most common histological patterns ▶ the ILD can be acute and aggressive (similar to AIP) with a mortality rate of up to 10%

HRCT Linear opacities (with a lower lung predominance) and irregular interfaces ▶ ground-glass opacification and areas of consolidation (histologically correlating with an organizing pneumonia and which may also be admixed with interstitial fibrosis)

- Parenchymal micro-nodules and honeycombing are less commonly seen

PEARLS

- Pulmonary complications are important determinants of the clinical course
- In some patients the lung disease is responsive to steroids or immunosuppression

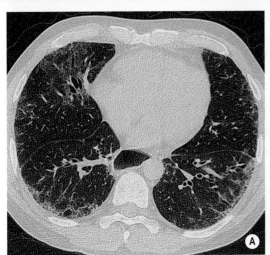
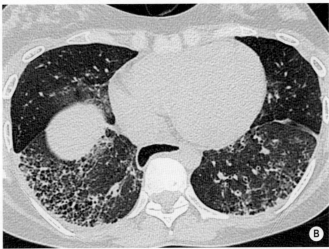

Scleroderma. (A,B) Two patients with scleroderma showing ground-glass opacification in association with traction bronchiectasis and a fine reticular pattern. The pattern of fibrosis is closest to that of non-specific interstitial pneumonia. Note the dilated oesophagus in both examples.*

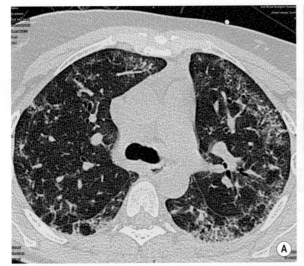
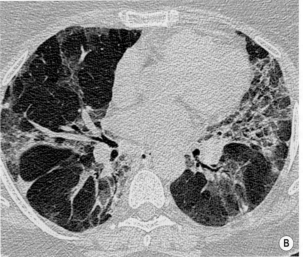

Polymyositis/dermatomyositis. HRCT features include (A) reticular opacities and (B) areas of ground-glass opacification. The appearances of (B) are compatible with organizing pneumonia being incorporated as fibrosis.*

SYSTEMIC LUPUS ERYTHEMATOSUS (SLE)

DEFINITION

- A chronic multisystem disease of unknown origin characterized by auto-antibodies against various cell nuclear antigens ▶ it is associated with widespread inflammatory changes in the connective tissues, vessels and serosal surfaces

CLINICAL PRESENTATION

- Butterfly facial rash ▶ arthralgias ▶ Raynaud's phenomenon ▶ renal involvement ▶ CNS disease
- This is typically a disease of young women

RADIOLOGICAL FEATURES

- Pleuropulmonary disease will occur in >50% of patients – pleuritis is the most common manifestation

Pleural effusions

- These are frequently bilateral and usually of small volume ▶ they are associated with pleuritic pain (unlike RA) which can lead to decreased diaphragmatic movement and lower lobe atelectasis
  - The pleural fluid has a normal glucose level (cf. decreased levels with RA)

Consolidation

- This can result from infection secondary to immunological abnormalities, steroid immunosuppression or respiratory muscle weakness ▶ it can also result from pulmonary oedema (secondary to renal disease or cardiac failure)

Acute lupus pneumonitis

- A rare manifestation characterized by fever, severe hypoxaemia and diffuse pulmonary infiltrates (secondary to a vasculitis and haemorrhage)

  HRCT Patchy consolidation with focal atelectasis seen predominantly within the lung bases

Chronic diffuse ILD

- This is not commonly associated with SLE

  HRCT Irregular linear and band-like opacities (in part due to atelectasis), ground-glass opacification and interlobular septal thickening ▶ honeycombing is extremely rare ▶ any lung volume loss can be prominent

Diffuse alveolar haemorrhage

- A rare but dramatic complication ▶ this is due to vascular thromboses related to the lupus anticoagulant

  HRCT Widespread ground-glass opacification and consolidation

PEARLS

- There is an increased risk of a pulmonary embolus (due to thromboembolic disease secondary to antiphospholipid antibodies)
- It is associated with an increased malignancy risk (particularly lymphoma)
- 'Shrinking lung' syndrome: secondary to diaphragmatic dysfunction, this can also lead to thick linear atelectasis at the lung bases

ANKYLOSING SPONDYLITIS

DEFINITION

- A chronic inflammatory disease affecting mainly the axial skeleton (costovertebral, apophyseal and sacroiliac joints)
- The majority of patients have mild airway and interstitial HRCT abnormalities

RADIOLOGICAL FEATURES

- **Apical fibrosis (1%):** upward retraction of the hila ▶ it is often associated with bullae formation and apical pleural thickening ▶ the changes are usually bilateral (but they may initially be unilateral and indistinguishable from tuberculosis) ▶ mycetomas may form within the upper lobe cavities

- **Dilatation of the ascending aorta** (with aortic insufficiency)

PEARL

- Occasionally pulmonary changes may antedate the spondylitis

Causes of bilateral upper lobe fibrosis*
Tuberculosis (including atypical mycobacterial infections)
Sarcoidosis
Histoplasmosis
Allergic bronchopulmonary aspergillosis
Chronic extrinsic allergic alveolitis
Ankylosing spondylitis
Progressive massive fibrosis (distinctive mass-like opacities)

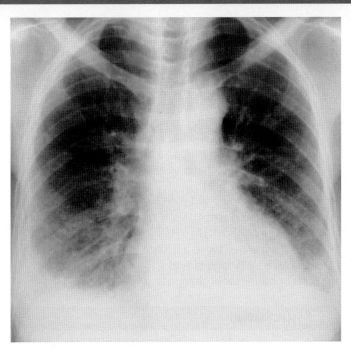

SLE. Bilateral pleural effusions.[†]

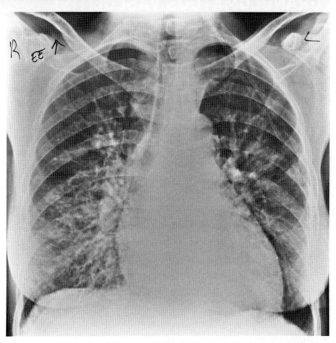

Acute lupus pneumonitis. Patchy consolidation is present in the right lung. Biopsy demonstrated vasculitis and haemorrhage.[‡]

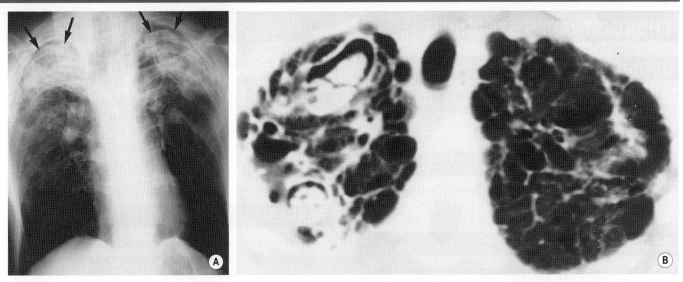

Ankylosing spondylitis. (A) PA CXR demonstrating bilateral apical mycetoma (arrows). (B) CT of ankylosing spondylitis in a different patient with mycetoma formation.[†]

WEGENER'S GRANULOMATOSIS (ANCA-ASSOCIATED GRANULOMATOUS VASCULITIS)

DEFINITION

- A multisystem disease of unknown aetiology characterized by a necrotizing granulomatous inflammation affecting the upper and lower respiratory tracts (the lungs are involved in 90%) ▶ it also leads to a focal necrotizing glomerulonephritis and a small vessel vasculitis affecting the arteries, capillaries and veins
  - *Limited (non-renal) Wegener's granulomatosis:* disease limited to the respiratory tract

CLINICAL PRESENTATION

- It can affect any age (M = F)
- *Nose, paranasal sinuses and upper respiratory tract:* nasal obstruction ▶ purulent nasal discharge ▶ sinusitis ▶ a saddle nose deformity (due to perforation of the nasal septum)
- *Chest:* cough ▶ haemoptysis ▶ malaise ▶ fever
- *Kidneys:* microscopic haematuria and proteinuria

RADIOLOGICAL FEATURES

CXR/HRCT

- *Pulmonary nodules:* these can measure a few mm to several cm in size ▶ a feeding vessel leading to the nodule may be identified ▶ can have a halo of ground-glass opacification (haemorrhage) ▶ there may be air bronchograms present within a nodule ▶ linear bands and pleural tags may be seen in relation to a nodule and there may be residual parenchymal scaring post resolution
  - There is no zonal predilection
  - Nodules are bilateral in 75%

- *Cavitation:* this usually occurs within larger nodules (≥ 2 cm) ▶ a cavitated nodule may have thin or thick walls
- *Consolidation:* this can take various forms: peripheral wedge-shaped lesions abutting the pleura (mimicking infarcts) ▶ peribronchial consolidation ▶ focal consolidation ± cavitation ▶ 'reverse halo' pattern
- *Diffuse bilateral ground-glass opacification:* this is due to pulmonary haemorrhage or necrotizing granulomatous inflammation
- *Mild bronchiectasis:* 40%
- *Fibrosing lung disease:* this is rarely seen and closest to a UIP-type pattern
- *Pleural effusions:* these are seen in 10% of patients ▶ they can be uni- or bilateral
- *Hilar or mediastinal adenopathy*

PEARLS

- Wegener's granulomatosis is due to a type IV mediated immune mechanism
- The upper and lower respiratory tracts are commonly involved (and most commonly causing a subglottic stenosis) ▶ bronchial narrowing can result in segmental or lobar atelectasis
- In adults consolidation and ground-glass opacification is less commonly seen than pulmonary nodules (the converse is seen in children)
- The disease is invariably fatal without treatment (usually from the renal disease) ▶ there is an improved outlook with cyclophosphamide and corticosteroids
- **The classic Wegener's triad:** sinusitis together with lung and renal parenchymal disease

CHURG–STRAUSS SYNDROME

DEFINITION

- An antineutrophil cytoplasmic antibody (ANCA) associated systemic necrotizing vasculitis affecting the small arteries and veins

CLINICAL PRESENTATION

- It is clinically characterized by the presence of asthma, fever and a blood eosinophilia

RADIOLOGICAL FEATURES

- The radiological appearances largely reflect the eosinophilic infiltrate and are largely non-specific

▶ up to 25% of patients have no imaging abnormalities

HRCT
Ground-glass opacification ▶ areas of airspace consolidation ▶ centrilobular nodules (some of which may cavitate) ▶ airway abnormalities attributable to the presence of asthma ▶ interlobular septal thickening (due to interstitial pulmonary oedema secondary to cardiac involvement)

PEARLS

- Predominantly small vessel involvement is rare – therefore diffuse pulmonary haemorrhage is uncommon

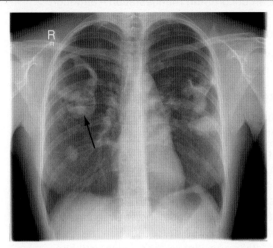

Wegener's granulomatosis. PA CXR demonstrating multiple large pulmonary nodules, the larger ones having cavitated (with residual thick walls). A mid-sized nodule demonstrates an air-fluid level (arrow).

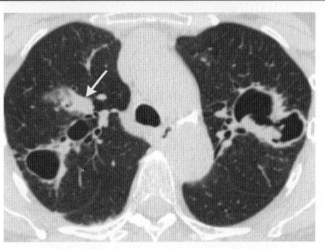

CT (lung windows) demonstrating Wegener's granulomatosis. Multiple irregularly thick-walled cavities are seen within both lungs. A smaller lesion (arrow) has yet to reach a sufficient size to undergo cavitation.

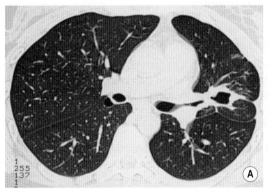

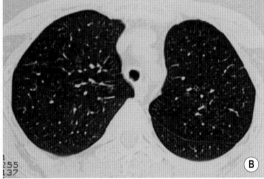

Wegener's granulomatosis. Images through the (A) mid and (B) upper zones in a patient with Wegener's granulomatosis. Thick-walled cavitating mass in the left upper lobe (A). Note also the focal narrowing of the mid intrathoracic trachea (B) reflecting focal involvement by Wegener's granulomatosis.*

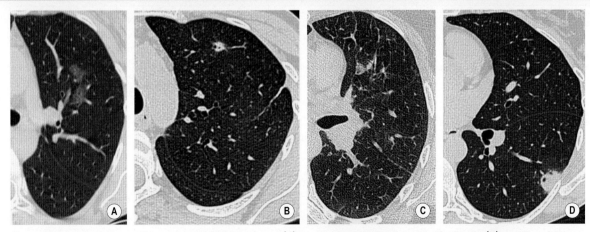

Churg–Strauss syndrome. Spectrum of HRCT features: (A) areas of ground-glass opacification ▶ (B) small cavitating nodules ▶ (C) thickened interlobular septa ▶ and (D) an area of airspace opacification, likely to be a peripheral infarct.*

DRUG-INDUCED LUNG DISEASE

DEFINITION

- Drug-induced lung disease can be the result of the pharmacological action of the drug in normal or excessive dosage, or caused by an allergic or idiosyncratic reaction
- The radiological manifestations are heterogeneous and non-specific – there is no specific radiological pattern of parenchymal change
    - In the early stages of the disease the CXR may be normal

RADIOLOGICAL FEATURES

Diffuse alveolar damage (DAD)

- This usually develops a few weeks or months after initiating therapy ▶ the onset is heralded by progressive dyspnoea
- The radiological features are similar to those seen in ARDS ▶ the diagnosis requires exclusion of other potential aetiologies (most importantly an opportunistic infection)

CXR Bilateral patchy and homogeneous airspace consolidation involving mainly the middle and lower lungs

HRCT Extensive bilateral ground-glass opacities with dependent areas of airspace consolidation

Hypersensitivity pneumonitis

- The radiological features are similar to those seen with a hypersensitivity pneumonitis secondary to organic dust inhalation

- This is an uncommon manifestation – although methotrexate is the most common offender it usually demonstrates a NSIP pattern

HRCT Bilateral ground-glass opacities ± small poorly defined centrilobular nodular opacities

Chronic interstitial pneumonia

- The radiological features are similar to those seen with an idiopathic NSIP, or less commonly UIP

HRCT Fibrosis and traction bronchiectasis with disease progression – the fibrosis is patchy in distribution and predominantly peribronchovascular (a pattern most commonly seen with nitrofurantoin)

- *The most common manifestation of amiodarone-induced lung disease:* NSIP is the most common manifestation ▶ ground-glass opacities in association with fine intralobular reticulation (which is predominantly peripheral) ▶ there may be occasional foci of consolidation representing an organizing pneumonia

Organizing pneumonia

CXR Patchy bilateral areas of consolidation, masses or nodules (which can be asymmetric or symmetric)

HRCT Patchy asymmetrical ground-glass opacities and areas of consolidation that often demonstrate a peripheral or peribronchiolar distribution

Eosinophilic pneumonia

CXR/HRCT Bilateral airspace consolidation (affecting mainly the peripheral and upper zones)

- A peripheral blood eosinophilia is seen in 40%

Histological pattern of drug-induced lung disease				
Diffuse alveolar damage	**Diffuse alveolar haemorrhage**	**Interstitial pneumonia**	**Organizing pneumonia**	**Eosinophilic pneumonia**
Amiodarone	Anticoagulants Amphotericin B	Amiodarone	Amiodarone Bleomycin Cyclophosphamide	Nitrofurantion Nonsteroidal anti-inflammatory drugs Paraaminosalicilyc acid Penicillamine Sulphasalazine
Bleomycin Cyclophosphamide Methotrexate	Cyclophosphamide Cytosine arabinoside (ara-c)	Carmustine Chlorambucil Cyclophosphamide Methotrexate Nitrofurantoin	Gold salts Penicillamine Methotrexate	
	Penicillamine			
Mytomycin Mephalan Gold salts			Nitrofurantion Sulphasalazine	

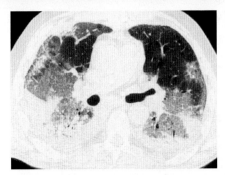
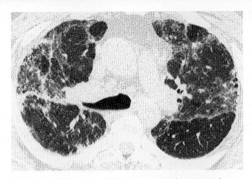
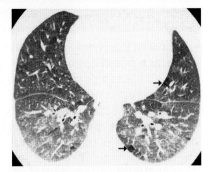

Diffuse alveolar damage secondary to amiodarone. There is extensive bilateral ground-glass opacification and airspace consolidation. Note also the bilateral pleural effusions.

Non-specific interstitial pneumonia secondary to bleomycin. The dominant abnormality is ground-glass opacification in association with a fine reticular pattern. The pattern of fibrosis most closely resembles non-specific interstitial pneumonia.

Hypersensitivity pneumonitis secondary to sertraline. HRCT shows extensive bilateral ground-glass opacification and lobular areas of air trapping (arrows).

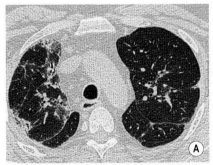
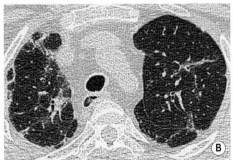
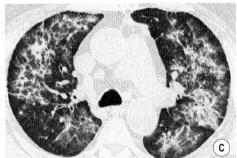

Organizing pneumonia secondary to (A,B) nitrofurantoin and (C) amiodarone. The HRCT features of ground-glass opacification and consolidation (A,C) and a perilobular pattern (B) are in keeping with organizing pneumonia. The areas of consolidation in (C) are both peribronchial and perilobular in distribution.

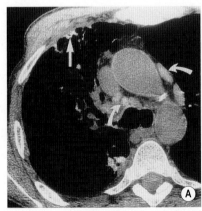
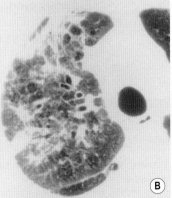
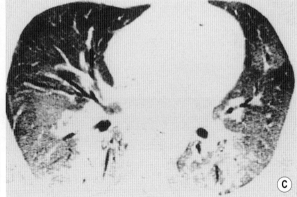

Amiodarone toxicity. (A) There are enlarged mediastinal lymph nodes (curved arrows). Note the area of dense peripheral consolidation due to amiodarone deposition (arrow). (B) On lung windows, coarse fibrosis is demonstrated. (C) ARDS reaction to methotrexate administration. Note the anterior posterior gradient of increase in lung density.[†]

SILICOSIS/COAL WORKERS' PNEUMOCONIOSIS

DEFINITION

- **Silicosis:** this is due to the inhalation of silicon dioxide (silica) ▶ hazardous occupations include those that disturb the earth's crust or expose the worker to the use or processing of silica-containing rock or sand (e.g. mining, stone cutting and foundry work)
- **Coal workers' pneumoconiosis (CWP):** this occurs as a consequence of coal dust inhalation

CLINICAL PRESENTATION

- Both coal mine dust and silica predispose workers to chronic bronchitis, simple pneumoconiosis and emphysema ▶ there is also an increased risk of lung cancer and tuberculosis
- It is rarely seen in patients < 50 years old ▶ M>F (as a result of the occupational risk)

RADIOLOGICAL FEATURES

Early changes

- The earliest changes of silicosis and CWP are nearly identical:
    - The lung disease is usually less severe in CWP (the nodules in CWP are often smaller than those seen in simple silicosis)

CT Small (1–3 mm) sharply defined, round nodules seen within the posterior aspects of the upper $\frac{2}{3}$ ▶ of the lung ▶ the nodules may be centrilobular or subpleural in location (subpleural nodules may become confluent forming a 'pseudo-plaque') ▶ with advanced disease the nodules increase in size and number to involve all the lung zones and are sometimes calcified ▶ hilar and mediastinal lymphadenopathy may demonstrate eggshell calcification in 5%

Progressive massive fibrosis (PMF)

- This is much more commonly seen in silicosis than in CWP and is due to the coalescence of larger nodules, leading to mass-like opacities:
    - These are typically seen in the posterior upper lobes with associated upper lobe contraction, hilar elevation and architectural distortion
    - They migrate towards the hila over time (leaving a peripheral rim of cicatricial emphysema)
    - Their outer margins often parallel the contour of the chest wall
    - Large lesions (>5 cm) often demonstrate necrosis but frank cavitation is infrequent (when this is present one should consider tuberculosis)
    - Unilateral disease may be distinguished from a lung cancer by the presence of lobar volume loss and peripheral emphysema

Acute silicoproteinosis

- This develops within weeks after exposure to high concentrations of crystalline silica ▶ the dominant feature is an alveolar proteinaceous exudate (similar to that seen in alveolar proteinosis)

CXR Widespread alveolar opacities with an upper and mid zone predominance ▶ air bronchograms may be seen initially ▶ hilar and mediastinal adenopathy can also occur

PEARLS

- Silica workers have an increased risk of IPF and an association with connective tissue disease is also seen (particularly silicosis and rheumatoid arthritis)
    - **Caplan's syndrome:** silicosis + rheumatoid arthritis + necrobiotic nodules
    - **Erasmus syndrome:** silicosis + systemic sclerosis
- With silicosis, fibrosis may continue after the exposure has ceased (unlike with CWP)

Patterns of disease caused by silica exposure*	
Clinical pattern	**Duration and level of exposure**
Acute silicoproteinosis	Occurs in response to a massive inhalation of silica (e.g. in sandblasting) ▶ usually occurs within a few weeks to 4–5 years after exposure
Accelerated silicosis	Develops less than 10 years after the first inhalation of high concentrations of silica. Its more rapid development than in simple silicosis indicates that the worker is at greater risk for the development of progressive massive fibrosis
Chronic simple silicosis	The most common manifestation, usually developing after 10–50 years of low level silica exposure

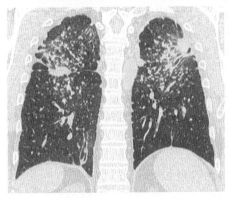

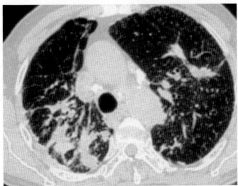

Progressive massive fibrosis in coalworker's pneumoconiosis. Mass-like opacities are seen bilaterally in the upper lobes in association with multiple small nodules and calcified mediastinal lymphadenopathy.*

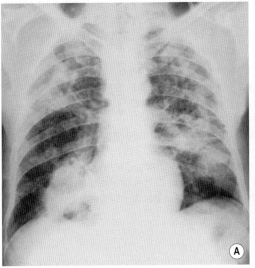

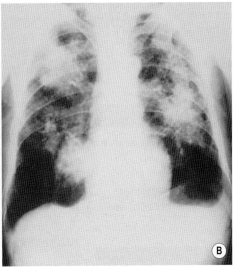

Progressive massive fibrosis. (A) nodular opacities are present throughout both lungs, and several areas of more confluent shadowing are present. (B) 4 years later, the lower zone masses have migrated centrally, leaving peripheral areas of emphysema. The upper lope opacities have enlarged.†

Silicosis. There is bilateral hilar adenopathy and many of the nodes are calcified, some of them demonstrating 'eggshell' calcification (arrowheads).†

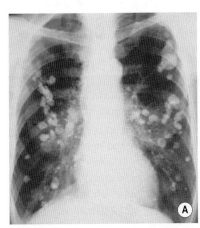

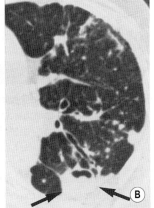

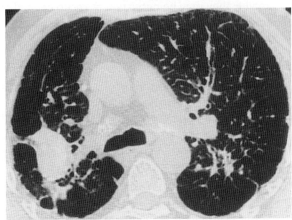

Caplan's syndrome. (A) Coal worker with rheumatoid arthritis. Multiple rounded opacities are present (some are calcified). (B) There is a left-sided cavitating pulmonary nodule (arrows) on a background of pneumoconiosis.†

Early complicated silicosis. CT demonstrating coalescence of pulmonary nodules into pulmonary masses.†

ASBESTOS-RELATED DISEASE

DEFINITION

- Asbestos is the generic term for a group of fibrous silicates that demonstrate heat resistance ▶ lung fibrosis is the result of physical and chemical irritation together with an autoimmune mechanism to the inhaled fibres ▶ the fibres can penetrate the pleura and will gravitate towards the lower lobes
- The fibres are classified into 2 groups: the serpentine (twisted and flexible) and amphibole (stiff and brittle) groups
  - The only commercially used serpentine asbestos is chrysolite ▶ this accounts for > 90% of the asbestos used in the USA
  - The amphibole group includes crocidolite – this group has a much greater pathogenicity (especially for inducing mesothelioma)
- High-risk occupations: construction ▶ pipe fitting ▶ asbestos mining

CLINICAL PRESENTATION

- Gradual onset of dyspnoea or a non-productive cough ▶ M>F (occupational exposure)
- Clinical manifestations typically do not appear until ≥ 20 years after the initial exposure (although asbestos-related pleural effusions may be present as early as 5 years post exposure)

RADIOLOGICAL FEATURES

Benign pleural effusions

- These are typically haemorrhagic exudates ▶ as they do not contain asbestos bodies their diagnosis is reliant on the exclusion of other causes ▶ the effusions are often small ▶ they may be persistent or recurrent and may be simultaneously or sequentially bilateral ▶ diffuse pleural thickening is the usual consequence

Pleural plaques

- These are the most common manifestation of asbestos exposure ▶ they are discrete foci of pearly white fibrous tissue (2–5 mm thick) ▶ calcification is seen in 10–15% ▶ pleural plaques are not associated with significantly impaired lung function as they are isolated discrete lesions

`CXR/HRCT` They almost exclusively involve the parietal pleura

- *Classic distribution:* along the posterolateral chest wall between the 7th and 10th ribs, the lateral chest wall between the 6th and 9th ribs, on the dome of the diaphragm and on the mediastinal pleura
- *'Holly leaf' appearance:* they may produce bizarre shapes on CXR

Diffuse pleural thickening

- The frequency increases with time from the 1st exposure and is dose related ▶ diffuse pleural thickening rarely calcifies ▶ it is not specific for asbestos exposure
  - It is caused by a more intense inflammatory response leading to extension of the interstitial fibrosis to the visceral pleura: the thickened and fibrotic visceral pleura fuses with the parietal pleura and therefore impairs lung function

Round atelectasis (folded lung)

- There is pleural fibrosis overlying the abnormal parenchyma as well as invaginations of fibrotic pleura into the region of collapse – subsequent retraction of the collagen within the pleura as it matures is the cause of the collapse (areas of atelectasis are therefore always adjacent to the visceral pleura)

`CXR/HRCT` Parenchymal collapse occurs in the peripheral lower lobes ▶ this 'mass' is never completely surrounded by lung and demonstrates a relatively stable appearance over time

- The collapsed lung has a rounded or oval shape (wedge and irregularly shaped masses can also occur) ▶ there is also volume loss of the affected lobe
- *'Comet tail' sign:* crowding of the bronchi and blood vessels extending from the border of the mass to the hilum

Asbestosis

- Defined as pulmonary parenchymal fibrosis secondary to asbestos inhalation (with a ≥20-year lag time)

`HRCT` Subpleural curvilinear lines and dots, pleurally based nodular irregularities, parenchymal bands, and septal lines ▶ the fine reticulation eventually progresses to a coarse linear pattern with honeycombing ▶ these changes are most severe within the subpleural regions of the lower lobes (as the fibres gravitate to the lower lobes) ▶ there is no associated hilar adenopathy

PEARLS

- Distinguishing asbestosis from idiopathic pulmonary fibrosis is desirable (as asbestosis is associated with a much slower rate of progression and hence a better prognosis) ▶ HRCT discrimination between the two is usually impossible and therefore a diagnosis of asbestosis is largely inferential (based on the radiology, an appropriate exposure history and exclusion of other plausible conditions)
- Malignant disease is an important complication of asbestos exposure: pleural and peritoneal mesothelioma ▶ tumours affecting the lung, oesophagus, pharynx and GI tract

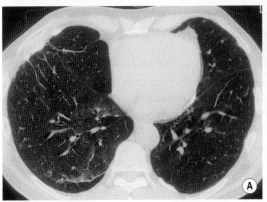
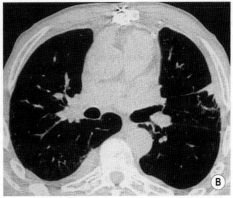

(A) Asbestos exposure has resulted in calcified pleural plaques. There are coarse parenchymal bands extending into the parenchyma from these plaques that are causing some distortion of the lung parenchyma. (B) In a different patient the result of asbestos exposure is the development of diffuse pleural thickening which predated the sternotomy.[†]

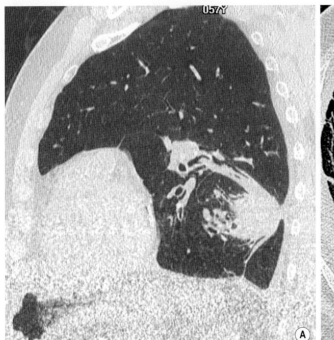
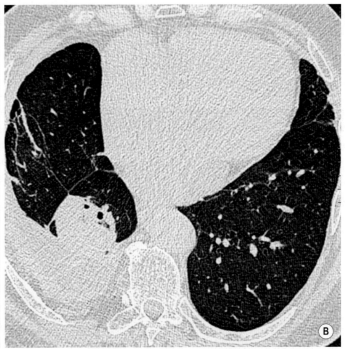

Atelectasis. Two examples of rounded atelectasis in association with (A)** pleural thickening and (B)* a pleural effusion. In both cases, there is evidence of lobar volume loss as seen by displacement of fissures. The most common location of rounded atelectasis is in the lower lobes.

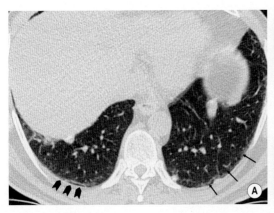
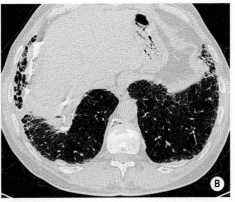

Asbestosis. (A) HRCT features of early asbestosis include subpleural lines (arrowheads) and fine reticulation (arrows). These subtle abnormalities persisted on prone sections. (B) In more advanced disease, a coarse reticular pattern with honeycombing, often indistinguishable from usual interstitial pneumonia on HRCT, is seen. Note the calcified pleural plaques in both examples.*

HYPERSENSITIVITY PNEUMONITIS (EXTRINSIC ALLERGIC ALVEOLITIS)

DEFINITION

- An immunologically mediated lung disease with an inflammatory reaction to specific organic dust antigens ▶ inhaled particles (< 10 μm) reach the alveoli causing damage by both type III (immune complex response) and type IV (cell-mediated) mechanisms
- *Causes:* avian proteins from exposure to pigeons/parakeets (bird fancier's disease) ▶ *Micropolyspora faeni* in mouldy hay (farmer's lung) ▶ *Thermoactinomyces vulgaris* in mouldy grain (malt worker's lung) ▶ various antigens (e.g. *T. vulgaris, M. faeni, Acanthamoeba*) in heated water reservoirs (humidifier or air conditioner lung)

CLINICAL PRESENTATION

- Fever, chills, dyspnoea and a cough – these characteristically occur approximately 6 hours after exposure ▶ an eosinophilia is not present

RADIOLOGICAL FEATURES

Acute disease

- An episode of illness with an acute onset with symptoms lasting < 1 month

`CXR/HRCT` This can be normal during an acute episode ▶ typical findings include diffuse ground-glass opacification and/or alveolar consolidation especially in the lower lung zones

- This reflects filling of the alveoli with polymorphonuclear leucocytes, eosinophils, lymphocytes and large mononuclear cells
- Consolidation may mimic pulmonary oedema ▶ this clears within hours to days
- The CXR may return to normal between attacks

Subacute disease

- Disease developing over weeks to 4 months and including episodic flare ups

`CXR` Fine nodular or reticulonodular pattern

`HRCT` Poorly defined centrilobular nodules (< 5 mm) with a mid to lower zone predominance ▶ ground-glass opacification can be seen in the acute phase but may also be seen in subacute or chronic hypersensitivity pneumonitis ▶ mosaic attenuation is common together with lobular areas of decreased vascularity with air trapping (representing coexisting bronchiolitis) ▶ small volume lymphadenopathy (< 2 cm) can be present ▶ thin-walled cysts are occasionally seen with subacute disease

- Nodular pattern corresponds to alveolitis, interstitial infiltration, small granulomas and bronchiolitis ▶ changes are most severe in peribronchiolar distribution

Chronic disease

- Indicates irreversible lung damage in general (or fibrosis specifically) ▶ it takes between 4 months and several years to develop

`CXR` Mid and upper lung fibrosis

`HRCT` Mid and upper lung fibrosis sparing the costophrenic angles (with volume loss, intralobular and interlobular interstitial thickening, traction bronchiectasis and honeycomb destruction) ▶ pulmonary arterial hypertension (enlarged pulmonary arteries)

- *Complications:* emphysema (farmer's lung) ▶ lung fibrosis (bird fancier's disease)

PEARLS

- Cigarette smoking has a suppressive effect
- *Treatment:*
  - In acute phase, identification and avoidance of antigen
  - Chronic disease: trial of corticosteroids
- *Differential:* RB–ILD: the distinction is usually made with a knowledge of a smoking history ▶ NSIP/UIP: an upper or mid zone predominance, ground-glass opacification and air trapping favours a hypersensitivity pneumonitis

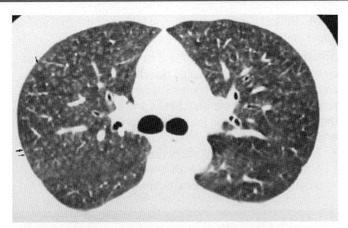

Hypersensitivity pneumonitis. Fish-plant worker. HRCT shows multiple ill-defined, low-attenuation nodules. In the subpleural zones the nodules occupy a centrilobular location 2 to 3 mm deep to the pleural surface (arrows).

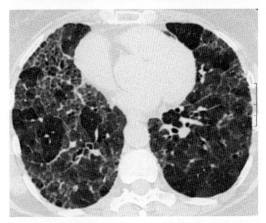

Chronic hypersensitivity pneumonitis. The reticular pattern with distortion of the lung parenchyma indicates established fibrosis in this case of chronic hypersensitivity pneumonitis.**

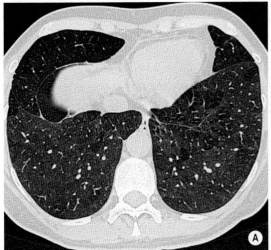

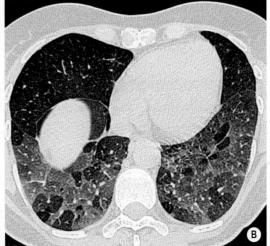

Hypersensitivity pneumonitis. (A) Inspiratory image shows patchy density differences, reflecting both the interstitial infiltrate of subacute hypersensitivity pneumonitis and coexisting small airways disease. (B) End-expiratory image enhances the density differences, revealing several secondary pulmonary lobules of decreased attenuation.**

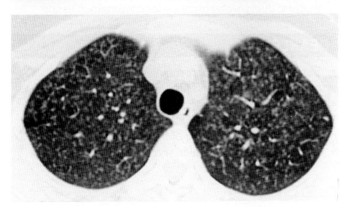

Subacute extrinsic allergic alveolitis. HRCT shows numerous poorly defined, relatively low attenuation nodules.*

Hypersensitivity pneumonitis		
Disease	**Antigen source**	**Antigen**
Bird fancier's disease	Avian excreta (e.g. pigeons, parrots)	Avian serum proteins (excreta/ feathers)
Farmer's lung	Mouldy hay	*Micropolyspora faeni*
Humidifier/air conditioner lung	Warm water/ contaminated air conditioners	*T. vilgaris, M. faeni,* acanthamoeba
Malt worker's lung	Mouldy malt	*Aspergillus* species
Furrier's lung	Animal fur	Animal fur proteins
Machine worker's lung	Metal-cutting fluid	*Mycobacterium* species, Gram-negative bacilli

LANGERHANS CELL HISTIOCYTOSIS

DEFINITION

- Formerly pulmonary histiocytosis X or eosinophilic granuloma of the lung.
- A granulomatous disorder characterized by the presence of large histiocytes (Langerhans cells) which cause destruction of the distal airways ▶ it is possibly an allergic reaction to inhaled cigarette smoke

CLINICAL PRESENTATION

- Dyspnoea ▶ cough ▶ constitutional symptoms ▶ spontaneous pneumothorax
- It is often asymptomatic during the early stages (4F:1M)

RADIOLOGICAL FEATURES

- Widespread bilateral and symmetrical pulmonary involvement ▶ cysts are more common than nodules

CXR Reticulonodular shadowing (affecting the mid and upper zones) ▶ normal or increased lung volumes

HRCT Nodules (a few mm to 2 cm) that are surrounded by normal lung ▶ the nodules can cavitate and demonstrate bizarre irregular shapes ▶ there is typical sparing of the extreme lung bases and anterior tips of the middle and lingular lobes (this is preserved even in end-stage disease)

- *There is a predictable sequence of nodule progression:* cavitation ▶ thin-walled cystic lesions ▶ emphysematous and fibro-bullous destruction

PEARLS

- **Hand–Schüller–Christian disease:** the chronic disseminated form
- **Letterer–Siwe disease:** the acute disseminated form

LYMPHANGIOLEIOMYOMATOSIS (LAM)

DEFINITION

- Non-neoplastic proliferation of atypical pulmonary interstitial smooth muscle cells of the bronchioles (wall thickening), pulmonary vessels (pulmonary hypertension and haemoptysis) and lymphatics (chylous effusions)
- There is ultimately cystic destruction of the lung parenchyma

CLINICAL PRESENTATION

- Pneumothorax ▶ chylothorax ▶ hemoptysis ▶ slowly progressive dyspnoea
- It presents between 20–40 years ▶ it is seen almost exclusively in women (particularly of child-bearing age), possibly due to oestrogen involvement

RADIOLOGICAL FEATURES

CXR/CT Generalized symmetrical reticular or reticulonodular opacities ▶ normal or increased lung volumes ▶ randomly distributed and numerous large regularly shaped thin-walled cysts with no zonal predilection (these eventually replace the entire lung) ▶ occasional interlobular septal thickening (pleuropulmonary lymphatic obstruction) or patchy ground-glass attenuation (pulmonary haemorrhage) ▶ pneumothoraces are seen in 50%

- *Chylous pleural effusions* (10–40%): these result from thoracic duct involvement by leiomyomatous tissue

PEARLS

- Similar pulmonary abnormalities are seen in 1% of tuberous sclerosis patients
- *Imaging features distinguishing LAM from LCH:* with LAM there is a more diffuse distribution of any cysts (typically with no sparing of the lung bases), and the cysts have a more regular shape

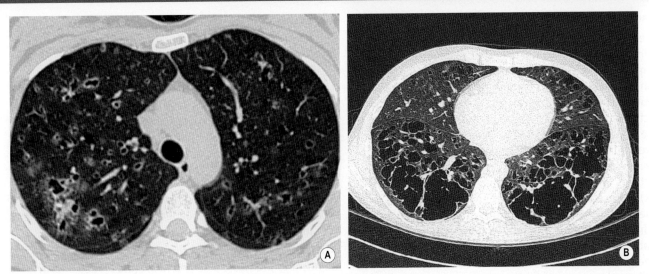

Langerhans cell histiocytosis. (A) The characteristic combination of thin-walled cysts and poorly defined nodules, some of which are just beginning to cavitate.* (B) Image from a patient with more advanced disease. There are numerous irregularly shaped cysts bilaterally.

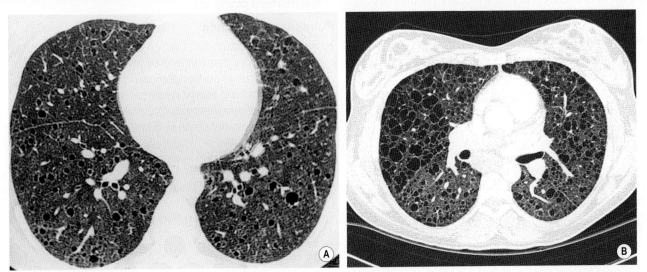

Lymphangioleiomyomatosis. (A) There is a profusion of thin-walled cystic airspaces scattered evenly throughout the lungs. The cysts are relatively uniform in size.* (B) A more advanced case of LAM.

1.8 CHEST TRAUMA

CHEST WALL AND LUNG TRAUMA

Rib fractures

- More than 50% of acute fractures are missed on the initial CXR ▶ additional lateral or oblique views are inappropriate in an acute trauma patient – the main priority is to detect complications such as a pneumothorax, haemothorax or a pulmonary contusion
- Fractures of the 1st to 3rd ribs imply a severe traumatic force and may be associated with vascular, brachial plexus, spinal or tracheobronchial injuries ▶ scapular injuries serve as a similar marker
- Fractures of the 10th to 12th ribs (often better seen on an AXR) are associated with injuries to the liver, spleen or kidneys ▶ further imaging of these organs is mandatory
- Rib fractures are uncommon in children due to their greater inherent elasticity (if present they are usually of the greenstick variety) ▶ there can therefore be significant intrathoracic injury without an associated rib fracture
  - Multiple fractures (particularly of the posterior ribs) should raise the possibility of non-accidental injury
- *Flail segment*: double fractures of ≥3 adjacent ribs (or adjacent combined rib, sternal and costochondral fractures) resulting in a segment of chest wall moving paradoxically during the respiratory cycle
  - This leads to impaired ventilation and atelectasis and there is usually a severe associated pulmonary contusion (contributing to the high mortality)

Sternoclavicular joint dislocation

- The less common posterior dislocation of the clavicle is potentially dangerous – there is potential for compression and injury of the trachea and the brachiocephalic vessels
- This injury is best appreciated on CT

Sternal fractures

- Mortality is high (25%) owing to the associated injuries (cardiac contusion, pulmonary contusion, haemothorax) ▶ diagnosis is made on a lateral CXR or CT

Fractures of the thoracic spine

- This typically occurs at the T9–T11 region (resulting from a hyperflexion ± an axial loading injury) ▶ around ⅓ will have associated spinal cord injuries with a neurological deficit

  CT   This is the imaging modality of choice (fractures can easily be initially missed when overshadowed by other injuries)

Pneumothorax

- This is commonly seen in major trauma victims (20–30%) ▶ it can result from a pulmonary laceration from a fractured rib fragment or due to a sudden rise in intra-alveolar pressure and rupture into the pleural space ▶ detection is important as a small pneumothorax

can rapidly increase in size with positive-pressure ventilation
- *Tension pneumothorax*: a 'flutter valve' allowing unidirectional air into the pleural space ▶ resultant mediastinal shift can lead to cardiovascular compromise

  CXR   The visceral pleura is visualized as a sharp thin line with absent lung markings peripherally

  CT   This is much more sensitive than a CXR

Pulmonary contusion

- Shock waves can lead to microvessel rupture with intra-alveolar and interstitial haemorrhage, as well as alveolar and interstitial oedema ▶ 'contre-coup' injuries can be seen

  CXR/CT   Non-segmental consolidation typically seen adjacent to the ribs, spine and heart (the kinetic energy tends to be absorbed by the lung at any tissue interfaces)
- Opacities appear within 6 h of impact and typically clear within 3–10 days (shadowing increasing over the days following admission is unlikely to be due to a simple contusion but may be due to infection, aspiration, fat embolism or ARDS)
- *Subpleural sparing*: there may be an outer 1–2 mm rim of uniformly non-opacified subpleural lung (this is because blood is forced out of the subpleural tissues at the moment of impact)

Pulmonary laceration

- Severe blunt trauma or sudden deceleration can induce shearing forces that can lead to parenchymal disruption (also can occur at aortic isthmus/right main bronchus)
- The inherent lung elastic recoil can leave a space that can fill with blood (haematoma) or air (pneumatocele) ▶ these are usually small (2–5 cm) and typically resolve over a few months

Lung herniation

- A rare complication of blunt chest trauma ▶ the lung herniates through a defect caused by either rib fractures or shoulder girdle dislocation ▶ most are treated conservatively

Lung torsion

- This is extremely rare and tends to occur in patients with a lobectomy

  CXR   Initially this shows an abnormal pulmonary vessel configuration – if the lung infarcts then complete opacification of the hemithorax will occur

Fat embolism

- Trauma can result in lipid emboli from the bone marrow entering the lungs (the CNS is also commonly affected)

  CXR/CT   Initially appears normal ▶ there is delayed development of poorly defined opacities at 48 h (which clears approximately 1 week later)

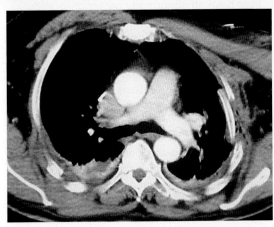

Flail chest. CT image of a left-sided flail chest with a segment of the chest wall pushed inwards. This is known as a 'stove-in-chest'.*

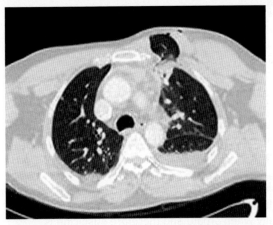

Lung herniation. CT image following blunt trauma to the left side of the chest demonstrates an anterior lung herniation.**

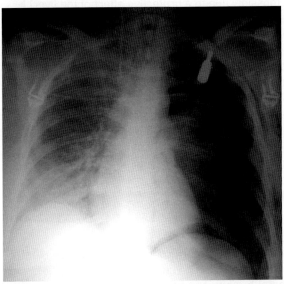

Left-sided pneumothorax seen on a supine chest radiograph demonstrating the deep sulcus sign and an unusually sharp left heart border.*

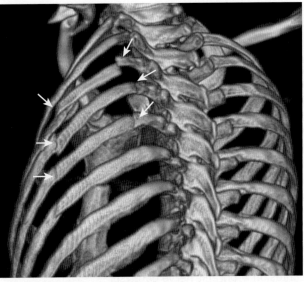

Flail segment. 3D CT reformat demonstrating double fractures of 3 posterior ribs (arrows).‡

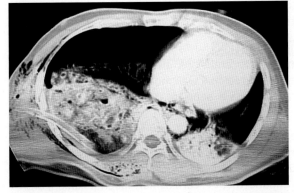

Pneumothorax. CT image demonstrating a post-traumatic pneumothorax. Despite the presence of an intercostal drain, a tension pneumothorax was developing as the drain was blocked with congealed blood. The right-sided pneumothorax is situated anteriorly and the mediastinum is displaced to the left due to the tension.*

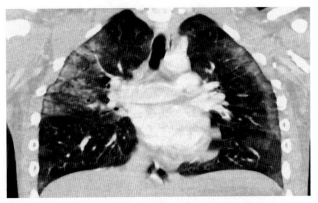

Pulmonary contusion. CT image in the coronal reformatted image illustrating bilateral post-traumatic pulmonary contusions. Note the subpleural sparing.*

TRAUMA TO THE DIAPHRAGM

Definition

- *Penetrating diaphragmatic injuries:* these are usually small (≤ 2 cm) ▶ imaging plays little part in their diagnosis
- *Major blunt thoraco-abdominal trauma:* the sudden rise in intra-abdominal pressure leads to a diaphragmatic rupture in 0.8–5% ▶ tears are usually ≥10 cm, radially orientated and commonly at the posterolateral musculotendinous junction (the weakest part of the diaphragm)

Clinical presentation

- 70% of diaphragmatic tears are missed initially (especially when small) and therefore suspicion is needed in all cases of trauma to the lower chest ▶ rupture is often diagnosed during surgery and prompt surgical repair is essential to reduce the risk of subsequent complications
- Patients undergoing positive-pressure mechanical ventilation may have a delayed presentation

Radiological features

CXR This is relatively insensitive (and normal in 25%)
- **Right-sided tear:** apparent elevation of the hemidiaphragm ▶ loss of the diaphragmatic contour ▶ leftward mediastinal displacement
- **Left-sided tear:** apparent diaphragmatic elevation ▶ hollow viscera seen within the hemithorax ▶ an obscured or discontinuous diaphragmatic contour ▶ rightward mediastinal displacement
  - A coiled nasogastric tube within the left hemithorax is characteristic
- *The following may mask or mimic a diaphragmatic tear:* associated atelectasis ▶ pleural effusions ▶ a lung contusion ▶ phrenic nerve paralysis
- *Delayed imaging (up to 6 h later) may be helpful:* especially in patients undergoing positive-pressure mechanical ventilation where any herniation may be delayed (barium studies may be helpful in the chronic stage)

Barium studies These are not permissible during an acute injury ▶ they may demonstrate intrathoracic bowel or an extrinsic narrowing where the stomach or bowel passes through the defect

US This has not gained widespread acceptance (as it is operator-dependent and there are practical difficulties)

CT The preferred modality (coronal and sagittal reformatted images should increase accuracy) ▶ the key findings:
- Discontinuity of the diaphragm
- Herniation of abdominal organs into the chest
- Thickening of the diaphragmatic crus
- *'Collar' sign:* constriction of the stomach or colon as it passes through a tear

- *'Dependent viscera' sign:* when organs such as the spleen or liver have an abnormally posterior location and are in contact with the posterior ribs (due to a lack of the normal diaphragmatic support)

MRI This is well suited to visualizing the diaphragm (particularly on the left side) ▶ IV gadolinium can be helpful (contused lung and adjacent atelectasis will enhance) ▶ cardiac and respiratory gating is required to minimize any motion artefact ▶ life support devices may not be MRI compatible
- **T1WI:** this will clearly show the diaphragm as a low SI line with high SI mediastinal and abdominal fat on either side ▶ tears are clearly depicted as defects in the low SI line with herniation of omental fat or upper abdominal organs

Pearls

- Clinical series show an increased incidence of left-sided tears (possibly due to a protective effect of the liver) ▶ however autopsy series show an equal incidence (many right-sided tears may be missed or are less clinically important)
- *Complications of a diaphragmatic rupture include:* atelectasis ▶ bowel herniation, strangulation or rupture (± a subsequent empyema)
- There are usually significant associated injuries:
  - *Left-sided tears:* splenic injuries ▶ thoracic injuries (e.g. haemothorax or a traumatic aortic injury)
  - *Right-sided tears:* hepatic and bowel lacerations

CARDIAC INJURY

Definition

- The myocardium is more commonly affected by blunt rather than penetrating injury (usually road traffic accidents) ▶ injury occurs usually due to crushing or deceleration, but cardiac damage can also occur due to over distension due to excessive hydrostatic pressure (combined with a reduced myocardial mass and anterior position) probably explains the increased right atrial and ventricular rupture

Clinical presentation

- Asymptomatic contusions; arrhythmias ▶ coronary artery injury, regional wall motion abnormalities ▶ pericardial tears ▶ papillary rupture ▶ valve dysfunction

CT

- Pericardial effusion; pneumopericardium ▶ haemopericardium (higher attenuation effusion) ▶ contusion represented by focal areas of myocardial hypo enhancement ▶ cardiac herniation (luxation) and is associated with torsion of the great vessels and represents the most severe complication of pericardial injury ▶ associated mediastinal injuries or sternal fractures

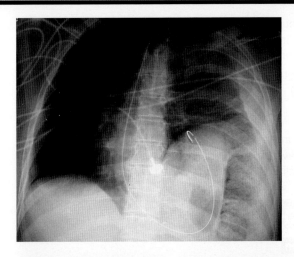

Diaphragmatic rupture. PA CXR showing a left-sided diaphragmatic rupture. Bowel can be seen herniating into the left hemithorax, the mediastinum is displaced to the right and there is a nasogastric tube seen coiled within an intrathoracic stomach.*

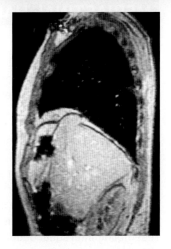

Diaphragmatic tear. Sagittal MRI showing a post-traumatic diaphragmatic tear.*

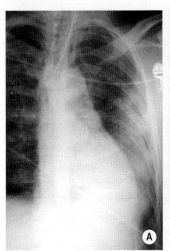
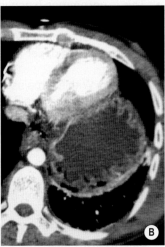
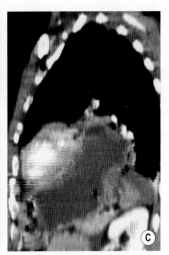

Rupture of the left hemidiaphragm following blunt trauma due to a road accident. (A) CXR reveals left mid-zone contusion. (B) Axial and (C) sagittal reformatted CT images reveal a ruptured diaphragm on the left side with the stomach herniating through into the thorax. The stomach is constricted as it passes through the diaphragmatic tear – the so-called 'collar sign'.*

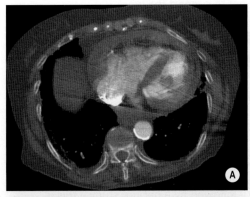
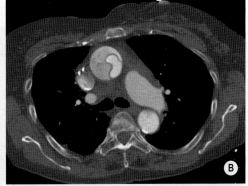
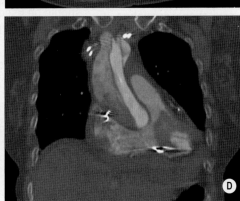

Haemopericardium and acute traumatic aortic injury. CT image following blunt trauma with a haemopericardium (A). The patient also sustained an acute traumatic injury with a dissection visible on axial images (B,C) and on a coronal reformatted image (D).**

MEDIASTINAL HAEMORRHAGE

Definition

- *Common causes:* arterial or venous trauma ▶ aneurysmal rupture ▶ aortic dissection ▶ as a complication of central venous catheterization

Radiological features

CXR An increased mediastinal diameter (which is maximal at the bleeding point) ▶ blood may run over the left lung apex producing a smooth and well-defined apical cap ▶ severe haemorrhage may rupture into the pleural cavity or dissect into the lung along the peribronchovascular sheaths resulting in an appearance resembling interstitial oedema

NECT High attenuation acute haemorrhage

MRI The appearance will vary with the age of the haemorrhage

MEDIASTINAL EMPHYSEMA (PNEUMOMEDIASTINUM)

Definition

- Extra-respiratory air seen within the mediastinum
- >95% of cases result from an air leak from a tear in a small intrapulmonary airway
  - *Causes:* asthma (most commonly) ▶ alveolar rupture (secondary to lung trauma) ▶ following positive-pressure ventilation
    - A pneumomediastinum occurs in up to 10% of cases of blunt chest trauma
    - In a minority of cases it can be caused by tracheobronchial or oesophageal rupture (e.g. secondary to vomiting)
    - Occasionally air can track into the mediastinum from a retroperitoneal air collection
  - *Macklin effect:* air dissects via the peribronchovascular sheaths through the lung and into the mediastinum via the hilum

Clinical presentation

- It may be responsible for substernal chest pain ▶ it can present with soft tissue swelling of the chest, neck and face ▶ precordial crackles (on auscultation) correlating with the heart beat

Radiological features

CXR Streaky translucencies outlining the mediastinal structures (most clearly seen adjacent to the left heart border, aortic knuckle, main pulmonary artery and adjacent left hilum) ▶ the air may elevate the mediastinal pleura

- Air often tracks into the neck, chest wall and retroperitoneum ▶ a lateral CXR is more sensitive

- *'Continuous diaphragm' sign:* air may track extraserosally on either side of the diaphragm, appearing as a continuous line of transradiancy

CT Similar signs as for a CXR (but CT is much more sensitive)

Pearl

- A pneumomediastinum is, in itself, of little significance – however, the condition causing the air leak may be of great clinical significance

TRACHEOBRONCHIAL RUPTURE

Definition

- This is uncommon (seen in up to 2% of cases of major blunt trauma) ▶ it is caused by sudden chest compression against a closed glottis and is commonly associated with upper rib, sternal and thoracic spine injuries
- *Location:* Within a mainstem bronchus (90%) ▶ involving the trachea and within 2 cm of the carina (10%)
- *Definitive investigation:* Bronchoscopy

Radiological features

CXR/CT Direct signs: tracheobronchial disruption, with surrounding extra-luminal gas ▶ indirect signs: pneumomediastinum and pneumothorax (typically failing to respond to a chest drain)

- *'Fallen lung sign':* the affected lung may sag to the pleural cavity floor with a complete mainstem bronchus rupture, usually the right (there are no longer intact airways present to support the lung)

OESOPHAGEAL RUPTURE

Definition

- This is usually iatrogenic (e.g. endoscopy ± therapeutic dilatation) ▶ it can also be caused by blunt or penetrating trauma

Radiological features

Contrast study Initially a water-soluble contrast agent should be used – followed by a barium study if this is negative ▶ extravasation of contrast will be seen at the site of rupture

CXR/CT A pneumomediastinum ▶ a left-sided pleural effusion

Pearl

- Prompt diagnosis and treatment is required to avoid a subsequent mediastinitis

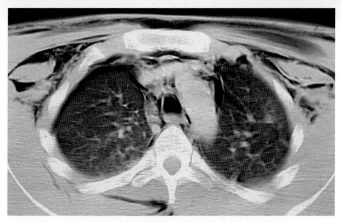

Extensive pneumomediastinum seen on CT following a high-speed road accident. Air can be seen around the trachea though no tracheal injury was seen at bronchoscopy.*

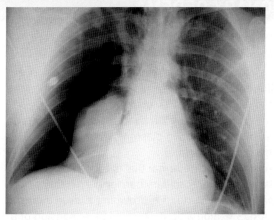

Fallen lung sign. CXR in a patient injured in a farming accident. The right lung is seen sagging to the floor of the right hemithorax (the 'fallen lung sign') and a completely ruptured right main bronchus was found at surgery.*

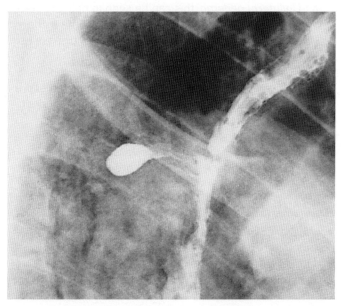

Oesophageal rupture following endoscopy. A localized perforation is shown on this water-soluble contrast swallow.†

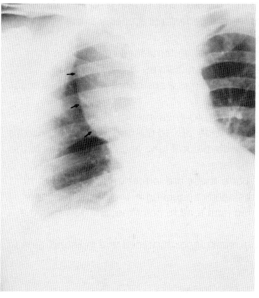

Mediastinal haematoma. Following an unsuccessful placement of a CVP line, a large extrapleural haematoma (arrows) is present.†

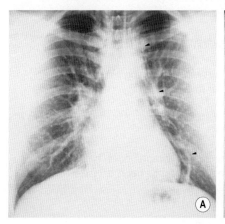

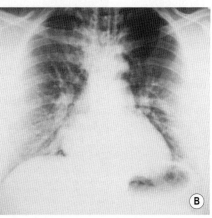

A ruptured trachea with dyspnoea and chest pain in a man suffering a deceleration injury. (A) Pneumoperitoneum with linear lucencies in the mediastinum and displacement of the pleura (arrowheads). (B) One hour later, following a bout of coughing, a left pneumothorax has developed. Bronchoscopy revealed a ruptured lobe.†

1.9 AIRSPACE DISEASE

PULMONARY OEDEMA

DEFINITION

- An excess of extravascular lung water
  - **Cardiogenic oedema:** increased hydrostatic pressure moves fluid out of the vascular compartment ▶ this is commonly caused by left heart failure ▶ it is rarely caused by a reduction in plasma osmotic pressure (e.g. hypoalbuminaemia)
  - **Non-cardiogenic oedema:** this is caused by an increased alveolar-capillary barrier permeability
    - *Causes:* fluid overload ▶ drowning ▶ drug induced ▶ ARDS ▶ high altitude ▶ rapid re-expansion of a collapsed lung ▶ intracranial disease

RADIOLOGICAL FEATURES

`CXR/CT` Fluid passes from the intravascular compartment into the interstitium and then into the alveoli (i.e. interstitial oedema precedes frank airspace opacification)

- **Interstitial oedema:** oedema fluid collecting in a subpleural space manifests as thickening of the interlobar fissures or as a costophrenic recess lamellar 'effusion'
  - *Kerley B lines:* thickened interlobular septa (1- to 2-mm wide, 30- to 60-mm long) ▶ this occurs within the sub-pleural lung and perpendicular to the pleural surface
  - *Kerley A line:* these are longer (up to 80–100 mm) and occasionally angulated ▶ they cross the inner ⅔ of the lung (and tend to point medially towards the hilum)
  - *Peribronchial cuffing:* thickened and indistinct airway walls
  - *Perihilar haze:* loss of conspicuity of the central pulmonary vessels
- **Alveolar oedema:** this generally spares the apices and extreme lung bases ▶ usually there is bilateral opacification (it can be unilateral) ▶ opacities may coalesce to produce a general 'white-out' (± air bronchograms) ▶ resolution of any airspace opacification may be rapid (over hours) ▶ the distribution of pulmonary oedema can vary with posture (dependent lung becomes more oedematous)
  - *'Butterfly' or 'bat's wing' distribution:* this occurs if the central lungs are predominantly affected
- **Additional signs:**
  - *Cardiomegaly:* this indicates chronic heart disease, compared with a normal cardiac size seen after an acute myocardial infarction
  - *Pleural effusions:* these are often bilateral
  - *Unilateral oedema:* this can be seen in patients placed in a lateral decubitus position for some time ▶ the distribution can be affected by coexisting disease (e.g. emphysema can lead to patchy oedema)
  - *Redistribution of blood to the upper zones:* this occurs with an elevated pulmonary venous pressure (when erect oedema accumulates in the dependent lung, compressing these vessels and increasing basal resistance to flow): the diameter of the upper lobe vessels > the lower lobe vessels ▶ diameter of pulmonary arteries > adjacent bronchi seen end on

PEARL

- Thickened interlobular septa are not diagnostic of pulmonary oedema – they may also be caused by fibrosis or malignant infiltration (e.g. lymphangitis carcinomatosa)

	Cardiogenic oedema	Non-cardiogenic oedema
Distribution	Central 'bat's wing'	Tends to be more peripheral
Septal lines	Common	Less common
Peribronchial cuffing	Common	Less common
Pleural effusions	Common	Less common
Cardiomegaly	Yes	No
Pulmonary vasculature	Upper lobe diversion	No redistribution

CT signs of pulmonary oedema
Common findings
- Ground-glass opacification (patchy or diffuse) ± consolidation
- Smooth interlobular septal thickening
- Peribronchovascular thickening
- Vascular dilatation
Ancillary findings
- Pleural effusions
- Enlargement of mediastinal lymph nodes/'hazy' opacification of mediastinal fat (in heart failure)—reversible

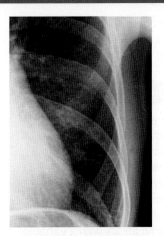

Magnified view of the left costophrenic region demonstrating multiple interstitial (Kerley B) lines. Each line is roughly perpendicular to the chest wall and extends to the pleural surface.*

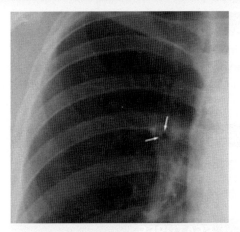

Peribronchial cuffing. The wall of the anterior segmental bronchus appears thickened and ill-defined (arrows) in early interstitial oedema due to (iatrogenic) fluid overload.*

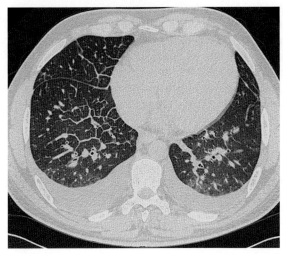

Pulmonary oedema on CT. There is diffuse ground-glass opacification, smooth thickening of multiple interlobular septa and peribronchovascular cuffing. Bilateral pleural effusions are also seen.*

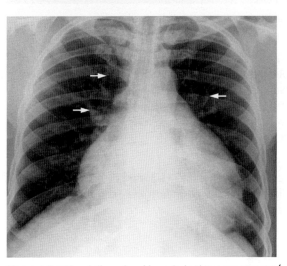

Upper lobe blood diversion. Vessels in the upper zones (arrows) are prominent in comparison to those in the lower lung zones.*

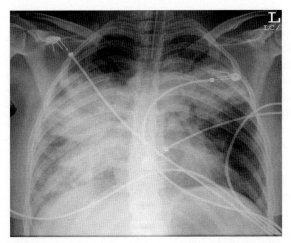

Pulmonary oedema on CXR demonstrating the characteristic 'bat's wing' distribution, with airspace opacification principally within the central lung.*

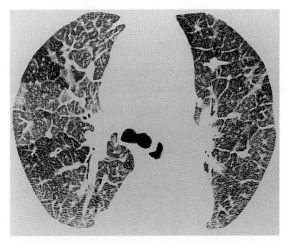

Generalized thickening of the interlobular septa on a background of ground-glass opacification in a patient with cardiogenic pulmonary oedema. ©2

DIFFUSE PULMONARY HAEMORRHAGE

DEFINITION

- Airspace bleeding is a surprisingly frequent event ▶ the severity can vary from small symptomless bleeds to life-threatening episodes
- Multiple causes (see table)

CLINICAL PRESENTATION

- Recurrent haemoptysis ▶ dyspnoea ▶ chronic cough ▶ intermittent pyrexia ▶ headache ▶ lethargy ▶ basal crackles ▶ clubbing

RADIOLOGICAL FEATURES

- Similar appearances regardless of cause

CXR

- *Acute phase:* widespread ground-glass opacification or consolidation (mainly affecting the perihilar regions of the mid and lower zones)
- *Chronic phase:* with repeated episodes ill-defined nodular or reticulonodular opacities are seen ± hilar lymph node enlargement

HRCT

- *'Subacute' phase:* nodules (1–3 mm) or ground-glass opacification (patchy or uniform) with no zonal predilection

- *'Crazy paving' appearance:* abnormal interlobular septal thickening within areas of ground-glass change
- *Fibrosis:* this follows repeated haemorrhage

PEARLS

- Compared to other causes of airspace opacification (except pulmonary oedema) the changes of diffuse alveolar oedema typically clear over a few days
- **Idiopathic pulmonary haemosiderosis:** a rare disorder of unknown aetiology presenting with episodic intra-alveolar haemorrhage, haemoptysis, iron-deficiency anaemia and airspace opacification ▶ it usually affects children or young adults with a variable prognosis (survival ranges from days to years) ▶ non-specific imaging features
- **Antibasement membrane antibody disease (Goodpasture's syndrome):** antibodies are directed against the components of the lung and kidney basement membrane ▶ it typically affects young men (3F:1M) ▶ pulmonary manifestations often dominate (although renal disease is present in the majority)

PULMONARY ALVEOLAR MICROLITHIASIS

DEFINITION

- This is due to the deposition of tiny (up to 3 mm) calcium and phosphate calculi (stones) within the alveoli ▶ the stones are of unknown origin

CLINICAL PRESENTATION

- It demonstrates a strong familial tendency and usually begins in early life
- It is usually asymptomatic

RADIOLOGICAL FEATURES

CXR/CT Innumerable discrete high-density opacities (resembling grains of sand) within both lungs ▶ there may be a 'white-out' appearance if profuse ▶ tell-tale line of black subpleural lung (caused by 5–10 mm small cysts or paraseptal emphysema) ▶ can be thickening and beading of the fissures ▶ changes are more pronounced in the lower zones and posteriorly

- There is a tendency for associated pulmonary fibrosis and cor pulmonale (the fibrosis is associated with apical bullae formation)

Scintigraphy Pulmonary activity is demonstrated on bone scintigraphy

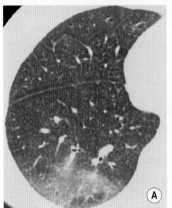
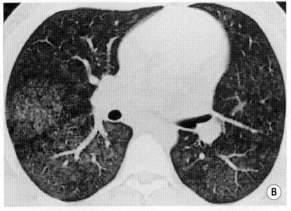

(A) Acute pulmonary haemorrhage. There is ground-glass opacification in the posterior aspect of the right lung due to alveolar haemorrhage. Note the generalized nodularity due to the effects of recent haemorrhage. (B) CT demonstrating the chronic phase of pulmonary haemosiderosis. There is diffuse ill-defined change, mainly in the posterior aspect of the lungs.[†]

Classification of diffuse pulmonary haemorrhage syndromes (according to a patient's immune status)		
Immunocompetent patient	*Immunologically mediated*	Antibasement membrane antibody disease (Goodpasture's syndrome)
	A presumed immunological basis (± nephropathy)	SLE ▶ rheumatoid arthritis ▶ systemic sclerosis ▶ systemic necrotizing vasculitis ▶ Wegener's granulomatosis ▶ microscopic polyarteritis
	Diseases with no known immune aetiology	Idiopathic pulmonary haemosiderosis ▶ rapidly progressive glomerulonephritis without immune complexes ▶ drug induced (e.g. anticoagulants, cocaine) ▶ valvular heart disease ▶ disseminated intravascular coagulation ▶ acute lung injury ▶ tumours
Immunocompromised patients		Blood dyscrasias ▶ infection ▶ tumours

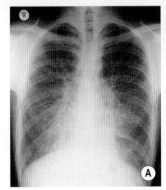
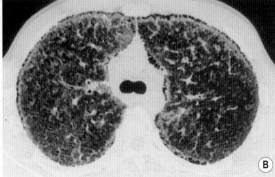
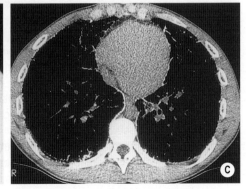

(A) Pulmonary alveolar microlithiasis. Multiple, fine, dense opacities are visible throughout the lungs. HRCT on (B) lung and (C) mediastinal windows demonstrates innumerable tiny nodules and there is a marked subpleural line. The high-density nature of the lesions is apparent adjacent to the mediastinum.[†]

EOSINOPHILIC LUNG DISEASE

Definition

- Historically this has been defined as pulmonary infiltration accompanied by a blood eosinophilia (pneumonia, hydatid disease, Hodgkin's disease and sarcoidosis must be excluded first)
- Simplified classification:
  - **Idiopathic:** simple, acute or chronic pulmonary eosinophilia
  - **Infective:** parasitic ▶ fungal ▶ bacterial ▶ viral
  - **Immunological:** Wegener's granulomatosis ▶ Churg–Strauss syndrome ▶ rheumatoid arthritis ▶ sarcoidosis)
  - **Drug induced:** NSAIDs ▶ captopril ▶ cocaine
  - **Neoplastic:** bronchogenic carcinoma ▶ bronchial carcinoid ▶ lymphoma

Radiological features

Simple pulmonary eosinophilia (Löffler's syndrome)

- This mimics a chronic eosinophilic pneumonia but with *transient* radiographic infiltrates (with resolution in days) ▶ there is minimal constitutional upset ▶ usually no cause is identified but it is associated with parasitic infections (e.g. *Ascaris*)
  - An elevated blood eosinophil count is present

CXR/CT Fleeting uni- or bilateral airspace or ground-glass opacification

Acute eosinophilic pneumonia

- This demonstrates a more fulminant course ▶ there is a brief history of a febrile illness followed by respiratory distress and marked hypoxia (occurring at any age) ▶ there is often a dramatic improvement with steroids (with resolution in days) ▶ spontaneous improvement is also possible
  - Elevated eosinophil levels are seen in the broncho-alveolar fluid

CXR Rapid progression of diffuse bilateral airspace opacification ± reticular infiltrates ▶ there is a lower lung predominance

HRCT Ground-glass opacification and consolidation ± smooth interlobular thickening ▶ pleural effusions are common

Chronic eosinophilic pneumonia

- The features are strikingly different from those above: there is a more protracted course and the symptoms are often more marked than in simple pulmonary eosinophilia (pyrexia, cough, breathlessness, weight loss, night sweats and occasionally haemoptysis or chest pain) ▶ lung function tests reveal a restrictive defect and impaired gas transfer ▶ there is a good prognosis with steroid therapy
  - Frequently eosinophilia is seen in the peripheral blood

CXR/HRCT Patchy, non-segmental areas of consolidation (affecting the mid and upper zones) ▶ pleural effusions are rare
  - *'The photographic negative of pulmonary oedema'*: notably these opacities are peripheral and parallel the chest wall

ALVEOLAR PROTEINOSIS

Definition

- Accumulation of surfactant within the alveoli (of unknown aetiology) ▶ it predisposes to pulmonary infection
  - *'Secondary' alveolar proteinosis*: occasionally it can be consequent on a pulmonary insult such as exposure to inorganic dusts or some infections
- There is a recognized link with some adult haematological malignancies (i.e. lymphoma and leukaemia) and immunodeficiency states in children

Clinical presentation

- A rare disease affecting adults (M>F) aged 20–50 years ▶ it has also been described in children (where the prognosis is worse)
- It commonly presents with exertional dyspnoea and a non-productive cough ▶ occasionally there is a pyrexia, chest pain and haemoptysis ▶ digital clubbing and inspiratory crackles may be present
  - There may be minimal clinical signs despite extensive radiographic changes

Radiological features

CXR Non-specific findings: bilateral airspace opacification (most pronounced centrally, sometimes producing a 'bat's wing' appearance) ▶ air bronchograms, pleural effusions and significant mediastinal lymphadenopathy are uncommon

HRCT *'Crazy-paving' pattern:* a striking geographical distribution of ground-glass opacification and thickened interlobular septa
- This pattern can also be seen with bronchioloalveolar carcinoma, exogenous lipoid pneumonia and diffuse haemorrhage

Pearl

- Although spontaneous resolution may occur, the majority require therapeutic (whole lung) saline bronchoalveolar lavage

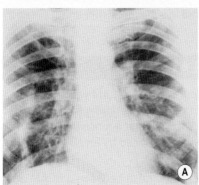
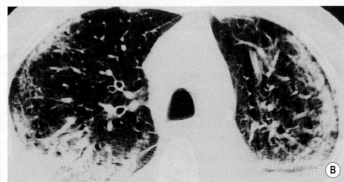

Chronic eosinophilic pneumonia. (A) CXR demonstrating alveolar opacities distributed peripherally. The vertical band in the right lung is characteristic (the photographic negative of pulmonary oedema). (B) CT demonstrating consolidation paralleling the chest wall bilaterally.[†]

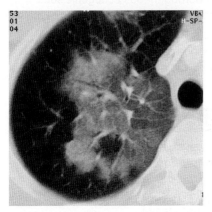

Simple pulmonary eosinophilia (Löffler's syndrome). CT demonstrating patchy areas of ground-glass opacification in both lung apices that cleared rapidly after steroid therapy.[†]

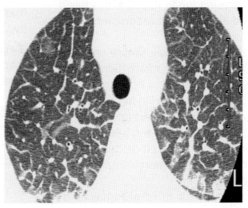

Acute eosinophilic pneumonia, CT demonstrating septal thickening, and patchy ground glass abnormality. ©1

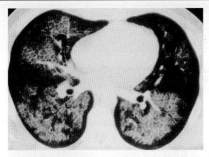

Alveolar proteinosis. CT demonstrating the typical 'crazy-paving' appearance with alveolar filling and septal wall thickening.[†]

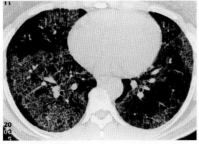

HRCT of the 'crazy-paving' pattern in alveolar proteinosis: patchy but geographical ground-glass opacification is seen and there are numerous thickened interlobular septa in areas of ground-glass opacification.*

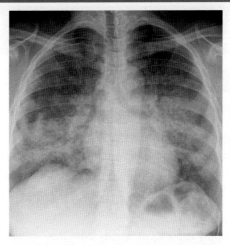

Alveolar proteinosis. CXR demonstrating bilateral symmetrical airspace opacification in the mid and lower zones with a predilection for the central lung, an appearance which can simulate the 'bat's wing' appearance of pulmonary oedema.*

1.10 PAEDIATRIC CHEST

CONGENITAL PULMONARY AIRWAY MALFORMATIONS (CPAM)

DEFINITION

- Previously known as congenital cystic adenomatoid malformation (CCAM)
- A rare lesion caused by hamartomatous proliferation of the terminal bronchioles at the expense of alveolar development ▶ it is characterized by a multicystic mass of pulmonary tissue with proliferation of the bronchiolar structures
- It is usually unilobar and communicates with a normal tracheobronchial tree ▶ it receives its blood supply from a normal pulmonary artery and vein ▶ it may compress the contralateral lung (resulting in hypoplasia)
  - *Type 1 – macrocystic (65%):* variable cysts with at least one dominant cyst present (up to 10 cm) ▶ this has a good prognosis (and an infrequent association with other congenital abnormalities)
  - *Type 2 – microcystic (10–15%):* smaller more uniform cysts (up to 2 cm) ▶ congenital malformations are common (50%)
  - *Type 3 – mixed (~8%):* solid-appearing microcysts (1.5 cm) with an associated mass effect (giving a ground-glass appearance on CT) ▶ it has a poor prognosis due to the associated congenital malformations and severe respiratory compromise ▶ nearly always mediastinal shift
  - *Type 4 (10–15%):* large cysts (up to 7 cm) ▶ may be a precursor of pleuropulmonary blastoma

CLINICAL PRESENTATION

- Neonatal respiratory distress or it can present in older children ▶ symptoms are due to a combination of obstructive emphysema, mediastinal shift and infection

RADIOLOGICAL FEATURES

- During the first few hours of life a CCAM will appear as a soft tissue mass (due to the retained lung fluid within it) which may cause mediastinal shift ▶ once this fluid has been reabsorbed it will be replaced by an air-filled cystic lesion

MRI (prenatal) This can distinguish between a CCAM and a congenital diaphragmatic hernia

Fetal USS Echogenic soft tissue mass ▶ multiple variable size anechoic cysts or a homogeneous echogenic solid mass ▶ large lesions can cause mediastinal shift (± lung hypoplasia)

Fetal MRI T2WI: hyperintense ▶ uni-/multilocular or solid ▶ over time the fluid can be replaced by air (± air–fluid levels)

PEARLS

- CPAMs can communicate with the airways ▶ infected (30%) ▶ blood supply from the pulmonary artery with drainage via pulmonary veins
- There is a variable natural history and prognosis (larger lesions have a worse prognosis)
- Lesions that are identified prenatally may involute in utero
- *Treatment:* early surgical removal may be required if there is severe pulmonary compromise (and if the contralateral lung is not hypoplastic)

SCIMITAR SYNDROME (HYPOGENETIC LUNG, PULMONARY VENOLOBAR SYNDROME)

DEFINITION

- This anomaly shares some features with sequestration except:
  - The lung is normally connected to the bronchial tree
  - The vein draining the affected lobe (usually the right lower lobe) drains into the IVC or portal vein (rather than the left atrium)
- There is usually an absent or small pulmonary artery perfusing the abnormal lung
  - The arterial supply is partly or wholly from the thoracic or abdominal aorta, or the coeliac axis

CLINICAL PRESENTATION

- It may be asymptomatic or present with features of a left-to-right shunt

RADIOLOGICAL FEATURES

- A small ipsilateral lung with ipsilateral mediastinal shift
- The abnormal pulmonary vein is seen draining down and enlarging towards the diaphragm in the shape of a 'scimitar' sword

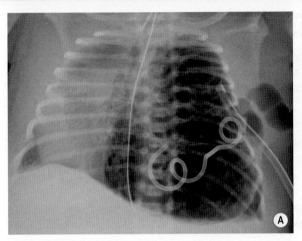
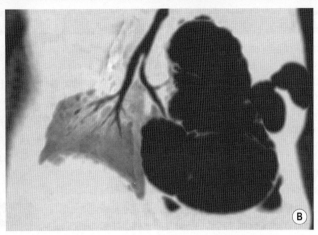

Type 1 CPAM. (A) CXR shows a large air-filled abnormality in the left lung causing marked contralateral mediastinal shift. Attempts have been made to insert intercostal drains. (B) Coronal CT reformat confirms the presence of a large multicystic mass. Note the narrowed and displaced left main bronchus.**

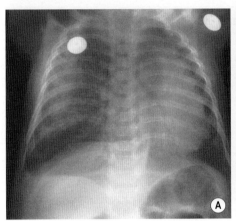
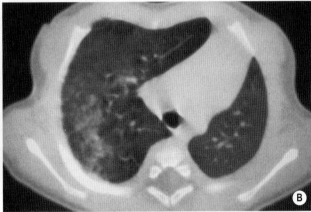

CCAM type 3. (A) CXR demonstrating extensive ground-glass opacification with gross overinflation of the right lung and herniation across the midline. (B) CT again demonstrates overexpansion of the right lung with ground-glass shadowing due to microcysts beyond CT resolution.†

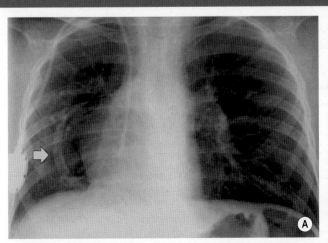
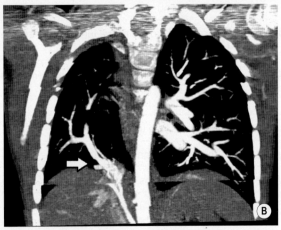

Congenital venolobar syndrome (scimitar syndrome). (A) CXR showing (1) shift of the heart into the right hemithorax, (2) a small right lung with an abnormal vessel (arrow) paralleling the right heart border and (3) overinflation (compensatory) of left lung. (B) Coronal CT reformat highlights the abnormal 'scimitar vein' (arrow) draining below the diaphragm into the systemic venous system bypassing the pulmonary veins.**

BRONCHOPULMONARY SEQUESTRATION

DEFINITION

- A congenital mass of aberrant pulmonary tissue that has no normal connection with the bronchial tree or pulmonary arteries ▶ lesions are defined as either intra- or extralobar
- It derives its arterial supply from either the thoracic or abdominal aorta ▶ its venous drainage can either be via the pulmonary or systemic veins

CLINICAL PRESENTATION

- It can present at birth or in an older child (depending on the type) with recurrent focal infections, bronchiectasis, haemoptysis or as an asymptomatic pulmonary mass

RADIOLOGICAL FEATURES

In utero US A solid well-defined highly echogenic mass ▶ the anomalous systemic arterial supply is difficult to visualize despite the availability of colour flow Doppler

CXR A persistent multicystic basal opacity which is frequently left sided

CTA/MRA This enables definition of the arterial and venous vascular anatomy

MRI Solid, well-defined hyperintense T2WI mass

PEARL

- Extralobar sequestration can be located below the diaphragm and mimic a neuroblastoma or adrenal haemorrhage

	Intralobar sequestration	Extralobar sequestration
Prevalence	75%	25%
Age at presentation	Older children ▶ adults	Neonates
Clinical presentation	Symptoms of pneumonia (recurrent or refractory to treatment)	Dyspnoea, cyanosis and feeding difficulties
Relationship to the native lung	Located within the native lung with no separate pleural lining	External to the native lung with its own pleural lining
Aeration of the affected segment	May be aeration of sequestered lung via collateral air drift (Kohn pores)	No aeration (due to its own pleural envelope preventing collateral air drift ▶ rarely air may be present due to communication with the GI tract)
Common location	Left lower lobe (60%)	Left sided (98%) between the lower lobe and diaphragm
Arterial supply	Thoracic > abdominal aorta	Thoracic > abdominal aorta
Venous drainage	Pulmonary veins	Systemic veins: IVC, azygous and portal veins
Anomalies	Uncommon (12%): skeletal deformities ▶ diaphragmatic hernia ▶ cardiovascular and renal anomalies	Common (65%): congenital lobar emphysema ▶ type 2 CCAM ▶ pulmonary hypoplasia ▶ bronchogenic cysts ▶ diaphragmatic hernia ▶ cardiovascular anomalies

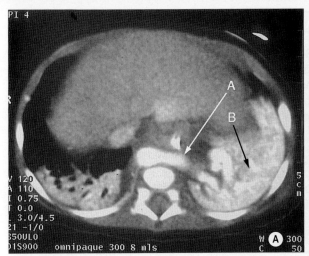
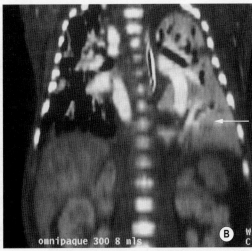

(A) Axial CECT through the lung bases with a large systemic vessel arising from the left side of the aorta (arrow A) supplying a very vascular left-sided extralobar sequestration (arrow B). (B) Coronal CT showing the normal lung and beneath this (arrow) the left-sided basal extralobar sequestration with a draining vein entering the azygous system below the diaphragm.†

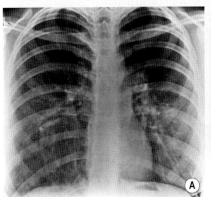
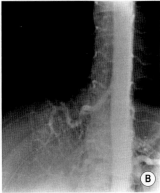
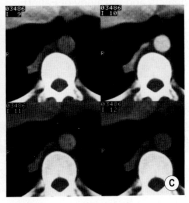

Intralobar sequestration (air-filled). (A) PA CXR. The pulmonary vessels at the right base display an abnormal course ▶ this suggests they may be draped around a space-occupying but air-filled lesion. The right hemidiaphragm is slightly depressed and the heart is shifted slightly to the left. (B) Aortogram demonstrates a large single vessel arising from the distal aorta supplying a portion of the right lower lobe. (C) CECT confirms the vascular supply.

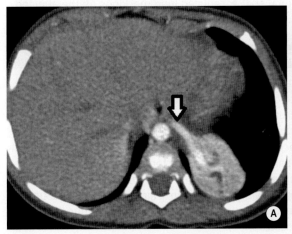
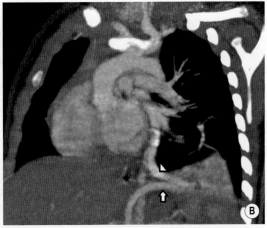

Pulmonary sequestration. (A) Axial CT shows an enhancing mass in the posterior left lower lobe with a large (enhancing) feeding vessel (arrow). (B) Oblique coronal reformat highlights the mass receiving arterial supply from a branch of the coeliac artery (arrow) with venous drainage occurring via a left pulmonary vein (arrowhead).**

CONGENITAL LOBAR OVERINFLATION

DEFINITION

- A congenital marked over-aeration of a single pulmonary lobe (usually an upper lobe and less commonly the middle lobe)
- It results from bronchial obstruction by a 'ball-valve' mechanism of unknown aetiology ▶ possible causes:
  - A congenital absence of bronchial cartilage (leading to bronchomalacia)
  - A primary alveolar abnormality (with an increase in size or number of alveoli in the affected lobe)
  - Compression of the bronchus by a vascular sling
  - A reduplication cyst
  - Secondary to inflammation

CLINICAL PRESENTATION

- Respiratory distress in the neonate (3M:1F)
- It is associated with congenital heart disease (e.g. ventricular septal defects and tetralogy of Fallot)

RADIOLOGICAL FEATURES

CXR Initially after birth the affected lobe is opaque ▶ this gradually becomes hyperlucent (due to a reduced pulmonary vascularity) with gross overinflation and compression of the remaining lobes of the lung (± contralateral mediastinal shift)

CT This is useful for indeterminate cases

V/Q scintigraphy This is useful for indeterminate cases
- *Early phase:* reduced perfusion with absent ventilation
- *Late phase:* delayed entry of isotope activity into the affected lobe with retention

PEARLS

- Urgent lobectomy is required for severe cases (some cases may resolve spontaneously)
- The term 'congenital lobar emphysema' is a misnomer as there is no alveolar wall destruction
- Left upper lobe is the most frequently affected (42%), followed by the middle lobe (35%)

PULMONARY AGENESIS AND HYPOPLASIA COMPLEX

DEFINITION

- This is due to an early insult to lung bud development or its vascular supply
- *Pulmonary agenesis:* this is associated with an absence of the pulmonary artery and bronchial development
- *Pulmonary aplasia:* blind-ending rudimentary bronchus without lung parenchyma or vasculature
- *Pulmonary hypoplasia:* rudimentary lung and bronchus, with decreased airways/alveoli/vessels
- *Pulmonary hypoplasia* secondary to lung compression during development (e.g. congenital diaphragmatic hernia/CCAM/pulmonary sequestration)

RADIOLOGICAL FEATURES

Pulmonary agenesis

CXR Ipsilateral mediastinal shift with absent lung markings on the affected side ▶ cross-herniation of the lung from the opposite side may cause confusion

Scintigraphy Absent perfusion or ventilation within the affected lung

Angiography A small or absent pulmonary artery

Pulmonary hypoplasia

CXR A 'bell-shaped' chest and slender ribs ▶ ipsilateral mediastinal shift ▶ reduced lung markings on the affected side

PEARL

- The acquired form overlaps with Swyer–James (Macleod) syndrome – but unlike Swyer–James syndrome pulmonary hypoplasia does not demonstrate air trapping
- *Bronchial atresia:* congenital obliteration of a segmental or lobar bronchus ▶ characteristically within the left upper lobe ▶ air enters the affected lobe by collateral channels with overinflation + air trapping ▶ mucous secretions accumulate in the atretic bronchus, forming a mucocele

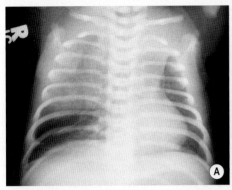
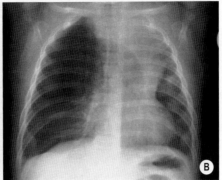

Congenital lobar overinflation. (A) Age 4 days: opacification in the right upper lobe. (B) Age 3 months: increased lucency and overinflation of the right upper lobe.*

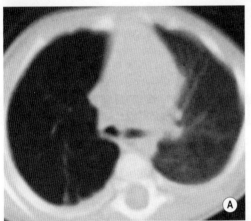
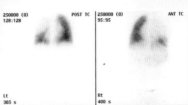
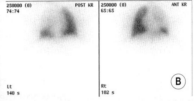

Congenital lobar overinflation (emphysema). (A) CXR shows hyperlucency in the LUL. (B) A V/Q shows limited ventilation but no perfusion within the overinflated segment.**

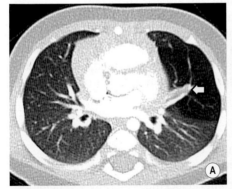
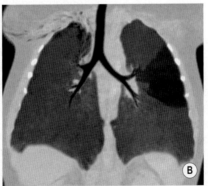

Bronchial atresia with mucocele. (A) Axial CT on lung windows shows segmental hyperlucency in LUL with a soft-tissue density at the left hilum in keeping with an atretic LUL segmental bronchus containing a mucocele. (B) Coronal MIP confirms the segmental hyperlucency.**

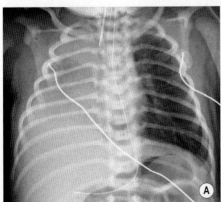
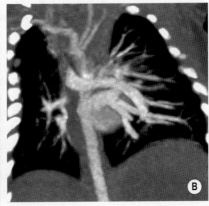

Lung hypoplasia. (A) Right lung hypoplasia in a child with complex congenital cardiac abnormalities. CXR shows complete white-out of the right lung with ipsilateral mediastinal shift. (B) Coronal CT reformat highlights the hypoplastic right pulmonary vein and paucity of pulmonary vessels on the right with a relatively normal left lung.**

TRANSIENT TACHYPNOEA OF THE NEWBORN (WET LUNG SYNDROME)

Definition

- This is due to impaired clearance of the amniotic fluid from the lungs ▶ it is commonly associated with a caesarean section, prematurity and some cases of maternal diabetes
  - Amniotic fluid is usually cleared by a combination of the thorax being squeezed in the birth canal ($\frac{1}{3}$), and fluid absorption by the pulmonary capillaries ($\frac{1}{3}$) and lymphatics ($\frac{1}{3}$)

Clinical presentation

- Tachypnoea soon after birth with mild to moderate hypoxia ▶ usually resolves by 48 hours

Radiological features

CXR Prominent pulmonary interstitial markings with slight overaeration ▶ fluid within the interlobar fissures and intrapleural spaces ▶ mild cardiomegaly

- *Severe cases:* alveolar oedema or a reticular granular appearance similar to that of respiratory distress syndrome of the newborn but with normal or hyperinflated lungs ▶ usually any changes are symmetrical (occasionally R>L)
- There is clinical and CXR resolution by 48–72 h of age
- May be a right-sided predominance (unexplained)

RESPIRATORY DISTRESS SYNDROME (HYALINE MEMBRANE DISEASE)

Definition

- This is due to a deficiency of alveolar surfactant (from the type II pneumocytes)
  - It is the most common life-threatening respiratory disorder of newborns ▶ most affected babies are premature (with an increasing incidence with increasing immaturity) – it is only occasionally seen in infants > 36 weeks' gestation
  - *Other risk factors:* infants of poorly controlled diabetic mothers ▶ fetal asphyxia ▶ maternal or fetal haemorrhage ▶ multiple gestations
    - It is more common and severe in black male children

Pathophysiology Surfactant deficiency results in the initial collapse of the smaller alveoli and hyperinflation of the larger alveoli ▶ increased respiratory effort is needed to inflate the resultant stiffened lungs ▶ there is progressive lung trauma with exudation of plasma from the pulmonary capillaries into the alveoli ▶ a secondary influx of white cells into the plasma exudate leads to the development of a thick inflammatory membrane (hyaline membrane disease)

Clinical presentation

- Respiratory distress which worsens during the first 18–24 h of life ▶ there is a gradual improvement (generally starting by the 3rd day)

Radiological features

CXR This will be abnormal at 6 h ▶ the lungs will be normal or small in size (a bell-shaped thorax) compared with TTN (transient tachypnoea of the newborn)

- Initially there is generalized fine reticular shadowing with air bronchograms – reticulogranular shadowing

becomes more confluent with the influx of plasma (together with a progressive loss of the clarity of the diaphragmatic and cardiac contours)

- Usually there is bilaterally symmetrical disease (there may be some gradation in the radiographic opacification between the upper and lower zones) ▶ pleural effusions are uncommon
- Asymmetric changes can be present if there is differential aeration (due to a misplaced ETT (endotracheal tube), asymmetric surfactant administration, or the presence of a localized pathology such as superimposed infection)
- Clearance of the lungs will depend on how quickly the individual baby is able to synthesize adequate amounts of endogenous surfactant and may take from 1–2 days to several weeks

Pearls

Prevention Antenatal corticosteroid administration (2 days prior to delivery)

Treatment Surfactant replacement therapy + ventilatory assistance ▶ >27 weeks' gestation: responds well to surfactant ▶ <27 weeks' gestation: prolonged ventilation may be required

- A patent ductus arteriosus is frequent in premature infants and contributes to the disease ▶ rigid lungs in *IRDS* and associated hypoxia may lead to left–right shunting
- Increasing use of continuous positive airway pressure (*CPAP*) ventilation in *IRDS* ▶ high-frequency ventilation also used to reduce the incidence of barotrauma (e.g. pneumothorax)
- Bronchopulmonary dysplasia (*BPD*) or chronic lung disease are long-term complications of *IRDS*

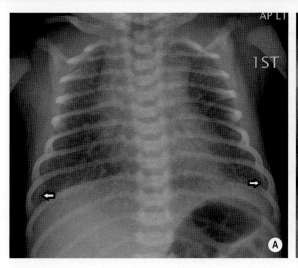
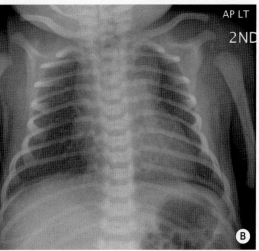

(A) Term infant. Radiograph shows mild hyperinflation, prominent vasculature, interstitial opacification most marked in the lower lobes and small pleural effusions (arrows) suggestive of TTN. (B) There is almost complete resolution at 24 hours.**

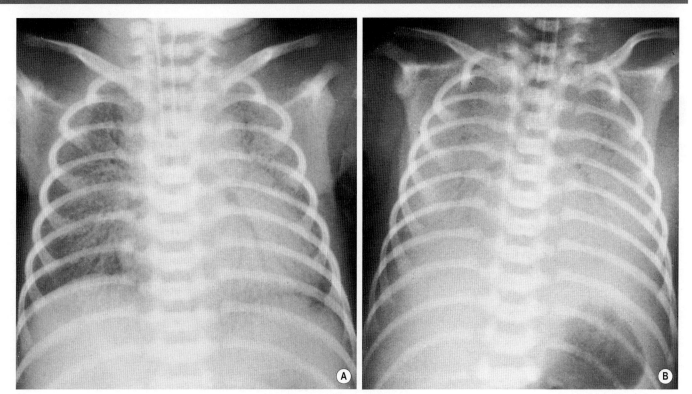

Respiratory distress syndrome. (A) Mild changes aged 1 day with fine reticulonodular shadowing with prominent air bronchograms. (B) Advanced changes aged 3 days – there is marked pulmonary opacification with loss of the diaphragmatic and cardiac contours.[†]

MECONIUM ASPIRATION SYNDROME

DEFINITION

- This occurs when infants who suffer a hypoxic stress in utero pass meconium into the amniotic fluid, which is then inhaled ▶ this results in patchy widespread collapse and consolidation combined with a severe inflammatory reaction
- Most common in postmature infants

RADIOLOGICAL FEATURES

CXR Patchy areas of collapse and consolidation (with a coarser appearance than seen in RDS) ▶ areas of peripheral hyperinflation (due to a complete bronchial obstruction or a partial occlusion with a 'ball valve' effect)

- A pneumothorax or pneumomediastinum are frequent complications which can result in hypoxia leading to: pulmonary artery vasoconstriction ▶ pulmonary hypertension ▶ a right-to-left shunt across the ductus arteriosus (a persistent fetal circulation)

PEARL

- 10% of term deliveries are accompanied by meconium staining of the amniotic fluid ▶ aspiration of this fluid in about half of these infants may result in presence of meconium below the level of the vocal cords (which is diagnostic) with clinical symptoms in about half of these cases

TREATMENT

- Airway suction using an ETT at the time of delivery ▶ otherwise the management is difficult with often a slow recovery ▶ it may require extracorporeal membrane oxygenation (ECMO)
- Inhaled nitric oxide can treat any severe pulmonary hypertension

NEONATAL PULMONARY INFECTION

DEFINITION

- Pneumonia acquired in utero or perinatally
- **Causes:**
  - *Transplacental infections:* TORCH (**T**oxoplasmosis, **R**ubella, **C**ytomegalovirus and **H**erpes) ▶ listeriosis ▶ tuberculosis ▶ congenital syphilis
  - *Peripartum:* inhalation of infected amniotic fluid or maternal tract secretions (group B streptococcus, *Escherichia coli, Chlamydia*) ▶ there is an increased risk with premature rupture of membranes
  - *Hospital acquired:* this occurs after the 1st week of life (Gram-negative organisms, *Staphylococcus aureus*, viral infections)

CLINICAL PRESENTATION

- Respiratory distress with tachnypnoea and metabolic acidosis

RADIOLOGICAL FEATURES

- Generally non-specific features
- Some pneumonias have characteristic patterns:
  - *Group B streptococcus:* pleural effusions
  - *E. coli, Haemophilus influenzae (and now less frequently S. aureus):* pneumatocele formation (which is usually uncommon in the neonate)
  - *Chlamydia:* overinflation with marked bilateral symmetric interstitial changes seen at 4–6 weeks ▶ conjunctivitis may present at 1–2 weeks

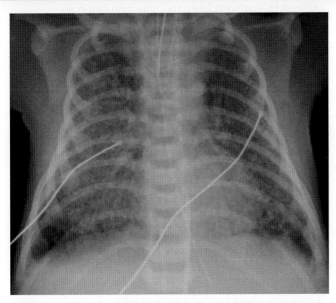

Infant born at 42 weeks' gestation. There is bilateral asymmetrical coarse opacification in the lungs in keeping with meconium aspiration.**

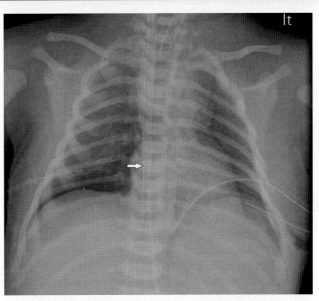

Term infant with meconium aspiration undergoing ECMO. Radiograph obtained immediately following insertion of a veno-venous catheter in the right atrium (arrow). There are bilateral pneumothoraces with chest drains in situ bilaterally.**

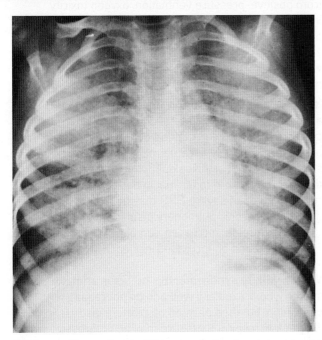

Pneumocystis pneumonia. Widespread alveolar shadowing.†

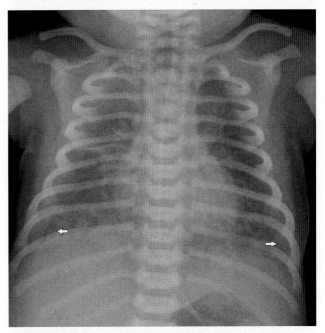

Infant with group B streptococcus infection. There is bilateral asymmetrical coarse pulmonary opacification and small bilateral pleural effusions (arrows). The appearances are similar to those seen in meconium aspiration syndrome.**

THE NORMAL PAEDIATRIC CHEST

- Sternal ossification centres may stimulate healing rib fractures or lung opacities
- The normal cardiothoracic ratio can be as large as 65% due to the presence of the thymus (a normal thymus does not compress or displace other structures) ▶ the thymus may involute rapidly with prenatal or postnatal stress or following exogenous steroids
- *CXR signs of a premature infant:* no subcutaneous fat ▶ no humeral ossification centres ▶ usually an ETT is present

COMMON ARTEFACTS

- Incubator holes may mimic a lung cyst or pneumatocele
- Redundant skin can result in a long vertical skin fold (mimicking a pneumothorax)
- Deep lower sternal retractions during respiratory distress can produce a central radiolucency that can mimic a pneumomediastinum

IDEAL POSITIONING OF TUBES AND LINES

- **Endotracheal tube:** its tip should lie approximately 1–1.5 cm above the carina ▶ the ET tube tip position may vary considerably with head/neck movement and this needs to be taken into account
- **Umbilical arterial line:** this courses inferiorly in the umbilical artery, into the internal and common iliac arteries to enter the aorta (just lateral to the left side of the spine)
  - Its tip should lie between T6 and T9 (avoiding the spinal arteries) or at L3–L5 (below the bowel and renal arteries)
- **Umbilical venous catheter:** this courses directly cephalad on the right side of the abdomen, entering the left portal vein (it may then enter the ductus venosus and then the IVC)
  - Its tip should lie above the liver without passing into a tributary vein ▶ ideal position is at the junction of the IVC and right atrium
- **Central venous lines/PICC lines**
  - Upper limb: superior vena cava
  - Lower limb: junction of IVC/right atrium

MECHANICAL VENTILATION

Early effects of mechanical ventilation

- **Air leak:** a premature infant's lungs are immature and vulnerable to damage with alveolar rupture leading to various air leak complications:
- **Pneumothorax:** this is often under tension with contralateral mediastinal shift ▶ frequently the pleural air lies anterior and medial to the lung and is more difficult to diagnose (with the only sign being an increased radiolucency of the ipsilateral hemithorax) ▶ often there is increased sharpness of the mediastinal border which, unlike with a pneumomediastinum, extends from the superior extent of the lung to the diaphragm ▶ a pneumothorax compresses the thymus (rather than being elevated as seen with a pneumomediastinum)
- **Pulmonary interstitial emphysema (PIE):** this is almost always secondary to positive-pressure ventilation with an air leak into the interstitial spaces and spread throughout the lymphatics and along the perivascular sheaths ▶ treatment is difficult with the risk of chronic lung disease

  CXR *Small* uniform bubbles of air radiating out from the hilum ▶ if these are peripheral they can rupture to produce a pneumothorax or extend medially to produce a pneumomediastinum ▶ if severe the overinflated lungs can cause cardiac compression

Late effects of mechanical ventilation

- **Bronchopulmonary dysplasia (BPD) or chronic lung disease of prematurity (CLD):** a chronic lung disease that develops in infants treated with positive-pressure mechanical ventilation and oxygen therapy ▶ defined as oxygen dependency at 28 days of age associated with an abnormal CXR ▶ the chronic lung inflammation is caused by a number of factors (e.g. barotrauma from positive-pressure ventilation, oxygen toxicity, infection, altered inflammatory response, a deficiency of antioxidant defences) ▶ areas of hyperexpansion and atelectasis are interspersed with patchy areas of fibrosis ▶ hyperexpansion may be so severe as to result in moderate-sized pulmonary cysts

  CXR A 'bubbly' appearance to the lungs (due to alveolar distension and scarred acini) with alternating cyst-like lucencies surrounded by curvilinear stranding of soft tissue density ▶ cardiomegaly may occur in severe cases and signifies pulmonary hypertension ▶ the CXR may return to normal in babies whose disease remains mild but severe BPD may be fatal or lead to debilitating chronic pulmonary insufficiency
  - **Late sequelae:** increased number of respiratory infections and an increased incidence of reactive airway disease
- **Wilson–Mikity syndrome:** this occurs in immature infants who are initially well and do not require ventilation, but then develop respiratory distress in the 2nd week ▶ respiratory failure may be progressive with symptoms persisting for many years

  CXR Diffuse streaky opacifications and small cystic lucencies

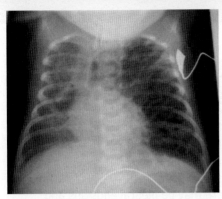

Pulmonary interstitial emphysema. Small bubbles of air radiate from the left hilum after leaking into the interstitial space. The left lung is overinflated.*

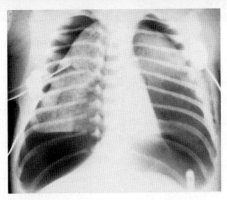

Bilateral pneumothoraces in hyaline membrane disease. A right intercostal drain is in situ.†

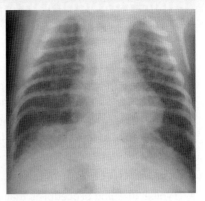

Chronic lung disease. The lungs are hyperexpanded with areas of hyperinflation interspersed with areas of fibrosis. Both lungs were equally affected.*

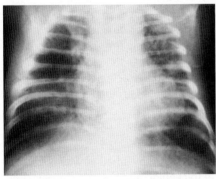

Bronchopulmonary dysplasia. Patchy shadowing from areas of volume loss and fibrosis, with areas of compensatory emphysema (especially in the right upper lobe).†

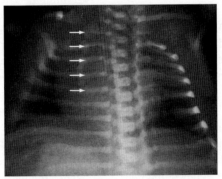

Rotated radiograph showing the sternal ossification centres simulating healing rib fractures (arrows).*

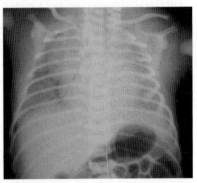

Prominent thymus in a premature baby with mild respiratory distress syndrome.*

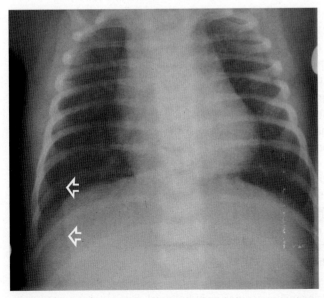

Skinfold (arrows) simulating a pneumothorax.*

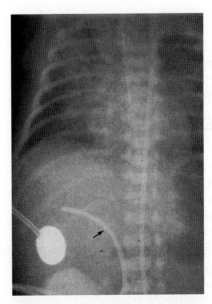

Tubes and lines. The tip of the umbilical arterial line is at T3, which is high and the top of the umbilical venous line (arrow) lies within the liver. The positions of both were altered following this radiograph.*

LUNG TRANSPLANTATION

Definition

Single lung transplantation This is indicated for non-suppurative lung disease: emphysema ▶ idiopathic pulmonary fibrosis ▶ sarcoidosis ▶ lymphangioleiomyomatosis

Bilateral sequential lung transplantation This is indicated for suppurative lung disease: cystic fibrosis ▶ bronchiectasis

PREOPERATIVE IMAGING

- Typical imaging procedures that are performed: PA and lateral CXR ▶ CT chest ▶ quantitative ventilation–perfusion scintigraphy
- This can determine the optimum side for a single lung transplant procedure, screen for potential cancer and assess for donor–recipient size matching

PERIOPERATIVE IMAGING

Reperfusion oedema (reimplantation syndrome)

Definition This is caused by increased capillary permeability and is nearly universally seen ▶ causes include interruption of the donor lung lymphatic drainage, underlying donor lung injury, surfactant deficiency and pulmonary capillary ischaemic damage

CXR/HRCT These are non-specific but will most commonly demonstrate airspace opacities (within the mid and lower zones) ▶ linear or reticular shadowing is also common ▶ peak shadowing is seen at day 4 and has usually cleared by day 10 post-op

- There is a poor correlation between the radiographic appearances and physiological measurements

EARLY GRAFT DYSFUNCTION

Definition A general term describing a range of early injuries (e.g. reperfusion oedema, ARDS or graft failure) with diffuse alveolar damage or an organizing pneumonia

CXR/HRCT The appearances range from mild airspace opacification (associated with reperfusion oedema) to complete lung opacification

POSTOPERATIVE IMAGING

Infection

Definition The lung transplant patient is vulnerable to infection due to a variety of causes: associated immunosuppressive therapy ▶ a lost cough reflex ▶ impaired mucociliary function (as the transplanted lung is denervated)

- The most common infecting organisms: *Cytomegalovirus* ▶ *Pseudomonas* ▶ *Aspergillus*

CT Consolidation ▶ ground-glass opacification ▶ septal thickening ▶ multiple or single nodules ▶ pleural effusions

- Imaging does not allow a specific organism to be identified

Acute rejection

Definition This occurs in virtually all transplanted lungs (usually within the first 3 months)

- The diagnosis is confirmed with a transbronchial biopsy (demonstrating perivascular and interstitial mononuclear infiltrates) ▶ the majority respond to IV methylprednisolone

CXR Non-specific appearances ▶ it can demonstrate new or persisting airspace opacities 5–10 days following transplantation ▶ there may be pleural effusions and interstitial lines without other signs of heart failure

HRCT This is similarly non-specific ▶ ground-glass opacification or septal lines may be the predominant finding

Bronchial anastomotic complications

Definition The bronchial anastamoses may be complicated by dehiscence or stenosis

- Dehiscence (or separation of the two anastamosed airway ends) tends to occur within the first few months and may be associated with infection
- *Contributing factors:* ischaemia ▶ acute allograft rejection ▶ low cardiac output ▶ prolonged postoperative ventilation

Obliterative bronchiolitis (OB)

Definition This is characterized by small airway fibrosis associated with intimal thickening and vessel sclerosis and is thought to represent a chronic allograft rejection ▶ episodes of acute rejection increase the likelihood of developing OB

- Long-term survival following lung transplantation is limited primarily by the development of OB
- Most cases are diagnosed 6–12 months following surgery (but can occur as early as 2 months)

CXR This may be normal (during the early stages) ▶ there can be signs of lung overinflation and subtle attenuation of the peripheral airways as the disease progresses

HRCT Areas of decreased lung attenuation associated with vessels of decreased calibre ▶ air trapping at end expiration ▶ mosaic perfusion ▶ bronchiectasis is commonly present

Post-transplantation lymphoproliferative disease (PTLD)

Definition This is thought to be caused by proliferation of donor B lymphocytes infected with the Epstein–Barr virus ▶ it usually occurs during the 1st year post transplant (affecting 5–20% of patients)

CT Multiple nodules (frequently demonstrating a peribronchovascular or subpleural distribution)

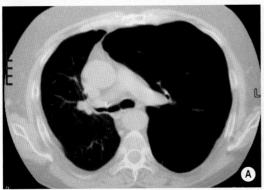
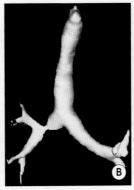

Post-transplant stenosis. (A) Axial plane and (B) 3D reconstruction showing a post-transplant stenosis of the distal right main bronchus.*

Post-lung transplantation obliterative bronchiolitis. The lungs are overinflated with mild cylindrical bronchiectasis and attenuation of pulmonary vessels. Areas of patchy ground-glass opacity in the periphery of the lung were thought to be due to cytomegalovirus pneumonitis.*

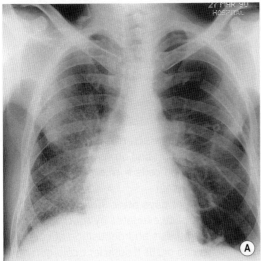
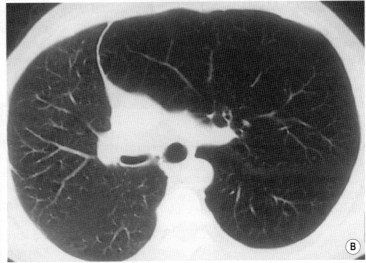

(A) CXR in a patient 2 weeks following a left lung transplant. Note the surgical defect in the posterior part of the left 5th rib. (B) HRCT of a different patient who has recently undergone a right lung transplant for emphysema related to α_1-antitrypsin deficiency. Note the displacement of the midline structures by the relatively large remaining left emphysematous lung.†

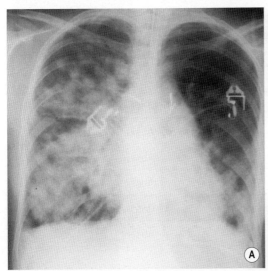
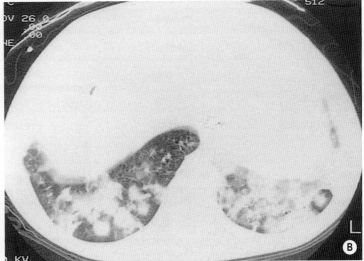

Post-transplantation B-cell lymphoma following a heart and lung transplant. The CXR (A) and CT (B) demonstrate widespread pulmonary nodules 2–3 cm in size which developed within 2 months of surgery. There was also mediastinal and hilar lymph node enlargement.†

135

ACUTE RESPIRATORY DISTRESS SYNDROME (ARDS)

DEFINITION

- A direct or indirect lung insult resulting in diffuse alveolar damage ▶ the increased pulmonary microvasculature permeability allows protein rich fluid to pass into the alveolar spaces at normal hydrostatic pressures
- ARDS and acute lung injury (ALI) describe the same clinicopathological process – the difference is merely one of severity
  - *ALI:* defined as a ratio of arterial to inspired fraction of oxygen of < 300 mmHg
  - *ARDS:* the more severe condition and defined as a ratio of arterial to inspired fraction of oxygen of < 200 mmHg

CLINICAL PRESENTATION

- Respiratory failure refractory to oxygen administration ▶ a diminished pulmonary compliance ▶ normal pulmonary capillary wedge pressures

RADIOLOGICAL FEATURES

CXR

- *Exudative phase:* patchy, ill-defined airspace opacities within both lungs – these may progress to more diffuse consolidation ▶ the opacities tend to have a more peripheral distribution than those seen with cardiogenic pulmonary oedema ▶ pleural effusions are seldom seen
- *Fibrotic phase:* after a week or so reticular opacities can be seen (corresponding to fibrosis)

CT

- **Typical features** (more strongly associated with extra-pulmonary causes): consolidation in the dependent, posterior parts of the lung with the density reducing more anteriorly (the density reduction is usually gradual with consolidation merging with areas of ground-glass opacity with normal lung in the most anterior part of the chest)
  - Dependent consolidation represents areas of atelectatic lung compressed by oedematous parenchyma – non dependent consolidation represents simple consolidation
- **Direct causes (e.g. pneumonia):** ground-glass opacities and consolidation are equally predominant ▶ asymmetrical consolidation ▶ patchy distribution of opacities, without gradation from dependent to non-dependent areas ▶ air bronchograms
- **Indirect (extra-pulmonary) causes (e.g. sepsis):** ground-glass abnormalities are dominant ▶ symmetrical ground-glass opacities ▶ cystic air spaces ▶ air bronchograms
- **Long-term survivors:** a reticular pattern indicating fibrosis with a striking anterior distribution (the more dependent lung is protected from any barotrauma related to mechanical ventilation)

PEARLS

- **Initial exudative phase:** characterized by interstitial oedema, capillary congestion and airspace filling with oedema and red blood cells ▶ microvascular thromboses are also present
- **Proliferative phase (7–14 days after the initial injury):** organization of the airspace exudates by macrophages and fibroblasts with synthesis and deposition of collagen
- **Fibrotic phase:** this can occur if sufficient collagen has been deposited ▶ parenchymal fibrosis with a striking anterior distribution may develop (although in many patients this resolves with no residual abnormality)

Comparison of the radiographic appearances in cardiac versus non-cardiac oedema*			
Signs	**Cardiac**	**Renal**	**ARDS**
Cardiomegaly	Present	Present	Absent
Vascular redistribution	Present	Present	Absent
Widened vascular pedicle	Present	Present	Absent
Interstitial lines	Present	Present	Absent
Peribronchial cuffing	Present	Present	Absent
Airspace opacification	Diffuse perihilar	Central perihilar	Patchy, peripheral
Pleural effusions	Present	Present	Absent
*relates to key in FM			

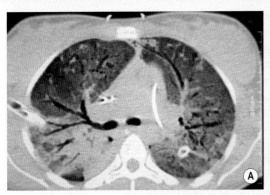 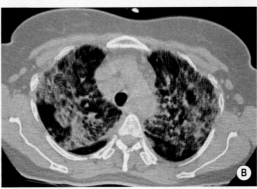

Acute respiratory distress syndrome (ARDS). CT images in two patients. (A) This patient's ARDS was due to an extrapulmonary cause and the CT shows increased opacification in the posterior, dependent portions of the lungs and ground-glass opacity more anteriorly. A right-sided intercostal tube is also present and part of a Swan–Ganz catheter can be seen in the left main pulmonary artery. (B) This patient's ARDS was related to pulmonary infection and there is patchy airspace opacity present with no gradation from dependent to non-dependent lung being seen.*

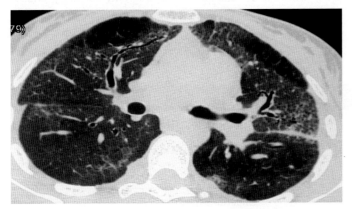

Post acute respiratory distress syndrome (ARDS) fibrosis. CT image following recovery from ARDS. Reticular opacities and traction bronchiectasis can be seen anteriorly indicating fibrosis.*

Causes of acute respiratory distress syndrome*	
Pulmonary causes	**Extrapulmonary causes**
Pulmonary contusion	Non-pulmonary injury (accidental and following surgery)
Aspiration of gastric acid contents	Burns
Smoke inhalation	Hypovolaemia
Near drowning	Hypoperfusion
Pneumonia	Massive blood transfusion
Fat embolism	Systematic sepsis

CT appearances of ARDS varies with the underlying cause		
	Direct (pulmonary) injury	**Indirect (non-pulmonary) injury**
Causes	Pneumonia, aspiration, near drowning	Sepsis, hypovolaemic shock, acute pancreatitis, non-thoracic trauma
Ground-glass opacification and consolidation	Equally prevalent. Asymmetrical consolidation. Consolidation tends to be patchily distributed throughout the lungs, without a graduation from the dependent to non-dependent areas	The dominant abnormality is ground-glass opacification. Symmetrical consolidation. Consolidation is seen in the dependent posterior parts of the lung with the density reducing anteriorly (eventually merging with any ground-glass opacification)
Air bronchograms	Almost universal	Almost universal

SUPPORT AND MONITORING APPARATUS

IDEAL POSITIONING

- **Endotracheal (ET) tube:** the ideal position is within the mid trachea about 5 cm cranial to the carina (this allows for a degree of movement with neck flexion without obstructing the right main bronchus)
  - *Neck flexion:* the ET tube descends 2 cm
  - *Neck extension:* the ET tube ascends 2 cm
- **Tracheostomy tube:** the tip of tube should lie between ½ and ⅔ of the distance between the stoma and carina (the tube does not move with neck flexion) ▶ the cuff should fill but not distend the tracheal wall
- **Central venous pressure (CVP) catheter:** the catheter tip should be projected between the medial end of the 1st rib (at the junction of the brachiocephalic vein and SVC), or within the SVC itself
- **Peripherally inserted central catheters (PICCs):** these should terminate within the SVC
- **Pulmonary capillary wedge pressure (PCWP or Swan–Ganz) catheter:** the tip should lie within the pulmonary artery about 5 cm distal to the main pulmonary arterial bifurcation (the tip should not extend beyond the proximal interlobar arteries as more distal positioning increases the risk of pulmonary infarction)
- **Intra-aortic balloon pump (IABP):** the tip should be located just distal to the left subclavian artery
- **Chest drain** (supine patient):
  - Anterosuperior (for a pneumothorax)
  - Posteroinferior (for a pleural effusion)
- **Nasogastric tube:** the tip should lie within the stomach fundus
- **Cardiac pacemaker lead position:**
  - *Single chamber:* within the right atrium near the SA node ▶ within the right ventricular apex ▶ within the right ventricular outflow tract
  - *Dual chamber:* within the right atrial appendage ▶ within the right ventricular apex
  - *Biventricular:* as for a dual chamber pacemaker but with the 3rd lead passing through the coronary sinus

Lines and tubes encountered on an ICU chest radiograph*		
Appliance	**Function**	**Optimum location of tip**
Endotracheal tube	Ventilatory support	3-8 cm above carina
Swan-Ganz catheter	Wedge and right heart pressures	Right or left pulmonary artery
Central venous pressure catheter	Central venous pressure	Superior vena cava
Left atrial catheter	Left atrial pressure	Left atrium
Peripherally inserted central catheter line	Intravenous therapy	Superior vena cava
Mediastinal drains	Mediastinal fluid evacuation	Anterior mediastinum or posterior pericardium
Pleural tubes	Pleural space evacuation	In pleural space via mid axillary line (6th to 8th rib spaces). Directed anteriorly for pneumothorax and posteriorly for effusion
Temporary pacing wires	Cardiac pacing	Over right heart
Nasogastric tube	Gastric evacuation	Left upper quadrant of abdomen, with side holes in stomach

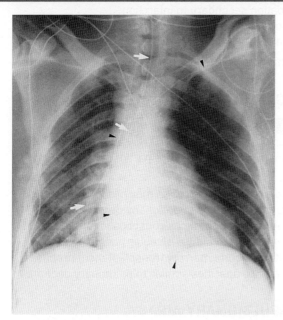

A PA CXR demonstrating a nasogastric tube (arrows) that has been placed within the right main bronchus. The patient has been 'fed' via the tube, causing patchy consolidation within the right lung. A temporary pacing electrode (arrowheads) is present.[†]

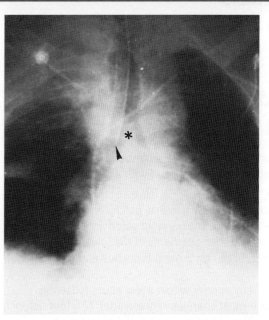

CXR demonstrating an endotracheal tube that has been placed too low. The tip of the endotracheal tube (arrowhead) is beyond the carina (asterisk) and in the right main bronchus. A well-positioned Swan-Ganz catheter is present.[†]

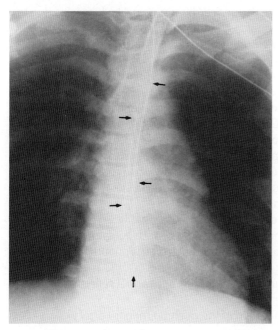

A nasogastric tube (arrows) has coiled within the oesophagus. The tube does not reach the stomach, but has folded back on itself.[†]

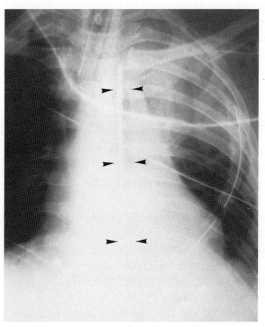

Intra-aortic ballon pump. Post-coronary artery bypass surgery. Bilateral pleural and mediastinal drains and an endotracheal tube are present. The pump is well sited and its balloon is seen to be inflated (arrowheads).

ATELECTASIS

Definition Retained secretions the most common cause

CXR Subsegmental atelectasis through to lobar collapse ▶ it usually affects the basal segments

ASPIRATION

Definition Patients with a reduced conscious level and an NGT (which disrupts the function of the oesophagogastric sphincter) are predisposed to aspiration

- It is usually more pronounced with acidic gastric contents – pH neutral fluids are less florid

CXR There are usually bilateral patchy and diffuse infiltrates ▶ these are mainly right sided and within the lung bases or superior segments of the lower lobes (due to the orientation of the right main bronchus and gravitational effects)

- They normally appear within a few hours following aspiration – most changes regress after 72 h (persistence suggests either infection or retained secretions)

PULMONARY OEDEMA

Causes Cardiac failure or overhydration

CXR Overhydration oedema may be radiologically indistinguishable from cardiogenic oedema (overhydration oedema tends to have a more central distribution with a wider vascular pedicle)

- *Upper lobe blood diversion:* this is a normal finding on supine XRs – therefore it is not a useful sign in an ITU patient

PNEUMONIA

Definition Hospital-acquired (nosocomial) pneumonia affects 10% of ICU patients

- Gram-negative bacteria ▶ *Staphylococcus aureus* ▶ fungi

CXR Appearances are non-specific – there may be lobar or segmental consolidation (± air bronchograms) or diffuse consolidation indistinguishable from pulmonary oedema ▶ cavitation is associated with infections causing necrosis or abscess formation ▶ loculation of pleural fluid is suggestive of an empyema

- *Haematogenous spread:* this can cause septic emboli – these appear as multiple rounded areas of consolidation (with a peripheral and basal predominance) which typically cavitate

PULMONARY EMBOLISM

Causes Trauma ▶ prolonged immobilization ▶ post-surgical patients

CXR This is non-specific and of limited value ▶ it may be normal or reveal non-specific atelectasis

- *'Hampton's hump':* a peripheral area of wedge-shaped consolidation secondary to infarction
- *Westermark sign:* regional oligaemia with a sharp cut-off due to a pulmonary embolism

CTPA This is the preferred technique in the ICU patient

HAEMORRHAGE

Definition This is commonly seen following thoracic interventional procedures (particularly following the coagulation disturbances that are part of cardiopulmonary bypass)

CXR Mediastinal haemorrhage may produce a widened mediastinum with displacement of any drains or tubes ▶ lung haemorrhage produces consolidation that can mimic a pneumonia ▶ diffuse alveolar haemorrhage (as a complication of bone marrow transplantation) produces bilateral airspace opacities similar to pulmonary oedema

EXTRAPULMONARY AIR

Causes Iatrogenic, blunt or penetrating trauma ▶ barotrauma

CXR/CT

- **Pneumomediastinum:** linear air densities streaking within the mediastinum ▶ a visible thymus ▶ air seen anterior to the pericardium ▶ ring-like lucencies due to air surrounding a pulmonary artery
  - *'Double bronchial wall' sign:* air on either side of a bronchial wall
  - *'Continuous diaphragm' sign:* air over a diaphragmatic surface
- **Pneumothorax:** this can be challenging to detect on a supine CXR ▶ there may be an unusually sharp heart border or mediastinal vascular structure
  - *'Deep sulcus' sign:* an unusually deep costophrenic sulcus (as air preferentially accumulates anterior to the lungs and also abuts mediastinal structures in the supine position)
- **Pneumopericardium:** this is usually seen following a cardiothoracic surgical procedure ▶ features indicating a pneumopericardium rather than a pneumomediastinum include:
  - air outlining a superior pericardial reflection around the great vessels
  - visualization of the main pulmonary artery

PLEURAL EFFUSIONS

Definition These are commonly seen and related to trauma, congestive cardiac failure, fluid overload, pneumonia or surgery

CXR Fluid tends to collect in a posterobasal position in a supine patient resulting in a diffuse, hazy increase in the lower lung density ▶ an elevated hemidiaphragm can be seen with a subpulmonary effusion

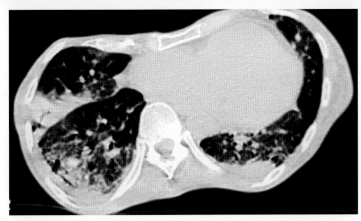

Recurrent aspiration. Axial CT image in a patient with oesophageal dysfunction due to systemic sclerosis. Multiple areas of airspace opacity in the lower zones of the lungs are due to recurrent aspiration.*

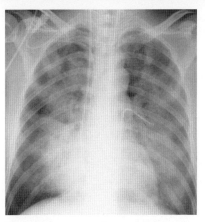

PA CXR demonstrating extensive bilateral basal and perihilar airspace shadowing following massive aspiration of gastric contents. Incidental note is made of a Swan–Ganz catheter with its tip projected more peripherally than is ideal within the left lung.†

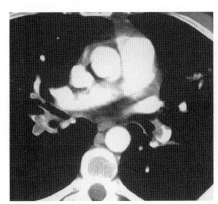

CTPA demonstrating multiple bilateral pulmonary emboli.†

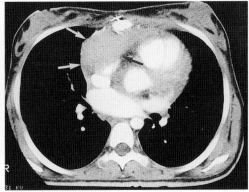

Mediastinal haematoma. CECT demonstrates a soft tissue density non-enhancing mass in the anterior mediastinum 3 days following cardiac surgery (arrows).†

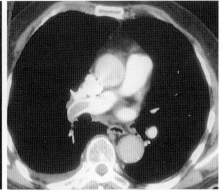

CTPA demonstrating a large filling defect (thrombus) within the right main pulmonary artery.†

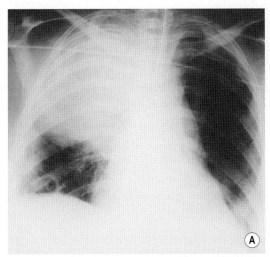
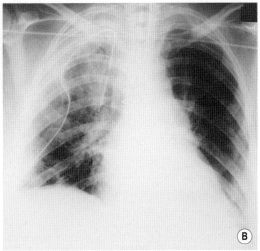

Haemorrhage following cardiac transplantation. (A) 4 h post surgery the CXR reveals opacification of the right upper zone. (B) After insertion of a chest drain there has been partial resolution of the appearances.†

CARDIOVASCULAR SYSTEM

2.1 CONGENITAL HEART DISEASE

CARDIAC DEVELOPMENT

- Between the 2nd and 7th week of intrauterine life the primitive cardiac tube grows in length more than the fetal trunk – as the ends of this tube are relatively fixed the rapidly elongating cardiac tube is compelled to bend into a loop and twist and rotate
- The formed curve is almost always convex to the right of the fetus (the D or dextro loop as viewed from the front)
- The axial rotation or twist is almost always clockwise (viewed from the caudal end of fetus) – this axial rotation results in the definitive orientation of the cardiac chambers after birth
  - *The right atrium is anterior and on the right ▶ the left atrium is posterior ▶ the right ventricle is anterior ▶ the left ventricle is posterior and on the left*

THE FETAL CIRCULATION

- The fetal right atrium receives blood from:
  - *The SVC:* desaturated blood from the head and myocardium
  - *The IVC:* partially oxygenated blood from the fetal placenta and systemic fetal veins
    - These two streams of blood remain reasonably distinct with a minimum of mixing
- There is no fetal blood flow through the fetal lungs (due to a very high pulmonary vascular resistance)
- The left fetal heart only receives blood from:
  - *A right atrium to left atrium shunt:* this occurs through a patent foramen ovale ▶ this allows partially oxygenated blood from the IVC to enter the left cardiac chambers (bypassing the pulmonary circulation) and thence into the aorta
  - *A fetal pulmonary artery shunt to the descending thoracic aorta:* this occurs through a patent ductus arteriosus (PDA) ▶ this allows poorly oxygenated blood from the SVC (via the right ventricle) to perfuse the lower half of the fetus (and also the placenta where it will become oxygenated)

CIRCULATORY CHANGES AT BIRTH

- Immediately after birth the placenta is shed (removing this oxygen source) and there is a major increase in the infant's pulmonary blood flow (the inhaled oxygen reduces the anoxic pulmonary vasoconstriction)
- This major increase in pulmonary blood flow distends the left atrium and closes the flap valve of the foramen ovale
- Within a few days the right-to-left shunt through the foramen ovale and PDA is abolished

DIAGNOSIS OF CONGENITAL HEART DISEASE

- The majority of cardiac developmental anomalies can be categorized as:

- **Abnormal communication between the right and left sides of the heart or their main vessels:** ASD ▶ VSD ▶ PDA
- **An obstruction involving or near a heart valve and within the pathway of blood flow:** tricuspid atresia ▶ pulmonary, mitral and aortic valve stenosis ▶ aortic coarctation
- **Common (combined right and left) chambers:** a common atrium, ventricle, or great artery (a common arterial trunk) receiving both oxygenated and desaturated blood
- **Abnormal connections (discordance) between the cardiac chambers and great arteries:** transposition of the great arteries (TGA)
  - The discordance may be congenitally uncorrected (UTGA) or congenitally corrected (CCTGA) by atrioventricular inversion (with the right atrium connecting to the left ventricle, and the left atrium connecting to the right ventricle)
- **Abnormal situs (position) of the heart chambers**

CAUSES OF A CENTRAL CYANOSIS

- **A direct right-to-left shunt of desaturated venous blood into an otherwise normal systemic circuit:** this entails a septal defect, plus a more distal right heart obstruction, which increases the proximal right-sided chamber pressure sufficiently to cause a right-to-left shunt (e.g. tetralogy of Fallot)
- **Transposition (discordance) of the great arteries:** see separate section
- **Common mixing situations:** at some point in the circulation, systemic venous (desaturated) and pulmonary venous (oxygenated) blood is obliged to mix
  - *Causes:* a common atria or ventricle ▶ a persistent truncus arteriosus

EISENMENGER'S SYNDROME

Definition

- Severe obstructive pulmonary arterial hypertension
  - This is due to an atheromatous hypertensive reaction and subsequent increased peripheral pulmonary arteriolar resistance as a response to a left-to-right shunt (and consequent increased pulmonary blood flow)
- Paradoxically, clearing of any initial pulmonary plethora in a left-to-right shunt may therefore represent worsening disease, with the development of a right-to-left shunt as a result of the pulmonary changes

CXR/CT

- Enlarged central pulmonary arteries with reduced calibre peripheral pulmonary arteries ▶ there can be possible central pulmonary arterial wall calcification – this is more marked if it complicates a previous long-standing severe left-to-right shunt

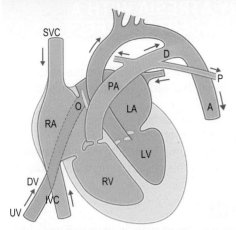

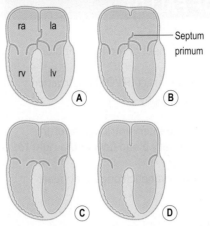

Normal fetal circulation. Oxygenated blood (red) is carried by the umbilical vein (UV) through the ductus venosus (DV) and inferior vena cava into the right atrium (RA) within which it is directed to pass through the flap valve foramen ovale (O) into the left atrium (LA) and thence into the left ventricle, aorta and finally the systemic arteries. Mixed venous blood (blue) from the superior and inferior caval veins (SVC and IVC) is passed into the RA, then via the right ventricle (RV) into the pulmonary artery (PA). The peripheral pulmonary arteries (P) are very small in the fetus due to the non-function of the fetal lungs and high resistance of the peripheral arterial circulation. Most of the output of the right ventricle therefore passes through the large valveless patent ductus arteriosus (D) and into the descending aorta (A) to supply the lower parts of the fetus and the fetal umbilical arteries, which supply the fetal placental plexus with poorly oxygenated blood for oxygenation in the placenta. The dark purple colour indicates blood having an oxygen content intermediate between mixed venous blood (blue) and fully oxygenated blood (red).

(A) Normal relationships of the interventricular and interatrial septa with the atrioventricular valves. The atrioventricular valves are inserted into the septum primum (thin line). ra = right atrium ▶ la = left atrium ▶ rv = right ventricle ▶ lv = left ventricle. (B) Ostium secundum ASD. The atrioventricular valves and left ventricular outflow tract are normal. (C) Ostium primum ASD. The septum primum is absent and the atrioventricular valves are inserted in a low position into the crest of the muscular interventricular septum. (D) Total AVSD. A large common valve separates the atrial cavities from the ventricular cavities. There is an ostium primum ASD and a large VSD in continuity.

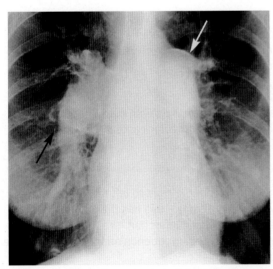

Obstructive pulmonary arterial hypertension (Eisenmenger's syndrome) complicating a large ASD with previous major left-to-right shunt. Very large central pulmonary arteries (arrows) with small peripheral vessels. Linear calcification of the central pulmonary arteries. Moderate cardiac enlargement.*

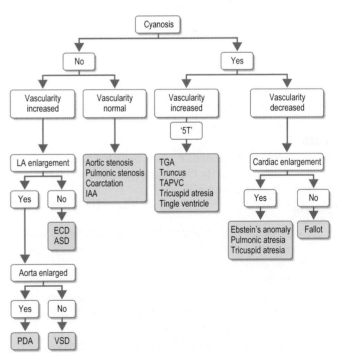

Flow diagram showing a differential diagnosis decision tree for cyanotic and non-cynanotic congenital heart disease.

TETRALOGY OF FALLOT

Definition

- This is caused by malalignment of the infundibular septum leading to:
  - Right ventricular outflow tract (RVOT) obstruction
  - Right ventricular hypertrophy
  - A large subaortic VSD
  - The aorta overriding the interventricular septum
- This results in low pulmonary blood flow and a right to left shunt
- This is the most common cyanotic congenital heart defect

Clinical presentation

- *Mild cases of pulmonary stenosis:* this forms the acyanotic end of the spectrum, behaving much like a simple VSD
- *Severe cases of pulmonary stenosis:* this presents with fainting spells on exertion ▶ cyanosis is due to the restricted pulmonary blood flow and this usually occurs by 4 months with earlier presentations with increasingly severe RVOT obstruction ▶ there is relief with squatting (the increased peripheral resistance directs more blood through the pulmonary circulation)

Radiological features

- The main role of cross-sectional imaging is the assessment of postoperative complications

CXR Pulmonary oligaemia or asymmetry ▶ a right-sided aortic arch (30%)

- *'Boot'-shaped heart:* this appearance is partly as a result of a concavity in the left heart border (hypoplastic main pulmonary artery) and an upward prominence of the cardiac apex (enlarged right ventricle)

Transthoracic echocardiography The investigation of choice

CMR

- Has a role in untreated or shunt palliated patients
- The gold standard for the assessment of the right ventricle in repaired TOF

Pearls

- Severe cases rely on alternative flow to the lungs via a PDA – as this closes shortly after birth, severe cyanosis will then develop
- **Treatment**
  - *Early:* a single-stage reconstructive surgical approach (VSD closure, relief of RVOT obstruction or possible transannular patch placement)
  - *Staged reconstruction:* this is required if there is significant central pulmonary hypoplasia ▶ there is initial placement of a modified Blalock–Taussig shunt – the shunt is taken down during the subsequent definitive repair
- **Trilogy of Fallot:** pulmonary artery stenosis + right ventricular hypertrophy + a patent foramen ovale
- **Pentalogy of Fallot:** tetralogy of Fallot (± ASD)

PULMONARY ATRESIA WITH A VENTRICULAR SEPTAL DEFECT

Definition

- A lack of continuity between the RVOT and the central pulmonary arteries (with a variable degree of hypoplasia of these structures)
- This is the more common variant – it is considered by some to be a severe form of tetralogy of Fallot
- The right ventricle can pump blood into the high pressure systemic circulation but this results in right ventricular hypertrophy

Radiological features

CXR A slightly enlarged heart with an upturned apex (due to an enlarged right ventricle) ▶ small pulmonary vessels with oligaemic lungs ▶ a right aortic arch (25% of cases)

CMR Its main role is the assessment of postoperative complications (as with tetralogy of Fallot) – this includes homograft stenosis and regurgitation, as well as conduit stenosis

Pearls

- The small pulmonary arteries initially receive blood via a PDA and subsequently through aorto-pulmonary collateral vessels (the multiplicity of these vessels can be mistaken for pulmonary plethora near the hilar regions)
- **Surgery:** this is similar to that with a severe tetralogy of Fallot

PULMONARY ATRESIA WITH AN INTACT VENTRICULAR SEPTUM

Definition

- There is no outlet for the right ventricle with no way for it to decompress ▶ this results in a very small cavity generating suprasystemic pressures
- Less common variant

Radiological features

CXR Small pulmonary vessels with pulmonary oligaemia ▶ a more rounded left ventricular contour (as this chamber receives all the cardiac flow)

Pearls

- Blood may shunt from the right to left through abnormal coronary communications – this has the potential for myocardial ischemia and infarction
- The type of surgical repair depends on the size and shape of the right ventricular cavity
  - The presence of a right ventricular infundibulum allows a biventricular repair
  - If the right ventricular cavity is small, then a single ventricular physiology is established (see the section on the single ventricle)

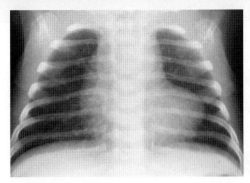

Tetralogy of Fallot. Boot-shaped heart, small hila and pulmonary oligaemia.*

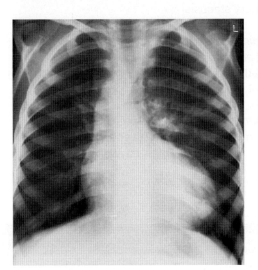

CXR of a child with pulmonary atresia and a VSD. There is a right-sided aortic arch indenting the trachea, which accentuates the concave pulmonary bay. The left heart border does not show an upturned apex as seen in the following CXR. (See adjacent figure.)[†]

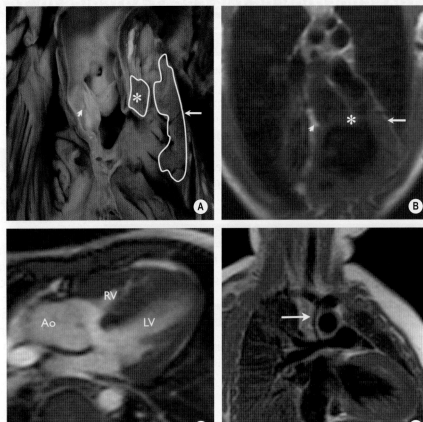

Tetralogy of Fallot. (A, B) Right ventricular outflow tract, morphological specimen and corresponding black-blood, spin-echo image in coronal view. The deviated outlet septum (asterisk), aortic root (arrowhead) and hypertrophied septoparietal trabeculations (arrow) are shown. (C) b-SSFP images of unrepaired tetralogy of Fallot: inflow/outflow view of the left ventricle (LV) shows a VSD with overriding aorta (Ao)—note the severe hypertrophy of the right ventricle (RV). (D) Black-blood, spin-echo image of right modified Blalock–Taussig shunt ▶ 3.5-mm gortex tube from innominate artery to right pulmonary artery (arrow).**

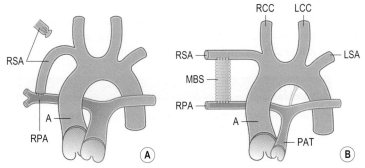

(A) The classic Blalock shunt. A = aorta ▶ RPA = right pulmonary artery ▶ RSA = right subclavian artery. (B) A modified Blalock shunt. MBS = modified Blalock shunt. RCC = right common carotid artery ▶ LCC = left common carotid artery ▶ LSA = left subclavian artery. PAT = pulmonary artery trunk.

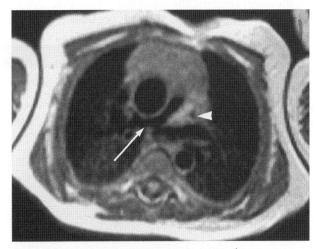

Axial CMR showing small pulmonary arteries (arrow and arrowhead) in a patient with pulmonary atresia.[†]

TRANSPOSITION OF THE GREAT ARTERIES (D-TGA)

DEFINITION

- A ventriculo-arterial discordance with an anterior aorta arising from the anterior right ventricle and the pulmonary artery arising from the posterior left ventricle
- It results in 2 independent circulations (there is a closed circulation of blood through the lungs and a separate closed circulation around the body)
- It is incompatible with life unless there is an associated anomaly to allow the mixing of blood (e.g. an ASD, VSD or PDA)

CLINICAL PRESENTATION

- Cyanosis and breathlessness in the first few weeks (the degree of mixing determines the degree of cyanosis)

RADIOLOGICAL FEATURES

CXR An 'egg on side' appearance: this is as a result of a narrow superior mediastinum (the main pulmonary artery is located directly behind the aorta) together with a slightly enlarged, rounded heart

Transthoracic echocardiography The imaging modality of choice
- Cross-sectional imaging is mainly used for assessing postoperative complications

PEARLS

- There is a normal ventricular D-loop
- A VSD is seen in 40% of patients (30% of these also have a subpulmonary stenosis)
- Treatment:
  - *PGE$_1$ administration:* to prevent PDA closure
  - *Rashkind procedure:* an atrial septostomy with a balloon catheter
  - *An arterial switch operation:* the aorta and main pulmonary artery are transected just above the coronary arterial origin, switched and then re-anastomosed to the correct ventricle) ▶ this is performed during the first few days of life

CONGENITALLY CORRECTED TRANSPOSITION (L-TGA)

DEFINITION

- There is both atrioventricular and ventriculo-arterial discordance resulting in independent circulations:
  - Through the right atrium, left ventricle and then the pulmonary artery
  - Through the left atrium, right ventricle and then the aorta
- Although anatomically abnormal the heart is physiologically normal – there is not usually cyanosis

CLINICAL PRESENTATION

- This may be asymptomatic – however many of the problems are similar to those seen with D-TGA
- It is rare

- It has a poor prognosis due to the associated cardiac abnormalities: VSD (>50%), pulmonary stenosis (50%), Ebstein's abnormality (20%)

RADIOLOGICAL FEATURES

CXR Many are normal ▶ however there may be a characteristic long curve to the left heart border (due to the abnormal leftward origin of the aorta)

CMR Its main role is the evaluation of any associated lesions, ventricular function quantification and postoperative complication assessment

PEARL

- Ventricular discordance results in a stereoisomer of a normal D-loop (the L-loop)

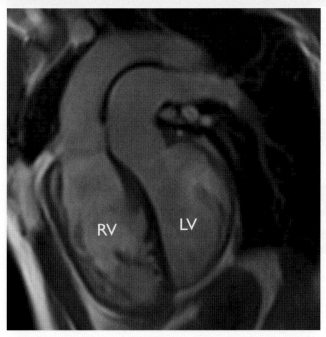

Transposition of the great arteries. b-SSFP CMR image showing an oblique sagittal outlet view of the aorta arising from the right ventricle (RV) and pulmonary artery arising posteriorly from the left ventricle (LV).**

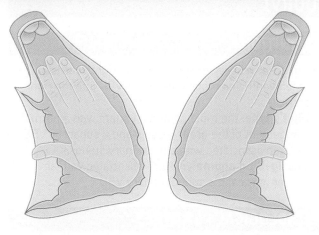

Right-hand topology   Left-hand topology

Looping (or topology). This term relates to the ventricular loop which has been formed during cardiac development. The normal ventricular D-loop can be understood most simply by using the analogy of the right-hand rule in which the morphological right ventricle is likened to a right hand. The inflow is represented by the thumb, the outflow is represented by the fingers and the interventricular septum will lie on the palmar side of the hand. D-loop and L-loop configurations are stereoisomers (mirror images) of each other.

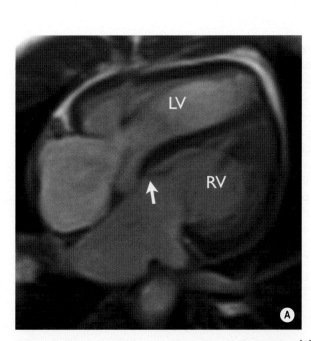

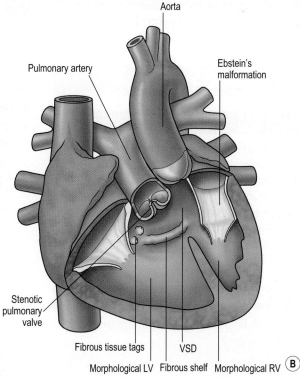

Congenitally corrected transposition of the great arteries. (A) b-SSFP CMR image of CCTGA showing the discordant atrioventricular connection, with anterior LV. Note the apical offset of the left-sided tricuspid valve. (B) Schematic drawing of CCTGA and frequent associated lesions.**

149

DOUBLE-OUTLET RIGHT VENTRICLE (DORV)

DEFINITION

- Both great vessels emerge from the right ventricle – the left ventricle empties through a VSD into the right ventricle
- **Fallot's type:** the most common variant with a normal arrangement of the great vessels and a subaortic VSD ▶ it is often associated with a pulmonary stenosis
- **Taussig–Bing anomaly:** DORV associated with an anterior aorta and a subpulmonary VSD

RADIOLOGICAL FEATURES

CMR   This plays an important role in preoperative assessment (it can demonstrate the 3D anatomy of the VSD and the arrangement of the great vessels)

PEARLS

- Surgical correction:
  - **Fallot's type:** VSD patch closure and correction of any pulmonary stenosis
  - **Taussig–Bing anomaly:**
    - *With pulmonary obstruction:* VSD patch closure and an arterial switch
    - *Without pulmonary obstruction:* Rastelli procedure: the left ventricular flow is tunnelled through the VSD to the aorta and a right ventricle – pulmonary artery pathway is established

EBSTEIN'S ANOMALY

DEFINITION

- A congenital tricuspid valve abnormality (there is a regurgitant valve with consequent atrialization of the proximal right ventricle) ▶ this results in gross right atrial enlargement, raised right atrial pressures and a relatively ineffective right ventricle
- It is usually associated with an ASD – thus there is right-to-left shunting at the atrial level with subsequent cyanosis

CLINICAL PRESENTATION

- **Severe cases:** right heart failure and poor pulmonary flow presenting in infancy

RADIOLOGICAL FEATURES

CXR   Pulmonary oligaemia ▶ a 'box-shaped' heart (due to gross cardiac contour enlargement with a prominent curved right atrial border)

CMR   This can assess the valve and right atrial morphology, and quantify the right ventricular function

PEARL

- It is associated with maternal lithium intake

ANOMALOUS CORONARY ARTERIES

DEFINITION

- Anomalous proximal and epicardial courses of the left coronary artery (LCA) and right coronary artery (RCA) – rarely anomalous *origin* of the left coronary artery from the pulmonary artery (ALCAPA)

CLINICAL PRESENTATION

- Chest pain or sudden death in an otherwise young asymptomatic patient ▶ it is one of the most frequent causes of sudden cardiac death in competitive young athletes

RADIOLOGICAL FEATURES

CXR/CT   A dilated left atrium and ventricle ▶ normal pulmonary vascularity

PEARL

- ALCAPA: following the postnatal fall in the pulmonary arterial pressure, the normal perfusion of the left coronary artery falls ▶ the heart muscle supplied by the left coronary artery then has to rely on a collateral circulation from the right coronary artery (with resultant flow reversal in the left coronary artery)
  - If there is inadequate collateral circulation, then the patient is at risk of infarction
  - If there is a large collateral circulation, then this essentially forms a large left-to-right shunt with increased volume overload of the heart
  - Can survive to adulthood with sufficient collateralization
  - Treatment = surgical reimplantation

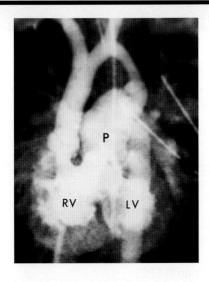

Taussig–Bing malformation. In this DORV a small bilateral conus is present with moderate subaortic stensois. The pulmonary artery (P) originates above the VSD. An aortic coarctation is associated with mild hypoplasia of the arch. The large VSD is the only outlet of the left ventricle (LV). RV = right ventricle.•

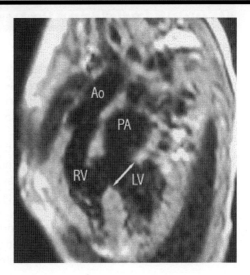

Double oblique spin-echo MRI of a Taussig–Bing anomaly to demonstrate the intracardiac anatomy. There is a double-outlet right ventricle (RV) with the VSD (arrows) lying in a subpulmonary position. The aorta (Ao) is distant from the left ventricle (LV) and 'anatomical repair' by VSD closure is not possible. PA = pulmonary artery.†

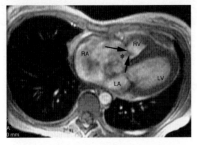

Ebstein's anomaly. Gradient-echo axial MRI. Due to adherence of the septal and posterior leaflets of the tricuspid valve to the right ventricle, the free portion of the leaflets (arrows) is located at a variable distance below the atrioventricular annulus within the right ventricle (RV) (downward displacement). The right atrium (RA) and the atrialized portion of the RV (asterisk) are enlarged with reduced functional RV chamber size.

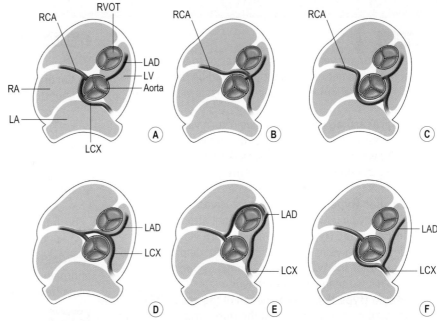

Coronary artery anomalies. Schematic diagram of the coronary arteries viewed in the axial oblique plane on CMR. (A) Anomalous LCX from RCA. (B) Anomalous RCA from left main stem (LMS), with interarterial course between pulmonary artery and aorta. (C) Anomalous RCA from LMS passing posteriorly between the aorta and atria. (D) Anomalous left coronary artery arising from RCA with interarterial course between the pulmonary trunk and aorta. (E) Anomalous left coronary artery arising from RCA passing anterior to pulmonary trunk. (F) Anomalous left coronary artery arising from RCA passing posteriorly between aorta and atria.** RA = right atrium, LA = left atrium, LV = left ventricle, RVOT = right ventricular outflow tract, LAD = left anterior descending artery, RCA = right coronary artery, LCX = left circumflex artery.

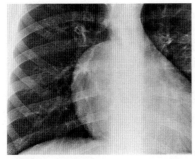

Ebstein's anomaly. The round right heart border is a massively enlarged right atrium. A large right ventricle contributes most of the left side and apex of the cardiac silhouette. The pulmonary arteries are slightly enlarged, reflecting the ASD. There is pulmonary oligaemia.

HYPOPLASTIC LEFT HEART (SHONE) SYNDROME (HLHS)

Definition

- Hypoplasia or atresia of the left heart components with a normal relationship to the great vessels ▶ it occurs if there is reduced flow through the aortic valve during development (e.g. due to atresia), leading to the failure of left ventricular development
  - *At birth:* the right ventricle supplies both the systemic and pulmonary circulations (via the pulmonary artery and a PDA) ▶ there is a diminutive ascending aorta with the coronary arteries supplied by retrograde flow through the PDA
  - *After birth:* the PDA closes and the presence of a restrictive patent foramen ovale leads to increasing cyanosis, heart failure and early death

Clinical presentation

- Neonatal congestive heart failure occurring soon after birth

Radiological features

CXR Pulmonary plethora and oedema ▶ a prominent right heart

CMR This assesses the 3D anatomy, complications, function and flow (at all stages)

Pearl

- **Treatment:** a surgical Norwood procedure (pulmonary artery to descending aorta conduit with pulmonary artery banding) with subsequent conversion to a total cavopulmonary connection (TCPC)

TOTAL ANOMALOUS PULMONARY VENOUS DRAINAGE (TAPVD)

Definition

- The pulmonary veins coalesce posterior to the left atrium but do not drain into it (as would be the case in a normal circulation) ▶ the venous return is via the right atrium:
  - **Supracardiac (type I):** venous return via a left ascending vein (a remnant of the left embryological SVC) which then connects with the left brachiocephalic vein and then the SVC
    - This is the most common type
  - **Cardiac (type II):** venous return via an enlarged coronary sinus directly into the right atrium
  - **Infracardiac (type III):** venous return via a descending vein, passing through the diaphragm and into either the IVC or portal venous system
    - This is the least common type
  - **Mixed (type IV):** a combination of the above (10%)
- Total cardiac mixing occurs at the right atrial level with a partial cyanosis ▶ a patent foramen ovale or an ASD is necessary to sustain life

Clinical presentation

Infracardiac type There is usually a degree of obstruction (as the descending vein passes through the diaphragm)

- There is therefore pulmonary congestion, tachypnoea, tachycardia, hepatomegaly, cyanosis, pulmonary oedema and respiratory distress and is more severe than the others
- This occurs several days after birth

Cardiac/supracardiac types These present with a left-to-right shunt and cardiac failure ▶ it is asymptomatic at birth

Radiological features

CXR

- **Cardiac/supracardiac:** pulmonary plethora (left-to-right shunt)
  - *Cardiomegaly*
  - *The supracardiac type can result in the 'snowman' or 'figure of eight' appearance:* the widened mediastinal shadow results from a dilated SVC, vertical vein and innominate vein
- **Infracardiac:**
  - A normal heart size
  - Interstitial oedema and heart failure (due to the pulmonary circulation obstruction)

CT/CMR These are often useful even though an anomalous pulmonary venous connection is usually easily visualized with echocardiography

Pearls

Associations Complex cardiac anomalies: e.g. heterotaxy syndromes (in particular right isomerism) ▶ AVSD ▶ pulmonary stenosis ▶ DORV ▶ HLHS ▶ a common arterial trunk ▶ transposition of the great arteries ▶ aortic coarctation

Partial anomalous pulmonary venous drainage (PAPVD)

- Some (but not all) of the pulmonary veins drain into either the right atrium, SVC or IVC
- It is commonly associated with an ASD (the sinus venosus type)

Scimitar syndrome An anomalous pulmonary vein drains down to the IVC below the level of the diaphragm (and is commonly right sided) ▶ it is associated with hypoplasia of the right lung

CXR A curved vessel is seen in the right lower zone (mimicking a scimitar sword), widening as it approaches the cardiophrenic angle

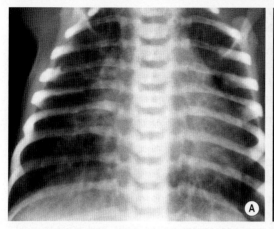

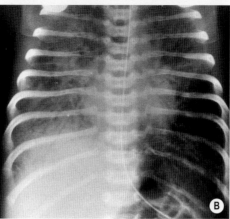

HLHS with mitral atresia. (A) The heart is enlarged and the pulmonary vessels are slightly hazy, suggesting minimal pulmonary oedema. (B) The heart is of normal size but severe pulmonary oedema exists. The difference between these two patients is that the patient in (B) has a restrictive ASD that prevents decompression of the left atrial hypertension.●

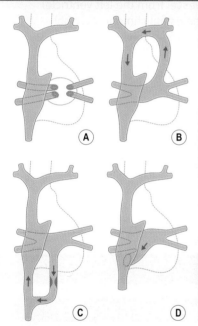

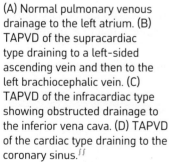

(A) Normal pulmonary venous drainage to the left atrium. (B) TAPVD of the supracardiac type draining to a left-sided ascending vein and then to the left brachiocephalic vein. (C) TAPVD of the infracardiac type showing obstructed drainage to the inferior vena cava. (D) TAPVD of the cardiac type draining to the coronary sinus.ʃʃ

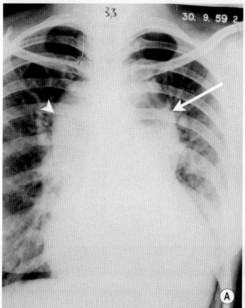

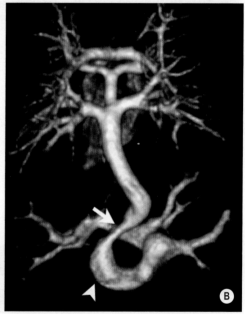

Total anomalous pulmonary venous drainage. (A) PA CXR in a patient with unobstructed supracardiac TAPVD. Note dilated ascending vein (arrow) returning all pulmonary blood to the brachiocephalic vein. The arrowhead shows the dilated SVC. (B) Volume-rendered 3D reconstruction of MR angiography showing total anomalous infracardiac drainage of the pulmonary veins. Note the narrowing of the veins as they pass through the diaphragm (arrow) before draining into the portal vein (arrowhead).**

COMMON ARTERIAL TRUNK (TRUNCUS ARTERIOSUS)

DEFINITION

- This describes a single arterial trunk (truncus) arising from both the ventricles and overriding a large misaligned VSD ▶ there is common mixing of blood across the VSD in all cases
  - It is due to a failure of formation of the spiral septum within the developing truncus arteriosus
- The pulmonary, systemic and coronary arteries originate from the single common arterial trunk ▶ the classification of the common arterial trunk relies on the pulmonary artery branching pattern:
  - **Type I:** a short main pulmonary artery arising from the common trunk and subsequently dividing (the most common type)
  - **Type II:** the right and left pulmonary arteries originate from the posterior wall of the common trunk with a negligible main pulmonary artery
  - **Type III:** the right and left pulmonary arteries emerge independently from the lateral wall of the common trunk

RADIOLOGICAL FEATURES

CXR Pulmonary plethora (due to increased blood flow through the pulmonary arteries at systemic pressures) ▶ an enlarged aortic shadow representing the truncus ▶ the heart is often moderately enlarged

CMR Its main role is in the assessment of any postoperative complications

PEARLS

- The truncal valve is often abnormal (with varying degrees of stenosis or insufficiency)
- 40% of truncal arches are on the right, and most truncal arches arise higher within the mediastinum than a normal aortic arch
- **Surgical repair:** reconstruction of the common trunk (producing a systemic vessel from the left ventricle) ▶ VSD patch closure and establishment of a right ventricle-to-pulmonary arterial conduit

COR TRIATRIUM

DEFINITION

- This is a rare congenital anomaly – the pulmonary veins and immediately related left atrium are separated from the main body of the left atrium by a perforated fibromuscular septum

CLINICAL PRESENTATION

- Symptoms depend upon the size of the septal orifice – it may present with a syndrome similar to that seen with a mitral valve stenosis with pulmonary venous congestion and oedema

RADIOLOGICAL FEATURES

CXR A normal-sized heart ▶ increased pulmonary vessel size (due to pulmonary venous hypertension) ▶ pulmonary oedema

Echocardiography This is the best method of diagnosis

PEARLS

- **Associated with:** septal defects ▶ anomalous pulmonary venous drainage ▶ tetralogy of Fallot
- **Treatment:** surgical excision of the septum

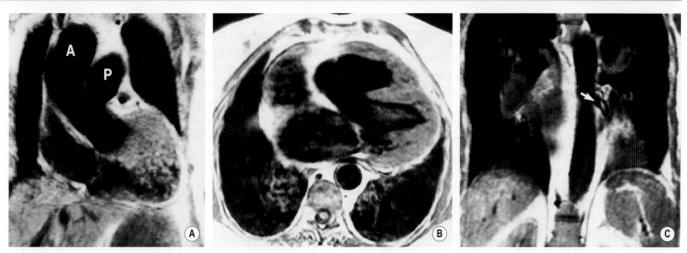

CMR of truncus arteriosus. (A) The coronal slice shows the large heart with the trunk originating as the single great artery from the heart. (B) The axial slice shows the 4 heart chambers and the large VSD. (C) The descending thoracic aorta has several aortopulmonary arteries (arrow) supplying the left lower lobe.

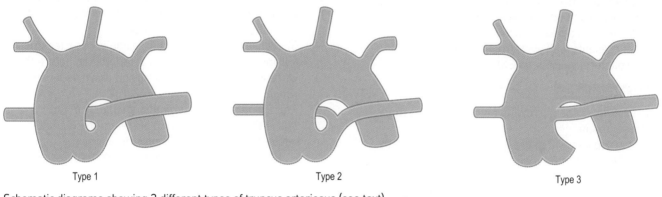

Type 1   Type 2   Type 3

Schematic diagrams showing 3 different types of truncus arteriosus (see text).

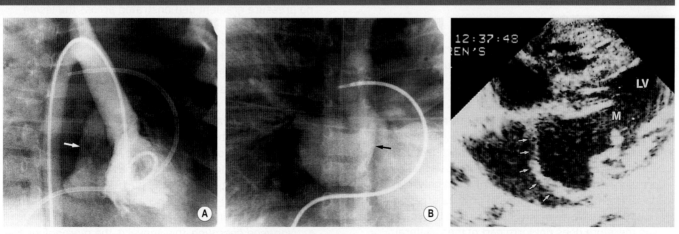

Cor triatrium. (A) Mitral regurgitation during a left ventriculogram outlines the left side of the membrane (arrow) of the cor triatrium and the appendage of the left atrium. (B) The venous phase of a right pulmonary arteriogram shows the right side of the membrane (arrow) and the connection with the pulmonary veins.

Subcostal echocardiogram of a patient with cor triatrium. A prominent membrane runs across the left atrium (arrows). M = mitral valve ▶ LV = left ventricle.

AORTIC COARCTATION

Definition

- An area of short thoracic aortic narrowing, with 95% occurring just beyond the origin of the left subclavian artery (the aortic isthmus) ▶ it rarely occurs within the more distal thoracic or abdominal aorta (where it can cause a 'mid aortic' syndrome)
- Occurs secondary to ductal tissue around the aortic isthmus contracting with the ductus arteriosus at birth ▶ compensatory mechanisms include renal (hypertension) + collateral formation
  - **Infantile type:** this usually occurs proximal to the ductus arteriosus ▶ as the ductus closes at birth this results in a reduced blood supply to the distal aorta with resultant heart failure (as no collateral pathways were required in utero) ▶ 50% are associated with other congenital heart defects
    - It presents with systemic hypertension and a failure to thrive
  - **Adult type:** this usually occurs distal to the ductus arteriosus and left subclavian artery – therefore collaterals are able to develop in utero
    - It presents with systemic hypertension and collateral vessels on CXR

Clinical presentation

- The severity of the narrowing helps determine the age of presentation:
  - It can present within the first few days of life with cardiac enlargement and failure
  - It is often asymptomatic in young adults (presenting with systemic hypertension and femoral pulses that are delayed and weakened compared to the carotid and upper limb pulses)
- It affects males in 80% of cases – in females it is associated with Turner's syndrome

Radiological features

Echocardiography This is used for the initial diagnosis in neonates ▶ it can be used for follow-up but MRI or CT are preferred as children grow older

CXR

- **A prominent left cardiac border:** this represents left ventricular hypertrophy
- **Inferior rib notching:** this is due to dilated collateral intercostal arteries bypassing the stenosis and causing pressure erosion of the inferior ribs ▶ it only involves ribs 3 to 8 (the first 2 intercostal arteries arise from the costocervical trunk which is proximal to the coarctation and therefore does not form part of the collateral circulation) ▶ usually bilateral but asymmetric
  - Rib notching is rare before 5 years of age
- **A unilateral absence of rib notching:** this can occur on the left with a stenosed or occluded left subclavian artery ▶ it can occur on the right in association with an anomalous origin of the right subclavian artery from below the coarctation
- 'Figure of 3' sign: this is due to prestenotic dilatation of the ascending aorta, indentation at the coarctation site and poststenotic dilatation of the descending aorta

Contrast-enhanced MRI This is the diagnostic study of choice ▶ 3D contrast-enhanced MRA may display the severity and extent of involvement ▶ MR flow mapping can define the stenosis severity by measuring the jet velocity at the level of the coarctation ▶ it can also assess any collateral flow or secondary pathologies (e.g. aortic root dilatation secondary to a bicuspid aortic valve)

Pearls

- **Associations:** coarctation is associated with a bicuspid aortic valve and a hypoplastic aortic arch ▶ it is the most common cardiac abnormality seen in Turner's syndrome
- **Treatment:**
  - *Resection and an end-to-end anastomosis:* if the lesion is short and the aorta can be mobilized ▶ this gives the best long-term result
  - *Subclavian patch repair:* the lesion is resected and a transected left subclavian artery (taken before the vertebral arterial origin) is turned down as a patch repair
  - *Percutaneous transluminal angioplasty (PTA):* this is the primary method of treatment in adults, adolescents and children outside of infancy
    - Post-surgical re-coarctation: a 90% success rate
    - A native coarctation: an 80% success rate
  - *Stent insertion:* this should be reserved for an initial failure of PTA due to elastic recoil ▶ this is not used in infants unless as a short-term measure in the critically ill (the stent will not stretch)
- **Pseudocoarctation:** an asymptomatic variant with no pressure gradient demonstrated across the lesion (thus although a 'figure of 3' sign is present, there is no associated rib notching)
- **Aortic atresia:** the ascending aorta is variable in size (but is usually very small and no larger than one of the brachiocephalic arteries) ▶ blood flow from the heart to the aorta is through the pulmonary trunk and ductus (with the aortic arch filling retrogradely) ▶ the brachiocephalic branches arise normally from the aortic arch and the coronary arteries are supplied via the diminutive ascending aorta) ▶ survival depends upon maintaining the patency of the ductus arteriosus (via prostaglandin E_1) ▶ it is associated with the hypoplastic left heart syndrome
  - *Norwood operation:* this converts the morphological right ventricle into a systemic ventricle by anastomosing the pulmonary trunk to the ascending aorta (with excision of the atrial septum) ▶ pulmonary arterial blood flow is maintained through a modified Blalock–Taussig shunt – the ductus is then closed

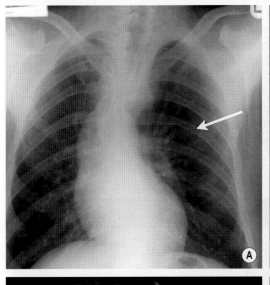

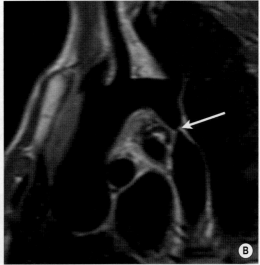

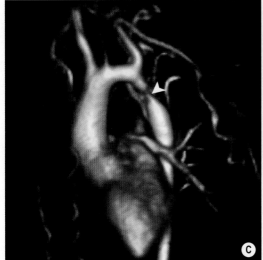

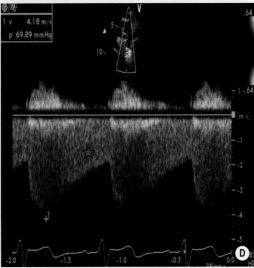

Severe coarctation of the aorta. (A) PA CXR showing characteristic bilateral rib-notching (arrow), secondary to the development of collateral circulation. (B) Black-blood, spin-echo, oblique sagittal image through the aorta showing a tight discrete coarctation (arrow). (C) Volume-rendered 3D reconstruction of MR angiography showing a tight coarctation (arrowhead), and multiple enlarged collateral vessels. (D) Echocardiographic continuous-wave Doppler profile of the coarctation region, demonstrating increased velocity across the stenosis, 4.18 m/s (blue cross), corresponding to a pressure gradient of 70 mmHg from the simplified Bernoulli equation. There is also markedly increased diastolic velocity, characteristic in coarctation, termed 'diastolic tail' (red star).**

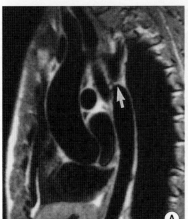

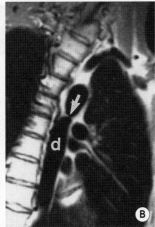

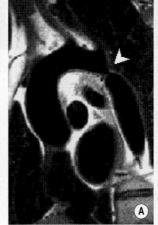

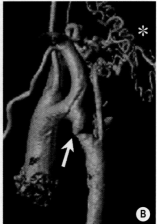

Post-ductal coarctation of the aorta showing a narrowed diaphragm (arrowed) on (A) sagittal-oblique and (B) coronal-oblique intermediate-weighted ECG-gated spin echo (SE 1000/21) scans. Note the dilated collateral vessels supplying the descending aorta (d) beyond the coarctation.[†]

Aortic coarctation. (A) Oblique sagittal CMR through a severe, discrete aortic coarctation (arrowhead). (B) 3D, volume-rendered MRA image of another severe aortic coarctation (arrow), with multiple collaterals (asterisk).*

VASCULAR RINGS AND AORTIC ARCHES

- **Vascular ring:** an anomalous aortic arch configuration (± involvement of the arch vessels) which completely or incompletely surrounds the trachea and oesophagus ▶ it is associated with compressive effects that can lead to respiratory distress (neonates) and stridor or dysphagia (older children)
  - *The most common complete vascular rings (85–95%):* a double aortic arch ▶ a right aortic arch with a left ligamentum arteriosum
- From about 4 weeks' gestation there are paired ventral aortas joined to paired dorsal aortas by 6 pairs of arterial arches (which are never all present simultaneously) ▶ the 4th arch is the most important when considering vascular rings:
  - *A normal left aortic arch:* the left 4th branchial arch persists
  - *A double aortic arch:* both the left and right 4th arches persist
  - *A right aortic arch:* the left 4th aortic arch involutes and the right 4th arch persists

DOUBLE AORTIC ARCH

- The persistence of both aortic arches, with the formation of a vascular ring
- The right arch is usually higher and larger than the left arch (which may be atretic or hypoplastic)
- The normal left arch (anterior to the trachea) joins the descending thoracic aorta after giving off the left subclavian artery (the posterior right aortic arch joins the thoracic aorta at the same level)
- The descending aorta is more commonly present on the left ▶ the ligamentum arteriosum is positioned normally
- The vascular ring, so formed, potentially compresses the trachea and oesophagus
  - *AP barium swallow / CXR:* bilateral oesophageal and tracheal indentations (with the right indentation usually higher than the left)
  - *Lateral barium swallow:* an anterior tracheal indentation and a posterior oesophageal impression

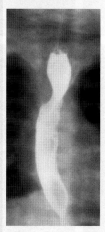

Barium swallow in a child with a double aortic arch. Note the constant impressions on either side of the oesophagus.

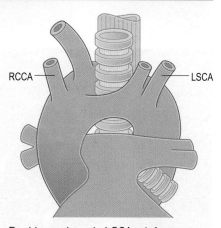

Double aortic arch. LSCA = left subclavian artery, RCCA = right common carotid artery.

RIGHT AORTIC ARCH WITH ABERRANT LEFT SUBCLAVIAN ARTERY AND LEFT LIGAMENTUM ARTERIOSUM

- The right arch first gives off the left carotid artery (which travels anterior to trachea), then the right carotid and subclavian arteries
- The final branch is the left subclavian artery which courses in a retro-oesophageal position and gives rise to the ligamentum arteriosum from its base – this completes the ring as it attaches to the pulmonary artery
  - *Lateral barium swallow:* an anterior tracheal indentation and a posterior oesophageal impression

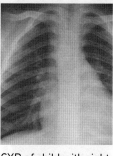

CXR of child with right aortic arch. Stridor in this situation suggests the presence of a vascular ring.

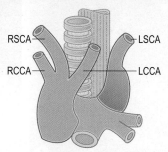

Diagram of right aortic arch with aberrant left subclavian artery and left ligamentum arteriosum. LCCA = left common carotid artery, LSCA = left subclavian artery, RCCA = right common carotid artery, RSCA = right subclavian artery.

RIGHT AORTIC ARCH WITH MIRROR-IMAGE BRANCHING AND A RETRO-OESOPHAGEAL LIGAMENTUM ARTERIOSUM

- The first vessel originating from the right arch is the left innominate artery (this branches into the left carotid and left subclavian arteries, which both course anterior to the trachea) ▶ the right carotid and subclavian arteries then arise
- The final structure arising from the arch is the ligamentum arteriosum (it originates from the Kommerell diverticulum, which represents the non-resorbed left 4th arch remnant) ▶ the ligamentum passes leftward and behind the oesophagus and then travels anteriorly to join the left pulmonary artery (completing the ring)
  - *Lateral barium swallow:* posterior oesophageal impression

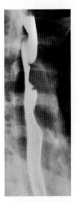
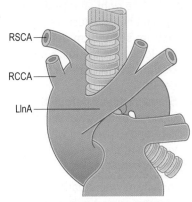

Barium swallow in a child with a vascular ring. Note the constant posterior impressions on the oesophagus.*

Diagram of right aortic arch with mirror-image branching and retro-oesophageal ligamentum arteriosum. LInA = left innominate artery, RCCA = right common carotid artery, RSCA = right subclavian artery.

LEFT AORTIC ARCH WITH RIGHT DESCENDING AORTA AND RIGHT LIGAMENTUM ARTERIOSUM

- The first arch vessel to exit the left aortic arch is the right common carotid, which passes anterior to the trachea ▶ this is followed by the left carotid, left subclavian artery and finally the right subclavian artery ▶ the latter arises more distally as a branch of the proximal right-sided descending aorta
- The ligamentum arteriosum arises from the base of the right subclavian artery or a nearby diverticulum and travels to the right pulmonary artery

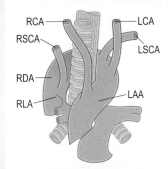

Diagram showing an example of a left-sided aortic arch with right descending aorta and right ligamentum arteriosum. LAA = left aortic arch, RLA = right ligamentum arteriosum, RDA = right descending aorta, RSCA = right subclavian artery, LSCA = left subclavian artery, LCA = left carotid artery, RCA = right carotid artery.

NORMAL LEFT AORTIC ARCH WITH AN ABERRANT RETRO-OESOPHAGEAL RIGHT SUBCLAVIAN ARTERY

- This is the most common congenital aortic arch anomaly (affecting 0.5% of the population) ▶ it is usually asymptomatic
- The right subclavian artery is the last brachiocephalic aortic branch arising from the descending aorta (it does not arise from an innominate trunk together with the right carotid artery)
- The majority run behind the oesophagus (a minority run between the oesophagus and trachea, or anterior to the trachea) ▶ oesophageal compression can cause dysphagia (dysphagia lusoria)
  - *Lateral barium swallow:* posterior oesophageal impression
    - *NB:* an aberrant left pulmonary artery will cause a posterior tracheal indentation and an anterior oesophageal impression

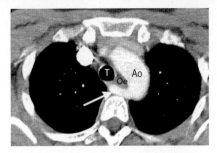
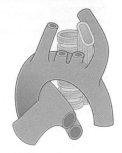

Aberrant right subclavian artery. Barium swallow: CECT confirms the presence of a left-sided aortic arch (Ao) with aberrant right subclavian artery (arrow) travelling posterior to the oesophagus (Oe) and trachea (T).†

Oblique diagram showing a normal left aortic arch with an aberrant retro-oesophageal right subclavian artery.

Atrial septal defect (ASD)

Definition A 'hole' or defect in the interatrial septum with a left to right shunt – this is the most common adult congenital heart defect

- **Ostium secundum defect:** the commonest type (80%) ▶ it is located in the fossa ovalis
- **Ostium primum defect:** a partial atrioventricular septal defect
- **Sinus venosus defect:** this is located at the junction of either of the caval veins and the right atrium ▶ it is rare and associated with partial anomalous pulmonary venous drainage

Clinical presentation

- Initially asymptomatic (the right ventricle can usually accommodate the low pressure left-to-right shunting)
- It can present during late childhood or early adulthood with volume overload (e.g. atrial dilatation and tachyarrythmias) ▶ it is associated with an increased risk of a paradoxical thromboembolic stroke (via the defect)

Radiological features

CXR This is usually normal if the pulmonary-to-systemic flow ratio is < 2:1 ▶ if it is greater than this then there can be mild pulmonary plethora and cardiac enlargement (the left atrium is normal unlike with a VSD)

Transoesophageal echocardiography This is the main imaging technique (although it cannot quantify any shunt accurately)

Transthoracic echocardiography Limited utility

CMR This is used if there remains doubt with regard to the anatomy or its functional significance

Pearls

- **Management:** transcatheter ASD mechanical closure devices or open surgical closure for larger defects
- **Holt–Oram syndrome:** an ostium secundum defect + absent or hypoplastic forearms and thumbs
- **Lutembacher's syndrome:** ASD + mitral stenosis

Atrioventricular septal defect (AVSD)

Definition Normally the membranous interventricular septum (derived from endocardial cushion tissue) is in contact with the atrial septum primum – this central structure is missing in all AVSD types, resulting in a large left-to-right shunt and admixing of the blood

- **Partial:** a defect of the atrial septum alone (also known as an ostium primum ASD)
- **Complete:** defects of both the atrial and ventricular septae
  - It is divided into **balanced** (relatively equal-sized atrioventricular valves and ventricles) or **unbalanced** (inflow through the atrioventricular valves is mainly into one ventricle)

Radiological features

CXR Cardiac enlargement and failure ▶ pulmonary plethora ▶ there are no specific features to differentiate it from an ASD or VSD

Echocardiography The usual method of diagnosis

Angiography A 'gooseneck' deformity of the left ventricular outflow tract with abnormal prolapsing of the anterior mitral valve leaflet during diastole

Pearls The atrioventricular valves are commonly malformed (allowing regurgitation)

- A partial defect is associated with Down's syndrome and other complex anomalies (e.g. atrial isomerism/Fallots/ subaortic stenosis/ventricular hypoplasia)
- **Treatment:** complex surgical atrioventricular valve reconstruction as well as closure of the septal defect

Ventricular septal defect (VSD)

Definition A 'hole' or defect within the ventricular septum – this is the most common congenital heart defect ▶ left → right shunt

- **Perimembranous defect** (80%): this involves the membranous septum (± the adjacent muscle close to the aortic root and tricuspid valve) ▶ the majority close spontaneously ▶ large lesions may remain open, leading to the development of Eisenmenger's syndrome
- **Muscular defect** (5–20%): lesions occur within the interventricular septum ▶ they can occur within the inlet, mid muscular, or outlet (conal) regions
- **'Restrictive' defect:** high-velocity shunt indicating preservation of pressure differences between LV + RV
- **'Unrestrictive' defect:** low-velocity jet indicating similar pressures between LV + RV

Clinical presentation

- **A small defect:** this has a late presentation ▶ it can be asymptomatic or present with a pansystolic murmur
- **A large defect:** this presents a few days or weeks after birth with breathlessness and feeding difficulties

Radiological features

CXR

- *Small shunt:* a normal CXR
- *Large shunt:* enlargement of the ventricles, left atrium and pulmonary vessels

Echocardiography This is used as the first assessment (particularly with Doppler flow) which can assess degree of shunting

CMR Left-to-right shunt quantification (using velocity-encoded phase-contrast MR) ▶ it is often better than echocardiography at demonstrating complex muscular defects ▶ it can assess additional cardiac abnormalities (such as aortic coarctation or stenosis) which can be seen in 50% of patients

Pearls

- **Surgical treatment:** patch closure (this can be difficult with some muscular defects)
  - 75% of defects close spontaneously by late childhood
- **Gerbode defect:** a communication through a small portion of the basal septum which separates the left ventricular outflow tract from the right atrium

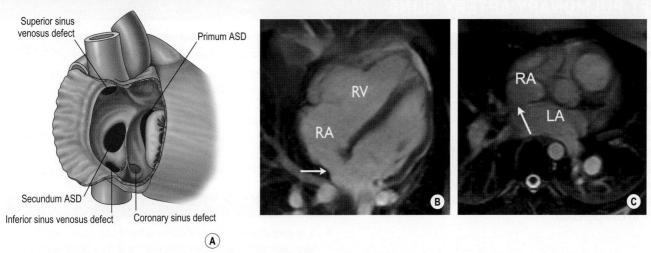

Atrial septal defects. (A) Schematic drawing of ASD positions. (B) b-SSFP CMR image. Four-chamber view showing a large secundum ASD with posterior extension. The absence of a posterior rim (arrow) precludes insertion of an ASD closure device. Note the dilated right atrium (RA), and right ventricle (RV), and flattened interventricular septum. (C) b-SSFP CMR image. Axial view showing a large superior sinus venosus defect, with PAPVD of the right upper and right middle pulmonary veins, straddling the deficient atrial septum (arrow).**

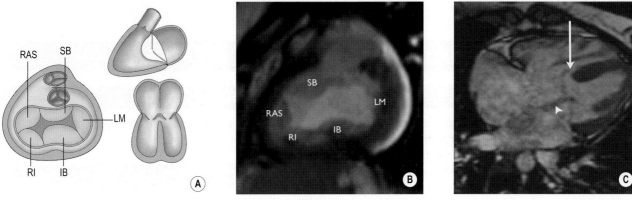

Atrioventricular septal defects. (A) Schematic drawing of orthogonal views of a common atrioventricular valve: short-axis view from below (left), long-axis (top right), 4-chamber (bottom right). (B) Valve view showing a complete AVSD in a patient with right atrial isomerism and double outlet RV. Valve leaflets: SB = superior bridging leaflet, RAS = right anterosuperior leaflet, RI = right inferior (mural) leaflet, IB = inferior bridging leaflet, LM = left mural leaflet. (C) b-SSFP CMR image showing 4-chamber view of a balanced complete AVSD. There are large atrial and ventricular components. Note the VSD (arrow) and moderate left AV valve regurgitation (arrowhead).**

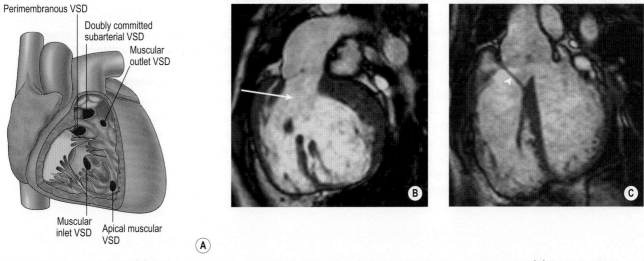

Ventricular septal defects. (A) Schematic drawing of VSD positions viewed from the right ventricular aspect. (B) b-SSFP CMR image of a VSD (arrow) with overriding aorta in a patient with tetralogy of Fallot. (C) Coronal oblique view following correction with VSD patch (arrowhead).**

LEFT PULMONARY ARTERY SLING

DEFINITION

- The left pulmonary artery arises from the proximal right pulmonary artery
- It then turns abruptly posteriorly and to the left (indenting and compressing the trachea anteriorly and the oesophagus posteriorly)
- It is associated with cardiovascular and tracheooesophageal anomalies
- The major respiratory abnormality is stenosis in the right main stem bronchus and the tracheal bifurcation due to compression

RADIOLOGICAL FEATURES

Barium swallow The aberrant left pulmonary artery appears as a mass between the trachea and the oesophagus CXR The right main bronchial stenosis can lead to air trapping:
- An opaque right upper lobe due to poor clearing of fetal fluid
- Lobar emphysema with a hyperlucent lung

PEARL

- It is one of the few conditions where the abnormal vascular structure runs anterior to the oesophagus

CONGENITAL AORTIC STENOSIS

DEFINITION

- Haemodynamic consequence is pressure loading of the left ventricle with secondary hypertrophy – aortic regurgitation is usually a manifestation of treated aortic stenosis (e.g. balloon angioplasty) or secondary to pathological dilatation of the aortic root
- **Subvalvular**
  - This ranges from a simple diaphragm to a more complex tubular narrowing ▶ least common form and usually secondary to hypertrophic cardiomyopathy
- **Valvular**
  - This is usually due to a bicuspid aortic valve – although these are not themselves stenotic they tend to calcify leading to an adult stenosis ▶ there is an association with coarctation of the aorta
  - *Other types*: a unicommissural (single horseshoe-shaped) valve or partial fusion of the valve leaflets
- **Supravalvular**
  - Rare ▶ this most commonly occurs with Williams' syndrome which is a genetic disorder of elastin formation (elastin is responsible for the normal aortic distensibility and recoil) ▶ reduced elastin and increased arterial wall, smooth muscle deposition leading to either a characteristic hourglass narrowing of the aorta (in 30% there is diffuse narrowing of the ascending aorta)

CLINICAL PRESENTATION

- Severe cases will present in infancy with heart failure and left ventricular dilatation

RADIOLOGICAL FEATURES

CXR Left ventricular hypertrophy ▶ aortic post stenotic dilatation is only seen with valvular causes

Doppler USS
- *Colour Doppler:* determine extension and width of regurgitant jet
- *Continuous-wave Doppler:* assess rate of decline of aortic regurgitant flow
- Transvalvular pressure gradients are flow dependent, and measurement of a combination of valve area transvalvular pressure gradient is preferred (+ ventricular function)
- A valve area < 1 cm^2 is considered severe

CMR Valvular stenosis can be identified by loss of signal on cine images (+ velocity mapping) ▶ CMR allows precise assessment of regurgitant volume and LV function (and regurgitant orifice area)

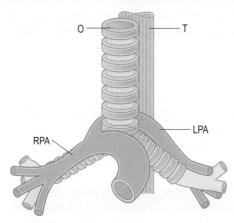

Pulmonary artery sling. The left pulmonary artery (LPA) originates from the right pulmonary artery (RPA) and passes between the trachea (T) and oesophagus (O). This location of the aberrant pulmonary artery frequently creates a stenosis in the trachea and left mainstem bronchus.

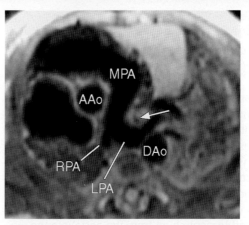

Pulmonary artery sling. CMR. The arrow indicates the severely compressed trachea, anterior to the left pulmonary artery (LPA). There is also significant mediastinal shift to the right chest.

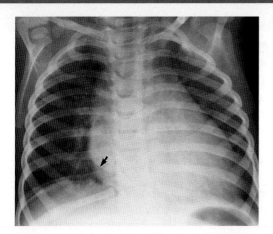

Aortic stenosis in the infant. The heart is globally enlarged with leftward dilatation of the apex. The large left atrium has a double density (arrow) which projects into the lung. The pulmonary hila have mild oedema.

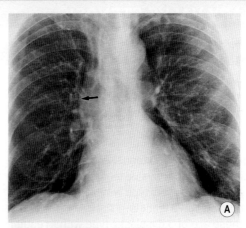

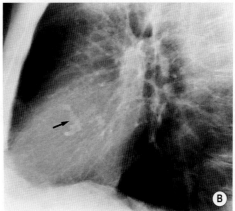

Aortic stenosis in the adult. (A) The ascending aorta is mildly dilated (arrow). (B) The aortic valve (arrow) is irregularly calcified.

PATENT DUCTUS ARTERIOSUS

DEFINITION

- A persisting communication between aorta and pulmonary artery (if the ductus arteriosus fails to close after birth)
- The ductus arteriosus is a normal fetal blood pathway (directing pulmonary arterial blood flow away from the non-functioning lungs and directly into the aorta) ▶ it usually closes spontaneously within the first few days of life in response to changes in blood gas composition (but remains open longer in premature infants especially if there is associated hyaline membrane disease)
- A large PDA will have similar effects to a large VSD as it permits a left to right shunt from the aorta into the pulmonary artery throughout the cardiac cycle ▶ this leads to pressure and volume overload of the pulmonary circulation (± Eisenmenger's syndrome)

CLINICAL PRESENTATION

- A continuous murmur

RADIOLOGICAL FEATURES

- **CXR**
  - *Small shunt:* this can be normal
  - *Large shunt:* identical features to those seen with a VSD (pulmonary plethora and cardiac enlargement) ▶ an enlarged aortic arch (cf. a small arch with a VSD) ▶ the ductus can calcify in later life
- **Echocardiography** This demonstrates a persistent communication

PEARLS

- **Treatment:** indomethacin (which inhibits PGE_1 which is a ductus dilator) ▶ closure may be via surgical ligation or a catheter device (closure reduces the infective endocarditis risk)
  - A PDA is usually surgically closed to avoid the risk of endocarditis

PULMONARY VALVE STENOSIS

DEFINITION

- Classified as valvular, subvalvular (infundibular) or supravalvular ▶ can occur as an isolated finding, or together with other lesions such VSDs or more complex lesions (e.g. tetralogy of Fallot)
- The most common form of pulmonary stenosis is an isolated pulmonary valve stenosis with fusion or thickening of the pulmonary valve leaflets
  - *Majority:* a 'dome-shaped' type with a small valve orifice and fused valve leaflets
  - *Minority:* these are of a dysplastic type with irregular thickened valve leaflets that are not fused
- There can also be infundibular stenosis with right ventricular hypertrophy causing systolic narrowing of the outflow tract as well as a distal pulmonary stenosis involving the main pulmonary artery or its branches

CLINICAL PRESENTATION

- It is usually asymptomatic (if severe it can present during the neonatal period)
- Breathlessness (± cyanosis and heart failure) may be features

RADIOLOGICAL FEATURES

- **CXR** Right ventricular hypertrophy ▶ a prominent main pulmonary artery due to post stenotic dilatation
  - Whilst the proximal left pulmonary artery is also dilated (as it lies in a direct line with the main vessel), the right pulmonary artery is not usually dilated (as it branches quite sharply from the main pulmonary artery)
- **Echocardiography** Doppler studies are the key to diagnosis (detecting high velocity through the stenosis)
  - *Mild stenosis:* peak velocity < 3 m/s (corresponding to a peak gradient < 36 mmHg)
  - *Moderate stenosis:* peak velocity 3–4 m/s (peak gradient 36–64 mmHg)
  - *Severe stenosis:* peak velocity > 4 m/s (peak gradient > 64 mmHg)
- **CT/CMR** These are used for post-surgical follow up

PEARLS

- It is frequently associated with an ASD or a patent foramen ovale ▶ a dysplastic pulmonary valve is often seen with Noonan's syndrome
- **Treatment**: balloon valvuloplasty in the first instance ▶ possibly surgical or transcatheter pulmonary valve implantation at a later date

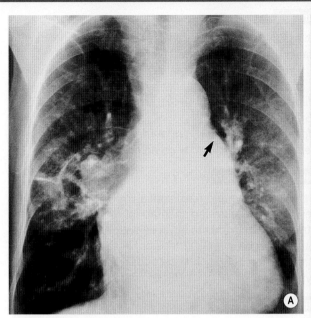
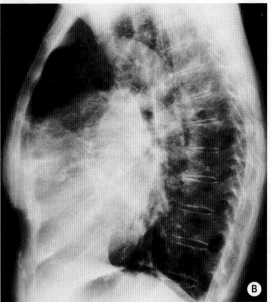

Calcified PDA (arrow). PA (A) and lateral (B) CXR. Moderate pulmonary hypertension has enlarged the hilar arteries and the right ventricle. The large aortic arch indicates the site of the shunt is extracardiac.

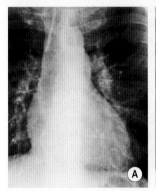
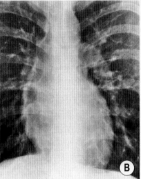
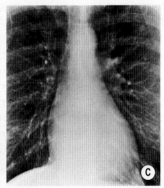

Pulmonary valve stenosis. Variations in appearance. (A) Typical appearance is a normal cardiothoracic ratio, convex main pulmonary artery segment and a dilated left pulmonary artery. (B) The main pulmonary artery is not enlarged with a straight segment. The left pulmonary artery is dilated and tapers rapidly. (C) An ASD and pulmonary stenosis create a mixed pattern of shunt vascularity plus a large left pulmonary artery. The main pulmonary artery segment is straight.●

Shunts: acyanotic left-to-right shunt and cyanotic right-to-left shunt*			
Acyanotic		**Cyanotic**	
Abnormal communication	Left-to-right shunt if no obstruction	Abnormal communication + distal right heart obstruction	Shunt reversal with distal obstruction. Right-to-left shunt
ASD	LA → RA	TS/PS/ER	RA → LA
VSD	LV → RV	PS/ER	RV → LV
PDA	Ao → PA	ER	PA → Ao
APW	Ao → PA	ER	PA → Ao
Ao = aorta, APW = aortopulmonary window, ASD = atrial septal defect, LA = left atrium, LV = left ventricle, PA = pulmonary artery, PDA = patent ductus arteriosus, PS = pulmonary stenosis or atresia, RA = right atrium, RV = right ventricle, TS = tricuspid stenosis or atresia.			

MITRAL REGURGITATION

Definition

- An incompetent mitral valve allowing regurgitant flow from the left ventricle (LV) into the left atrium (LA) during systole (mid-to-late systolic murmur) ▶ maintaining an adequate stroke volume requires an increased ventricular stroke volume and ejection fraction

Clinical presentation

- *Acute regurgitation* (e.g. ruptured chordae tendineae): sudden volume loading with acute pulmonary oedema/heart failure
- *Chronic regurgitation* (e.g. hypertrophic cardiomyopathy): volume overload with dilated left cardiac chambers ± cardiac failure

Radiological features

CXR Selective left atrial enlargement may be absent, slight or moderate (the left atrial appendage is usually not enlarged)

- *Acute severe non-rheumatic disease:* a normal heart size ▶ pulmonary oedema
- *Later stages:* compensatory left ventricular dilatation

Echocardiography It can assess coaptation of the valve leaflets and any regurgitant jet direction (with Doppler assessment)

CMR mitral regurgitation seen as a retrograde jet through the mitral orifice secondary to turbulent flow and spin dephasing ▶ CMR can also quantify the degree of regurgitant flow (e.g. phase contrast velocity flow mapping)

Pearls

- **Mitral valve prolapse:** systolic bowing of the mitral leaflet >2 mm beyond the annular plane into the atrium (due to rupture or elongation of the chordae tendineae) ▶ most common cause of non-ischaemic mitral regurgitation
- **Chordal rupture:** following bacterial endocarditis or MI leading to eversion of the valve leaflet into the atrium during systole and preventing full closure
- **Functional mitral regurgitation:** occurs in dilated cardiomyopathy or ischaemic failure, with a normal valve
- **Mitral annulus calcification:** this rarely occurs before 70 years of age (F>M) ▶ it is seen with hypercalcaemic states (e.g. end-stage renal disease) ▶ it may lead to mild mitral regurgitation (but rarely stenosis) ▶ there is a possible increased risk of infective endocarditis ▶ it is also associated with transient ischaemic attacks (due to emboli)
  - **CXR** it is seen as a C-shaped open ring (the gap occurs where the anterior mitral valve leaflet base is in contact with the posterior aortic valve ring)
- **Dystrophic calcification of the mitral valve:** unlike mitral annulus calcification this is very suggestive of a rheumatic aetiology

MITRAL STENOSIS

Definition

- This is usually due to chronic rheumatic fever (leading to leaflet thickening/nodularity/commissural fusion)
  - The most common result is a mixture of stenosis and regurgitation (both cannot be severe at the same time)
- *Mild stenosis:* mitral area >1.5 cm^2 ▶ mean gradient <5 mmHg
- *Moderate stenosis:* 1–1.5 cm^2 ▶ mean gradient 5–10 mmHg
- *Severe stenosis:* <1 cm^2 ▶ mean gradient >10 mmHg

Clinical presentation

- It is usually asymptomatic until a critical stenosis develops (e.g. following an attack of rheumatic fever)
- Atrial fibrillation (due to atrial dilatation) ▶ dyspnoea (pulmonary venous hypertension) ▶ sequelae of atrial thrombus embolization ▶ secondary pulmonary arterial hypertension

Radiological features

CXR

- **Left atrial enlargement:** the left atrial appendage is particularly affected (suggesting a rheumatic aetiology) ▶ simple straightening of the left heart border to a large bulge at the appendage ▶ a grossly dilated left atrium can enlarge to the right and also posteriorly (causing oesophageal displacement and dysphagia)
  - A 'double density' behind the heart
  - Widening of the subcarinal angle
  - Left ventricular enlargement is not a feature (cf. mitral regurgitation)
- **Parenchymal lung changes of haemosiderosis and intrapulmonary ossification:** these may appear after several years of pulmonary venous congestion
- **Curvilinear calcification:** this may occur within the left atrial wall or within the clot lining the wall

Echocardiography Standard for diagnosis ▶ evaluates mitral valve morphology and valve mobility

CMR Can show restricted mitral valve opening ▶ thickened leaflets ▶ commissural fusion ▶ antegrade jet due to turbulent flow across a stenotic valve ▶ 'fish mouth' appearance on short axis images ▶ 'hockey stick' appearance due to bowing of a thickened/fibrotic anterior leaflet during diastole ▶ can directly measure the orifice area ▶ mitral valve area can be calculated via mitral flow velocity analysis

Pearls

- Congenital mitral stenosis is rare
- **Treatment:** valve replacement or valvuloplasty for severe stenosis

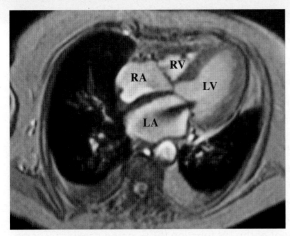

Mitral regurgitation. Axial CMR shows a jet-like signal void in the left atrium due to moderate mitral regurgitation. LA = left atrium, LV = left ventricle, RA = right atrium, RV = right ventricle.*

Causes of mitral regurgitation	
Valve abnormalities	**Supporting structure abnormalities**
Acute rheumatic mitral valve disease	Chordal rupture (e.g. post MI)
Mitral valve prolapse	Papillary muscle rupture dysfunction
Bacterial endocarditis	Functional mitral regurgitation
Prosthetic valve leaks	Mitral annular calcification
Connective tissue diseases (e.g. SLE/RA)	Atrial myxoma

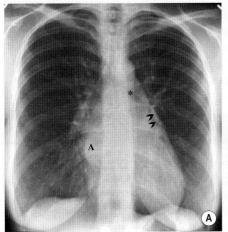

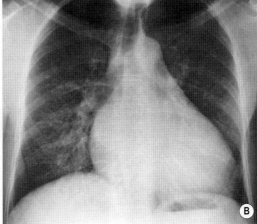

(A) Classical appearance of rheumatic mitral stenosis. PA CXR. The heart size is normal. The enlarged left atrium (A) displaces the left bronchus upwards (asterisk) and creates a right retrocardiac double density. The left atrial appendage is enlarged (arrowheads). There is severe pulmonary venous hypertension. (B) Severe mitral valve disease. Pulmonary haemosiderosis in mitral stenosis. Long-standing severe mitral stenosis. The heart and left atrium are enlarged. Bilateral nodular interstitial prominence is due to pulmonary haemosiderosis.

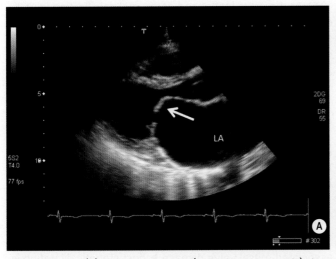

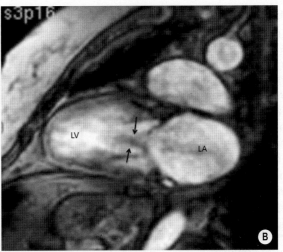

Mitral stenosis. (A) Echocardiography (parasternal long axis) shows marked thickening of mitral leaflets with restricted mitral valve orifice (doming anterior leaflet). Left atrial (LA) enlargement is evident. (B) Cine-MRI frame of mitral stenosis. A small flow void directed from left atrium (LA) to left ventricle (LV) is visible (arrows), due to mild mitral stenosis. Left atrium is enlarged.**

AORTIC REGURGITATION

Definition This may result from aortic valve cusp or aortic wall disease

- **Acute aortic regurgitation:** causes include bacterial endocarditis or rarely occurring after trauma or aortic dissection (with acute avulsion of a leaflet into the left ventricle) ▶ it develops rapidly with increasing left ventricular end-diastolic pressure and acute heart failure
- **Chronic aortic regurgitation:** congenital deformities (e.g. bicuspid aortic valve or Marfan's syndrome) ▶ rheumatic heart disease ▶ syphilitic aortitis ▶ ankylosing spondylitis ▶ a descending aortic aneurysm

Radiological features

Acute

CXR A normal heart size or minor left ventricular enlargement depending on the speed of onset ▶ pulmonary oedema with left heart failure (an important cause of pulmonary oedema with a normal-sized heart) ▶ an unremarkable aorta (unless there is associated aortic disease causing dilatation – e.g. Marfan's syndrome)

Transoesophageal US The technique of choice for displaying aortic vegetations, cusp perforation or aortic root abscesses ▶ regurgitant flow is seen with Doppler imaging

CMR This allows for detection of any aortic regurgitation as well as assessing the aortic valve morphology

Chronic

CXR There may be severe left ventricular enlargement (paralleling the disease severity) ▶ moderate thoracic aortic enlargement (or severe enlargement with aortitis or chronic dissection) ▶ there is infrequent valve calcification ▶ if mitral valve disease is also present then left atrial enlargement may dominate the picture

CMR Precise assessment of regurgitant volume can be estimated from the degree of signal loss ▶ it also allows assessment of the LV function (ECG-gated cardiac CT is an alternative if MRI is contraindicated)

Pearls

- **Chronic disease:** this allows the left ventricle to dilate with an increased compliance ▶ end-diastolic pressures remain low and the patient remains asymptomatic until heart failure develops ▶ once failure develops the prognosis is markedly worsened
- **Acute disease:** ventricular compliance cannot compensate ▶ it is associated with a very large rise in ventricular end-diastolic pressures (limiting regurgitant flow)

AORTIC STENOSIS

Definition Stenosis with a valve area < 1.0 cm^2 is severe ▶ stenosis can be:

- **Supravalvular:** a rare lesion associated with Williams–Beuren syndrome (genetic disorder of elastin which is responsible for aortic recoil) – characteristic hourglass aortic narrowing (or diffuse tubular narrowing of the ascending aorta in 30%)
- **Valvular:**
  - **Calcific aortic stenosis:** this is most commonly due to degenerative calcium deposition on normal aortic cusps (cf. mitral stenosis where calcium is deposited on an already stenosed valve) ▶ it was previously commonly due to calcification of a congenitally deformed bicuspid valve
  - **Rheumatic aortic stenosis:** this causes inflammatory fusion of the commissures of the aortic valve cusps and is often associated with aortic regurgitation and mitral valve involvement ▶ associated with pronounced dyspnoea due to the associated mitral valve disease
- **Subvalvular** (least common): commonly caused by hypertrophic cardiomyopathy

Radiological features

Calcific aortic stenosis

CXR can be normal with significant disease

- Rounding of the cardiac apex (suggesting left ventricular hypertrophy – however there is usually cardiac dilatation which may be marked with aortic regurgitation)
- Localized prominence of the ascending aorta (representing post-stenotic dilatation) ▶ in older patients the whole thoracic aorta may be dilated from atherosclerosis
- Aortic valve calcification (the extent of calcification is only loosely related to the stenotic severity)

Echocardiography Thickened echogenic valve leaflets with reduced mobility

CT Aortic valve leaflet and aortic root calcification is well shown ▶ ultrafast CT can assess the severity of aortic stenosis by imaging the valve opening

CMR Calcified valves appear as a signal void

- It can demonstrate impaired aortic valve opening (and degree of stenosis), the valve morphology and any left ventricular function ($\pm$ hypertrophy)
- Systolic flow dephasing within the aortic root has a loose relationship to the severity of the stenosis
- Diastolic flow dephasing within the left ventricular outflow tract can assess any associated aortic regurgitation
- Phase-contrast systolic gradient echo sequences compare favourably with US

Rheumatic aortic stenosis

CXR The appearances are commonly dominated by any associated mitral valve disease ▶ post stenotic dilatation is rare; gross valvular calcification is rare

Pearls There is a frequent association with coronary artery disease – coronary angiography is therefore necessary prior to valve replacement surgery

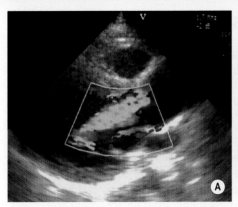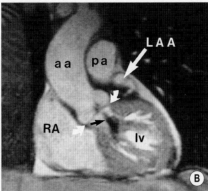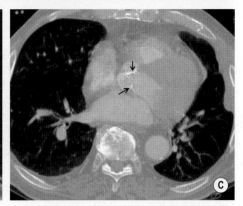

(A) Colour flow Doppler image taken in the parasternal long-axis view. A broad-based jet in a patient with severe aortic regurgitation. (B) Coronal MRA. Oblique breath-hold cine-MRA in a patient with mild aortic regurgitation indicated by the black area of signal loss (black arrow). The left atrial appendage (LAA) is embedded in epicardial fat. There is mild dilatation of the ascending aorta (aa) as a result of the aortic regurgitation. Between curved arrows = aortic valve. lv = left ventricle, pa = pulmonary artery, RA = right atrium. (C) Aortic valve calcification. Axial CT at aortic valve level shows calcification of the aortic leaflets (arrows).

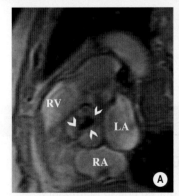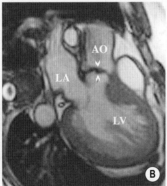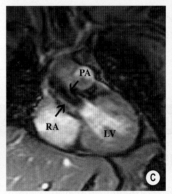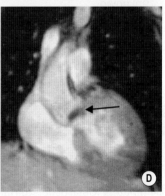

Tricuspid aortic stenosis. CMR of (A) aortic valve view, diastolic image, (B) left ventricular outflow tract (LVOT) view, systolic image, and (C) coronal, ascending aorta view. In the aortic valve view (A), fusion of the commissures of a markedly thickened valve is noted (arrowheads). Doming of the valve leaflets is noted in the LVOT projection (arrowheads) (B). The systolic image demonstrates the turbulent jet (arrows) from aortic stenosis (C). (D) Coronal gradient-echo MRI image (ECG gated) through the left ventricular outflow tract and aortic valve in a patient with calcific aortic stenosis. There is calcification of the aortic valve, which produces a signal void (arrow). AO = ascending aorta, LA = left atrium, LV = left ventricle, PA = pulmonary artery, RA = right atrium, RV = right ventricle.*

TRICUSPID VALVE DISEASE

TRICUSPID REGURGITATION

Causes Usually functional and secondary to: rheumatic disease (less commonly causing stenosis) ▶ endocarditis (often as a complication of IV drug abuse) ▶ pulmonary hypertension (caused by the associated dilated right ventricle) ▶ previous mitral valve replacement ▶ Ebstein's anomaly ▶ endomyocardial fibrosis

Clinical presentation High venous pressures with a big 'v'-wave and a pulsating enlarged liver

CXR An enlarged right atrium (with an increased curvature of the right heart border)

- This appearance has a single margin unlike the 'double heart border' seen with left atrial enlargement (as the IVC limits right atrial expansion)

Echocardiography The definitive method of investigation ▶ a low pressure drop across the valve is seen with severe disease ▶ easily detects retrograde flow in the right atrium

CMR Regurgitant velocities may be so low that they do not cause aliasing and therefore may not immediately be recognized

PEARLS

- Rheumatic tricuspid valve calcification is almost unknown
- Metastatic carcinoid can produce toxic metabolites causing deformity and regurgitation of the tricuspid and pulmonary valves

TRICUSPID STENOSIS

Causes Rheumatic heart disease (usually) ▶ carcinoid syndrome ▶ tumours (especially right atrial myxoma) ▶ endocarditis

- It can result in right atrial and right ventricular enlargement

CXR
- Non-specific cardiac enlargement ▶ there may be dilatation of the superior and inferior vena cava
- In rheumatic heart disease the features of mitral stenosis predominate (left atrial enlargement and pulmonary arterial enlargement)
- Tricuspid valve calcification may be seen (dystrophic degeneration from ageing as well as chronic severe right ventricular hypertension)

Echocardiography Thickened valve leaflets with limited motion ▶ Doppler can measure any jet present

PEARL

- Congenital causes include Ebstein's anomaly or isolated tricuspid stenosis (very rare)
- Usually associated with tricuspid regurgitation and mitral stenosis

PULMONARY VALVE DISEASE

PULMONARY STENOSIS

Definition Obstruction to right ventricular emptying occurs at the valvular, subvalvular or supravalvular level
- Most causes are congenital (see separate section)

Acquired causes

- *Valvular:* carcinoid ▶ rheumatic heart disease (very rare)
- *Subvalvular:* right ventricular hypertrophy ▶ tumour
- *Supravalvular:* carcinoid ▶ rubella ▶ tumour ▶ thrombus ▶ surgical banding ▶ Takayasu's aortoarteritis ▶ Behcet's disease

CXR Valvular stenosis causes post-stenotic dilatation of the main ± left pulmonary artery (the right pulmonary artery is normal size) ▶ right ventricular hypertrophy

PULMONARY REGURGITATION

Definition This is usually acquired due to pulmonary arterial hypertension ▶ pre- and post-stenotic dilatation occurs with dilatation of the right ventricle and central pulmonary arteries
- A congenital cause is the absence of the pulmonary valve in tetralogy of Fallot – characterized by large pulmonary arteries and a narrow pulmonary annulus resulting in stenosis

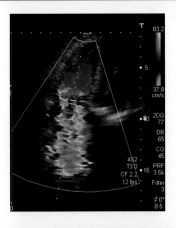

Tricuspid regurgitation. Echo colour Doppler demonstrates severe tricuspid insufficiency with mosaic effect occupying entirely the right atrium.**

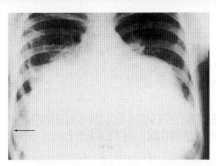

Tricuspid valve disease. Gross right atrial enlargement (arrow), extending to the right, developing in a patient with severe mitral valve disease.*

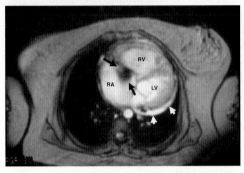

Axial systolic gradient-echo acquisition from a 24-year-old woman with primary pulmonary hypertension. The free wall right ventricular (RV) myocardium is hypertrophied. The heart is rotated toward the left and the interventricular septum is nearly in the coronal plane. The broad signal void jet (black arrows) of tricuspid regurgitation extends into the dilated right atrium (RA). Notice the small pericardial effusion (white arrows). LV = left ventricle. RV = right ventricle.*

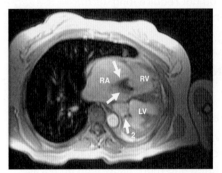

Axial early systolic gradient-echo acquisition from a 24-year-old woman with pulmonary hypertension and agenesis of the left pulmonary artery. The heart is markedly rotated into the left chest. The right ventricular myocardium is moderately hypertrophied. The signal void jet of tricuspid regurgitation (arrows) extends into the dilated right atrium (RA). Also notice the dilated left ventricle (LV) and small jet (arrow 2) of mitral regurgitation. At this anatomic level, the enlargement of the left atrium cannot be appreciated.*

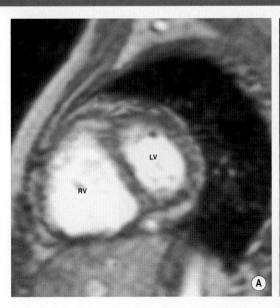

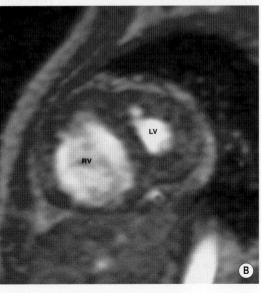

Short-axis gradient-echo acquisition through the mid-heart from a 39-year-old man with primary pulmonary hypertension. (A) End-diastolic image shows dilatation of the right ventricle (RV) with straightening of the interventricular septum. (B) End-systolic image shows thickening of both the right (RV) and left (LV) ventricular myocardium, and straightening of the interventricular septum.*

PROSTHETIC CARDIAC VALVES

- Mechanical valves and bioprostheses are currently available for both aortic and atrioventricular positions
- Postoperative complications tend to be valve-type specific ▶ 5% of patients with an aortic valve replacement die within 5 years

CARDIAC VALVE PROSTHESES IN CURRENT USE AND OF HISTORICAL INTEREST

- **Variety of different prosthetic valves:** central ball occluder valve/eccentric monocuspid disc valve/bileaflet disc valve/bioprosthesis
- **Bioprostheses** (e.g. Carpentier–Edwards porcine prosthesis): these do not require long-term anticoagulation (unlike synthetic valves)

DIAGNOSTIC IMAGING FOLLOWING VALVE IMPLANTATION

Echocardiography The primary method of evaluation, providing a postoperative baseline

PA CXR An aortic valve prosthesis is orientated in partial profile along the direction of flow ▶ a mitral valve is usually more vertically orientated and more likely than an aortic valve to be visualized en face (as mitral flow is towards the cardiac apex)

CMR Artefacts caused by prosthetic valves limits their evaluation

COMPLICATIONS

- **Infective endocarditis:** this is an infrequent complication (up to 4.4%), and occurs most frequently within 6 months of implantation ▶ it is usually due to coagulase-negative staphylococci, streptococci or *Candida albicans*
  - ▪ **Potential sources of infection:** contaminated blood and surgical products ▶ pre-existing infection

▶ indwelling catheters ▶ endotracheal tubes ▶ pacemakers ▶ previous endocarditis ▶ post-surgical wound infection
  - ▪ Infection typically develops within the coronary ostia, ascending aorta and aortic annulus ▶ local abscesses, pannus and vegetations can obstruct valve flow or limit occluder motion ▶ sinus of Valsalva and perivalvular pseudoaneurysms may develop ▶ paravalvular insufficiency can develop as tissue fragments and sutures loosen with infection
- **Valve regurgitation:** minor regurgitation is a normal finding – major regurgitation occurs with sewing ring dehiscence, thrombus, disc wear and valve vegetations ▶ it can lead to sudden cardiac enlargement and pulmonary oedema (with a regurgitant murmur in 80%)
  - ▪ Perivalvular leak occurs more frequently after mechanical valve implantation than with a bioprosthesis
- **Thromboembolism:** thrombosis is more commonly seen involving mitral rather than aortic prostheses ▶ thrombosis reduces the excursion of the occluding ball, disc or leaflet ▶ the risk is decreased with the introduction of cloth-covered prostheses and diminishes with time after implantation
  - ▪ *A surgical emergency:* requiring immediate valve replacement or intervention by catheter remobilization and intracardiac thrombolysis
- **Porcine bioprostheses:** although stent fracture is rare, the major problem is poor durability (cusp tears, degeneration, perforation, fibrosis and calcification appear by the 5th postoperative year) ▶ 20% have failed by year 10 and require reimplantation

PEARL

TAVI: transcatheter aortic valve replacement implantation ▶ technique for non-operable symptomatic critical aortic stenosis ▶ an auto- or balloon-expandable stent with valve delivered percutaneously (transfemoral)

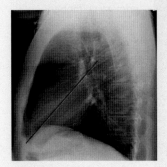

The aortic and pulmonary valves are generally above the red line and the mitral and tricuspid valves generally lie below it.

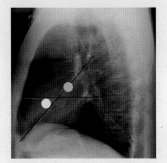

Lateral chest radiograph. A second line is drawn which bisects the cardiac silhouette. Blue = aortic valve, pink = mitral valve, green = pulmonary valve, yellow = tricuspid valve.

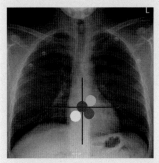

Frontal chest radiograph. A longitudinal line bisects the sternum and a perpendicular line is drawn thereafter. Blue = aortic valve, pink = mitral valve, green = pulmonary valve, yellow = tricuspid valve.

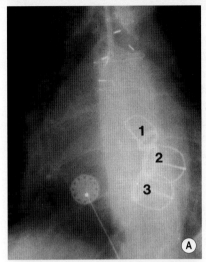

Three Starr–Edwards prostheses in a 53-year-old patient with rheumatic valvular disease. CXR in (A) PA and (B) lateral views. Note the perpendicular orientation of the atrioventricular valves to the aortic valve. 1 = Aortic position, 2 = mitral position, 3 = tricuspid position.

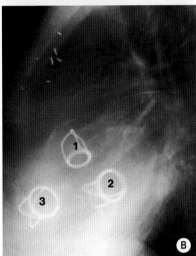

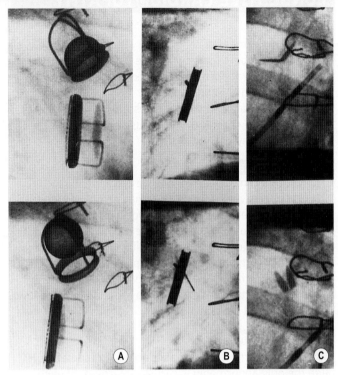

Cine-fluoroscopic findings with commonly implanted prosthetic valves. (A) Starr–Edwards aortic valve in the closed position during diastole and a Beall mitral valve in the open position (upper panel). The lower panel shows the Starr–Edwards valve in the open position during systole and the mitral central occluding the disc Beall valve in the closed position. (B) Upper panel shows a Bjork–Shiley valve in the closed mitral position. Lower panel shows the disc to be 50° from the horizontal baseline (ring) during systole in the open position. (C) In the upper panel, the St Jude aortic bileaflet valve is in the closed position during diastole. In the lower panel, it is in the open position during systole, permitting two blood streams at the outer sides of the leaflets and one stream between the leaflets.*

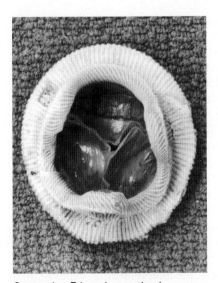

Carpentier–Edwards prosthesis. Photography from the outlet aspect.*

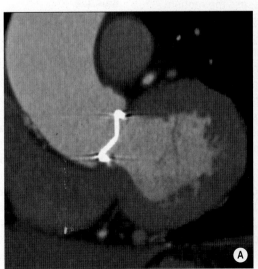

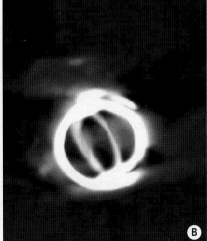

Cardiac CT of mechanical valvular prosthesis. (A) Coronal reformatted image. (B) Axial reformatted image of the valve.**

DILATED CARDIOMYOPATHY (DCM)/ CONGESTIVE CARDIOMYOPATHY

Definition
- Global impairment of contractility with dilatation of all cardiac chambers (particularly the left ventricle) in the absence of an abnormal loading condition ▶ this is the most common cardiomyopathy
- **Causes**: idiopathic (the commonest) ▶ post-viral myocarditis ▶ chronic alcohol abuse ▶ endocrine disturbance (hyperthyroidism)

Clinical presentation
- It presents clinically as congestive cardiac failure (chest pain is very unusual) ▶ it may be noticed after an acute influenza like illness (myocarditis may be underlying cause) ▶ there may be accompanying mitral regurgitation (due to mitral ring dilatation) ▶ pericardial effusions can be present, but tamponade is rare
- There is a variable illness course with often a good response to the initial drug therapy ▶ ultimately the low cardiac output leads to death

Radiological features
CXR This is almost always abnormal at presentation ▶ often the only abnormality is cardiac enlargement (with a left ventricular predominance) with variable degrees of pulmonary oedema

Echocardiography Increased left ventricle end-diastolic diameter (>112%) after age and body surface correction ▶ ejection fraction < 45% ▶ regional diffuse hypokinesis ▶ decreased forward flow velocities

CMR This is the best imaging method to categorize various cardiomyopathies and to distinguish them from ischaemic myocardial disease or myocarditis ▶ it allows the estimation of cardiac function (including measurements of end-diastolic and systolic volumes together with wall thickness) ▶ myocardial tagging can assess the motion of individual wall segments ▶ allows detection of any thrombus
- Delayed enhancement technique can differentiate between ischaemic and non-ischaemic DCM:
  - *Ischaemic:* subendocardial or transmural scars
  - *Non-ischaemic:* late enhancement is faint and limited to mesocardial layers (diffuse or septal)
  - *Active myocarditis:* this may demonstrate delayed enhancement but there will be normal perfusion

Pearls
- The right ventricle is usually affected to a lesser degree (due to its lower working pressures), therefore severe right ventricular dilatation is a poor prognostic sign
- Aortic stenosis needs to be excluded from DCM as both have similar clinical presentations

HYPERTROPHIC CARDIOMYOPATHY (HCM)

Definition
- Excessive hypertrophy of the myocardium (symmetrical/asymmetrical/apical/mass-like/midventricular/non-contiguous) not explained by other causes ▶ there is good or hyperdynamic contractility – the myocardium may outgrow its blood supply causing angina (and rarely infarction) ▶ variable amount of associated interstitial fibrosis
- It is much less common than dilated cardiomyopathy ▶ the right ventricle may also be involved ▶ autosomal dominant

Clinical presentation
- It is an important cause of sudden death in young adults (due to arrhythmias caused by the abnormal wall thickness) ▶ it is often familial

Radiological features
CXR This can be normal through to varying degrees of abnormal left ventricular shape (the dilated phase will resemble DCM) ▶ the left atrium is sometimes enlarged

Echocardiography HCM is well displayed (especially SAM of the mitral valve) ▶ septal thickness >15 mm ▶ ratio between septal thickness and inferior wall of left midventricle >1.3

MRI Precise measurement of wall thickness ▶ quantifies right ventricular involvement ▶ myocardial tagging can demonstrate the pattern of hypertrophy and assess the left ventricular mass ▶ serial measurements of the left ventricular mass assesses the natural history of the disease
- Delayed enhancement can detect interstitial fibrosis ('bright' myocardium with impaired washout)
- Detection of fibrosis is important as it is related to prognosis (increased risk of severe arrhythmias/sudden cardiac death in young patients/heart failure in older patients)

Pearls
- HCM must be distinguished from ventricular hypertrophy resulting from left ventricular outflow obstruction (e.g. hypertension or aortic stenosis)
- Increased myocardial thickness can be due to other cardiomyopathies (storage disease such as Anderson–Fabry disease, amyloidosis and sarcoidosis) ▶ these have different delayed enhancement patterns c/w HCM
- **Asymmetric septal hypertrophy/idiopathic hypertrophic subaortic stenosis (IHSS):** the upper interventricular septum is the most affected region resulting in a subvalvular obstruction ▶ this affects up to 25% of patients
- **Systolic anterior motion (SAM) of the mitral valve:** slackened mitral valve chordae (due to the very small end systolic left ventricular volume) allows the tip of the anterior leaflet to float towards the septum and stray into the left ventricular outflow tract ▶ the flow of blood slams it against the interventricular septum partially obstructing the subaortic region ▶ the resultant end-systolic gradient gives a further stimulus to left ventricular hypertrophy

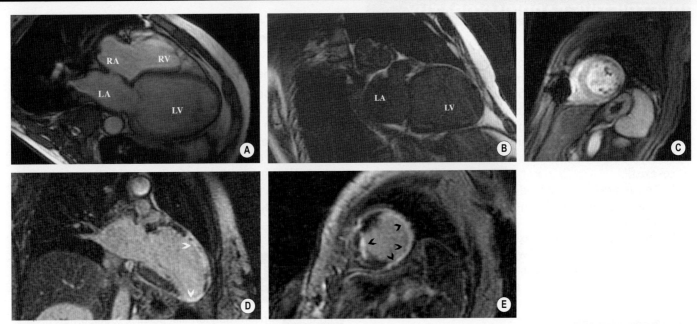

Differentiation of (A,B) dilated and (C–E) ischaemic cardiomyopathy using CMR. (A) Four-chamber projection shows dilatation of all four chambers with greater involvement of the left ventricle (LV). (B) Same patient, post-gadolinium administration delayed image, two-chamber projection. There is no regional hyperenhancement of the left ventricular myocardium. (C) Short-axis, mid-ventricular level pre-contrast gradient-echo image. (D,E) Post-contrast medium, delayed inversion recovery sequence. Before injection of contrast medium, left ventricle wall thinning involving the posterior wall is seen. Post-contrast medium delayed images show extensive hyperenhancement involving anterior, apical, septal and posterior segments (arrowheads). LA = Left atrium, RA = right atrium, RV = right ventricle.*

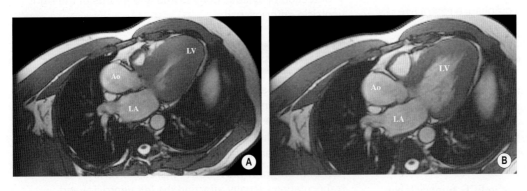

Hypertrophic cardiomyopathy. CMR, left ventricular outflow tract view of (A) systolic and (B) diastolic phases show massive hypertrophy of the left ventricle, with near complete obliteration of the left ventricle (LV) cavity in systole (A). Ao = Ascending aorta, LA = left atrium.*

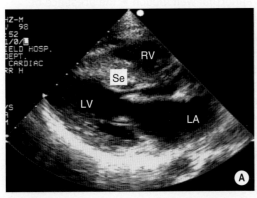
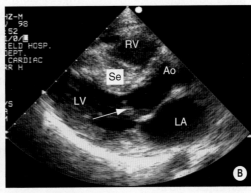

Hypertrophic cardiomyopathy with SAM of the mitral valve. Cross-sectional echocardiogram, long-axis parasternal view. (A) Diastole – the increase in septal thickness (Se) is apparent. (B) Systole – the anterior leaflet of the mitral valve has moved forward to touch the septum and obstruct the outflow tract (arrow). Se = septum, RV = right ventricle, LV = left ventricle, LA = left atrium, Ao = aorta.

RESTRICTIVE CARDIOMYOPATHY

Definition

- Heart failure due to impaired ventricular diastolic filling ▶ normal wall thickness with a rapid pressure increase with only a small volume increase
- Familial restrictive cardiomyopathy (autosomal dominant) is very rare ▶ non-familial forms include amyloidosis/sarcoidosis/haemochromatosis
- Two general mechanism are responsible (both can co-exist):
  1. The ventricle(s) may have stiff walls which fail to relax requiring high filling pressures (e.g. myocardial infiltrative conditions)
  2. There may be a fixed maximum ventricular volume which is easily achieved with normal filling pressures, but beyond which there is an abrupt rise in pressure but no further ventricular expansion (similar to a constrictive pericarditis)

Radiological features

Echocardiography/CMR There is rapid, early diastolic filling (due to the volume restriction) ▶ the stiffened (low compliance) ventricles demonstrate low velocity and protracted filling ▶ there is accentuation of the atrial contraction wave (the 'a' wave)

Pearls

Amyloid heart disease A low-compliance restrictive cardiomyopathy

- *Primary (AL) amyloidosis:* the most common and severe form involving the kidneys, liver, heart and peripheral nerves
- *Familial amyloidosis:* an uncommon autosomal dominant disease causing cardiac (± neurological) dysfunction
- *Senile systemic amyloidosis:* this is almost exclusively limited to cardiac involvement ▶ it is more prevalent with an ageing population

Clinical presentation A low-voltage ECG ▶ intractable low-output cardiac failure ▶ cardiac involvement in all forms indicates a poor prognosis and a poor tolerance to high-dose chemotherapy and stem cell transplantation

Echocardiography The non-invasive test of choice ▶ however it lacks specificity

CMR T1WI: low myocardial SI ▶ T1WI + Gad: qualitative global and subendocardial delayed enhancement ▶ both echocardiography and MRI can demonstrate systolic and diastolic dysfunction

Sarcoidosis

- Myocardial sarcoid granulomas can cause cardiac arrhythmias as well as a restrictive cardiomyopathy (papillary muscle involvement can cause mitral regurgitation)

CMR T2WI (+fat sat): sarcoid granulomas appear as high SI areas ▶ T1WI + Gad: granulomas appear as hyperenhancing areas

Haemochromatosis

Definition Iron deposition within the liver and spleen ▶ there can also be a restrictive cardiomyopathy

- *Primary:* an inherited autosomal recessive condition which spares the spleen
- *Secondary:* due to repeated blood transfusions, long-term haemodialysis or alcohol abuse

CMR T1WI + T2WI: signal loss (the degree of SI loss correlates with the tissue iron level) ▶ increased signal loss on in phase imaging

ARRHYTHMOGENIC RIGHT VENTRICULAR CARDIOMYOPATHY

Definition Uncommon familial disease (autosomal dominant) ▶ right ventricular myocardial replacement with fatty and fibrous tissue, resulting in right ventricular dysfunction (± left ventricular involvement) ▶ frequent cause of sudden cardiac death in young people

CMR Can demonstrate extensive fatty infiltration within the 'triangle of dysplasia' (outflow tract/inflow tract/apex) ▶ assessment of ventricular size and functional assessment ▶ detection of systolic bulging and aneurysms of the right ventricle anterior wall

UNCLASSIFIED CARDIOMYOPATHY

Left ventricular non-compaction (LVNC) A congenital disorder due to arrested intrauterine myocardial development ▶ it can be subdivided into isolated (more common in adults) or non-isolated (associated with other congenital heart defects such as Ebstein's anomaly) forms

Echocardiography/CT/CMR Increased ventricular trabeculation (usually affecting the left ventricle) and deep intertrabeculae recesses ▶ segments of thickened myocardium ▶ abnormal wall motion ▶ the presence of two myocardial layers

Takotsubo CMP (transient left ventricular apical ballooning syndrome) A reversible regional systolic dysfunction, associated with chest pain and negative invasive coronary angiography ▶ typical presentation is an acute coronary syndrome, more common in post-menopausal women following physical or emotional stress

Echocardiography Detects abnormal function and ballooning

CMR Detects functional ballooning but also myocardial oedema without delayed enhancement (indicating absence of necrosis and reversibility)

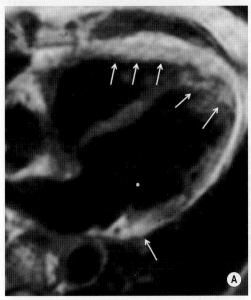
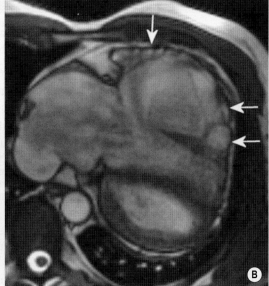

Arrhythmogenic right ventricular cardiomyopathy. (A) Black-blood axial image shows a complete fatty substitution of right ventricle free wall (high signal intensity tissue); similar foci are evident in left ventricle apex and basal lateral wall (arrows). (B) Cine-MRI axial image shows huge right ventricle dilation with small free-wall bulges (arrows).**

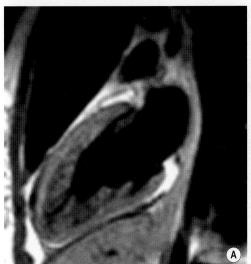
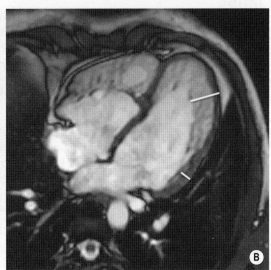

Left ventricular non-compaction. (A) T1w black-blood vertical long-axis image shows increased number and thickness of myocardial trabeculae in mid and apical left ventricle regions. (B) Cine-MRI frame in horizontal long axis with measurement of non-compacted and compacted myocardium.**

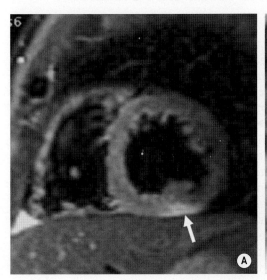
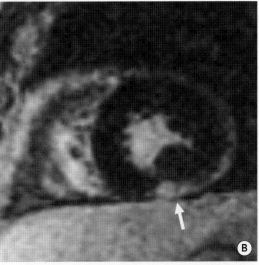

Acute myocarditis. (A) T2w STIR short-axis image shows a subepicardial hyperintense area in inferior wall; (B) late enhancement image in corresponding plane shows contrast uptake with a non-ischaemic pattern. Patient presented 36 h before in emergency unit with chest pain and slight increase in cardiac enzymes; emergency coronary angiography was negative.**

PRIMARY CARDIAC TUMOURS

Definition These are rare tumours (the majority are benign – 75%) ▶ myxoma >>> rhabdomyoma > fibroma

Clinical features Arrhythmias ▶ intracavity tumours are commonly pedunculated and may impact on or occlude the valves or fill the cardiac chambers ▶ pericardial tumour extension may produce a haemorrhagic pericardial effusion (± tamponade) ▶ lesions can compress the heart/great vessels

Echocardiography This is the imaging technique of choice ▶ it can demonstrate tumour mobility and distensibility

CT Features suggestive of malignancy: wide wall attachment ▶ wall destruction ▶ >1 chamber involved ▶ pericardial invasion ± nodular thickening ▶ right atrial location ▶ delayed enhancement

CMR This provides better soft tissue characterization than CT as well as functional information

BENIGN CARDIAC TUMOURS

Cardiac myxoma

Definition This is the commonest benign primary cardiac tumour ▶ the tumour tends to be solitary (90%), pedunculated or polypoid ▶ it is attached to the interatrial septum (near the fossa ovalis) in 85% of patients

- **Location:** left atrium (75%) > right atrium (20%) – the remainder are within either ventricle

Clinical presentation F > M ▶ it is asymptomatic or presents with a triad of:
- Peripheral embolic phenomena
- Symptoms and signs of mitral valve obstruction
- Constitutional symptoms: fever ▶ anaemia ▶ a raised ESR ▶ finger clubbing

CXR/CT An atrial filling defect (the tumour is calcified in 14%) ▶ left atrial enlargement (rarely an enlarged appendage which would otherwise suggest rheumatic disease) ▶ pulmonary venous hypertension, pulmonary oedema and pulmonary arterial hypertension

Echocardiography A rounded, hyperechoic mobile mass which often prolapses through the mitral orifice during diastole (unlike a sarcoma or metastases)

CMR This is ideal for demonstrating muscle invasion ▶ T1WI: hypointense to myocardium ▶ T2WI: high SI (intratumoral haemorrhage appears as high or heterogeneous SI on T1WI + T2WI) ▶ T1WI + Gad: mild or heterogeneous enhancement ± delayed enhancement

Pearls
- **Familial myxoma:** <10% of all myxomas ▶ presents earlier more likely to be multiple / recurrent / atypical locations
- **Carney complex:** familial myxomas + primary pigmented nodular adrenocortical disease + skin pigmentation + testicular tumours

Lipoma

- **Location:** right atrium (interatrial septum) with a narrow attachment + growth into the pericardial space

Clinical presentation Rarely symptomatic

CT A low attenuation mass (–50 to –150 HU)

MRI T1WI/T2WI: high SI ▶ no enhancement

Rhabdomyoma

Definition The commonest paediatric cardiac tumour ▶ associated with tuberous sclerosis (50%)
- **Location:** usually intramural, starting within the interventricular septum

Clinical presentation Arrhythmias (can be fatal)

CT/MRI It may be pedunculated and obstructive + enhancement

Pearl Spontaneous resolution is common – however, they are often inoperable ▶ 3–4 cm, rarely up to 10 cm

Fibroma

- **Location:** usually a single tumour of the ventricular wall (generally on the left)

CT They may calcify (with characteristic whorls)

MRI T1WI: intermediate to high SI compared with skeletal muscle ▶ T1WI and T2WI: low SI relative to myocardium (due to the fibrous component) ▶ poor enhancement

MALIGNANT CARDIAC TUMOURS

Sarcomas

Definition This accounts for nearly all the primary malignant cardiac neoplasms (commonly an angiosarcoma)
- **Location:** mainly intramural and infiltrating (and may encroach on the chamber cavity) ▶ it usually affects the right atrium ▶ metastases usually present

Clinical presentation M>>F (arising in childhood) ▶ intractable arrhythmias and relentless cardiac failure

CT/MRI It can obstruct the vena cava, tricuspid or pulmonary valves ▶ large infiltrative broad-based mass ▶ heterogeneous ▶ heterogeneous enhancement ▶ haemorrhagic pericardial effusions (± tamponade)

CARDIAC METASTASES

- Metastatic tumours are 20–40 times more common than primary heart tumours ▶ pericardial metastases are a sign of advanced disease
- **Metastatic involvement can be by:**
  - *Direct mediastinal infiltration:* lung cancer ▶ breast cancer ▶ lymphoma
  - *Intralymphatic dissemination:* lung ▶ breast ▶ mesothelioma
  - *Haematogenous metastasis:* malignant melanoma ▶ lymphoma ▶ leukaemia ▶ sarcoma
  - *Transvenous spread:* via the IVC (renal or hepatic tumours), SVC (lung cancer) or pulmonary veins
- **CT features suggestive of malignancy:** a wide attachment to the cardiac wall ▶ cardiac chamber wall destruction ▶ involvement of >1 cardiac chamber ▶ pericardial invasion (especially with haemorrhage) ▶ extension into the pulmonary artery, pulmonary vein, or vena cava

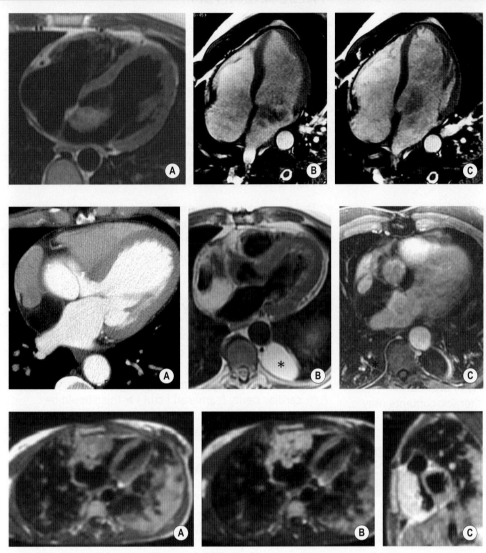

Atrial myxoma of fossa ovalis. (A) Axial T1 and T2 images show heterogeneity in signal intensity of the lesion. (B) and (C) are systolic and diastolic frames of cine-MRI: prolapse of the pedunculated myxoma through the mitral orifice is evident.**

Atrial septum lipoma. (A) Cardiac CT shows a marked hypodense well-defined lesion. (B) T1w image demonstrates marked hyperintensity of the lesion. Post-contrast T1 GRE image does not demonstrate enhancement (C). Furthermore, in the MR images, a subpleural lipoma is evident (*).**

Angiosarcoma of right ventricle. (A) Axial T1w image shows a large tumour with irregular margins, involving free wall of right ventricle, right atrioventricular groove, tricuspid annulus and right atrium wall; furthermore, multiple nodules are visible in both lungs, with large consolidation in left inferior lobe. (B) T2w image demonstrates high signal intensity of the tumour. (C) Post-contrast T1w short-axis image shows strong enhancement of the tumour and the lung metastasis. Biopsy confirmed the suspected angiosarcoma.**

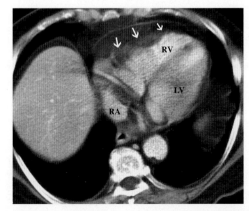

Metastasis to the right ventricular myocardium from carcinoma of the vulva. CECT of the chest. There is irregular infiltration of the anterior free wall of the right ventricle (arrows). LA = left atrium, LV = left ventricle, RA = right atrium, RV = right ventricle.*

Distinguishing thrombus from an atrial myxoma		
	Myxoma	**Thrombus**
Contrast enhancement	Yes	No
Morphology	Sessile or pedunculated	Usually sessile
Atrial fibrillation	Uncommon	Likely to be present
Atrial location	Commonly attached to the intra-atrial septum	Usually occurs in an enlarged chamber and the atrial appendage is commonly involved

PENETRATING TRAUMA

- Gunshot and knife wounds that penetrate the heart usually lead to haemorrhage and pericardial tamponade ▶ pericardial tamponade is assumed if there is a suspicion of cardiac penetration and resuscitation has not been successful with an adequate blood transfusion
- Penetrating injuries require emergency surgical exploration without any delay introduced by additional imaging
- After the acute phase, retained foreign bodies are located by CT or angiocardiography before attempts are made to remove them

BLUNT TRAUMA

- Clinical effects may be delayed, causing an insidious deterioration of cardiac function
- Blunt trauma may result in:
  - Traumatic pericarditis with haemorrhage, or traumatic haemorrhage with associated myocardial necrosis (large areas of necrosis may be fatal – such lesions resemble a myocardial infarction)
  - A disrupted pericardium allows the herniation and subsequent strangulation of parts of the heart ▶ alternatively, the abdominal or thoracic contents may enter the torn pericardium

INJURIES COMMON TO BOTH TYPES OF TRAUMA

PERFORATION OF THE VENTRICULAR SEPTUM

- This is more common with a penetrating trauma ▶ it can present as a pansystolic murmur following chest trauma (often with a subacute clinical presentation) ▶ the ventricular septal defect tends to be low or apical within the ventricular septum ▶ haemodynamically significant shunts should be surgically repaired

FALSE ANEURYSM

- This may occur if the rupture or perforation of the myocardial wall is held in check by the pericardium – such an aneurysm will increase in size and commonly rupture (either early or after many years)

CXR An abnormal cardiac contour (which may calcify if chronic)

CT A post-traumatic aneurysm will have a narrow neck, whereas a post-infarct aneurysm will have a wide neck

VALVE DISRUPTION

- The aortic valve is the most commonly affected with subsequent incompetence (although any valve can rupture) ▶ tricuspid incompetence may be asymptomatic but traumatic mitral incompetence usually requires urgent correction

CORONARY ARTERY TRAUMA

- Traumatic thrombosis may lead to myocardial infarction ▶ false aneurysms may develop after coronary artery trauma
  - Rarely, trauma may lead to a coronary artery to cardiac cavity (cameral) fistula ▶ this should be suggested by a continuous murmur developing for the 1st time after major chest trauma

PERICARDIAL TRAUMA

- Pericardial tamponade is one of the most common causes of death after cardiac trauma ▶ traumatic pericarditis may calcify but rarely leads to constriction

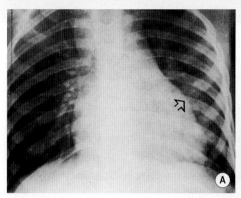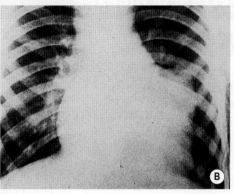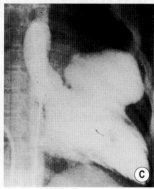

Traumatic false aneurysm. Plain CXRs (A) immediately after a car accident involving chest trauma, showing an insignificant bulge on the left heart border (arrow), and (B) 16 months later, a large bulge has developed in the mid-left heart border. (C) Left ventriculogram shows that the bulge is a narrow-necked false aneurysm filling from the upper left ventricular cavity.*

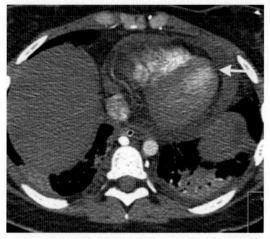

CECT showing pericardial effusion of intermediate attenuation (arrow) that developed acutely following traumatic removal of central venous catheter in keeping with a haemopericardium.

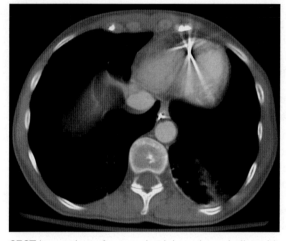

CECT in a patient after gunshot injury shows bullet with streak artefacts lodged in the right side of the interventricular septum.*

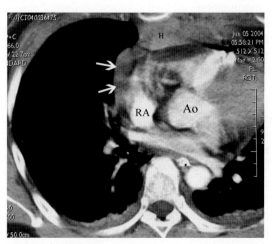

Blunt chest trauma causing rupture of right atrial appendage. There is a large anterior mediastinal haematoma (H) and haematoma surrounding the right atrial appendage (arrows). At surgery, rupture of the right atrial appendage near its junction with the right atrium was noted. Ao = aortic root, RA = right atrium.*

Blunt cardiac trauma●
Pericardium
Laceration laterally with communication with the pleural space
Laceration of the diaphragmatic pericardium with herniation of the abdominal contents into the pericardium
Tamponade
Myocardium
Rupture
Cardiac chamber into the pericardium
Interventricular septum
Papillary muscle
Cardiac valve
Laceration or contusion
Ventricular aneurysm
True aneurysm from coronary occlusion or from contusion
False aneurysm from penetrating trauma
Coronary arteries
Laceration
Occlusion
Fistula

PULMONARY THROMBOEMBOLIC DISEASE

DEFINITION

- A pulmonary embolus (PE) usually arises from a thrombus within a pelvic or lower limb vein (>90%)
  - *'Saddle' embolus:* a thrombus lodged at the main pulmonary arterial bifurcation
  - *Pulmonary infarction:* This is relatively rare as there is a second 'systemic' arterial supply to the lungs from the bronchial arteries
- **Risk factors for a pulmonary embolism:** increasing age ▶ hypercoagulable state ▶ orthopaedic surgery ▶ immobilization ▶ malignancy ▶ medical illness ▶ pregnancy ▶ oestrogen use
- **d-Dimers:** these are a measure of fibrinolytic activity ▶ it is a highly sensitive but non-specific test (with a high false-positive rate but a very high negative predictive value) ▶ false-negative tests can occur (particularly with subsegmental emboli) ▶ false positive tests with inflammation/pregnancy/malignancy

CLINICAL PRESENTATION

- Dyspnoea ▶ chest pain (which may be pleuritic) ▶ haemoptysis ▶ cough ▶ hypotension ▶ tachycardia ▶ pulmonary oedema (due to left ventricular failure precipitated by a large PE)

RADIOLOGICAL FEATURES

CXR

- This has a low sensitivity and specificity – however it may exclude other causes (e.g. a pneumothorax)
- **The most common signs (without infarction):**
  - *Westermark's sign:* localized peripheral oligaemia secondary to an embolus lodging in a peripheral artery ▶ this may be associated with proximal arterial dilatation
  - *Peripheral airspace opacification:* this represents pulmonary haemorrhage
  - *Linear atelectasis:* ischaemic injury to type II pneumocytes leads to surfactant deficiency
  - *Pleural effusions:* these are often small
  - *Central pulmonary arterial enlargement:* this is secondary to chronic repeated embolic disease
- **Signs associated with infarction:**
  - *Hampton's hump:* a pleurally based, wedge-shaped opacity normally seen within the lateral or posterior costophrenic sulcus ▶ the apex of the triangle points toward the occluded feeding vessel with its base against the pleural surface ▶ it rarely contains air bronchograms ▶ it is a rare and non-specific sign
  - *Consolidation* (which may be multifocal): this predominantly affects the lower lobes ▶ it can be seen from 12 h to several days post embolism

- *Cavitation:* this follows secondary infection at the infarction site or following a septic embolus
- *Haemorrhagic pleural effusions:* this is seen in 50% of patients
- *Serial CXRs:* rapid resolution of any parenchymal changes is associated with a non-infarcting PE – infarction normally heals with scarring and localized pleural thickening

Computed tomography pulmonary angiography (CTPA)

- *Technical considerations:*
  - The imaged area encompasses the central and segmental pulmonary arteries (i.e. from the aortic arch to the inferior pulmonary veins)
  - Contrast medium concentrations > 120–250 mg/ml can be associated with significant streak artefacts (particularly adjacent to the SVC)
  - Accurate timing of data acquisition (post IV contrast administration) is essential in order to achieve optimum pulmonary arterial opacification
  - Contrast density < 300–350HU usually implies a non-diagnostic study
    - *Patient-related factors affecting opacification:* a SVC thrombosis ▶ persistent intracardiac shunts ▶ pregnancy (the increased cardiac output may result in the majority of the contrast residing beyond the pulmonary arteries when imaging)
- CTPA may reliably detect emboli in up to 4th-order vessels (which are 7 mm in diameter)
  - **Acute emboli:** an intravascular filling defect ▶ it may appear as an expanded unopacified vessel
    - *'Tram track' appearance:* contrast medium flows around or is adjacent to a clot if the vessel is within the image plane
  - **Chronic emboli:** a crescentic thrombus adherent to the arterial wall (which may also be calcified or show evidence of recanalization) ▶ enlargement of the bronchial vessels (representing the collateral supply) ▶ a prominent mosaic attenuation pattern ▶ right heart strain
  - **Infarction:** a peripheral wedge-shaped region of consolidation (analogous to a Hampton's hump on CXR) ▶ this is only a specific sign if the vessel can be traced to the apex of the wedge
- Can be combined with CT venography from calves to IVC
- **CTPA in pregnancy:** leg USS first choice ▶ radiation dose to fetus at *any* stage is negligible with CTPA or V/Q scintigraphy (CTPA protocol should still be adapted to reduced dose and to hypercirculatory state of patient) ▶ check thyroid function (iodine in CT contrast may reduce thyroid function) ▶ breast radiation dose is an issue, but reduced with perfusion scintigraphy (with slightly increased fetal dose)

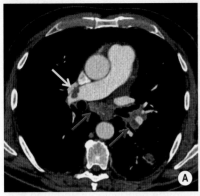 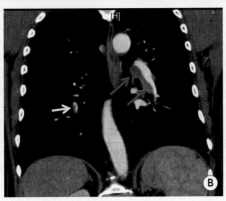 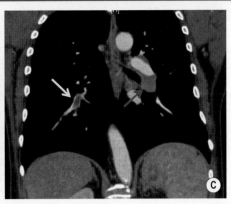

(A) Central thrombus (yellow arrow) with smooth margins, centrally located and acute angles with the vessel wall, and lymphadenopathy (red arrows). Coronal reconstructions (B, C) may aid in the differentiation between endoluminal clots (yellow arrows) and lymphadenopathy (red arrows). Note the central position of the clot surrounded by contrast medium.**

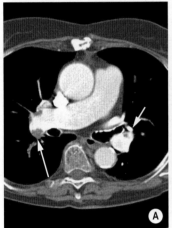 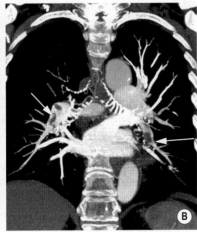 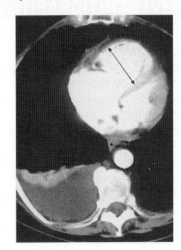

CTPA identifying additional features that can be detected supporting a diagnosis of pulmonary embolism. There is a right-sided pleural effusion and dilatation of the right ventricle (arrow).[†]

(A) CTPA demonstrating multiple filling defects (arrows) within both main pulmonary arteries consistent with multiple pulmonary emboli. (B) Coronal CTPA reformat again demonstrating these filling defects (arrows).

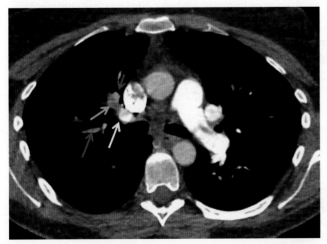 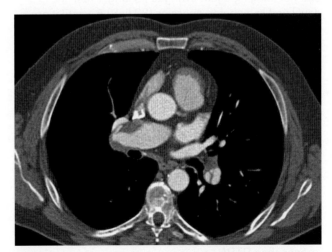

Beam-hardening artefact in the right upper lobe pulmonary artery (yellow arrow) due to dense contrast medium in the superior caval vein. Thrombus (blue arrow) more peripherally. Red arrows, non-opacified pulmonary veins.**

CTEPH. Eccentric thrombus with obtuse angles in the right pulmonary artery and a web in the left lower lobe pulmonary artery.**

PERFUSION (Q) SCINTIGRAPHY

- This assesses the distribution of the pulmonary blood flow ▶ particles microembolize within the lung, providing a map of the pulmonary blood flow (only approximately 2% of the capillaries are occluded) ▶ the effective dose is <1 mSv
  - *Technique:* it is performed using injected microparticles (10–100 μm) of ^{99m}Tc microaggregate albumin (MAA) and performed supine to maximize blood flow to the lung apices ▶ the preparation should not be 'backflushed' with blood in order to prevent coagulation and 'hot spots' forming on the lungs
- A normal perfusion study rules out a PE with almost 100% certainty

VENTILATION (V) SCINTIGRAPHY

This assesses the distribution of the inhaled air
- **Technique:** this is performed by the inhalation of krypton-81m, xenon-133, ^{99m}Tc-DTPA or 'technegas' ▶ 8 images are conventionally acquired (anterior, posterior, oblique and lateral projections on both sides)
- **^{81m}Kr:** this is the optimal imaging agent, emitting high-energy photons (190 keV) ▶ its higher photon energy allows the ventilation images to be obtained after the perfusion images as well as allowing matching of both image sets without moving the patient ▶ owing to its short half-life (13 s) it can be continuously administered (including during perfusion imaging) although it means that no washout images are possible
  - *Disadvantages:* there is decreased resolution due to collimator penetration by the high-energy photons ▶ it is expensive
- **^{133}Xe:** although it is cheaper than ^{81m}Kr, it is a less optimal imaging agent owing to its longer half-life (5.3 days) and low photon energies (80 keV) ▶ ventilation studies need to be performed prior to any perfusion studies (thus preventing Compton scatter from the ^{99m}Tc into the lower ^{133}Xe photopeak)
  - *Single breath inhalation image:* a cold spot is abnormal
  - Equilibrium phase: tracer activity corresponds to aerated lung
  - *Washout phase:* tracer retention corresponds to areas of air trapping (e.g. COPD)
- **^{99m}Tc-DTPA and technegas aerosols:** these are administered via a nebulizer during inspiration ▶ the aerosol imaging provides a non-physiological static image of lung ventilation with central airway deposition demonstrated (^{81m}Kr allows dynamic imaging) ▶ technegas aerosols and ^{81m}Kr both provide better images than DTPA
  - *Disadvantage:* it cannot be administered during perfusion (as both aerosols and MAA are labelled with ^{99m}Tc)

- **V/Q 'mismatches':** a defect on perfusion imaging that appears normal on ventilation imaging and refers to a region of underperfused lung ▶ it suggests the presence of a non-infarct causing pulmonary embolus (despite the interruption of perfusion, the ventilation still remains intact)
  - If an infarct develops, a defect may be seen on both perfusion and ventilation studies (i.e. it will become matched as the area will no longer be ventilated) ▶ the ventilation defect is smaller than the perfusion defect as the peri-infarct lung remains ventilated
- **Matched ventilation and perfusion defects:** these are caused by pulmonary hypoxic vasoconstriction reducing the blood flow to the poorly ventilated lung ▶ it is commonly seen with obstructive airways disease (e.g. asthma, COPD)
- **Reversed mismatch:** the ventilation defect is more prominent than the perfusion defect ▶ this can be seen with lobar collapse, pneumonic consolidation, a large pleural effusion and obstructive airway causes
- **A normal V/Q study:** this has a negative predictive value of 100%
- **A high probability (>85%) V/Q study:** this can be confidently treated as a PE
- **An intermediate (15–85%) or low (<15%) probability V/Q study:** this requires further imaging if there is a strong clinical suspicion
- **Causes of a false-positive results:**
  - *Pulmonary arterial wall causes:* vasculitis ▶ infection ▶ irradiation
  - *Vascular malformations:* arterial agenesis ▶ arteriovenous malformations ▶ surgical shunts
  - *Extrinsic compression of the pulmonary vasculature:* hilar adenopathy ▶ tumour
  - *Pulmonary arterial luminal block:* non-thrombotic material ▶ tumour
  - *A prior pulmonary embolus that has not completely resolved*

PEARLS

- **The terminology of segmental involvement:**
  - *Non-segmental:* it does not conform to a lung segment
  - *Subsegmental:* it involves 25–75% of a bronchopulmonary segment
  - *Segmental:* it involves > 75% of a bronchopulmonary segment

Causes of non-segmental defects[§§]	
Pacemaker artefact	Cardiomegaly
Tumours	Hilar adenopathy
Pleural effusion	Atelectasis
Trauma	Pneumonia
Haemorrhage	Aortic ectasia or aneurysm
Bullae	

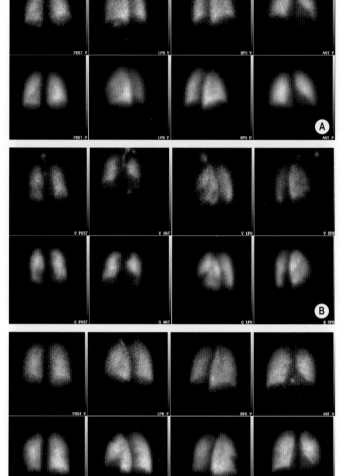

Pulmonary thromboembolism. (A) Normal V/Q study (ventilation (v) images on top row and perfusion (p) images beneath). No defects are seen in either series. (B) Matched defects – multiple foci of non-tracer uptake seen in ventilation and perfusion series. Scrutiny of the images reveals that the defects are well matched for position on both series. (C) Perfusion defect (wedge-shaped peripherally) seen on perfusion imaging which is not replicated on ventilation imaging. This suggests a high probability for the presence of pulmonary embolus.*

Ventilation-perfusion terminology[§§]	
V/Q matched defect	Both scans abnormal in same area and of equal size
V/Q mismatch	Abnormal perfusion in an area of normal ventilation or a much larger perfusion defect than ventilation abnormality
Triple-match	V/Q matching defects in a region of chest X-ray abnormality where the X-ray abnormality is of the same size or smaller than the radiographic lesion
Segmental defect	Characteristically wedge-shaped and pleural based and conforms to segmental anatomy of the lung. May be caused by occlusion of pulmonary artery branches • Large: > 75% of a lung segment • Moderate: 25–75% of a lung segment • Small: < 25% of a lung segment
Non-segmental defect	Does not conform to segmental anatomy or does not appear wedge-shaped

Modified PIOPED criteria for pulmonary embolus diagnosis	
High probability scan ≥ 80%	2 or more large mismatched segmental defects or equivalent moderate/large defects with a normal chest X-ray Any perfusion defect substantially larger than a radiographic abnormality
Intermediate probability scan (20–79%)	Multiple perfusion defects with associated X-ray opacities Greater than 25% of a segment and less than 2 mismatched segmental perfusion defects with a normal radiograph – one moderate segmental – one large or two moderate segmental – one large and one moderate segmental – three moderate segmental – solitary moderate/large matching segmental defect with matching X-ray (triple match) Difficult to characterize as high probability or low probability
Low probability scan (<20%)	Non-segmental defects: small effusion blunting the costophrenic angle, cardiomegaly, elevated diaphragm, ectatic aorta Any perfusion defect with a substantially larger radiographic abnormality Matched ventilation and perfusion defects with a normal chest X-ray Small subsegmental perfusion defects with a normal chest X-ray
Normal scan	No perfusion defects

PULMONARY VENOUS HYPERTENSION (PVH)

DEFINITION

- PVH is caused by increased resistance in the pulmonary veins (>12 mmHg), usually due to aortic left-sided heart disease (only an elevated end diastolic left ventricular pressure leads to PVH) ▶ less commonly due to mediastinal disease
  - *Mild PVH* – Vascular redistribution (grade I): PVH 12–20 mmHg
  - *Moderate PVH* – Interstitial oedema (grade II): PVH 20–25 mmHg
  - *Severe PVH* – Alveolar oedema (grade III): PVH > 25–30 mmHg

RADIOLOGICAL FEATURES

Vascular redistribution (grade I)

- Upper lobe venous distension (reversing the normal gravity dependent pattern)

Interstitial oedema (grade II)

- *'Kerley A' lines:* deep septal lines (representing lymphatic channels) radiating from the periphery (not reaching the pleura) into the central lung ▶ approx 4-cm long ▶ usually indicate acute or more severe oedema
- *'Kerley B' lines:* short (<1 cm) interlobular septal lines ▶ usually found in the lower zones peripherally and parallel to each other but at right angles to the pleura
- *Perihilar haze:* a loss of clarity of the lower lobe and hilar vessels
- *Peribronchial cuffing:* proximal bronchial wall thickening due to interstitial fluid accumulating within their walls

Alveolar oedema (grade III)

- Kerley B lines ▶ airspace nodules ▶ bilateral symmetric consolidation (mid to lower zones) ▶ pleural effusions
- *'Perihilar Bat's Wing' pattern:* a pattern of airspace consolidation most commonly seen in left ventricular and renal failure
  - *Alveolar oedema localised to the right upper zone:* severe mitral regurgitation
  - *Predominantly upper lobe odemea:* neurogenic head injury

CT findings of oedema

- *Interstitial oedema:* smoothly thickened interlobular septa ▶ thickened peribronchovascular interstitium ▶ subtle increased parenchymal density
- *Alveolar oedema:* peribronchovascular airspace nodules progressing to diffuse ground-glass or dense airspace opacification
- Chronic pulmonary venous hypertension: additional signs of pulmonary arterial hypertension ± a fine nodular pattern (representing haemosiderin deposition)

PEARLS

- *Septal lines vs. blood vessels:* the latter are not visible in the outer 1 cm of lung, septal lines do not branch uniformly and are seen with greater clarity
- Septal lines can persist in chronic disease (e.g. chronic PVH with fibrosis) or idiopathic interstitial fibrosis, lymphangitis carcinomatosis and pneumoconiosis
- Pre-existing lung disease influences the pattern/ distribution of oedema (e.g. extensive emphysema)

PULMONARY ARTERIAL HYPERTENSION (PAH)

DEFINITION

- A systolic pulmonary artery pressure > 35 mmHg or a mean pulmonary artery pressure > 25 mmHg at rest or > 30 mmHg with exercise

RADIOLOGICAL FEATURES

CXR/CT

- Right atrial/ventricular enlargement ▶ enlarged central pulmonary arteries ▶ tapering of peripheral arterial branches ('peripheral pruning') ▶ atheroma calcification within central pulmonary arteries in chronic cases (not seen in non-hypertensive pulmonary arteries)
- Central arterial enlargement may mimic adenopathy (lymph nodes are typically more lobulated)
- Flattening/bowing of the cardiac septum/RV dilatation
- Main pulmonary artery (at its bifurcation) > 29 mm ▶ pulmonary artery to aortic ratio > 1.1 ▶ dilatation of bronchial arteries (> 1.5 mm) ▶ hepatic vein reflux
- Mosaic perfusion (peripheral vascular obstruction)

MRI

- Assessment of ventricular dysfunction/stroke volume/ cardiac output ▶ MR angiography to assess pulmonary vasculature ▶ MR perfusion techniques can distinguish between PAH and CTEPH

PEARLS

- *Other useful techniques:* transthoracic USS/ventilation– perfusion lung scintigram/traditional pulmonary angiography/right heart catheterization

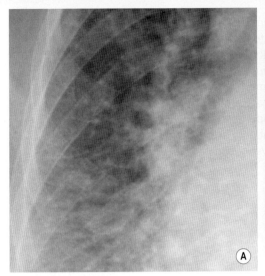

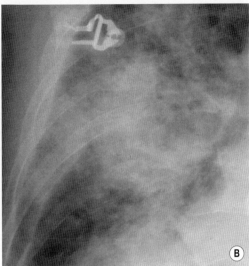

Magnified view of interstitial (A) and alveolar oedema (B). Note the sharp thickened interlobular septa in (A) versus the opacification ranging from ground-glass to dense consolidation in (B).**

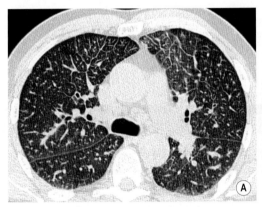

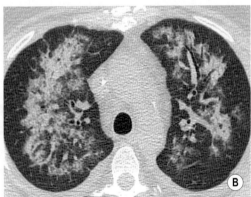

Interstitial oedema (A) is characterized by thickened interlobular septa and focal areas of increased density. Alveolar oedema (B) causes dense consolidations which can be diffuse or more patchy in distribution. The subpleural area may be spared.**

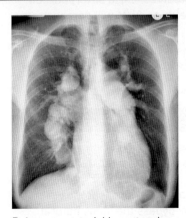

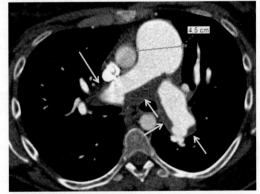

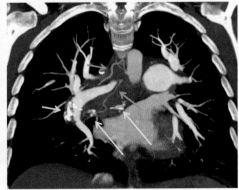

Pulmonary arterial hypertension. Chest X-ray demonstrates gross dilatation of the main, left and right pulmonary arteries in a patient with Eisenmenger's atrial septal defect.*

CT in a patient with CTEPH demonstrating an enlarged pulmonary trunk and enlarged main pulmonary arteries when compared to the ascending aorta. There is eccentric thrombus with irregular margins and obtuse angles to the vessel wall (arrows).**

Coronal maximum intensity projection showing dilatation of bronchial arteries (blue arrows) and a thrombus with calcifications (yellow arrows) in the central pulmonary arteries.**

ASYMMETRIC PULMONARY VASCULARITY

DEFINITION

- Pulmonary hypoxia results in local vasoconstriction causing diversion of blood to regions of better ventilation (although contrary to the effect seen within the rest of the body, this mechanism serves to protect the alveolar–arteriolar PO_2 balance)
  - This is responsible for the 'matched defects' seen with pneumonic consolidation on V/Q imaging
- **Uneven pulmonary vascularity:** this may be 'apparent' or 'real':

- *Apparent causes:* patient rotation ▶ a unilateral mastectomy ▶ atrophy or congenital absence of the pectoral muscles
- *Real causes:* bullae ▶ emphysema ▶ Macleod's syndrome ▶ previous pulmonary resection ▶ pulmonary embolism ▶ previous cardiovascular shunt operations (e.g. a Blalock–Taussig shunt) ▶ pulmonary artery stenosis ▶ pulmonary arteriovenous fistula

PULMONARY ARTERIOVENOUS MALFORMATION (PAVM)

DEFINITION

- An abnormal (congenital or acquired) communication between a pulmonary artery and vein
- Two types of PAVM:
  1) Simple: single feeding artery and 1 or more draining veins (80%)
  2) Complex: more than 1 feeding artery and 1 or more draining veins (20%)
- They can take the following forms:
  - A single fistula
  - Multiple discrete fistulas with one or a few predominant lesions
  - Multiple discrete fistulas of a similar size
  - Diffuse telangectasia – 50% of congenital cases have hereditary haemorrhagic telangiectasia (Osler–Weber–Rendu disease)

CLINICAL PRESENTATION

- Systemic arterial desaturation with signs of dyspnoea, hypoxia, cyanosis and heart failure
- Most cases do not clinically manifest until the 3rd or 4th decade ▶ multiple lesions are seen in 50% of cases
- Massive haemoptysis and haemothorax with rupture

RADIOLOGICAL FEATURES

CXR Round, oval or lobulated opacities with an associated prominent vascular shadow ▶ these are most commonly seen within the lower lobes

CT The feeding and draining vessels are more easily seen than with CXR ▶ they may demonstrate a change in size with respiratory manœuvres (e.g. a size reduction during a Valsalva manœuvre) ▶ an AVM will demonstrate intense enhancement

Selective angiography This is the 'gold standard' – it will demonstrate the feeding artery and vein (draining into the left atrium)

PEARLS

- Acquired forms may be seen in conjunction with liver cirrhosis, schistosomiasis and metastatic thyroid carcinoma
- There is an increased stroke incidence (paradoxical embolism) – the AVM may bypass the lungs natural embolic filtering properties

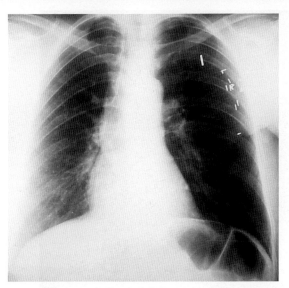

Left mastectomy. The left hemithorax is more transradiant than the right.

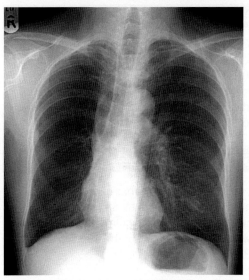

Uneven vascularity. In a patient with Macleod's syndrome a hypoplastic right main pulmonary artery leads to a reduction in vascular markings and a small right hemithorax is seen.*

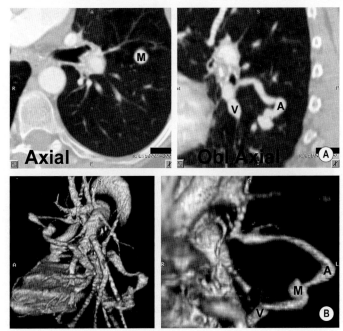

Pulmonary arteriovenous malformation. (A) Axial and oblique axial CT images (lung window) shows a malformation in the left lower lobe. (B) Shaded surface display images clearly delineate the angioarchitecture of the lesion prior to embolotherapy. M, malformation ▶ A, feeding artery ▶ V, draining vein.©1

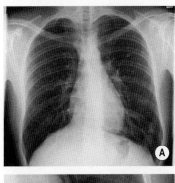

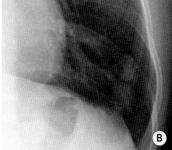

Pulmonary arteriovenous malformation. (A) CXR shows a band-like opacity leading to a nodular opacity in the left lower lobe. (B) A close-up of (A).*

PULMONARY OVERCIRCULATION (PLETHORA)

DEFINITION

- This results from an increased blood flow through the lungs ▶ it is most commonly secondary to a left-to-right cardiac shunt
  - It can also be seen with bidirectional shunts or increased cardiac output states (e.g. in well-trained athletes or pregnant women)

RADIOLOGICAL FEATURES

`CXR` Central pulmonary arterial enlargement (requiring a left-to-right shunt of at least 2:1 to be apparent on CXR)
- *'Pulmonary plethora'*: peripheral pulmonary vessels that are visible within the outer third of the lung (cf. arterial pruning in PAH)

PEARLS

- With associated cyanosis, pulmonary plethora is commonly due to a bidirectional shunt
- In the absence of cyanosis, it is most commonly due to a left-to-right shunt

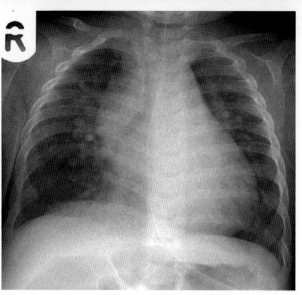

Pulmonary plethora. There is a marked increase in the size and number of visible vessels in both lungs (seen in a patient with an atrioventricular septal defect). The prominent right superior mediastinum is due to normal thymus.*

PULMONARY OLIGAEMIA

DEFINITION

- This describes decreased blood flow within the lungs
- It is usually due to right ventricular outflow tract obstruction (which is often seen in association with a right-to-left shunt)

RADIOLOGICAL FEATURES

`CXR` Fewer and smaller vascular markings ▶ a small pulmonary trunk

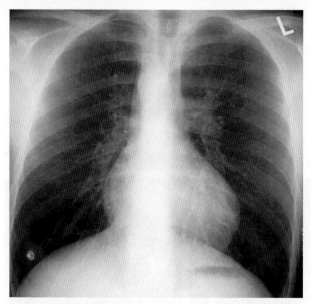

Pulmonary oligaemia. The peripheral vascular pattern is diminished in a patient with tetralogy of Fallot and a right aortic arch.*

CONGENITAL ABNORMALITIES OF THE PULMONARY ARTERY

CONGENITAL ABSENCE OF THE PULMONARY ARTERY

Definition This is a short segment atresia of the proximal left or right pulmonary artery (the more distal segments are usually present) ▶ it usually occurs on the side opposite to the aortic arch
- It is associated with various congenital cardiac defects (e.g. tetralogy of Fallot)

CXR A small volume ipsilateral lung without air trapping (cf. Macleod's syndrome) ▶ a small ipsilateral hilum ▶ occasionally opacities are seen within the affected lung (representing systemic–pulmonary collaterals)

PULMONARY VALVE ABNORMALITIES

Congenital absence of the pulmonary valve This is associated with aneurysmal dilatation of the main pulmonary artery and hilar vessels (especially the left pulmonary artery) ▶ it is almost always associated with cyanotic heart disease (typically tetralogy of Fallot)

Pulmonary valve stenosis See acyanotic heart disease – other anomalies (Section 2 Chapter 1)

PULMONARY ARTERY STENOSIS

Definition This occurs in three forms:
- *Central form*: involving the main pulmonary arterial bifurcation
- *Peripheral form:* this involves the origin of the lobar segmental or subsegmental pulmonary arteries
- *Diffuse form*: general hypoplasia of the entire pulmonary arterial system

CXR/CT There may be no discernible abnormality ▶ there may be sausage-shaped arteries produced by the proximal stenosis and post-stenotic dilation

Associations Rubella syndrome ▶ William's syndrome ▶ Ehlers–Danlos syndrome (⅔ have additional cardiac lesions)

PULMONARY ARTERY ANEURYSMS

Definition Aneurysms rarely occur within the pulmonary circulation (if present they usually involve the main, lobar or segmental arteries)
- They are most commonly mycotic aneurysms (due to septic embolization or direct extension of a parenchymal infection) ▶ they require monitoring as they have a propensity to enlarge rapidly and rupture
- *Rasmussen's aneurysm*: a pulmonary arterial aneurysm seen in association with tuberculosis

CXR/CT Fusiform or saccular arterial dilatations

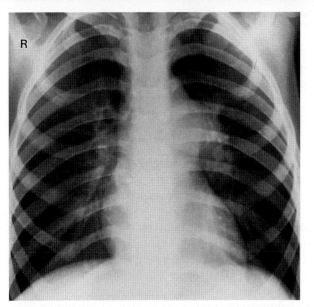

CXR of a child with pulmonary valve stenosis. The main pulmonary artery and left pulmonary artery are considerably enlarged, but pulmonary vascularity is otherwise normal.[†]

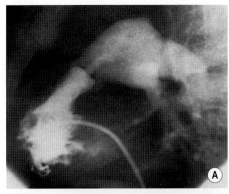

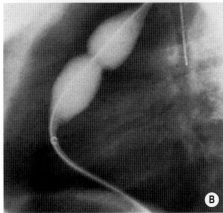

(A) Lateral view of a right ventricular angiogram in a child with pulmonary valve stenosis. The doming of the stenotic valve and the central jet of contrast medium are seen. There is post-stenotic dilatation of the main pulmonary artery. (B) Lateral view of pulmonary valve dilatation in the same patient. The indentation in the balloon indicates that the valve is not yet fully dilated.[†]

2.4 THE AORTA

TRAUMATIC AORTIC INJURY (TAI)

Definition

- This occurs as a result of a rapid deceleration injury generating shearing forces at the aortic isthmus ▶ other mechanisms of injury include an AP compression force displacing the heart to the left (a torsion stress)
  - *Incomplete rupture:* the adventitia remains intact (maintaining the aortic integrity) in the majority of survivors ▶ the saccular outpouching that can develop is known as a pseudoaneurysm
  - *Complete rupture:* the adventitia is disrupted and is normally associated with mediastinal haemorrhage ▶ if the patient survives it may progress to apical pleural capping or a haemothorax (99% mortality at 24 hrs)
- **Classification of aortic injuries:** (A) intimal haemorrhage ▶ (B) intimal haemorrhage with a laceration ▶ (C) medial laceration ▶ (D) complete laceration ▶ (E) false aneurysm formation ▶ (E) periaortic haemorrhage
- **Contributory factors:** tethering by the ligamentum arteriosum ▶ an 'osseous pinch': compression of the heart and aorta between the anterior chest wall and the thoracic spine during impact

Clinical presentation

- 80–90% of patients die at the scene of the trauma due to a complete aortic rupture ▶ survivors tend to have either a simple intimal lesion/IMH/false aneurysm
- *There should be a high index of suspicion with:* road traffic accidents (RTAs) at speeds greater than 30 mph (particularly involving unrestrained occupants of vehicles or pedestrians involved in an RTA) ▶ falls from a height of greater than 10 ft (3 m) ▶ severe crush injuries to the chest

Radiological features

CXR This is rarely normal with a traumatic aortic rupture ▶ the signs include:

- *Mediastinal widening:* this can be problematical as in the trauma setting the patient is usually imaged in the supine position ▶ signs include:
  - A mediastinal width above the level of the carina of ≥ 8 cm
  - The mediastinum forms > 25% of the width of the chest above the level of the carina (i.e. a mediastinal-to-cardiac ratio of 0.25)
  - NB: a subjective impression of a wide mediastinum should override these measurements
- *Blurring of the aortic arch contours*
- *Filling-in of the aortopulmonary window*
- *A left apical pleural cap:* due to an extrapleural haematoma
- *Tracheal or nasogastric tube deviation:* to the right
- *Depression of the left mainstem bronchus*
- *Widening of the right paratracheal stripe* (or the presence of paraspinal lines)

CT/angiography This is a second-line investigation (after a CXR) ▶ images can be degraded by streak artefact from the shoulders

- *Direct signs:* pseudoaneurysm formation ▶ an intimal flap ▶ an intramural haematoma ▶ contrast extravasation ▶ focal calibre change or contour abnormality
- *Indirect sign:* periaortic mediastinal haematoma (haematoma that is not adjacent to the aorta and is without direct signs of an aortic injury can be ascribed to mediastinal venous bleeding)
- *Minimal aortic injury:* this is represented by a small intramural haematoma or an intimal thrombus – these can be treated conservatively
- *A false-negative result:* poor contrast enhancement ▶ partial volume effects
- *A false-positive result:* the presence of severe atheroma or a ductus diverticulum ▶ young patients with residual thymic tissue

DSA This is now seldom performed as a result of improved CT imaging

- *Signs:* irregularity of the aortic isthmus ▶ pseudoaneurysm formation ▶ the presence of an intimal flap ▶ aortic dissection ▶ pseudocoarctation (uncommon) ▶ acute margin at junction of normal and abnormal aortic wall, differentiating a pseudoaneurysm from a ductus diverticulum (with classically a smooth symmetrical contour)
- *False positives:* presence of a prominent ductus diverticulum ▶ severe aortic atheroma ▶ double densities from overlapping adjacent vessels

Pearls

- **Aortic isthmus:** this is the junction between the relatively mobile arch and the relatively fixed descending thoracic aorta, tethered by the ligamentosum arteriosum ▶ it is located just distal to the left subclavian artery and at the site of the ligamentum arteriosum
  - In clinical series 90% of ruptures occur at the isthmus
  - Ascending aortic injuries account for 20–25% of cases ▶ as these are usually rapidly fatal (due to exsanguination, haemopericardium and cardiac tamponade) they only account for 5% of clinical cases
- 'Osseous pinch': mechanical compression of the aortic arch and branch vessels between the thoracic spine and sternoclavicular junction
- 'Water hammer' effect: increased intravascular pressure within the aorta as a direct result of compression causing injuries at the isthmus and root
- 'Red flag' signs indicative of a need for urgent aortic repair:
  - *Pseudocoarctation syndrome:* partial aortic compression by the pseudoaneurysm sac just distal to the aortic wall injury site leading to aortic lumen reduction
  - *Circumferential lesion:* a traumatic aortic wall injury >270° ▶ a strong predictor of impending rupture

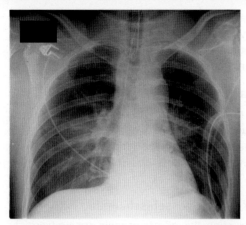

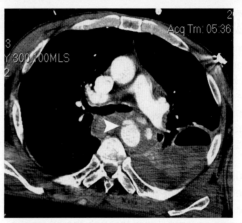

Supine CXR of a patient involved in a road traffic accident demonstrates signs of traumatic aortic injury. There is widening of the superior mediastinum. The right paratracheal stripe is widened and there is deviation of the trachea and the nasogastric tube to the right of the midline. The contour of the aortic knuckle is enlarged and partially obscured by mediastinal haematoma.*

Pseudoaneurysm. CT following blunt trauma demonstrates a pseudoaneurysm at the aortic isthmus (arrowhead) but in addition there is some extravasation of contrast indicating that there has been a complete disruption of the aortic wall.*

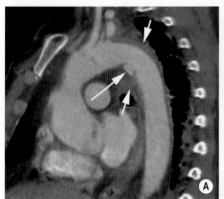

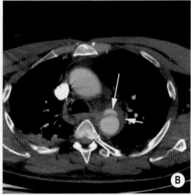

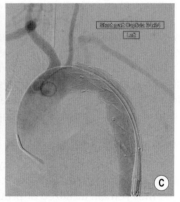

Aortic trauma. (A, B) Typical appearances of blunt traumatic incomplete aortic injury with irregularity of the external aortic contour in the region of the ligamentum arteriosum (long arrow) and periaortic blood (short arrow) from damage to vasavasorum and mediastinal vessels. (C) Stent-graft repair with coverage of the site of aortic injury with a short device.**

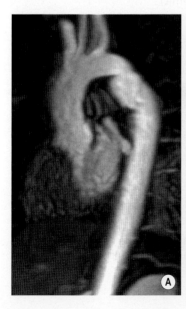

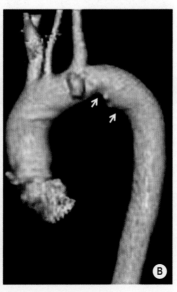

Difference between a traumatic pseudoaneurysm and a normal ductus diverticulum. (A) The pseudoaneurysm is asymmetric and has an acute proximal margin with the normal aorta (MRA image). (B) The ductus diverticulum (MDCT VR image) has a smooth symmetrical contour with obtuse margins at its junction with the 'normal' aorta (arrows).**

AORTIC DISSECTION

DEFINITION

- A dissection is initiated by an intimal tear – this allows blood to penetrate into and split the medial layer in a longitudinal fashion (the cleavage plane is produced between the inner $\frac{2}{3}$ and outer $\frac{1}{3}$ of the media)
- Arterial pressure extends the dissection for a variable distal distance, producing a false channel (or lumen) ▶ this can also sometimes extend proximal to the entry tear
- The 'false' lumen is separated from the 'true' lumen by an intimomedial flap ▶ an additional communication between the 2 lumens can be caused by either shear forces producing re-entry tears through the adventitia or back through the intima into the true lumen, or by an avulsion of the flap attachment at a branch vessel origin (producing a natural fenestration within the flap)
  - The 'false' lumen is prone to aneurysmal dilatation due to the reduced elastic tissue within its wall ▶ it can thrombose completely or partially over time
- Associations: uncontrolled hypertension ▶ Marfan's syndrome
- The aetiology is frequently unknown (most dissections are spontaneous) ▶ almost all will originate within the thoracic aorta with extension into the abdominal aorta ▶ many dissections can occur in non-aneurysmal aortas
- Prognosis: poor (1% mortality per hour for the 1st 48 hours) ▶ greater mortality for type A dissections

Potential dissection precursors

- *Intramural haematoma:* this results from a hypertensive rupture of the vasa vasorum within the aortic media ▶ the haematoma may remain localized or propagate and rupture through the intima

  NECT A hyperdense subintimal haematoma (a mural thrombus will lie on top of the intima)
- *A penetrating atherosclerotic ulcer:* ulceration of an atheromatous plaque can disrupt the internal elastic lamina (exposing the media to pulsatile arterial flow with the subsequent development of a haematoma within the media)

CECT A focal contrast medium-filled outpouching surrounded by intramural haematoma (an atheromatous plaque will not extend beyond the intima and an intramural haematoma will be absent)

Predisposing factors

- *Cystic medial degeneration due to:* coarctation ▶ aortitis ▶ a bicuspid aortic valve ▶ pregnancy ▶ blunt chest trauma ▶ advancing age (± hypertension) ▶ connective tissue disorders (e.g. Marfan's and Ehlers–Danlos syndromes)

Mechanisms of branch vessel ischaemia

- *Dynamic obstruction:* this affects vessels arising from the true lumen – bowing of the dissection flap across the true lumen can cause collapse of the true lumen and restriction of branch vessel ostial flow
- *Static obstruction:* this results from extension of the dissection into a branch vessel without a re-entry point ▶ the increased pressure or thrombus formation within the branch vessel false lumen produces a focal stenosis (± end-organ ischaemia)
  - Both dynamic and static obstruction can coexist – the identification of the mechanism of ischaemia is vital (as the endovascular management differs)

Classification

- *Acute dissection:* < 14 days
  - *Subacute:* > 14 days to 2 months
  - *Chronic:* >2 months

CLINICAL PRESENTATION

- Chest (± back pain) ▶ branch vessel occlusion can lead to neurological deficits as well as blood pressure differences between the extremities (which may ultimately become ischaemic)
- A dissection commonly occurs in middle-aged to elderly hypertensive patients

Classification systems for aortic dissection

Site of dissection	Classification system		
	Crawford	DeBakey	Stanford
Both ascending and descending aorta	Proximal dissections	Type I	Type A
Ascending aorta and arch only	Proximal dissections	Type II	Type A
Descending aorta only (distal to left subclavian artery)	Distal dissections	Type III IIIa – limited to thoracic aorta IIIb – extends to abdominal aorta	Type B

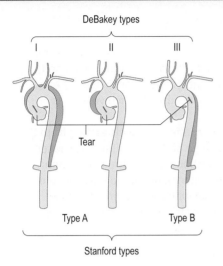

DeBakey types

I II III

Tear

Type A Type B

Stanford types

Schematic diagram showing the DeBakey and Stanford classification of aortic dissection.

Axial CT image of a type B aortic dissection. There is a circumferential intimal flap seen on CT as a hypodense linear image inside the aorta. The true lumen is very small and completely surrounded by the false lumen (intimal intussusception).**

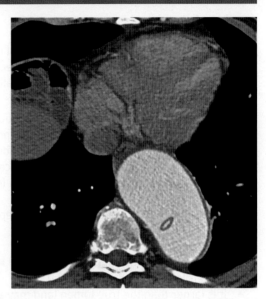

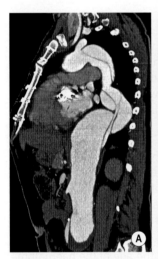
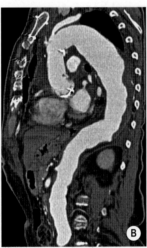
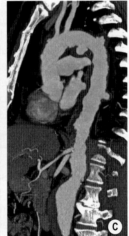

MDCT sagittal oblique MPR images of a type B dissection (A) and an aneurysm with mural thrombus (B). Note the spiralling shape of the intimal flap and the true lumen in the descending aorta, while the thrombus maintains its relationship with the posterior aortic wall. The internal border of the thrombus is irregular, different from aortic dissection and the calcifications are on the external border. (C) Penetrating atherosclerotic ulcers. MDCT sagittal oblique MPR image shows diffuse multiple finger-like ulcers of descending thoracic aorta. Severe and diffuse aortic wall atheromas are present.**

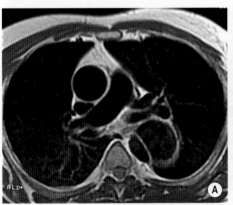
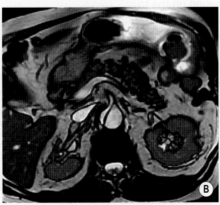
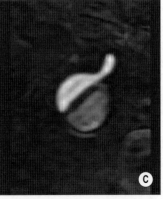

(A) Axial BBFSE image of chronic type B aortic dissection. The intimal flap is well depicted as a straight hyperintense line dividing the true and false lumen at the level of descending aorta. (B) Axial SSFP image of type B dissection at the level of the abdominal aorta. Note the optimal contrast resolution between aortic lumen and wall with an excellent depiction of the intimal flap and its relationship with the origin of SMA. (C) MR angiography of type B aortic dissection. Axial image displays clearly the relationships of true and false lumen with coeliac trunk, superior mesenteric artery (SMA), right and left arteries, respectively. Note that true lumen is the smaller and best enhanced one.**

AORTIC DISSECTION

Radiological features

NECT This may demonstrate any intramural haematoma (as areas of increased attenuation) ▶ the dissection flap may be visible as a linear track of high attenuation (from intimal calcification) within the aortic lumen

CECT This is the primary imaging investigation ▶ images are acquired just cephalad to the aortic arch and extend inferiorly down to the aortic bifurcation or femoral heads ▶ avoid injecting via the left arm (as this may cause a potential streak artefact across the aortic arch from the left brachiocephalic vein)

- *Dissection flap:* a band of low attenuation separating the contrast enhanced true and false lumens
- *False lumen:*
  - *Location:* anterolateral (ascending aorta) ▶ posterolateral (descending aorta)
  - It is larger than the true lumen (and may also compress the true lumen)
  - It will demonstrate delayed opacification (due to its slower flow)

MRI Sensitivity and specificity approaching 100% ▶ with BBFSE sequences the bright flap is seen within the black vessel lumen

- *False lumen:* higher SI than the true lumen (due to slower flow)
- *False lumen:* cobwebs adjacent to the outer wall (representing residual strands within the dissected media)
- Sagittal FSE sequence can define any dissection extent ▶ MRI + Gad for assessing detailed anatomy ▶ SSFP sequences can give high contrast between the lumen and wall

Transoesophageal echocardiography This provides real-time imaging ▶ it can localize the site of any intimal tears ▶ it provides haemodynamic information on the true and false lumen flows ▶ it can assess the functional status of the aortic valve and coronary arterial involvement for type A dissections

- *Disadvantage:* it only provides poor views of the distal ascending aorta and some of the aortic arch

Intravascular ultrasound (IVUS) This provides intraluminal cross-sectional vessel images ▶ it can demonstrate the entry tear and the extent of the dissection ▶ it can differentiate between a true and false lumen ▶ it can demonstrate dynamic obstruction

- *Disadvantage:* transducers (12.5 MHz) are expensive and generally there is limited experience in most departments

Pearls

- This represents the most common non-traumatic acute aortic emergency with an overall in-hospital mortality of 15–20%

- *Visceral malperfusion:* suggested by a thread-like true lumen or an intimal flap showing a convexity towards the true lumen ▶ can lead to renal ischaemia or GI ischaemia (mesenteric oedema/thickened and decreased bowel enhancement – 'shock bowel') ▶ restriction of flow into the aortic branch vessels is caused by:
  1. *Dynamic obstruction:* affects vessels arising from the true lumen ▶ collapse of the true lumen is caused by bowing of the dissection flap into the true lumen
  2. *Static obstruction:* extension of the dissection into the branching vessel without a re-entry point ▶ increased pressure or thrombus within the false lumen produces focal stenosis

Acute aortic syndrome

- A general term used to encompass: aortic dissection/ intramural haematoma/penetrating atherosclerotic ulcer

Intramural haematoma
Definition

- A lesion confined to the aortic wall and therefore subintimal ▶ it can be spontaneous or from a penetrating aortic ulcer or following trauma ▶ there can be symmetric or asymmetric wall thickening (3 mm – 1 cm) ▶ there are smooth walls (cf. irregular walls with plaque or thrombus)

Radiological features

CT Hyperdense on NECT (acute) ▶ no enhancement (cf. a false lumen) ▶ constant circumferential wall relationship (cf. a spiralling relationship with a false lumen) ▶ no luminal reduction (cf. a compressed true lumen with a false lumen)

MRI This can help differentiate the age of the haematoma

Penetrating atherosclerotic ulcer (PAU)
Definition

- An aortic ulcer disrupting the internal elastic lamina + haematoma with a focal contrast filled outpouching surrounded by an intramural haematoma (an atheromatous plaque does not extend beyond the intima, is frequently calcified and lacks intramural haematoma) ▶ this can evolve into a localised dissection or pseudoaneurysm ▶ mainly located within the descending aorta but also seen within the aortic arch

Radiological features

- CT/MRI: a crater like, contrast filled outpouching with jagged edges

Pearl

- PAU and IMH are potential precursors of dissection ▶ IMH can evolve into PAU

Differentiation of a dissection (with a thrombosed false lumen) and an aneurysm with calcified mural thrombus		
	Dissection (thrombosed false lumen)	**Aneurysm (calcified mural thrombus)**
NECT	High attenuation within the false lumen	No high attenuation within the false lumen
Morphology	Usually an extensive lesion spiraling as it passes along the aorta	A more focal lesion maintaining a constant relationship to aortic wall
Border	An irregular internal border	A smooth internal border
Calcification	Intimal calcification can be seen within the aorta	Intimal calcification can be seen at the periphery of the thrombus
Aortic lumen	This is often normal	This is large

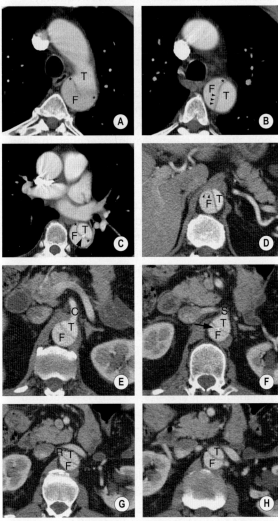

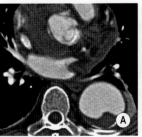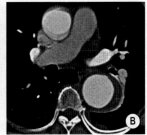

CT cross-sectional images of a thrombosed aneurysm (A) and an IMH (B) of descending thoracic aorta. Note that IMH has a typical semilunar shape with smooth borders, while the thrombus margins are irregular.**

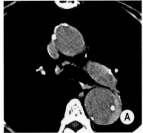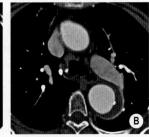

Typical CT appearance of an acute IMH. The crescent-like wall thickening is hyperdense in relation to the lumen on unenhanced CT image (A), while the density reverses after contrast administration (B).**

Differentiating the true and false lumen on CT. The false lumen usually tracks around the convexity of the aortic arch (A) and is more often than not the larger of the two lumens (B–E). The outer wall of the false lumen produces an acute angle at its junction with the dissection flap (asterisk) (A–C,H). Occasionally, linear strands of low attenuation may be seen within the false lumen (cobweb sign). These represent residual strands of media incompletely sheared away at the time of dissection (arrowheads) (B,D). Finally, the true lumen can be correctly identified by its continuity with the non-dissected aorta. Intimal calcification can be seen along the dissection flap (arrows) (C,F). C = coeliac axis, F = false lumen, R = right renal artery, S = superior mesenteric artery, T = true lumen.*

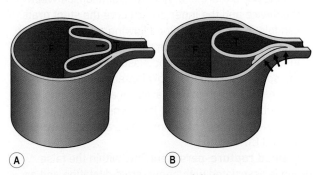

Diagram of branch vessel ischaemia. (A) Dynamic obstruction. The intimomedial flap bows across the true lumen (arrow) and obstructs flow into the branch vessel. (B) Static obstruction. The dissection extends into the branch vessel and may thrombose (arrowheads), causing stenosis of the vessel origin. F = false lumen, T = true lumen.**

THORACIC AORTIC DISSECTION

Management

- **Initial:** medically reduce the systolic blood pressure (< 100–200 mmHg) and reduce the rate of rise of the left ventricular systolic pressure
- **Type A dissection** (75%): emergency surgical repair is required in all patients due to involvement of the aortic root ► generally unsuitable for endovascular repair (common involvement of the aortic valve and coronaries)
- **Type B dissection** (25%): treatment is based on a complication-specific approach
  - **Uncomplicated disease** (no rupture or branch vessel ischaemia): medical treatment
  - **Complicated disease** (or failed medical management): surgical or endovascular intervention (there is a reduced morbidity and mortality with endovascular techniques) ► the aim is to treat the complications of the pathology and prevent aneurysm formation and rupture ► early surgery is recommended in Marfan's syndrome

Endovascular treatment of a type B dissection

- Restoration of flow is achieved by closure (stent coverage) of the dissection entry tear to depressurize the false lumen and allow true lumen re-expansion ► ideally the false lumen should collapse entirely and thrombose – ongoing false lumen perfusion can occur via uncovered fenestrations, retrogradely from the distal dissection or from branch vessel backbleeding ► 'cheese-wiring' the flap can also be used to eradicate the false lumen
- Stent grafts for acute dissection should not be oversized (cf. TAA) as the vessel wall is very friable (converting a type B to a type A)
- Requires enough disease free aorta proximally (15–20 mm) to achieve a seal ► the left subclavian artery can be covered by the device without significant morbidity ► more proximal seals can be achieved with prior carotid-carotid bypass
  - Excessive aortic arch angulation is a problem where it is not a smooth curve – this can lead to a type 1 endoleak – if there is a marked 'stand-off' between the device and the inner aortic curve the stent graft can fold in on itself by blood flowing around the graft rather than through it ► preferably seal zones will be in straight segments ► endovascular repair can risk the spinal cord blood supply (anterior spinal artery which is a branch of the vertebral artery arising from the subclavian artery, and the dominant radicular artery – the artery of Adamkiewicz arising between T8 and L1)
- **Contained rupture:** persistent flow within the false lumen is associated with aneurysmal dilatation and an increased risk of rupture ► stent graft placement across the entry tear can promote thrombosis of the false lumen (reducing the rupture risk) ► the dissection flap in a chronic dissection may become thickened and rigid

reducing the chance of a complete false lumen exclusion
- **Branch vessel ischaemia:**
  - **Dynamic obstruction** (resulting from true lumen collapse): sealing the entry tear with stent graft placement directs the blood flow back into the true lumen (increasing the true lumen size and moving the dissection flap away from any branch vessels)
  - **Static obstruction:** direct stent insertion into the compromised vessel (via the true lumen) or the deliberate formation of holes in the flap ('fenestration') may be required
- **Percutaneous fenestration:** this is less frequently employed since the introduction of endovascular techniques ► both the lumens are accessed and a stiff guidewire is passed from the true into the false lumen with a large balloon inflated across the flap to produce the fenestration
  - If multiple, debate exists as to whether all fenestrations or just the 'primary' entry tear should be covered – the hope being that covering the proximal tear only alters the haemodynamics enough to allow true lumen re-expansion

Abdominal aortic aneurysm

- Most AAA stent-graft systems comprise a main body with a long limb on one side and a short limb ('gate') on the other – once the main body is deployed the short limb is catheterized from the opposite side with a second limb inserted over a wire into the short limb (sealing inside the main body)
- The distal 'landing zone' is usually the common iliac artery – if not suitable then extension to the external iliac artery is possible (with embolization of the internal iliac artery to prevent a significant type II endoleak, but which can be associated with buttock claudication and erectile dysfunction)
- Surgical management of AAAs < 5.5 cm is associated with greater mortality than conservative management ► endovascular repair has a 30-day mortality one-third that of open repair (2 vs. 6%)
  - Possibly increased rate of secondary intervention with EVARs (type 1 and 2 endoleak), not all patients are anatomically suitable, and possible increased EVAR cost
- Emergency AAA (eEVAR) repair – trade-off between increased delay by scanning a haemodynamically compromised patient for stent planning vs. benefits of minimally invasive repair in a critically ill patient
  - eEVAR may be associated with reduced cost, transfusion requirements, intensive care and hospital stay
- 'Hybrid' repair: insertion of a stent graft with mesenteric and renal arteries surgically reimplanted onto a conduit from the iliac arteries
- Some endovascular grafts have fenestrations (holes) or branches to allow aortic side branch perfusion

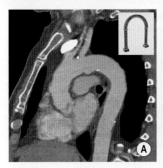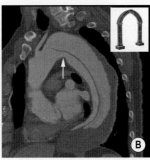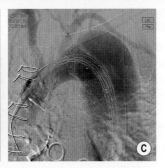

Aortic arch configurations for thoracic EVAR. (A) Norman arch configuration with a shallow ulcer on the inner curve at its apex. Note the smooth curve around the arch without a focal angle (inset: architectural drawing of a Norman arch). (B) Gothic arch configuration with an aortic dissection. Note the angle (arrow) at the apex of the arch (inset: architectural drawing of a Gothic arch). (C) Complication of stent-grafting into a short neck around the apex of a Gothic arch. The device has dislocated out of the short neck at the point of arch angulation, resulting in a significant type 1 endoleak. A new device is being deployed (arrow: delivery system nosecone), extending the stent-graft more proximally in the arch (covering the left subclavian artery) to seal the leak.** (Architectural images courtesy of Redwood Stone, West Horrington, Well, UK.)

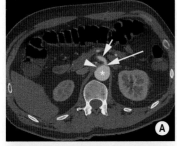

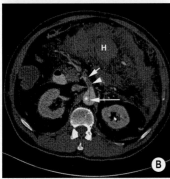

Static and dynamic branch vessel occlusion. (A) Dynamic branch vessel occlusion. The true lumen (arrowhead) is markedly compressed by the false lumen (asterisk). The dissection flap (long arrow) is seen to prolapse across the ostium of the superior mesenteric artery (SMA) (short arrow), compromising its inflow (though the SMA is still filling). The patient had abdominal pain, rising lactate and thickening of small bowel loops (not shown) consistent with small bowel ischaemia. (B) Static vessel occlusion. The dissection flap (long arrow) has extended into the SMA (short arrow) and there has been thrombosis of the false lumen in the SMA (arrowhead). The true lumen (asterisk) is obliterated distally in the SMA by the combination of the dissection and the thrombus. A large intraperitoneal haematoma is evident (H) due to bleeding from infarcted bowel.**

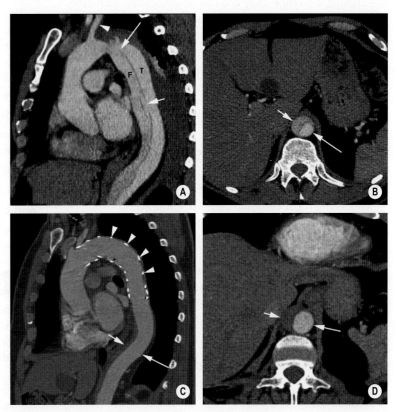

Coverage of proximal entry tear of a dissection with false lumen thrombosis and collapse. (A) Acute type B dissection. The entry tear (long arrow), a more distal fenestration (short arrow) and the dissection flap are clearly visualized. Arrowhead: left common carotid artery; F: false lumen; T: true lumen. (B) Representative aortic cross-section at the level of the diaphragmatic crura. The true lumen (long arrow) and false lumen (short arrow) both opacify with contrast, indicating patency. (C) Following stent-graft (arrowheads) placement in the true lumen, covering (and sealing) the proximal entry tear. The false lumen (short arrow) has thrombosed and partially collapsed. The true lumen (long arrow) remains patent. (D) Representative aortic cross-section (same level as B), demonstrating thrombosis of the false lumen (short arrow) and retained patency of the true lumen (long arrow).**

AORTIC ANEURYSMS

DEFINITION

- A common multifactorial condition characterized by the degeneration and remodelling of the aortic wall, which leads to abnormal dilatation ▶ an aneurysm is defined as a vessel diameter ≥ 1.5 times the normal diameter at the involved site

  True aneurysm This will contain all 3 arterial wall layers ▶ it will tend to have a fusiform shape and is commonly atherosclerotic in nature

  False aneurysm (pseudoaneurysm) The wall is represented by the adventitial layer only ▶ it will tend to have a saccular shape and can be post-traumatic or mycotic in nature

  Abdominal aortic aneurysm (AAA) (95%) This is defined as a vessel diameter ≥ 3 cm (rupture is uncommon with aneurysms < 5 cm) ▶ they are can be associated with other aneurysms (e.g. a popliteal aneurysm)
  - 90% are infrarenal in location

  Thoracic aortic aneurysm (15%) This is defined as a vessel diameter within the ascending aorta of ≥ 5 cm, and within the descending aorta of ≥ 4 cm (rupture is uncommon with aneurysms < 5 cm) ▶ they are commonly associated with abdominal aortic aneurysms

PATHOLOGICAL ANEURYSM TYPES

Atherosclerotic aortic aneurysms

- This is the most common cause of a thoracic or abdominal aneurysm ▶ 95% affect the abdominal aorta ▶ the circumferential atherosclerosis results in a fusiform aneurysm
  - The natural history is progressive remodelling, expansion and eventual rupture (this is a major cause of death as only 14% are symptomatic prior to rupture)
- Haemorrhage following rupture can mimic an inflammatory aneurysm
- Patients will usually have major associated co-morbidities (e.g. coronary disease, COPD, diabetes and renal disease)

Inflammatory aneurysms

- These are more commonly seen within abdominal aneurysms (accounting for 3–10% of all abdominal aortic aneurysms)
  - The underlying pathology is aortic dilatation with a thickened aneurysm wall, marked perianeurysmal and retroperitoneal fibrosis and dense adhesions to the adjacent abdominal organs ▶ they have a similar aetiology to atherosclerotic aneurysms but have a more marked inflammatory component (the risk of rupture remains)
- The age range at presentation is generally 5–10 years younger than that seen with atherosclerotic aneurysms (M > F)
  - These are more commonly symptomatic than a non-inflammatory aneurysm (e.g. abdominal or back pain) ▶ they can also present with weight loss and an elevated ESR
- Surgical management is technically difficult due to the adherence of adjacent structures (e.g. the ureters) to the inflammatory mass

Aneurysms commonly affecting the aortic root, ascending aorta and aortic arch

Mycotic aneurysms

- These result from infective thrombosis of the vasa vasorum with consequent destruction of the aortic intima and media ▶ they can be caused by emboli from infective endocarditis, septicaemia, or local spread
  - They are usually eccentric saccular aneurysms with an atypical position

Infective aneurysms

- Causes include a syphilitic aneurysm or as a delayed manifestation of tertiary syphilis

Connective tissue diseases

- Marfan's and Ehlers–Danlos syndromes

Aortitis

- Takayasu's arteritis ▶ collagen vascular diseases (e.g. rheumatoid arthritis and ankylosing spondylitis)

CLINICAL PRESENTATION

- *Thoracic aneurysm:* these are usually asymptomatic ▶ however they can present with pain, hoarseness or dysphagia
- *Abdominal aneurysm:* they are usually asymptomatic but can present with:
  - Back pain ▶ an expansile abdominal mass ▶ clinical signs of distal embolization ▶ congestive heart failure or haematemesis (due to an aortocaval fistula)
  - Cardiovascular collapse ± death (following rupture)
  - An abdominal aortic aneurysm <5.5 cm which is not rapidly enlarging and asymptomatic requires nothing more than regular US follow-up
  - Rupture risk: 5.5 cm AAA (annual rupture risk of 6%) ▶ 8 cm AAA (annual rupture risk of 25%)

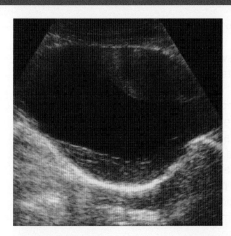

Ultrasound demonstrating a large 9 cm AAA (containing thrombus).[†]

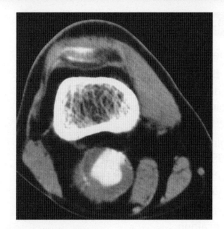

Axial CT demonstrating a right popliteal artery aneurysm.[†]

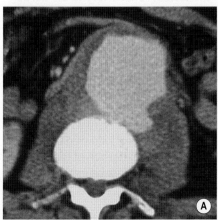

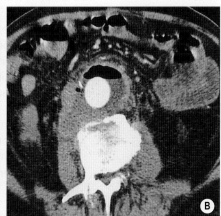

CT. (A) An aortic abdominal aneurysm with a contained leak into the left psoas muscle. (B) An infected aortic bifemoral Dacron graft with a gas–fluid level in the sac of the aneurysm.[†]

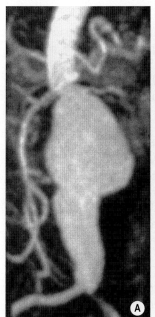

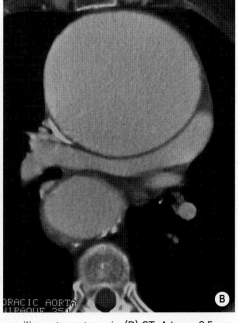

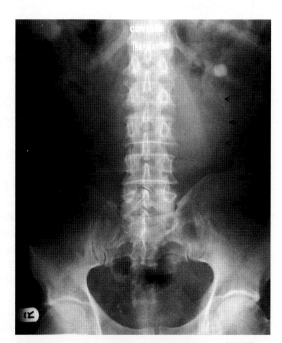

(A) MRA. An AAA and left common iliac artery stenosis. (B) CT. A large 9.5 cm ascending thoracic aortic aneurysm.[†]

Control image from IVU requested because of left renal colic. Curvilinear calcification (arrowheads) is consistent with a significantly sized calcified abdominal aortic aneurysm.[*]

AORTIC ANEURYSMS

RADIOLOGICAL FEATURES

CXR A soft tissue mediastinal mass (± calcification)

AXR Mass effect on the surrounding structures (e.g. small bowel) ▶ curvilinear aortic wall calcification

- A lateral lumbar spine view may reveal anterior scalloping of the vertebral bodies

US Abdominal imaging is the method of choice for screening ▶ regular US follow up is appropriate for abdominal aneurysms <5.5 cm (which are not rapidly enlarging or symptomatic)

CT This is being increasingly used with the introduction of endovascular stent grafting

- **Rupture:** discontinuous aortic wall ▶ contrast extravasation ▶ periaortic haematoma
- **Impending rupture:** haemorrhagic pleural effusion ▶ periaortic haematoma ▶ periadventitial enhancement or acute inflammation are signs of potential instability
- **Haemorrhage**: this appears as poorly defined retroperitoneal tissue planes (making identification of any inflammatory component difficult) ▶ fresh blood has a higher CT attenuation than muscle, and usually tracks into the pararenal fat away from the aneurysm ▶ there may be contrast extravasation
- **Peri-aortitis:** this appears as a thick cuff of enhancing inflammatory soft tissue around the aorta (a liposarcoma and bladder cancer can also cause a similar strong inflammatory fibrous reaction) ▶ enhancement of the periaortic cuff

MRI Standard BBSE sequences can evaluate the aortic wall and periaortic space ▶ MRI + Gad is also helpful

Imaging features to be addressed with a thoracic aneurysm

- The size and morphology of the aneurysm
- Its position superiorly in relation to the great vessels (>15 mm): a left subclavian artery can be covered if both the vertebral arteries are patent
- The diameter of any potential stent graft 'drop zone' superiorly
- The amount of atheroma at the proximal and distal graft site (which can potentially affect the seal)
- The distal extent of the aneurysm and its relationship to the visceral arteries (>15 mm) – these may require bypassing or stenting if they have to be covered
- The abdominal aorta must be of a satisfactory size and condition to allow passage of the stent graft delivery system
- There must not be a large radicular artery supplying the spinal cord (this can be potentially covered by a stent graft)

Imaging features to be addressed with an abdominal aneurysm

- The AP and transverse size of the aneurysm
- The aortic diameter at and just below the level of the visceral arteries
- The aneurysm neck length from the lowest renal artery to the aneurysm origin (this needs to be at least 15 mm)
- The neck shape (a conical neck may lead to a poor proximal seal and a late endoleak)
  - Significant atheroma within the neck may prevent the formation of a perfect seal
- The neck angulation (AP and lateral) ▶ if this is > 60° a satisfactory seal may be difficult to achieve or the stent graft may dislodge
- The distance from the lowest renal artery to the aortic bifurcation (this determines the graft length)
- Any accessory renal arteries that may have to be covered (a preoperative assessment of split renal function may be required)
- The size, tortuosity and calcification of the common femoral and external iliac arteries (a stenosis precludes stent delivery)
  - If the common iliac artery is aneurysmal then the possibility of buttock claudication following internal iliac artery embolization and extension of the stent graft into external iliac artery must be explained to the patient

PEARLS

Treatment

- **Thoracic aortic aneurysm:** endovascular repair should be considered when an asymptomatic descending thoracic aneurysm reaches 5.5 cm (6 cm for open repair due to the higher risks) ▶ rapidly expanding or symptomatic aneurysms require treatment regardless of size
- **Atherosclerotic aneurysms**: open surgical repair ▶ endovascular stent grafting (this is associated with lower blood loss and a quicker recovery)
- **Inflammatory aneurysms:** steroid therapy can be used to control the inflammatory process ▶ a conventional surgical approach is technically difficult making endovascular grafting an attractive option (the ureters can be involved in the inflammatory process, and the duodenum and left renal vein are often adherent to the aneurysm)
  - The repair of an inflammatory aneurysm halts progression of any retroperitoneal fibrosis but does not cure it
- **Mycotic aneurysms:** the results of surgical treatment can be poor ▶ stent grafting gives mixed results

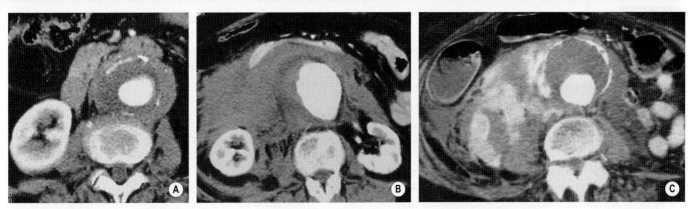

CT. (A) An inflammatory AAA with calcification in its wall. (B) A leaking AAA with a retroperitoneal haematoma. (C) A leaking AAA with active retroperitoneal bleeding (indicated by the high attenuation contrast within the haematoma).[†]

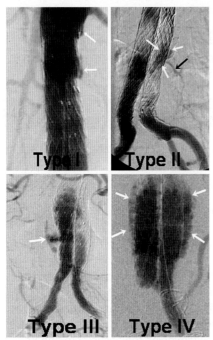

Four types of endoleak are identified which can complicate the exclusion of an aneurysm by stent graft. Type I is the most dangerous and is due to failure to obtain a seal either proximally or distally. This should not be left and is usually solved with a moulding balloon and/or a cuff. Type II is caused by retrograde flow into the sac from lumbar or inferior mesenteric arteries. Mostly these resolve themselves but if they do not and the sac continues to enlarge they have to be embolized retrogradely. Type III is due to a failure of the stent graft material. This can be due to a manufacturing problem or long-term wear and tear and changes in aneurysm morphology causing holes in the graft or dislocations of modular components. They can be fixed either by repeat stent grafting or open surgery. Type IV is unimportant and rarely occurs now. It was due to graft porosity. The term endotension (type V) is applied where there is sac expansion in the absence of a recognizable type I–IV endoleak. The white arrows in types I–III indicate the site of leak for each type. The black arrow in type II indicates a supplying lumbar artery.*

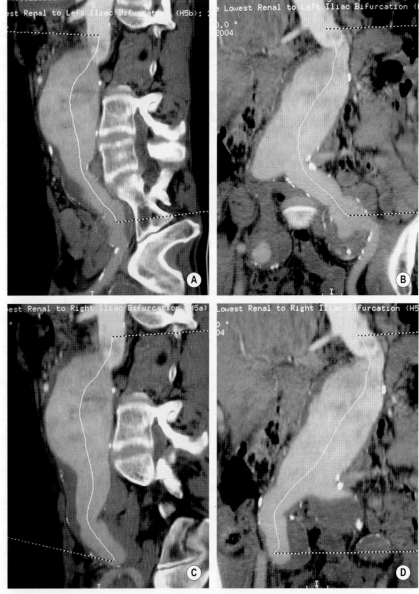

(A,C) Sagittal and (B,D) coronal reconstructions of an axially acquired CECT with measurements. Such reconstructions and measurements are vital to the successful use of stent grafts to treat significantly sized abdominal and thoracic aortic aneurysms.*

203

MID-AORTIC SYNDROME

Definition

- This is characterized by segmental narrowing of the proximal abdominal aorta and ostial stenosis of its major branches ▶ causes include:

von Recklinghausen's disease (type 1 neurofibromatosis)

- A genetic disorder associated with chromosome 17 ▶ it is distinguished from other causes of a mid-aortic syndrome by the presence of café au lait skin lesions and neurofibromas
- Vascular abnormalities include renal, aortic and mesenteric stenoses (affecting 2% of patients) ▶ vessels are surrounded by neurofibromatous and ganglioneuromatous adventitial tissue

Alagille's syndrome

- A multisystem autosomal dominant disorder caused by mutations in the *JAG1* gene (chromosome 20p12)
- It often presents during infancy and early childhood with clinical symptoms involving the liver (e.g. cholestasis)

- Mid-aortic coarctation is one of several heart, bone and ocular defects that can also occur
- Patients have distinctive facial features: deep set eyes ▶ frontal bossing ▶ a bulbous tip of the nose ▶ a down-turned mouth ▶ a small mandible ▶ a pointed chin

Williams' syndrome

- A rare genetic condition ▶ patients have characteristic facial features and metabolic problems (particularly hypercalcaemia)
- Mid-abdominal or thoracic coarctation commonly causes hypertension

Congenital aortic coarctation   This can involve the mid-thoracic or abdominal aorta and is a very uncommon cause of mid-aortic syndrome

Clinical presentation

- It is usually diagnosed in young adults (it may present in childhood) ▶ hypertension is a feature in all cases

GRANULOMATOUS VASCULITIS (TAKAYASU'S DISEASE)

Definition

- A chronic inflammatory disease involving the aorta, its branches and the pulmonary arteries ▶ there can be varying degrees of stenosis, occlusion, or dilatation of the involved vessels ▶ the aetiology is unknown
  - Initially there is inflammation around the vasa vasorum of the media and adventitia which progresses to nodular fibrosis of all the wall layers
- The infrarenal aorta, IMA and iliac vessels are not usually involved ▶ intercostal collaterals rarely occur as the disease also affects the ostia of the intercostal vessels (cf. aortic coarctation)

Clinical presentation

- It is predominantly a disease of young adults (it can affect children but is very rare in infancy) ▶ F>M (up to 9:1) ▶ it is commonly seen in Ashkenazi Jews

Radiological features

Angiography   Features occur late in the disease and include luminal irregularity, vessel stenosis, occlusion, dilatation and aneurysms within the aorta or its primary branches
- *Type I:* involving the aortic arch and its branches
- *Type II:* involving the thoracoabdominal aorta and its branches
- *Type III:* lesions of both type I and II
- *Type IV:* pulmonary arterial involvement in addition to any of the above types

US/CT/contrast-enhanced MRI   These are beginning to replace angiography ▶ aortic intimal calcification may be seen

- FDG-PET may demonstrate increased uptake in affected vessels

Pearls

- The major morbidity and mortality result from stenosis and occlusion of the aorta, renal and carotid arteries
- Saccular or fusiform aortic aneurysms occur in 2–26% of cases and usually coexist with stenotic lesions ▶ aneurysms without a stenosis, pseudoaneurysms or an aortic dissection are rare
- There can be differing patterns of vessel involvement according to the geographical area:
  - *Japan:* it commonly involves the aortic arch and its branches
  - *Korea/India:* the thoracoabdominal aorta is mainly involved

Treatment

- *Surgical treatment is not preferred because of the diffuse, inflammatory and progressive nature of the disease*
- **Acute phase:** corticosteroids ± cytotoxic drugs (for resistant cases)
- **Angioplasty of stenosed segments:** this is preferably performed during the chronic phase of the disease (but may be performed acutely)
  - *Renal artery:* this is successful in up to 90% of cases ▶ restenosis may occur in 20–25% ▶ renal artery stents are not usually required
  - *Aorta:* this is highly effective even in diffuse, long segment stenoses (90%) ▶ restenosis may occur in 14–20% of cases ▶ stents should not be used in children

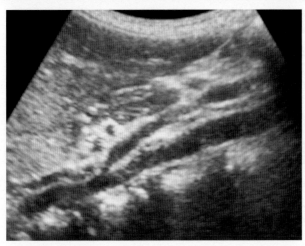

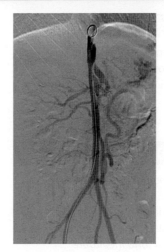

Right oblique abdominal aortogram in a hypertensive patient with the cutaneous stigmata of neurofibromatosis. Note the mid-aortic stenosis and the coeliac axis and superior mesenteric artery stenoses with collateral supply from the inferior mesenteric artery.*

Longitudinal abdominal US. There is stenosis at the origin of the superior mesenteric artery and narrowing and irregularity of the aorta. This is characteristic of mid-aortic syndrome. The patient had café au lait spots consistent with the diagnosis of neurofibromatosis.*

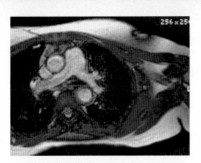

Takayasu's disease. MRI shows thickening of all layers of the descending thoracic aortic wall and is also seen in the left subclavian origin.*

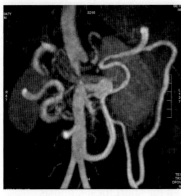

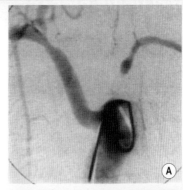

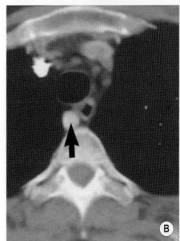

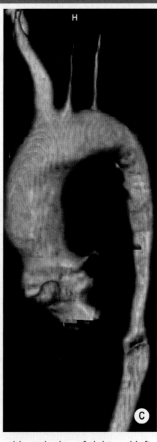

A contrast-enhanced MRA confirms mid-aortic syndrome with focal occlusion of the juxtarenal aorta. The distal aorta is perfused by the mesenteric arteries. There is a grossly hypertrophied inferior mesenteric artery together with hypertrophied marginal artery and arc of Riolan. The source images (not shown) demonstrated a high-grade right renal artery stenosis but normal left renal and superior mesenteric arteries. Axial FISP images (not shown) confirmed a thickened aortic wall at the level of the occlusion consistent with Takayasu's disease.*

(A) DSA. (B) CT. Takayashu's disease with occlusion of right and left common carotid and left subclavian arteries, but patent aberrant right subclavian artery (arrow) with stenosis.† (C) MDCT VR reconstruction of a 20-year-old woman presenting with right arm ischaemia and hypertension with diagnosis of Takayasu's disease. Thickening of all layers of the proximal and mid descending thoracic aorta wall produced segmental lumen reduction.**

ACUTE AORTIC OCCLUSIVE DISEASE

DEFINITION

- A vascular emergency resulting from either
  - A saddle embolus of the aortic bifurcation
  - An in situ thrombosis of an aortic stenosis or aneurysm
  - A traumatic dissection

CLINICAL PRESENTATION

- A neurological deficit (including paralysis) of the lower limbs – this can be confused with a spinal cord compression and potentially delay the diagnosis
- An absence of the femoral pulses
- *Signs of irreversible ischaemia (and inevitable amputation):* major tissue loss ▶ absent capillary return with marbling ▶ profound paralysis and sensory loss ▶ absent Doppler signals

RADIOLOGICAL FEATURES

Catheter angiography/MRA The purpose of imaging is to differentiate an embolic from a thrombotic occlusion, confirm the proximal extent of the occlusion and determine the state of the run-off (a poor run-off mitigates against percutaneous intervention)

PEARLS

Treatment

- *Bypass grafting or surgical embolectomy:* if it is due to a thrombotic or an embolic acute event
- *Endovascular thrombolysis:* if the severity of the ischaemia allows for this
- *Following successful revascularization:* a treatable cause must be excluded (e.g. cardiac echocardiography to exclude an embolic source or angioplasty of any underlying vascular stenosis)

CHRONIC AORTIC OCCLUSIVE DISEASE

DEFINITION

- Aortic occlusive disease that is predominantly secondary to atherosclerosis (>90%) – Takayasu's disease accounts for the rest
- The infrarenal aorta and iliofemoral arteries are hypoplastic ▶ the infrainguinal arteries are 'protected' by the aortic lesion and are characteristically disease free

CLINICAL PRESENTATION

- Chronic lower limb ischaemia (± absent femoral pulses and a reduced ABPI) ▶ symptoms of critical limb ischaemia are unusual at presentation and are associated with supra- and infrainguinal disease
- It tends to affect younger patients than for lower limb arterial disease ▶ patients are typically female, heavy smokers and demonstrate hyperlipidaemia

RADIOLOGICAL FEATURES

Angiography This is currently the investigation of choice

MRA This offers major advantages as it is non-invasive ▶ it provides excellent images of the aortic lesion and any associated run-off ▶ unlike CT it avoids the need for large volumes of iodinated contrast medium

- *Considerations to be addressed:*
  - The upper limit of the lesion (infrarenal or juxtarenal?)
  - The lower limit of the lesion (is there involvement of the aortic bifurcation?)
  - Are the coeliac axis and superior mesenteric arteries normal? – this is important as intervention compromises the inferior mesenteric artery and collateral supplies are therefore important

PEARLS

Management

- **Traditional treatment:** surgical aortic bypass surgery or aortic endarterectomy (with primary patencies of 75–90% and 90–95%, respectively)
  - However there is an appreciable morbidity (9–27%) and mortality (1–7%)
- **Endovascular techniques:** this is now the treatment of choice, consisting of angioplasty with selective or primary stenting
  - *Angioplasty:* this is used for short focal stenosis (<2 cm)
  - *Stenting:* this is usually reserved for a flow limiting dissection or a residual stenosis following angioplasty ▶ primary stenting is advocated for occlusions and complex lesions (eccentric, ulcerated or calcified plaques) where there is a risk of distal embolization

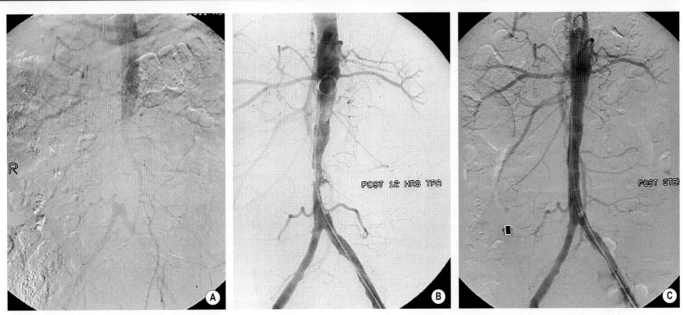

Acute aortic occlusion. (A) Infrarenal aortic occlusion with meniscus sign suggests that this is an embolic occlusion. (B) However, following successful thrombolysis, an underlying stenosis is revealed which appears secondary to extrinsic compression of the aorta. (C) A good angiographic result is achieved after stent placement.*

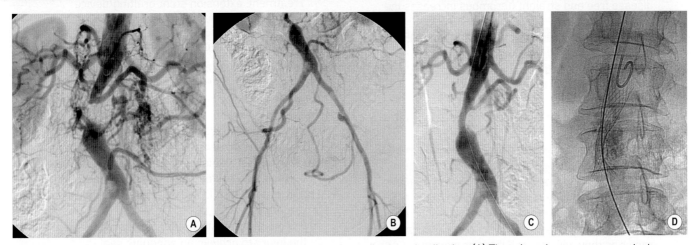

Chronic aortic occlusion in a 56-year-old woman presenting with short-distance claudication. (A) There is a short-segment occlusion of the infrarenal aorta. The aorta proximal to this is also diseased and narrowed. The lumbar arteries are markedly hypertrophied. (B) A plaque is seen at the aortic bifurcation, but the iliac arteries are relatively disease free. (C) Following primary stenting of the occlusion the patient's symptoms subsided, despite underdilatation of the lesion. (D) The extreme calcific nature of the lesion is seen on the native image.*

INTERVENTIONAL ENDOVASCULAR MANAGEMENT

Aortic intervention

- The cohort of patients requiring aortic surgery are often those least able to withstand it (medical co-morbidities/ diseased and friable aortic tissue) – hence the development of minimally invasive endovascular therapies
- *Stent-graft:* a fabric tube (woven polyester or Gore-Tex) with circular or crown shaped metal struts providing support to the fabric ▶ the stent graft is held in place by the radial force of the ring stents (some devices have small hooks to engage with the aortic wall) ▶ some devices are uncovered at one end to provide additional anchorage ▶ complex devices (fenestrated or branched) can be made to order ▶ stent grafts are supplied preloaded on a deployment system constrained within a sheath – when this is removed the stent expands under its own radial force (some systems allow partial deployment and repositioning prior to release)
  - Proximal 'seal' point: neck
  - Distal 'seal' point: landing zone
- *Stent considerations:*
  - A stent graft is usually oversized relative to the aorta by 10–20% to give a good 'seal'
  - The aortic neck/landing zone should be relatively disease free and straight (thrombus increases the risk of endoleak)
  - Most stent grafts require a neck length of 8–15 mm to achieve a seal
  - A sharply angulated neck risks the stent not deploying truly perpendicular to the aortic wall (increased leak risk)
  - Barrel or conical shaped necks increase the risk of a poor seal
  - 'Windsock' effect: systolic pressure forcing a partially deployed stent distally from its intended position
  - Patients with narrow access vessels may require adjunctive angioplasty/stenting/placement of a temporary surgical conduit – heavily calcified or tortuous access vessels may preclude endovascular repair as they will not straighten or expand sufficiently to allow passage of the delivery system

Endovascular repair complications

- ***Endoleak***
  - *Type 1:* poor sealing between the device and the aortic wall (proximal and distal seals) resulting in the leakage of blood between the aortic wall and device
    - Associated with adverse neck morphology/device migration/errors in sizing ▶ poor long-term outcome (risk of rupture), requiring treatment
    - *Therapeutic options:* insertion of extension cuffs/ balloon moulding/restenting of the seal zones/

transcatheter embolization of the endoleak/device explantation and repair
  - *Type 2:* retrograde blood flow into the diseased aorta via small aortic side branches (not usually occluded during endovascular repair)
    - Often spontaneously cease and do not require treatment in the absence of ongoing expansion ▶ treatment is usually side branch embolization
  - *Type 3:* graft defects and fabric tears
    - Requires treatment (balloon moulding any joints/ relining defects with a second device/operative repair)
  - *Type 4:* transient graft 'porosity'
    - Rare ▶ does not require treatment
  - *Type 5:* ongoing sac expansion in the absence of a demonstrable cause
    - Treatment may be required (can be difficult and complex)
- ***Device migration***
  - Migration occurs especially where the proximal seal zone is short or diseased (suboptimal device apposition) ▶ migration can result in limb kinking (predisposing to occlusion or thrombus/embolus) ▶ migration can result in a type 1 or 3 endoleak
  - Treatment: extension stent grafting/device reinforcement/device explantation

Traumatic Aortic Injury (TAI)

- Patient outcome is related as much to associated injuries as to the TAI itself, therefore it has been suggested to delay surgical repair until these other life-threatening conditions are managed (definitive repair may be delayed by days or weeks)
  - Controlled hypotension is mandatory (systolic < 70 mmHg), β-blockers to reduce rate of systolic ejection, decreasing shear forces on aortic wall
- Thoracic stent graft (TSG) is a less-invasive alternative to surgery
  - It requires at least 15 mm of aortic wall proximal to the injury to achieve an adequate seal
  - As the isthmus is the most common site of TAI and usually close to the site of origin of the left subclavian artery (LSA), this proximal distance can be insufficient – this 'landing zone' can be lengthened by intentionally covering the LSA and extending the graft to the origin of the left common carotid artery (most patients have an adequate collateral supply to the left arm via the circle of Willis and left vertebral artery)

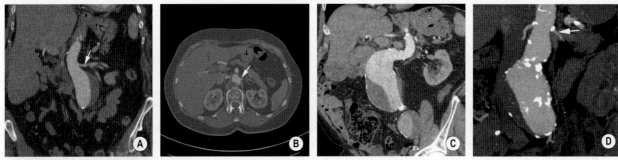

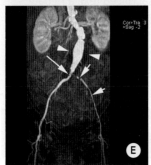

Adverse anatomy for EVAR. (A) Short neck between the renal artery (short arrow) and the aneurysm. (B) Significant atheroma/thrombus in the aneurysm neck (posteriorly) at the level of the renal artery (short arrow). (C) Markedly angulated neck with 90° bends between the suprarenal aorta and the neck (which runs horizontally in the image) and between the neck and the aneurysm itself. (D) Conical neck below the renal artery (short arrow). (E) Stenosed access vessels precluding passage of a device delivery system. There is a right common iliac artery origin stenosis (long arrow) and multifocal left iliac stenoses (short arrows). The true diameter of the AAA (between the arrowheads) is discernible from the dark bands of thrombus outwith the flowing lumen.**

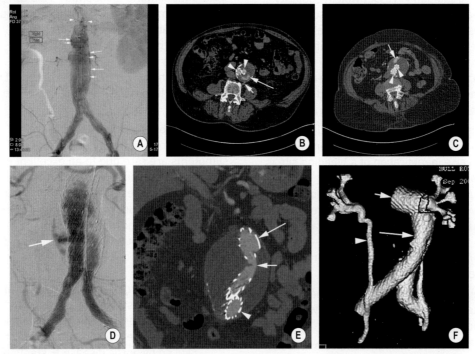

Complications of EVAR. (A) Type 1 endoleak. Pigtail aortogram immediately following stent-graft deployment. The outer margins of the stent-graft are indicated by the lateral edges of the ring stents (short arrows). Contrast can be seen outside the stent-graft in the aneurysm sac and neck (long arrows). The lumbar vessels were filling antegradely, indicating this was not a type 2 leak. The proximal markers on the stent-graft fabric (arrowheads) are evident just below the proximal bare metal stent. (B) Type 2 endoleak from a lumbar vessel. A pool of contrast (long arrow) is evident posteriorly in the aneurysm sac outside the stent-graft limbs (arrowheads). It lies in close association with a prominent lumbar vessel (short arrow). (C) Type 2 endoleak from the inferior mesenteric artery. A pool of contrast (arrow) is evident anteriorly in the aneurysm sac outside the stent-graft limbs (arrowheads). It lies in close association with the inferior mesenteric artery (not shown). (D) Type 3 endoleak. A defect in the graft fabric has resulted in leakage of contrast from the graft lumen into the aneurysm sac (arrow). (E) Limb kinking. A fold of stent-graft fabric (short arrow), causing significant stenosis in one of the limbs of a bifurcated device (reformatted oblique image), is evident. The other limb (arrowhead) and proximal main body (long arrow) are unremarkable as they course through the image plane. (F) Device dislocation. Morphological changes in the aneurysm post EVAR have resulted in marked dislocation of a proximal extension cuff (short arrow) out of the main body (long arrow) of this bifurcated device. The renal collecting systems have been opacified by iodinated contrast media at the time of scan (arrowhead).**

MESENTERIC HAEMORRHAGE

Upper gastrointestinal (GI) haemorrhage This is defined as bleeding proximal to the duodenal–jejunal flexure (most commonly from the left gastric artery)
- *Causes:* peptic ulceration ▶ pancreatitis ▶ gastro-oesophageal varices ▶ as a complication of endoscopic, surgical, or percutaneous biliary procedures

Lower GI haemorrhage This is defined as bleeding distal to the duodenal–jejunal flexure and is less commonly seen
- *Causes:* colonic angiodysplasia ▶ diverticular disease ▶ neoplasms ▶ haemorrhoids

DSA This can detect active bleeding at a rate of 0.5 ml/min ▶ it is performed if an endoscopy is negative or if it is not possible to control the site of haemorrhage
- Selective catheterization of the coeliac axis, superior mesenteric and inferior mesenteric arteries is required
- *Direct sign of haemorrhage:* contrast medium extravasation into the bowel lumen (this may not be visible if the bleeding is intermittent or too slow)
- *Indirect signs of haemorrhage:* the presence of a pseudoaneurysm ▶ early venous return ▶ vascular lakes or tumour circulation ▶ vessel wall irregularity
- *Angiodysplasia:* a focal area of increased vascularity with dilated arterioles and an early prominent draining vein
- *Diverticulitis:* bleeding is often venous and difficult to demonstrate
- *Meckel's diverticulum:* a feeding vitelline artery extending beyond the mesenteric border and with no side branches (ending in a corkscrew appearance)

Embolization This is more difficult within the lower GI tract – as there is a poorer collateral supply than within the upper GI tract ▶ precise identification of a bleeding site is required to avoid ischaemia or infarction
- *Upper GI tract:* use particulate emboli (the good collateral supply means that ischaemia is rare)
- *Lower GI tract:* use coils (due to the poor collateral supply)
- Consider Gelfoam embolization for self-limiting lesions (thus allowing recanalization)

Red cell scintigraphy This is more sensitive and can detect bleeding rates as low as 0.1 ml/min ▶ however it cannot precisely localize a bleeding site

CT angiography This is increasingly used as a first line non-invasive investigation to evaluate and localize acute active GI bleeding ▶ it can detect bleeding rates as low as 0.3 ml/min ▶ an unenhanced CT scan is first performed followed by CT imaging in the arterial and portal venous phase ▶ high attenuation material within the bowel lumen at CTA not present on the unenhanced CT is diagnostic for acute GI haemorrhage ▶ active bleeding seen during the arterial phase will also increase or pool during the venous phase

VISCERAL ARTERY ANEURYSMS

- These are uncommon and usually involve the splenic artery (followed by the hepatic and superior mesenteric arteries)
- They are found incidentally on imaging or when they rupture
  - Rupture can be precipitated by trauma, atherosclerosis, arteritis, collagen vascular disorders, or infection

Endovascular treatment Embolization (coils, glue or particles) or stent graft insertions used alone or in combination
- If the involved vessel can be sacrificed (e.g. a hepatic artery aneurysm with patent portal vein) coils may be placed across its neck
- 'Flow-diverting stent': a new type of stent that occludes the aneurysm neck whilst maintaining patency of side branches

MESENTERIC OCCLUSIVE VASCULAR DISEASE

Acute mesenteric ischaemia This can present as an acute abdomen (with a metabolic acidosis) and is often diagnosed at laparotomy
- *Causes:* thrombosis ▶ embolization ▶ dissection ▶ vasculitis
- *Treatment:* surgical bowel resection if the bowel is not viable ▶ thrombolysis is an option if the bowel remains viable

Chronic mesenteric ischaemia This is due to chronic atherosclerosis of the mesenteric vessels ▶ clinical symptoms are rare due to an excellent mesenteric collateral vessel supply (at least two of the three mesenteric arteries must be significantly stenosed for symptoms to occur) ▶ it can present with postprandial abdominal pain and weight loss
- *Diagnosis:* colour Doppler US, CT or MRI (angiography is reserved for confirmation before or at the time of intervention)
- *Treatment:* surgical resection of the affected bowel or angioplasty (± stenting)
  - Stenting is preferred over angioplasty as most stenoses are found at an arterial origin and are caused by aortic disease ▶ stenting of more than one vessel improves the long-term outcome and may reduce the restenosis rate

Pearls
- Most lesions occur at vessel origins and are treated by primary stenting
- It is important to exclude extrinsic compression of the coeliac axis by the median arcuate ligament of the diaphragm (MALC) as this requires surgery
  - MALC causes a non-ostial asymmetric narrowing on the superior aspect of the coeliac axis, accentuated on expiratory angiography

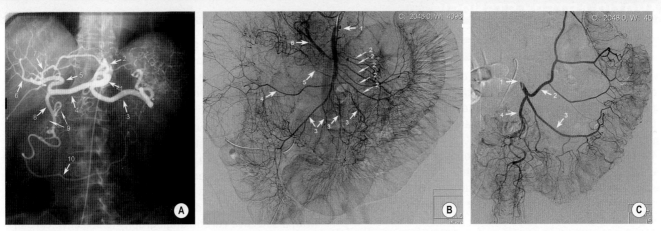

Mesenteric anatomy. (A) Coeliac artery: 1 = coeliac axis, 2 = left gastric artery, 3 = splenic artery, 4 = common hepatic artery, 5 = proper hepatic artery, 6 = right hepatic artery, 7 = left hepatic artery, 8 = gastroduodenal artery, 9 = superior pancreaticoduodenal arteries, 10 = right gastroepiploic arteries. (B) Superior mesenteric artery: 1 = sidewinder catheter in the superior mesenteric artery, 2 = jejunal arteries, 3 = ileal arteries, 4 = ileocolic artery, 5 = right colic artery, 6 = middle colic artery. (C) Inferior mesenteric artery: 1 = catheter in the inferior mesenteric artery, 2 = left colic artery, 3 = sigmoid artery, 4 = superior rectal artery.*

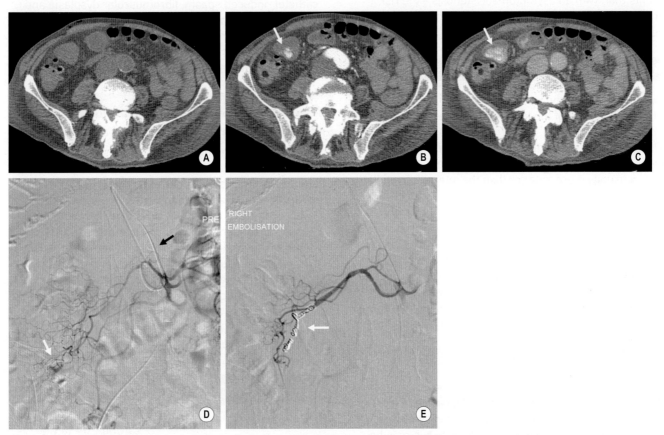

Acute lower gastrointestinal haemorrhage on MDCTA and catheter embolization. (A) Unenhanced axial CT image shows no evidence of high attenuation in relation to the bowel wall or lumen. (B) Arterial phase shows contrast material extravasation into the lumen of the ascending colon. (C) There is pooling of contrast in the bowel lumen on portal-venous phase. (D) Superselective angiogram performed via a coaxial microcatheter (black arrow). Contrast extravasation is seen from a right colic branch (white arrow). (E) After embolization with microcoils (white arrow), there is no further bleeding.**

CAROTID ARTERY STENOSIS

DEFINITION

- A reduction in the luminal diameter of the internal or common carotid artery – this is determined by the ratio of the luminal diameter at the point of the maximal stenosis to the luminal diameter in an adjacent normal internal carotid arterial segment
- The carotid bifurcation is the commonest extracranial vessel location for atheroma deposition: >90% of carotid artery stenoses are found at the bifurcation of the common carotid artery or within the proximal internal carotid artery
- An internal carotid arterial stenosis > 50% is an important cause of an ischaemic stroke or a transient ischaemic attack (TIA)
- Patients with a symptomatic carotid stenosis are at higher risk of developing further ischaemic cerebral events than with an asymptomatic stenosis – the risk of developing a cerebral infarction after an ischaemic neurological event is highest within the first 6 months

RADIOLOGICAL FEATURES

Doppler US This is the first-line investigation and allows reliable identification of the key stenosis levels of a 50% and 70% diameter reduction

- *The external carotid artery can be distinguished from the internal carotid artery by the following:*
  - It is usually more anterior than the internal carotid artery
  - It has visible branches (the internal carotid artery does not have any branches within the cervical region)
  - It has less diastolic flow than the internal carotid artery
  - Tapping the superficial temporal artery as it passes over the zygoma induces fluctuations in the waveform of the external carotid artery (but not the internal carotid artery)
- A 50% diameter reduction is equivalent to a 75% cross-sectional area reduction
- Flow through a stenosis is first accelerated, and only decreases when the lumen is severely narrowed
- Distal to a stenosis, the waveform broadens with a loss in amplitude and eventually pulsatility ▶ it may be difficult to distinguish a critical stenosis (with very slow distal flow) from a total occlusion

CTA/MRA This demonstrates a >90% sensitivity and specificity for the detection of a haemodynamically significant carotid stenosis (i.e. a >50% reduction in luminal diameter)

- **CT:** calcified plaque will exaggerate any stenosis on a MIP
- **TOF MRA:** this is a flow-sensitive technique prone to artefactual signal loss due to changes in vessel orientation and high-grade stenoses ▶ it has been superseded by contrast-enhanced MRA (CEMRA)
- **CEMRA:** this can use 2D time-of-flight sequences or 3D sequences with gadolinium ▶ it may have a tendency to exaggerate the degree of carotid stenosis

DSA This is not routinely used (it has been replaced by non-invasive methods such as duplex US and MRA/CTA) ▶ it is occasionally used as a problem-solving tool if the non-invasive methods are discordant

- An arch aortogram is performed first – there is less chance of producing distal embolic complications than with a selective carotid angiography (a selective carotid angiography is associated with a 1% risk of a stroke)
- Vessel narrowing can be underestimated if a plaque is partially obscured on frames acquired when there is maximal contrast density
- Irregularity due to atheroma must be distinguished from catheter-induced spasm, fibromuscular dysplasia and spontaneous or iatrogenic dissection
  - *Fibromuscular dysplasia:* this causes extensive concentric corrugation of the artery, is frequently bilateral and rarely extends above the skull base

PEARLS

Endovascular treatment of a carotid arterial stenosis

- The standard non-medical treatment is a surgical carotid endarterectomy ▶ carotid angioplasty and stenting is increasingly used
  - Unlike angioplasty at other sites, this requires predilatation to avoid any arterial wall trauma and subsequent embolization of material on stent advancement (cerebral protection devices are also usually used to catch any released embolic debris)
- All methods show a benefit if there is a 70–99% stenosis
  - A symptomatic 50–69% stenosis of the internal carotid artery may be a suitable target for intervention but requires good patient selection
  - Carotid intervention should not be considered for a stenosis < 50% (even if the patient is symptomatic)

US evaluation of an internal carotid arterial stenosis			
Lesion severity	PSV (cm/s)	EDV (cm/s)	Ratio of the internal carotid PSV to the middle/distal common carotid PSV
≥ 50%	150	60	2.5
≥ 60%	175	70	2.75
≥ 70%	225	90	3.75
≥ 80%	300	100	5
PSV, peak systolic velocity ▶ EDV, end diastolic velocity			

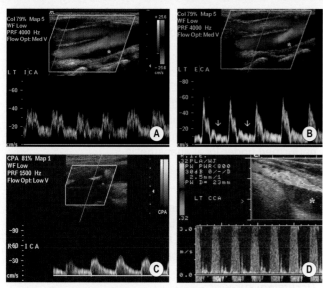

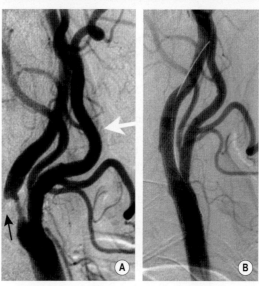

The carotid bifurcation shows (A) higher diastolic flow in the internal carotid artery compared with (B) the external carotid artery – the normal region of reversed flow in the bulb is also seen (*). In addition, the external carotid waveform shows fluctuations (arrows) induced by tapping the superficial temporal artery. A branch artery can also be seen arising from the external carotid artery. (C) Power Doppler image of a critical ICA stenosis showing the narrow residual lumen. (D) A dissection of the common carotid artery, showing the thrombosed channel posteriorly (*) and the tapered stenosis anteriorly.†

Carotid stenting. (A) Lateral projection angiogram following selective injection into the common carotid artery. There is a tight stenosis at the origin of the internal carotid artery (black arrow). The external carotid artery is marked (white arrow). (B) DSA following self-expanding stent deployment.*

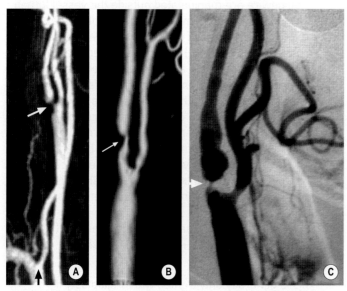

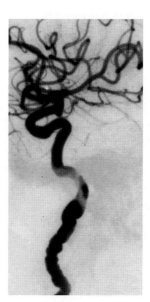

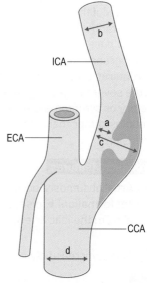

Carotid bifurcation atheroma. Examples of internal carotid artery stenoses (arrows) from different patients on (A) CEMRA MIP, (B) CTA volume rendering and (C) DSA. Note the right vertebral artery origin is clearly demonstrated in A (black arrow).*

Fibromuscular dysplasia ► internal carotid arteriogram, lateral projection. The cervical portion of the artery shows regular concentric corrugations: appearances were similar on the other side.*

Different ways of measuring the percentage of carotid artery stenosis. (A) NASCET method = [1–(a/b)] × 100 ► (B) ESCT method = [1–(a/c)] × 100 ► common carotid method = [1–(a/d)] × 100.
a, Minimum residual lumen.
b, Distal internal carotid lumen.
c, Original internal carotid lumen.
d, Common carotid lumen.

213

LOWER EXTREMITIES

Definition

- The most common condition affecting the lower extremity arteries is ischaemia due to atherosclerotic occlusive disease ▶ this is common in the elderly population where a stenosis or occlusion is almost always due to atherosclerosis
  - *Acute occlusion:* this is due to an embolism or acute thrombosis
  - *Acute-on-chronic occlusion:* this is due to an acute occlusion occurring on a background of chronic stenosis or occlusion
  - *Chronic occlusion:* this is due to progressive atherosclerosis
- Less common causes (tending to affect younger patients): trauma ▶ vasculitis (including vasospastic disorders and Buerger's disease) ▶ popliteal artery entrapment
  - *Diabetic patients:* arterial occlusive disease involves mainly the distal vessels of the calf and feet
  - *Pelvic radiotherapy:* patients can develop occlusive lesions of the common and external iliac arteries due to a radiation-induced ischaemic vasculitis

Clinical presentation

- The presentation depends on the type, location and number of arterial lesions:
  - *Asymptomatic*
  - *Intermittent claudication:* this is only invasively treated if the claudication distance is very short or if it substantially limits lifestyle
  - *Rest pain or tissue loss* (including ulceration and gangrene): the patient is at risk of limb loss and requires urgent angioplasty, stenting, or surgery
- Acute severe pain within the lower leg with no previous history or symptoms probably represents an acute embolus rather than a long-standing atherosclerotic occlusion

Radiological features

DSA Arterial stenosis, occlusion or dilatation (i.e. aneurysm formation) ▶ disease can affect the arteries at any level from the iliac arteries to the small vessels of the foot

CTA This is increasingly used as an alternative

Pearls

Treatment

Iliac artery disease

- *Stenosis:* the angioplasty technical success rate approximates 100% (with 4-year patency rates of 60–70%) ▶ stents are used if an angioplasty is unsuccessful or if a lesion recurs rapidly ▶ patients with diffusely stenotic disease respond less well to angioplasty and are often treated with stents

- *Occlusion:* primary stent insertion is favoured (a distal angioplasty carries a risk of calf vessel embolization) ▶ stent insertion has similar treatment durabilities to that seen with a stenosis

Common femoral artery

- *Stenosis:* angioplasty (with access from the contralateral groin) with similar success rates as with the iliac arteries ▶ an endarterectomy may be performed under local anaesthesia
- *Occlusion:* surgery

Profunda femoris

- *Stenosis:* angioplasty is performed if the SFA is occluded as the profunda becomes the main route for blood flow – if the SFA is patent or salvageable by interventional means, profundal angioplasty is not usually performed
- *Occlusion:* surgery

Superficial femoral artery (SFA)

- *Stenosis:* angioplasty provides 50% patency rates at 4 years ▶ there is a reduced angioplastic success if there is diffuse stenosis or a reduced number of calf run-off vessels ▶ spares the long saphenous vein (may be needed for bypass)
- *Occlusion:* this is usually treated by angioplasty (which has a lower morbidity than surgery)
  - *Subintimal angioplasty:* the catheter and guidewire are manipulated outside the vessel lumen (underneath the intima and into the subintimal space) ▶ they are advanced down the occluded vessel (via the subintimal space) until the catheter and guidewire re-enters the lumen at the level of the patent vessel beneath the occlusion (this creates a false lumen that communicates with the true lumen via the entry and re-entry sites) ▶ the catheter is then replaced with a balloon catheter and dilated in the normal manner
    - Although it is claimed that this has better long-term patency rates it can be technically difficult to re-enter the vessel and there is a high incidence of perforation and collateral vessel occlusion
- Drug-eluting balloons and stents are available (inhibit neointimal hyperplasia + vessel restenosis)

Popliteal artery

- This is generally only treated with angioplasty if there is critical limb ischaemia or very short distance claudication

Calf vessels (tibial and peroneal vessels)

- This is only performed in the setting of critical limb ischaemia and requires small-calibre catheters and guidewires
- Angioplasty is the main method of treatment for focal or diffuse lesions (stenoses or occlusions)

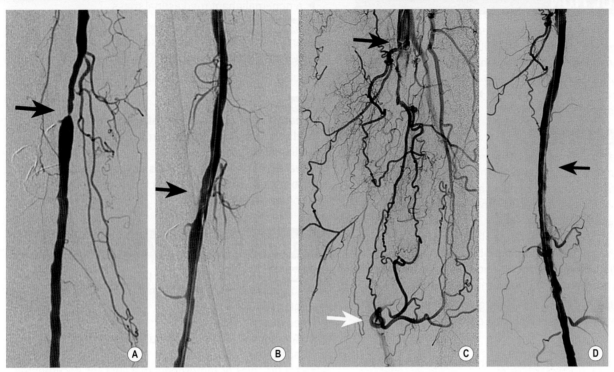

SFA angioplasty. (A) Tight distal SFA stenosis (arrow) in a patient with claudication. (B) Appearance after angioplasty with a 5-mm balloon (arrow). (C) Occlusion of the SFA in another patient (black arrow). There is reconstitution of the popliteal artery via collaterals (white arrow). (D) The occlusion has been crossed subintimally with hydrophilic guidewire and a 5-mm PTA performed, restoring flow.*

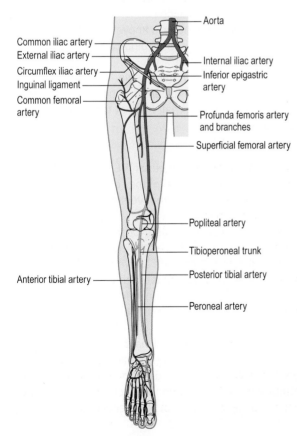

Diagram of lower limb anatomy.**

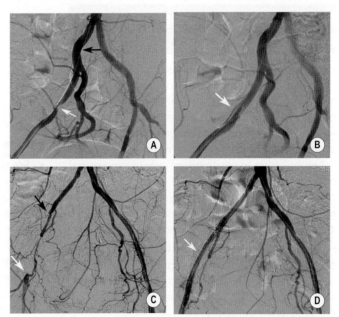

Iliac angioplasty and stenting. (A) Left anterior oblique iliac angiogram performed with a 4F flush catheter (black arrow) inserted via the right common femoral artery. There is a 90% stenosis of the mid external iliac artery (white arrow). (B) Improved lumen dimensions following 8-mm balloon angioplasty. Note the fissuring, which is a normal post-angioplasty appearance (arrow). (C) Flush angiogram in another patient. There is occlusion of the right external iliac artery just after the iliac bifurcation (black arrow). The external iliac artery reconstitutes distally via collateral vessels (white arrow). (D) A guidewire has been passed retrograde through the occlusion from the right and a 9-mm self-expanding stent deployed. This has resulted in successful recanalization of the occluded segment (arrow).*

LOWER EXTREMITY VENOUS OBSTRUCTION

Definition The main pathology affecting the lower extremity venous system is thrombosis ▶ 90% of pulmonary emboli originate from a lower limb deep venous thrombosis (DVT)

- *Causes:* procoagulant factors (e.g. patient immobility, dehydration, thrombocythaemia) ▶ an underlying iliac vein stenosis or occlusion

Radiological features

US The traditional method of investigation (reduced sensitivity for iliac and calf venous thrombosis)
- *Direct signs:* non-compressible veins ▶ echogenic material within the venous lumen ▶ an enlarged vein (if acute) ▶ a lack of Doppler flow
- *Indirect signs:* absence of respiratory variation within the proximal veins (indicating a possible iliac thrombosis)
- *False negatives:* acute-on-chronic disease ▶ thrombosis within an additional profunda femoris vein

CT venography This has an emerging role and is performed after a suitable delay (e.g. 3 min) following a CTPA

Pearls
- **Treatment:** anticoagulation for above-knee thrombosis

May–Thurner syndrome Lower limb venous thrombosis and oedema due to a common iliac occlusive lesion

UPPER EXTREMITY VENOUS OBSTRUCTION

Thoracic outlet syndrome (Paget–Schroetter syndrome)
- Obstructing thoracic outlet musculature and bony structures can cause venous obstruction and thrombosis within the subclavian and axillary veins
  - It is associated with neurological symptoms (due to concomitant brachial plexus compression) and distal arterial emboli (due to concomitant subclavian arterial compression)
  - It is initially treated by thrombolysis ▶ the 1st rib can be resected to create additional space ▶ there may be a need for angioplasty of any residual stenosis

Occlusive disease related to a dialysis fistula
- This occurs due to the resultant high pressure within the upper extremity veins ▶ it can be treated by angioplasty (± stenting) – however there are frequent recurrences and a poor long-term durability

SUPERIOR VENA CAVA (SVC) OBSTRUCTION

Definition
- **Malignant causes:** neoplasm (95%) – of these 80% are due to a lung carcinoma and 20% due to lymphoma

- **Benign causes:** fibrosing mediastinitis (5%) ▶ aneurysm ▶ a non-malignant mediastinal mass

Clinical presentation Venous engorgement of the head, neck and arms ▶ treatment is usually aimed at palliation

CT/DSA/radioisotope scanning This will confirm any caval obstruction ▶ CT will identify the cause

Pearls
- **Treatment of an uncomplicated stenosis or occlusion:** angioplasty (or primary stenting for malignant causes)
- **Treatment of a SVC stenosis complicated by thrombosis:** primary stenting (± initial thrombolysis and thrombectomy)

INFERIOR VENA CAVA (IVC) FILTERS

Definition These are placed to prevent a further fatal pulmonary embolism (PE) in a patient with a documented PE
- Unequivocal indications
  - A recurrent PE (or thrombus progression) despite adequate anticoagulation
  - An IVC, iliac or femoropopliteal DVT (or documented PE) which cannot be treated with anticoagulation
- Relative indications
  - Pregnant women with a proven DVT during Caesarean section or childbirth
  - Preoperative placement for a known iliofemoral DVT if anticoagulation is contraindicated or pelvic manipulation is expected
  - A spinal cord injury with paraplegia
  - A PE and severely limited cardiorespiratory reserve
- Temporary filters have a small hook at their apex to allow snare retrieval

Pearls
- **Ideal filter position:** the infrarenal IVC with the filter apex at or just below the level of the renal veins ▶ the IVC diameter, anatomy and renal vein position requires vena cavography prior to insertion
  - *Indications for suprarenal filter positioning:* IVC thrombosis extension above the renal veins ▶ a renal vein thrombosis ▶ thrombus above a previously placed filter ▶ for pregnant women where there will be infrarenal IVC compression ▶ for a PE following a gonadal vein thrombosis ▶ if there are anatomical variants (e.g. a double IVC)
- **Technique:** the filter is inserted via a femoral or jugular venous route (depending on the site and extent of thrombus) ▶ it can be retrieved via the right jugular vein
- **Complications:** IVC perforation ▶ incorrect deployment ▶ IVC thrombosis ▶ structural filter failure

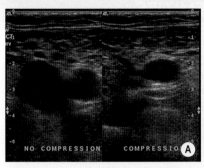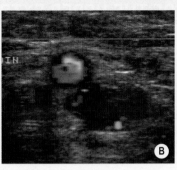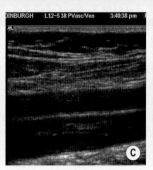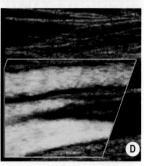

(A) Normal compression of the left common femoral vein (the vein is to the left of the artery). (B) Thrombus occupying the majority of the common femoral vein with only a small amount of flow around the periphery. (C) A tail of fresh thrombus is seen extending up a superficial femoral vein, with its appearance shown using power Doppler (D).†

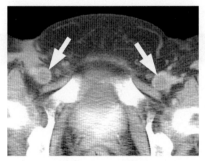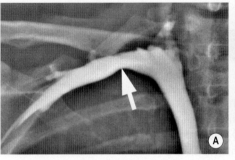

Acute CFV thrombosis. CECT shows enlarged CFV bilaterally (arrows) with low attenuation centres and enhancement of the vein wall.¶¶

(A) Venogram with the arms in a neutral position shows minimal inferior indentation (arrow) of the subclavian vein with no collateral veins. (B) With the arm abducted there is partial compresion (arrows). Again there are no collaterals.¶¶

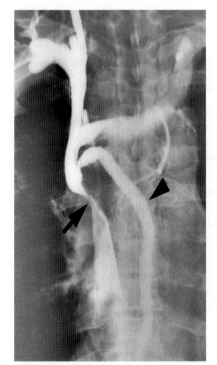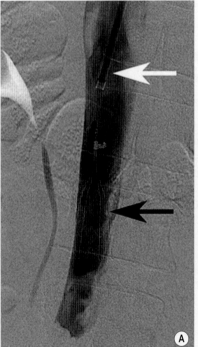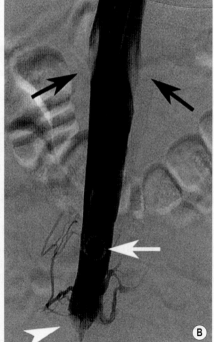

Collateral pathways in SVC obstruction. Venogram showing severe stenosis of the central SVC (arrow) with collateral drainage via the azygous vein (arrowhead).¶¶

Inferior vena cava filter. (A) Post Gunther tulip filter (black arrow) deployment. The delivery catheter is marked (white arrow). (B) Cavogram performed with a pigtail catheter (white arrow) placed from the right internal jugular vein. Unopacified blood from the renal veins creates a void (black arrows) in the column of contrast medium and thus delineates their position. Thrombus is seen as a filling defect distally (white arrowhead).*

PERIPHERAL VASCULAR DISEASE OF THE UPPER EXTREMITIES

Definition

- Most lesions are secondary to atherosclerosis
  - Other disease processes account for a greater proportion of lesions seen within the upper extremities: Takayasu's arteritis ▶ thoracic outlet syndrome ▶ thromboembolism ▶ other vasculitides

Pearls

Endovascular treatment

- *Subclavian arterial stenosis:* lesions usually occur at the subclavian arterial origin and are amenable to angioplasty (± stent insertion) ▶ most interventionalists would treat with stent insertion
- *Subclavian artery occlusion:* these can be recanalized but with a substantially reduced technical success rate
- *Occlusive lesions distal to the subclavian artery:* angioplasty or stenting can be used (these are usually only treated if there is limb-threatening ischaemia)
- *Acute thromboembolism:* thrombolysis has a limited role – surgery remains the treatment of choice

CAROTID BODY TUMOUR

Definition

- This is located within the adventitia of the posterior medial common carotid arterial bifurcation ▶ it is composed of neural tissue and is very vascular ▶ 5% are bilateral, up to 50% are malignant and 5% are endocrinologically active

Radiological features

US A hypoechoic mass splaying the bifurcation of the common carotid artery ▶ colour Doppler: very hypervascular

CECT Vivid homogeneous enhancement

DSA A vascular mass

Pearl

Carotid artery aneurysm

- These can be spontaneous, as a result of a penetrating neck injury, or following a hyperextension injury

BRONCHIAL ARTERY EMBOLIZATION

Definition

- Bronchial arterial embolization is used for the treatment of a significant haemoptysis ▶ the source of the haemorrhage lies within the bronchial arteries in up to 90% of cases – the pulmonary arteries are rarely the cause of a massive haemoptysis
  - *Massive haemoptysis:* this is defined as > 300 ml of blood loss over 24 h
  - *Moderate haemoptyis:* this is defined as >3 episodes of 100 ml/day within 1 week
  - *Causes of haemoptysis:* tuberculosis ▶ cystic fibrosis ▶ malignancy ▶ bronchiectasis ▶ aspergilloma ▶ lobar pneumonia

Radiological features

- There is a highly variable bronchial arterial anatomy:
  - The bronchial arteries arise anterolaterally from the descending thoracic aorta (T5/T6 level) and the most common configurations are:
    - An intercostobronchial trunk (ICBT) on the right and two bronchial arteries on the left
    - One ICBT on the right and one bronchial artery on the left
    - One ICBT, one right bronchial artery and two left bronchial arteries
  - Selective arterial catheterization is performed using preshaped catheters (e.g. cobra or sidewinder catheters)
  - **Angiographic signs of abnormality:** hypertrophy ▶ bronchial to pulmonary arterial or venous shunting ▶ peribronchial vascularity ▶ aneurysm formation ▶ contrast medium extravasation

Treatment

- Bronchial artery embolization is effective at stopping haemorrhage (and preserving the lung parenchyma) but it will not treat the underlying cause and therefore rebleeding is likely
  - Embolization is usually performed using polyvinyl alcohol particles of 300–500 μm ▶ this provides immediate relief of symptoms (in 75% of cases)
  - *Complications:* broncho-oesophageal fistula ▶ oesophageal embolization (leading to dysphagia or necrosis) ▶ spinal cord ischaemia (causing a myelitis or paraplegia) ▶ retrograde aortic embolization

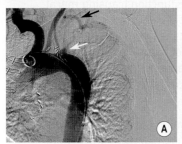
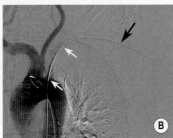
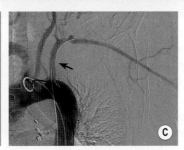

Subclavian artery occlusion. (A) Left anterior oblique projection flush aortogram performed via a pigtail catheter in the ascending aorta. There is left subclavian artery occlusion in this patient, who presented with arm claudication. Note that the left vertebral artery (the 3rd vessel from the right) arises directly from the aortic arch, rather than off the left subclavian. The stump of the left subclavian is marked (white arrow). There is reconstitution of the distal left subclavian artery (black arrow). (B) A guidewire (black arrow) has been placed across the occlusion from the left brachial artery. A balloon expandable stent (white arrows) is seen in position ready for deployment. (C) After deployment of a 7-mm stent (arrow). Continuous flow has been restored.*

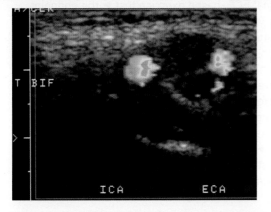

Transverse view of carotid bifurcation with an hypoechoic carotid body tumour splaying the two major branches.†

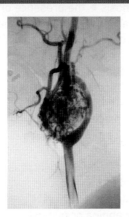

Lateral common carotid DSA showing a hypervascular mass splaying the internal and external carotid arteries.¶¶

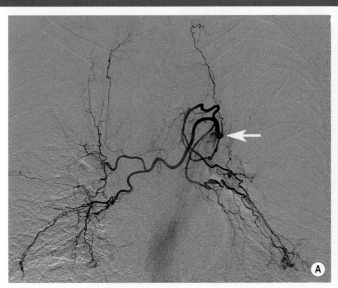
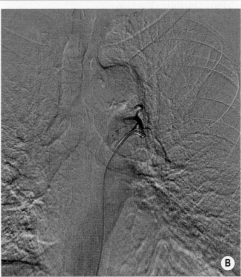

Bronchial embolization. (A) Bronchial angiogram in a patient with lower lobe bronchiectasis who presented with haemoptysis. A large abnormal bronchial artery has been selected with a cobra catheter (arrow). It is providing supply to both lower lobes. (B) DSA after embolization with 355–500 μm polyvinyl alcohol particles.*

CONVENTIONAL CORONARY ANGIOGRAPHY

- This involves the selective injection of contrast medium into the right and left coronary arteries and the left ventricle (while recording the resultant moving images)
- Being replaced by non-invasive CCT and CMR

Technique

- A percutaneous femoral arterial catheterization is the usual approach (an alternative percutaneous route is the radial artery) ▶ at least 3 shaped catheters are required – one for each coronary artery and one for the left ventricle) ▶ low osmolality contrast media is used with rapid filming at 25+ frames/s ▶ images are acquired in multiple orientations with very short exposures (5–10 ms) to freeze cardiac motion

Considerations during coronary angiography

- The severity and length of a stenosis ▶ the presence of a complete occlusion (± collateral vessels) ▶ the number of affected vessels ▶ the vessel diameter and stenosis configuration
  - Significant (>50% diameter reduction) accessible stenoses in 1 or 2 vessels (with a diameter > 2 mm) are treated by angioplasty or stenting
  - Left main coronary artery disease or significant disease affecting all 3 coronary arteries is usually best treated with a CABG
- Poor ventricular function is associated with an increased risk, but a greater potential benefit (the prognosis is related to the degree of ventricular dysfunction)
- High-risk patients with unstable angina or non-ST elevation myocardial infarction may benefit from early angioplasty or stenting
- May miss mild or non-stenotic disease
- A normal coronary angiogram does not exclude disease, and a stenotic plaque may be the tip of the iceberg

ECHOCARDIOGRAPHY

2D echocardiography This allows imaging of the heart and great vessels through a limited chest wall acoustic window ▶ transoesophageal echocardiography can also image the heart

Doppler echocardiography This can estimate blood flow and pressure gradients

Contrast medium echocardiography This uses IV microbubble contrast ▶ it improves the definition of the margins of the ventricular cavity and enhances the accuracy of echocardiography for assessing ventricular function in poor echocardiography patients ▶ it can also assess myocardial perfusion

Indications

- Demonstration of the effects of IHD on ventricular function
  - A large infarct will appear hypoechoic, whereas fibrotic scar tissue is stiffer than normal myocardium and appears hyperechoic

- Detecting structural complications such as a VSD, papillary muscle dysfunction (causing mitral regurgitation) and ventricular thrombus
- Demonstrating the origins of the main coronary arteries (especially with transoesophageal echocardiography) ▶ demonstrating any anomalous origins and coronary artery aneurysms (e.g. Kawasaki's disease)

Stress echocardiography

- This detects reversible wall motion abnormalities (indicating reversible ischaemia) using the same stimulants as for CT or MR stress imaging
- It enables risk stratification for patients with known or suspected IHD (a normal study indicates a very good prognosis)
- It enables preoperative risk assessment (this determines myocardial viability)
- It is more sensitive for detecting ischaemia than a conventional ECG-based exercise test ▶ the endpoint of the test is the appearance of new wall motion abnormalities (chronic ischaemia causes diffuse dysfunction, an acute myocardial infarction causes more localized changes)
- *Factors affecting the accuracy of the technique:* the threshold for defining a significant stenosis ▶ whether there is single or multivessel disease ▶ whether an adequate stress is achieved (especially for exercise-based protocols) ▶ the presence of other disease processes which affect myocardial function (such as cardiomyopathy, microvascular disease, or hypertrophy)

Complications of cardiac angiography*	
Vascular	Haematoma
	False aneurysm
	Arteriovenous fistula
	Mycotic aneurysm
	Retroperitoneal haematoma
	Acute occlusion
	Arterial dissection
Cardiac	Arrhythmias (catheter manipulation)
	Myocardial infarction
	Coronary dissection
	Systemic embolus (including stroke)
	Myocardial perforation
Contrast medium	Heart failure (reduced with low-osmolality contrast agent)
	Arrhythmias (sinus bradycardia, sinus arrest, ventricular fibrillation in 0.1-1.0%)
	ECG changes (wide QRS, long QT, ST changes, change in QRS axis)
	Hypotension (reduced with low-osmolality contrast agent)
	Allergic/idiosyncratic (reduced with non-ionic contrast agent)
	Renal impairment (possibly reduced with low-osmolality contrast agent)

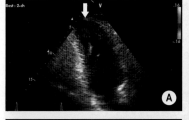
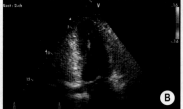
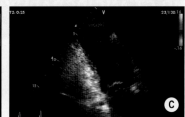
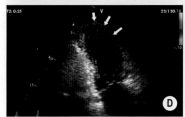
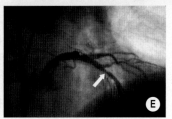

Stress echocardiography. (A) End-diastolic apical two-chamber view at rest shows thinning of the apical myocardium (arrow). (B) End-systolic apical two-chamber view at rest shows concentric contraction of left ventricle, except for the cardiac apex. (C) End-diastolic apical two-chamber view during stress (dobutamine infusion) shows dilatation of the left ventricle when compared with (A). (D) End-systolic apical two-chamber view during stress (dobutamine infusion) shows dilatation of the left ventricle due to akinesia of the anterior wall to contract (arrows). (E) Selective coronary arteriogram (right anterior oblique with cranial angulation) in the same patient shows a significant left anterior descending coronary artery stenosis (arrow).*

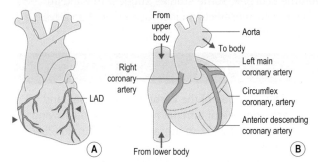

Normal coronary anatomy. (A) Anterior view of the heart showing the left anterior descending (LAD) and right coronary arteries (black arrowheads). (B) Diagrammatic depiction of the three coronary arteries. The dotted lines represent the atrioventricular (AV) and interventricular grooves *posteriorly*. The continuous parallel lines represent the same grooves *anteriorly*. The interventricular groove for the left anterior descending artery is the more vertical of the two grooves.

ACC/AHA guidelines for coronary angiography*

- Severe resting left ventricular dysfunction (LVEF <35%)
- High-risk treadmill score (score ≥ 11)
- Severe exercise left ventricular dysfunction (exercise LVEF <35%)
- Stress-induced large perfusion defect (particularly if anterior)
- Stress-induced moderate size multiple perfusion defects
- Large, fixed perfused defect with left ventricular dilatation or increased lung uptake (^{201}Tl)
- Stress-induced moderate-size perfusion defect with left ventricular dilatation or increased lung uptake (^{201}Tl)
- Echocardiographic wall motion abnormality (involving more than two segments) developing at a low dose of dobutamine or at a low heart rate
- Stress echocardiography evidence of extensive ischaemia

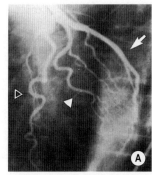
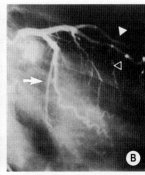
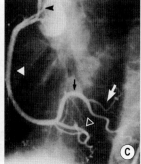
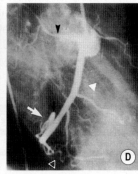

Normal coronary arteriography. (A,B) Left coronary artery: the normal coronary artery has a smooth, gently tapering outline. (A) Left anterior oblique (LAO) projection ▶ (B) right anterior oblique (RAO) projection. Open arrowhead = left anterior descending artery (LAD), solid arrowhead = diagonal, branch arrow = circumflex/obtuse marginal vessels. In (B) the LAD and its diagonal branch overlap but the LAD may be identified by its septal branches and its extension to the apex of the heart. The small circumflex branch (arrow) has the characteristic straight appearance which suggests that it is running in the left atrioventricular (AV) groove. The larger obtuse marginal branch has left the AV groove and is running on the surface of the left ventricle. (C,D) Right coronary artery: (C) LAO projection ▶ (D) RAO projection. Solid white arrowhead = right coronary artery, open arrowhead = posterior descending coronary artery, black arrowhead = sinus node artery, black arrow = inverted U at the crux, white arrow = posterolateral left ventricular branch. In (C) the entire right coronary artery is seen in profile as it passes around the heart in the right side of the AV groove. The posterior descending branch is the last branch before the crux. Beyond the crux (marked by the inverted U) are posterolateral left ventricular branches supplying the free wall of the left ventricle. In (D) both the origin and the terminal part of the right coronary artery are foreshortened but the sinus node artery (black arrowhead) can be distinguished from the conus and other right ventricular (RV) branches. As seen in (D) it runs posteriorly to the atria, whereas the conal and RV branches run anteriorly to the right ventricle.*

CARDIAC CT AND CT ANGIOGRAPHY (CTA)

- 3D imaging technique – any imaging plane can be reconstructed with a slice thickness down to 0.5 mm
- Single heart beat acquisition with wide volume detectors (up to 16 cm) or high pitch helical scanning (flash scanning) ▶ multiple (3-4) heart beat acquisition with narrow detector coverage (4 cm) and step-and-shoot 'sequential' acquisition
- ECG-gating and heart rate control (oral or IV β-blocker, target heart rate <65 bpm) are used to minimize cardiac motion artefact ▶ sublingual nitroglycerin immediately prior to the scan is used for coronary vasodilatation
- *Prospective ECG-gating:* image acquisition at a certain time point of the cardiac cycle (R-R interval), either diastole (70-80%) or systole (30-40%) or systole and diastole (30-80%) ▶ it is used for coronary artery assessment depending on the heart rate
  - Higher or unstable heart rates require imaging in systole or both systole and diastole
- *Retrospective ECG-Gating:* data acquisition throughout the cardiac cycle (0-100% of R-R interval) only for functional assessment
  - Higher radiation dose due to longer exposure ▶ dose modulation reduces radiation doses
- *Temporal resolution:* 75-175 msec depending on the scanner type ▶ best temporal resolution of 75 msec with dual source cardiac CT scanner
  - 2 X-ray tubes and 2 sets of detectors ▶ only $\frac{1}{4}$ rotation for data acquisition
- *Coronary CTA:* dual-head injection pumps allow contrast injection to be followed by saline injection (or a mixture of contrast and saline) using biphasic or triphasic injection protocols (cf. single-head pumps) ▶ volume of contrast ranges depending on the scanner type from 60-100 ml with an injection rate of 4-6 ml/s
  - Radiation doses range significantly (0.5-8 mSv) depending on the protocol, scanner type, body habitus and heart rate

3D IMAGE RECONSTRUCTION

- *Multiplanar reconstruction (MPR):* this enables the viewing of any 2D section from a 3D dataset (the spatial resolution is the same for any orientation with near isometric voxels) ▶ a curved MPR can follow any tortuous anatomy
- *Maximum intensity projection (MIP):* the highest attenuation voxels (CTA) or highest signal voxel (MRA) along any ray (line) are identified and projected onto a 3D image
- *Surface shaded display (SSD):* all voxels with an attenuation or signal above a certain threshold are represented as a 3D image (which can be rotated in any direction) ▶ an imaginary source of illumination is used to provide 3D perspective

- *Volume-rendered techniques:* volumes with a certain range of attenuations or SI are assigned a colour or grey scale density ▶ 3D reconstructions can benefit from the removal of areas of a certain attenuation or SI (e.g. bone for CTA or fat for MRA)

CORONARY CALCIFICATION

- *Agatston calcium score:* this quantifies the presence of high attenuation material within the coronary arteries ▶ the amount of coronary calcium roughly correlates to the plaque extent, but is not related to plaque stability (weakly related to the degree of luminal stenosis) ▶ tissue densities ≥ 130 HU are used as an attenuation level for calcified plaque ▶ alternatively the actual volume of plaque is quantified (CVS: total calcium volume score) ▶ some studies suggest that a high calcium score predicts an increased risk of an adverse coronary event

CORONARY CTA

- It can detect plaque of the coronary artery wall and assess the degree of luminal narrowing ▶ narrowing may be severe (>70%), moderate (50-69%), mild (25-49%) or minimal (<25%)
  - CT fractional flow reserve (FFR) and CT perfusion are emerging applications for assessment of haemodynamic significance of stenosis, increasing the accuracy of CTA (a purely anatomical test)
- It has a very high negative predictive value for coronary artery disease (95-99 %) when images are diagnostic
  - Non-diagnostic images mainly due to cardiac motion artefact (caused by high heart rate), blooming artefact (caused by heavy calcification, stents, metallic clips)
  - In addition (in up to 10% of cases) MDCT can detect significant non-cardiac diagnoses (e.g. pneumonia, lung cancer, PE)
- *Coronary artery dominance:* the artery that gives rise to the posterior descending artery
  - Right dominant (85%) ▶ left dominant (7%) ▶ co-dominant (8%)

OTHER CARDIAC CT INDICATIONS

- Assessment of anatomy and patency of grafts post CABG
- Assessment of suspected coronary artery anomalies
- Evaluation of aortic pathology
- Evaluation of congenital heart disease and pericardial disease pathology
- Evaluation pre and post procedures:
  - TAVI (trans-catheter aortic valve implantation) ▶ TMVI (trans-catheter mitral valve implantation) ▶ AF ablation
- Assessment of valvular heart disease in selected cases
- Assessment of myocardial scarring and ventricular function are feasible but of limited use in clinical practice

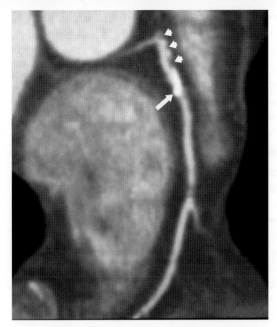

Coronary CTA. Curved MIP reconstruction from ECG-gated MDCTA of a complex left anterior descending artery stenosis showing both eccentric low attenuation plaque (arrowheads) and high attenuation calcified plaque (arrow).*

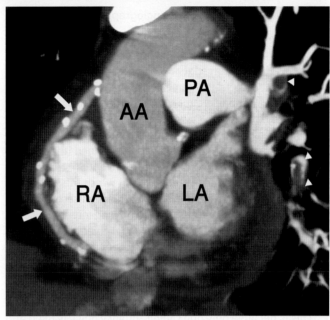

CTA of coronary artery bypass grafts. Thin maximum intensity projection (MIP) showing a patent saphenous vein bypass graft (arrows) to the distal right coronary artery. Also note thrombus in the left pulmonary arteries (arrowheads). AA = aortic arch, PA = pulmonary artery, RA = right atrium, LA = left atrium.*

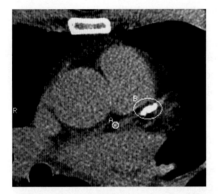

EBCT screening. EBCT image with conventional soft tissue windowing and with a threshold set at 130 HU. An area of dense calcification (circled) is identified in the proximal left anterior descending artery (LAD) – the calcium score was high (total score 887 ▶ LAD score 227).*

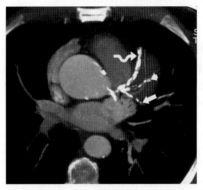

Heavy coronary calcification. Axial thin MIP reconstruction from a coronary CTA shows multiple areas of dense calcification which prevent visualization of most of the arterial lumen in the left anterior descending (LAD) (curved arrow), ramus intermedius (arrowhead), and circumflex (arrow) coronary arteries. An area of low attenuation in the ramus intermedius represents an area of clear occlusion by fatty plaque.*

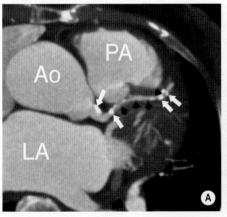
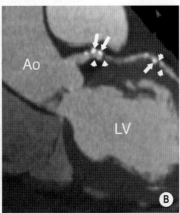

Multiplanar visualization of complex coronary stenoses. (A). Oblique axial thin MIP reconstruction from coronary CTA and orientated along the left anterior descending artery (LAD) shows multiple high attenuation (calcified, arrows) and low attenuation (fatty, black arrowheads) lesions. Ao = aortic root, LA = left atrium, LV = left ventricle, PA = pulmonary artery. (B) Oblique coronal thin MIP reconstruction from coronary CTA shows more of the length of the LAD and multiple high attenuation (calcified, arrows) and low attenuation (fatty, arrowheads) lesions from a different perspective.*

Cardiac MRI (CMR) and MR angiography (MRA)

Spin-echo imaging *'Black blood' imaging:* the myocardium and vascular wall appear bright and the blood dark ▶ useful for high spatial resolution static anatomical imaging (but rather slow to perform)

- 180° inverting pulse applied to the imaging volume followed by a slice selective 180° 'de-inversion' pulse: net result is inverted spins outside the imaged slice but spins within the imaged slice are unchanged (they have experienced both inversion and de-inversion) ▶ the time at which this is applied is the time at which the longitudinal magnetization of blood has reached zero from the initial inversion – therefore blood flowing into the slice will generate no signal ('black blood') ▶ variable signal from slow or in-plane blood flow (producing artefacts)

Gradient-echo imaging

- *'Bright blood' imaging:* blood produces a higher SI than that seen with spin-echo sequences
- This is because only one radiofrequency pulse is used and there is less time for the blood to move out of the imaging plane between slice selection and image acquisition (turbulent blood flow will produce areas of signal loss)
- The gradient-echo sequence can be repeated more rapidly with a reduced RF flip angle, allowing the acquisition of cine loops ▶ this also allows quantification of ventricular stroke volumes (comparing end-systolic and end-diastolic volumes)

Phase shift velocity mapping

- This allows quantification of flow velocities
- **Positive velocity encoding:** if a gradient is applied in the direction of blood flow for a finite time and then turned off, the relationship of phase will change in relation to the two ends of the gradient (the protons at the stronger end of the gradient precess at a faster rate during its application than those at the weaker end)
- **Negative velocity encoding:** when the gradient is turned off, the rate of precession becomes constant again in the slice, but the phase relationship has changed and the phase signature remains ▶ when the gradient is reversed and applied for the same period of time as the original gradient, the phase signature of still material is cancelled, but flowing blood moving during the gradients to a different phase territory retains a phase change proportional to its velocity
  - Simple subtraction of the images obtained with positive and negative velocity encoding will generate a phase image whose pixel value is directly proportional to the blood flow velocity

Myocardial perfusion imaging

- T1WI: the heart is imaged during the bolus administration of a gadolinium contrast agent
- Ischaemic areas will demonstrate delayed enhancement

Contrast-enhanced MRA

- T1WI: accurately determines CABG patency-possibly that of the infarct-related artery after coronary thrombolysis

- It has an equivalent accuracy to MDCTA (however MDCTA is quicker and easier to use)

Myocardial tagging Prior to a GE cine loop a special selective excitation pulse produces a 2D grid structure within the myocardium (narrow planes of very low SI appearing as a latticework)

- This moves and deforms throughout the cardiac cycle allowing assessment of movement

Cardiac gating

- *Prospective gating:* the QRS complex of the ECG triggers the imaging such that the image is formed from a specific part of the cardiac cycle
- *Retrospective gating:* the imaging sequence is repeated continuously with a constant repeat time while the ECG is monitored ▶ the data are sorted at the completion of the sequence and adjusted to give images at specific parts of the cardiac cycle
  - Prevention of respiratory motion (breath holding) is important

CMR imaging planes Usually obtained in orientation to the axes of the heart (as for echocardiography)

Cardiac MRI (CMR)

CMR indications and applications

- **Myocardial function at rest:** end-diastolic and end-systolic volumes can be calculated from the endocardial outlines using fast cine GE imaging
- **Myocardial function during stress:** this allows stress assessment for inducible ischaemia and reversible dysfunction using dobutamine or adenosine infusions
- **Myocardial perfusion and viability:** it is possible to measure the myocardial perfusion from the peak myocardial enhancement ▶ delayed hyperenhancement identifies infarcted or non-viable myocardium
- **Coronary arteries and bypass grafts:** useful for assessing anomalous coronary arteries and graft patencies
- **Valvular heart disease:** velocity mapping allows measurements of peak velocities across stenoses ▶ it provides quantification of regurgitation (GE sequences show turbulent blood flow as areas of signal loss) ▶ phase contrast imaging allows assessment of the stenosis severity
- **Acute myocarditis:** focal wall motion with abnormal high signal on T2WI and contrast enhancement on T1WI
- **Cardiac infiltration:**
  - *Sarcoidosis:* T2WI: high SI ▶ T1WI + Gad: enhancement ▶ delayed contrast-enhanced MRI: enhancement
  - *Amyloidosis:* thickening of the myocardium, interatrial septum, valves, leaflets and papillary muscles ▶ atrial dilatation ▶ pleural and pericardial effusions ▶ T2WI: high SI ▶ T1WI + Gad: enhancement
  - *Myocardial iron overload:* a diffuse reduction in contraction ▶ reduced myocardial SI
- **CMR can also assess:** the pericardium ▶ cardiac thrombus and tumours ▶ cardiomyopathies ▶ congenital heart disease

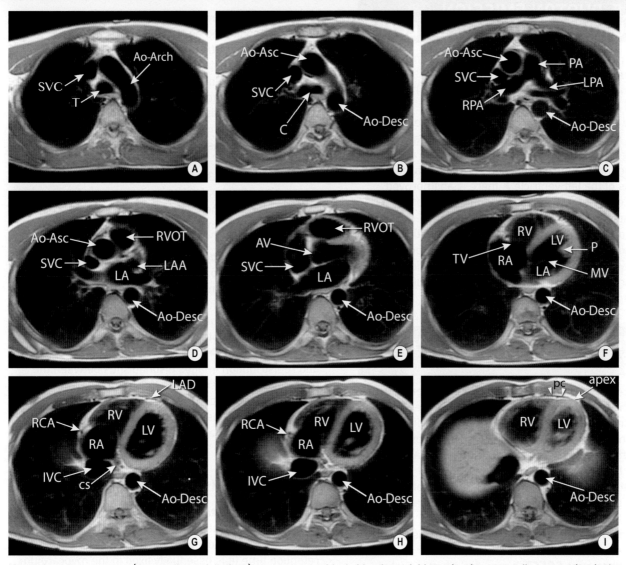

Normal cardiac anatomy (descending axial slices) on transverse black-blood acquisitions. Ao-Asc, ascending aorta; Ao-Arch, aortic arch; Ao-Desc, descending aorta; RA, right atrium; LA, left atrium; RV, right ventricle; LV, left ventricle; RVOT, right ventricular outflow tract; PA, main pulmonary artery; RPA, right pulmonary artery; LPA, left pulmonary artery; LAA, left atrial appendage; TV, tricuspid valve; MV, mitral valve; P, papillary muscle; LAD, left anterior descending coronary artery; cs, coronary sinus; pc, pericardium; T, trachea; C, carina; IVC, inferior vena cava; SVC, superior vena cava.**

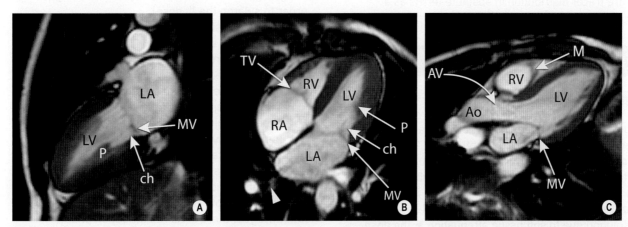

Normal cardiac anatomy on bright blood; two-, four- and three-chamber views. RA, right atrium; LA, left atrium; RV, right ventricle; LV, left ventricle; P, papillary muscle; TV, tricuspid valve; MV, mitral valve; AV, aortic valve; Ao, aorta; M, moderator band; ch, chordae tendineae.**

SINGLE-PHOTON EMISSION COMPUTED TOMOGRAPHY (SPECT)

- This is a nuclear medicine tomographic imaging technique using gamma rays
- A gamma-emitting radioisotope (radionuclide) is first injected intravenously
- Multiple planar projections are acquired as the gamma camera rotates around the patient and the images are reconstructed into tomograms and presented as images in orthogonal planes parallel and perpendicular to the long axis of the left ventricle ▶ there is an improved image contrast because of the elimination of any overlying structures
- When combined with CT, it allows for attenuation correction and the provision of anatomical information ▶ it provides a true 3D display of the distribution of radionuclide ▶ there is the potential for quantification of tracer uptake

POSITRON EMISSION TOMOGRAPHY (PET)

- Positrons travel a very short distance in matter before an annihilation reaction with an electron causes the emission of two gamma photons in opposite directions ▶ the photons sensed simultaneously by opposing detectors are presumed to come from annihilation along the line between the detectors ▶ this inherent spatial information allows construction of a tomographic image without the need for collimators (leading to a higher sensitivity)
  - Rubidium-82 can assess flow ▶ FDG can assess glucose metabolism
- *Advantages over SPECT:* it provides a better spatial resolution and higher sensitivity (no collimators are required) ▶ it is able to use most physiological molecules as tracers (carbon, nitrogen and oxygen can all be labelled with positron emitters) ▶ it has the ability to measure tracer distribution in absolute terms as a function of time

PERFUSION AGENTS

THALLIUM

- The original myocardial perfusion agent ▶ it is cyclotron produced and decays by electron capture
- *Advantages:* it has higher myocardial accumulation than ^{99m}technetium (and also provides redistribution images)
- *Disadvantages:* low photon energies (71 keV) result in poor resolution due to soft tissue attenuation ▶ the dose

is limited by the long $t_{1/2}$ (3 days) ▶ there is an associated high cost and limited availability

- *Uptake & distribution:* intracellular uptake via the Na-K ATPase with its distribution proportional to the regional myocardial blood flow (approximately 90% is cleared by first-pass hepatic metabolism with 4% localizing within the myocardium) ▶ the myocardial clearance is proportional to the regional perfusion (zones of initial high uptake will wash out faster than zones of lower uptake)
- *Stress images (5-30 min post injection):* the tracer distribution after peak exercise is relatively fixed and is proportional to the myocardial blood flow ▶ a defect suggests the presence of a coronary artery stenosis or infarction
- *Redistribution image (2-4 h post injection):* this represents the map of the equilibrium phase between the tracer uptake and tracer efflux ▶ thallium washes out of the myocardium at a slower rate in underperfused than normally perfused myocardium – areas with decreased initial uptake appear to have a relative increase in uptake ▶ comparison between the stress and redistribution images distinguishes between the reversible defect of inducible hypoperfusion and the fixed defect of myocardial necrosis ▶ as redistribution can be slow in areas of reduced perfusion, delayed (up to 72 h) imaging may avoid underestimation of myocardial viability

^{99m}TECHNETIUM MIBI (SESTAMIBI)

- *Uptake & distribution:* this demonstrates high myocardial accumulation (proportional to the regional perfusion) with a slow washout and a long myocardial retention time (it is essentially fixed in the myocardium with no redistribution) – therefore imaging requires separate injections for stress and rest studies
- *Protocols:*
  - *1-day protocol:* rest images are followed by stress images 4 h later (the 2nd dose needs to be larger in order to swamp the 1st dose)
  - *2-day protocol:* stress images on the 1st day are followed by rest images on the 2nd day (if the original stress images are abnormal) ▶ a 2-day protocol allows for the decay of activity from the 1st injection
  - *A combined ^{99m}technetium and thallium approach:* an initial thallium injection is followed by an immediate ^{99m}technetium injection (as its higher-energy photons are unaffected by any residual thallium)
- *Advantages:* shorter $t_{1/2}$ (6 h) allows larger doses with less radiation exposure ▶ there is improved resolution due to its higher photon energies (140 keV) ▶ it is associated with a low cost and easy availability
- *Disadvantages:* there is no redistribution phase, allowing for the assessment of viability

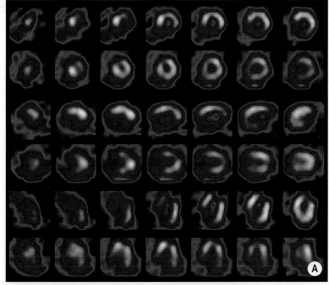

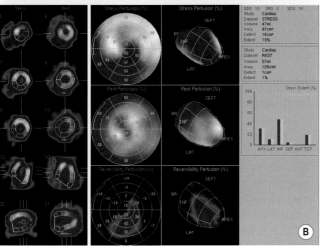

Inferior wall ischaemia. (A) Exercise [99m]sestamibi and rest [201]thallium myocardial perfusion. Marked hypoperfusion of the entire inferior wall and inferior apex post stress, which normalizes on rest images consistent with a large region of severe ischaemia. (B) Polar map and volume quantitative display. The reversibility perfusion (%) box shows the extent and severity of the reversible perfusion defect as a polar map and 3D volume display. At the right, the stress extent (%) and reversibility (%) are shown in graphical form.[§§]

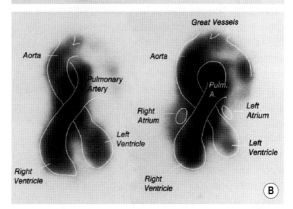

Anatomy at end systole and end diastole and correlation with a MUGA study. (A) End-diastolic images. Anterior (top left), left anterior oblique (top right) and left posterior oblique (bottom) views are the most commonly obtained. (B) Drawings over the left anterior oblique end-diastolic (left) and end-systolic (right) frames, indicating the position and relationships of the major structures.[§§]

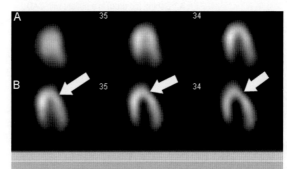

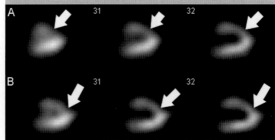

Attenuation artefact. There are several causes of artefactual reduction of activity on cardiac scintigraphy. Increased overlying tissue, as with the female breast (shown here), breast augmentation, or a high diaphragm, can reduce activity and mimic a fixed perfusion defect (arrows ▶ row A stress, row B rest). The imaging agent is ^{99m}Tc-tetrofosmin.[§§]

NUCLEAR CARDIAC IMAGING

PEARLS

- Myocardial perfusion imaging depends on the differences in flow delivering different amounts of activity to normal and ischaemic myocardium
  - *Fixed perfusion defect:* a defect seen with rest and stress imaging ▶ it indicates myocardial infarction, scarring or an area supplied by a very severe (> 85%) stenosis ▶ the depth of the defect indicates the degree of myocardial loss
  - *Reversible perfusion defect:* a perfusion defect seen on stress imaging which normalizes on rest imaging ▶ this indicates reversible (inducible) ischaemia
  - *Partially reversible defect:* this occurs if the ischaemia is superimposed on a partial-thickness infarction
  - *Reverse distribution:* a defect on thallium redistribution images that is less apparent on stress imaging ▶ it usually represents an artefact but may be due to rapid tracer washout
  - *Abnormalities not resulting from coronary artery disease:* coronary spasm ▶ anomalous arteries ▶ muscle bridges ▶ small vessel disease (e.g. diabetes) ▶ cardiomyopathies ▶ infiltrative disorders such as sarcoidosis and amyloidosis ▶ connective tissue disorders ▶ conduction defects (LBBB, left bundle branch block)
  - *Artefacts:* these are due to motion or attenuation (e.g. reduced anterior wall counts from breast attenuation)

Stress testing This can be achieved with physical exercise or alternatively pharmacologically induced if the patient is unable to tolerate exercise

- *Adenosine:* this activates coronary receptors that produce vasodilation ▶ it has a very short half-life and is commonly associated with side-effects

- *Dipyridamole:* this blocks the reuptake mechanism of adenosine and therefore raising endogenous adenosine levels
- *Dobutamine:* a β_1 agonist that can be used in patients with asthma or other contraindications to dipyridamole or adenosine ▶ serious complications are uncommon
  - As coronary vessels with significant stenoses cannot increase blood flow to the same degree as normal vessels, vasodilator stress results in vascular regions of relative hypoperfusion similar to exercise-induced ischaemia

Multiple gated acquisition (MUGA) study This is also known as a cardiac blood pool study and enables the assessment of ventricular function by displaying the distribution of radioactive tracer within the heart ▶ it can assess ventricular ejection fractions and regional ventricular wall motion ▶ it can be performed at rest and during the application of stress

- *First-pass studies:* all data are collected during the initial transit of the tracer bolus through the central circulation ▶ any ^{99m}Tc agent may be administered as a bolus
  - *Advantage:* it provides a more accurate quantification of right ventricular function (the left and right ventricles overlap in equilibrium studies)
  - *Disadvantage:* it provides low counting statistics
- *Equilibrium studies:* data are collected over many cardiac cycles (100–300 cardiac cycles provides sufficient counting statistics) ▶ using ECG gating the cardiac cycle is usually divided into 16 frames ▶ it requires a tracer that remains within the blood pool (e.g. ^{99m}technetium-labelled autologous red blood cells)

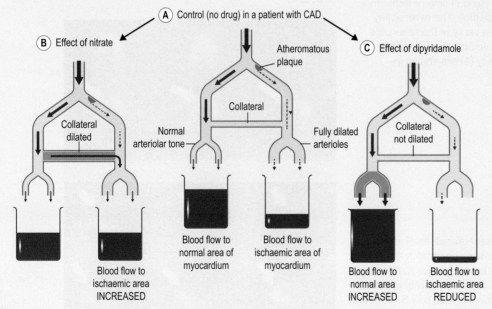

Comparison of the effects of organic nitrates and an arteriolar vasodilator (dipyridamole) on the coronary circulation. (A) Control. Nitrates dilate the collateral vessel, thus allowing more blood through to the underperfused region (mostly by diversion from the adequately perfused area). Dipyridamole dilates arterioles, increasing flow through the normal area at the expense of the ischaemic area (in which the arterioles are anyway fully dilated). (CAD, coronary artery disease.)

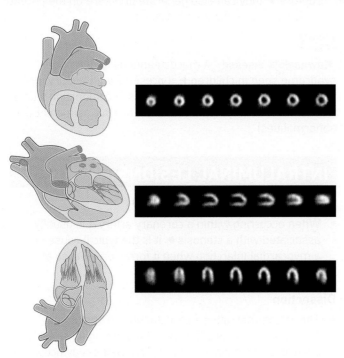

Standard display of SPECT cross-sectional images correlated with cardiac anatomy. Top row: short axis ▶ middle row: vertical long axis ▶ bottom row: horizontal long axis. The left ventricle is best seen due to its greater myocardial mass. The atria are not visualized.

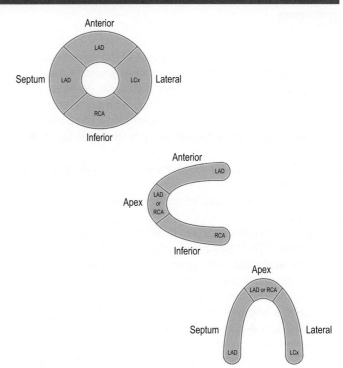

Planar scintigraphy: relationship of the coronary artery vascular supply to the ventricular wall segments. Anterior, left anterior oblique, and left lateral projections. LAD, left anterior descending artery. LCx, left circumflex branch. RCA, right coronary artery.

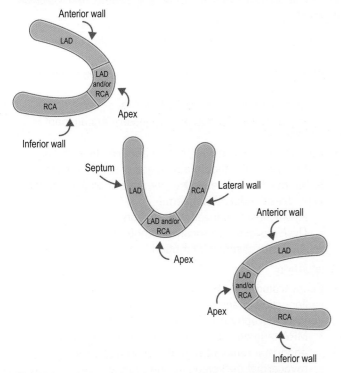

SPECT schematic correlation of myocardial wall segments and vascular supply. Short-axis, vertical long-axis and horizontal long-axis SPECT views. LAD, left anterior descending artery. RCA, right coronary artery.

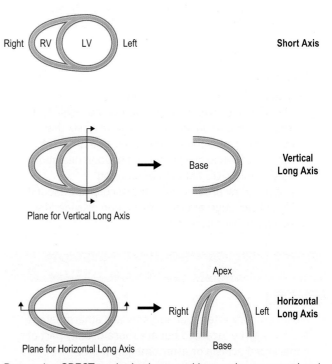

Processing SPECT to obtain short- and long-axis cross-sectional cuts. Schematic diagram displays the standard orientation along the short and long axis of the heart.

CORONARY ARTERY STENOSIS

Definition

- The normal lumen is preserved as atherosclerosis develops with increasing thickness of the vessel wall accompanied by an increased outer diameter – it is only during the late stages that a stenosis develops ▶ calcification indicates the presence of atherosclerosis (with a directly proportional relationship to stenosis severity, although not necessarily at the same place) ▶ hence:
  - CT screening uses coronary arterial calcification as an endpoint
  - Arteriography tends to underestimate the stenosis severity
- Significant coronary artery disease: major vessel stenosis ≥70% (≥50% in the left main)
- **Acute occlusion:** this is due to plaque rupture with subsequent thrombosis ▶ unless an arterial stump is identified, caution must be exercised as absent flow beyond a 'stenosis' may be caused by collateral (or CABG) flow ▶ in the presence of coronary arterial obstruction, anastamoses can form:
  - *'Ring of Vieussens':* an anastomosis around the right ventricular conus (between the RCA and the anterior descending artery)
  - *'Kugel's' artery:* an anastomosis between an atrial branch and an atrioventricular nodal artery
  - *Septal anastomoses:* these develop within the ventricular septum between branches of the anterior descending and posterior descending arteries, or between atrial branches proximally and distally
  - Anastomoses may also occur by direct terminal communications of large arteries

Treatment

- Percutaneous coronary intervention
  - The ideal lesion is a short, discrete, non-calcified lesion with a relatively concentric stenosis that does not involve the vessel origin or a branch ▶ recanalization is possible using balloon dilatation, atherectomy, US ablation or stenting
  - Doppler flow probes and intravascular ultrasound (IVUS) can augment the information provided by coronary arteriography

CORONARY ARTERY ANEURYSMS

Definition

- Most coronary arterial aneurysms are atheromatous ▶ they may be localized but are more usually part of a generalized ectasia or arteriomegaly (M>F)
  - A false aneurysm can complicate percutaneous coronary intervention procedures

- They may be symptomatic or cause sudden death due to rupture ▶ they can also generate pressure on the parent artery or cause distal embolization

Pearl

Kawasaki's disease A mucocutaneous lymph node syndrome seen in children ▶ it presents with aneurysms and strictures of the coronary arteries in conjunction with a fever and swollen lymph nodes (± ischaemic pain and ECG abnormalities)

INTRALUMINAL LESIONS

Thrombus

- When occurring within a coronary artery it is usually associated with a stenosis ▶ it is the typical cause of a myocardial infarction when it forms on an area of unstable ruptured plaque

Dissection

- This is common after a percutaneous transluminal coronary angioplasty (PTCA) – it is only significant if it obstructs flow ▶ spontaneous dissections may occur (either associated with aortic dissection or in isolation) and can cause chest pain or sudden death

IMPAIRED VENTRICULAR FUNCTION

Definition

- The degree of ventricular emptying is reflected by the ejection fraction (the stroke volume divided by the end-diastolic volume) ▶ the normal ejection fraction is approximately 66%
  - Significant impairment = 30–50% ▶ severe impairment = 10–30% ▶ very severe impairment = <10%
- Abnormal localized wall motion abnormalities occur within areas of ischaemia or areas of scarring from ischaemic heart disease ▶ reversible changes can occur with stress-induced ischaemia
  - *Hypokinesia:* reduced wall motion
  - *Dyskinesia:* paradoxical wall motion
  - *Akinesia:* absent wall motion

Evaluation

- Echocardiography ▶ first-pass or gated blood-pool radionuclide imaging ▶ conventional left ventriculography ▶ MDCT or cine-MRA
  - MRA tagging sequences can be used to highlight abnormal regional wall motion and reduced myocardial thickening during systole

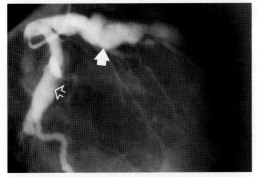

Coronary artery ectasia. Left coronary arteriogram (right anterior oblique) shows marked dilatation of the left anterior descending (LAD, solid arrow) and circumflex (open arrow) coronary arteries. Notice the poor opacification of the distal LAD due to the effect of gravity in preventing flow of the heavy contrast medium into the more anterior segment of the vessel.

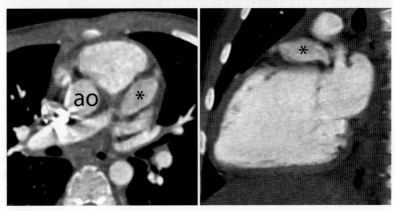

CCT images showing aneurysm of the left anterior descending coronary artery in a young patient with Kawasaki's disease. Presence of a fusiform aneurysm (*) (36 × 15 mm) in the proximal part of the left anterior descending coronary artery. No evidence of thrombus formation in the aneurysm. ao, aorta.**

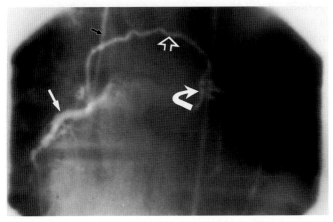

Vieussens' ring. Anterior view following injection into an occluded right coronary artery (arrow) shows a collateral vessel, Vieussens' artery (open arrow) is opacifying the left coronary artery (curved arrow) distal to a severe proximal stenosis. The black arrow indicates the aortic catheter.*

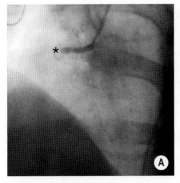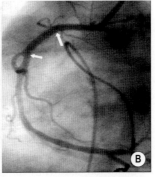

Acute myocardial infarction treated by mechanical thrombolysis and stenting. (A) Left anterior oblique coronary arteriogram shows thrombotic occlusion (asterisk) of the proximal right coronary artery. (B) Subsequent coronary arteriogram in the same orientation shows a patent vessel following mechanical thrombolysis.*

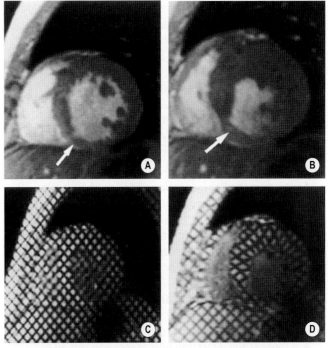

Inferior myocardial infarction shown by short-axis breath-hold cine-MRA and breath-hold tagging. (A) End-diastolic image shows minor narrowing of the inferior wall and the lower part of the interventricular septum (arrow). (B) End-systolic image shows normal thickening of the posterior and upper septal myocardium. There has been little thickening of the inferior wall and the lower part of the interventricular septum (arrow) representing the area affected by the inferior myocardial infarction. (C) End-diastolic, breath-hold tagging image shows no displacement of the orthogonal grid lines applied immediately before this image at the end of diastole. (D) End-systolic tagging image shows deformation of the tagging grid applied to the posterior and upper septal myocardium, indicating normal motion and thickening. There has been little distortion of the tagging grid, indicating poor contraction and thickening, in the region of the inferior myocardial infarction.*

231

MYOCARDIAL INFARCTION

- Most patients usually have obstructive coronary artery disease (involving 1 artery or multiple lesions in all 3 arteries) ▶ whereas infarction can occur with apparently normal arteries, the majority are caused by plaque rupture involving a <50% stenosis (the infarct-causing lesion is not always the most severe stenosis)
  - Plaque fissuring occurs within a cholesterol-rich atheromatous lesion with thrombosis developing on the exposed intima – this leads to infarction or unstable angina
- Thrombus may resolve spontaneously or after thrombolysis ▶ if the underlying plaque causes significant stenosis, then angina or reinfarction may occur – it therefore requires treatment
- In addition to infarct size, infarct transmurality is important (related to lack of inotropic reserve/impaired function/aneurysm formation)

Coronary angiography

- Thrombus is visualized as an intraluminal filling defect ▶ it is used for the anatomical assessment of disease severity and deciding whether surgery or percutaneous intervention is appropriate (as well as providing a surgical roadmap)
  - It will indicate the number and site of stenosed vessels to be bypassed and the state of the vessel at the insertion site ▶ small and irregular vessels beyond the stenosis may indicate diffuse disease and a difficult graft procedure

MRI

- *Acute myocardial infarction:* T2WI: high SI (within 30 min of coronary artery occlusion) ▶ slowly fades with healing
- *Recent myocardial infarction:* this shows poor perfusion with first-pass contrast medium imaging
- *Healed infarcts:* similar or decreased SI to normal myocardium
- *Late gadolinium enhancement (LGE) CMR:* this uses an inversion recovery technique (which nulls the signal from normally perfused viable myocardium) ▶ a myocardial infarction and associated region of non-viable myocardium will demonstrate delayed hyper-enhancement
- *LGE-MRI or high SI (T2WI):* this is not a specific finding and can be seen in other conditions causing myocardial damage, such as sarcoidosis or myocarditis
- Intramyocardial haemorrhage reflects microvascular injury and serves as a marker for reperfusion injury

MYOCARDIAL INFARCTION COMPLICATIONS

CARDIAC RUPTURE

- Myocardial rupture is followed by pericardial tamponade and death

LEFT VENTRICULAR ANEURYSM

- This is defined as a large thin-walled fibrous sac (bulging from the left ventricular lumen and external surface of the heart), clearly demarcated from the normal myocardium

ECG Persisting Q waves and ST segment elevation

CXR A normal cardiac silhouette ± diffuse left ventricular enlargement ± an obvious left ventricular focal bulge ▶ curvilinear calcification can develop within the aneurysm wall after several years

CT/MRI *The aneurysm has a wide neck*

- **DCE-MRI:** non-viable myocardium within the wall of a true aneurysm will demonstrate enhancement

FALSE OR PSEUDOANEURYSM

- This results from a localized perforation of the ventricular myocardium following an infarction or trauma ▶ they have a tendency to rupture and should be excised

CT/MRI *It will generally have a narrow neck ▶ it will fill and empty slowly with contrast medium ▶ there is an abrupt change in wall thickness often with an abrupt angulation at the aneurysm mouth ▶ as aneurysms are fibrous and akinetic, there may be paradoxical motion*

- **MRI+GAD:** a false aneurysm has no myocardium within its wall and will therefore not demonstrate enhancement

POST-INFARCTION VENTRICULAR SEPTAL DEFECT (VSD)

- Defects may occur anywhere within the muscular septum but are most frequently seen towards the apex ▶ the resultant acute volume overload may precipitate severe cardiac failure in association with a systolic murmur ▶ it has a poor prognosis, requiring immediate surgery

CXR Cardiomegaly + pulmonary oedema

Echocardiography The usual method of diagnosis

POST-INFARCTION MITRAL REGURGITATION

- This is caused by papillary muscle dysfunction or chordal rupture ▶ the clinical presentation and timing are similar to a septal perforation ▶ it is usually diagnosed with echocardiography

VENTRICULAR THROMBUS

- This occurs following infarction or with the cavity dilatation seen with congestive cardiomyopathy or a ventricular aneurysm ▶ fresh thrombus is mobile but later it may become flattened against the ventricular wall and become more echogenic with organization ▶ thrombus is commonly apical and less commonly seen on the posterior wall or proximal septum
  - It can be demonstrated with CECT, CMR and echocardiography (particularly transoesophageal)

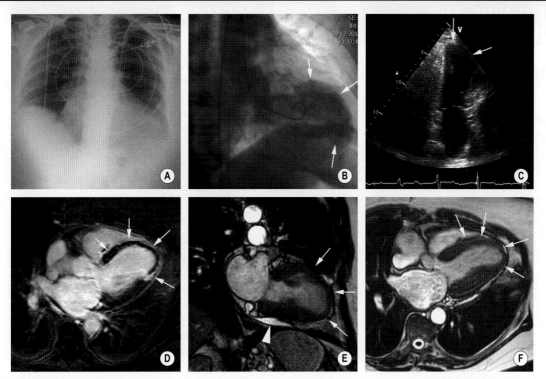

Comparison of imaging techniques in assessing patients with an acute myocardial infarction. Conventional chest film (A), cardiac catheterization (B), cardiac ultrasound (C) and CMR using LGE CMR (D), and cine CMR in vertical long-axis (E) and horizontal long-axis (F). Conventional CXR (bedside radiograph) shows moderate cardiomegaly without evidence of pulmonary oedema. LV contrast ventriculography (RAO position, end-systolic time frame) shows extensive area of decreased contractility involving the anterior wall, apex and the apicoinferior LV wall (arrows, B). Cardiac ultrasound (longitudinal parasternal view) reveals similar information (arrows, C). LGE CMR shows extensive myocardial infarction involving the majority of the ventricular septum, apical two-thirds of the anterior wall, apex, and apical inferolateral wall (arrows, D). While the periphery of the infarct is strongly enhanced, centrally an extensive zone of microvascular obstruction remains on LGE CMR, reflecting severe microvascular damage. The functional consequences of the infarction can be well appreciated on cine CMR (arrows, E, F). Small amount of pericardial fluid (arrowhead, E).**

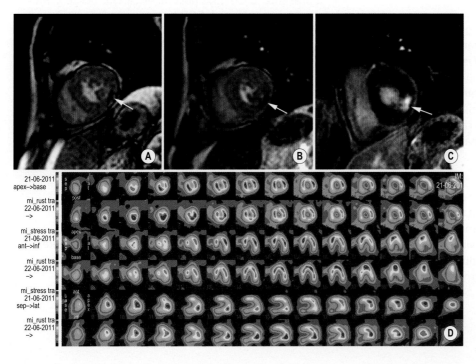

Small inferolateral myocardial infarct, MIBI SPECT versus CMR. History of PCI with stent placement in LAD coronary artery in 45-year-old man. MIBI SPECT shows reversible defect in mid/apical LV anterior wall (± 10% of LV myocardium) and decreased tracer activity in mid/basal inferolateral wall. Rest perfusion (A) and stress perfusion (B) CMR show focal hypointense appearance of the mid/basal LV inferolateral wall during first pass of contrast (arrow, A, B). On LGE CMR, this area shows a focal, almost completely transmural enhancement (arrow, C), compatible with healed myocardial infarction. No evidence of myocardial ischaemia in LAD territory in stress perfusion CMR (D).** (MIBI SPECT courtesy of O. Gheysens, Department of Nuclear Medicine, UZ Leuven, Leuven, Belgium.)

MYOCARDIAL STUNNING AND MYOCARDIAL HIBERNATION

MYOCARDIAL STUNNING

Definition

- Prolonged but temporary ventricular dysfunction following a period of ischaemia (there is abnormal ventricular function but the myocardium is viable and can regain normal function with revascularization) ▶ it can be seen after the relief of ischaemia by thrombolysis, percutaneous coronary interventions, coronary bypass grafting, reversal of vasospasm or after exercise

Radiological features

- It is identified by the recovery of left ventricular function during extended pharmacological stress testing with imaging by echocardiography, radionuclide imaging or cine-MRA
- Myocardial perfusion imaging using contrast echocardiography, radionuclide imaging or first-pass MRI can identify areas of perfused but ischaemic myocardium that demonstrates impaired function but which may benefit from revascularization
  - *Infarcted non-viable myocardium:* this can be identified as it fails to recover systolic function on extended pharmacological stress testing, retains contrast on DCE-MRI and does not recover function after reperfusion

MYOCARDIAL HIBERNATION

Definition

- A more chronic condition resulting from months or years of ischaemia causing ventricular dysfunction that persists until normal blood flow is restored (and is reversible with revascularization)
- The affected myocardium shows contractile reserve allowing differentiation from ischaemia during stress assessment with echocardiography, radionuclide imaging, cine-MRA and perfusion imaging

Pearl

Dobutamine stress MRI imaging

- Dobutamine will increase myocardial contractility ▶ a viable myocardial segment will demonstrate a wall motion abnormality at rest but this will improve with low-dose dobutamine ▶ high-dose dobutamine will induce ischaemia and cause the segment to cease contraction

ANGINA PECTORIS

Definition

- This is caused by reversible myocardial ischaemia, and presents with a crushing central chest pain characteristically radiating to the left arm or jaw ▶ it can occur in coronary artery disease, valvular heart disease, hypertrophic cardiomyopathy and tachyarrhythmias
  - *Prinzmetal's angina:* pain of spontaneous onset associated with ST segment elevation
  - *Syndrome X:* angina with apparently completely normal coronary arteries

Radiological features

- It can be investigated using stress ventriculography (echocardiography, first-pass or equilibrium radionuclide imaging or cine-MRA) or stress perfusion imaging (contrast agent, echocardiography, radionuclide scintigraphy or contrast CMR)
  - *Radionuclide imaging* (e.g. thallium-201): reversible ischaemia will demonstrate perfusion defects on stress that fill in on rest

DRESSLER'S SYNDROME

Definition

- A triad of pleuritis (with a small pleural effusion) + pneumonitis (ill-defined basal lung shadows) + pericarditis (rarely progressing to a pericardial tamponade)

Clinical presentation

- It presents 10–30 days post MI or cardiac surgery with chest pain and a high ESR ▶ it may remit and relapse over weeks to months

MRI Pericardial enhancement

Myocardial viability imaging

- Reversible LV dysfunction may benefit from revascularization
- Only viable myocardium (stunned/ischaemic/hibernating) can recover function ▶ non-viable myocardium (necrotic/scarred) cannot

PET Viable myocardium (mismatch pattern) vs. non-viable (match pattern)

Echocardiography Assess any improvement in myocardial contractility with dobutamine

- **CMR** Viable = normal wall thickness ▶ non-viable = reduced wall thickness (<6 mm) ▶ also can perform low-dose dobutamine stress function CMR late gadolinium enhancement (LGE) CMR to assess size of any healed infarct and transmural depth

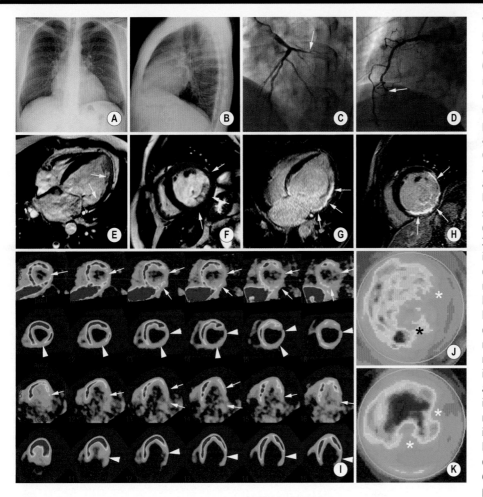

Viability imaging. Viability imaging in 57-year-old patient presenting ischaemic cardiomyopathy and increasing dyspnoea (NYHA III). Chest film (A, B) shows moderate cardiomegaly with redistribution of the pulmonary vascularization to the upper lung fields, reflecting increased pulmonary venous pressures. Coronary angiography shows complete occlusion of the proximal left circumflex coronary artery (arrow, C), and mid right coronary artery (arrow, D). Cine CMR in horizontal long axis (E) and short axis (F) shows severely dilated left ventricle end-diastolic volume 453 ml, (ejection fraction 36%) with severe thinning of the entire inferolateral wall (arrows, E, F). Presence of a severe mitral regurgitation due to mitral valve enlargement secondary to LV dilatation (regurgitant fraction 37%). LGE CMR shows presence of transmural enhancement in the inferolateral wall reflecting a healed extensive inferolateral myocardial infarction (arrows, G, H). PET imaging with perfusion imaging (NH$_3$ as tracer) and myocardial metabolism imaging (fluorodeoxyglucose (FDG) as metabolic tracer). Reconstructed slices in short axis and horizontal long axis (I), NH$_3$ (J) and FDG (K) polar maps. Presence of an extensive perfusion defect in the entire inferolateral wall (*, J) that matches perfectly with the lack of metabolism on FDG-PET (*, K). This match pattern reflects irreversibly damaged myocardium. The PET and CMR abnormalities correlate perfectly.** (FDG/NH$_3$ PET courtesy of O. Gheysens, Department of Nuclear Medicine, UZ Leuven, Leuven, Belgium.)

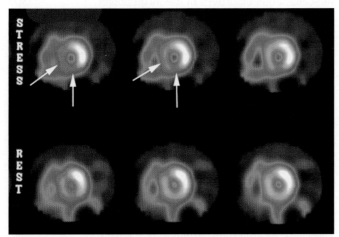

A ^{99m}technetium myocardial perfusion scan showing SPECT images. This study is performed after exercise stress of the myocardium (top images) and a later study was performed at rest (bottom images). The images are through the short axis of both the left and right ventricle and demonstrate a partially reversible perfusion defect in the interventricular septum and posterior wall of the left ventricle (arrows).[†]

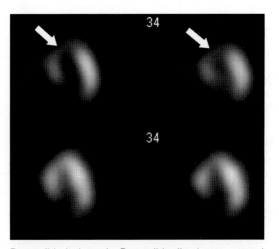

Reversible ischaemia. Reversible distal anteroseptal and apical myocardial ischaemia on vertical long-axis views. Upper-row images are during stress (dipyridamole) with an area of reduced activity (arrows) not seen on resting images (lower-row images). This suggests ischaemia in the distal left anterior descending artery (LAD) territory. The imaging agent is ^{99m}Tc-tetrofosmin.*

GASTROINTESTINAL

3.1 OESOPHAGUS

HIATUS HERNIA

Definition

- Protrusion of part of the stomach through the diaphragmatic oesophageal opening
  - **Type 1 – sliding hernia** (the commonest type): the gastro-oesophageal junction (GOJ) slides proximally through the diaphragmatic hiatus to assume an intrathoracic position ▶ it is accompanied by reflux and oesophagitis
    - The squamocolumnar junction is seen at ≤38 cm (the normal is 40 cm) from the incisors at endoscopy
  - **Type 2 – rolling hernia:** the GOJ is in a normal position below the diaphragm – the proximal stomach (usually the fundus) herniates through the hiatus/focal defect ▶ this is more prone to incarceration and obstruction, and it may undergo torsion, resulting in strangulation, infarction or perforation
    - The squamocolumnar junction maintains its normal position
  - **Type 3 – combined hernia:** features of both are present
  - **Type 4 – intrathoracic stomach** (± organoaxial rotation)

Clinical presentation

- Asymptomatic or gastro-oesophageal reflux (± reflux oesophagitis) ▶ symptoms are more commonly seen with a sliding hernia

Radiological features

Barium swallow

- **Sliding hiatus hernia:** the Schatski or B ring is demonstrated above (>2 cm) the diaphragmatic hiatus ▶ gastric rugae traversing the diaphragm
- **Rolling hiatus hernia:** a part of the stomach (usually the gastric fundus) is prolapsed into the chest anterior or lateral to the oesophagus

Pearls

- **Schatski or B ring:** a ring of mucosal tissue at the lower border of the phrenic ampulla marking the junction between the squamous and columnar epithelium (the 'Z line')
- *The 'A' ring or inferior oesophageal sphincter:* about 2-4 cm proximal to the B ring is a thicker ring produced by active muscular contraction
- The Schatski ring is always associated with a small sliding hiatus hernia ▶ it can be congenital or secondary to gastro-oesophageal reflux (with associated inflammation and fibrosis)
- The Schatski ring is usually no more than 2–3 mm in thickness ▶ despite being mucosal it can be symptomatic (requiring dilatation)
- If the B ring is incomplete, part of it can sometimes be demonstrated as the incisural notch (which is inevitably seen on the greater curve aspect of the stomach)

GASTRO-OESOPHAGEAL REFLUX DISEASE (GORD)

Definition

- GORD follows lower oesophageal sphincter dysfunction ▶ this initially leads to reflux (with minor irritation and inflammation) but can then proceed to ulceration, fibrosis and stricture formation ▶ it may also be associated with a hiatus hernia

Clinical presentation

- Heartburn or dysphagia ▶ the major long-term complications are peptic oesophagitis (± stricture formation or Barrett's oesophagus)

Radiological features

Barium swallow

- *Reflux:* this may be demonstrated but alone is of questionable significance – minor amounts can occur in the normal population ▶ gross reflux (up to the level of the aortic knuckle or above and not cleared by a stripping wave passing down the oesophagus) is likely to be symptomatic
  - Associated features: a wide gastro-oesophageal junction (> ⅔ of the maximally distended thoracic oesophagus) ▶ an inflammatory gastro-oesophageal polyp (seen as a single linear polyp straddling the GOJ)
- *Reflux oesophagitis:* this can demonstrate mucosal oedema, erosive disease or frank ulceration ▶ initially the collapsed oesophagus shows thickened longitudinal folds (>3 mm) ▶ multiple fine ulcers give the mucosa a punctate or granular appearance ▶ larger discrete punched-out ulcers can develop ▶ ulceration is most pronounced immediately above the GOJ and local circular muscle spasm may produce transverse folds ▶ scarring produces permanent folds that radiate from the ulcer margins
- *Long-term sequelae:* stricture formation (typically a short stricture above a hiatus hernia with smooth tapered margins) ▶ the development of Barrett's oesophagus (in 10% of cases)

Radionuclide study Reflux of ^{99m}Tc-sulphur colloid labelled scrambled egg can demonstrate gastro-oesophageal reflux

Pearls

- 24-hour pH measurement is the 'gold standard' in the assessment of reflux
- There is no direct relationship between a hiatus hernia and GORD: many patients have a hiatus hernia but no GORD (but most patients with GORD will have a hiatus hernia)

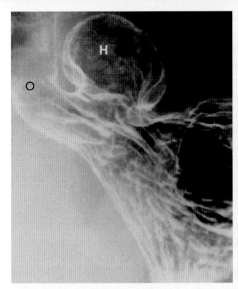

Rolling (paraoesophageal) hiatus hernia. The gastric fundus (H) lies alongside the lower oesophagus (O).[†]

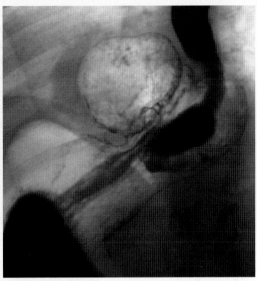

Contrast study demonstrating a combined-type hiatus hernia. Note the rolling component with a large portion of stomach above the diaphragm, but in addition the gastro-oesophageal junction has also migrated cranially.*

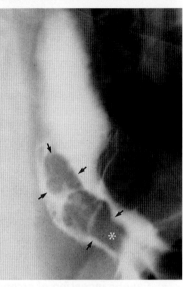

Inflammatory polyp (arrows) lying at end of gastric fold (asterisk).[†]

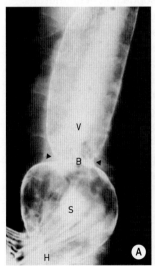

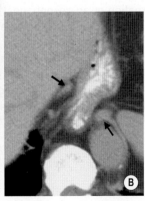

Sliding hiatus hernia. (A) Barium swallow shows a hiatus hernia (H), more than 3-cm wide with at least 3 gastric folds seen extending across it ▶ S = stomach forming the hernia ▶ B = B ring, the gastro-oesophageal junction ▶ V = vestibule. The A ring is not visible. (B) CT scan showing the crura of the diaphragm (arrows) separated by 28 mm (normal is <15 mm). The fundus of the stomach is seen herniating through the diaphragmatic hiatus.[†]

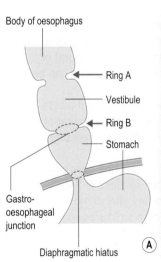

Body of oesophagus
Ring A
Vestibule
Ring B
Stomach
Gastro-oesophageal junction
Diaphragmatic hiatus

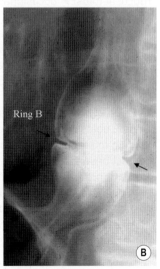

Ring B

The lower end of the oesophagus. (A) The B ring may normally be within 2 cm above (as shown here) or below the hiatus. Thus the oesophageal vestibule may normally be above, or straddle the diaphragmatic hiatus. (B) Small sliding hiatus hernia with normal B ring (between arrows).[†]

OESOPHAGITIS AND BENIGN STRICTURES

DEFINITION

- Oesophageal inflammation (± subsequent smooth benign stricture formation) can be caused by the following:
  - **GORD** (see separate section)
  - **Infection:** especially in the immunocompromised patient *Candida albicans* ▶ herpes simplex virus (HSV) ▶ cytomegalovirus (CMV) ▶ human immunodeficiency virus (HIV) ▶ tuberculosis
  - **Drugs:** potassium chloride tablets ▶ tetracycline ▶ clindamycin ▶ doxycycline ▶ NSAIDs
  - **Radiation:** this is often self-limiting
  - **Crohn's disease:** this is very rare and usually accompanied by extensive GI disease elsewhere
  - **Iatrogenic:** following prolonged placement of a nasogastric tube (NGT)
  - **Caustic ingestion of strong acids or alkalis**

CLINICAL PRESENTATION

- Odynophagia ▶ dysphagia ▶ haematemesis

RADIOLOGICAL FEATURES

Barium swallow

- **Candidiasis:** initially there is dysmotility and atony of the oesophagus ▶ eventually classic plaque-like filling defects with ulceration and pseudomembrane formation are seen (there are also irregular and thickened mucosal folds) ▶ occasionally pseudo-ulcerations may appear as aphthous ulcers
- **HSV:** vesicles in the upper and mid-oesophagus appear as sessile filling defects ▶ when they burst they leave punched-out superficial ulcers on a background of normal mucosa ▶ in advanced disease there can be diffuse ulceration
- **CMV/HIV:** presents with giant oesophageal ulcers
- **Drugs:** potassium chloride causes deep ulceration leading to stricture formation ▶ NSAIDs can cause contact oesophagitis
- **Radiation:** >20 Gy results in a transient oesophagitis with aperistalsis or tertiary contractions ▶ >45 Gy results in obliterative endarteritis after 6 months with severe oesophagitis and smooth strictures – deep ulcers can also form (which may fistulate to the trachea)

- **Crohn's disease:** this can present with aphthoid ulcers or frank ulceration
- **Nasogastric tube:** this renders the lower oesophageal sphincter incompetent, resulting in a reflux oesophagitis and a long tapered stricture within the lower oesophagus ▶ this may occur only 48 h post placement ▶ the strictures are often long and extensive
- **Caustic ingestion:** this can lead to mucosal necrosis with ulceration and mucosal sloughing ▶ the oesophagus may perforate within the 1st 2 weeks or result in fistulation to the pleural cavity or pericaridium ▶ it heals with fibrosis and stricture formation ▶ strictures occur at the normal sites of oesophageal compression (e.g. at the level of the aorta, left main bronchus or diaphragmatic hiatus)

PEARLS

Epidermolysis bullosa dystrophica

- A hereditary skin disease affecting children where minor trauma produces bullae formation ▶ the oesophagus may be involved (leading to stricture formation)

Pemphigoid

- A benign mucous membrane disease of middle age, involving the conjunctiva and mucosa of the oral cavity and skin ▶ the upper oesophageal mucosa may be involved with ulcers, webs and stricture formation

Intramural pseudodiverticulosis

- The excretory ducts of the oesophageal deep mucous glands dilate and fill with barium ▶ they are seen on barium studies as multiple, flask-shaped mucosal outpouchings ▶ this disease is usually diffuse, but may be localized if it is associated with peptic stricture formation or an oesophageal carcinoma
- Fistulation may occur between these pseudodiverticula ▶ intramural abscesses may develop which can rarely perforate through the oesophageal wall ▶ long tapered strictures may arise
- It is associated with oesophagitis (usually due to reflux) ▶ other underlying disorders include diabetes, candidiasis and alcoholism

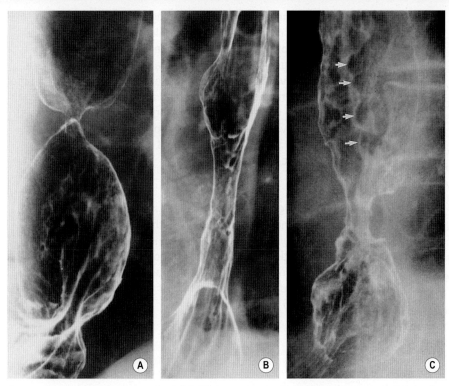 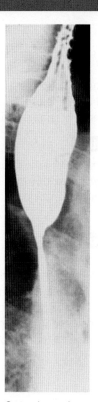

An annular peptic stricture at the GOJ. (A) An area gastricae pattern is present below the stricture. (B) Benign peptic stricture above a hiatus hernia. The stricture has smooth tapered margins. (C) Benign peptic stricture. Asymmetric ulceration and scarring has produced a stricture with irregular and shoulder margins resembling a carcinoma. Erosions on the oesophageal folds give them a lobular margin resembling varices (arrows).[†]

Corrosive stricture. A long stricture extending up to the mid-oesophagus (resulting from swallowing lye as child).[†]

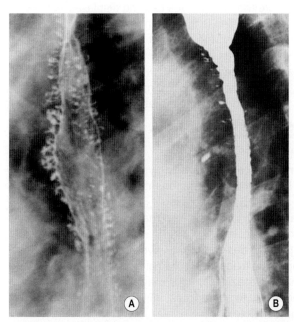 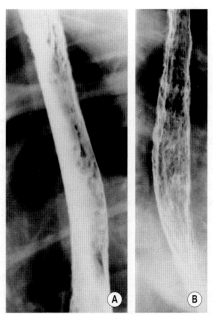 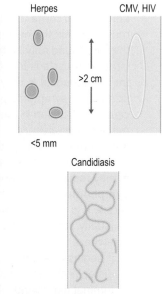

Intramural pseudodiverticulosis. (A) Multiple flask-shaped projections produced by barium entering dilated oesophageal glands. (B) Mid-oesophageal stricture with small flask-shaped projections.[†]

Candida oesophagitis (A) Mucosal plaques. (B) Extensive mucosal nodularity.[†]

Diagrammatic representation of oesophageal ulceration.

BENIGN TUMOURS

Definition

- Benign tumours arising from the oesophageal mucosa or submucosa:
  - *Mucosal origin:* papilloma
  - *Submucosal origin:* leiomyoma (the commonest type) ▶ neurofibroma ▶ lipoma ▶ fibrovascular polyp

Clinical presentation

- These can be asymptomatic or present with dysphagia
  - *Fibrovascular polyp:* this may be regurgitated into the mouth and even, on occasion, aspirated (resulting in asphyxia)

Radiological features
Barium swallow

- **Papilloma:** these are usually small (2–5 mm) ▶ larger papillomas may trap barium within the interlacing fronds that cover their surface
- **Leiomyoma:** these are usually found within the lower ⅓ of the oesophagus ▶ they appear as a smooth submucosal wide-based filling defect covered by an intact mucosa ▶ they may calcify and can be multiple
- **Neurofibroma/lipoma:** these may be difficult to distinguish from a leiomyoma and are extremely rare
- **Fibrovascular polyp:** these are usually found within the proximal oesophagus ▶ they are pedunculated (the stalk forms due to repeated passage of food with peristalsis) ▶ they may expand the oesophageal lumen but rarely cause significant barium hold-up (due to their very pliable nature)

Pearls

- **Glycogenic acanthosis:** this results from the accumulation of glycogen within the squamous epithelium (and is therefore not a tumour as such) ▶ its aetiology is unclear (but possibly age related) ▶ it demonstrates no malignant potential
  - *Endoscopy:* small white or yellow plaques measuring 2–5 mm in size

MALIGNANT TUMOURS

Definition

- Malignant tumours arising from the oesophageal mucosa or submucosa
  - **Oesophageal carcinoma**: the commonest malignant tumour (see separate section)
  - **Leiomyosarcoma** (1%): these arise from the *smooth* muscle within the oesophageal wall – therefore they are found only within the distal oesophagus (*striated* muscle is found within the proximal ⅓ of the oesophagus) ▶ they can grow to an extraordinary size before symptoms present due to their failure to cause obstruction ▶ they are relatively indolent and metastasize late
  - **Melanoma** (1%): these are rare tumours (melanoblasts are uncommon within the oesophagus) ▶ they metastasize early with a very poor prognosis
  - **Lymphoma** (1%): oesophageal involvement is very rare ▶ it is usually of the non-Hodgkin's type and is usually associated with lymphomatous disease elsewhere
    - It begins as a submucosal lesion (usually in the distal ⅓ of the oesophagus) resulting in a smooth luminal narrowing with an intact overlying mucosa ▶ later ulceration can develop
    - Secondary involvement by contiguous spread from adjacent nodal disease is more common but rarely results in dysphagia
  - **Spindle cell carcinoma**: a rare tumour containing both carcinomatous and spindle cell elements
  - **Metastases**: these are usually due to direct extension from tumours within the thoracic cavity (notably carcinoma of the bronchus) ▶ involved nodes may also infiltrate the oesophagus causing displacement and occasionally fistula formation between the oesophageal lumen and the adjacent bronchus ▶ carcinoma of the pancreas (particularly the tail) may involve the distal oesophagus or gastro-oesophageal junction
    - Breast carcinoma is the most common distant cause of oesophageal metastases

Radiological features
Barium swallow/CT

- **Leiomyosarcoma:** a large polyploid mass ▶ there can be a large exophytic component which may be seen on a CXR as a mediastinal mass
- **Melanoma:** a large polyploid mass (which will appear black on endoscopy)
- **Lymphoma:** this commonly involves the distal oesophagus following spread of lymphoma from the stomach ▶ the oesophagus may show widespread changes due to submucosal infiltration (presenting as multiple nodules)
- **Spindle cell carcinoma:** a bulky, polyploid tumour within the mid-oesophagus
- **Metastases:** involvement of the distal oesophagus and GOJ by carcinoma of the pancreas may lead to a right-angled bend of the distal oesophagus
  - Breast carcinoma usually causes submucosal masses

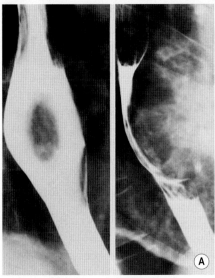
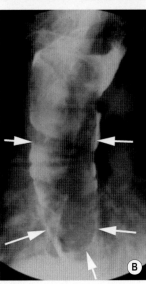
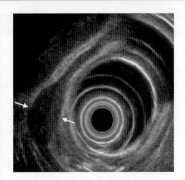

Leiomyoma. Endoscopic ultrasound demonstrating an echo-poor mass (between arrows) that is continuous with the layer of the muscularis propria.†

Leiomyoma of the oesophagus. (A) Two views showing features typical of an intramural or extrinsic lesion. There is a broad-based filling defect bulging into, and widening, the lumen of the oesophagus.† (B) Barium swallow image demonstrating a grossly dilated oesophagus with a large filling defect (arrows) consistent with a fibrovascular polyp.** (Image courtesy of Dr DJM Tolan, Leeds Teaching Hospitals.)

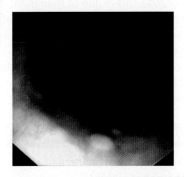

An endoscopic view of glycogenic acanthosis showing the typical small, smooth plaques of this condition.*

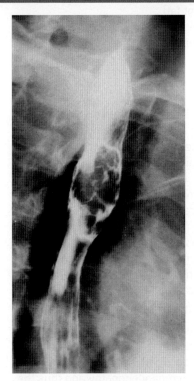

Spindle cell sarcoma. A bulky polypoid tumour arising in the mid-oesophagus.†

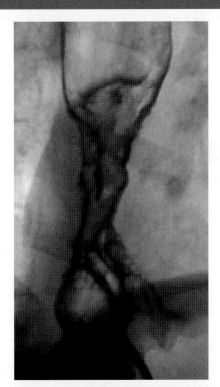

Barium study of a stricturing adenocarcinoma situated just above the gastro-oesophageal junction, as demonstrated by irregularity and an abrupt transition to normal mucosa on its cranial side.*

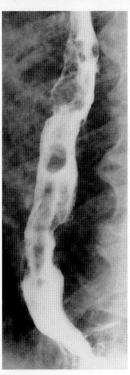

Oesophageal carcinoma with submucosal extension simulating varices, however (unlike varices) the width of the elongated filling defect was not influenced by the degree of oesophageal distension.

OESOPHAGEAL CARCINOMA

DEFINITION

- A malignant tumour of the oesophagus:
  - *Squamous cell carcinoma (>70%):* this arises from the squamous epithelium ▶ it is commonly found within the mid-oesophagus (50%), but rarely invades the stomach (cf. an adenocarcinoma)
    - It is associated with smoking, alcohol and tobacco consumption
    - Less common associations include: achalasia ▶ Plummer–Vinson syndrome ▶ head and neck tumours ▶ coeliac disease ▶ radiation change
  - *Adenocarcinoma (<30%):* this is due to malignant degeneration of columnar metaplasia ▶ the majority (90%) are found within the distal ⅓ of the oesophagus ▶ there is an increasing frequency relative to squamous carcinoma due to an increasing prevalence of Barrett's oesophagus and scleroderma (the patulous oesophagus leads to reflux)

CLINICAL PRESENTATION

- It is rare under the age of 40, with an increasing incidence with age thereafter (3M:1F)
  - It is often advanced with a poor prognosis at presentation: the lack of oesophageal serosa does not provide a barrier to tumour spread ▶ there are multiple mediastinal structures that are close by
- *Presenting features:* dysphagia (indicating unresectable disease) ▶ weight loss ▶ recurrent aspiration ▶ early satiety (with distal adenocarcinomas) ▶ fistula formation with the tracheobronchial tree (seen in up to 10% of squamous cell carcinomas)

RADIOLOGICAL FEATURES

- There are a wide range of morphological appearances: nodular, polypoid, ulcerative or irregular structuring
  - There can also be an uncommon varicoid (or superficial spreading) type

Barium swallow

- **Early:** stiffened mucosa ▶ a failure to collapse completely following a peristaltic wave
- **Late:** an irregular stricture with nodular or rolled margins ▶ the ulcerative type usually has a firm irregular tumour rim
- **Varicoid carcinoma:** this follows submucosal spread of tumour ▶ it results in tortuous thickened folds that can mimic varices
- **GOJ tumours:** an achalasia-like picture due to infiltration and destruction of the myenteric plexus ▶ nodules and irregular margins can be seen at the GOJ
- **Advanced cases:** fistulation with the tracheobronchial tree (leading to recurrent aspiration) ▶ total dysphagia

CT

- Asymmetric oesophageal wall thickening (≥5 mm) ▶ a dilated oesophagus cranial to the tumour (due to obstruction)
- The tumour may extend through the serosa into the peri-oesophageal fat with loss of the sharp interface, together with the formation of a high attenuation mass ▶ it may invade any adjacent structures (e.g. the aorta)
- Rarer polypoid tumours are shown as intraluminal filling defects that may expand the overall oesophageal diameter
- CT is excellent at assessing local gastro-hepatic nodes ▶ however it is poor at assessing the extent of tumour invasion of the oesophageal wall (i.e. differentiating between T3 and T4 tumours)
  - Ill-defined para-oesophageal fat suggests T3 disease
  - Tumour contact >90° with the aorta/loss of the triangular fat between the oesophagus, aorta and spine/nodular protrusion into the airways suggests T4 disease

MRI

- Like CT, it is also unable to distinguish between T1 and T2 disease
- T1WI: tumour is isointense to the normal oesophagus (extra-oesophageal invasion is suggested by loss of the high SI from the adjacent fat)
- T2WI: intermediate to high SI tumour mass
- T1WI + Gad: enhancement

EUS

- A hypoechoic tumour disrupting the normal 5 oesophageal wall layers
  - This is the only modality that can currently differentiate between a T1 (just involving the mucosa) and a T2 (invading the muscularis propria) tumour ▶ a T3 lesion will demonstrate adventitial infiltration
- It can identify malignant local nodes: these are well marginated, spherical, hypoechoic and demonstrate loss of their internal structure
  - Elongated nodes are more likely to be benign
- *Limitations:* it cannot pass a tight stricture ▶ it may overestimate the tumour extent (due to peritumoral inflammation) ▶ it may not be able to distinguish reactive from metastatic lymph nodes

FDG PET and FDG PET-CT

- Oesophageal carcinomas are FDG avid ▶ PET cannot usually identify T1 tumours, and often not T2 tumours
- This is more sensitive, specific and accurate than CT in identifying loco-regional lymphadenopathy and thus the overall staging ▶ PET-CT is more sensitive than PET alone
- It can define the craniocaudal tumour extent and also can assess any chemotherapeutic response (particularly the differentiation of malignant disease from residual oesophageal thickening)

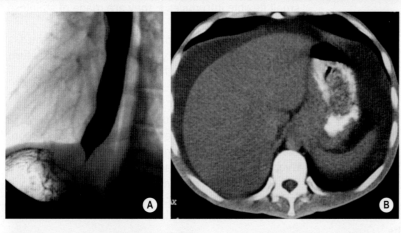

Pseudo achalasia appearance. Note the tapered appearance of the distal oesophagus which superficially resembles an achalasia, but the clue to the sinister nature of this lesion is from the impression on the gastric fundus.[†]

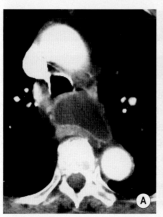
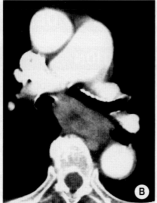
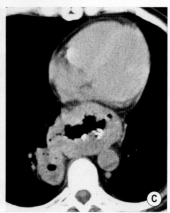

Typical CT appearances of oesophageal carcinoma. Note the dilated oesophagus (A) situated cranial to an area of wall thickening (B). (C) CT showing gross thickening of the oesophageal wall due to an extensive carcinoma that has also extended into the right lung base, producing an associated thick-walled cavity.*

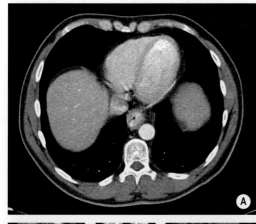
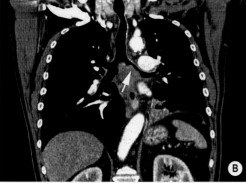
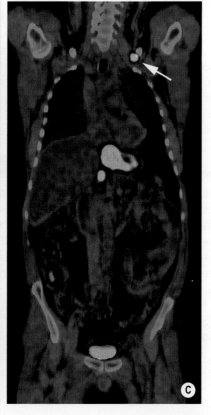

(A) CT image of a lower oesophageal adenocarcinoma. There are no features of invasion of adjacent organs such as the aorta. Statistically this tumour is most likely to be a T3 tumour, but a T2 could look identical; hence the requirement for EUS. (B) Coronal CT image of a patient with a lower oesophageal adenocarcinoma. There is nodular protrusion of soft tissue from the tumour into the left main bronchus (arrow), in keeping with T4 invasion. (C) Coronal PET-CT image of an FDG-avid left supraclavicular lymph node (arrow) metastasis in a patient with a distal oesophageal adenocarcinoma.**

OESOPHAGEAL CARCINOMA

PEARLS

Normal oesophageal wall layers on Endoscopic Ultrasound (EUS)

- Superficial mucosa: *hyperechoic*
- Muscularis mucosae: *hypoechoic*
- Submucosa: *hyperechoic*
- Muscularis propria: *hypoechoic*
- Adventitia: *hyperechoic*

Mechanisms of tumour spread

- **Lymphatic spread:** malignant nodes are not usually enlarged, and may first arise some distance from the primary tumour ▶ nodal involvement occurs at the same level as the tumour (± paratracheal, hilar and para-aortic adenopathy) ▶ frequent non-regional nodes include left supraclavicular + retroperitoneal abdominal
  - Cranial longitudinal spread can occur to the internal jugular, cervical and supraclavicular nodes
  - Caudal longitudinal spread can occur to the left gastric and coeliac nodes
  - Coeliac axis and perioesophageal cervical nodes are classified as regional nodes rather than metastases
- **Haematogenous spread:** this occurs early and is commonly to the lungs, liver, adrenals (and less commonly to bone)
- **Direct invasion**
  - *Aortic invasion:* surgical resectability of the primary tumour is less likely to be successful if there is ≥90° of contact with the aortic circumference, or if there is obliteration of the small triangle of fat between the oesophagus, aorta and spine
  - *Tracheobronchial invasion:* there is inward bowing of the posterior tracheal wall (which normally has a convex appearance) ▶ there is tracheal or bronchial displacement away from the spine ▶ there is obliteration of the fat plane between the oesophagus and the upper respiratory tract

Treatment and palliation of oesophageal cancer

- **Treatment:** endoscopic mucosal resection (EMR) for T1 tumours ▶ primary surgical resection (with gastric conduit/pull through) if the tumour involves the mucosa or submucosa ▶ neoadjuvant therapy if there is extension into the muscularis propria (or beyond)
- **Palliation for advanced disease:** stents are used when there is progressive dysphagia with an inability to swallow saliva
  - *Stent delivery:* either at endoscopy (via the endoscope biopsy channel) or under direct radiological control

- *Self-expanding metal stents:* these are delivered on a small flexible introducer ▶ they are made of stainless steel or nitinol
  - Nitinol: a compound of nickel and titanium which has an inbuilt memory feature allowing it to return to a preset size and shape following delivery
- *Covered stents* (coating of polyurethane): these are useful to reduce tumour overgrowth and for dealing with fistulae ▶ they are unsuitable for deployment across the GOJ (as there can be significant migration)
- *Complications:* oesophageal perforation ▶ distal stent migration into the stomach ▶ gastro-oesophageal reflux (if a stent is placed across the GOJ) ▶ possible tracheal compression or a persistent sensation in the throat (with high stent placement)

BARRETT'S OESOPHAGUS

DEFINITION

- Chronic gastro-oesophageal reflux causes a specialized non-secretory columnar epithelium to grow cranially into areas previously covered by squamous epithelium
  - Usually 2 cm or more of columnar epithelium is required before the term is used

RADIOLOGICAL FEATURES

- **Barium swallow:** there is a wide patulous hiatal segment (associated with a hiatus hernia) ▶ there is a dilated segment of oesophagus above the hernia (lined by columnar epithelium) which often appears to be 'bell' or 'tent' shaped
  - The junction of the two mucosal types is marked by a ring (which is often slightly contractile) where ulceration and secondary strictures may form ▶ this may be some way above the hiatus (at the level of the aortic knuckle or above)

PEARLS

- It is ultimately diagnosed with endoscopy and biopsy
- Barrett's oesophagus is associated with up to a 40-fold increased risk of developing oesophageal carcinoma (15% of patients with a Barrett's oesophagus develop an adenocarcinoma) ▶ the precursor is a high-grade dysplasia and therefore regular endoscopic screening is required
- If >2 cm, surveillance endoscopy (2 yearly) is offered

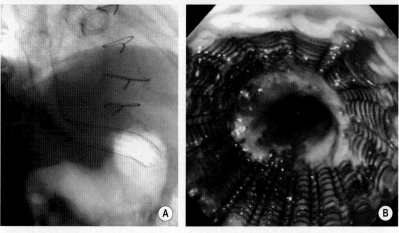

(A) An oesophageal stent in situ across a junctional tumour. (B) Endoscopic view of an oesophageal stent in position. Note the tumour ingrowth through the mesh of the distal part of this stent.*

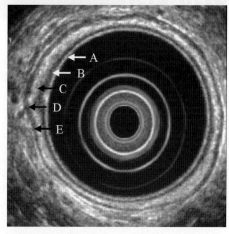

EUS of the oesophagus showing the wall layers. A = mucosa, B = muscularis mucosae, C = submucosa, D = muscularis propria, E = adventitia.†

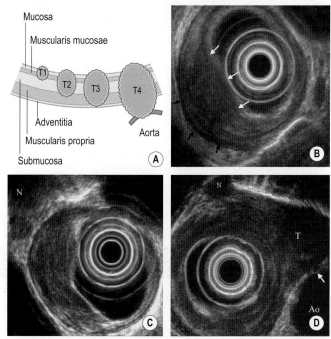

EUS staging of oesophageal carcinoma. (A) T staging: T1 (limited to the mucosa and submucosa), T2 (involves the muscularis propria), T3 (involves the adventitia), T4 (invades adjacent structures). (B) T2 tumour – the muscularis propria has not been breached (black arrows). The luminal tumour border is indicated by the white arrows. (C) T2N1 tumour. The muscularis propria has not been breached but there are adjacent involved lymph nodes (N). Malignant nodes are round, hypoechoic and well defined with a loss of their internal structure. (D) T4 – tumour has breached the muscularis propria and is invading the aortic wall (arrow). Ao = aorta, T = tumour, N = metastatic lymph node.†

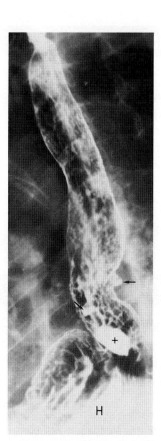

Barrett's oesophagus. Ulceration (arrows) at the squamocolumnar junction, below which is a fine reticular pattern. This resembles the areae gastricae pattern of the stomach, and is produced by islands of columnar mucosa. + = pool of barium, H = hiatus hernia.†

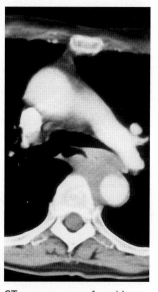

CT appearances of a mid-oesophageal carcinoma, which demonstrates extensive soft tissue involvement around the adjacent aorta, thus rendering it inoperable.*

ACHALASIA

Definition

- A motor disorder of the oesophagus caused by the degeneration of the neurones of Auerbach's plexus (which is situated between the oesophageal longitudinal and circular muscle coats)
  - This leads to a failure of relaxation of the GOJ

Clinical presentation

- The onset occurs between 20 and 40 years of age
- It presents initially with dysphagia for both solids and liquids (cf. strictures which initially only cause dysphagia for solids)
  - There is a recurrent aspiration and pneumonia risk (10%)

Radiological features

Barium swallow

- *Early:* defective distal peristalsis is associated with a slight narrowing at the GOJ

- *'Vigorous achalasia':* marked non-propulsive contractions may occur
- *Late:* the body of the oesophagus becomes progressively dilated and aperistaltic with a subsequent huge oesophageal residue of food and fluid debris (this can be seen as a fluid level on a CXR and is a significant aspiration risk)
  - *'Rat's tail' or 'bird's beak' appearance:* a characteristic appearance of the gastro-oesophageal junction

Pearls

- Oesophageal squamous cell carcinoma is a likely complication with severe long-standing (> 20 years) disease
- In patients with early achalasia, drinking hot water in the erect position during fluoroscopy produces an immediate and pronounced relaxation of the GOJ
  - The diagnosis still needs to be confirmed by manometry (± scintigraphy) ▶ endoscopy will exclude a carcinoma as a cause of secondary achalasia

DIFFUSE OESOPHAGEAL SPASM

Definition

- A dysmotility disorder of the oesophagus (it is five times less common than achalasia)
- It is characterized by strong repetitive non-propulsive contractions which may be interspersed with normal peristaltic waves ▶ these marked contractions may completely obliterate the oesophageal lumen

Clinical presentation

- Chest pain (it may or may not be associated with swallowing)

Radiological features

Barium swallow

- Strong non-propulsive contractions may lead to a 'corkscrew' or 'curling' oesophagus
- There may be marked oesophageal wall thickening (which may extend to a depth of up to several cm)
- Occasionally there can be oesophageal diverticula (as a consequence of the high pressure contractions)

OTHER CAUSES OF DYSMOTILITY

GORD This is probably the commonest cause of oesophageal dysmotility

Presbyoesophagus An age-related (>70 years) oesophageal dysmotility which is not attributable to a specific condition

Scleroderma This is the commonest systemic disease to cause oesophageal dysmotility ▶ it is a collagen vascular disorder of unknown aetiology characterized by smooth muscle atrophy followed by collagen deposition and fibrosis involving the oesophagus, stomach and small bowel

Barium swallow Initially there is diminished peristalsis (or tertiary contractions in the distal ⅓ of oesophagus) – this is then followed by absent peristalsis ▶ the GOJ becomes wide and patulous resulting in GOR, reflux oesophagitis and stricture formation ▶ oesophageal stasis

may result in *Candida* colonization and an increased risk of adenocarcinoma

Chagas disease This is caused by *Trypanosoma cruzi* which produces a neurotoxin destroying the ganglion cells within the myenteric plexus ▶ it can affect the oesophagus, colon (megacolon or sigmoid volvulus), stomach (megastomach), duodenum (megaduodenum), heart (cardiomyopathy) and CNS (encephalitis)

Barium swallow Initially the oesophagus will demonstrate hypercontractility and distal muscular spasm ▶ during the later stages an appearance similar to achalasia can present when denervation has occurred
- Oesophageal complications include ulceration, perforation and carcinoma

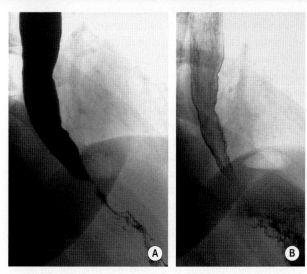

Classical appearances of achalasia. Note the tapered appearance of the GOJ with the column of barium above (A). As soon as hot water has been drunk, the whole barium column falls through into the stomach (B).*

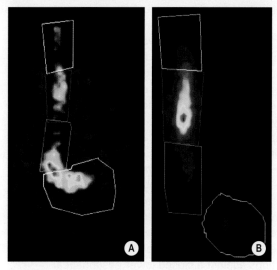

Radio-isotope study also demonstrating achalasia. A normal examination is shown with isotope in the stomach (A), whereas in achalasia the isotope is retained in the oesophagus (B).*

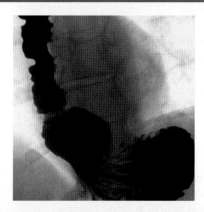

View of a large sliding hiatal hernia that demonstrates gross spontaneous gastro-oesophageal reflux when the patient lifts the left side while in the supine position. Note also the marked oesophageal incoordination produced by the reflux.*

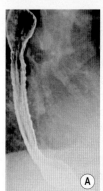 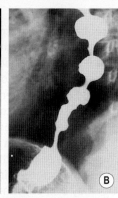

Tertiary contractions of the oesophagus seen as (A) a rippling of the oesophageal wall or (B) a series of indentations resembling a corkscrew (hence the description 'corkscrew oesophagus').†

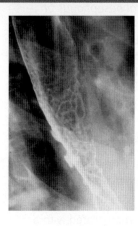

Scleroderma. Incompetence of the gastro-oesophageal sphincter resulting in severe reflux oesophagitis with stricturing, oedematous mucosa (mosaic pattern) and deep ulceration.†

Differentiating scleroderma from achalasia		
	Scleroderma	**Achalasia**
Oesophageal dilatation	Mild	Significant
GOJ	Wide and patulous	Characteristic 'rat's tail' or 'bird's beak' appearance
Complications	Reflux ± late stricture formation ± Barrett's oesophagus	Aspiration

Oesophageal diverticula

Pulsion diverticulum This results from high intraluminal pressures acting on a potential oesophageal wall weakness

- **Zenker's diverticulum (pharyngeal pouch):** a false diverticulum originating within the posterior midline of the hypopharynx and above cricopharyngeus (Killian's dehiscence) ▶ it presents with dysphagia, retention of food debris within the diverticulum, halitosis and possibly a neck mass
  - *Complications:* ulceration ▶ aspiration pneumonia ▶ carcinoma
- **Killian–Jamieson diverticulum:** this is located off the midline and below cricopharyngeus (arising from the lateral cervical oesophageal wall) ▶ it is smaller and less symptomatic than a Zenker's diverticulum
- **Epiphrenic diverticulum:** this is located within the distal oesophagus and is the result of oesophageal contractions against a closed lower oesophageal sphincter
- **Intramural pseudodiverticulosis:** the dilated mucous glands within the oesophageal wall can simulate true diverticula on contrast studies

Traction diverticulum These result from an adjacent external inflammatory process generating pulling forces on the oesophageal wall (e.g. inflamed adjacent lymph nodes)

Varices

Definition Dilated oesophageal submucosal veins act as a collateral venous drainage pathway in the presence of an obstruction elsewhere ▶ it is very rarely idiopathic

- **Uphill varices:** these affect the lower oesophagus ▶ they are caused by cirrhosis of the liver – portal blood flow is rerouted (via the oesophagus) to the SVC
- **Downhill varices:** these affect the upper ⅔ of the oesophagus ▶ SVC obstruction causes blood to be rerouted from the head and neck (via the oesophagus) into the azygos vein ▶ if the azygos vein is also blocked then downhill varices may also be found within the lower oesophagus (taking blood to the coronary and portal vein)

Barium swallow Characteristic serpiginous filling defects best appreciated on the prone swallow examination (after administration of an IV anti-peristaltic agent)

CT Enhancing vascular venous structures around the oesophagus

Oesophageal webs

Definition These are common shelf-like (1–2 mm thick) mucosal infoldings protruding into the oesophageal lumen ▶ they can be semicircular or form a complete ring ▶ they are usually found at the anterior aspect of the proximal cervical oesophagus

- They are usually asymptomatic but may cause dysphagia

Barium swallow A thin transverse filling defect (which may be circumferential)

Pearl As well as being spontaneous, they can be associated with: pemphigoid ▶ epidermolysis bullosa ▶ graft-versus-host disease ▶ reflux oesophagitis (a web within the distal oesophagus) ▶ Plummer–Vinson syndrome (a web + iron deficiency anaemia + dysphagia)

Extrinsic lesions

- **Thyroid masses**
- **Lymph node masses:** these are usually secondary to a bronchial carcinoma or lymphoma, affecting both the superior and mid-oesophagus
- **Fibrotic changes at the lung apices:** these can pull the oesophagus sideways, which may then form an acute angle within the superior mediastinum
- **Carcinoma of the bronchus**
- **Vascular causes**
  - *Aberrant right subclavian artery:* this gives rise to the classic appearance of a posterior impression on the proximal oesophagus or a band-like impression as the vessel ascends posterior to the oesophagus (AP view) ▶ dysphagia lusoria
  - *A right-sided aortic arch:* an impression on the right side of the oesophagus
  - *Descending thoracic aortic aneurysm:* the aorta may erode into the oesophagus with catastrophic haematemesis
  - *An enlarged left atrium:* this displaces the distal ⅓ of the oesophagus
- **Cricopharyngeal spasm**
  - The cricopharyngeus normally relaxes during swallowing – if it remains contracted it forms a smooth posterior impression at the pharyngo-oesophageal junction (C5/6 level) ▶ this may cause dsyphagia and lead to a Zenker's diverticulum

Trauma

Definition This is usually iatrogenic and commonly due to an oesophageal perforation following an endoscopy (due to an unsuspected pharyngeal pouch) ▶ other causes:

- *An ingested foreign body:* this can also cause an intramural haematoma or an oesophageal dissection
- *Severe vomiting affecting the distal oesophagus or proximal stomach:*
  - *Mallory–Weiss tear:* a mucosal tear where the wall integrity is maintained (with no pneumomediastinum)
  - *Boerhaave's syndrome:* a full-thickness tear (usually on the left posterolateral side) presenting with severe chest and epigastric pain ▶ immediate surgery is required

Radiological features of a full-thickness tear

CXR Surgical emphysema within the neck ▶ pneumomediastinum ▶ a left pleural effusion

CT This can detect free gas adjacent to the oesophagus

Contrast swallow A leak is best demonstrated with a decubitus film (a horizontal X-ray beam)

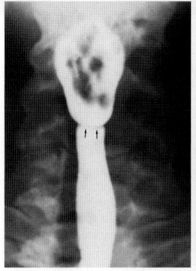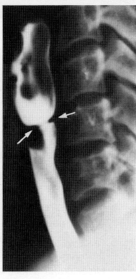

A concentric upper oesophageal web seen in both the frontal and lateral projections (arrows). The way in which the web narrows the lumen is well seen in the lateral view.[†]

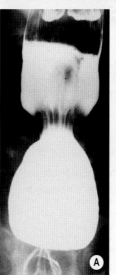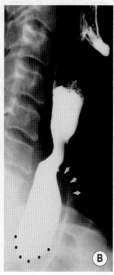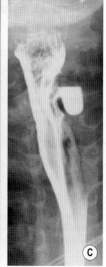

Zenker's pharyngeal diverticulum. (A) Frontal view. (B) Lateral view. Barium fills the diverticulum and then spills over into the anteriorly displaced oesophagus (arrows). (C) Lateral cervical oesophageal diverticulum (Killian–Jamieson diverticulum).[†]

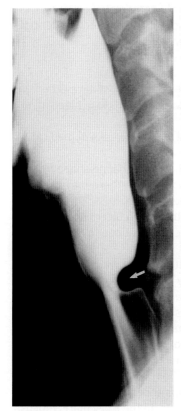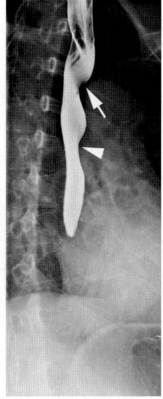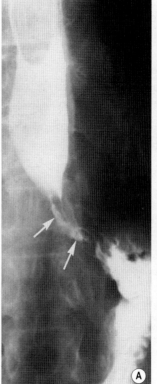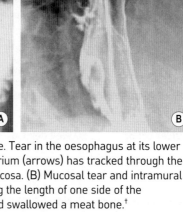

Barium swallow showing the cervical oesophagus. Lateral view. The posterior impression (arrow) is produced by failure of the cricopharyngeus muscle to relax.[†]

Single-contrast barium swallow image of a patient with dysphagia lusoria. Note the normal impression made by the left main bronchus (arrowhead), and the deeper oblique impression superior to this (arrow) made by the aberrant right subclavian artery.** (Image courtesy of Dr A Husainy, Leeds Teaching Hospitals.)

(A) Mallory–Weiss syndrome. Tear in the oesophagus at its lower end caused by vomiting. Barium (arrows) has tracked through the defect to lie beneath the mucosa. (B) Mucosal tear and intramural haematoma spreading along the length of one side of the oesophagus. The patient had swallowed a meat bone.[†]

BENIGN GASTRIC ULCERS

Definition

- Gastric ulcers penetrate the stomach wall through the mucosa and into the submucosa (and frequently also into the muscularis propria) ▶ 95% are benign and they can also be multiple

CAUSES

- *Helicobacter pylori* infection (70%) ▶ NSAIDs ▶ alcohol abuse ▶ steroid use ▶ emotional stress ▶ smoking ▶ hereditary factors

Radiological features

Location Distal stomach > proximal stomach ▶ lesser > greater curvature ▶ posterior wall > anterior wall ▶ benign ulcers are rarely seen within the fundus and along proximal half of the greater curvature ▶ ulcers here should always be suspicious for malignancy

- *Ulcers due to NSAIDs /alcohol:* these often affect the distal greater curvature (particularly the antrum) ▶ they are often multiple
- *Ulcers in the elderly:* these are more evenly distributed throughout the stomach (particularly affecting the proximal lesser curve)

Double-contrast barium studies (en face)

- The primary sign is a collection of barium on the dependent wall ▶ benign ulcers are usually round, oval or linear in shape ▶ a ring shadow may be seen if the ulcer is located on a non-dependent surface (as barium coats the edge of the ulcer crater)
- A smooth mound of surrounding oedema is seen as a circular filling defect ▶ the presence of normal areae gastricae extending to the ulcer crater is a good sign of a benign lesion

Double-contrast barium studies (in profile)

- A benign ulcer will project beyond the stomach lumen
  - *Hampton's line:* a thin lucent line crossing the ulcer base (representing preserved gastric mucosa with undermining of the more vulnerable submucosa) ▶ although rarely seen, this is virtually diagnostic of a benign ulcer
  - *Ulcer collar:* more commonly there is a thicker smooth rim of lucency at the ulcer base
  - *Ulcer mound:* with increasing oedema a symmetrical gently sloping mass can be seen
- Virtual CT gastroscopy: smooth, regular, round or oval shape ▶ even base ▶ sharply demarcated or round edges ▶ converging gastric folds with smooth tapering + radiation ▶ no excessive enhancement

Pearls

- **'Giant' ulcers (>3 cm):** these are almost always benign but have a higher rate of complications (e.g. bleeding or perforation)
- **Healing ulcers:** >95% heal within 8 weeks of medical treatment
  - As benign ulcers heal they may change shape from round or oval to linear crevices ▶ there may be a residual central pit or depression
  - Radiating folds seen with healing ulcers should be smooth, thin, symmetric and continue to the edge of the crater
  - There may be subtle retraction or wall stiffening ▶ a healed antral ulcer may form prominent transverse folds or significant antral narrowing with the deformity leading to obstruction
- **Features suspicious for malignancy:** location within the fundus or proximal ½ of the greater curvature ▶ incomplete healing ▶ irregularity of the radiating folds ▶ a residual mass ▶ loss of the mucosal pattern
- **Gastric erosions (aphthous ulcer):** these are shallow ulcerations that do not penetrate the muscularis mucosa ▶ they are usually seen with *H. pylori* infection, alcohol and NSAID ingestion, stress (e.g. severe trauma), or Crohn's disease ▶ they heal without scarring

Double-contrast barium studies 1–2 mm shallow collections of barium ▶ short linear or serpentine lines or dots of barium

  - *'Complete' (varioloform) erosions:* a complete radiolucent rim of surrounding oedema is present
  - *'Incomplete' erosions:* the oedema halo is lacking

Benign vs malignant ulceration**		
	Benign	**Malignant**
Location	Usually the antrum (75% on the lesser curve)	Usually the antrum (but can occur anywhere)
Size	5–10 mm, >3 cm	>10 mm, <3 cm
Fold convergence	To the crater edge	Stops short of the crater edge
Fold shape	Normal or uniformly swollen	Amputated, fused or clubbed folds
Projection beyond gastric wall	Yes	No
Ulcer collar	Well defined	If present, it is irregular
Multiplicity	Common	Uncommon
Carman meniscus sign	No	Yes
Hampton's line	Yes	No
Response to therapy	Yes	No

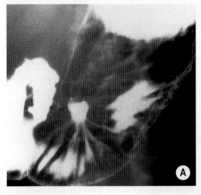
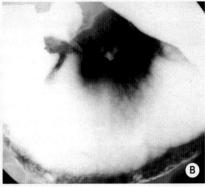

En face appearance of benign gastric ulcer. (A) The posterior wall ulcer is nearly filled with barium in this RPO projection. Thin regular radiating folds (best seen around the inferior border of the ulcer) are seen converging to the ulcer. (B) Unfilled benign ulcer crater is outlined by a 'ring' shadow. This ulcer is surrounded by a prominent ring of oedema – the lucent area around the crater.*

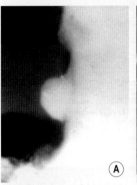
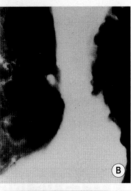
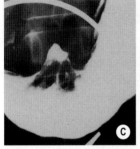
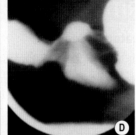

Profile views of benign gastric ulcer. (A) Hampton's line, a thin line of radiolucency crossing the opening of an ulcer, a virtually infallible sign of a benign ulcer. (B) Lesser curvature ulcer with a clearly visible ulcer collar. (C) Large lesser curvature ulcer niche, its projection from the lumen of the stomach strongly suggesting a benign lesion. (D) Smooth, straight radiating folds converge at the ulcer crater.*

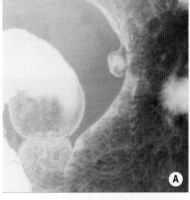
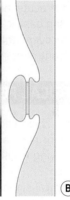

Benign gastric ulcer. (A) Mid lesser curvature ulcer in profile. The ulcer crater projects outside the wall of the stomach. (B) Diagram of a benign ulcer with an oedematous collar. Beneath the collar, a thin lucent line (Hampton's line) may be seen across the mouth of the ulcer.†

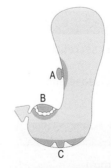

Graphical description of three types of gastric ulcer (the shading represents barium): A = benign, projecting, lesser curvature ulcer with collar (broken lines = Hampton's line) ▶ B = malignant, intraluminal ulcer with irregular nodular tumour rim which traps a lenticular barium collection that is convex relative to the gastric lumen (Carman meniscus sign) ▶ C = non-projecting benign greater curvature ulcer.†

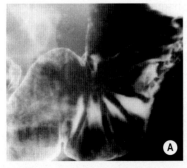
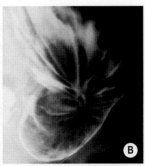
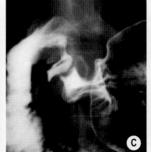
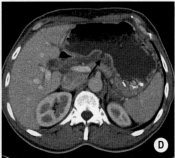

Healing gastric ulcer. (A) Focal retraction along the incisura angularis with small residual outpouching is present. Converging smooth folds no longer fill an ulcer crater. (B) Radiating folds converging to a linear scar. (C) Scarred antrum with constriction at site of previous ulcer causing narrowing and deformity. (D) Axial CT image showing benign ulcer (arrow) along the lesser curvature with a crater and surrounding smooth mound.**

GASTRITIS DUE TO *HELICOBACTER PYLORI* INFECTION

DEFINITION

- *H. pylori* is a Gram-negative, flagellated, spiral bacterium ▶ it is more prevalent in developing countries, tending to affect the lower socioeconomic groups
- The gastric cancer risk is 6 times higher in patients with *H. pylori* infection ▶ associated with MALT lymphoma of the stomach

Pathophysiology The enzyme urease converts urea into ammonia and bicarbonate – the resultant alkaline 'microenvironment' protects the bacterium from the effects of gastric acid ▶ acute infection initially injures the parietal cells (decreasing gastric acid production) – once parietal cell function recovers, the resultant abnormally high acid output causes antral gastritis and duodenitis

RADIOLOGICAL FEATURES

Barium meal There can be diffuse or focal changes including: thick or nodular gastric folds ▶ erosions ▶ ulcers ▶ antral narrowing ▶ inflammatory polyps ▶ prominent areae gastricae
- The radiological signs are non-specific – similar appearances can be seen with gastritis due to NSAID and alcohol ingestion

HYPERTROPHIC GASTRITIS

DEFINITION

- Glandular hyperplasia and increased acid secretion (inflammation is not prominent)
  - The differential includes Ménétrier's disease and lymphoma

RADIOLOGICAL FEATURES

Barium meal Thickened folds (often >10 mm) predominantly located within the fundus and body of the stomach (the acid-producing regions) ▶ prominent areae gastricae – these can be up to 4–5 mm in size and more angular and polygonal than their usual round or oval configuration
- There is a high prevalence of duodenal and gastric ulcers

ATROPHIC GASTRITIS

DEFINITION

- Atrophy of the gastric glands with associated histological inflammatory changes ▶ it is associated with pernicious anaemia and is more common with advancing age
  - *Pernicious anaemia:* this is caused by decreased intrinsic factor and vitamin B_{12} production (characterized by parietal and chief cell loss leading to achlorhydria and atrophy of the mucosa and mucosal glands)
    - 90% of patients will also have atrophic gastritis
    - There is also an association with gastric polyps, carcinoma, benign and malignant ulcers
- It is also associated with intestinal metaplasia (which is a premalignant condition) – radiographically this is suggested by enlargement of the areae gastricae

RADIOLOGICAL FEATURES

Barium meal A loss of the rugal folds (± the areae gastricae) ▶ a tubular and featureless narrowed stomach

OTHER TYPES OF INFECTIOUS GASTRITIS

Granulomatous infections

- Including tuberculosis, histoplasmosis and syphilis

Barium meal Ulceration ▶ thick folds ▶ mucosal nodularity ▶ antral narrowing is a late finding

Moniliasis

- This is usually associated with severe oesophageal disease

Barium meal Prominent aphthous ulcers

Immunocompromised patients

- Infection with cytomegalovirus (CMV), toxoplasmosis or cryptosporidiosis
  - Cryptosporidiosis primarily affects the small bowel rather than the oesophagus ▶ it causes severe diarrhoea with thickened small bowel folds

Barium meal Deep ulceration and fistulization (CMV) ▶ antral narrowing and rigidity (cryptosporidiosis)

Strongyloides

- A parasitic infection affecting the upper gastrointestinal tract, duodenum and proximal small bowel

Barium meal Advanced cases will cause thickened effaced folds with associated narrowing

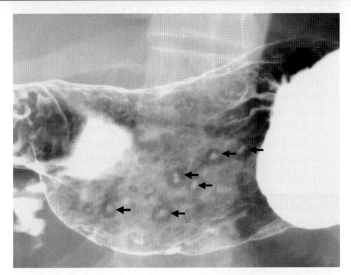

Acute erosive gastritis. There are numerous erosions in the stomach (arrows). Each erosion consists of a small central collection of barium surrounded by a translucent ring (a small 'target' lesion).[†]

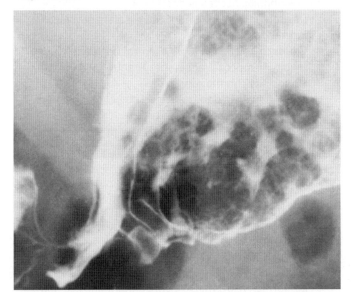

Severe antral gastritis. Conical narrowing of the antrum with multiple thickened gastric folds.[†]

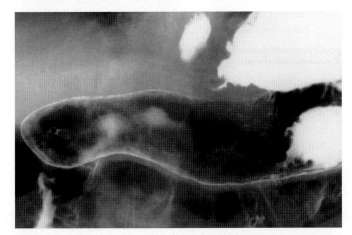

Atrophic gastritis. Featureless narrowed stomach. Note pyloric channel seen 'end on'.*

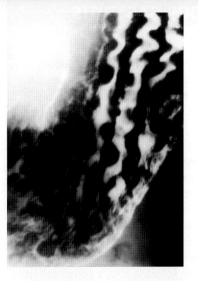

Diffuse erosive gastritis with thick nodular folds. Erosions are scattered along the folds.*

Prevalence of *Helicobacter pylori* infection with upper GI disease*	
Disease	**Prevalence (%)**
Active chronic gastritis	100
Duodenal ulcer	95
Gastric cancer (body or antrum)	80–95
MALT lymphoma	90
Gastric ulcer	60–80
Non-ulcer dyspepsia	35–60
Asymptomatic population	20–55

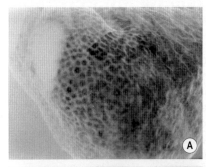

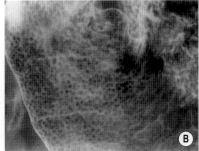

H. pylori gastritis with lymphoid hyperplasia. (A) and (B). In both patients, enlarged lymphoid follicles are seen as innumerable tiny, round nodules that carpet the mucosa of the gastric antrum. In (A) note how many of the nodules have central umbilications with punctate collections of barium seen en face in the lesions.©20

255

GRANULOMATOUS GASTRITIS

Definition

- Granulomatous inflammation of the gastric mucosa can be secondary to: Crohn's disease ▶ sarcoidosis ▶ tuberculosis ▶ syphilis ▶ fungal disease

Pearl
Crohn's disease

- Gastroduodenal involvement is seen in up to 20% of patients (usually with an associated ileocolitis) ▶ if the upper GI tract is involved both the stomach and duodenum are usually involved (isolated duodenal involvement is more common than isolated stomach involvement) ▶ the radiographic findings of gastric disease usually always involve the stomach antrum and body ▶ a gastrocolic fistula is a rare complication (usually involving the transverse colon)
  - *Early (non-stenotic) phase:* aphthous ulcers ▶ larger discrete ulcers ▶ thickened and distorted folds ▶ a nodular 'cobble-stoned' mucosa
    - These features are indistinguishable from aphthous ulcers or erosions due to other causes
  - *Late (stenotic) phase:* a 'rams-horn' or 'pseudo post-Bilroth I' appearance: this is caused by scarring and fibrosis of the gastric antrum and pylorus – it can foreshorten the stomach enough to simulate a partial gastrectomy
    - This appearance can also be seen with other granulomatous disorders such as tuberculosis, syphilis, sarcoid and eosinophilic gastroenteritits
    - The antral narrowing can also mimic a scirrhous gastric carcinoma

ZOLLINGER–ELLISON SYNDROME

Definition

- A gastrin-secreting gastrinoma (a non-beta islet cell tumour) stimulates excessive gastric acid secretion ▶ this leads to prominent ulcer formation, often in locations distal to the normal ulcer distribution
  - *Ulcer location:* duodenal bulb > stomach > post-bulbar duodenum
  - *Gastrinoma location:* pancreas (75%) ▶ duodenum (15%)
  - *Gastrinoma metastases:* these are primarily to the liver (up to 50% of tumours are malignant)
  - 10% of tumours are associated with the type 1 multiple endocrine neoplasia (with associated parathyroid, pituitary and adrenal tumours)

Radiological features

Barium meal Thickened gastric and duodenal folds ▶ single or multiple ulcers (10%) ▶ reflux oesophagitis

EOSINOPHILIC GASTRITIS

Definition

- This follows a focal or diffuse infiltration of the GI tract with eosinophils ▶ it is associated with atopy, asthma and often a peripheral eosinophilia (there is possibly an atopic aetiology)
  - Any segment of the GI tract can be affected ▶ however, it commonly involves the stomach (particularly the antrum) and the proximal small bowel

Clinical presentation

- Crampy abdominal pains ▶ diarrhoea ▶ distension and vomiting

Radiological features

- These will depend upon which layers of the GI tract are affected (involvement may be predominantly mucosal, muscular or serosal) ▶ if the disease is panmural then an eosinophilic ascites is often seen
  - *Oesophagus:* involvement can result in stricture formation
  - *Stomach:* thickened folds ▶ antral narrowing and rigidity ▶ mucosal nodularity ▶ antral and pyloric stenosis is common
  - *Small bowel:* fold thickening ▶ bowel stenosis

CORROSIVE GASTRITIS

Definition

- Inflammation of the gastric mucosa due to acid or alkali ingestion ▶ acids are more injurious (the already acidic gastric contents have no residual ability to neutralize strong acids)
  - *Initially:* there is necrosis with sloughing of the mucosal and submucosal layers
  - *Moderate cases:* there is subsequent fibrosis and stricture formation – the resultant contracted (± obstructed) stomach may require a gastrectomy
  - *Severe cases:* there can be subsequent full-thickness necrosis with perforation

Radiological features

Barium meal A swollen, irregular gastric mucosa (occasionally with visible blebs)
- As this sloughs barium can flow beneath it (the mucosa is then seen as a thin radiolucent line paralleling the outline of the stomach)
- After a few weeks fibrotic contraction of the stomach can occur – this can be severe enough that the stomach lumen is no larger than the duodenal bulb

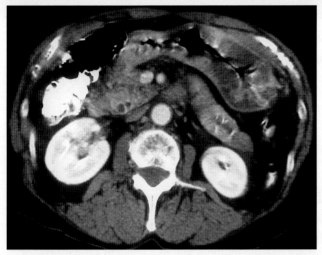

CT shows diffuse thickening of the gastric wall in a patient proven to have eosinophilic gastroenteritis. No ascites was present. Symptoms resolved with steroid therapy.*

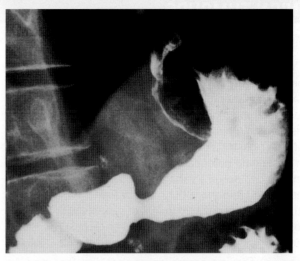

Corrosive gastritis following the ingestion of household bleach. The distal stomach has undergone considerable scarring and contraction in a manner similar to syphilitic gastritis or linitis plastica.*

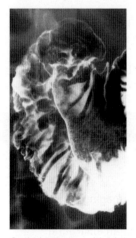

Crohn's disease. Multiple aphthous erosions are present on the antrum. Duodenal folds are thick and nodular.*

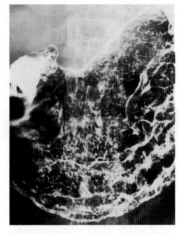

Hypertrophic gastritis in a patient with a recently healed lesser curvature gastric ulcer. This characteristic enlargement and prominence of the areae gastricae can be correlated with an increased incidence of gastric hypersecretion and peptic ulcer disease (PUD).*

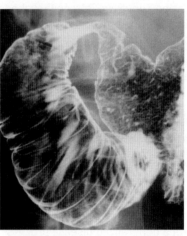

Crohn's disease. Antral erosions and a tapered stricture involving the first part of the duodenum. The second part of the duodenum is dilated as a result of a further stricture of the third part.†

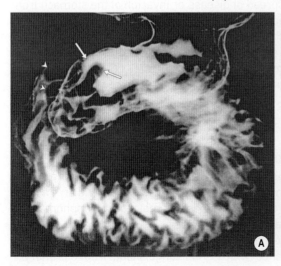

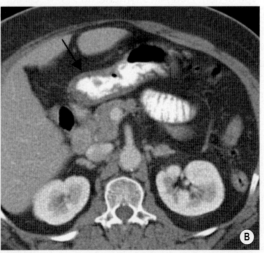

(A) Prominent thickened antral folds in a patient with antral gastritis. (B) Axial CT in this patient shows thickened antral wall (arrow) secondary to inflammation.••

BENIGN TUMOURS

Definition

Mucosal polyps

Hyperplastic polyps The commonest benign gastric neoplasm (accounting for 80% of all polyps) ▶ with a low premalignant potential but they do occur more commonly in patients with other risk factors for gastric malignancy (e.g. atrophic gastritis or bile reflux gastritis) ▶ excised if >2 cm (malignant potential)

- *Fundic gland polyp:* a variant representing a hyperplastic fundal gland (therefore they are not found in the antrum) ▶ they can be seen in up to 40% of patients with familial adenomatous polyposis coli (FAPC) or chronic PPI therapy ▶ usually <0.5 cm, multiple and sessile

Adenomas This is a premalignant neoplasm that may develop into a gastric carcinoma (malignancy is detected histologically in 50% of adenomas that are >2 cm) ▶ it is also often found in FAPC (along with hypertrophic polyps) ▶ redefined as non-invasive intraepithelial neoplasia (NiN) ▶ solitary, sessile or pedunculated ▶ common in antrum

Hamartomas/inflammatory polyps Along with hyperplastic polyps, these are found in various polyposis syndromes (e.g. Peutz–Jeghers, Cronkhite–Canada and Cowden's disease)

Submucosal lesions

Gastrointestinal stromal tumour (GIST)

- A benign mesenchymal tumour arising within the submucosa (and previously designated as a leiomyoma, leiomyoblastoma or leiomyosarcoma)
- 70% of GISTs occur within the stomach, accounting for 1–3% of all gastric malignancies ▶ 70–90% of GISTs are benign
- See Section 3 Chapter 4, Small bowel

Radiological features

Barium meal

Hyperplastic polyps A round, smooth sessile lesion ▶ they are usually multiple and of a uniform similar size (5–10 mm) ▶ they are commonly found within the fundus or body of the stomach

- They can rarely present as an isolated large, irregular lesion

Adenoma A polypoid sessile or pedunculated lesion ▶ they are usually solitary and >1 cm in size ▶ they are commonly found within the antrum

- Villous adenomas can have frond-like projections and are associated with a very high risk of malignancy

MALIGNANT TUMOURS

Definition

Histological types

Lymphoma Lymphoma is usually due to primary disease, as a result of direct extension from adjacent lymph nodes, or as part of a generalized disease process

- The GI tract is the commonest site of primary extra-nodal lymphoma, with the stomach the most frequent site of a GI lymphoma (accounting for 3% of all gastric malignancies) ▶ most lymphomas involving the stomach are of the non-Hodgkin's type
  - *MALT lymphoma:* a type of non-Hodgkin's lymphoma occurring within the stomach (its commonest location), lung, thyroid, salivary glands and intestine ▶ it usually arises within the mucosa-associated lymphoid tissue which has been acquired in response to a *H. pylori* infection (there is normally no lymphoid tissue present within the gastric mucosa)
  - *Hodgkin's type:* this mimics a scirrhous carcinoma (with a strong associated desmoplastic reaction)

GIST Suspect malignancy if it is >5 cm in size ▶ see Section 3 Chapter 4, Small bowel

Metastases The most common primary tumours to metastasize to the stomach are breast, malignant melanoma and lung

- There can also be contiguous spread from the colon (via the gastrocolic and gastrosplenic ligaments), the liver (via the gastrohepatic ligament) or the pancreas (direct spread)

Radiological features

Lymphoma

Barium meal/CT There is no typical imaging appearance and it may mimic the appearances of any gastric carcinoma

- The most common appearance is of an infiltrating lesion extending over a large area of the stomach with diffuse gastric fold thickening (± ulceration) ▶ it may also appear as a bulky polypoid mass or a malignant ulcer
- Lymphoma is more likely to spread across the pylorus and into the duodenum than is a gastric carcinoma
- Direct spread of disease or invasion of the stomach from enlarged regional lymph nodes may be a helpful sign
- Stomach remains pliable, and the lumen is preserved, even in severe lymphoma (gastric outlet obstruction is uncommon)
- NHL can however cause linitis plastica

FDG-PET Evaluation of gastric lymphoma can be challenging (variable uptake) ▶ can help evaluate treatment response

Haematogenous metastases

Barium meal Initially there will be small intramural masses (these may have central ulceration and are most frequently seen with metastatic melanoma, lymphoma and Kaposi's sarcoma)

- Breast carcinoma may produce a linitis plastic type appearance (which is indistinguishable from a primary gastric carcinoma)

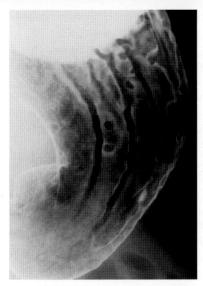

Hyperplastic polyps in the body of the stomach – small, sessile and uniform in size.*

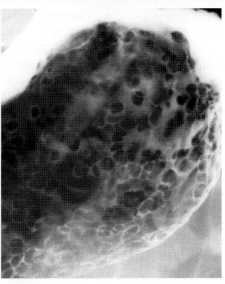

Fundic gland polyps morphologically identical to hyperplastic polyps predominate in the fundus as shown in this image. This is a patient with familial adenomatosis coli.*

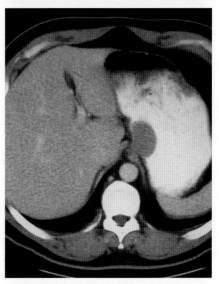

Leiomyoma adjacent to the gastro-oesophageal junction shown on CT as a smooth soft tissue mass in the contrast-filled stomach.*

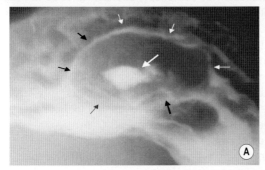

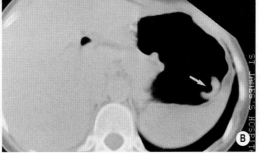

Gastric 'target' lesion. (A) An ulcerating (large arrow) tumour in the gastric fundus (small arrows). This appearance is typical of an ulcerating submucosal metastasis from a malignant melanoma. (B) CT shows the same tumour (arrow).†

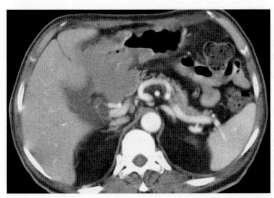

Gastric lymphoma. CECT. Note the marked thickening of the gastric antrum.*

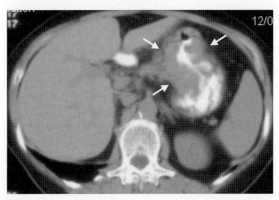

MALT lymphoma. Multifocal tumour (arrows) thickening the gastric wall.†

GASTRIC CARCINOMA

Definition A malignant tumour arising from the gastric mucosa (it is an adenocarcinoma in 95% of cases, the remainder are lymphoma/GIST/NET)

- *Japan:* this has the highest prevalence (dietary)
- *Western countries:* it is usually detected at an advanced stage (due to its non-specific symptoms)
- The disease results from a progression through chronic inflammation (gastritis), to intestinal metaplasia and then carcinoma
  - There is a demonstrable link between *H. pylori* colonization and a *distal* gastric carcinoma
  - The incidence of gastric cardia tumours has increased – the incidence elsewhere has decreased or remained stable
- **Other risk factors:** diet ▶ familial factors ▶ smoking ▶ chronic atrophic gastritis ▶ pernicious anaemia ▶ Ménétrier's disease ▶ a low socioeconomic status ▶ obesity ▶ a Billroth partial gastrectomy ▶ gastric polyps
  - *Gastric polyps:* adenomas have the highest malignant potential (40%) ▶ hyperplastic and hamartomatous polyps have a low malignant potential
- **Histological types:**
  - *Diffuse type (40%):* the undifferentiated form ▶ signet ring cells are present ▶ there is a worse prognosis and greater dissemination
  - *Intestinal type (60%):* the differentiated form (tubular or papillary glands are present)

Radiological features

Barium meal
- **Early gastric carcinoma** (confined to the gastric mucosa and submucosa without muscle layer invasion)
  - A polypoid, superficial or excavated tumour (which is frequently irregular) ▶ converging folds (which are often thickened, irregular or nodular) ▶ nodularity is frequently seen around the central portion of a lesion

Ulcers*		
Findings	**Benign**	**Malignant**
Hampton's line	Present	Absent
Extends beyond the gastric wall	Yes	No
Folds	Smooth, even	Irregular, nodular, may fuse
Associated mass	Absent	Present
Carman meniscus	Absent	Present
Ulcer shape	Round, oval, linear	Irregular
Healing	Heals completely	Rarely heals

- **'Carmen meniscus' sign**: A large flat ulcer with heaped up edges – the edges of the ulcer trap a lenticular barium collection that is convex relative to the lumen
- **Advanced gastric carcinoma** (involving muscularis propria with outward spread)
  - A large irregular mass (± ulceration) ▶ an irregular mucosal surface ▶ the mass margin may exhibit a shelf (forming an acute angle with the gastric wall)
  - Antral involvement can lead to narrowing and obstruction
  - *A 'malignant ulcer':* this indicates an ulcer within a gastric mass
  - *Linitis plastica:* diffuse stomach infiltration with tumour and fibrosis, resulting in a narrowed rigid stomach ('leather bottle' stomach)

CT This requires good distension with water
- **Abnormal signs:** focal wall thickening (± ulceration) ▶ a focal mass or diffuse wall thickening ▶ T1 lesion: focal thickening of inner layer ▶ enhancing ▶ visible low attenuation outer layer ▶ clear perigastric fat plane
  - A wall thickness >1 cm is considered abnormal in a well-distended stomach (except at the GOJ where the transverse imaging plane complicates assessment)
  - There may be abnormal contrast enhancement of the gastric wall or loss of the normal multilayered wall pattern
  - Linitis plastica may complicate assessment due to the associated difficulties with gastric distension
  - Serosal involvement is indicated by an irregular border to the external gastric wall (± perigastric fat stranding)
- Virtual CT gastroscopy: irregular/angulated shape ▶ uneven base ▶ asymmetric edge ▶ bulbous enlargement ▶ fusion/disruption of gastric folds towards crater edge
- **Metastatic spread**
  - *Direct invasion:* involving the pancreas, left liver lobe, spleen or transverse colon
  - *Haematogenous spread to the liver:* this is seen with 25% of cases at presentation
  - *Intraperitoneal seeding:* to the rectosigmoid colon, caecum and small bowel ▶ ascites can also be present
  - *Kruckenberg tumours:* bilateral drop metastases to the ovaries (especially with the signet ring cell tumour type)

EUS This is able to resolve the individual layers of the gastric wall, allowing the determination of the T staging (more accurately than with CT)
  - Carcinoma appears as a hypoechoic lesion with irregular margins
- *Nodes:* it can assess the perigastric nodes only (due to its limited depth of view of approximately 6 cm) ▶ it will allow FNA biopsy of any affected nodes

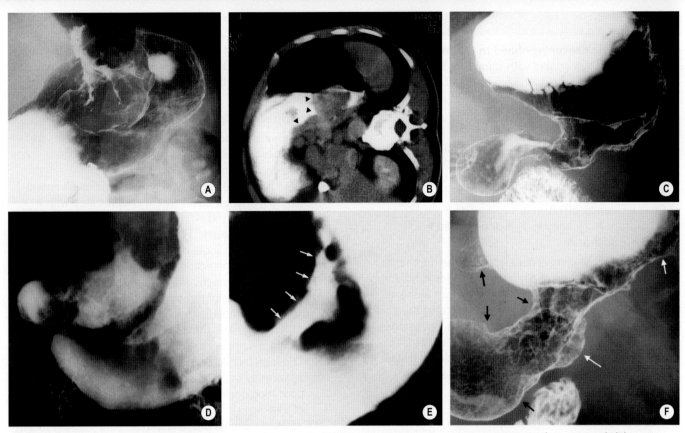

Advanced gastric cancer. (A) Large polypoid mass of the cardia. (B) Polypoid mass of the cardia shown on CT (arrowheads). (C) Large circumferential mass in the body of the stomach with a shelf at the proximal margin sharply demarcating the cancer from the proximal stomach. (D) Large ulcerated mass in the antrum. This is often referred to as a 'Carman' ulcer. (E) Malignant gastric ulcer. Single contrast examination. The ulcer is situated close to the lesser curvature and near the incisura. The arrows indicate the base of the ulcer, which is in line with the lesser curvature, i.e. the crater is non-projecting. Tumour at the margin of the crater appears translucent and nodular, creating a pool of barium, convex one side and concave the other (arrows) ('meniscus' sign). (F) Infiltrating and ulcerative gastric carcinoma. The proximal half of the stomach is involved with thickening of the wall, destruction of mucosa and narrowing of the lumen (black arrows). Ulceration is present on the greater curve (white arrows).*

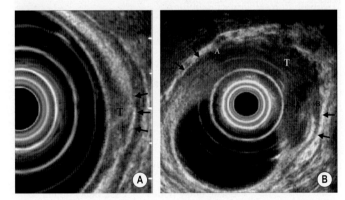

Gastric carcinoma. (A) T1 stage. The echogenic submucosal layer has not been breached (black arrows) by the tumour (T). (B) Tumour stage T3. Tumour (T) has breached muscularis propria between points A and B. Intact muscularis propria can be seen at the margins of the tumour (black arrows).†

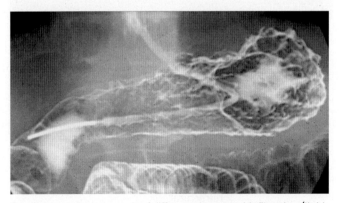

Small stomach as a result of diffuse submucosal infiltration (linitis plastica).

GASTRIC CARCINOMA

PEARLS

- **Early gastric cancer (confined to the mucosa or submucosa)**: associated with significant lymph node involvement at presentation (up to 15% of cases) ▶ the degree of lymph node involvement increases with the depth of submucosal invasion
- Japanese classification:
  - *Type I polypoid*: >5 mm protruding into lumen
  - *Type II superficial*: IIa elevated (<5 mm) ▶ IIb flat ▶ IIc depressed
  - *Type III*: excavated
- Peak incidence: 50-70 years
- ⅓ antrum ▶ ⅓ body ▶ ⅓ fundus/cardia ▶ 10% diffusely infiltrative

Lymph nodes   Staging is dependent on the number rather than the location of any involved nodes ▶ a node is considered abnormal if it measures ≥8 mm along its short-axis diameter (the usual issues regarding the ability to differentiate between enlarged benign reactive nodes and non-enlarged metastatic nodes of course remain):

- Compartment III and IV nodes are considered distant metastases (except for the splenic arterial nodes)
- **Surgical dissection:**
  - *D1 lymphadenectomy*: compartment I
  - *D2 lymphadenectomy*: compartments I–II
    - A D2 resection confers improved survival over a D1 resection (but with an increased morbidity)
  - *D3 lymphadenectomy*: compartments I–III
  - *D4 lymphadenectomy*: compartments I–IV

Staging   Preoperative tumour staging is usually by CT, and occasionally by EUS for evaluating the depth of any gastric wall invasion ▶ the role of FDG PET in locoregional staging is limited at present as mucinous, signet ring and poorly differentiated adenocarcinomas are not FDG avid ▶ often intense FDG uptake in normal stomach ▶ spatial resolution can limit differentiation of primary mass from adjacent nodes

Treatment and prognosis

- Two important factors influence the survival rates for resectable gastric cancer:
  - The depth of invasion
  - Whether there is regional lymph node involvement (compartment II involvement is associated with a worse prognosis)
- **Resectable tumours:** T1, T2 or T3 tumours (without metastases) ▶ a single resectable liver metastasis may permit possible resection
- **Treatment approach:** gastrectomy (total or subtotal depending on site of tumour) ± lymphadenectomy (limited or extended) ± neoadjuvant chemotherapy
  - Although gastric tumours are chemosensitive there is a minimal impact on long-term survival rates
  - The high incidence of local recurrence, even after apparently complete resection, contributes to the poor long-term prognosis (with a 5-year survival rate of 5%)
  - >50% of patients present with an unresectable locally advanced tumour or metastatic disease ▶ options then include palliative surgery (± chemotherapy)

Nodal locations	
Compartment I (perigastric)	Pericardial (left or right) ▶ lesser or greater curvature ▶ supra- or infrapyloric
Compartment II	Left gastric ▶ common hepatic, coeliac or splenic arterial ▶ splenic hilum
Compartment III	Hepatoduodenal ligament ▶ posterior to the pancreatic head ▶ mesenteric root ▶ splenic artery (if the tumour is within the lower ⅓ of the stomach)
Compartment IV	Middle colic vessels ▶ para-aortic ▶ retrocrural

Lymphoma vs gastric carcinoma	Lymphoma	Gastric carcinoma
Wall thickening	Very thick	Less thick
Perigastric fat planes	Usually preserved	May be obliterated
Regional adenopathy	Common	Common
Extent of adenopathy	May extend below renal vein Large bulky nodes	Does not extend below renal vein Less bulky nodes
Extent	May involve duodenum	Does not commonly involve duodenum

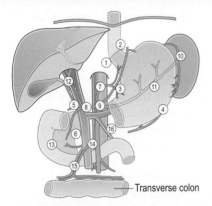

Drawing illustrates lymph node locations according to the Japanese Research Society for Gastric Cancer, *1* = right paracardium, 2 = left paracardium, 3 = lesser curvature, 4 = greater curvature, 5 = supraylorum, 6 = infrapylorum, 7 = left gastric artery, 8 = common hepatic artery, 9 = coeliac artery, 10 = splenic hilum, 11 = proximal splenic artery, 12 = hepatoduodenal ligament, 13 = posterior surface of the pancreatic head, 14 = superior mesenteric vessels (SMA = superior mesenteric artery, SMV = superior mesenteric vein), 15 = middle colic vessels, 16 = abdominal aorta (modified from RadioGraphics 2006 ▶ 26:143–156).

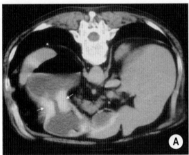
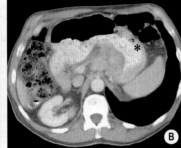
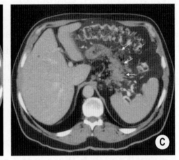

(A) Gastric carcinoma constricting the stomach body (arrows). Stomach distended with water. Prone image demonstrating that the fat plane between the stomach and pancreas is preserved, excluding pancreatic invasion. (B) Gastric carcinoma (asterisk) extending beyond the serosa to encase the coeliac axis vessels. (C) Extension into the transverse mesocolon (arrows) from an antral carcinoma.[†]

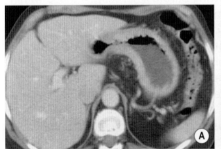
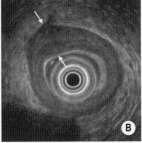

Linitis plastica – (A) diffuse gastric wall thickening demonstrated on CT. (B) EUS demonstrates diffuse thickening of all layers of the gastric wall (between arrows).[†]

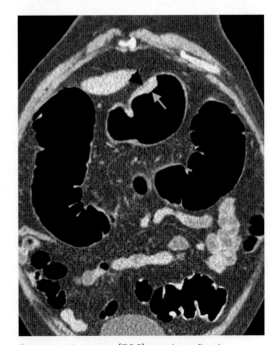

Early gastric cancer (EGC) type I, confined to mucosa (T1 lesion). Coronal MPR CT image shows a type 1 polypoid lesion (arrow) in the lesser curvature of the stomach. These post-contrast images show abnormal focal mucosal hyperenhancement with preservation of the outer hypodense stripe (arrowhead), which represents submucosa.**

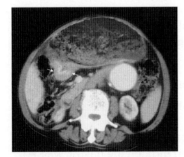

Gastric carcinoma. The tumour is enhancing and thickening the wall of the antrum (arrows). The stomach is distended with food debris as a result of gastric outlet obstruction.[†]

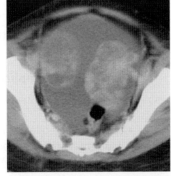

Kruckenberg tumours. Bilateral partly cystic ovarian tumours and malignant ascites.[†]

GASTRIC SURGERY

SURGERY TYPES

Billroth

- A partial gastrectomy (historically performed for peptic ulcer disease) consisting of an antrectomy, vagotomy and creation of either a gastroduodenostomy (Billroth I) or gastrojejunostomy (Billroth II)

Gastric bypass surgery

- The creation of a proximal small pouch from the upper stomach with a surgical bypass of the remaining larger distal stomach remnant (the surgical reconstruction allows drainage of both of the stomach segments)
  - *It commonly uses a 'Roux-en 'Y' reconstruction:* the proximal small bowel is divided, with the distal segment attached to the small stomach pouch ▶ the proximal small bowel segment (draining the distal stomach pouch via the duodenum) is anastomosed to a segment of mid small bowel

Laparoscopic adjustable gastric band

- A silicon band is placed around the fundus, 3 cm from the GOJ creating a small pouch ▶ there is still a connection to the remaining stomach via a stoma ▶ the size of the pouch and stoma can be varied by accessing a port anterior to the left rectus sheath

Sleeve gastrectomy

- A large portion of the greater curvature is removed (creating a tubular stomach)

Fundoplication

- The gastric fundus is wrapped around the inferior oesophagus to prevent gastro-oesophageal reflux ▶ it produces a characteristic deformity of the gastric cardia

Partial gastrectomy and gastroenterostomy

- This is performed with either a cholecysto- or choledochojejunostomy for pancreatic carcinoma

COMPLICATIONS

Acute

- *Leakage:* from the duodenal stump or the anastomosis after gastrojejunostomy is the most common cause of postoperative death
- *Submucosal haemorrhage:* this is associated with gastric outlet obstruction (and is self-limiting)
- *Gastric outlet obstruction:* this is due to anastomotic oedema
- *Efferent loop obstruction:* this is due to spasm or inflammation with delayed transit in the efferent loop

(again this is self-limiting) ▶ it manifests between the 5th and 10th postoperative day

Acute or chronic

- *Afferent loop obstruction:* this follows afferent loop herniation through a surgically created defect behind the gastroenteric anastomosis or because of preferential gastric emptying into the afferent loop ▶ it presents with intermittent bilious vomiting, weight loss or malabsorption
  - **Barium studies:** there is preferential filling of the afferent loop or afferent loop barium retention on delayed films
- *Efferent loop obstruction:* usually caused by spasm and inflammation (5–10 days post op)
- *Prolapse and intussusception:* this is commonly jejunogastric, occurring at the anastomotic site (usually affecting the efferent loop)

Chronic

- *Marginal ulcerations:* these follow peptic ulcer surgery and are usually located within 2 cm of the anastomosis (on the jejunal side)
  - They are usually caused by an inadequate vagotomy
- *Phytobezoars (due to a poor diet):* these can be gastric (following Billroth I surgery) or found within the small bowel (following Bilroth II surgery) ▶ those within the small bowel may cause obstruction
- *Primary gastric carcinoma:* this occurs within the gastric remnant (patients have a relatively high incidence of atrophic gastritis)
  - There is a variable appearance: a lack of distensibility of the gastric remnant ▶ an intra-luminal mass or ulcer
- *Gastric outlet obstruction:* this is due to anastomotic stricture or stenosis formation
- *Gastric ischaemia leading to necrosis and fistula formation (e.g. gastrogastric or enterocutaneous):* this is associated with significant mortality
- *Internal herniation:* this can be transmesenteric or transmesocolonic
  - The Roux limb or small bowel herniates through a surgical defect within the mesentery or transverse mesocolon

Gastric band complications

- *Early*: band misplacement ▶ perforation ▶ early slippage
- *Late*: pouch dilatation ▶ band herniation ▶ spontaneous volume variation ▶ erosion through the gastric wall ▶ migration/slippage of the band

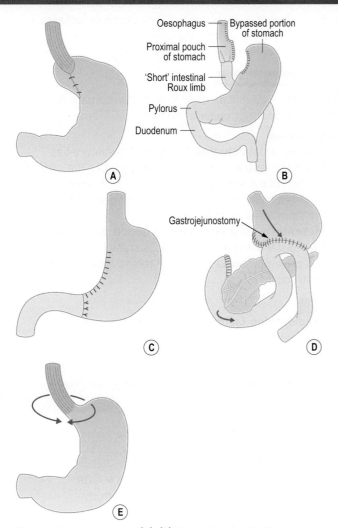

Types of gastric surgery. (A), (E) Nissen fundoplication. (B) Roux-en-Y gastric bypass. (C) Billroth I. (D) Billroth II (gastrojejunostomy).

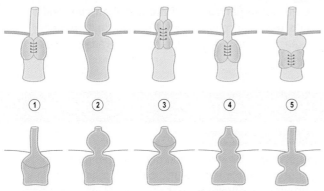

Appearance of a failure of a fundoplication. Anatomical drawings top row, barium meal appearances bottom row. 1, Normal postoperative appearance ▶ 2, complete disruption of wrap with recurrence of hiatus hernia ▶ 3, wrap intact but herniates through diaphragmatic hiatus ▶ 4, stomach slips up through wrap and bulges above diaphragm ▶ 5, stomach slips up through wrap but remains below diaphragm.

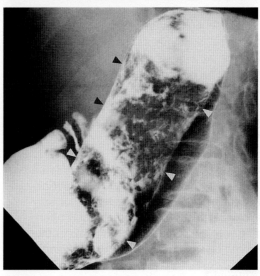

Bezoar – a large phytobezoar (arrowheads) within the stomach.[†]

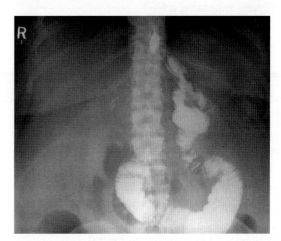

Gastric bypass. Single-contrast upper GI status post gastric bypass.[*]

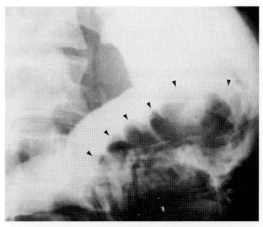

Retrograde jejunogastric intussusceptions following gastrojejunostomy. The loops of jejunum within the stomach (arrowheads) have a characteristic 'coiled spring' appearance.[†]

GASTRIC VOLVULUS

Definition

- The stomach twists on itself between its points of normal anatomical fixation ▶ it is usually associated with a large sliding or para-oesophageal hiatus hernia and a stomach that is partially or totally within the thoracic cavity
  - **Organo-axial volvulus:** the stomach rotates by 180° along its long axis (a line drawn between the cardia and pylorus)
    - *Complications are rare*
  - **Mesentero-axial volvulus:** the stomach rotates around its short axis (the axis of its mesenteric omental attachments – this is perpendicular to the long axis) ▶ this is less common but is often associated with a traumatic diaphragmatic rupture
    - *There can be significant clinical consequences*

Clinical presentation

- Violent retching with little vomitus ▶ severe epigastric pain ▶ difficulty in passing a NGT

- It may result in gastric outlet obstruction or ischaemia (resulting in a surgical emergency)
- It is most commonly seen in the elderly

Radiological features

Erect XR A double air-fluid level of the stomach within the mediastinum or upper abdomen

Barium meal

- **Organo-axial volvulus:** the greater curvature lies above the lesser curvature (occurring when the original position of the stomach is horizontal) or it is seen as a right-left twist (occurring when the original position of the stomach is vertical)
- **Mesentero-axial volvulus:** an 'upside down stomach' – the distal antrum and pylorus is cranial to the fundus and proximal stomach with the torsed area as a site of obstruction

Pearls

- **Predisposing factors:** phrenic nerve palsy ▶ diaphragmatic eventration ▶ traumatic diaphragmatic hernia ▶ gastric distension

HYPERTROPHIC PYLORIC STENOSIS

Definition

- Hypertrophy and hyperplasia of mainly the circular muscle results in lengthening and narrowing of the pyloric channel

Clinical presentation

- It is a relatively frequent congenital disorder diagnosed in infancy (commonly affecting first-born males and peaking between 3 and 6 weeks after birth)
- It presents with non-bilious projectile vomiting and a hypokalaemic hypochloraemic metabolic alkalosis

Radiological features

US This usually gives the definitive diagnosis

- Single wall pyloric thickness: >3 mm
- Pyloric length: >16 mm
- Transverse pyloric diameter: >11 mm

Barium meal Delayed gastric emptying ▶ GOR

- *'Tit' sign:* the canal indents the distal antrum
- *'String' sign:* pyloric canal elongation
- *'Shoulder' sign:* the hypertrophied muscle bulges retrogradely into the antrum

Pearl

- **Acquired hypertrophy of the distal antrum and pylorus:** this occurs in peptic or other inflammatory disease in adults ▶ there is no retrograde muscular bulge

MÉNÉTRIER'S DISEASE

Definition

- This is characterized by gastric gland hypertrophy, achlorhydria or hypoproteinaemia ▶ it is associated with gastric carcinoma
  - A protein-losing enteropathy occurs due to protein loss from the hyperplastic mucosa into the gastric lumen (with an associated increase in small bowel fluid)

Radiological features

Barium meal Bizarre, markedly enlarged gastric folds (most prominent within the proximal stomach and along the greater curvature) ▶ poor mucosal coating with barium (due to the increased fluid) ▶ gastric wall and small bowel fold thickening (due to the hypoproteinaemia)

- Although classically not involved, the antrum can be involved in up to 50% of cases
- The thickened folds remain pliable (cf. a rigid stomach with carcinoma)

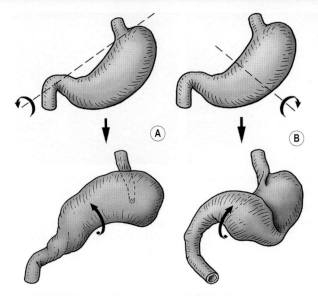

Organoaxial volvulus. (A) Rotation occurs around an axis connecting the pyloris to the oesophagogastric junction, with the greater curve folded upward and to the right. (B) Mesenteroaxial volvulus. Rotation occurs around an axis connecting the middle of the greater curve to the middle of the lesser curve. Generally this type of volvulus is partial as a result of excess mobility of the antrum and duodenum and so the stomach often kinks and obstructs between the body and the antrum.

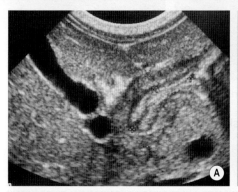

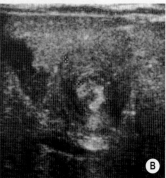

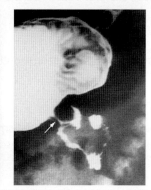

Hypertrophic pyloric stenosis. Barium meal showing the narrow pyloric canal with a double track of barium. The hypertrophied pylorus indents the base of the duodenal cap.*

Hypertrophic pyloric stenosis. Longitudinal US image (A) showing an elongated thickened pylorus, muscle length 17 mm and width 4 mm. Transverse image (B) with muscle width 6 mm.†

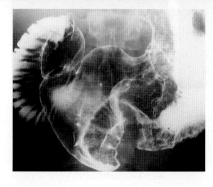

Ménétrier's disease. Classic appearance with massively distended folds in the body without abnormality in the antrum.*

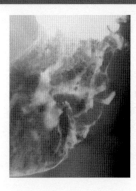

Ménétrier's disease. Gross thickening of the folds of the upper two-thirds of the stomach. These patients often weep a protein-rich exudate from the stomach wall, and this excess of fluid in the stomach may impair barium coating.†

AIR WITHIN THE GASTRIC WALL

Definition

- Disrupted gastric mucosa allows air entry into the gastric wall
  - **'Gastric emphysema':** this occurs without any underlying infection (e.g. secondary to corrosive ingestion, a gastric ulcer, gastric outlet obstruction, COPD, ischaemia or trauma)
  - **'Emphysematous gastritis':** this is due to an acute infection with a gas-forming organism (e.g. *Escherichia coli* or *Clostridium perfringens*)
  - **'Phlegmonous gastritis':** acute panmural infection with a non-gas-forming organism

Radiological features

AXR/CT It is characterized by thin curvilinear lines of radiolucent gas paralleling the gastric wall

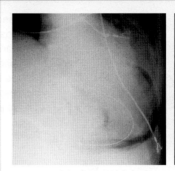

Gastric emphysema on AXR in a patient with ischaemic gastritis after extensive abdominal surgery.*

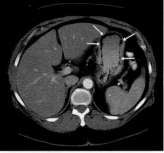

Computed tomographic scan shows a rounded collection of contrast material (arrows) arising from the posterior gastric fundus - this represents a fundal diverticulum.••

PRE-PYLORIC WEB (ANTRAL MUCOSAL DIAPHRAGM)

Definition

- A congenital thin diaphragm-like, exaggerated fold of gastric mucosa perpendicular to the long axis of the stomach (demarcating the distal antrum into a third small chamber between the proximal antrum and duodenal bulb)

Clinical presentation

- It can be asymptomatic or can cause gastric outlet obstruction

Radiological features

Barium meal A thin persistent circumferential smooth band within 3-4 cm of the pylorus

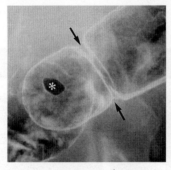

An antral diaphragm (between arrows). The pyloric canal is seen end on (asterisk).†

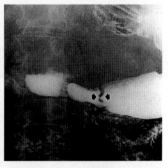

Upper gastrointestinal (UGI) study shows a thin, incomplete, web-like structure in the antrum of the stomach representing an antral web (arrows).••

GASTRIC DISTENSION

Obstructive causes

- This is usually due to peptic ulcer disease (duodenal, pyloric or antral ulcers) ▶ carcinoma of the antrum or pylorus is the 2nd commonest cause
  - *Rarer causes:* Crohn's disease ▶ pancreatitis ▶ pancreatic cancer

Non-obstructive causes

- Paralytic ileus (commonly seen in elderly patients) ▶ abdominal surgery ▶ acute trauma ▶ peritonitis ▶ chronic diabetes

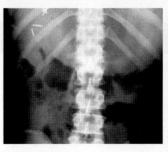

Supine AXR shows the transverse colon depressed by a distended, fluid-filled stomach. (Surgical clips are present in the right upper quadrant from prior cholecystectomy.)*

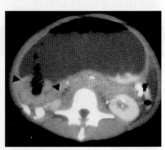

Gastric outlet obstruction – cancer of the antrum. Markedly distended stomach with air-fluid level on CT. In this case, a mass in the distal antrum is seen (arrowheads).*

GASTRIC DIVERTICULA

Definition

- This is a true diverticulum (containing muscularis propria) – thus it will demonstrate peristalsis ▶ it is usually several cm in size and readily fills with barium
  - It is most commonly seen within the posterior aspect of the fundus (near the lesser curvature) ▶ it can be confused with a left adrenal lesion

Pearl

Intramural or partial gastric diverticula These are due to invagination of the gastric mucosa into the gastric wall ▶ they are usually <1 cm in size with a lenticular shape (in profile) and a small opening into the gastric lumen ▶ they usually occur along the greater curvature ▶ they can be mistaken for an ulcer or pancreatic rest ▶ they are usually asymptomatic

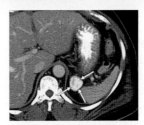

Computed tomographic scan shows air in gastric wall (arrows) after instrumentation.••

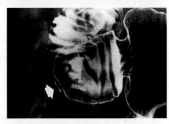

On UGI examination, a small, shallow protrusion along the greater curvature of the stomach (arrow) was diagnosed to be a shallow gastric ulcer. Note the absence of inflammatory changes around the area. Endoscopy showed no evidence of inflammation or ulceration and a small antral diverticulum.••

GASTRIC VARICES

Definition

- These usually occur in patients with portal hypertension and oesophageal varices (as the gastric veins are an additional collateral pathway)
  - The presence of gastric varices, in the absence of oesophageal varices, is a sign of a splenic thrombosis (which is usually associated with pancreatitis or pancreatic cancer)

Radiological features

Barium study/CT Widened effaceable polypoid enhancing folds – these can be nodular-appearing, 'grape-like' or mass-like (the latter mimicking gastric cancer) ▶ they are usually seen at the fundus and around the GOJ (the antrum is rarely involved without fundal involvement)

- *Differential diagnosis of thick polypoid gastric folds:* hypertrophic gastritis ▶ Ménétrier's disease ▶ lymphoma

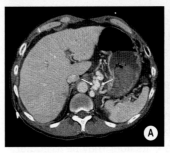
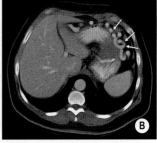

(A) Large serpentine varices (arrows) are seen in the gastric fundus. (B) Coiled serpentine varices are also seen along this patient's greater curvature (arrows) of stomach.••

ECTOPIC PANCREAS (PANCREATIC REST/ABERRANT PANCREAS)

Definition

- Pancreatic tissue located within the submucosa of the luminal GI tract
  - This is most commonly seen along the greater curvature of the antrum (also within the 1st and 2nd parts of the duodenum) ▶ it is usually a solitary lesion

Radiological features

Barium meal A sharply defined submucosal nodule (<2 cm) ▶ 50% have a central depression or umbilication (representing a rudimentary duct)

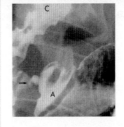

Ectopic pancreatic rest. These are generally found in the distal antrum on the greater curve. The small diverticulum results from barium entering the primitive duct system (arrow). A = distal antrum ▶ C = duodenal cap.†

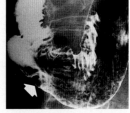

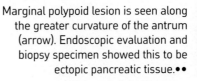

Marginal polypoid lesion is seen along the greater curvature of the antrum (arrow). Endoscopic evaluation and biopsy specimen showed this to be ectopic pancreatic tissue.••

3.3 DUODENUM

PEPTIC ULCERATION

Definition

- Mucosal ulceration occurring within an acidic part of the GI tract ▶ it is often associated with *H. pylori* infection ▶ duodenal ulcers are 2–3x more common than gastric ulcers
  - **Bulbar ulcers** (95%): these are usually benign
    - *Location:* anterior wall > posterior wall
  - **Postbulbar ulcers** (5%): these are usually malignant (95%) and fail to heal on medical treatment
    - *Location:* these are usually seen on the concave border of the 2nd part of the duodenum or within the immediate postbulbar area ▶ frequently spasm of opposite wall
- *Risk factors:* surgery ▶ severe head injury ▶ steroids ▶ COPD

Radiological features

Barium studies A duodenal ulcer appears as a sharply defined constant collection of barium (± surrounding oedema or radiating folds)

- *Postbulbar ulcer:* a typical crater is seen – often with spasm of the opposite wall (± thickened mucosal folds and a narrowed lumen) ▶ scar formation may obscure the ulcer crater
- *Kissing ulcers:* this describes two ulcers opposite each other on the anterior and posterior walls
- *Giant duodenal ulcer:* a benign ulcer crater measuring >2 cm ▶ it is constant in size and shape and often has a sharp round or oval outline ▶ its floor may be irregular (particularly when the ulcer is penetrating an adjacent organ) ▶ due to its size it may simulate a deformed duodenal bulb or diverticulum
- *A 'cloverleaf' or 'hourglass' deformity:* this can occur when an ulcer heals with scarring

Pearls

- Multiple postbulbar ulcers occur in the Zollinger–Ellison syndrome
- **Ulcer complications:** perforation ▶ bleeding ▶ stenosis ▶ penetration of any adjacent organs
  - *Perforation:* this can be localized or 'walled off' with marked duodenal deformity due to the adjacent inflammatory reaction

GASTRIC HETEROTOPIA

Definition

- Gastric mucosa occurring in various ectopic locations within the bowel (e.g. the duodenum, small bowel or rectum) ▶ it is found in a small percentage of normal people

Radiological features

Barium meal Irregular filling defects (varying in size from 1 to 6 mm) seen within the duodenal cap, extending from the pylorus distally

Pearls

- This should be differentiated from lymphoid hyperplasia of the duodenal bulb

DUODENAL DIVERTICULA

Definition

- Serosal and mucosal herniations through the muscular wall of the duodenum (seen in 2–5% of barium studies)

Clinical presentation

- It is usually an asymptomatic incidental finding (symptoms may occur due to the retention of food or a foreign body) ▶ it is a rare cause of haemorrhage or perforation
- Occasionally it may contain aberrant pancreatic, gastric or other functioning tissue – it then becomes a possible site of ulceration, perforation or gangrene
- Cholangitis or pancreatitis may result from the aberrant insertion of the common bile duct or pancreatic duct into an intraluminal diverticulum (with associated impaired biliary drainage)

Radiological features

- It is usually found within the 2nd part of the duodenum with most (85%) arising from the medial periampullary surface ▶ the diverticulum is frequently in contact with the pancreas (and may be embedded in its surface)

Pearl

- Duodenal ulceration with spasm or scarring may deform the duodenum, producing a pseudodiverticulum – these are deformable (unlike an ulcer)

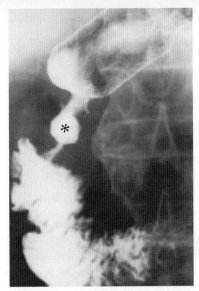

Postbulbar duodenal ulcer. Characteristic appearance with an ulcer crater (asterisk) in the middle of a stricture produced by spasm and oedema.[†]

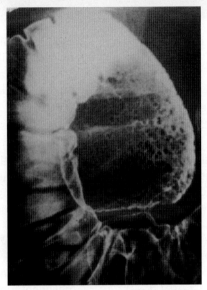

Gastric heterotopia. Multiple small irregular filling defects of varying size are seen in the duodenal cap.[*]

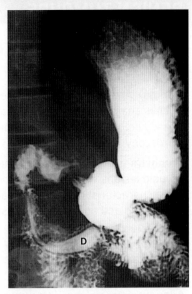

UGI study demonstrates intraluminal diverticulum or wind sock configuration (D).[••]

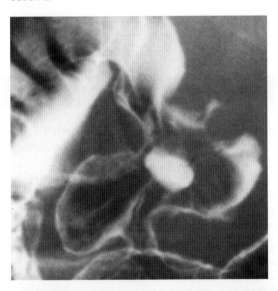

Duodenal ulceration. The duodenal cap is deformed and a moderate-sized ulcer crater is outlined with barium.[†]

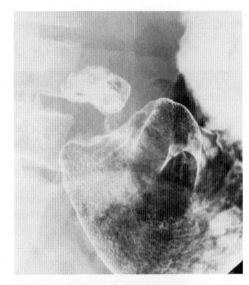

Giant duodenal ulcer replacing the duodenal cap.[*]

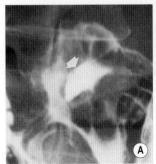 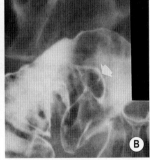

Anterior wall duodenal ulcer. (A) prone projection. The ulcer (arrow) is dependent, and so fills with barium. (B) supine projection. The ulcer, which is now on the non-dependent wall of the cap, is outlined with a ring of barium (arrow).[†]

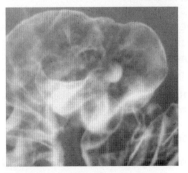

Duodenal ulcer. Barium collects in an ulcer on the dependent (posterior) wall of the duodenal cap.[†]

BENIGN TUMOURS

TYPES AND APPEARANCES ON BARIUM STUDIES

Lipoma An intraluminal filling defect (3-4 cm in size) which is sharply marginated, solitary and sessile ▶ it is easily deformed by peristalsis or compression on fluoroscopy

Brunner's gland hyperplasia These are single or multiple polypoid lesions within the 1st part of the duodenum (often with a characteristic cobblestone appearance) ▶ a single Brunner's gland adenoma is occasionally seen as a 1 cm smooth polypoid mass
- The Brunner's glands normally produce alkaline secretions to protect the duodenal mucosa from gastric acid

Adenomatous polyps Intraluminal filling defects (<1 cm) which can be solitary, sessile or polypoid ▶ they are seen as a soft tissue mass on CT

Villous adenomas These have a characteristic 'cauliflower' or 'soap bubble' appearance (caused by trapping of barium in the crevices between the multiple frond-like tumour projections) ▶ they are often 2–3 cm in size

Benign lymphoid hyperplasia This is seen as multiple small rounded filling defects of uniform size
- This may be a normal finding in children ▶ in adults it can be associated with hypogammaglobulinaemia and giardiasis

Carcinoid This is seen especially within the peripapillary region of the 2nd part of the duodenum as a discrete smooth polyp or an irregular infiltrating lesion

Other benign tumours Periampullary adenoma ▶ gastrointestinal stromal tumour (GIST) ▶ neurogenic tumour (e.g. neurofibroma) ▶ hamartoma

PEARL

- Benign duodenal tumours are more common than malignant tumours ▶ they are often asymptomatic
  - The commonest tumour types are lipomas and leiomyomas

MALIGNANT TUMOURS

TYPES AND APPEARANCES ON BARIUM STUDIES

Primary tumours

Adenocarcinoma of the papilla of Vater This appears as an enlarged papilla of Vater with irregular borders (sometimes with spiculation and ulceration)
- This is the most commonly encountered malignant duodenal tumour ▶ it usually presents with jaundice

Non-papillary adenocarcinomas of the duodenum These appear as ulcerative, polypoid or annular lesions
- **CT:** focal masses with asymmetric mural thickening and luminal narrowing ▶ co-incident adenopathy or hepatic metastases may be present
- It usually presents with obstruction

GIST/lymphoma These can also be found within the duodenum

Secondary tumours

Carcinoma or lymphoma of the stomach These can spread directly across the pylorus to involve the duodenum (seen in 25% and 40% of cases, respectively)

Carcinoma of the head of the pancreas A widened duodenal loop ▶ a double duodenal contour (± irregularity of the inner border) ▶ stricturing or distortion of the valvulae conniventes ▶ a reversed '3' sign of Frostberg
- Carcinoma of the tail of the pancreas may compress or invade the duodenum (resulting in mucosal destruction, bleeding or obstruction)

Carcinoma of the colon (particularly the hepatic flexure) This may cause destruction of the mucosal pattern, stricturing or the formation of a postbulbar ulcer ▶ a duodenocolic fistula may also form

Carcinoma of the gallbladder This may displace, compress or infiltrate the distal ½ of the 1st part of the duodenum

Enlarged neoplastic retroperitoneal lymph nodes These may also invade the duodenum

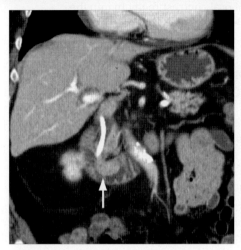

Periampullary adenoma (coronal reconstruction). CECT with water used as oral contrast shows a sharply defined mass (arrow) within the lumen of the second duodenal part extending to the infrapapillary area. A biliary stent is also seen.*

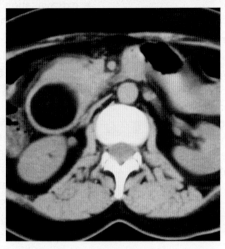

Lipoma. CT shows the lesion to be a well-defined, round mass with low attenuation values, characteristic of fat.*

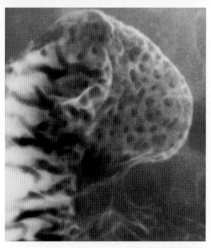

Lymphoid hyperplasia. Multiple small filling defects characteristic of lymphoid hyperplasia are shown on a double-contrast view of the duodenal cap.*

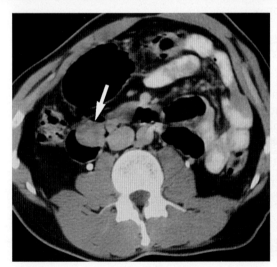

Ampullary carcinoma. CT scan showing a soft tissue intraluminal mass (arrow) arising from the medial aspect of the descending duodenum.©20

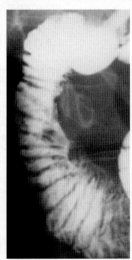

Carcinoma of the pancreas. Barium examination of the duodenum shows the characteristic reversed '3' sign of Frostberg with effacement and distortion of the mucosal pattern on the medial wall of the second portion of the duodenum.*

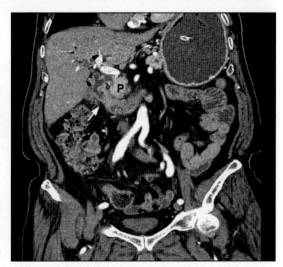

Primary duodenal adenocarcinoma. CECT with water used as oral contrast shows asymmetric mural thickening and encroachment of the lumen at the second portion of the duodenum (arrow). Dilatation of the common bile duct is also seen. The head of pancreas (P) appears normal.*

CROHN'S DISEASE

Definition Crohn's disease affects the duodenum in 4% of cases ▶ the radiological appearances are similar to those seen within the more distal small intestine

Barium meal The valvulae conniventes are frequently thickened ▶ with advanced disease there may be stricture formation with eccentric or concentric narrowing ▶ cobblestoning, asymmetry and skip lesions may be seen (fissure ulcers, sinuses and fistulae are uncommon)

- *A 'pseudo post-Billroth I' appearance:* this can result from continuous tubular narrowing of the antrum and proximal duodenum

TUBERCULOSIS

Definition This rarely affects the duodenum (if it does it is usually the 2nd part)

Barium meal A narrowed lumen (± mucosal destruction and ulceration)

- Tuberculous mesenteric lymphadenitis (in the absence of intrinsic duodenal tuberculosis) may produce extrinsic pressure on the duodenum leading to obstruction

RADIATION DAMAGE

Definition Duodenal damage is very uncommon – if it does occur, it will usually affect the 2nd part

Barium meal Ulceration ▶ thickened mucosal folds ▶ stricturing

PROGRESSIVE SYSTEMIC SCLEROSIS

Definition The duodenum is frequently involved

Barium meal Gross dilatation (which is often more pronounced in the 2nd, 3rd and 4th parts of the duodenum) ▶ the dilated duodenum can be slow to empty (the atonic organ can produce a sump effect)

INTRAMURAL HAEMATOMA

Definition This is usually due to blunt abdominal trauma

Barium meal Intramural haematoma is usually seen as a concentric obstructive lesion within the duodenum ▶ thickened valvulae conniventes can result from infiltration by blood and oedema

CT This will demonstrate the extent of any haematoma and will be seen as a mixed attenuation mass surrounding the duodenum

TRAUMATIC RUPTURE

Definition The most frequent site of rupture is at the junction of the 2nd and 3rd parts of the duodenum

CT Retroperitoneal air adjacent to the duodenum ▶ extravasation of oral contrast medium into the retroperitoneum ▶ duodenal wall oedema ▶ peripancreatic fat stranding

SUPERIOR MESENTERIC ARTERY COMPRESSION SYNDROME

Definition This is a rare form of high intestinal obstruction due to narrowing of the normal angle between the aorta and the superior mesenteric artery (through which the 3rd part of the duodenum passes) ▶ there is a possible association with marked weight loss

Barium meal Strong to-and-fro peristalsis and proximal duodenal dilatation due to compression of the 3rd part of the duodenum ▶ there will be a sharp cut-off seen in the right anterior oblique position with compression and proximal dilatation persisting when the patient is prone

CT This can measure the angle between the aorta and superior mesenteric artery (on sagittal views)

AORTIC ANEURYSMAL COMPRESSION

Definition An aortic aneurysm may compress the 3rd part of the duodenum and can occasionally cause duodenal obstruction

Pearl A faintly opacified duodenum can stretch around an aneurysm and mimic a contained leak or perianeurysmal inflammation

AORTODUODENAL FISTULA

Definition This is an abnormal communication between the aorta and the duodenum which is usually seen in patients who have undergone aortic graft surgery ▶ it usually involves the 3rd part of the duodenum

Clinical presentation Patients can present with gastrointestinal haemorrhage

CT Abnormal passage of IV contrast medium from the aorta into the duodenum (endoscopy can also be used for detection)

BOUVERET'S SYNDROME

Definition Following erosion of a gallstone through the gallbladder wall into the duodenum, the gallstone may travel retrogradely and become impacted within the duodenal cap (cf. a gallstone ileus with impaction at the terminal ileum following antegrade movement)

Barium meal A radiolucent mass within the duodenal cap with a thin coat of barium between the stone and duodenal wall

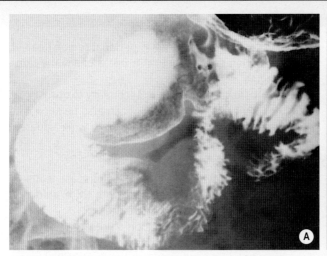
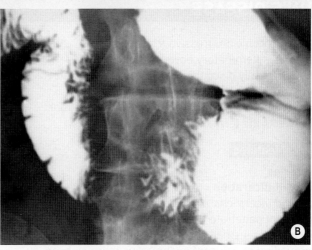

Superior mesenteric artery syndrome caused by carcinoma of the pancreas involving the root of the mesentery. (A) Supine position. Compression of the 3rd part of the duodenum. (B) Prone position. The compression persists and dilatation of the proximal duodenum is accentuated.[†]

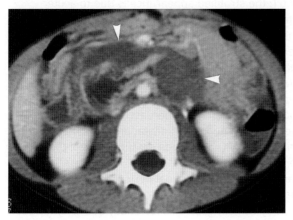

Intramural haematoma. CT shows a mass of mixed attenuation, characteristic of haematoma, surrounding the 3rd portion of the duodenum (arrowheads).*

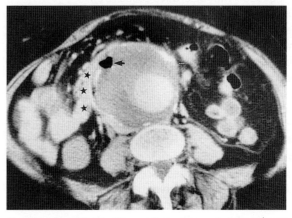

Aortoduodenal fistula. Recent haematemesis. The 3rd part of the duodenum (stars) is stretched over the aortic aneurysm, which contains thrombus. A fistula accounts for the gas within the aortic wall (arrow).[†]

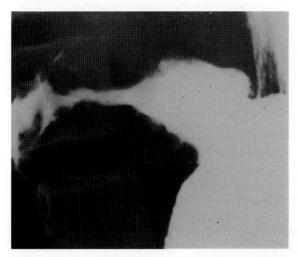

Crohn's disease. Marked irregular narrowing of the antrum and first portion of the duodenum, giving the 'pseudo post-Billroth I' appearance.*

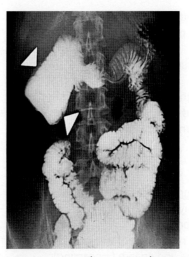

Megaduodenum (arrowheads) in a patient with scleroderma.••

3.4 SMALL BOWEL

CROHN'S DISEASE

Definition A chronic progressive *transmural* granulomatous inflammatory bowel disease
- There are typically discontinuous ('skip') lesions with asymmetrical bowel wall involvement
- It can affect any part of the GI tract – however it almost always affects the terminal ileum (in 95% of cases)

Radiological features

Barium studies
- **Bowel wall ulceration**
  - *Aphthoid ulcers:* characteristic superficial ulcers that do not penetrate the muscularis mucosa ▶ they appear as small collections of barium with surrounding radiolucent oedematous margins ▶ en face they appear as a dense amorphous barium pool with a surrounding black halo
    - They are typical of Crohn's disease (CD) (but are not seen with ulcerative colitis [UC])
  - *Fissuring 'rose thorn' ulcers:* deep ulcers with penetrating thorn-like cuts into the thickened intestinal wall ▶ they may lead to abscess formation, sinuses or fistulae
  - *Longitudinal ulcers:* these run along the ileal mesenteric border
  - *'Cobblestone' mucosa:* a combination of longitudinal and transverse ulceration separating intact portions of mucosa
- **Inflammatory polyps (pseudopolyps):** small, discrete round filling defects ▶ these are not a frequent finding
- **Thickened valvulae conniventes:** they can also be distorted, blunted or flattened (they are due to hyperplasia of the lymphoid tissue which causes an obstructive lymphoedema)
- **Bowel wall thickening**
  - Thickened bowel wall segments will displace adjacent barium-filled loops
  - Occasionally a smooth featureless outline will replace the normal mucosal pattern without a significant calibre change
  - *'Skip lesions':* discontinuous involvement of the bowel wall
  - *'Pseudodiverticula':* these are due to asymmetrical wall involvement and represent small patches of normal intestine in an otherwise severely involved segment
- **Strictures/stenoses**
  - These may be short, long, single or multiple (the latter is virtually diagnostic of CD) ▶ solitary strictures are common and may be accompanied by proximal (prestenotic) dilatation
  - *'String sign':* tubular narrowing of the intestinal lumen secondary to oedema and spasm (± scarring)
- **Fistulae formation:** this can involve adjacent loops of ileum, caecum or sigmoid colon

- *Other sites:* urinary bladder ▶ perianal region (leading to a 'watering can' perineum) ▶ occasionally the skin and vagina
- **Bowel wall sacculation:** this is secondary to fibrosis within healing eccentric ulcers ▶ it can also be seen with ischaemic strictures or scleroderma (with wide 'square'-shaped diverticulae)

CT
- **Thickened bowel wall:** the transmural disease leads to greater wall thickening than seen with UC ▶ mild reactive adenopathy (<1 cm) can be present
- *'Dirty fat':* transmural inflammation of the small bowel usually involves the adjacent mesentery
- *'Target' or 'halo' sign:* a homogeneous or stratified appearance is seen on both NECT and CECT:
  - *NECT:* the stratified appearance is due to a thickened muscularis mucosae and submucosal fatty infiltration
  - *CECT:* the stratified appearance is due to acute inflammation with submucosal oedema and enhancement of the mucosa and muscularis propria
- *Mesenteric fibrofatty proliferation:* this results in increased CT attenuation ▶ it is the most common cause of bowel loop separation in CD
- *'Creeping fat':* fat accumulates on the serosal surfaces
- *'Comb' sign:* mesenteric hypervascularity manifested as tortuosity, prominence and dilatation of the mesenteric arterial branches with a wide arrangement of the vasa recta
- **Advanced disease:** intestinal perforation may lead to mesenteric phlegmon or interloop abscess formation ▶ these may contain gas – this is usually due to enteric or cutaneous fistulae and sinus tracts rather than due to a gas-producing bacteria

Magnetic resonance enterography/enteroclysis
This is an emerging technique which is able to assess disease activity and which is comparable with conventional enteroclysis (but it can also demonstrate extramural manifestations)
- *It can demonstrate:* bowel wall thickening ▶ ulceration ▶ cobblestoning ▶ a 'target' appearance ▶ fibrofatty proliferation ▶ vascular engorgement ▶ adenopathy ▶ luminal narrowing and stenosis ▶ sinus/fistulous tracts (high SI on T2WI)
- *MR rectum:* this can assess any perianal fistulae (with fat suppressed T2WI and STIR sequences)

Pearls
- **Complications:** there is an increased incidence of GI tract tumours, lymphoma and toxic megacolon
- **Extraintestinal findings:** gallstones ▶ spondylitis ▶ symmetrical sacroiliitis ▶ renal stones ▶ complications of steroid treatment (e.g. avascular necrosis) ▶ primary sclerosing cholangitis
- **Clinical presentation:** abdominal pain (can present as an acute abdomen) ▶ diarrhoea ▶ weight loss

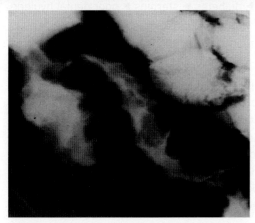

Cobblestoning of the terminal ileum, thickening of the wall of the terminal ileum, and an enlarged ileocaecal valve in Crohn's disease (CD).*

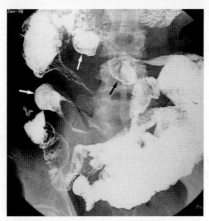

Advanced Crohn's disease with several characteristic pseudodiverticulae (arrows).†

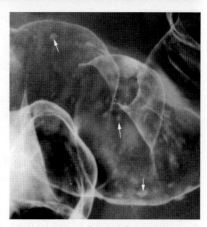

Aphthoid ulcers (arrows) in CD.*

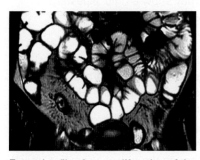

Extensive fibrofatty proliferation of the mesentery, accompanying involved ileal segments, is demonstrated on a coronal true FISP image.*

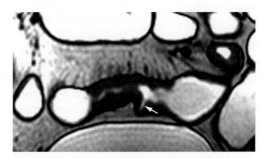

Active CD. Coronal true FISP spot view demonstrates luminal narrowing and wall thickening in a segment of distal ileum. A fissure ulcer (arrow) penetrating the thickened wall and increased mesenteric vascularity are also disclosed.*

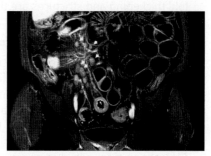

Active CD. Coronal 2D FLASH image + Gad, showing multilayered mural enhancement of distal ileal loops (small arrow) and multiple enhancing mesenteric lymph nodes (arrowheads). Vascular engorgement is also present.*

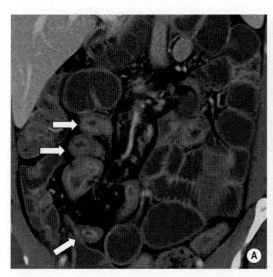

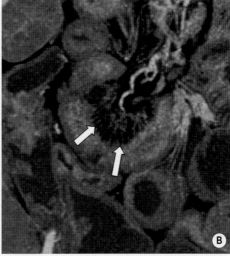

CD. (A) Coronal reconstruction image of CT enterography shows thickened distal ileal loops and mural stratification resulting in a 'target' appearance (arrows). Prestenotic dilatation is also seen. (B) A coronal, three-dimensional projection of the same patient showing the vascular engorgement (arrows) of an involved ileal loop (comb sign).*

Tuberculosis (TB)

Definition Up to 5% of patients with *Mycobacterium tuberculosis* infection have GI involvement ▶ it used to be secondary to pulmonary disease but is now more likely to be of primary bovine origin (from drinking unpasteurized milk)

- *Affected sites:* GI tract ▶ liver ▶ spleen ▶ lymph nodes ▶ peritoneum ▶ female genital tract

Clinical presentation

- Abdominal pain ▶ fever ▶ weight loss ▶ diarrhoea ▶ intestinal obstruction ▶ bowel perforation (rare)

Radiological features

- Although any part of the GI tract can be involved, the ileum is the commonest involved site (esp. the terminal ileum and ileocaecal junction) ▶ there are often multiple bowel lesions
- Discrete transverse and circumferential ulcers, mucosal fold thickening and strictures are the main radiological features

Barium follow through (ileocaecal tuberculosis)

- Ulcerative, hypertrophic or fibrotic forms are described:
  - *Ulcerative:* there are discrete ulcers with a 'shaggy' edge – these tend to be large and circumferential
  - *Hypertrophic:* this presents as an inflammatory mass with associated bowel stenosis ▶ it may be difficult to distinguish from lymphoma
- **Fleischner sign:** a thickened patulous ileocaecal valve seen in conjunction with a narrowed terminal ileum
- **Stierlin's sign:** this is due to rapid emptying of contrast through a gaping incompetent ileocaecal valve and into a conically contracted caecum

CT Bowel wall thickening with homogeneous attenuation and lack of mural stratification ▶ there may be enlarged rim-enhancing low-density mesenteric nodes (due to caseous liquefaction)

- *TB peritonitis:* this is suggested by diffuse omental and mesenteric infiltration, nodules, peritoneal thickening and high attenuation ascites

Yersinia

Definition Infection with the Gram-negative bacilli *Yersinia enterocolitica* and *Yersinia pseudotuberculosis* ▶ acute inflammation of the terminal ileum is often indistinguishable clinically from an acute appendicitis

Barium follow through (BaFT) Disease is limited to the distal 20 cm of ileum ▶ tortuous, thickened mucosal folds with small discrete nodular filling defects of lymphoid hyperplasia ▶ there can be mural thickening

Actinomycosis

Definition Infection with *Actinomyces israelii*, a common saprophyte in the mouth, throat and GI tract ▶ the appendix is the most commonly affected site

- *Risk factors:* GI perforation ▶ previous surgery ▶ neoplasms ▶ diabetes ▶ steroids ▶ poor dental hygiene

BaFT and CT Appendix mass causing ileocaecal compression (± sinus tracts and fistulae)

Giardiasis

Definition A tropical infection with *Giardia lamblia* (a flagellate protozoon parasite of the upper small intestine) ▶ it is contracted through contaminated drinking water

BaFT Irregular thickening of the valvulae conniventes within the duodenum and proximal jejunum ▶ small well-defined nodular lymphoid hyperplasia in patients who also have dysgammaglobulinaemia

Strongyloidiasis

Definition A tropical small intestine infection with *Strongyloides stercoralis* (roundworm)

BaFT Delayed barium passage ▶ thickened or absent valvulae conniventes within the duodenum and proximal jejunum ▶ severe cases may show a rigid 'pipestem' stenosis with irregular narrowing

Anisakiasis

Definition Infection with *Anisakis* larvae (found within affected raw, pickled or salted fish): it can cause eosinophilic granuloma formation within the GI tract, affecting the stomach, terminal ileum

BaFT Concentric narrowing of the involved segment of ileum (± proximal dilatation) ▶ it may be indistinguishable from Crohn's disease (although the mucosa remains intact)

Ascariasis

Definition Infection with *Ascaris lumbricoides* (a roundworm) can cause intestinal or biliary obstruction, or oriental cholangiohepatitis ▶ it is very commonly seen in the tropics

BaFT Single or multiple smooth longitudinal or coiled filling defects within the small bowel (a thin central track of barium outlining the worm's intestinal tract may be seen)

Cytomegalovirus

Definition Infection usually occurs in immunocompromised patients (especially AIDS)

BaFT Diffuse small bowel narrowing, ulcerations and fold effacement ▶ there can be associated oesophagitis, gastritis or colitis

Cryptosporidiosis

Definition A protozoal infection causing enteritis in AIDS patients

BaFT Small bowel dilatation ▶ thickened small bowel folds

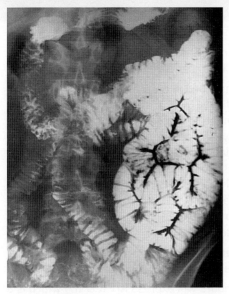

Giardiasis. Diffuse, irregular small bowel fold thickening is seen.••

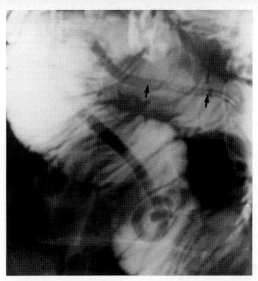

Roundworm. Tubular intraluminal filling defect in the jejunum represents an ascaris worm. The thin white line bisecting part of the length of the worm (arrows) indicates barium in the worm's gastrointestinal tract.••

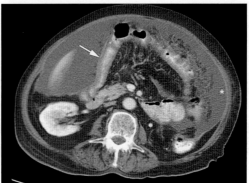

Colonic TB with thickening of the transverse colon (arrow) and extensive tuberculous ascites (asterisk).

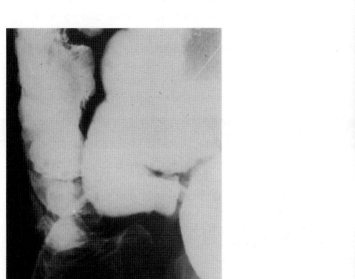

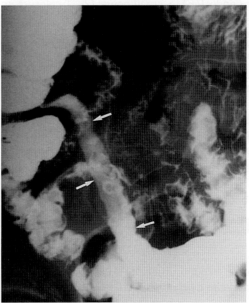

Tuberculosis. A short, irregular stricture, about 4 cm long, is shown to involve the terminal ileum and ileocaecal valve. The narrowing caused considerable delay in the passage of barium, and dilatation of the ileum proximal to the stricture can be seen. The patient presented with intestinal obstruction.*

CMV enteritis in a patient with AIDS. Tubular distal ileum (arrows) is seen.••

GASTROINTESTINAL STROMAL TUMOURS (GISTS)

Definition

- A submucosal mesenchymal (non-epithelial) tumour appearing to arise from the muscularis propria ▶ GISTs may arise from the interstitial cells of Cajal (these serve a gastric pacemaker function)
  - They are not related to a leiomyoma or leiomyosarcoma
- The commonest gastrointestinal mesenchymal tumour (< 1% of all GI tract tumours)
- *Location:* stomach (40–70%) > small intestine (20–50%) > large intestine and rectum (5%) ▶ leiomyomas and leiomyosarcomas are rare at these sites
  - *Oesophagus:* a leiomyoma is more common than a GIST

Clinical features It usually presents during the 6th to 7th decades (M = F)

- Asymptomatic (10–30%) ▶ abdominal pain ▶ abdominal mass ▶ ileus ▶ GI bleeding ▶ weight loss

Radiological features Malignant GISTs (10%) are radiographically indistinguishable from their benign counterparts (if >5 cm, malignancy should be considered)

Barium meal Usually a small incidental and discrete submucosal mass (preserved overlying areae gastricae pattern) ▶ the border of the smooth mucosal surface forms right or obtuse angles with the adjacent mucosa

- Ulceration if it outstrips its blood supply (>2 cm)
- *'Bulls-eye' or 'target' lesion:* this results from contrast collecting within the ulcer cavity

CT A well-circumscribed submucosal mass extending exophytically from the GI tract (± an intra- and extraluminal 'dumb-bell' component) ▶ coarse mottled calcifications (25%) ▶ occasionally pedunculated (and may obstruct the pylorus or duodenum/act as a lead point for an intussusception) ▶ hypo- or hypervascular

- Lymphadenopathy is rare (its presence should suggest an alternative diagnosis such as lymphoma)
- The liver and peritoneum are the most common sites of distant metastases

MRI T1WI: intemediate SI ▶ T2WI: low to intermediate SI ▶ T1WI + Gad: variable heterogeneous enhancement

Pearls 90% of tumours will express KIT (CD 117) which is a tyrosine kinase growth factor receptor ▶ this differentiates a GIST from other gastrointestinal mesenchymal tumours (e.g. leiomyoma or leiomyosarcoma)

- Increased prevalence of GIST with NF-1
- *Unfavourable prognostic signs:* tumour size >5 cm ▶ infiltration into adjacent organs ▶ metastases ▶ a high mitotic and proliferation index
- **Carney's triad:** a genetic syndrome of young women
  - Multiple stomach GISTs + a functioning extra-adrenal paraganglioma + a pulmonary chondroma

CARCINOID TUMOURS OF THE GASTROINTESTINAL TRACT

Definition A low-grade malignant neoplasm arising from submucosal neuroendocrine enterochomaffin cells

- It has a relatively indolent course with a prolonged survival (even with metastases)
- *Location:* appendix (45%) > small bowel (25%), colorectum (25%) ▶ it is multiple in ⅓ of cases

Clinical presentation The primary tumour rarely produces symptoms (due to its small size and deep mucosal location) ▶ it can present with abdominal pain, obstruction, or an abdominal mass ▶ GI haemorrhage is very rare

- **Carcinoid syndrome:** seen in ⅓ of jejunoileal carcinoids that have metastasized to the liver ▶ tumour secretion of serotonin can cause recurrent diarrhoea, bronchospasm, flushing, tricuspid insufficiency and pulmonary valvular stenosis
  - It can produce ACTH (Cushing's syndrome)

Radiological features

BaFT

- *Primary lesion:* a round, smoothly outlined intraluminal filling defect (it can be multiple)

- *Secondary mesenteric mass:* there is stretching, rigidity and fixation of the ileal loops
- Thickened valvulae conniventes (due to chronic ischaemic changes)
- A stellate, spoke-like arrangement of adjacent bowel loops or a sharp angulation of a bowel loop (due to the associated desmoplastic reaction)

CT Secondary mesenteric changes including a discrete soft tissue mass (± stippled dystrophic calcification due to tumour necrosis) ▶ displaced adjacent bowel loops ▶ hypervascular liver metastases (which may calcify) ▶ mesenteric adenopathy (± dystrophic calcification)

- *Desmoplastic reaction:* this is incited by local serotonin release ▶ it can cause a radiating 'stellate' pattern of linear strands into the surrounding fat ▶ it may encase the mesenteric vessels with resultant chronic ischaemia and segmental bowel wall thickening

Pearls Small bowel carcinoids commonly metastasize ▶ gastric and appendiceal tumours rarely metastasize

- ¹²³I- or ¹³¹I-MIBG scintigraphy can be used to localize and treat tumours
- 30% of small bowel carcinoids are multicentric

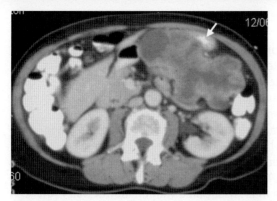

Malignant gastric stromal tumour. CT. This predominantly exophytic tumour is compressing the stomach (arrow).[†]

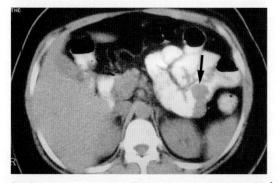

Benign stromal tumour. The tumour is visible on CT (arrow).[†]

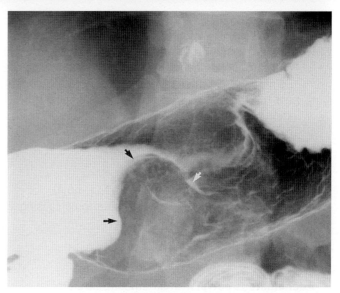

Benign GIST. The margins of this submucosal tumour make an obtuse angle with the adjacent normal mucosa.[†]

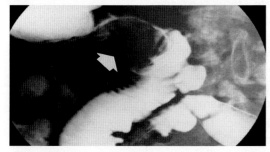

Carcinoid tumour. A round, well-defined, intraluminal filling defect (arrow) is seen in the distal ileum of a patient who presented with symptoms of intermittent obstruction but without any manifestations of the carcinoid syndrome.[†]

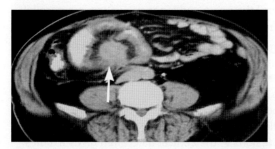

CT shows a carcinoid mass (arrow) with a characteristic stellate radiating pattern and thickening of the adjacent intestinal wall.

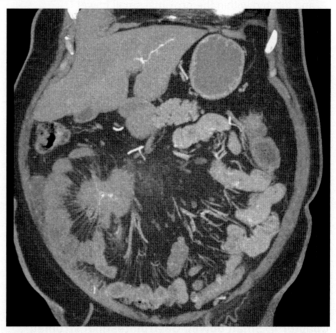

Coronal reformat CECT showing a secondary mesenteric soft tissue mass containing dystrophic calcification and demonstrating surrounding desmoplastic reaction with radiating 'stellate' pattern of linear strands into the surrounding fat.

BENIGN TUMOURS

Definition

- These arise from mucosa or submucosa (up to 2% of all GI tract neoplasms)
  - *Common:* adenoma (polyp or villous) ▶ leiomyoma
    - Only types with definite malignant potential
  - *Less common:* lipoma (3ʳᵈ commonest tumour) ▶ a vascular or neurogenic tumour ▶ hamartoma (these are developmental anomalies – multiple lesions are seen in Peutz–Jeghers syndrome)

Clinical presentation

- Acute GI bleeding (commonly with a leiomyoma)
- Abdominal pain (commonly with a hamartoma causing a recurrent intussusception)

Radiological features

BaFT

- **Adenomatous polyp:** a small, smooth, intraluminal filling defect (often of different sizes and may be pedunculated) ▶ often solitary and sessile (if multiple it will usually affect a single segment)
- **Villous adenoma:** a broad-based, lobulated cauliflower-like filling defect with multiple radiolucent striations and frond-like projections ▶ usually >3 cm in size

- **Leiomyoma:** these can lead to a tenting deformity of the intestinal wall, ulceration (± bleeding) and intussusception
  - *Intraluminal tumour:* a broad-based, smooth, round or semilunar filling defect
  - *Extraluminal tumour:* there is displacement and distortion of the neighbouring bowel loops
  - *Bidirectional or dumb-bell tumour:* both of the above
    CT A round or semilunar, homogeneous soft tissue mass associated with the bowel wall ▶ there is homogeneous or rim contrast enhancement (± peripheral crescent-shaped necrosis)
    DSA Well-defined, lobulated hypervascular mass
- **Hamartomatous polyp:** multiple round or lobulated filling defects present in large numbers in Peutz–Jeghers syndrome ▶ often pedunculated (intussusception is frequent)
- **Lipoma:** a sharply marginated, solitary, sessile, intraluminal filling defect (3-4 cm in size) ▶ it is easily deformed by peristalsis or compression on BaFT
    CT It will demonstrate fat attenuation

MALIGNANT TUMOURS

Definition

- An adenocarcinoma is the most common malignant neoplasm of the small intestine ▶ it is usually solitary and located within the proximal small bowel

Clinical presentation

- It is almost always symptomatic (but with a non-specific presentation) ▶ there is a dismal prognosis due to the late diagnosis

Radiological features

Adenocarcinoma

BaFT An infiltrative tumour with circumferential narrowing, mucosal destruction and shouldering of its margins ▶ it can also appear as a filling defect or as a polypoid mass (± ulceration)

CT Mural thickening (not > 1.5 cm) with either concentric or asymmetric luminal narrowing ▶ homogeneous or heterogeneous with moderate enhancement ▶ advanced tumours can infiltrate the mesentery ▶ lymphadenopathy (50%)

Carcinoid/lymphoma/malignant GIST: see Section 3 Chapter 4, Small bowel, Gastrointestinal stromal; Section 8 Chapter 2, Lymphoma

Pearls

Secondary neoplasms arise by:

Direct invasion e.g. primary neoplasms of the ovary, colon, prostate, uterus and kidney
- These appear as a mass invading the adjacent intestine (often over a considerable length) ▶ there is mucosal destruction, luminal narrowing (± obstruction) and tethering of the mucosal folds

Lymphatic extension This is rare (e.g. spread of a caecal carcinoma to the terminal ileum)

Peritoneal seeding These frequently localize within the right lower quadrant (stasis within the lower recesses of the distal mesentery allows deposition and growth)

  CT Mesenteric infiltrates ▶ peritoneal implants ▶ omental 'caking' ▶ ileal loop separation with angled tethering of the mucosal folds
- *'Palisading':* the narrowed loops may align in a parallel configuration

Blood borne embolic metastases These are rare ▶ the common primaries are the lung, breast, kidneys and melanoma ▶ the resultant intraluminal soft tissue masses may lead to intussusception
- Small, focal, nodular or infiltrating obstructive lesions
- Metastatic melanomas appear as multiple submucosal polypoid lesions ▶ the central ulceration gives a 'bull's eye' or 'target' appearance on a BaFT

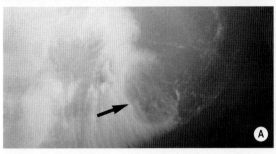
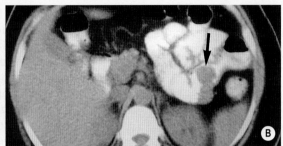

Benign stromal tumour. (A) BaFT reveals an intraluminal mass (arrow) on compression. (B) The tumour is also visible on CT (arrow).†

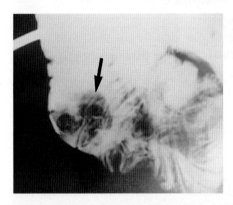

BaFT reveals an ileal hamartoma (arrow) in Peutz–Jeghers syndrome.

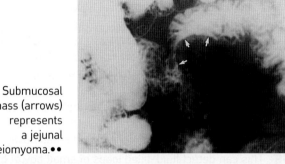

Submucosal mass (arrows) represents a jejunal leiomyoma.••

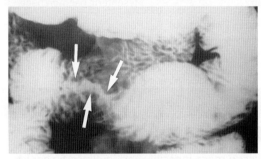

Small bowel adenocarcinoma (between arrows).†

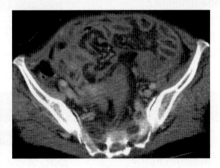

Peritoneal carcinomatosis involving the small bowel wall. CT enteroclysis demonstrates irregular thickening of the small bowel wall—more pronounced at the right lower abdomen—confluent and adhered intestinal loops and lumen narrowing or lack of distensibility due to numerous, small, malignant peritoneal implants from ovarian carcinoma, 'covering' the surface of the small bowel wall. Mesenteric infiltration is also present.**

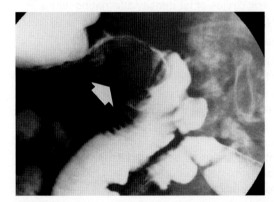

Carcinoid tumour. A round, well-defined, intraluminal filling defect (arrow) is seen in the distal ileum of a patient who presented with symptoms of intermittent obstruction but without any manifestations of the carcinoid syndrome.*

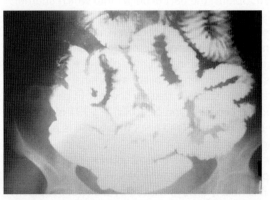

Lymphoma. Diffuse fold thickening and nodularity.†

MECHANICAL SMALL BOWEL OBSTRUCTION

Causes

- **Mural lesions:** tumour ▶ Crohn's stricture ▶ irradiation ▶ ischaemia
- **Luminal lesions:** bezoar ▶ gallstone ▶ *Ascaris lumbricoides* bolus ▶ intussusception
- **Extrinsic lesions:** volvulus ▶ abdominal malignancy
  - *Adhesions:* this accounts for 75% of cases in developed countries
  - *Hernias:* this accounts for 75% of cases in underdeveloped countries

Radiological features

Erect AXR This is not routinely performed ▶ >2 fluid levels within dilated (> 2.5 cm) small bowel loops

Supine AXR Small bowel dilatation (this can be gas or fluid filled, fluid-filled loops are not easily seen) ▶ collapsed colon ▶ a cause may be identified (e.g. an inguinal hernia may appear as a gas-filled viscus below the level of the inguinal ligament)

- *'String of beads' sign:* a line of gas bubbles trapped between the valvulae conniventes within almost completely fluid-filled and very dilated small bowel

US This can detect fluid-filled loops of small bowel but is rarely used

CT Adhesions are suggested by angulated and tethering of the bowel loops ▶ a cause may be identified (e.g. neoplasm)

- *'Transition point':* the definite point of obstruction, with dilated small bowel loops proximally and collapsed loops distally

- *Small bowel 'faeces sign':* presence of faeces-like material within small bowel proximal to an obstruction (stasis + water reabsorption)
- *Simple obstruction:* a transition zone may be seen with dilated small bowel loops proximal to the obstruction, and collapsed loops distally
- *Closed-loop obstruction:* a U- or V-shaped configuration of the dilated loops with a fixed radial distribution
- *Strangulated bowel:* this represents incarceration of the two limbs of the mechanical small bowel obstruction with subsequent ischaemia

CT signs*	
Closed-loop intestinal obstruction	**Strangulating obstruction**
Dilated fluid-filled loops	Wall thickening of affected loop
U- or C-configuration	High attenuation* in bowel wall
Thickening of mesenteric vessels	Gas in bowel wall
Radial spread of mesenteric vessels	Gas in mesenteric veins
Tapering of the loop ('beak' sign)	Mesenteric congestion
Triangular loop	Mesenteric haemorrhage
Twisted mesentery ('whirl' sign)	Poor or no contrast enhancement
*Representing haemorrhage	

INTUSSUSCEPTION

Definition

- Telescoping of a segment of proximal bowel into a segment of distal bowel
  - *Intussuscipiens:* the part of bowel into which another part is prolapsed
  - *Intussusceptum:* the part of bowel that has prolapsed
- **Children:** a common surgical emergency a (peak incidence between 5 and 9 months of age) ▶ presents with intermittent colicky abdominal pain and 'redcurrant jelly' stools ▶ usually ileocolic (it can also be ileo-ileocolic, ileo-ileal and colocolic) ▶ >90% of children have no demonstrable lead point (the cause is often lymphoid hypertrophy)
  - *Other causes:* Meckel's diverticulum ▶ intestinal polyp ▶ duplication cyst ▶ lymphoma
- **Adults:** it is nearly always caused by a bowel neoplasm ▶ a colonic lipoma, lymphoma and melanoma metastases are other causes

Radiological features

AXR A soft tissue mass (possibly part-outlined by gas) ▶ if orientated end-on a target sign may be seen (consisting of two concentric circles of fat density alternating with soft tissue density) ▶ small bowel obstruction

US A 'pseudotumour' or 'kidney' sign

CT The intussusceptum brings the mesenteric fat into the lumen of the intussuscipiens ▶ an intussusception appears as a sausage-shaped mass or as a 'target' mass (depending on its orientation)

Pearls

- **Treatment:** pneumatic air reduction under fluoroscopic guidance or hydrostatic reduction under US control ▶ this is contraindicated if there is free gas present, septicaemic shock or peritonitis
- **Pneumatic reduction:** this should only use a maximum pressure of 120 mmHg
  - 3 attempts for 3 minutes is recommended (initially at a pressure of 60–80 mmHg)

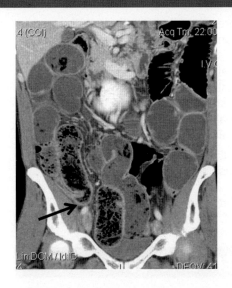

Small bowel obstruction. Contrast-enhanced CT, coronal reformation image demonstrates the small bowel 'faeces sign' proximal to the transition zone (arrow).**

Adhesive small bowel obstruction. Coronal reformat CECT shows the transition zone (white arrow), distended, fluid-filled proximal jejunal loops and collapsed distal loops (black arrow). No mass is seen. *If the bowel becomes oedematous (e.g. ischaemia) these folds may become thickened and difficult to distinguish from colonic haustra.*

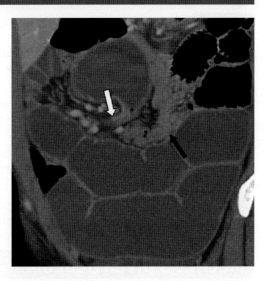

Distiniguishing features of small and large bowel dilatation		
	Small bowel dilatation	**Large bowel dilatation**
Number of bowel loops	Usually numerous	Fewer loops
Distribution of bowel	Central abdomen	Peripheral abdomen
Size of bowel	Rarely >5 cm	Often >5 cm
Fold pattern	Valvulae conniventes: thin complete bands across the small bowel ▶ the folds are closer together than colonic haustra ▶ they are most prominent in the jejunum	Colonic haustra: these are usually thick incomplete bands ▶ they may be absent from the descending and sigmoid colon
Bowel contents	Fluid and gas	Faeces and gas

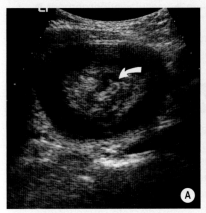 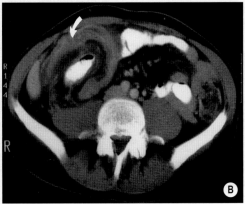

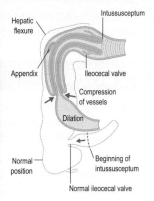

Schematic representation of an ileocolic intussusception.

Ileocolic lymphoma leading to ileocolic intussusception. (A) US image of the right iliac fossa showing the 'pseudotumour' or 'kidney' sign. The ileum can be seen centrally (arrow), surrounded by mesenteric fat that is hyperechoic, all within the thickened ascending colon. (B) CT showing oral contrast medium in the ileal lumen, the surrounding mesenteric fat accompanying the intussusceptum and the thickened ascending colon, which is the intussuscipiens (arrow).*

JEJUNAL DIVERTICULA

Definition Mucosal herniation through the jejunal wall ▶ these are uncommon
- *Ileal diverticula:* these are rarer still (affecting the mesenteric border of the terminal ileum) ▶ they are also smaller and fewer in number

Clinical presentation The 'blind loop' syndrome (due to bacterial overgrowth): abdominal pain + distension + weight loss + a megaloblastic anaemia
- *Less common complications:* acute diverticulitis ± perforation ▶ a mesenteric abscess ▶ bleeding or small bowel obstruction

BaFT A relatively large narrow-necked outpouching affecting the mesenteric border ▶ they are usually multiple

MECKEL'S DIVERTICULUM

Definition An ileal outpouching following failure of the yolk sac to close during fetal life ▶ they are found in up to 3% of the population
- *Location:* the antimesenteric border of the ileum (30–90 cm from the ileocaecal valve and measuring between 0.5 and 13 cm)
- Ectopic gastric mucosa can be found within a diverticulum in 20% of adults and 95% of children presenting with bleeding
- *Complications:* ulceration ▶ bleeding ▶ perforation ▶ inflammation ▶ intussusception ▶ internal herniation ▶ volvulus ▶ adhesions

⁹⁹ᵐTc-pertechnetate Increased uptake if gastric mucosa is present ▶ this is more accurate in children

Enteroclysis A blind-ending sac arising from the antimesenteric border of the ileum ▶ a triradiate pattern of mucosal folds may be seem at the diverticulum base

Angiography It can demonstrate a persistent vitelline artery in patients presenting with chronic bleeding

WHIPPLE'S DISEASE

Definition A rare chronic bacterial infection with *Tropheryma whippelii* (a Gram-positive bacillus) causing abdominal pain, diarrhoea, malabsorption, adenopathy and polyarthritis

BaFT Thickened valvulae conniventes (often with a micronodular appearance within the proximal small intestine)

CT Non-specific bowel wall thickening ▶ low-density retroperitoneal and mesenteric lymphadenopathy (due to an increased amount of fat and fatty acids)

SMALL BOWEL FISTULAE

Definition These are associated with Crohn's disease, diverticulitis, malignancy (e.g. colorectal cancer) and in the postoperative patient
- *Enterocolonic:* small bowel to colon
- *Enteroenteric:* small bowel to small bowel
- *Enterocutaneous:* small bowel to skin
- *Enterovaginal:* small bowel to vagina
- *Enterovesical:* small bowel to bladder

Fistulogram This allows assessment via the use of water-soluble contrast injected into the fistula (using a small catheter)
- *Alternative methods of diagnosis:* a small bowel FT or barium enema ▶ CT or MRI (with oral contrast medium)

ACUTE MESENTERIC ISCHAEMIA

Definition A compromised small intestinal blood supply due to mesenteric arterial embolism or thrombosis, mesenteric venous occlusion or low flow states

Clinical presentation Severe abdominal pain (which can be out of proportion to the clinical signs) ▶ a lactic acidosis (due to infarcted tissue)

CT Dual-phase imaging with oral (water) and IV contrast medium is required for accurate mesenteric vessel evaluation
- *Thrombus:* a filling defect within a mesenteric artery or vein
- *Acute transmural infarction:* mural thinning ▶ small bowel dilatation ▶ reduced/absent mural enhancement
- *Non-occlusive mesenteric ischaemia:* mural thickening ▶ mucosal hyperenhancement
- *Ischaemia due to mesenteric venous thrombosis:* marked mural thickening ▶ mucosal hyperenhancement ▶ mesenteric stranding ▶ vascular engorgement ▶ ascites
  - *Late signs:* pneumatosis ▶ mesenteric or portal venous gas represents irreversible ischaemia

NODULAR LYMPHOID HYPERPLASIA

Definition This is a normal finding within the terminal ileum in children or young adults
- In older adults it is associated with immunoglobulin deficiency (particularly late-onset hypogammaglobulinaemia)

BaFT Multiple small (1–3 mm) discrete round lesions throughout the small intestine (increasing in number as one travels distally) ▶ the colon is frequently involved throughout its length

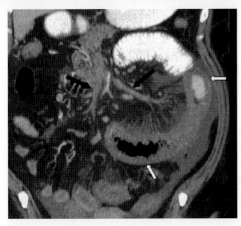

Mesenteric venous thrombosis. CECT, coronal reformation image shows circumferential thickening of distended jejunal loops (white arrows) and haziness of the adjacent mesentery. Non-opacification of superior mesenteric and jejunal branches is noted (black arrows). Ascites is also present.*

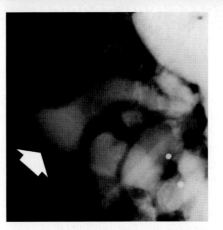

Meckel's diverticulum. Follow through study demonstrating a blind-ending sac is shown arising from the antimesenteric border of the distal ileum (arrow).*

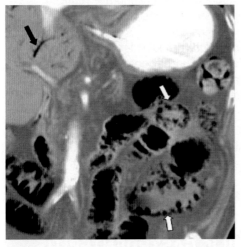

Small bowel infarction. CECT shows pneumatosis of small bowel loops (white arrows) and hepatic portal vein gas (black arrow).

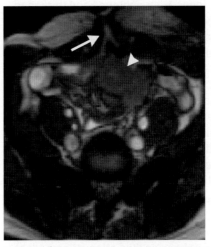

Enterocutaneous fistula. Axial true FISP showing a high SI fistula extending from an inflamed loop of small bowel (arrowhead) to skin (arrow) in a patient with Crohn's disease.*

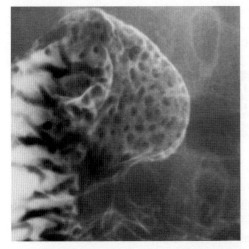

Lymphoid hyperplasia. Multiple small filling defects characteristic of lymphoid hyperplasia are shown on a double-contrast view of the duodenal cap.*

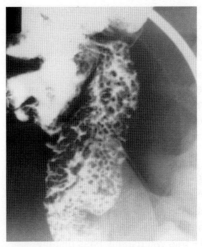

Follow through study demonstrating terminal ileum nodular lymphoid hyperplasia.

COELIAC DISEASE (NON-TROPICAL SPRUE/GLUTEN-SENSITIVE ENTEROPATHY)

Definition

- *Non-tropical sprue (coeliac disease):* a disorder of the small intestinal mucosa caused by intolerance to α gliaden (a component of gluten) ▶ it tends to affect the more proximal small bowel
  - Genetically susceptible individuals are usually children or young adults
- *Tropical sprue:* a malabsorption state seen within tropical countries and which affects the entire small bowel ▶ there is a possible infective aetiology (it is distinct from coeliac disease)

Clinical presentation Symptoms are secondary to malabsorption: diarrhoea ▶ weight loss ▶ steatorrhoea ▶ malnutrition ▶ anaemia ▶ abdominal pain

BaFT Dilated bowel loops ▶ straightened and thickened jejunal valvulae conniventes

- *Flocculation:* a coarse appearance of small clumps of disintegrated barium (due to the increased intestinal fluid)
- *Segmentation:* of a normally continuous barium column
- *'Moulage' sign:* mucosal atrophy and absence of valvulae
- *'Jejunization' of the ileum:* the presence of numerous mucosal folds within the ileum (reversal of the normal jejunoilieal fold pattern)
- *'Colied spring' appearance:* due to a transient non-obstructive intussusception

CT As above but also: bowel wall thickening ▶ small volume ascites ▶ vascular engorgement ▶ low attenuation mesenteric lymphadenopathy ▶ cavitating mesenteric lymph nodes (thin rim-enhancing fluid attenuation nodes)

Pearls

- **Diagnosis:** this is based upon an abnormal villous pattern detected with a peroral jejunal biopsy (radiological investigation is generally reserved for those with a normal biopsy or suspected complications)
- **Associated disorders:** dermatitis herpetiformis ▶ IgA deficiency ▶ hyposplenism
- **Complications:** there is an increased risk of GI T-cell lymphoma or oesophageal and jejunal carcinoma
  - *Ulcerative jejunoileitis:* segments of bowel wall thickening with irregularity and ulceration

GALLSTONE ILEUS

Definition A rare condition caused by a gallstone eroding through an inflamed gallbladder and passing into the adjacent duodenum – this will usually pass distally until it impacts at the narrowed terminal ileum (causing obstruction)

- *Bouveret's syndrome:* the gallstone passes proximally into the stomach

AXR/CT Small bowel obstruction ▶ an obstructing gallstone within the pelvis ▶ gas within the biliary tree (due to retrograde passage of air from the duodenum through the fistula)

- *Gas within the liver parenchyma:* biliary gas tends to normally be centrally located (portal venous gas will tend to have a more peripheral distribution)

PROGRESSIVE SYSTEMIC SCLEROSIS (SCLERODERMA)

Definition A collagen vascular disease of unknown aetiology – smooth muscle atrophy is followed by collagen deposition and fibrosis ▶ it affects the skin, joints, blood vessels and viscera

BaFT A dilated duodenum and jejunum ▶ reduced peristalsis with an increased transit time ▶ pneumatosis intestinalis

- *Sacculations (pseudodiverticula):* large broad-based outpouchings with a squared contour seen on the antimesenteric small bowel border
- *'Hidebound' appearance:* an increased number of mucosal folds

Associations A dilated oesophagus and reflux oesophagitis (± stricture) ▶ soft tissue calcification ▶ pulmonary interstitial fibrosis ▶ acro-osteolysis

SMALL BOWEL DISORDERS DUE TO CELLULAR INFILTRATION: EOSINOPHILIC GASTROENTERITIS

Definition Eosinophilic infiltration of the walls of the stomach and small intestine

BaFT Thickened valvulae conniventes and mural thickening (± bowel obstruction) ▶ gastric nodularity ▶ a narrowed pyloric antrum

SMALL BOWEL DISORDERS DUE TO CELLULAR INFILTRATION: MASTOCYTOSIS

Definition This is due to mast cell infiltration of the small intestine ▶ skin infiltration causes a typical skin rash (urticaria pigmentosa)

- It is a associated with hepatomegaly, dense bones and peptic ulcer disease

BaFT Thickened valvulae conniventes ▶ 2–5 mm nodular mucosal defects – these are usually seen within short jejunal segments (they can also be seen within the ileum)

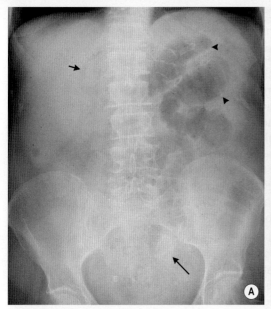

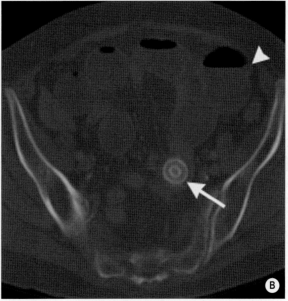

(A) Plain AXR demonstrating a pelvic gallstone (long arrow), small bowel obstruction (arrowheads) and gas within the biliary tree (short arrow). (B) CT confirming the laminated pelvic gallstone (arrow) and small bowel obstruction (arrowhead).

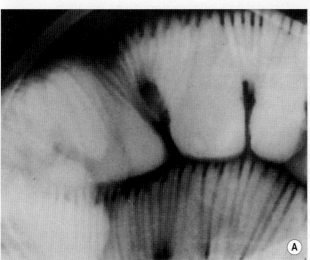

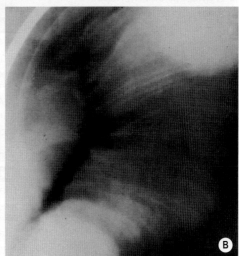

Systemic sclerosis. (A) Sacculation shown as broad-based outpouchings. (B) Dilatation of a segment of intestine with the 'hide-bound' appearance of the valvulae conniventes seen on a spot compression view.*

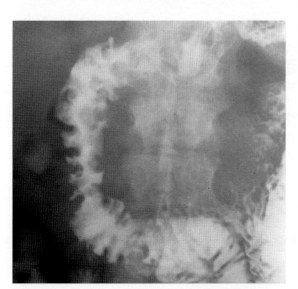

Mastocytosis. Nodular asymmetrical fold thickening of the duodenum is seen. Note sclerotic bones.••

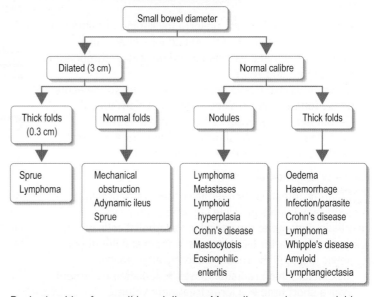

Basic algorithm for small bowel disease. Many diseases have a variable appearance.

Intestinal lymphangiectasia

Definition

- *Primary disease:* part of a generalized lymphatic channel hypoplasia (with generalized lymphoedema, chylous pleural effusions, malabsorption and lymphocytopenia) which is seen in children or young adults
- *Secondary disease:* lymph flow is obstructed by retroperitoneal fibrosis or malignant infiltration of the mesenteric and retroperitoneal lymph nodes

Radiological features

BaFT Non-specific uniformly thickened, closely set and parallel valvulae conniventes (± a micronodular mucosal surface pattern)

CT Mural thickening

AIDS

Definition The small bowel is affected in 50% of patients by opportunistic infections (commonly *M. avium-intracellulare* and cryptosporidiosis), Kaposi's sarcoma and AIDS-related lymphoma

Radiological features

BaFT Thickened (± nodular) valvulae conniventes within the proximal small intestine

CT Bulky retroperitoneal and mesenteric nodal masses are seen that are often indistinguishable from Kaposi's sarcoma or lymphoma

Graft-versus-host disease

Definition

- This develops following an allogenic bone marrow transplantation – the foreign donor lymphoid graft tissue mounts an immunological reaction against the hosts skin, liver and GI tract

Radiological features

BaFT

- *Acute phase (4–15 days):* uniform thickening or flattening of the mucosal folds ▶ a thickened intestinal wall ▶ ribbon-like luminal narrowing and ulceration throughout the jejunum and ileum
- *Subacute phase (13–96 days):* this is similar to the acute phase (often with a striking segmental distribution)
- *Resolution phase:* improvement is demonstrated (with no mucosal fold abnormality) but there is mural thickening confined to the terminal ileum

Chronic radiation enteritis

Definition Intestinal ischaemia secondary to previous radiotherapy (with a possible lag time of 25 years) ▶ it results in damage to the vascular endothelial cells which leads to an endarteritis obliterans ▶ the distal ileum (esp. its pelvic loops) is the most frequently affected region

- *Risk factors:* high radiation doses ▶ radiation treatment over a short time ▶ a large treatment volume

Clinical presentation Colicky abdominal pain ▶ diarrhoea ▶ malabsorption ▶ intermittent small intestinal obstruction

Radiological features

BaFT Thickened valvulae conniventes ▶ mural thickening ▶ effacement of the mucosal pattern ▶ ulceration, fixation and angulation of the small intestinal loops ▶ luminal narrowing and stenosis ▶ sinus and fistulae formation (uncommon) ▶ linear streaks of increased attenuation within the mesenteric fat (secondary to oedema)

- *'Mucosal tacking':* spiking and distortion of antimesenteric mucosal folds (caused by adhesions to inflamed and thickened mesentery) ▶ mesenteric retraction

CT This is best for assessing any mural thickening

- *Acute phase:* a target configuration (due to oedema and inflammation)
- *Chronic healing fibrotic phase:* homogeneous mural thickening

Non-steroidal anti-inflammatory drugs (NSAIDs)

Definition Patients may develop non-specific small intestinal ulceration (with blood and protein loss) on long-term treatment

Radiological features

BaFT Concentric, circumferential diaphragm-like narrowings (submucosal fibrosis secondary to focal ulceration) ▶ this may progress to stricture formation

Amyloidosis

Definition Infiltration of the GI tract with amyloid occurs in the majority of patients with primary amyloidosis

Radiological features

BaFT Amyloid deposition can cause symmetrical thickening or effacement of the valvulae conniventes (as well as atrophy) ▶ intraluminal masses of amyloid ▶ bowel dilatation

CT Non-specific symmetric wall thickening

Behçet's disease

Definition A chronic multisystem vasculitis involving the mucocutaneous, ocular, cardiovascular, gastrointestinal and central nervous systems

Radiological features It resembles ileocaecal tuberculosis or Crohn's disease

BaFT Deep discrete ulceration leading to haemorrhage or perforation

CT A polypoid mucosa with wall thickening and marked enhancement ▶ there is little adenopathy, fibrofatty change or pericolonic inflammation unless perforation has occurred (cf. Crohn's)

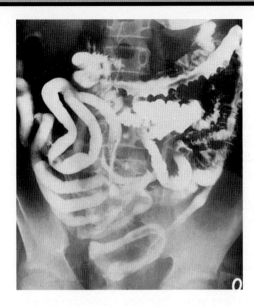

Graft-versus-host disease. Diffuse effacement of small and large bowel folds are seen. Note the ribbon-like appearance of small bowel.••

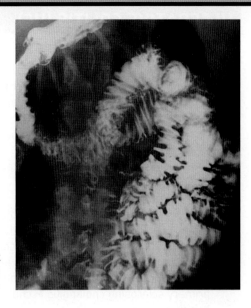

M. avium-intracellulare in a patient with AIDS. Diffuse small bowel fold thickening is seen.••

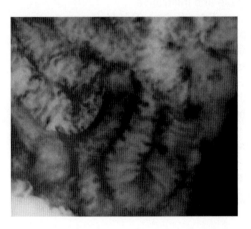

Lymphangiectasia. Diffuse small bowel fold thickening is seen.••

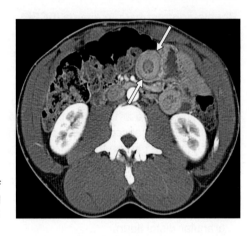

Patient with AIDS and involvement of the small bowel. Note the thickened wall (arrows).••

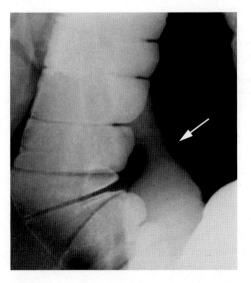

Radiation stricture. This spot view of a barium infusion examination shows a short, tight stricture of the terminal ileum in a patient who 4 years earlier had undergone radiotherapy for carcinoma of the uterus.*

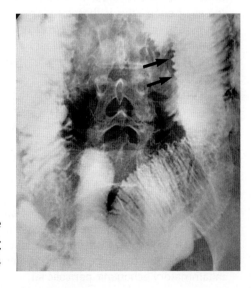

BaFT in a patient with extensive radiation enteritis reveals strictures, dilatation and a 'picket-fence' appearance (arrows).†

3.5 COLON

ULCERATIVE COLITIS (UC)

Definition

- A relapsing and remitting inflammatory bowel disease predominantly involving the colorectal mucosa and submucosa ▶ there is symmetrical colonic involvement (cf. asymmetrical Crohn's disease)
- It always involves the rectum – any remaining colitis is in continuity with its proximal extent
  - *Proctitis:* inflammatory changes limited to the rectum

Clinical presentation

- Bloody diarrhoea (± constitutional symptoms) in young adults ▶ an acute fulminating colitis with a risk of perforation (15%) ▶ extracolonic manifestations:
  - Synovitis ▶ ankylosing spondylitis ▶ sacroiliitis ▶ erythema nodosum ▶ pyoderma gangrenosum ▶ primary sclerosing cholangitis ▶ cholangiocarcinoma ▶ iritis

Radiological features

Double-contrast barium enema (DCBE)

- **Crypt abscesses:** may erode through the muscularis mucosae and spread laterally within the submucosa:
  - *En face appearance:* linear, transverse, serpiginous or rounded
  - *Tangential appearance:* undercutting of the mucosal edge can give a 'T' or 'collar stud' shape
- Ruptured crypt abscesses lead to superficial erosions which fill with barium to produce a typical granular mucosal pattern (producing continuous ulceration on a background of diffusely abnormal mucosa – discrete ulceration with normal intervening mucosa is not seen)
- **Reflux ileitis:** there is a patulous ileocaecal valve and a granular distal ileum
- **Postinflammatory polyps:** when an acute attack remits, the granulation tissue forming at the ulcer base undermines the residual oedematous mucosal flap at the ulcer edge – this is therefore prevented from sealing down, resulting in sessile, filiform, frond-like polyps (less commonly found in Crohn's disease)
- **Chronic colitis:** a tubular, shortened, featureless ('lead-pipe') colon
- **Strictures:** chronic hypertrophy of the muscularis mucosa (and submucosal thickening with fat) can cause generalized colonic shortening as well as localized left-sided colonic strictures (10–20%) ▶ the strictures are smooth, tapering and symmetrical (cf. asymmetrical strictures in Crohn's disease)

US

- Wall thickening (≥4 mm) ▶ a stratified appearance with differentiation between the submucosa and muscularis propria ▶ ulceration (with focal disruption of the bowel wall layers which may be outlined by intracolonic gas) ▶ inflammatory echogenic pericolic fat

CT

- *Acute disease:* wall thickening (≥4 mm) tending to be less marked than with Crohn's disease ▶ absence of formed faecal residue within any affected segments ▶ normal pericolonic tissues (unless perforation has occurred)
- *Chronic disease:* a widened presacral space due to fibrofatty proliferation
- *'Target' sign:* due to chronic muscularis mucosae thickening and fatty submucosal infiltration (visible even with NECT)
- Increasing wall thickness and contrast enhancement (particularly in a layered pattern) correlate with disease activity

Pearls

- There is an increased risk of colorectal carcinoma (due to dysplastic changes within diseased epithelium rather than from a prior adenoma) – this is more common with an extensive colitis of >10 years duration ▶ tumours are frequently multiple and infiltrative
  - *Dysplasia-associated lesions (DALMs):* representing severe dysplasia and are a very high risk marker for cancer (similar to a villous adenoma)
  - *Early infiltrative carcinoma:* this presents with a fixed, irregular, in-drawn base
  - *Strictures:* these are usually benign ▶ malignancy is suggested by an irregular raised area, shouldering or asymmetry
- **Complications:** toxic megacolon ▶ perforation

TOXIC MEGACOLON

Definition

- A fulminating colitis: transmural inflammation and ulceration extends deep into the muscular layers with neuromuscular degeneration ▶ it accounts for most UC-related deaths
- It can also occur in any other cause of colitis but is less frequently seen in Crohn's disease, bacterial colitis, pseudomembranous colitis or ischaemic colitis

Radiological features

- It usually affects the transverse colon (the least dependent part of the colon where intraluminal gas collects) ▶ perforation is frequent
  - **Dilatation:** if >5 cm it is associated with deep ulceration into the muscular layers (>8.5 cm in established cases) ▶ the haustra are always absent, and toxic megacolon should not be diagnosed if they are present
- A daily plain AXR is important for assessing and monitoring the colitis extent (barium studies are contraindicated due to the perforation risk)

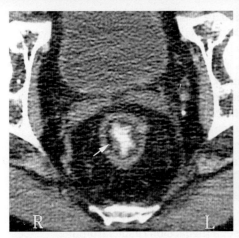

Chronic UC with mesorectal lipohyperplasia causing widening of the post-rectal space. There is increased submucosal fat (arrow) creating a target sign in this NECT.*

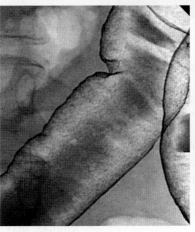

The granular mucosa typical of UC. Note the intact mucosal line.*

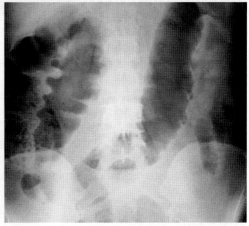

Toxic megacolon. Luminal dilatation, abnormal haustration, mural thickening and mucosal islands. Mucosal islands represent oedematous mucosal remnants.†

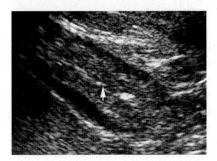

Stratified wall thickening in UC on US. The outer low reflective muscle layer is well defined, but the thickened mucosa/ submucosa are poorly distinguished. The mucosal surface is indicated by the bright central reflective line (arrow).*

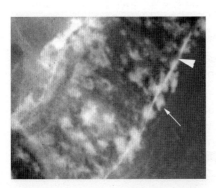

DCBE in an acute attack of UC with collar stud ulcers (arrow) protruding through the mucosal line (arrowhead).*

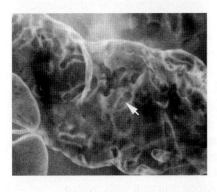

Filiform postinflammatory polyposis (arrow) following an acute attack of UC. The mucosal surface and haustration are normal as the colitis was inactive.*

Distinguishing features between ulcerative and Crohn's colitis*		
Radiographic feature	**Ulcerative colitis**	**Crohn's disease**
SB involvement	Reflux ileitis only	+++
Rectal involvement	Always	50%
Multiple anal fistula	–	+
Aphthoid ulceration	–	+++
Fissuring ulceration	–	++
Granularity	+++	+
Transverse symmetry	Symmetric	Asymmetric
Longitudinal extent	In continuity	Discontinuous
Free perforation	+	–
Toxic megacolon	+	–/+
Cancer risk	+	–/+
Entero-enteric fistula	–	+
Submucosal inflammation	++ in chronic disease	–
Mesenteric inflammation	–/+	++
Enlarged lymph nodes	–	+
Fibrofatty proliferation	Mesorectal only	++
Pathological process	Limited to mucosa	Transmural inflammation

ISCHAEMIC COLITIS

Definition This is a common cause of colitis in the elderly, often involving the splenic flexure or proximal descending colon (the 'watershed' areas) ▶ it is associated with bacterial superinfection

- *Mild disease:* initially the mucosa is the most susceptible to vascular compromise (with oedema, haemorrhage or necrosis) ▶ recovery is usually complete
- *Severe disease:* necrosis of the submucosal and muscle layers leads to fibrosis and stricture formation ▶ transmural necrosis is life-threatening (due to the risk of perforation)

Clinical presentation Disease commonly affects the SMA or IMA distributions:

- *SMA:* these are very unwell patients (they are acidotic ± abdominal pain) ▶ it often requires surgery
- *IMA:* this has a less acute presentation (and can mimic diverticulitis) ▶ it can be treated conservatively

AXR A narrowed colon (secondary to stricture formation) ▶ mucosal thumb-printing (due to submucosal haemorrhage and oedema) ▶ free air (secondary to perforation) ▶ colonic sacculation

CT Colonic wall thickening (this is more marked with venous occlusion but does not correspond with the extent of necrosis) ▶ submucosal oedema can cause a 'target' sign

- *Transmural necrosis:* mesenteric fat stranding ▶ free fluid ▶ pneumatosis ▶ portomesenteric gas
- *'Shock' bowel:* there is increased mural enhancement (due to the generalized low perfusion state) ▶ there can be a 'slit-like' IVC (as a result of the low intravascular volume)

Pearls Causes of ischaemic colitis:

- *Mesenteric occlusion:* this can be arterial or venous in origin
- *Mechanical obstruction:* secondary to bowel strangulation or obstruction
- *Low flow states*

INFECTIOUS COLITIS

- **Salmonella:** there may be a marked ileus during the acute stage ▶ a toxic megacolon has been reported
- **Shigella:** this usually affects the sigmoid colon (with aphthoid-type ulceration)
- **Campylobacter:** this affects the distal colon
- **Gonococcus:** this usually affects the rectum
- **Amoebiasis:** this usually affects the right colon and caecum
  - It leads to a segmental or diffuse colitis with granular or ulcerated mucosa (± aphthoid-type ulceration)
  - An amoeboma (an inflammatory granulation mass) is seen in 10% of cases – it can cause irregular stricturing (mimicking a carcinoma)
  - Disease is limited to the caecum in 3% of cases, producing a characteristic conical caecum and a shaggy ulcerated mucosa ▶ it may be complicated by appendicitis
  - Embolic liver spread is seen in 15% of cases

- **Cytomegalovirus:** this demonstrates an ileocolic distribution ▶ there is a thick-walled vasculitis with large bleeding ulcers ▶ mesenteric adenopathy and often ascites is present
- **Herpes simplex virus:** this leads to a proctitis with multiple superficial ulcers
- **Chlamydia trachomatis:** this causes lymphogranuloma venereum, which is a chronic proctitis complicated by fistula formation, extensive fibrosis and eventual stricturing

PARASITIC COLITIS

- **Strongyloides stercoralis:** this may simulate UC
- **Chagas' disease:** a megacolon results from the neurotoxic effect of the protozoon *Trypanosoma cruzi*
- **Schistosomiasis:** ova are deposited within the large bowel submucosa ▶ the inflammatory response results in polyp formation ▶ fibrosis may later cause stricture formation (± bowel wall calcification)

RADIATION COLITIS

Definition This is caused by a radiation-induced occlusive endarteritis with thrombosis and fibrosis ▶ it is a late complication (often presenting years after radiotherapy when the total dose is >45 Gy)

- *Acute stage:* mucosal injury with an acute colitis
- *Chronic stage:* proctitis (± ulceration) ▶ strictures are usually smooth and symmetrical unless there is superimposed ulceration ▶ fistula formation is commonly to the bladder or vagina ▶ perforation is rare

CT Wall thickening ▶ increased mesorectal fat and a thickened mesorectal fascia ▶ a widened presacral space

NEUTROPENIC COLITIS

Definition This is usually due to chemotherapy with bone marrow transplantation

CT A thickened right-sided bowel wall (usually less than pseudomembranous colitis) ▶ pneumatosis ▶ mesenteric stranding and small bowel involvement is common

- *Typhlitis:* changes limited to the caecum

PSEUDOMEMBRANOUS COLITIS

Definition A left-sided or pancolitis due to cytoplasmic endotoxin produced by overgrowth of *Clostridium difficile* ▶ it is usually as a result of broad-spectrum antibiotic therapy and may be life-threatening

XR A generalized ileus and nodular haustral thickening ▶ mucosal thumbprinting

CT Gross colonic wall thickening (average 1.5 cm) ▶ ascites ▶ small bowel dilatation ▶ marked mucosal enhancement + low attenuation from submucosal oedema

- There is minimal pericolonic fat stranding (cf. IBD)
- *'Accordion' sign:* the appearance of contrast between thickened low attenuation mucosal folds, with a prominent target sign

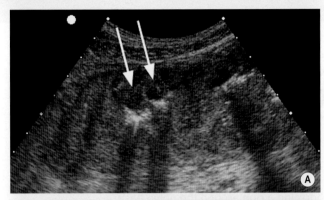

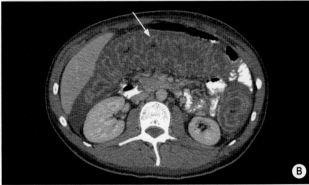

(A) Ultrasound showing florid bowel wall and haustral fold thickening (arrows) secondary to pseudomembranous colitis. (B) The corresponding CT confirms marked colonic thickening and mucosal hyperenhancement (arrow).**

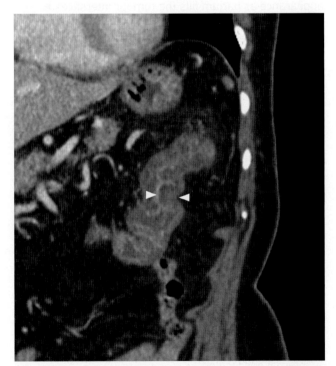

Coronal CT shows mural thickening (arrowheads) due to acute ischaemic colitis extending from around the splenic flexure distally. The entire descending colon was affected (not shown). The mucosa retains brisk enhancement.**

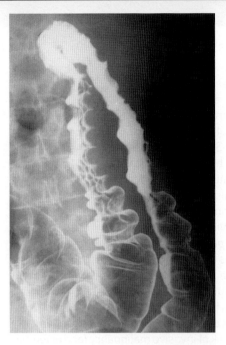

Classical splenic flexure 'thumb-printing' due to ischaemic colitis.†

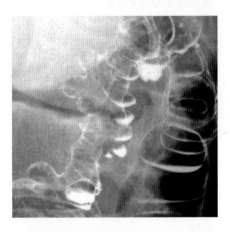

Ischaemic stricture at the splenic flexure with prominent sacculation.*

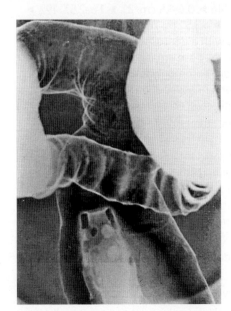

Rectosigmoid spot film in a patient with chronic radiation proctitis and sigmoiditis. There is general loss of haustral pattern with tubular appearance of the bowel.••

POLYPS

Definition An elevated colonic mucosal lesion

Types

Epithelial adenoma

- This is defined as a circumscribed area of dysplastic epithelium (an intraepithelial neoplasia) ▶ they are found in 25% of the population over 50 years old (they are rare in patients under 30 years of age)
- An adenoma can be tubular (65%), tubulovillous (25%) or villous (10%) in nature ▶ villous adenomas may present with electrolyte disturbances due to excessive mucous production ▶ villous adenomas are higher risk than tubular or tubulovillous lesions
  - *Pedunculated polyp:* extrusion of a stalk of mucosa and muscularis mucosae may occur as the adenoma is pulled by the faecal stream ▶ considered cured if resected and tumour confined to the stalk
  - *Sessile polyp:* a broad-based lesion (base must be at least twice that of its height) ▶ roughly hemispheric ▶ intermediate risk of invasive malignancy for a given size
  - *Flat polyp:* a lesion with a height that is no more than twice the height of the adjacent normal mucosa ▶ it is categorized into a slightly elevated, completely flat, or slightly depressed lesion ▶ flat depressed lesions carry a higher risk for invasive cancer for a given size – other subtypes are generally less aggressive ▶ can be challenging to detect on endoscopy and imaging
- *Location:* rectosigmoid colon (50%) ▶ descending colon (25%) ▶ transverse colon (10%) ▶ ascending colon and caecum (15%)
  - Adenomas tends to be larger when present within the left colon ($\frac{2}{3}$ of polyps >2 cm are within the rectosigmoid colon)
- Size is the most important single indicator for the likelihood of malignancy:
  - <5 mm: negligible ▶ 0.6–1.5 cm: 2% ▶ 1.6–2.5%: 19% ▶ 2.6–3.5 cm: 43% ▶ >3.5 cm: 76%
  - Flat adenomas with a depressed centre may be invasive even if they are small (<1 cm)
    - They are more commonly found within the right colon and in association with hereditary non-polyposis colorectal cancer (HNPCC) ▶ they may demonstrate a more rapid progression to overt cancer than a polypoid tumour

Non-epithelial Carcinoid ▶ leiomyoma ▶ lipoma ▶ fibroma

- *Lipoma:* a well-defined submucosal lesion ▶ it is usually a solitary right colonic lesion (and may cause pain, bleeding or intussusception if >4 cm)
  - *The 'squeeze' sign:* it is easily deformable during compression
    - **CT** This will easily demonstrate the inherent fat attenuation

Non-neoplastic Juvenile or postinflammatory polyps

Unclassified Hyperplastic polyps – these are usually small with a characteristic 'saw-toothed' epithelial lining ▶ they are common within the rectum ▶ there is no malignant potential unless they demonstrate a 'serrated' appearance

Radiological features

DCBE appearances of polyps

- Localized areas of increased attenuation (the incident X-ray beam passes through more than 2 barium layers and consequently less gas)
- A thin layer of contrast medium covers the mucosa, forming a ring around the polyp base
  - *Viewed en face:* this creates a ring shadow with a sharp inner border and an outer margin fading into the normal surface coating (cf. the opposite appearance with an ulcer)
  - *Viewed obliquely:* this produces the 'hat' sign
- *Pedunculated polyps:* the axis of the stalk usually runs obliquely to the lumen axis (making it easy to distinguish from a haustral fold)
  - *'Stalk' sign:* two parallel lines of barium
  - *'Target' sign:* the head and stalk are superimposed
- *Juvenile polyps:* these are smooth and pedunculated with a thin stalk (affecting patients <40 years old)
- *Postinflammatory polyps:* these have a filiform configuration (i.e. finger-like submucosal projections covered by mucosa on all sides)
- *Villous polyps:* these demonstrate a lace-like or mosaic appearance as barium fills the tumour interstices ▶ some may present as a flat, nodular, carpet-like growth (with minimal elevation) within the rectosigmoid colon or caecum

CT colonography (CTC) appearances of polyps

- CTC is equivalent to colonoscopy in the detection of polyps >7 mm in size
- Technique: full bowel preparation is standard, although reduced preparation regimens with faecal tagging are being developed ▶ CO_2 distension is used (and improved with IV Buscopan) ▶ oral contrast agents to tag residual colonic contents as higher attenuation ▶ supine and prone sequences are reviewed to reduce the chance of any collapsed or fluid-filled segments hiding a lesion ▶ the original datasets and 3D reformatted images (which are useful for problem solving) are reviewed
  - *Pitfall:* an inverted diverticulum may simulate a polyp on 3D images (on 2D images it will contain gas)
- *Distinguishing a polyp from faecal residue:*
  - A polyp demonstrates homogeneous attenuation similar to bowel wall (unless it is a lipoma, when it will be of fat density) ▶ faecal residue often contains internal gas locules
  - A polyp tends to have a fixed position on the bowel wall (colon movement between supine and prone acquisitions may suggest polyp movement) – faecal residue will tend to fall onto the dependent colonic surface

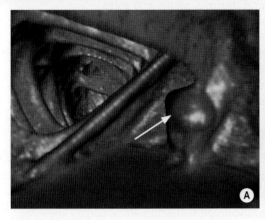 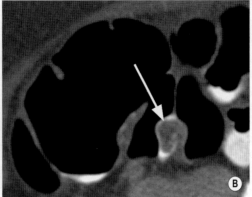

(A) Endoluminal CTC image depicts a polyp (arrow) growing on a haustral fold just above residual colonic fluid. (B) The corresponding 2D image shows a stalked lesion (arrow) coated by a thin rim of tagged fluid.**

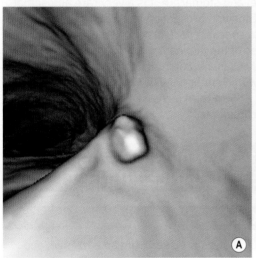 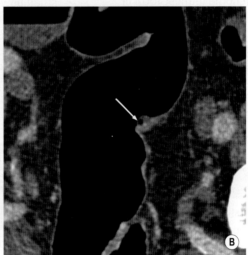

(A) 3D view from CT colonogram shows a polypoid lesion that might be mistaken for a sessile polyp. However, the 2D view (B) shows a tiny locule of gas (arrow), demonstrating that this is, in fact, retained faecal residue.**

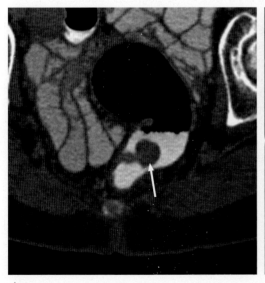 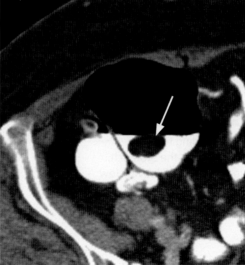

2D axial CT colonogram image shows a pedunculated rectal polyp (arrow) bathed by tagged fluid. Axial CT colonogram image with faecal tagging shows a smooth, lobulated fat-density polypoid lesion (arrow), diagnostic of a lipoma.**

FAMILIAL ADENOMATOUS POLYPOSIS (FAP)

DEFINITION

- An autosomal dominant condition (caused by an APC tumour suppression gene mutation on chromosome 5q21) ▶ it is characterized by multiple (500–2500) colonic adenomas and requires at least 100 adenomas to be present for the diagnosis to be made
  - The polyps develop by the early teens – all patients will eventually develop colorectal cancer (accounting for 1% of all colorectal cancers) ▶ a restorative proctocolectomy is recommended once the condition is diagnosed
  - *Associations:* hamartomatous stomach polyps (>50% of patients) ▶ duodenal adenoma (almost 100% of patients) ▶ periampullary carcinoma (5% of patients)

GARDNER'S SYNDROME

- This forms part of the FAP spectrum ▶ extracolonic manifestations include multiple skull and mandible osteomas, epidermoid cysts, soft tissue tumours, abnormal dentition and desmoid tumours

DESMOID TUMOUR

A benign fibromatous tumour involving the abdominal wall or small bowel mesentery ▶ it is only locally invasive and is often precipitated by surgery

CT Ill-defined mesenteric infiltration with small bowel tethering (giving a 'whorled' appearance) ▶ this occurs prior to the development of an overt mass ▶ it can cause ureteric or small bowel obstruction

MRI T2WI: high SI suggests active growth

PEUTZ-JEGHERS SYNDROME

DEFINITION

- An autosomal dominant condition leading to the presence of multiple hamartomas within the stomach, small bowel and colon (colonic polyps are relatively few but are larger, often pedunculated and may bleed)

  - *Associations:* mucocutaneous pigmentation of the lips, oral mucosa, palms and soles
  - There is no intrinsic malignant potential (although the overlying mucosa may become dysplastic with an increased risk of an upper GI tract cancer)
    - *There is an increased risk of an extraintestinal cancer:* ovary ▶ thyroid ▶ testis ▶ pancreas ▶ breast

JUVENILE POLYPOSIS

DEFINITION

- Smooth pedunculated hamartomatous polyps are found within the colon (50–200 polyps) as well as the small bowel and stomach ▶ it is a very rare autosomal dominant condition presenting in infancy
  - *'Swiss cheese' effect:* cystic epithelial tubules in excess of the lamina propria
- Epithelial dysplasia is common in young adults, occurring within either juvenile polyps or co-existing adenomas – there is an increased risk of developing a colorectal carcinoma

HEREDITARY NON-POLYPOSIS COLORECTAL CANCER (HNPCC)

DEFINITION

- With HNPCC, polyps are seen from an early age, and cancers occur at an earlier age than those seen in non-HNPCC patients ▶ autosomal dominant ▶ lifetime risk of CRC is 70–85% ▶ the diagnosis requires ('3-2-1' rule):
  - ≥3 relatives with colorectal cancer (one of which is a 1st-degree relative)
  - Cases over 2 or more generations
  - A colorectal carcinoma diagnosed before the age of 50 years
- *Location:* most lesions are within the proximal colon (70%) ▶ multiple tumours are common
- *Associations:* cancers of the breast, endometrium, ovary and pancreas

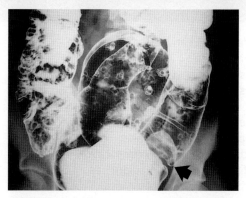

FAP – there are innumerable colonic adenomas. The patient refused surgery, with the inevitable consequence of a cancer (arrow).[†]

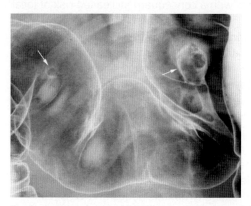

Peutz–Jeghers syndrome with a large pedunculated and smaller sessile polyp proximally (arrows).*

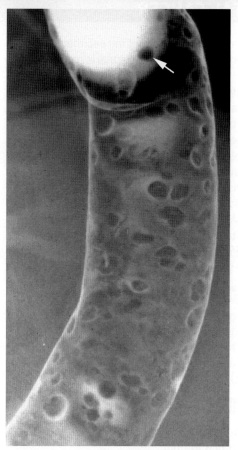

DCBE view of the descending colon in FAP with multiple small polyps about 5 mm in size, creating ring shadow menisci around their bases, or as a filling defect in the barium pool (arrow).*

Other rare polyposis syndromes		
Syndrome	**Inheritance**	**Manifestations**
Turcot's syndrome	Autosomal recessive	An association between colonic carcinoma, polyps and medulloblastoma
Cowden's syndrome	Autosomal dominant	Hamartomatous intestinal polyposis and lesions of the skin, mucous membranes, breast and thyroid
Muir–Torre syndrome	Autosomal dominant	Benign cutaneous sebaceous adenomas and keratoacanthomas ▶ it is associated with GI polyps and cancers in various sites
Cronkhite–Canada syndrome	Non-hereditary	Diffuse intestinal polyposis (usually colonic although the stomach and small bowel can be affected) ▶ it is associated with alopecia, skin hyperpigmentation and nail atrophy secondary to malabsorption ▶ it is rapidly fatal

Classification of polyps and polyposis syndrome*		
Histological type	**Single or few in number**	**Polyposis**
Epithelial	Adenoma – tubular, villous, tubulovillous Adenocarcinoma	Familial adenomatous polyposis, Turcot's syndrome, Cowden's disease
Harmatomatous	Juvenile Metaplastic	Juvenile polyposis Peutz–Jeghers syndrome Metaplastic polyposis
Inflammatory	Postinflammatory polyp	Postinflammatory polyposis
Non-epithelial	Lipoma, carcinoid, GIST, benign lymphoid, neurofibroma	Lymphomatous polyposis, metastatic neurofibromatosis
Miscellaneous	Endometriosis	Cronkhite-Canada syndrome

COLORECTAL CANCER

Definition Extension of a malignant intraepithelial neoplasia (adenoma) through the muscularis mucosae into the submucosa

- It generally develops from a polypoid adenoma over many years via a multistep accumulation of genetic faults (the adenoma to carcinoma sequence)
  - Familial Adenomatous Polyposis (FAP): 1%; Hereditary Non Polyposis Colorectal Cancer (HNPCC): 5–10%
  - There is also an increased risk with inflammatory bowel disease, obesity, red meat consumption, smoking and excess alcohol consumption
  - Aspirin/NSAIDs/low red meat diets + high in fibre may be protective
- Lifetime risk: 1 in 15 (men) ▶ 1 in 19 (women) ▶ 65% of cases are >60 years

Clinical presentation

- Change in bowel habit ▶ rectal bleeding ▶ abdominal pain ▶ bowel obstruction (<20% of cases)
  - *Generally:* fresh blood = a distal lesion ▶ altered blood or anaemia = a proximal lesion (e.g. involving the caecum)

Radiological features

Double-contrast barium enema This only demonstrates the luminal aspect of a tumour

- *Early:* sessile (plaque-like) lesion, or a pedunculated lesion
- *Late:* polypoid cancers have an irregular in-drawn base ▶ carpet lesions seen with malignant villous tumours
  - *'Apple-core' lesion:* an annular or semi-annular lesion with abrupt shouldered margins and an irregular narrow lumen

CT *This is generally used for assessing the presence of any metastatic disease and not for determining the local T staging*

- It demonstrates luminal and extraluminal disease, the extent of any wall thickening (normal colonic wall is <4 mm) and luminal narrowing ▶ tumour may appear as a focal soft tissue mass (± necrosis)
- *Extramural infiltration* (T3): suggested by (but not pathognomonic for): irregular projections from the serosal surface ▶ clouding of pericolic fat ▶ loss of normal fat planes ▶ thickened contiguous fascial reflections ▶ colonic segments with a mesentery are enveloped by visceral peritoneum and are more likely to be T4 tumours
- Extramural vascular invasion (EMVI) is suggested by nodular or undulating colic vein expansion
- *Tumour enhancement:* this is usually homogeneous ▶ heterogeneous enhancement can be seen with an abscess, large adenocarcinoma or a mucinous tumour
- *Intratumour calcification:* this is seen with mucinous adenocarcinomas

- *Enlarged nodes:* these can be due to reactive hyperplasia or metastatic involvement
  - A metastasis is suggested if a node measures >1 cm diameter (short axis) or if there is a cluster of >3 nodes
- *Intraperitoneal spread is indicated by:* ascites ▶ peritoneal deposits ▶ omental cake
- *Frail elderly patients:* a minimal preparation CT (1.5L 1% Gastrografin 48 h prior to imaging) has an 85% sensitivity for detecting CRC

MRI *This is used for the local staging of rectal cancer* (considered a separate entity to colon cancer as its pelvic location reduces the ability to obtain wide resection margins with a consequent increased risk of local recurrence)

- *It can assess for:* extramural spread ▶ peritoneal infiltration ▶ extramural venous involvement ▶ nodal involvement ▶ response to chemoradiotherapy
- **Bowel wall layers (T2WI):** *muscularis mucosa:* a fine low SI line ▶ *submucosa:* a thicker high SI layer ▶ *muscularis propria:* inner circular and outer longitudinal layer with an irregular grooved appearance ▶ *perirectal fat:* high SI ▶ *mesorectal fascia:* a fine low SI layer enveloping the perirectal fat
- **Mesorectal fascia:** encloses the mesorectum (which contains the draining lymphatic nodes and vessels) ▶ nodal spread usually occurs cranially within this compartment ▶ caudal spread and pelvic side wall involvement is unusual (caudal spread and associated inguinal lymph node involvement can occur if there is some impairment of the normal drainage pattern) ▶ total mesorectal excision (TME) without breach of the mesorectal fascia minimizes local recurrence
  - *Positive circumferential resection margin (CRM):* if there is tumour within 1 mm of the mesorectal fascia this requires preoperative chemotherapy
- **Local nodal involvement:** small nodes may still be involved by tumour ▶ malignant nodes tend to have an irregular border and demonstrate internal mixed SI ▶ it is important to record whether a suspicious node lies within 1 mm of the CRM
- **Extramural vascular invasion:** this describes the presence of tumour cells beyond the muscularis propria and within endothelial-lined vessels ▶ any extramural vascular invasion is further classified according to the number of vessels involved and whether they can be identified anatomically
- **Poor prognostic features:** increasing depth of extramural invasion ▶ nodal involvement ▶ involvement of the circumferential resection margin ▶ extramural vascular invasion
  - Low rectal tumours extending into the intersphincteric plane are high risk

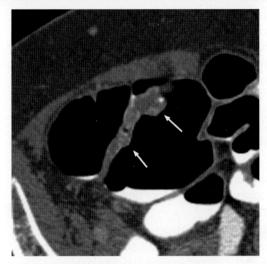

2D axial CT colonogram demonstrating a flat cancer manifesting as lobulated fold thickening (arrows).**

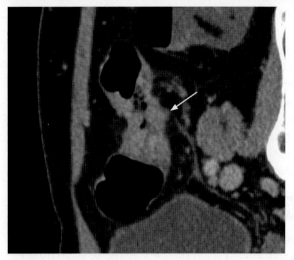

Sagittal oblique CT through a mid-sigmoid cancer shows an irregular outer margin (arrow) with soft tissue extending into the pericolic fat, indicating T3 disease.**

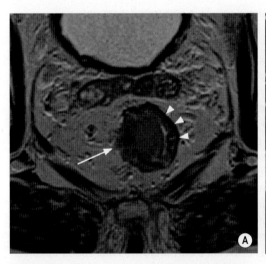

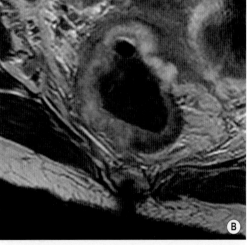

Axial T2-weighted MR through a mid-rectal cancer. The normal low-signal muscularis propria (arrowheads) is intact on the left but breached by intermediate signal tumour (arrow) between 8 and 9 o'clock, indicating T3 disease. The tumour is well away from the circumferential resection margin (A). Conversely, (B) shows a different patient, with tumour abutting the resection margin. Surgery will almost certainly leave a positive margin, and hence increase the risk of local recurrence.**

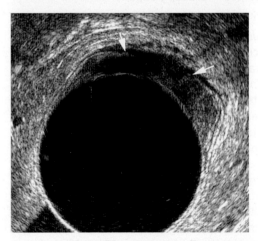

Endorectal US of a T2 rectal cancer. The submucosa is breached (white arrows) but the muscularis propria is intact.

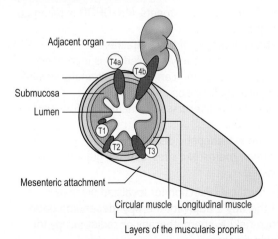

The layers involved in T1–T4 colorectal cancers according to the TNM, 7th edition. Note how the mesenteric attachments determine the likelihood of T3 versus T4a disease status.**

COLORECTAL CANCER

FDG PET-CT

- This is useful for detecting extracolonic disease (lesions >1 cm) ▶ it is the most accurate modality for detecting recurrent pelvic cancer (scar tissue does not demonstrate increased FDG PET uptake)

Endorectal US

- This allows for better differentiation of the rectal wall layers than MRI ▶ it is used to assess early tumour involvement and select T1N0 cases for local excision

PEARLS

Approximate distribution Rectum (35%) ▶ sigmoid colon (25%) ▶ descending colon (10%) ▶ transverse colon (10%) ▶ ascending colon (10%) ▶ caecum (10%)

- Right-sided tumours are more common in the elderly
- A primary scirrhous carcinoma with a pronounced desmoplastic reaction is very rare (and is indicated by long circumferential spread)

Liver metastases

- *Colon and upper rectum:* drainage is via the portal vein and therefore commonly leads to liver metastases (however metastatic deposits derive their blood supply from the hepatic artery and will therefore appear hypoattenuating on portal phase imaging)
- *Lower rectum:* drainage is via the portal vein as well as directly into the IVC (via the pelvic veins) ▶ metastases can therefore be to the liver but can also produce isolated pulmonary metastases (without liver involvement)
- *Mucinous tumours:* these produce cystic or calcified liver metastases ▶ there can be widespread peritoneal deposits
- *Liver-specific MR contrast agents:* Mn-DPDP is taken up by functioning hepatocytes
  - T1WI: the conspicuity of any metastases (demonstrating relatively reduced SI) is increased
- A partial hepatic resection can remove all anatomically resectable liver metastases as long as:
  - sufficient normal liver tissue remains to allow normal hepatic function
  - there is no extrahepatic disease
- *Other common metastatic sites:* adrenal glands ▶ bone (lytic deposits)

Treatment Surgical resection for localized disease ± neoadjuvant therapy ± adjuvant therapy (depending upon the recurrence risk) ▶ chemotherapy or radiotherapy for non-resectable disease

- Early T1 + T2 tumours can be treated with transanal endoscopic microsurgery (TEM) without the need for a full total mesorectal excision (TME)

- TME: en bloc resection of the rectal tumour, rectum and mesorectum – the dissection plane extends along the mesorectal fascia, constituting the circumferential resection margin (CRM)
  - Likely to have an involved CRM post surgery: preoperative downstaging with chemoradiotherapy
  - Intermediate risk not threatening the CRM: operative therapy ± preoperative radiotherapy
  - Low-risk tumours: surgery only

Differential Diverticulitis (which can appear very similar to a colonic tumour, especially if a tumour has perforated) ▶ ischaemic colitis ▶ inflammatory bowel disease ▶ local colonic spasm

Complications Colonic obstruction (with advanced disease) ▶ tumour perforation (with an adverse prognostic effect due to tumour dissemination and any local peritonitis) ▶ colonic intussusception (the tumour acts as the lead point) ▶ appendicitis presenting in the elderly (due to appendiceal obstruction by a caecal tumour)

Disease recurrence This commonly presents with pelvic pain ▶ rising CEA levels should prompt a search for recurrence ▶ it leads to a poor prognosis as most cases are unresectable

- *Common sites:* at the anastomotic site ▶ within the presacral region with soft tissue thickening ▶ a growing mesorectal nodule ▶ nodular thickening of the pelvic side wall ▶ peritoneal seeding (which is commonly seen within the pouch of Douglas or the lower right small bowel mesentery)
- **MRI:** T2WI: recurrence demonstrates higher SI than fibrosis (image after the first 6 months to allow for post-surgical resolution) ▶ there is possibly increased enhancement (and washout) demonstrated by tumour recurrence vs fibrosis
- **FDG-PET:** recurrence demonstrates increased uptake (fibrosis does not) ▶ probably superior to MRI

Dissemination of other tumours to the colon via

- *Direct invasion:* a gastric carcinoma may invade the transverse colon via the gastrocolic ligament and a pancreatic cancer via the transverse mesocolon
  - *Serosal involvement:* there is mass effect with a spiculated fold pattern due to the associated desmoplastic response
- *Intraperitoneal seeding:* affects surface of pelvic bowel loops/right paracolic gutter/colon ▶ omental caking is typical
- *Haematogenous spread:* breast carcinoma and melanoma tumour cells have a propensity to spread to the colon ▶ tumour cells embolize to the colonic vasa recta capillaries (presenting as submucosal masses on the antimesenteric border) ▶ these can be polypoid or umbilicated (due to a differential growth pattern between the centre and the periphery)
- *Along the mesenteric planes ▶ via lymphatic spread*

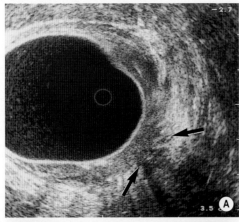

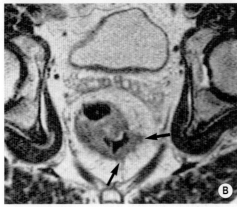

(A) Transrectal US reveals a T3 posterior tumour that has penetrated the muscularis propria to reach the surrounding tissue (arrows). (B) T2WI confirms the rectal wall penetration (arrows).

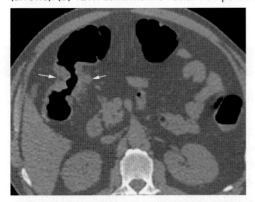

CTC of an annular carcinoma revealing the irregular lumen and thickened bowel wall (arrows).

MRI T staging of rectal cancer	
T1	Intermediate SI involving mucosa/submucosa
T2	Intermediate SI within the muscularis propria
T3	Intermediate SI nodularity projecting beyond the muscularis propria and into the perirectal fat
T4	Abnormal SI projecting beyond the serosa into an adjacent organ or structure, or tumours that have perforated the peritoneum

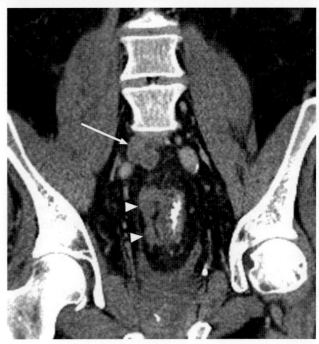

Coronal CT in this patient with a low rectal cancer demonstrates undulating expansion of a draining rectal vein (arrowheads), which is filled by abnormal soft tissue, typical of EMVI. There are abnormal lymph nodes (arrow) just below the aortic bifurcation.**

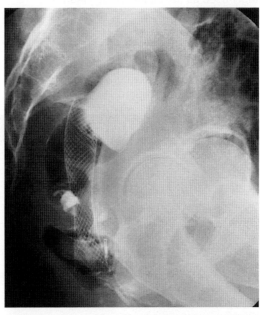

Self-expanding metal stent crossing a low rectal tumour.

Duke's classification	Description	5-year survival
A	Tumour limited to the rectal wall	85–95%
B	Tumour spread to the extrarectal tissues, no nodal spread	60–80%
C	Nodal spread	30–60%

DIVERTICULOSIS

Definition

Diverticulum A pouch of mucous membrane with a very thin covering of longitudinal muscle ▶ it arises between the mesenteric and antimesenteric taeniae at the points of weakness where the vasa recta penetrate the circular muscle layer

Diverticulosis The presence of colonic diverticula

Diverticulitis Inflammatory changes within one or more colonic diverticula (10% of patients with diverticulosis)

- It is caused by faecal retention within a diverticulum – this leads to ischaemic necrosis (± perforation)
- *Complications:* faecal peritonitis (rare) ▶ colonic bleeding due to weakening of the vasa recta walls – this can be profuse ▶ wider mouthed diverticulae in proximal colon appear more predisposed to haemorrhage ▶ abscess and fistula formation

Location Diverticulosis is commonest within the sigmoid colon ▶ localized to the proximal colon in only 10% (right-sided diverticulae tend to be larger with wider mouths)

- It is extremely rare within the rectum

Radiological features

CT Increasingly used as the initial investigation:
- *Diverticulosis:* multiple outpouchings from the bowel wall (± bowel wall thickening)
- *Diverticulitis:* diverticulosis + inflammation: mural thickening ▶ pericolic 'fat stranding' and oedema producing a generalized increase in attenuation ▶ colonic obstruction (10% perforation)

- *Mild disease:* minimal wall thickening (4–5 mm) ▶ inflammatory changes within pericolic fat only
- *Moderate disease:* abscess formation
- *Severe disease:* wall thickening >5 mm ▶ perforation ▶ large abscess (>5 cm) formation ▶ inflammatory extension into the pelvis
- *Pericolic abscess* (35%): a localized fluid collection with enhancing walls – communication with the bowel lumen is confirmed by gas within the abscess (± extravasation of any luminal contrast)
- *Fistula formation:* this is usually with the bladder (with focal bladder wall thickening)

Pearls

- It can be difficult to distinguish diverticulitis from a colonic cancer: diverticulitis will tend to demonstrate pericolic inflammation and colonic involvement >10 cm ▶ cancer will tend to demonstrate enlarged nodes and a discrete mass
- **Giant sigmoid diverticulum:** a large gas-filled structure that is rarely seen within the lower abdomen
  - *Complications:* diverticulitis ▶ small bowel obstruction ▶ perforation ▶ volvulus
- **Epiploic appendagitis:** this follows infarction of an epiploic appendage, causing acute pain similar to that seen with appendicitis or diverticulitis ▶ it usually resolves spontaneously in about 2 weeks
  - **US:** a non-compressible pericolic hyperechoic ovoid mass immediately under the abdominal wall
  - **CT:** a focal area of hyper-attenuation with a central area of fat density

LARGE BOWEL STRICTURES

Definition

- Colonic strictures (narrowing) can be due to various causes (see Table):
  - It is important to distinguish a stricture from a functional narrowing – 7 'physiological sphincters' exist within the colon (e.g. Cannon's point within the mid-transverse colon)

Radiological features

Double-contrast barium enema

- *Fibrotic strictures:* classically this has a smooth lumen with tapering ends
- *Malignant strictures:* classically this has an 'apple-core' configuration: an irregular lumen with shouldered ends involving a short colonic segment
- *Diverticular disease:* narrowing is common ▶ it is distinguished from a malignant stricture by retention of its mucosal folds and demonstration of the spiculated necks of compressed diverticulae

Further clues to the underlying aetiology (on DCBE and CT)

- *Wall thickening:* minimal and symmetric (with ischaemia) ▶ marked (with an inflammatory mass) ▶ eccentric (with tumour)
- *Sacculation:* only with ischaemia or Crohn's disease
- *Contraction of the mucosal folds:* crenation with a mass effect is characteristic of a desmoplastic response with endometriosis or carcinoma
- *Site of the stricture:* rectosigmoid (radiotherapy) ▶ anterior rectosigmoid wall (endometriosis) ▶ splenic flexure (ischaemia) ▶ disease elsewhere (Crohn's disease)
- *Extraluminal components:* associated fibrosis (radiotherapy) ▶ lack of a discrete extraluminal component (ischaemia)
- *Malignant potential:* mesenteric stranding suggests a likely benign cause ▶ nodal enlargement suggests a likely malignant cause

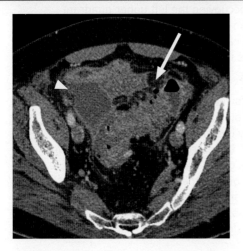

Axial CT shows acute diverticulitis manifest by a thickened sigmoid with diverticula and adjacent inflammatory fat stranding (arrow). A pelvic abscess (arrowhead) has formed next to the inflamed sigmoid.**

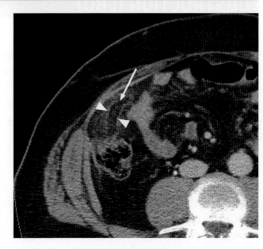

Axial CT of epiploic appendagitis showing the typical, central ovoid fat-density mass (arrow) with peripheral enhancement (arrowheads).**

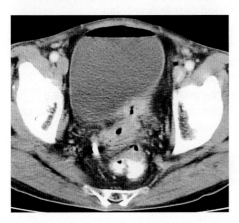

CT of a bladder fistula secondary to diverticulitis. Note the gas in the bladder indicating a fistulous communication to the bowel, the presence of sigmoid diverticular disease with inflammatory thickening of the base of the bladder at the site of the fistula.*

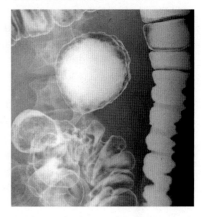

A giant sigmoid diverticulum with sigmoid diverticular disease.*

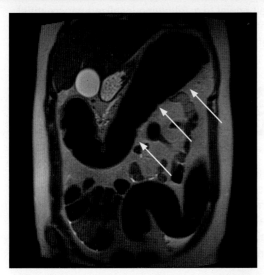

Coronal T2-weighted MRI showing gross dilatation of the transverse colon (arrows). In the correct clinical setting, a haustral appearance and florid dilatation allows the diagnosis of toxic megacolon.**

Causes of large bowel strictures	
Physiological	Distended bladder ▶ spasm
Surgical	Anastomosis ▶ site of colostomy
Malignant	Annular ▶ scirrhous ▶ metastatic carcinoma ▶ lymphoma
Diverticular disease	Pericolic abscess
Ischaemia	Sacculation common as with Crohn's strictures
Radiation colitis	In radiation field so usually rectosigmoid
Inflammatory bowel disease	Ulcerative colitis ▶ Crohn's disease ▶ tuberculosis ▶ lymphogranuloma venereum ▶ amoebiasis
Miscellaneous	Extrinsic masses ▶ endometriosis ▶ pelvic lipomatosis ▶ trauma

MECHANICAL LARGE BOWEL OBSTRUCTION (LBO)

Definition

- There are numerous causes: colonic carcinoma (the commonest cause) ▶ diverticulitis (the 2ⁿᵈ commonest cause) ▶ colonic volvulus
  - Obstruction more commonly involves the left colon
  - Adhesive large bowel obstruction is very unusual (cf. small bowel obstruction)

Radiological features

AXR/instant unprepared barium enema/CT Appearances depend on the site of the obstruction and whether the ileocaecal valve remains competent:

- *A competent ileocaecal valve:* this affects a minority of patients ▶ in spite of increasing intracolonic pressure and marked caecal distension, the small bowel is not distended
- *An incompetent ileocaecal valve:* there is marked small bowel dilatation ▶ the caecum and ascending colon are not unduly distended

Pearls

- If both small and large bowel dilatation is present then the appearances can mimic a paralytic ileus
- As large bowel obstruction can mimic a pseudo-obstruction, any patient with a suspected large bowel obstruction therefore requires further imaging (e.g. an instant unprepared enema) to confirm the diagnosis
- There is a risk of perforation if the caecum measures >9 cm (and the transverse colon >6 cm)

LARGE BOWEL VOLVULUS

Definition

- Twisting of a colonic segment around its mesenteric attachment – it can therefore only occur in those parts of the colon that have a long freely mobile mesentery (sigmoid colon > caecum > transverse colon)
- **Caecal volvulus:** this can only occur when the caecum and ascending colon are on a mesentery (this is not seen in all patients) ▶ it affects a younger age group (30–60 years) than a sigmoid volvulus
- **Sigmoid volvulus:** the sigmoid colon twists around its mesenteric axis ▶ it is usually chronic with intermittent acute attacks ▶ it tends to occur in old age or in patients with a mental handicap or institutionalization

Radiological features

Caecal volvulus

AXR/CT A gas-filled distended caecum ▶ the haustra are still visible (cf. sigmoid volvulus) ▶ often there is small bowel distension (the left side of the colon is usually collapsed)

- The caecum can twist and invert with the caecal pole and appendix occupying the left upper quadrant
- The caecum can twist in the axial plane without inversion – the caecum then occupies the right lower quadrant ▶ this is associated with vascular compromise

Sigmoid volvulus

AXR/CT A massively air distended inverted U-shaped loop ▶ proximal colonic dilatation is typical ▶ the apex of the loop usually lies above T10 and under the left hemidiaphragm ▶ the margins of the loops are devoid of haustra ▶ there is generally an air:fluid ratio of >2:1

- *'Inferior convergence':* the two limbs of the loop converge inferiorly on the left at the level of the upper sacral segments
- *'Liver overlap' sign:* the ahaustral margin overlaps the lower liver border
- *'Left flank overlap' sign:* the ahaustal margin overlaps the haustrated dilated descending colon
- *'Pelvic overlap' sign:* the ahaustral margin overlaps the left side of the pelvis

Contrast enema/CT The mucosal folds can show a 'screw' pattern at the point of twisting

- *'Bird of prey' sign:* the point of torsion appears as a smooth, curved tapering of the colonic lumen, which can look like a hooked beak

PARALYTIC ILEUS

Definition

- Peristalsis ceases with accumulation of fluid and gas within the bowel

Radiological features

AXR The appearances can vary from dilatation of a short length of small bowel (e.g. following localized pancreatitis) to dilatation of the entire intestine (e.g. following peritonitis) ▶ it can be difficult to differentiate from a low large bowel obstruction

PSEUDO-OBSTRUCTION (OGILVIE'S SYNDROME)

Definition

- This usually occurs in elderly patients and is often due to cathartic abuse ▶ there is no mechanical obstruction but it will mimic intestinal obstruction clinically and radiologically
- Mechanical obstruction needs to be excluded with a contrast enema, CT or colonoscopy

Pearls

- The caecum may exceed the critical diameter of 9 cm with the risk of imminent perforation – a caecostomy or right-sided colostomy may be urgently required

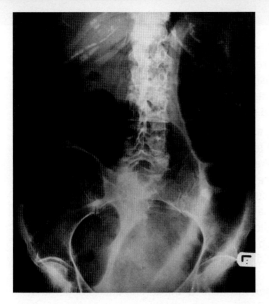

Large bowel obstruction in sigmoid carcinoma: supine position. Gas-filled, distended large bowel and caecum. A competent ileocaecal valve has resulted in no dilatation of small bowel.*

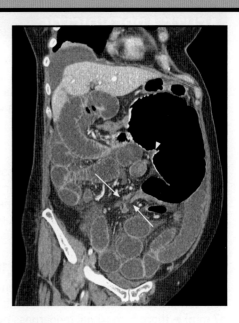

Coronal oblique CT shows a dilated caecum in the left upper quadrant (arrowhead shows part of the ileocaecal valve). At the site of the twist there are two overlapping transition points (arrows), sometimes called the 'X-marks-the-spot' sign.**

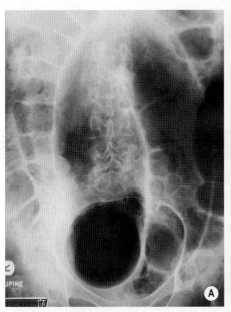

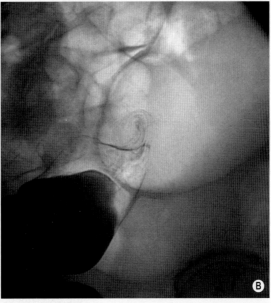

Sigmoid volvulus. (A) Massively dilated distended gas-filled loop of sigmoid colon. (B) Contrast enema showing the twisted sigmoid colon (bird of prey sign).*

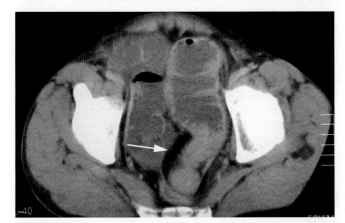

Large bowel obstruction. CT demonstrating dilated fluid-filled large bowel due to a stricture of the sigmoid colon (arrow). Histology of resection specimen showed stricture due to diverticulitis.*

Causes of a paralytic ileus	
Peritonitis	Congestive heart failure
Surgery	Pneumonia
Trauma	Renal colic
- *spine*	Renal failure
- *ribs*	Leaking abdominal aortic
- *hip*	aneurysm
- *retroperitoneum*	Low serum potassium
Inflammation	Drugs (e.g. morphine)
- *appendicitis*	Spinal lesions
- *pancreatitis*	General debility or infection
- *cholecystitis*	Vascular occlusion
- *salpingitis*	

ACUTE APPENDICITIS

Definition Inflammation of the appendix following obstruction of the appendix lumen by an appendicolith, hypertrophied lymphatic tissue or tumour

- Venous obstruction causes ischaemia with necrosis and bacterial invasion

Radiological features

AXR A localized paralytic ileus ▶ an associated abscess may lead to indentation of the medial border of the caecum (± loss of the lower part of the properitoneal fat line and right psoas muscle shadow) ▶ the small bowel may become stuck to the inflamed appendix leading to small bowel obstruction

- An appendicolith can be seen in up to 10% of cases

US The appendix appears as a blind-ending non-compressible tubular structure (with a diameter ≥7 mm) ▶ there is maximal tenderness over the appendix ▶ an appendicolith will appear as a hyperechoic focus casting an acoustic shadow ▶ there may also be a hyperechoic inflammatory mass, abscess or free fluid around the appendix

- *A false-negative examination:* focal appendicitis of the appendiceal tip ▶ a gangrenous or perforated appendicitis

- ⅔ of appendices have a retrocaecal location (and are therefore difficult to see with US)
- *A false-positive examination:* a dilated Fallopian tube ▶ peri-appendicitis ▶ inflammatory bowel disease ▶ inspissated stool

CT The appendix measures >6 mm in diameter ▶ the appendix will fail to fill with oral contrast medium or air up to its tip ▶ an appendicolith will appear as a calcified 'stone' ▶ there may be an enhancing appendiceal wall, local adenopathy, surrounding inflammatory change, an abscess or extraluminal gas (indicating perforation)

- An appendicolith can be seen in up to 30% of cases
- *'Arrowhead sign':* luminal contrast or air within the caecum and pointing towards the obstructed appendix origin
- *A caecal bar:* focal caecal thickening due to oedema at the appendix origin

Pearl **Appendix mucocele:** accumulation of mucus within an appendix due to an aseptic obstruction

- This results in cyst formation (± mural calcification) ▶ the cyst may rupture, resulting in pseudomyxoma peritonei

ANAL FISTULA

Definition This is secondary to Crohn's disease or cryptogenic anal gland infection:

- Discharge of an abscess creates a track through part of the sphincter (usually the longitudinal layer) to the perianal skin ▶ the internal opening is usually situated posteriorly (at 6 o'clock) and at the level of the dentate line
- **Park's classification:** 'SITES': **S**uperficial ▶ **I**ntersphincteric ▶ **T**rans-sphincteric ▶ **E**xtrasphincteric ▶ **S**uprasphincteric
- **Goodsall's rule** (on axial imaging):
  - A fistula with an external opening *posterior* to a plane passing horizontally through the centre of the anus: a curved track with its internal opening within the dorsal midline
  - A fistula with its external opening *anterior* to a plane passing horizontally through the centre of the anus: a linear track directly to the nearest anal crypt
  - An external opening adjacent to the anal margin suggests an intersphincteric tract whilst a more laterally located opening suggests a trans-sphincteric tract
  - Openings seen on both sides of the anal canal are likely to arise from a midline posterior crypt with a horseshoe type of fistula
- **Superficial perianal fistula:** the superficial fistula tracks below both the internal anal sphincter and the external anal sphincter complex
- **Intersphincteric fistula (70%):** the intersphincteric fistula tracks between the internal anal sphincter and the

external anal sphincter complex in the inter-sphincteric space ▶ the external opening is at the natal cleft/perianal skin ▶ the internal opening is usually in the midline posteriorly in the anal canal at the level of the dentate line

- **Trans-sphincteric fistula (25%):** a trans-sphincteric fistula tracks through the internal anal sphincter, inter-sphincteric space and external anal sphincter complex ▶ the external opening is through the ischioanal fossae to the perianal skin ▶ the internal opening is into the anal canal at the level of the dentate line
- **Extrasphincteric fistula (1%):** an extrasphincteric fistula tracks outside both internal and external anal sphincters ▶ it penetrates the levator ani muscle with an internal opening at the level of the rectum
- **Suprasphincteric fistula (5%):** a suprasphincteric fistula travels upwards in the intersphincteric space over the top of puborectalis and penetrates levator ani muscle – it then tracks down to the perianal skin ▶ the internal opening is into the anal canal at the level of the dentate line

Radiological features

MRI (axial, coronal, sagittal STIR) ▶ this can demonstrate
  - The primary and secondary tracks (high SI on STIR images)
  - The internal and external openings
  - Any supralevator extension or associated abscess

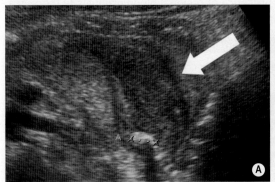

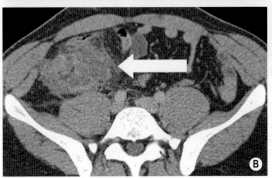

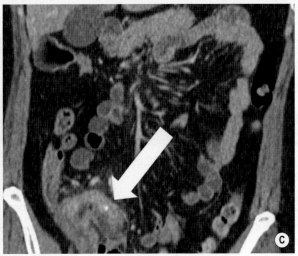

Appendicitis. (A) US demonstrating a thickened appendix wall (arrow), with an appendicolith at its tip. (B) CT demonstrating an appendix mass (arrow). (C) CT demonstrating an inflamed appendix, with a tiny appendicolith as its cause (arrow).

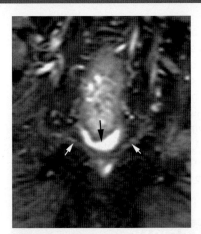

STIR coronal MRI of a supralevator horseshoe abscess (black arrow) above the levator ani (white arrows).*

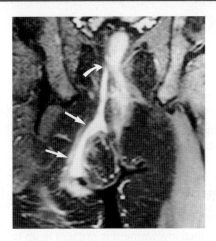

Coronal STIR MRI reveals a right-sided extrasphincteric fistula (straight arrows) with its enteric communication in the rectum (curved arrow).†

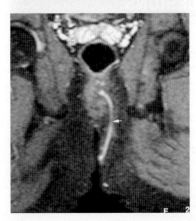

Coronal STIR image of a trans-sphincteric fistula (arrow).*

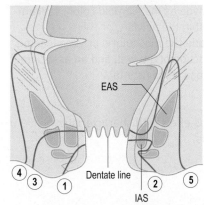

A classification of fistula-in-ano. EAS: external anal sphincter. IAS: internal anal sphincter. (1) Superficial. (2) Intersphincteric. (3) Transsphincteric. (4) Extrasphincteric. (5) Suprasphincteric.

CHRONIC MEGACOLON

Definition A long-standing dilated colon ▶ there are various causes:

- Hirschsprung's disease ▶ chronic laxative abuse ▶ colonic pseudo-obstruction (Ogilvie's syndrome) ▶ Chagas' disease ▶ hypothyroidism ▶ an electrolyte imbalance ▶ diabetes ▶ scleroderma ▶ amyloidosis

PELVIC LIPOMATOSIS

Definition A rare condition of unknown aetiology leading to the proliferation of pelvic adipose tissue

Radiological features

XR Increased radiolucency of the pelvis with exceptionally good sacral delineation

CT/MRI A diffuse increase in the pelvic fat with associated bladder and rectal compression

SOLITARY RECTAL ULCER SYNDROME

Definition This forms part of the spectrum of rectal prolapse – it is an area of reddening or ulceration on the anterior rectal wall with associated lamina propria fibrosis ▶ it presents with difficulty in evacuation, rectal bleeding and excess mucus production

Radiological features

DCBE Bowel wall deformity at the ulcer site ▶ mucosal irregularity or nodularity due to the associated granulation tissue

- *Colitis cystica profunda:* polypoid change (due to retention cysts) that may be seen at the ulcer margin

Evacuation proctography Frequently this will show an intra-anal intussusception (which is the cause of the anal trauma)

ENDOMETRIOSIS

Definition Gastrointestinal involvement is present in up to ⅓ of cases ▶ it mainly involves the sigmoid colon, caecum or small bowel loops within the pelvis

- Serosal implants invade the muscularis propria leading to fibrosis with contraction of the wall and an associated mass effect (the mucosa remains intact)

Radiological features

DCBE A localized mass effect with characteristic contracted mucosal folds

MRI T1WI (FS): high SI ▶ T2WI: high SI with 'shading' due to the presence of residual blood products (if there is a cystic component)

Differential diagnosis

- Metastatic disease ▶ chronic pelvic inflammation

LOCAL COMPLICATIONS IN THE POSTOPERATIVE COLON

Definition Local complications following colonic surgery: anastomotic breakdown or stricture formation ▶ postoperative abscess or haematoma formation ▶ recurrent tumour formation

Radiological features

Water-soluble contrast enema This is performed at about the 12th postoperative day ▶ it can demonstrate a leak of contrast at the anastomosis or the formation of a stricture

- *Benign stricture:* a smooth outline
- *Malignant stricture:* an irregular outline

CT This can also demonstrate a leak with water-soluble colonic contrast

- *Postoperative abscess:* a rim enhancing fluid collection (± internal locules of air)
- *Haematoma:* a high attenuation fluid collection

Pearls

- Colonic resection with anastomosis formation is covered by a defunctioning colostomy – this does not reduce the incidence of a leak but does mitigate against the effects of any associated abscess ▶ an anastomotic leak warrants delay in closing the colostomy
- A defunctioned colon always has a low-grade bacterial colitis (causing narrowing and loss of haustration)
- Stricture formation is a long-term consequence of anastomotic breakdown
- Anastomotic leakage is a poor prognostic factor for long-term function

RETRORECTAL LESIONS

Definition

- These present as a mass that may be complicated by infection, bleeding, or malignant change
  - *Developmental cysts:* epidermoid cyst ▶ dermoid cyst ▶ enteric cyst
  - *Sacral lesions:* teratoma ▶ anterior sacral meningocele ▶ chordoma ▶ lymphangioma
  - *Anorectal lesions:* lipoma ▶ GIST ▶ anal gland cyst

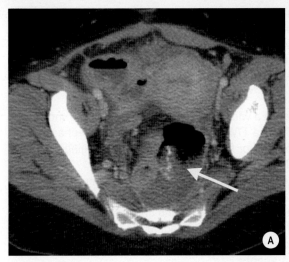

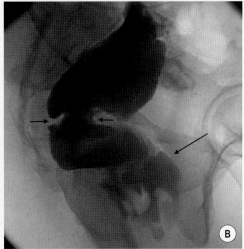

Patient with anastomotic leak following anterior resection. (A) CECT showing large pelvic collection (arrow) at the site of anastomosis. (B) Corresponding water-soluble enema showing extraluminal leak of contrast from the rectum (long arrow). There appears to be a stricture proximal to this (short arrows).

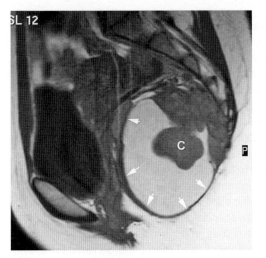

Sagittal MRI of a large tailgut cyst (arrows) with cystic and solid (C) components, the latter due to the development of a carcinoid tumour within the cyst.*

Axial T2-weighted MR of the pelvis shows low signal obliteration of the pouch of Douglas (arrow) with tethering and angulation of the rectal wall (arrowhead) due to advanced endometriosis with deep colonic involvement.**

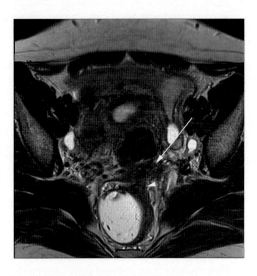

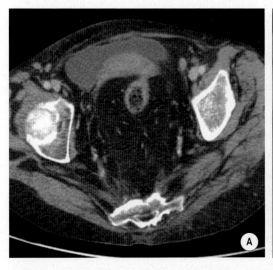

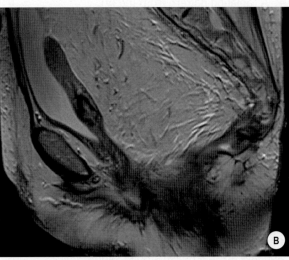

Pelvic lipomatosis. (A) Axial CT and (B) sagittal T1WI demonstrating abundant pelvic fat.

3.6 LIVER

ANATOMY

Couinaud classification

- The liver is subdivided anatomically into 8 segments; segments II – VIII are divided anatomically via the portal and hepatic veins
- *The caudate lobe (segment I):* this is autonomous, receiving vessels from both the left and right portal vein branches and the hepatic artery ▶ it has an independent venous drainage directly into the IVC

Vascular anatomy

- *Blood supply to liver:* $2/3$ is from the portal vein ▶ $1/3$ is from the hepatic artery
- *Venous drainage:* this is via the 3 hepatic veins into the IVC (30% of patients have accessory draining veins) – usually an accessory inferior RHV draining of segments VI or VII
- Aberrant gastric venous drainage of segments I and IV: this is correlated with focal fatty change within this segment

Riedel's lobe

- A normal variant where there is extension of the inferior tip of the right lobe to or beyond the costal margin

LIVER IMAGING TECHNIQUES

US

Normal texture Homogeneous (and slightly more reflective than the renal cortex)

Hepatic artery
- *Doppler:* a pulsatile vessel with continuous forward flow

Portal vein branches A radiating pattern from the porta hepatis (with reflective vessel walls)
- *Doppler:* monophasic flow is seen in a hepatopetal direction (cf. hepatofugal flow with cirrhosis) ▶ there is a mean peak velocity of 15–25 cm/s with slight respiratory variation

Hepatic vein branches A radiating pattern from the IVC (with non-reflective vessel walls)
- *Doppler:* there is a triphasic flow pattern with reversal of flow during the cardiac cycle (reflecting transmitted right heart pressure changes)

Contrast-enhanced US This gives improved lesion characterization during the arterial and portal phases of enhancement (after an IV injection of a microbubble contrast agent)

CT

NECT This can detect diffuse changes (e.g. fat and iron deposition) and focal changes (e.g. calcification and haemorrhage) ▶ the liver usually has attenuation values of 54–60 HU (8–10 HU greater than the spleen)

CECT This can detect and characterize focal lesions using a combination of early and late arterial phase studies along with portal, late and delayed imaging

- The majority of pathological solid liver lesions have a predominantly arterial supply (normal liver parenchyma receives up to 80% of its blood supply from the portal vein) ▶ they will therefore appear low attenuation on portovenous imaging.

MRI

- There are a wide range of protocols available, including breath-hold T1WI and T2WI, in- and out-of-phase sequences (for fat detection), diffusion imaging and T1WI + Gad
  - The biliary system can be imaged using a dedicated heavily T2W MRCP technique
  - Hepatic steatosis, iron and fibrosis can be quantified using chemical shift imaging, T2 + T2* relaxometry and elastography

Contrast agents
- **Gadolinium-based agents:** these will generate enhancement (T1WI) ▶ tend to give better enhancement profiles than hepatocyte specific agents as larger doses used
- **Hepatobiliary specific agents:** the target includes the reticuloendothelial system or hepatocyte
  - *Iron oxide particles:* these are superparamagnetic causing susceptibility induced proton dephasing (with a reduced SI) within normal tissues on T1WI and particularly T2WI ▶ larger particles (50–100 nm) are taken up by the Kupffer and endothelial cells and are rapidly cleared from the circulation ▶ smaller particles are retained within the circulation for a longer period providing a prolonged 'intravascular' phase of enhancement (and therefore providing an angiographic effect as a blood pool agent)
  - *Hepatocyte-specific paramagnetic agents* (e.g. gadoxetate disodium [Primovist]) ▶ these accumulate within hepatocytes, and then undergo renal (50%) and biliary (50%) excretion ▶ they will cause enhancement of normal liver parenchyma and the biliary tree (T1WI) – a low SI indicates an abnormal area
    - used to differentiate between FNN + adenoma ▶ also used for increased lesion conspicuity (e.g. liver metastases)

Normal imaging appearances The liver demonstrates the same (or slightly higher) SI than adjacent muscle (for all sequences except for inversion recovery techniques which are designed to null the liver signal)
- T1WI: spleen < liver
- T2WI: spleen > liver

Liver scintigraphy
- This provides a global view of the liver and helps characterize a lesion if CT or MRI is not available
- ^{99m}Tc-sulphur colloid or albumin colloid is usually used – 90% is taken up by the Kupffer cells (10% is taken up by the spleen) ▶ ^{99m}Tc-labelled red blood cells can be used if a haemangioma is suspected
- FDG-PET has a relatively limited role (as normal liver takes up FDG)

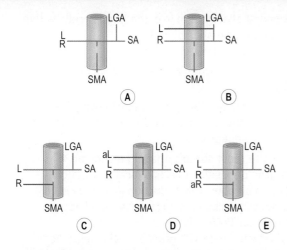

Hepatic artery normal variants. The normal arrangement is shown in (A). The commonest four variations are: replaced left hepatic artery (B), replaced right hepatic artery (C), accessory left hepatic artery (D), accessory right hepatic artery (E). R = right hepatic artery, L= left hepatic artery, LGA = left gastric artery, SMA = superior mesenteric artery, SA = splenic artery, a = accessory.

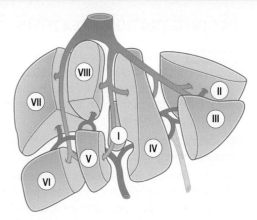

Surgical segments of the liver.

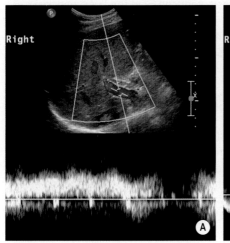

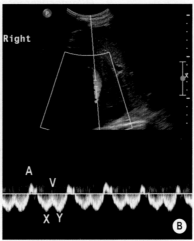

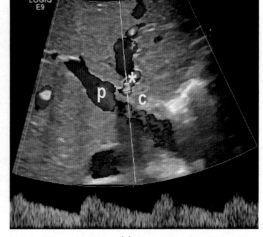

(A) Normal portal vein on duplex US. Flow is normally continuous towards the liver (hepatopetal) with slight undulation related to the cardiac cycle and respiration. (B) Normal hepatic vein on duplex US. The spectral tracing reflects the normal right heart pressure changes leading to flow reversal occurring normally during the 'A' wave (right atrial contraction) and occasionally during the 'V' wave. The 'X' and 'Y' descents are also normally demonstrated.

Normal hepatic artery (*) demonstrating pulsatile flow. p = portal vein, c = common bile duct.

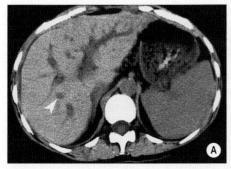

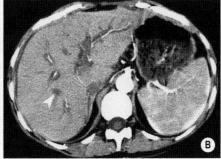

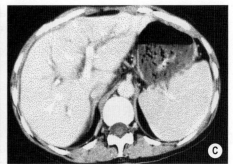

Biphasic CT examination. Axial sections at the same location following a bolus of IV contrast medium demonstrating clearly the hepatic vessels and phases of enhancement, (A) NECT, (B) early arterial phase and (C) portal phase. The patient has mild intra-hepatic bile duct dilatation emphasizing the anatomical relationships. Note the hepatic vein appears as a focal lesion on the arterial phase but normally fills in during the portal phase (arrowheads).*

FAT INFILTRATION/STEATOSIS

Definition Diffuse hepatocyte triglyceride loading
- *Causes:* acute and chronic alcohol abuse ▶ obesity ▶ diabetes mellitus ▶ cystic fibrosis ▶ malnourishment ▶ total parenteral nutrition ▶ tetracyclines ▶ steroids ▶ ileal bypass surgery

US An increased echoreflectivity, which obscures the portal vein margins

CT The attenuation decreases by approximately 1.6 HU per mg of triglyceride increase per gram of liver substance ▶ the liver architecture is preserved ▶ there will be uniform enhancement post IV contrast medium administration
- *Moderate fat infiltration:* liver attenuation < spleen attenuation
- *Severe fat infiltration:* liver attenuation < blood attenuation (the hepatic vasculature appears 'enhanced')

MRI Chemical shift or 'in- and out-of-phase' imaging allows for diagnosis and quantification ▶ steatosis causes relative signal loss on out of phase imaging

HEPATITIS

Definition Acute or chronic liver inflammation
- **Infection:** this is usually due to hepatitis
  - *Hepatitis A:* this is usually benign and self-limiting
  - *Hepatitis B:* this can present as an asymptomatic carrier state, or with acute or chronic hepatitis, fulminant hepatic failure, and hepatocellular carcinoma
  - *Hepatitis C:* an acute or chronic hepatitis with possible subsequent cirrhosis
- **Other causes:** alcohol ▶ drugs (e.g. methotrexate)

US
- *Acute hepatitis:* non-specific reduced reflectivity with echogenic portal vein walls ▶ gallbladder wall thickening
- *Chronic hepatitis:* an increased echogenicity with loss of the portal vein wall echogenicity

Colloid scintigraphy There are similar appearances to early cirrhosis but with uneven and reduced uptake

CT/MRI/angiography This is of limited value until cirrhosis develops

HAEMOCHROMATOSIS AND HAEMOSIDEROSIS

Haemochromatosis An autosomal recessive condition causing iron deposition within the hepatocytes (leading to subsequent cirrhosis) and other organ tissues (including the myocardium, skin and pancreas)
- *There is an increased risk both of developing a malignancy in general (and HCC in particular)*

Haemosiderosis This is due to hepatic iron overload resulting from multiple transfusions ▶ uptake occurs via the reticuloendothelial system (e.g. the Kupffer cells within the liver, bone marrow and spleen)
- *There is less risk of liver damage*

US This may demonstrate increased parenchymal echogenicity

NECT Increased liver attenuation values (HU>75) ▶ previous amiodarone treatment and Thorotrast exposure may give similar appearances

MRI This is the most specific imaging technique ▶ intracellular iron deposition exerts a local susceptibility effect leading to an abnormal reduction in liver SI ▶ NB: normal hepatic parenchyma is brighter than adjacent skeletal muscle on T1W1 + T2W1
- It is best detected with T2* gradient-echo sequences (moderate accumulation will cause changes on T2WI – severe accumulation will cause changes on T1WI)
- *Haemochromatosis:* reduced SI in the liver, pancreas and heart
- *Haemosiderosis:* reduced SI in the liver and spleen
- Relative signal loss in affected organs on in phase imaging

NEONATAL HEPATITIS

Causes *Idiopathic* (the majority) ▶ *antenatal infections* (e.g. CMV, rubella, enterovirus, toxoplasmosis, herpes simplex and spirochaete) ▶ *metabolic disorders* (e.g. cystic fibrosis, α_1-antitrypsin deficiency, tyrosinaemia and galactosaemia)

US There are non-specific features, but may include: hepatomegaly ▶ a heterogeneous coarse liver parenchyma ▶ a visible gallbladder (>1.5 cm) without the triangular cord sign (cf. biliary atresia)

99mTc-DISIDA Extraction into the liver is often reduced and excretion into the bowel may be reduced proportional to the degree of cholestasis and hepatocellular dysfunction ▶ if cholestasis is severe, reduced extraction and excretion may make it difficult to distinguish this from biliary atresia

Pearls 5–10% will develop persistent fibrosis
- Diagnosis: percutaneous liver biopsy

WILSON'S DISEASE

Definition An autosomal recessive condition causing copper deposition within the liver, cornea and lenticular nucleus of brain ▶ this is hepatotoxic and triggers an inflammatory response that progresses to cirrhosis

US Non-specific features ▶ generalized cirrhotic changes

CT There is rarely increased hepatic attenuation (more often there is reduced attenuation secondary to fatty infiltration)

MRI T1WI: possibly high SI ▶ T2WI: low SI

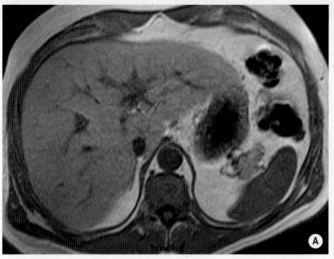 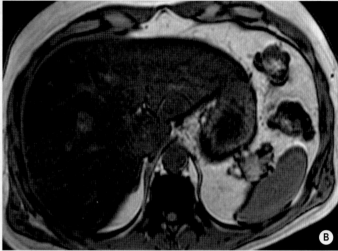

Liver steatosis. (A) In-phase imaging. (B) Out-of-phase imaging. The signal loss demonstrated by the hepatic parenchyma on out-of-phase imaging indicates significant liver steatosis.

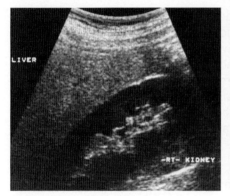 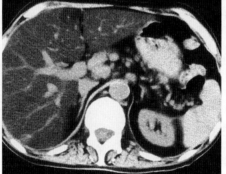 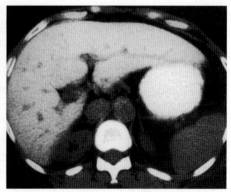

Diffuse fat infiltration. The liver is abnormally echoreflective when compared with the cortex of the adjacent right kidney.*

Diffuse fat infiltration. NECT in which the liver parenchyma is markedly reduced in attenuation, reversing the normal relationship with the spleen and blood vessels. The shape and vascular architecture of the liver are normal.*

Haemochromatosis. NECT section through the liver of a patient with haemochromatosis showing diffuse increased attenuation of the liver compared with the spleen.*

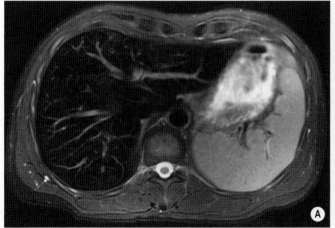 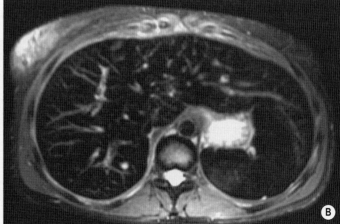

T2WI images demonstrating abnormally low liver signal in (A) haemochromatosis and (B) haemosiderosis. Note the spleen is abnormally low signal in haemosiderosis as the reticuloendothelial system becomes iron loaded compared with predominantly hepatocyte accumulation in haemochromatosis.*

CIRRHOSIS

DEFINITION

- This represents the endpoint of a wide variety of chronic disease processes that cause hepatocellular necrosis and ultimately lead to hepatic fibrosis and nodular regeneration:
  - Alcohol abuse ▶ hepatitis B ▶ storage disorders (e.g. haemochromatosis and Wilson's disease) ▶ biliary cirrhosis ▶ certain drugs

RADIOLOGICAL FEATURES

US

- *Early cirrhosis:* there is increased reflectivity (due to fat infiltration and fibrosis)
- *Advanced cirrhosis:* a nodular liver margin (this is seen especially with a high-frequency transducer and if ascites is present) ▶ a coarse heterogeneous echotexture ▶ hypoechoic regenerating nodules
  - Attenuated hepatic veins can be seen with end-stage disease (due to the liver atrophy)
  - Pure hepatic fibrosis increases liver reflectivity (resulting in loss of the portal vein branch margins) but will not significantly alter its attenuation – this can be used to discriminate fibrosis from fatty infiltration

Doppler US Damping of the normal right-heart waveforms within the hepatic veins ▶ reduced main portal venous blood flow (<10 cms^{-1} mean peak) or hepatofugal portal venous flow ▶ collateral vessel development (e.g. left gastric, splenorenal, paraoesophageal or retroperitoneal collaterals) including a recanalized para-umbilical vein

- Increased hepatic arterial flow can be seen with advanced cirrhosis (due to a reduced portal venous contribution to the hepatic blood supply)
- Increased flow in a large recanalized para-umbilical vein may 'steal' blood from the right portal vein branch – this can lead to reversed flow within the right portal vein but normal hepatopetal flow within the main and left portal veins
- Ultrasound elastography:
  - The technique uses either an external mechanical device generating an external mechanical impulse whose speed is measured by an USS probe (Fibroscan), or inducing shear waves in the liver tissue by generating an internal acoustic radiation force (ARFI) or via Shear Wave Elastography (SWE); shear wave propagation velocity is then measured using USS imaging to determine tissue stiffness; usually 10 different ROI are assessed and the median value taken
  - Advanced Fibrosis: > 15kPa (2.2 m/sec)

CT This is relatively insensitive for early cirrhosis
- *Advanced cirrhosis:* a nodular liver margin ▶ lobar atrophy or hypertrophy ▶ ascites ▶ portal vein thrombosis
  - Heterogeneous attenuation: this is often due to coexisting fibrosis (with reduced attenuation) and hepatocyte iron deposition (with increased attenuation)

MRI This is relatively insensitive for early cirrhosis
- *Early cirrhosis:* T2WI and delayed T1WI + Gad: subtle parenchymal heterogeneity
- *Advanced cirrhosis:* morphological changes as seen with CT ▶ it can assess portal vein patency, flow direction and bulk flow volume
- MR elastography can quantify liver stiffness in a similar fashion to USS

Colloid scintigraphy

- *Early cirrhosis:* there is uneven radionuclide uptake (and lobar morphological changes with progression)
  - *'Colloid shift':* with the development of portal hypertension there is splenomegaly and a reduced activity halo around the liver
- *Advanced cirrhosis:* less sulphur colloid is taken up by the liver and increased extrahepatic activity is seen within the heart, and the reticuloendothelial cells of the bones and lungs

Angiography

- This can assess any vascular complications and portal hypertensive changes
- *Hepatic arteriography:* there is increased tortuosity of the intrahepatic branches ('corkscrew vessels'), reflecting hepatic lobar shrinkage

PEARLS

Advanced cirrhosis There is atrophy of the posterior segments of the right lobe (VI and VII), hypertrophy of the caudate lobe (I) and hypertrophy of the lateral segments of the left lobe (II and III)
- This is thought to be caused by altered hepatic blood flow dynamics, including an increased overall hepatic blood flow (due to intrahepatic arteriovenous shunts) and areas of reduced hepatic blood flow (due to increased intrahepatic vascular resistance)

Complications Hepatocellular carcinoma (10%) ▶ portal hypertension (± variceal bleeding)

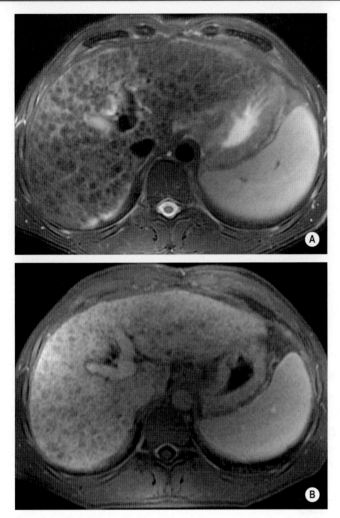

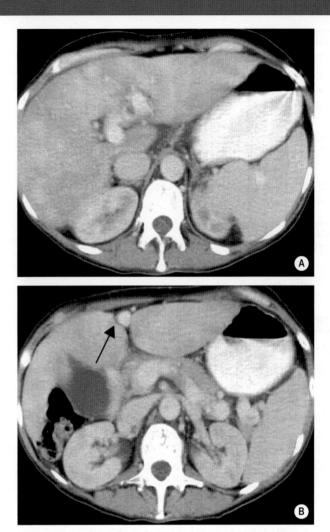

Cirrhosis. On MRI marked heterogeneity may occur in cirrhotic livers on (A) multi-shot T2W FSE imaging due to the combination of increased signal from fibrosis and reduced signal from iron accumulation within nodules and for similar reasons on delayed post-gadolinium T1W imaging (B).**

CT appearances of cirrhosis (A, B) Patchy irregular enhancement of the hepatic parenchyma due to altered portal blood flow in cirrhosis with portal hypertension. Recanalization of the umbilical vein in the falciform ligament is arrowed.†

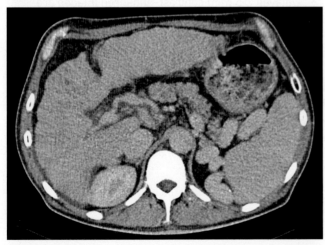

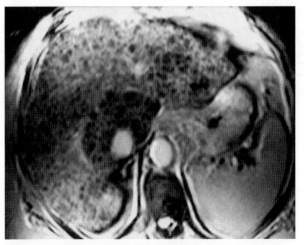

Cirrhosis. On portal phase CECT the nodular margin, atrophy of the hepatic right lobe and large splenorenal varices are all indicators of cirrhosis.*

Cirrhosis. SPIO-enhanced T2 image illustrates the nodular architecture of the cirrhotic liver. Nodules of regenerating liver tissue show SPIO uptake giving low signal, while interstitial bands of fibrosis show relatively high signal.†

HEMANGIOMA

Definition

- These are composed of vascular channels of varying size (cavernous to capillary) which are endothelium lined ▶ there is often intervening fibrous tissue of varying amounts
  - *Capillary haemangioma:* the usual form
  - *Cavernous haemangioma:* this accounts for most neonatal and infantile haemangiomas (and some adult lesions)
- It is the commonest benign hepatic tumour (it can be multiple in <10% of cases)

Clinical presentation

- They are usually asymptomatic ▶ larger lesions may rarely cause discomfort or undergo spontaneous rupture (F>M)
- They may enlarge during pregnancy

Radiological features

US

- *Capillary haemangioma:* a well-defined lobular homogeneous hyperechoic lesion (large lesions can be heterogeneous) ▶ there is no Doppler signal (due to the very slow vascular flow through the dilated channels) ▶ it can appear very similar to some metastases (e.g. from a GI primary)
- *Cavernous haemangioma:* a hypoechoic lesion (due to the larger vascular channels) ▶ a Doppler signal is usually detectable (there are more rapid flow rates)

CT
A well-defined lobulated lesion ▶ thrombi, calcification, fibrosis and scarring are variably present
- *NECT:* there is a similar attenuation to blood
- *CECT:* there is centripetal enhancement – the lesion eventually merges with the background parenchyma

MRI
A well-defined lobulated lesion ▶ characteristic imaging features are demonstrated if a lesion is between 2 and 4 cm in size.
- *T2WI:* there is increasingly high SI with extended echo times (malignant lesions are typically less prominent with later echo times)
  - *'Lightbulb' sign:* homogeneously high SI (greater than that of the spleen and approaching that of cyst fluid)

- *T1WI + Gad:* centripetal enhancement from the periphery to the centre over a period of minutes ▶ there are three distinct enhancement patterns:
  1. A well-circumscribed hepatic mass with peripheral, nodular and interrupted enhancement progressing centripetally to uniform enhancement (most common)
  2. Immediate uniform enhancement (small capillary haemangiomas <1.5 cm).
     - This will also show persistent delayed enhancement
  3. Peripheral nodular enhancement with centripetal progression but persistent central hypointensity (giant haemangiomas >5 cm).
  - *Small (<1.5 cm) lesions:* these may fail to demonstrate characteristic T2WI signal changes (due to partial volume effects) or the typical enhancement pattern
  - *Larger (>4 cm) lesions:* these often have atypical internal features such as an area of central fibrosis that can prevent complete infilling during contrast enhancement
- *DWI:* hyperintense (T2 shine through)

Sulphur colloid studies Lesions appear as photopenic areas

Blood pool studies (e.g. ^{99m}Tc-labelled red cells) Lesions demonstrate increased uptake

DSA A characteristic 'cotton wool' appearance: normal-sized arteries supply groups of peripherally arranged vascular spaces that opacify gradually and retain contrast for 20 s or longer

Pearls

- Haemangiomas are more T2 hyperintense than are most metastases, although hypervascular metastases can mimic haemangiomas because of their marked T2 hyperintensity
  - Delayed (>5 min) contrast-enhanced images are helpful in these cases because small, uniformly enhancing haemangiomas retain contrast material and remain hyperintense, whereas hypervascular metastases will show 'washout' of contrast material

Diagnosis This may require a core needle biopsy in adults if the diagnosis is in doubt

Kasabach–Merritt syndrome A large haemangioma may sequester thrombocytes, leading to a thrombocytopenia

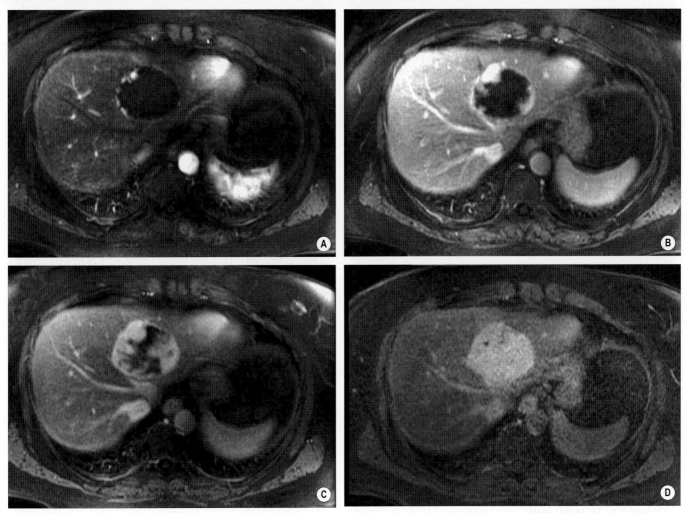

Haemangioma. Typical appearance of enhancement following IV gadolinium with initial peripheral nodular high signal vessel signal followed by progressive infilling of the lesion. Images obtained at 40 s (A), 120 s (B), 5 min (C) and 15 min (D) following injection.*

Typical imaging features of common liver lesions					
	Adenoma	**FNH**	**Haemangioma**	**HCC***	**FLC****
Sex	F > M	F > M	F > M	M > F	M = F
Capsule	Yes	No	No	Thin	Thin
Central scar	Uncommon	Yes High SI (T2WI)	No	Uncommon	Yes Low SI (T1WI and T2WI)
Calcification	No	No	Yes	7%	50%
Enhancement	Uniform arterial	Uniform arterial ▶ delayed scar enhancement	Centripetal	Arterial (may be mosaic) ▶ portovenous washout	Uniform arterial ▶ there is no scar enhancement
Colloid scintigraphy	Reduced uptake	Normal uptake	Reduced uptake	Reduced uptake in less well-differentiated tumours	Reduced uptake

FNH, focal nodular hyperplasia
*Hepatocellular carcinoma
**Fibrolamellar carcinoma

FOCAL NODULAR HYPERPLASIA (FNH)

Definition

- An underlying congenital vascular lesion composed of normal liver elements (hepatocytes, bile ducts, Kupffer cells and intervening fibrous septa) ▶ however, there is a lack of normal liver architecture (e.g. there are absent portal tracts)
  - It may enlarge in response to hormone stimulation (e.g. oral contraceptives)
- It is the 2nd commonest benign hepatic tumour

Clinical presentation

- It is usually asymptomatic (it may present with pain or hepatomegaly)
- It occurs most commonly in women aged 20–50 years (and is multiple in 20% of cases)

Radiological features

- A central stellate fibrovascular scar is seen in 50% of cases ▶ there is no true capsule ▶ calcification, necrosis and haemorrhage are extremely rare (even large lesions do not usually outgrow their blood supply)

US There are non-specific features with lesions demonstrating a similar reflectivity to the adjacent liver (but demonstrating mass effect) ▶ the central scar is rarely seen

- Doppler signals can be seen within and at the edge of the lesion

NECT A well-defined mass which often exhibits a mass effect (with vessel displacement) ▶ the lesion demonstrates the same attenuation as the surrounding liver ▶ there is a central low attenuation scar

CECT

- *Arterial phase:* uniform enhancement (except for the scar) ▶ there can be large peripheral feeding vessels
- *Portal phase:* the attenuation is identical to normal liver (the scar remains low attenuation)
- *Delayed imaging:* there is slow scar enhancement

MRI The same enhancement pattern is seen as for CT ▶ the specificity increases with iron oxide agents (which are taken up by the Kupffer cells)

- *T1WI:* intermediate or minimal low SI ▶ a low SI central scar
- *T2WI:* intermediate to high SI ▶ a high SI central scar
- *T1WI + Gad:* marked, homogeneous arterial phase enhancement that becomes isointense during the portal venous phase ▶ there can also be a peripheral, ring-type delayed enhancement pattern on delayed images obtained 1 h after hepatocyte selective gadolinium chelate administration
  - The central scar usually demonstrates delayed enhancement
- *DWI:* generally isointense

Sulphur colloid This is usually normal (due to Kupffer cell activity within the lesion)

DSA A vascular mass with a large tortuous central supplying artery ▶ radiating vessels spread out to supply the lesion

Pearls

- *Other lesions with a central scar:* hepatocellular adenoma (HCA) ▶ hepatocellular carcinoma ▶ haemangioma
- *Other lesions demonstrating Kupffer cell activity:* HCA ▶ a well-differentiated hepatocellular carcinoma
- MR imaging with a hepatocyte-specific contrast agent may help confirm the hepatocellular origin of the mass (taken up by hepatocytes and partially excreted into the biliary system):
  - Primovist (disodium gadoxetate): iso- to hyperintense on 1-h to 3-h delayed images, unlike an adenoma (which is hypointense)
- Occasionally surgical excision is required for symptomatic lesions

FOCAL CONFLUENT FIBROSIS

Definition

- A focal manifestation composed of massive confluent fibrosis and associated atrophy of the affected liver segment
- It occurs uncommonly in established cirrhosis, typically affecting the anterior segment of the right lobe or the medial segment of the left lobe

Radiological features

NECT The involved atrophic segment is of low attenuation (often with retraction of the overlying capsule)

CECT The attenuation of the affected region is the same or lower than normal liver

MRI Similar morphological changes are evident
- *T1WI:* low SI
- *T2WI:* high SI
- *T1WI + Gad:* delayed enhancement

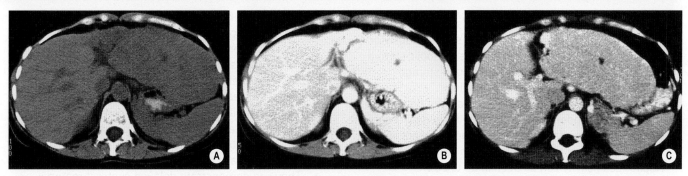

FNH. A large lesion (homogeneous except for a low attenuation central scar) expands and replaces much of the left lobe. The attenuation is almost identical to normal liver on the unenhanced section (A) but the lesion demonstrates transient avid and even enhancement during the arterial phase (B), becoming indistinguishable on the portal phase section (C).*

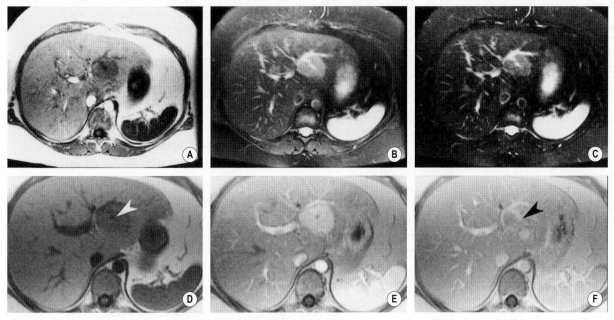

FNH. A well-defined lesion in the left lobe that is homogeneous except for a central scar, low signal on T1WI (A, D) and increased signal on T2WI (TE 60 ms [B], TE 120 ms [C]). Following IV gadolinium the whole lesion enhances transiently in the arterial phase (E) with the exception of the scar, which enhances on delayed sections (F) (arrowhead).*

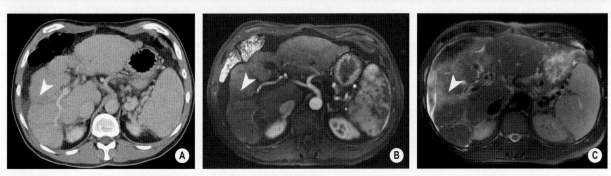

Focal confluent fibrosis. (A) Portal phase CECT. The right lobe has contracted and confluent bands of fibrosis are present (arrowheads). These appear of low attenuation and may mimic malignant lesions when focal. (B) On T1WI + Gad imaging there is no enhancement. (C) On T2WI the fibrosis is usually of increased signal and can mimic HCC.

HEPATIC ADENOMA

Definition

- A rare benign hepatic tumour arising spontaneously or in association with oral contraceptives, anabolic steroid use, Klinefelter's syndrome and glycogen storage disease type 1 (when it is often multiple)
- It is a vascular lesion composed primarily of hepatocytes which have a tendency to accumulate fat and glycogen ▶ there are no portal tracts or bile ducts present and no bilirubin excretion ▶ although Kupffer cells are absent, Kupffer cell activity can be seen in up to 20%
- It may demonstrate a fibrous pseudocapsule and a central scar (like FNH) ▶ there is a tendency to outgrow its blood supply, resulting in haemorrhage, thrombosis and necrosis

Clinical presentation

- It is usually asymptomatic ▶ if rupture occurs there can be pain or life-threatening haemorrhage

Radiological features

US An isoechoic or hyperechoic (if there is a significant fat component) mass lesion

CT Uncomplicated lesions are usually homogeneous with a well-defined margin ▶ it will be of similar attenuation to normal liver (or lower attenuation if there is a substantial fat component) ▶ intraparenchymal haemorrhage will appear as high attenuation thrombus on unenhanced images (which may extend through the capsule and into the peritoneum)
- *Arterial phase:* there is marked uniform enhancement
- *Portal phase:* a lesion merges with the surrounding liver
  - Necrosis: minimally enhancing low attenuation regions

MRI An uncomplicated adenoma has similar appearances to a region of FNH

- T1WI: a well-defined isointense or slightly high SI lesion ▶ there can be hyperintense foci secondary to haemorrhage or intracellular fat
- T2WI: variable signal intensity but are often mildly hyperintense relative to the liver ▶ haemorrhage or necrosis: this leads to a heterogeneous appearance
- T1WI + Gad: uniform marked enhancement (arterial phase), equilibrating with the liver parenchyma (portal phase) ▶ heterogeneous enhancement in complex lesions ▶ they are typically not as vascular as FNH
  - They can demonstrate delayed contrast material washout with or without a delayed-enhancing pseudocapsule
  - They are hypointense on 1-h to 3-h delayed images obtained with Primovist (absence of biliary ducts)
  - An adenoma may demonstrate venous washout – it is the only 'benign' hypervascular mass that may do so (cf. delayed isoenhancement with FNH)
  - Persisting delayed enhancement with the telangiectatic histological variant
- DWI: variable signal intensity depending on the presence of blood or necrosis

Sulphur colloid Reduced activity

HIDA There is uptake within a lesion but no excretion (due to the absent bile ducts)

DSA The lesion is usually hypervascular

Pearls

- Large lesions are resected due to the bleeding risk
- As there is a 1% risk of malignant change, resection is usually preferred to conservative management
- **Liver adenomatosis:** multiple, progressive, symptomatic adenomas (these are not steroid dependent) ▶ there is a risk of liver dysfunction, haemorrhage and HCC formation

ATYPICAL REGENERATIVE NODULES

Definition

- These occur with chronic cirrhosis ▶ some regenerative nodules may appear more prominent than others, causing diagnostic confusion with a HCC
- Form part of the spectrum of HCC development (regenerative nodule → dysplastic nodule → HCC)

Radiological features

US A well-defined, homogeneous lesion of reduced reflectivity

T1WI Iso- to hyperintense (high SI due to fat and glycogen accumulation)

T2WI Iso- to hypointense ▶ low SI if there is accumulation of iron ('siderotic nodules')
- A malignant focus within a nodule appears as a region of high SI

T1WI + Gad Multiple small, similar-sized enhancing nodules are demonstrated during the hepatic arterial phase ▶ these nodules then fade to isointensity (differentiating from HCC)

DWI Generally isointense

Pearl

- Increasing SI on T2WI or increasing washout on T1WI + Gad is worrying for developing dysplasia

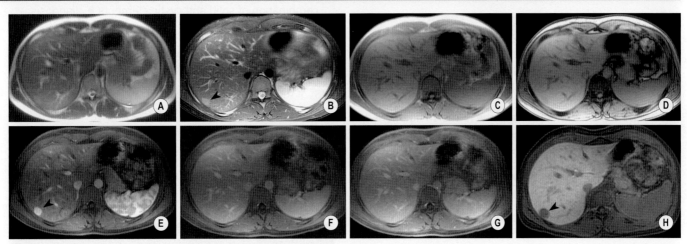

Adenoma MRI. A subtle posterior right lobe lesion is barely visible on single-shot T2W FSE (A) but more obvious (arrowhead) on the fat-suppressed multi-shot T2W FSE (B). (C) In- and (D) out-of-phase imaging demonstrate no fat accumulation. There is avid homogeneous enhancement in the arterial phase T1W imaging (E) and rapid equilibration in the portal (F) and delayed phase (G). On a separate occasion the lesion is low signal on the hepatobiliary phase following gadoxetic acid administration (H).**

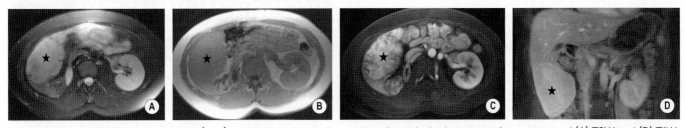

Telangiectatic adenoma. These lesions (star) exhibit features similar to that of a typical adenoma on fat-suppressed (A) T2W and (B) T1W imaging, but demonstrate persistent enhancement in the delayed phase following contrast enhancement (C, D). Owing to the arterial heterogeneity and patient symptoms, the lesion was biopsied and then resected.**

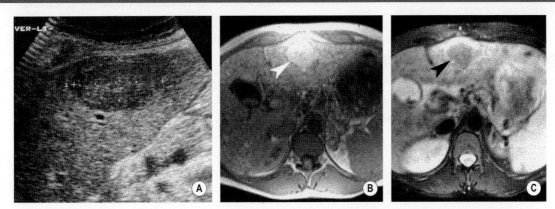

Atypical regenerative nodule. Regeneration in cirrhosis often results in heterogeneity of the parenchyma. Occasionally nodules may become large, 'atypical' or 'dominant' as in this patient. US (A) demonstrates a reduced echoreflectivity lesion in the left lobe, initially interpreted as a probable tumour. However, on MRI, the relatively homogeneous lesion (arrowheads) is of increased signal on T1WI (B) and decreased signal on T2WI (C) (arrowhead).

FOCAL FAT

DEFINITION

- Focal fat variation within the liver parenchyma is due to alterations in the underlying blood supply and venous drainage ▶ it can cause diagnostic confusion with a tumour
  - *Common sites:* either side of the falciform ligament ▶ the cranial aspect of the gallbladder fossa ▶ the posterior aspect of segment IV

RADIOLOGICAL FEATURES

MRI – 'chemical shift' or 'in- and out-of-phase' imaging
This detects the presence of fat and water within the same image voxel ▶ fat and water protons have different resonant frequencies – over time these will alternatively be in and out of phase with each other ▶ imaging at specific predetermined times will give either in- or out-of-phase images (they are out of phase 2.2 ms after an excitation pulse and in phase 4.4 ms after excitation)
- Water and fat signal intensities will combine on the in-phase imaging, but cancel out on the out-of-phase imaging ▶ as both image sets use a different TE, one needs to compare any signal change with a non-fat-containing organ (e.g. spleen) or correct for T2 signal changes using T2 mapping
- Lesions containing significant amounts of fat will lose SI on the out-of-phase images (relative to the in-phase images)
- *Out-of-phase images:* these can be identified as the intra-abdominal viscera are outlined by an 'inky black' line ▶ this occurs because at the organ–intra-abdominal fat interface the imaged voxel contains both fat and water and will therefore lose signal intensity (voxels located internally within the organ or intra-abdominal fat will tend to contain predominantly fat or water only and therefore not lose signal intensity)

NECT/US A large area of regional fat variation has a geographic appearance with a lack of mass effect and preservation of the vascular architecture

BILIARY HAMARTOMAS

DEFINITION

- A rare benign malformation of the bile ducts ('von Meyenburg complexes')

- Typically they are small lesions (3–5 mm) with a combination of solid and cystic elements ▶ diagnosis usually requires biopsy

RADIOLOGICAL FEATURES

US If multiple they often range from 1 to 3 mm in size and are often interpreted as diffuse malignant infiltration

CT There can be cystic or solid components ▶ they will enhance (but remain low attenuation on unenhanced and portal phases)

MRI T1WI: low SI ▶ T2WI: there is a characteristic appearance of multiple high SI lesions

PEARL

- They may be indistinguishable from small metastases on US and CT and are often the cause of 'indeterminate' or 'too small to characterize' lesions

MESENCHYMAL HAMARTOMA

DEFINITION

- This is a lesion containing a mixture of bile ducts and mesenchyme
- Although rare, it is the 2nd commonest benign liver tumour or developmental lesion occurring in children

CLINICAL PRESENTATION

- It is usually seen at <2 years of age (with a peak incidence at 15–22 months)

RADIOLOGICAL FEATURES

- It is usually a large lesion (5–30 cm) ▶ it can appear as a mixed solid or cystic mass (appearing more solid when small) ▶ it can be multiseptated with a cystic and gelatinous composition

CT A low attenuation lesion ▶ there is variable septation with fluid loculation
- Although the tumour is hypovascular, atrioventricular shunting can occur through the enlarged irregular tortuous feeding vessels

MRI Multiseptated fluid areas ▶ T1WI: low SI ▶ T2WI: high SI
- A lesion can displace major vessels

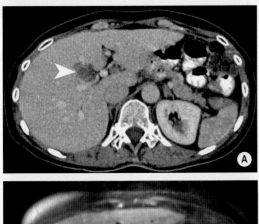

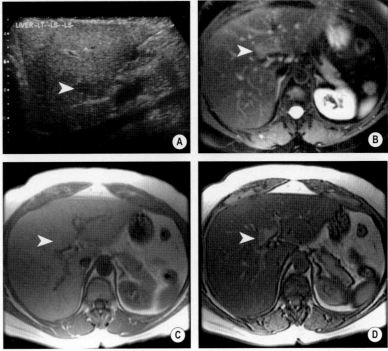

Focal fat sparing. On US (A) an area of focal fat sparing (arrowheads) in the posterior aspect of the left lobe medial segment (Couinaud IV) in an otherwise fatty liver has a similar appearance to a metastasis. On T2WI FS (B) this will appear of increased signal, suggesting a malignant lesion but the use of in- (C) and out- (D) -of-phase gradient-echo imaging indicates that the 'lesion' is in fact normal liver surrounded by fatty liver that has reduced in signal on the out-of-phase image (D).*

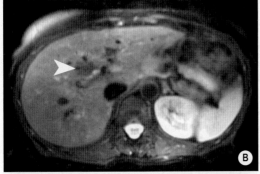

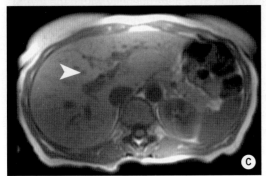

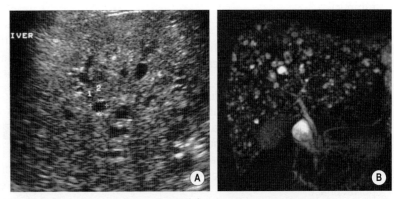

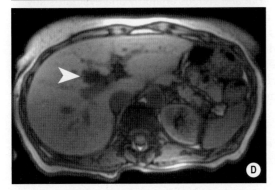

Focal fat infiltration. On portal phase CT (A) focal fat infiltration (arrowheads) in the posterior aspect of the left lobe medial segment (Couinaud IV) has a similar appearance to a metastasis. On T2WI FS (B), the low signal makes metastasis unlikely but does not characterize the lesion. However the demonstration of signal loss (relative to the spleen) on in- (C) and out- (D) -of-phase gradient-echo imaging is diagnostic.*

Multiple biliary hamartomas. On US (A) only the larger cystic lesions are seen clearly and the background texture of the liver is heterogeneous and often misinterpreted as malignant infiltration. With MRCP type T2WI (B) imaging the extent and number of the multiple cystic lesions is more obvious. The solid components may be indistinguishable from metastases.*

HEPATOCELLULAR CARCINOMA (HCC) / HEPATOMA

Definition

- The commonest primary malignant neoplasm of the liver, typically occurring within an abnormal (e.g. cirrhotic) liver
  - *Risk factors:* direct carcinogens (e.g. aflatoxin) ▶ chronic hepatitis B and C ▶ cirrhosis (particularly postnecrotic cirrhosis and haemochromatosis)
  - *Types:* solitary ▶ multifocal (accounting for up to 40% of cases in the Far East) ▶ diffuse
- It is unclear whether HCC arises from a regenerative nodule (via a dysplastic intermediate state) or as a de novo lesion

Radiological features

- Imaging has limited sensitivity for detecting small (≤1 cm) HCC in cirrhotic livers
- *Larger lesions (>3 cm):* these may contain fat ▶ they may demonstrate haemorrhage, thrombosis or necrosis
  - *Vascular invasion:* this can involve the portal vein (35%) or hepatic veins (15%)

US

- A hypo-, iso- or hyperechoic lesion in relation to the adjacent parenchyma (± a hypoechoic outer margin representing a fibrous capsule) ▶ larger lesions can be heterogeneous (due to any haemorrhage, necrosis or fat)
- *Colour Doppler:* internal high-velocity signals can be due to arterioportal shunting) ▶ a portal vein filling defect represents either thrombosis or intravascular tumour (arterial signals will only be demonstrated within tumour)

CT

- *NECT:* ill-defined low attenuation lesions ▶ focal areas of internal calcification (7% of cases) ▶ there may be a hypoattenuating capsule
- *CECT:* enhancement is seen during the arterial phase, as it is a hypervascular tumour supplied via the hepatic artery ▶ it may demonstrate a mosaic enhancement pattern (with an enhancing grid-like pattern around a central lower area of attenuation) ▶ it will become hypoattenuating to the liver parenchyma during the portal phase
  - *Portal venous invasion:* arterioportal fistulae ▶ periportal streaks of high attenuation ▶ dilatation of the main portal vein (or its major branches) ▶ enhancement of any thrombus or detection of intrathrombus arterial flow
- *Lipoidal CT:* HCC foci will retain lipoidal (as there is no biliary drainage) and will be clearly seen when imaged 7–14 days later

MRI

- *T1WI:* lesions less than 1.5 cm are often isointense, whereas larger lesions may be hyperintense secondary to lipid, copper or glycogen

- Fatty metamorphosis in a cirrhotic nodule is suspicious for HCC
- *T2WI:* mild to moderate high SI (and possibly heterogeneous). Most lesions are hyper- or isointense
- *T1WI + Gad:* lesions <2 cm in diameter can demonstrate homogeneous intense enhancement during the arterial phase, whereas larger lesions more often demonstrate heterogeneous enhancement
  - During the portal venous and equilibrium phases, a HCC will show rapid loss of enhancement (becoming iso- or hypointense relative to the liver) – this feature is very suggestive of malignancy
  - *Atypical regenerative nodules:* these may cause confusion as they can also enhance during the arterial phase ▶ often high signal on T1WI ▶ however they will be low SI on T2WI (due to iron accumulation – the so-called 'siderotic nodules') ▶ venous washout is not displayed by regenerative and dysplastic nodules
    - The development of malignant foci within these nodules is suggested by the development of focal areas of high SI or heterogeneity within the low SI nodule ('nodule in nodule' appearance)
- *DWI:* variable appearance that depends on their histologic make-up
  - Well-differentiated tumours are often isointense
  - Moderately to poorly differentiated tumours are more often hyperintense
- *FDG PET:* this is relatively non-specific for HCC and is not widely used
- *DSA:*
  - This is used for preoperative assessment ▶ it defines the arterial and venous anatomy and evaluates any portal or caval involvement
  - HCC is usually a vascular lesion demonstrating dilated feeding arteries, abundant abnormal vessels or arteriovenous shunting
    - *Portal vein invasion:* a 'threads and streaks' appearance

Pearls

- The incidence parallels the prevalence of local predisposing conditions (in particular chronic hepatitis B and C)
- Serum α-fetoprotein (AFP) may or may not be elevated in HCC ▶ AFP may also be elevated with simple cirrhosis ▶ AFP may fluctuate with flares of HBV or HCV infection ▶ only a proportion of early tumours have elevated AFP levels
- It commonly metastasizes to the lungs and bone
- Non-invasive diagnosis
  - Nodule 1–2 cm: CT *or* MRI showing enhancement and washout ▶ CT *and* MRI showing enhancement and washout in non-specialist centres
  - Nodule >2 cm: CT *or* MRI showing enhancement and washout

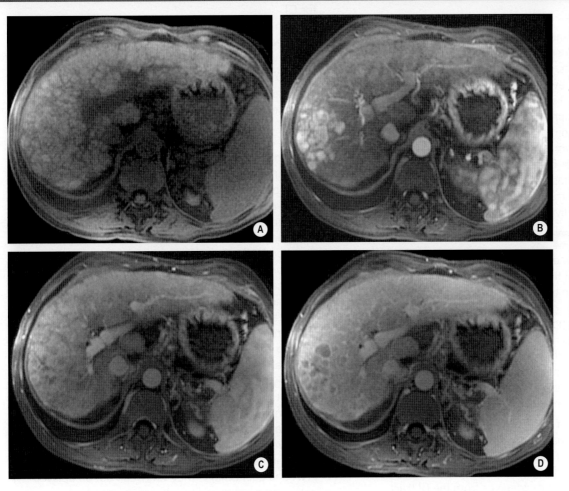

Multifocal hepatocellular carcinoma. 3D T1W MRI (A) unenhanced demonstrates widespread multiple increased signal nodules, (B) arterial enhancing multifocal HCC is clearly visible in the right lobe, (C) the HCC lesions become isointense in the portal phase and (D) the HCC demonstrates washout on the 5-min delayed image. Note that a protocol providing only (A) and (C) would likely result in the diagnosis being missed.**

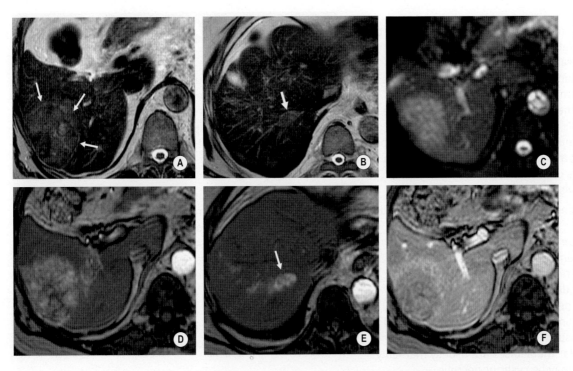

HCC. (A) T2WI showing a heterogeneous high SI HCC (arrows). (B) T2WI. The right hepatic vein is expanded by high SI tumour extension (arrow). (C) DWI confirms restricted diffusion (also within the right hepatic vein - not shown). (D) Following IV gadolinium, there is heterogeneous enhancement. (E) The tumour within the right hepatic vein also enhances (arrow). (F) The HCC demonstrates washout on delayed imaging.

METASTASES

Definition

- The liver is a common site for metastases from many primary cancers (usually due to haematogenous spread)
  - *GI tract tumours:* these metastasize via the portal vein ▶ there is evidence for blood flow separation within the portal vein as right–sided colon cancers are more likely to spread to the right lobe (with left–sided tumours spreading to either the right or left lobes)
  - *Non-GI tract tumours:* these metastasize via the hepatic artery ▶ both lobes are equally affected
- Although a metastasis will derive its vascular supply from the hepatic artery it will usually be less vascular than the adjacent liver parenchyma

Radiological features

- Metastases can be difficult to radiologically detect and characterize if they measure less than 5 mm in size (particularly in distinguishing them from a biliary hamartoma)
  - FDG PET does not improve the sensitivity (as there is a relatively high normal background liver uptake) but is useful in detecting extrahepatic metastases
- Metastases can demonstrate a wide range of appearances but they will usually demonstrate growth on serial imaging, multiplicity and a variation in size

US Homogeneous or heterogeneous mass lesions ▶ they can be hyperechoic (mimicking a haemangioma) or hypoechoic (mimicking a simple cyst) ▶ central necrosis can cause a partly cystic appearance ▶ calcification can be seen in mucin-secreting metastases from the GI tract

- *'Target' appearance:* there may be a surrounding rim of reduced reflectivity

CT The majority of metastases are of low attenuation on unenhanced and portal phase imaging ▶ hypervascular tumours may show transient arterial enhancement, becoming isoattenuating to liver during the portal phase ▶ central necrosis, rim enhancement and calcification (in mucin-secreting metastases of GI origin) can also be demonstrated

- A <5 mm low attenuation lesion within the liver is more likely to represent a simple cyst (unless a metastasis is purely cystic it is unlikely to be of low enough attenuation to be visible at such a small size)

MRI The signal intensity of a metastasis roughly parallels that of the spleen

- T1WI: hypervascular metastases are moderately hypointense ▶ haemorrhagic metastases can demonstrate hyperintensity
  - Perilesional fat deposition has been specifically described with hepatic metastases from a primary pancreatic insulinoma and is thought to be related to the effects of insulin
- T2WI: hypervascular metastases are usually markedly hyperintense and may be cystic or necrotic

- T1WI + Gad: similar enhancement characteristics as for CT
  - With paramagnetic iron oxide agents the normal liver parenchyma is of low SI (due to Kupffer cell uptake) – this will make a metastatic lesion more obvious
- DWI: hyperintense

Colloid scintigraphy There is reduced activity (metastases lack Kupffer cells)

Pearls

- *Cystic metastases:* ovarian tumours (the most common) ▶ carcinoma of the colon ▶ teratoma ▶ metastatic squamous tumours
- *Hypervascular metastases:* breast ▶ renal ▶ thyroid ▶ neuroendocrine tumours ▶ melanoma
- *Calcified metastases:* mucinous tumours of the GI tract ▶ endocrine pancreatic carcinoma ▶ osteosarcoma
- *Haemorrhagic metastases:* colon ▶ thyroid ▶ breast ▶ choriocarcinoma ▶ melanoma ▶ RCC
- After the initiation of chemotherapy, metastases can exhibit a less aggressive enhancement pattern that can mimic a haemangioma (including early peripheral nodular enhancement and delayed retention of contrast material)
  - A key distinguishing feature of chemotherapeutically treated metastases is an early, intact peripheral rim of enhancement (unlike the discontinuous peripheral enhancement seen with a haemangioma)
- Hypervascular metastases classically show marked T2 hyperintensity and restricted diffusion (compared with FNH and adenoma) ▶ they will wash out on delayed enhanced images (unlike a haemangioma)

ANGIOSARCOMA

Definition

- A rare malignant vascular hepatic neoplasm derived from the endothelial cells and which can form vascular derivatives, cavernous spaces, or solid masses
- It is associated with exposure to polyvinylchloride, arsenic and Thorotrast contrast medium

Radiological features

CT It can appear as an infiltrating mass demonstrating heterogeneous enhancement ▶ it can occasionally present in a diffuse form that is not easily detected with imaging

- Background Thorotrast exposure causes heterogeneously increased attenuation within the liver, perihepatic lymph nodes and spleen

MRI It can present as a large mass or as multiple nodules

- T1WI: low SI ▶ T2WI: high SI ▶ T1WI + Gad: heterogeneous enhancement

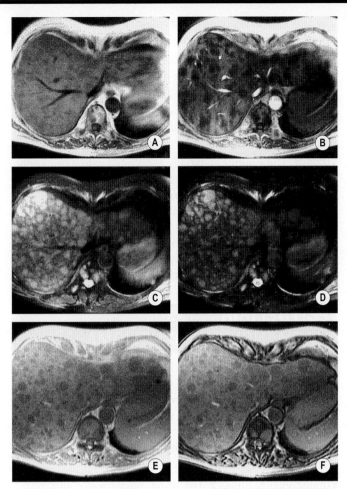

Multiple metastases. MRI demonstrates lesions within both the liver and the vertebral bodies. They are of reduced SI on T1WI (A) gradient-echo images (B), moderately increased SI on T2WI images (C, D), and do not significantly change in relation to the splenic signal on in- (E) and out- (F) of-phase gradient-echo imaging, indicating the lack of any lipid content.

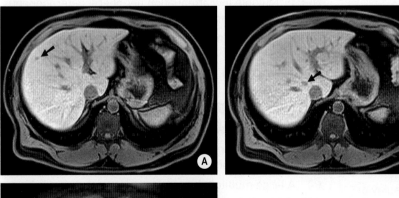

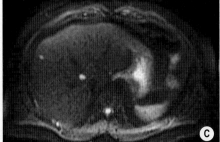

Hepatic colorectal cancer metastases MRI. (A, B) Two small (arrows) low signal metastases on adjacent thin sections of 3D T1W imaging in the hepatobiliary phase following gadoxetic acid. (C) Both lesions are clearly shown on DWI imaging (b = 500).**

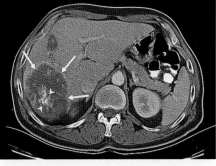

Hepatic metastatic lesion (arrows) from a mucinous adenocarcinoma of the rectum shows calcifications within the centre (arrowheads).**

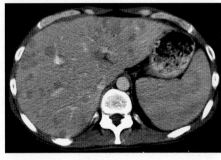

Liver metastases. Portal phase CT study demonstrates multiple low attenuation lesions, most likely multiple metastases, in a patient with known colorectal malignancy.*

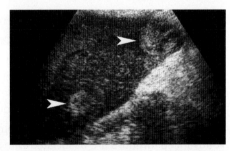

Echoreflective liver metastases. Metastatic carcinoid lesions of typical increased echoreflectivity (arrowheads). These lesions are usually of increased vascularity and can demonstrate arterial phase enhancement on CT and MRI.*

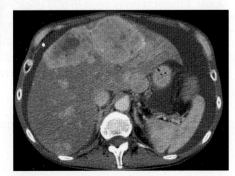

CECT of the liver demonstrating multiple hypervascular liver metastases. Ascites is also present.

329

FIBROLAMELLAR CARCINOMA (FLC)

Definition A hepatic tumour composed of sheets of fibrosis and numerous eosinophilic hepatocytes ▶ it arises spontaneously with no predisposing factors, and occurs within an otherwise normal liver (cf. HCC) ▶ there are no elevated AFP levels ▶ 5–35 years

- It was previously classified as a variant of HCC – it is now considered a separate entity

Radiological features It is often a large, lobulated, well-defined tumour containing a central fibrous scar (with punctate calcification in >50% of cases) ▶ it is usually a solitary lesion

US Increased reflectivity (with a central scar of high reflectivity and a related acoustic corridor if calcification is present)

CT A low attenuation well-defined lesion with an even lower attenuation central scar (demonstrating radial components) ▶ there is punctate calcification of the central scar in ⅔ of cases (this is rare in FNH)

CECT There is moderate enhancement (± delayed scar enhancement)

MRI T1WI/T2WI: there is a low SI scar (cf. FNH with a high SI scar on T2WI)

Pearls There is a higher 5-year survival rate than seen with HCC (60% vs 30%) ▶ this is possibly due to a younger age at presentation and a lack of background liver disease

HEPATOBLASTOMA

Definition A hepatic tumour composed of primitive hepatocytes (often with mesenchymal components)

- It is the 3rd commonest childhood abdominal tumour (after neuroblastoma and Wilms tumour)

Clinical presentation Many are asymptomatic masses ▶ advanced tumours are associated with anorexia, weight loss, pallor, anaemia and abdominal pain ▶ 20% of patients have metastases at presentation

- Patients are usually <3 years at presentation (M:F 2:1)

Radiological features

AXR Calcification is seen in 50% of cases

US A heterogeneous mass of mixed high and low reflectivity ▶ it may demonstrate calcification, cystic areas of necrosis, or a pseudocapsule ▶ the lesions can be small, large, single or multiple ▶ the tumours can splay or infiltrate the IVC, hepatic or portal veins

CT Presents as a large heterogeneous mass but may also be composed of multiple confluent nodules – a mixed low attenuation lesion (± calcification) ▶ there can be peripheral rim enhancement

MRI T1WI: heterogeneous low SI (haemorrhage may demonstrate high SI) ▶ T2WI: high SI with hypointense fibrous septae

Scintigraphy 99mTc-sulphur colloid scintingraphy demonstrates activity during the angiographic phase and a photopenic area on delayed imaging

Pearls The tumour is usually associated with a markedly elevated serum AFP level (in over 75% of cases)

- **Associations:** Beckwith–Wiedemann syndrome (chromosome 11) ▶ familial adenomatous polyposis (chromosome 5)
- **Diagnosis:** percutaneous needle biopsy
- **Differential:** haemangioma ▶ metastatic neuroblastoma ▶ mesenchymal hamartoma ▶ hepatocellular carcinoma

EPITHELIOID HAEMANGIOENDOTHELIOMA

Definition A malignant tumour of vascular origin composed of 'epithelioid' endothelial cells

- It predominantly affects female adults and is associated with oral contraceptive pill use and vinyl chloride exposure
- It is not to be confused with an infantile haemangioendothelioma

Radiological features The lesion appears as multiple peripherally situated nodules that may coalesce and cause capsular retraction, with compensatory hypertrophy of the un-involved liver segments ▶ may lead to hepatic vein occlusion

US Solid hypoechoic lesions

NECT Multiple low attenuation peripheral heterogeneous areas (± calcification)

CECT Nodular rim enhancement with a surrounding low attenuation 'halo'

MRI T1WI: low SI ▶ T2WI: moderate high SI

HEPATIC LYMPHOMA

Definition Primary hepatic lymphoma is rare ▶ the liver is a common site of secondary involvement

CT A large multilobulated mass ▶ central necrosis ▶ poor enhancement

- Secondary involvement is commonly diffuse infiltration or micronodular ± non-specific hepatomegaly

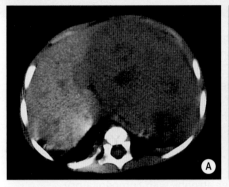 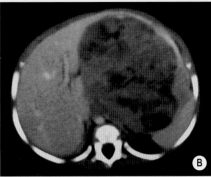 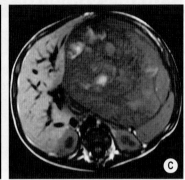

Hepatoblastoma. (A, B) Large, low-density solid heterogeneous mass seen on CT without calcification and with patchy enhancement in a 17-month-old boy. (C) MRI. T1WI: low-SI large mass with areas of increased SI consistent with blood ▶ low-signal internal septae are also seen.*

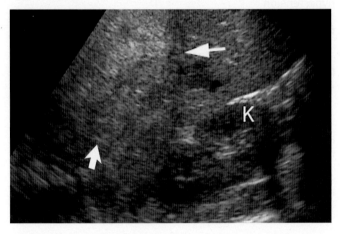

Hepatoblastoma. Parasagittal view through the right lobe of the liver showing a solid echogenic mass (arrow) compressing the IVC (thick arrow). K = kidney.*

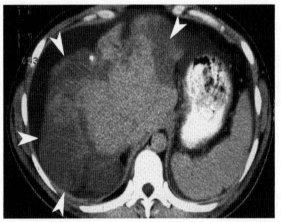

Epithelioid haemangioendothelioma. CT demonstrates peripheral low-attenuation lesions (arrowheads) that have coalesced to form a rind of tumour enclosing the central normal liver parenchyma. The patient presented with Budd–Chiari syndrome secondary to the tumour, diagnosed on needle biopsy and confirmed at subsequent liver transplantation.*

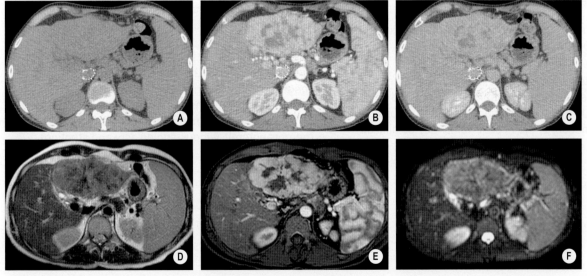

Fibrolamellar carcinoma. The large heterogeneous lesion with a fibrous central region with limited enhancement post contrast medium is demonstrated on CT pre (A), arterial (B) and delayed phase (C), as well as on MR single-shot T2W FSE (D), arterial phase T1W (E) and on DWI b500 imaging (F).**

BUDD–CHIARI SYNDROME

DEFINITION

- A syndrome of global or segmental hepatic venous outflow obstruction which is secondary to obstruction of the IVC (usually by a membrane or thrombus), or by occlusion of the major hepatic vein branches (usually by thrombus)
  - *Type I:* occlusion of the IVC (± hepatic veins)
  - *Type II:* occlusion of the major hepatic veins (± IVC)
  - *Type III:* occlusion of the small centrilobar veins
- **Other causes:** congenital membranes or webs within the IVC (webs can also occur following a long-standing IVC thrombosis) ▶ oral contraceptive use or pregnancy ▶ coagulopathies (e.g. polycythaemia, thrombotic thrombocytopenic purpura or sickle cell disease) ▶ tumour-induced hepatic vein compression ▶ hepatic vein trauma or surgery ▶ constrictive pericarditis ▶ right heart failure

CLINICAL PRESENTATION

- Acute hepatic vein obstruction can present with hepatomegaly, abdominal pain and ascites
- There can be a more insidious presentation with features of secondary portal hypertension and jaundice

RADIOLOGICAL FEATURES

Acute

US Hepatomegaly ▶ thrombus within the major veins (this can give an unequivocal diagnosis during the acute phase) ▶ abnormal collateral veins passing between the major hepatic veins ▶ poor visualization of the hepatic veins or of the flow within them
- A damped hepatic venous waveform (a non-specific sign)
- A continuous reversal of flow within a main hepatic vein
- An enlarged portal vein
- Gallbladder wall thickening

CT The caudate lobe is often preserved with a normal attenuation and enhancement pattern (it has not had time to enlarge) ▶ there may be hepatic vein thrombus (± collateral formation) ▶ the hepatic veins may be difficult to identify

- NECT: the enlarged, congested peripheral liver is of a lower attenuation than normal
- CECT: a 'flip flop' enhancement pattern:
  - *Early:* prominent central and weak peripheral liver enhancement
  - *Delayed:* washout of the central liver, with enhancement of the liver periphery

Chronic

CT Peripheral liver atrophy with compensatory hypertrophy of the caudate lobe (the caudate lobe usually drains via separate veins directly into the IVC and inferior to the normal hepatic venous confluence) ▶ secondary portal hypertension

Other investigations

MRI T1WI/T2WI: a heterogeneous and congested peripheral liver ▶ a normal or hypertrophied caudate lobe
- MRA: this can assess vascular patency and direction of flow

Sulphur colloid A normal or increased caudate lobe activity (there is reduced activity within the remainder of the liver) ▶ colloid shift to the spleen

DSA The venographic appearances are characteristic, resembling a 'spider's web'

Cavography This can identify any IVC abnormality

PEARLS

- Collateral venous channel development can allow some regeneration within the peripheral liver and caudate lobe, leading to variable findings (Budd–Chiari syndrome can be mistaken for extensive tumour involvement)
- The diagnosis in a patient with underlying cirrhosis is difficult – the related lobar and regenerative changes may distort the hepatic veins, making their visualization difficult
- A core needle biopsy is frequently required to exclude tumour and confirm the presence of central venous congestion and venous thrombi
- **Treatment:** liver transplantation ▶ some cases can be treated by interventional techniques (e.g. venous membranotomy, venous angioplasty and stenting)

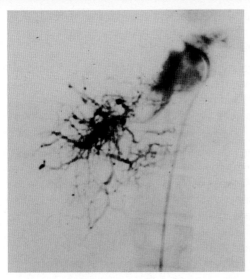

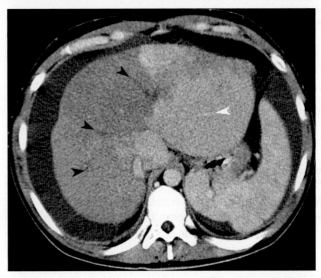

Budd–Chiari syndrome. A catheter has been passed retrogradely into a right hepatic vein. Injection of contrast medium has outlined an extensive fine network of collateral vessels. This 'spider web' appearance is pathognomonic of the Budd–Chiari syndrome.*

Acute Budd–Chiari syndrome. On portal phase CT most of the caudate and left lobe of the liver has enhanced normally and the left hepatic vein can just be seen (white arrowhead) but the right lobe is abnormally low attenuation and the middle and right hepatic vein branches are attenuated and have failed to opacify (black arrowheads). Ascites is present.**

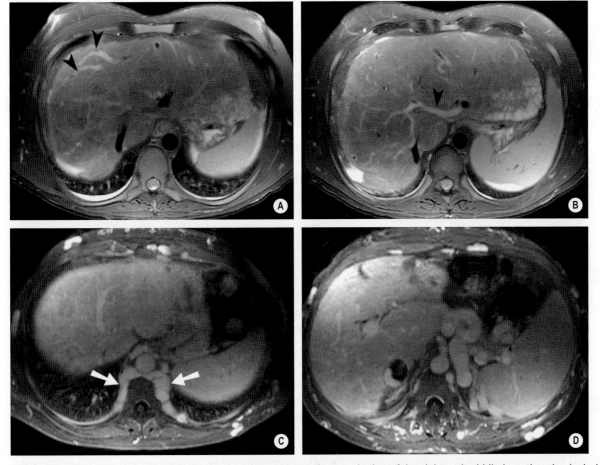

Chronic Budd–Chiari syndrome. Changes in a patient with previous occlusion of the right and middle hepatic veins include hypertrophy of the left lobe and numerous abnormal curved venous channels (arrowheads) shown on multi-shot T2W FSE imaging at two different levels (A, B). In a separate patient following occlusion of the IVC by thrombus (C, D) there are enlarged retroperitoneal and azygos system veins (arrows) as well as numerous superficial collateral veins shown on post-gadolinium T1W MRI.**

PORTAL VENOUS HYPERTENSION (PH)

Definition

- A corrected sinusoidal pressure difference between the wedged (occluded) hepatic vein and IVC of >8 mmHg (it is normally 4–8 mmHg) ▶ causes can be defined as:
  - *Prehepatic:* portal vein thrombosis (this may cause PH or be the consequence of it)
  - *Hepatic:* cirrhosis
  - *Posthepatic:* Budd–Chiari syndrome ▶ congestive heart failure

Radiological features

US Ascites and distended mesenteric veins ▶ an oedematous gallbladder, stomach and small bowel wall

- *Portal vein diameter:* this is >15 mm (a normal diameter does not exclude the diagnosis)
- *Main portal vein mean peak velocity:* <10 cm/s ▶ there is initially oscillating flow within the portal vein progressing to reversed (hepatofugal) flow
- *Splenomegaly:* this depends upon the degree of porto-systemic shunting, and an absence of splenomegaly does not exclude the diagnosis
- *Portosystemic venous collaterals:* splenogastric ▶ gastro-oesophageal ▶ splenorenal ▶ a recanalized paraumbilical vein
  - *Recanalized paraumbilical vein:* unusual portal venous patterns may emerge due to the increased

paraumbilical flow 'stealing' blood from the right portal vein (and resulting in hepatopetal right and hepatofugal left portal venous flow)

CT This is ideal for detecting the extrahepatic changes of portal venous hypertension, such as portosystemic shunts, and small bowel and gastric wall oedema

- Pre- and postcontrast images can assess the portal vein patency

MRI This is the non-invasive technique of choice if US is technically inadequate

- MRI and MRA: these can assess any GI tract changes as well as the hepatic and portal venous vasculature (± the presence of any shunt vessels)
- T1WI + Gad multiphase volumetric studies: this confirms the findings and also allows assessment of the flow direction (with breath-hold phase contrast or bolus tracking)

DSA This has been largely replaced by non-invasive techniques

Pearls

- Imaging is often used to assess the patency of surgical shunts (e.g. between the splenic and left renal vein, and between the portal vein and IVC)
- A radiologically placed transjugular intrahepatic portosystemic stent shunt (TIPSS) is increasingly used for palliating portal hypertension

PORTAL VEIN THROMBOSIS

Definition

- Thrombus formation within the portal vein can be idiopathic or due to: hepatic cirrhosis ▶ infection (portal pyaemia and acute cholecystitis) ▶ inflammation (pancreatitis and necrotizing colitis) ▶ tumour (HCC and pancreatic carcinoma) ▶ trauma ▶ coagulopathy ▶ surgery (liver transplantation)

Clinical presentation

- A patient can present with acute abdominal pain or with secondary complications (e.g. bowel infarction and ascites)
- There may be an occult presentation if there is already established cirrhosis (± portal hypertension and portosystemic shunt vessel formation)

Radiological features

Early An avascular solid lesion occluding and often expanding the portal vein

Late Contraction of the portal vein (which is often fibrotic or calcified)

- *Cavernous transformation:* multiple collateral vessel formation around the occluded portal vein
- Recanalization may make the discrimination between a tumour and pure thrombus difficult (a thrombosed portal vein or branch vein that remains enlarged is suspicious for tumour involvement)

US Acute thrombus is hypoechoic ▶ arterial signals within a thrombus is suggestive of tumour involvement (but may represent recanalization of the thrombus)

- Severe cirrhosis or fat infiltration may attenuate the acoustic beam to the extent that Doppler assessment is unreliable

MRI Time-of-flight and contrast-enhanced techniques can accurately demonstrate any portal vein thrombosis

CT Unenhanced and portal phase imaging will visualize a portal vein thrombus and any underlying structural causes (e.g. tumour or pancreatitis)

Pearl

- Assessment of portal vein patency in a cirrhotic patient is important as it will influence the choice of surgical or radiological shunt procedure

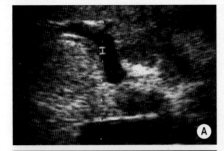

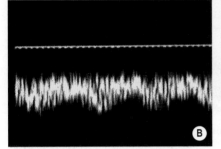

Portal venous hypertension: reversed portal vein flow. Duplex examination of the portal vein (A) demonstrates continuous reversed (hepatofugal) flow in the portal vein (B), usually reflecting underlying severe cirrhosis and portal venous hypertension with varices.*

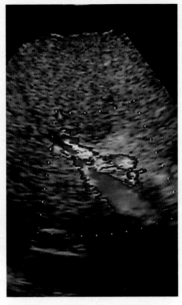

Note the irregular liver margin, coarse echoreflectivity and ascites in this cirrhotic liver, with normal forward flow (encoded red) within the hepatic artery and reversed flow (encoded blue) within the portal vein.

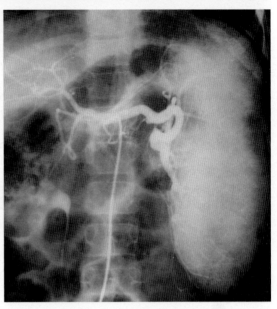

Coeliac angiogram in portal hypertension. Sparse liver arteries. Enlarged tortuous splenic artery with aneurysms on the main trunk and its divisions. Intrasplenic branches are stretched within a grossly enlarged spleen.†

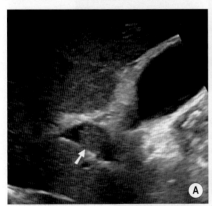

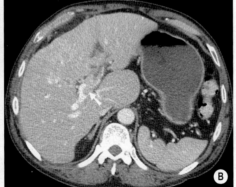

Portal vein thrombosis. A partial thrombosis is visible on ultrasound (A) as echo-reflective material within the portal vein (arrow). (B) This is shown as a filling defect on the matching portal phase CT (arrow).**

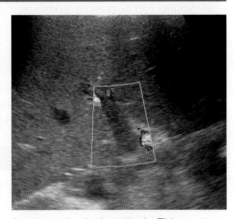

Acute portal vein thrombosis. This patient deteriorated 48 h after liver transplantation.**

VENO-OCCLUSIVE DISEASE (VOD)

DEFINITION

- This results from obliteration of the central draining veins of the hepatic lobules by an inflammatory fibrotic process
- It usually occurs following chemotherapy for bone marrow transplantation (resulting in secondary portal hypertension)
  - Cirrhosis is uncommon in bone marrow transplant patients – therefore suspect the onset of VOD

RADIOLOGICAL FEATURES

- Imaging is used to exclude other causes of abnormal liver function
- It demonstrates non-specific features: hepatomegaly ▶ portal hypertension (the major hepatic veins are not usually involved)

PEARL

Diagnosis Biopsy (coagulation markers may be an effective alternative)

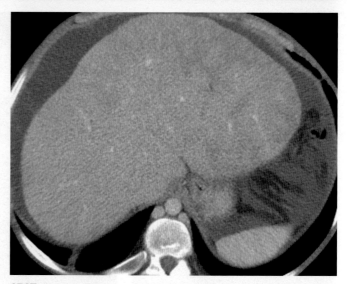

CECT showing hepatomegaly and ascites in a patient with veno-occlusive disease.

VASCULAR SHUNTS: ARTERIOPORTAL

DEFINITION

- A direct communication between branches of the hepatic artery and portal vein
  - Shunts can be misinterpreted as malignant lesions ▶ large shunts require embolization

CAUSES

- A penetrating liver injury (e.g. percutaneous diagnostic and interventional procedures) ▶ cirrhosis ▶ portal hypertension ▶ tumours (e.g. a large HCC)

RADIOLOGICAL FEATURES

US An area of increased flow on colour Doppler imaging (± arterialization of the portal venous flow if the shunt is large enough) ▶ a lesion may appear rounded or wedge shaped

CECT/DSA An early enhancing focal lesion with early filling of the portal vein ▶ hepatic arterial blood entering a portal vein branch produces a cone-shaped segmental portal 'blush' within the surrounding parenchyma

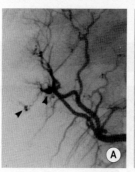 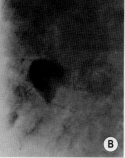

Hepatic arteriogram in a patient who had undergone percutaneous cholangiography 2 days earlier. (A) Arterial phase: arrowheads point to small arterioportal fistulae. (B) Capillary phase: dense 'blushes' due to early portal venous staining.*

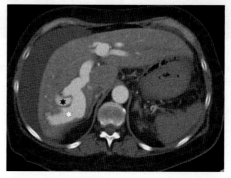

Arterioportal shunt. Portal phase CT demonstrates ascites and an atrophic right liver lobe. The enlarged artery is visible (black *) which connected almost directly into the portal vein (white *), creating a large volume shunt. The portal venous system has enlarged as a result and the shunting led to the right lobe atrophy and liver failure.**

VASCULAR SHUNTS: INTRAHEPATIC PORTOSYSTEMIC

DEFINITION

- A direct communication between the branches of the portal venous system and systemic hepatic veins

RADIOLOGICAL FEATURES

- *Congenital cases:* multiple small portovenous shunts (1–2 mm in diameter) within the periphery of an otherwise normal liver ▶ it may present with unexplained hepatic encephalopathy ▶ it is only detected with angiography
- *In association with portal hypertension and cirrhosis:* these are larger shunts typically between the right main portal vein and IVC ▶ their larger size allows detection with angiography, US and CECT

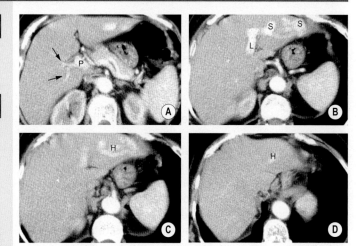

Intrahepatic portosystemic shunt. (A) The main portal vein (P) has fairly atrophic right branches (arrows). (B) This is because the left portal vein (L) is engorged as it directs the majority of flow through a portosystemic shunt (S). (C, D) The shunt directs flow into an early-filling left hepatic vein (H).

VASCULAR SHUNTS: ARTERIOVENOUS

DEFINITION

- A direct communication between arteries and veins without an intervening capillary bed
  - *Causes:* trauma ▶ tumours ▶ hereditary haemorrhagic telangiectasia (Osler–Weber–Rendu disease with multiple small intrahepatic arteriovenous shunts)

CLINICAL PRESENTATION

- They are often asymptomatic, but large shunts can lead to heart failure ▶ vascular dilatation can cause biliary obstruction and recurrent cholangitis ▶ ultimately hepatic necrosis may occur (and can be exacerbated by attempts at arterial embolization)

RADIOLOGICAL FEATURES

- Dilated hepatic arteries, hepatic and portal veins and with a tortuous vascular channel providing an intraparenchymal communication
  - *Small lesions:* these are only evident on DSA
  - *Larger lesions:* these are demonstrated with US (particularly Doppler studies), CECT and MRI

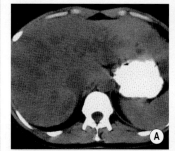
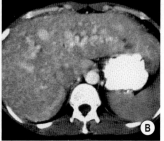
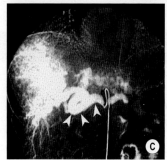

Hereditary haemorrhagic telangiectasia. Arteriovenous shunts result in enlarged vascular channels throughout the liver at CT (A), which enhance rapidly (B). The increased volume of shunted blood results in further enlargement of the vessels (C), including the supplying hepatic artery (arrowheads).*

HEPATIC TRAUMA

Definition Blunt or penetrating trauma may lead to an intraparenchymal laceration or haematoma, a subcapsular haematoma, or capsular rupture (with associated intraperitoneal haemorrhage)

Radiological findings

US This is more useful for follow-up rather than for diagnosis

- *Acute injury:* a parenchymal laceration with a related haematoma appears as an elliptical or irregularly shaped area of mixed low and high reflectivity (very recent haemorrhage may be relatively hyperechoic) ▶ free intraperitoneal fluid indicates a capsular rupture ▶ a subcapsular haematoma is well demonstrated

CT This is the investigation of choice ▶ it is able to assess the type of lesion and its anatomical relationship to the major hilar structures, the confluence of the hepatic veins and the IVC ▶ intraparenchymal lacerations and haematomas are again usually elliptical or linear in shape

- *NECT:* a low attenuation laceration ▶ high attenuation subcapsular and free intraperitoneal blood (recent haemorrhage is of higher attenuation than normal blood due to clot retraction)

- *CECT (arterial phase):* this is suggestive of a major vascular injury if a laceration involves the hilum or if there is a major perfusion deficit
- *CECT (portal phase):* this is mandatory to detect subtle lesions

Angiography This is only required when there is continuing haemorrhage (suggesting a major vessel laceration of a degree that is not immediately life-threatening) ▶ it can identify the source of any bleeding and permits embolization

MRI This is not routinely used ▶ it can demonstrate a parenchymal or subcapsular haematoma (especially when it is subacute as methaemoglobin increases the SI on T1WI) ▶ MRCP can assess the biliary system

Pearl

Unless the injury is life-threatening there is a trend towards conservative management

Complications Ischaemia and necrosis of the liver ▶ abscess formation ▶ haemobilia ▶ focal fibrosis ▶ calcification ▶ lobar or segmental atrophy

LIVER ABSCESS

Definition

- A localized intrahepatic collection of pus
- It is usually secondary to portal pyaemia (e.g. pyogenic, fungal, or mycobacterial) ▶ immunocompromised patients are at an increased risk
- **Early:** It can mimic a solid tumour (e.g. metastases) ▶ it may require aspiration or biopsy for diagnosis
- **Late:** There is progressive central liquefaction with a surrounding inflammatory wall

Radiological features

US *Early:* a solid ill-defined lesion of low reflectivity ▶ *Late:* there is a thickened irregular wall ▶ the necrotic centre generates sparse echoes

CT An ill-defined low attenuation lesion demonstrating rim enhancement (which may not be apparent once antibiotic treatment is started) ▶ when the central abscess liquefies it may be of water attenuation (and fail to enhance), appearing similar to a necrotic or cystic metastasis

MRI T1WI: low SI ▶ T2WI: high SI (often with a higher SI outer margin)

- With progressive liquefaction the central region will demonstrate increasingly low SI (T1WI) and high SI (T2WI)

Pearl

Treatment Image-guided aspiration or drainage (+ medical therapy) ▶ surgery is rarely required

AAST liver injury grading system	
Grade	**Description**
I	***Haematoma:*** subcapsular, <10% surface area Laceration: capsular tear, <1 cm in parenchymal depth
II	***Haematoma:*** subcapsular, 10–50% surface area ▶ intraparenchymal, <10 cm in diameter Laceration: 1–3 cm in parenchymal depth, <10 cm in length
III	***Haematoma:*** subcapsular, >50% surface area or expanding or ruptured subcapsular haematoma with active bleeding ▶ intraparenchymal, >10 cm or expanding or ruptured Laceration: >3 cm in parenchymal depth
IV	***Haematoma:*** ruptured intraparenchymal haematoma with active bleeding Laceration: parenchymal disruption involving 25–75% of a hepatic lobe or one to three Couinaud segments within a single lobe
V	***Laceration:*** parenchymal disruption involving >75% of a hepatic lobe or more than three Couinaud segments within a single lobe Vascular: juxtahepatic venous injuries (i.e. retrohepatic vena cava or central major hepatic veins)
VI	***Vascular:*** hepatic avulsion

© 19

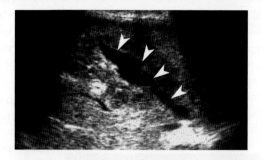

Intrahepatic laceration. Blunt hepatic trauma from a horse hoof has resulted in a linear laceration of the parenchyma clearly visible on US.*

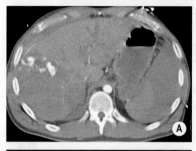

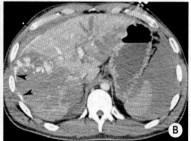

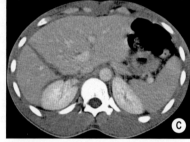

Traumatic hepatic laceration. A complex laceration and active haemorrhage is demonstrated in a road traffic accident patient on (A) arterial phase and (B) portal phase. Note the ongoing accumulation of contrast medium in the laceration and around the liver capsule (arrowheads). The patient went to immediate laparotomy. In a separate patient stabbed with a 15-cm knife a deep laceration is clearly demonstrated on portal phase imaging (C). Remarkably no major vessel was damaged and there was minimal haemorrhage.**

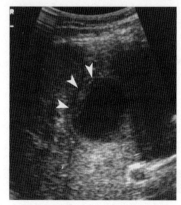

Liver abscess. An abscess, with typically reduced echoreflectivity and a thickened irregular wall (arrowheads).

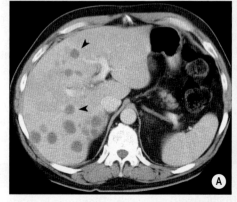

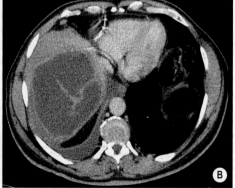

Liver abscess. Portal phase CT examinations in two different cases. (A) Multiple low attenuation lesions with ring enhancement (arrowheads) ▶ these appearances are often non-specific on CT and often overlap with those of metastatic deposits. (B) The presence of septae, central low attenuation, along with a sympathetic pleural effusion, aid the diagnosis.*

LIVER CYSTS

DEFINITION

- True hepatic cysts arise from abnormal development of the bile duct precursors (Meyenburg's complexes) which are lined by cuboidal epithelium
  - *Rare causes:* as a long-term sequelae of a parenchymal haematoma ▶ abscesses or if multiple as part of the spectrum of adult polycystic disease

CLINICAL PRESENTATION

- They are rarely symptomatic
- Large cysts may cause pain, become infected, or suffer internal haemorrhage

RADIOLOGICAL FEATURES

US

- **Simple cyst:** spherical anechoic structures with an imperceptible wall ▶ there is posterior acoustic enhancement ▶ there is no internal flow on Doppler settings
- **Complex cyst:** there can be internal echoes, thick septations, perceptible wall, or solid components ▶ this needs CT or MRI to characterize further

- *Causes:* haemorrhagic cyst ▶ abscess ▶ cystic metastasis (e.g. ovarian) ▶ biliary cystadenoma (or cystadenocarcinoma) ▶ hydatid disease

CT A homogeneous (0–10 HU) lesion with an imperceptible wall ▶ there is a lack of enhancement (internally or within the wall) ▶ there can be increased attenuation if it is a proteinaceous, infected, or haemorrhagic cyst

- Partial voluming may efface the characteristics of small lesions

MRI T1WI: low SI ▶ T2WI: very high SI (similar to CSF) ▶ T1WI + Gad: no enhancement

Scintigraphy Non-specific photopenic regions ▶ hepatobiliary iminodiacetic acid (HIDA) imaging may distinguish this from a choledochal cyst (which will show increased activity)

PEARL

Peliosis hepatis This is related to androgenic anabolic steroid use, and HIV with associated cutaneous bacillary angiomatosis (vascular proliferation containing bacteria) ▶ it is rare but increasing in frequency ▶ it affects the liver and other sites (e.g. the spleen)

- It is characterized by multiple small cystic lesions which demonstrate centrifugal or centripetal enhancement

HYDATID DISEASE

DEFINITION

- This follows liver infection with *Echinococcus granulosus* – a parasitic tapeworm transmitted to humans from dogs, sheep, foxes and other wild animals
- The larvae migrate from the gut and embed within the liver (and subsequently the lungs) where they encyst and develop, slowly provoking a surrounding inflammatory reaction ▶ they may remain occult for several years
  - *Endocyst:* the parasitic component – an inner germinative layer giving rise to the daughter vesicles
  - *Ectocyst:* the cyst membrane
  - *Pericyst:* the protective host fibrotic granulation tissue

RADIOLOGICAL FEATURES

XR Crescentic calcification within the pericyst ▶ complete calcification of all the cyst layers implies parasitic death

US The appearances can range from a simple cyst to a complicated cyst with any of the following features:

- *A heterogeneous mass:* the most common appearance
- *'Hydatid sand':* internal echogenic foci formed from dead dependent scolices
- *'Cyst with a cyst' appearance:* multiple daughter cysts
- *'Double rim' sign:* the pericyst and endocyst are seen as echogenic lines
- *Partial or complete detachment of the endocyst from the pericyst:* a floating membrane (partial) or the 'water lily' sign (complete)

CT A well-demarcated low-density cyst of fluid attenuation ▶ there is enhancement of the cyst wall ▶ wall calcification

MRI T1WI: low SI cyst contents with a low SI rim ▶ T2WI: high SI cyst contents with a low SI rim

- MRI is insensitive to any calcification

PEARL

- Diagnosis is made with serological testing ▶ the risk of anaphylaxis with aspiration is less than previously thought

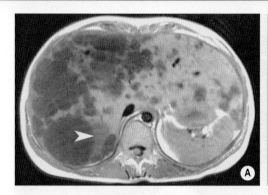

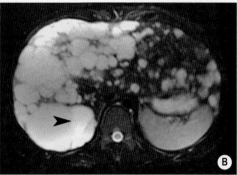

Polycystic liver disease. Multiple simple liver cysts are present and typically low signal on T1WI (A), and increased signal (greater than that of the spleen) on T2WI (B). Confusion may occur in the presence of haemorrhage, as this may increase the signal on T1WI (white arrowhead). In these circumstances the lack of enhancement following IV gadolinium DTPA may be diagnostic.*

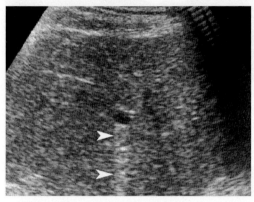

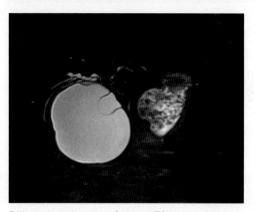

Simple liver cyst. On US simple cysts are well-defined areas of reduced echoreflectivity with no perceptible wall and posterior acoustic enhancement (arrowheads).

Biliary cystadenoma. Coronal T2 image demonstrating a large biliary cystadenoma with some simple septation seen medially.

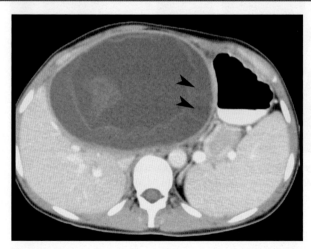

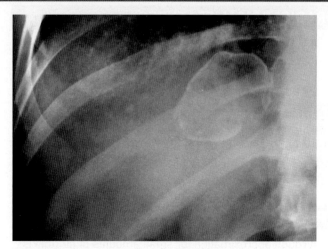

Hydatid disease. Portal phase CT demonstrates a large cystic structure with a discrete wall, separated internal membranes and several 'daughter cysts' (arrowheads).*

Typical egg shell calcification of an hydatid cyst.*

HEPATIC CALCIFICATION

DEFINITION

- Focal benign parenchymal calcification is relatively common
- *Causes:* tuberculosis ▶ sarcoidosis ▶ pyogenic abscesses ▶ parenchymal haematoma ▶ giant haemangioma ▶ metastatic mucin-secreting adenocarcinomas (e.g. colonic) ▶ hepatoblastoma ▶ fibrolamellar hepatoma ▶ Pneumocystis infection (with widespread focal calcification)

RADIOLOGICAL FEATURES

- Parenchymal calcification is usually well demarcated and surrounded by normal parenchyma

AXR Calcific densities

US Increased areas of reflectivity with a posterior acoustic shadow

NECT A high attenuation focus

MRI This is insensitive to calcification

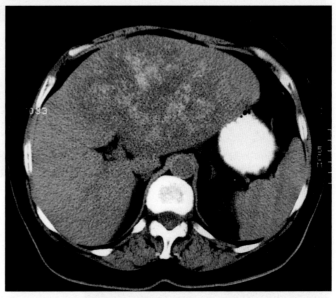

Liver calcification. NECT showing a large metastatic deposit in the left lobe of the liver from a primary colonic adenocarcinoma. Faint calcification is visible in the metastasis, which could be masked following IV contrast medium enhancement.[†]

AEROBILIA

DEFINITION

- Gas present within the biliary tree
- *Causes:* a sphincterotomy ▶ a Roux loop procedure (allowing reflux of intestinal gas into the biliary tree)

RADIOLOGICAL FEATURES

- A linear distribution of gas radiating from the hilum ▶ there is a gravity dependence with air predominantly located within the non-dependent parts of the biliary tree

US The biliary ducts are apparent as echogenic linear structures ▶ there is movement of any gas with respiration or patient position

CT This is extremely sensitive for the detection of air (which will measure –1000 HU)

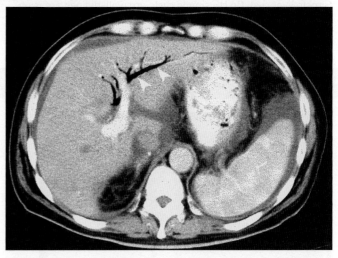

Biliary duct gas. CT demonstrates clearly the low attenuation gas (arrowheads) in the non-dependent biliary tree.[*]

PEARL

- A rough approximation for small amounts of air (this is not valid for large amounts of air):
  - Biliary air tends to be more centrally located within the liver (due to centripetal biliary flow)
  - Portal venous gas tends to be more peripherally located within the liver (due to centrifugal portal venous flow)

PORTAL VEIN GAS

DEFINITION

- Gas within the portal vein and its branches ▶ this arises when intestinal permeability increases together with an increase in the intestinal luminal pressure
- *Causes:* neonatal necrotizing enterocolitis ▶ gastric emphysema ▶ intestinal volvulus ▶ infection ▶ ischaemic bowel ▶ blunt abdominal trauma ▶ invasive abdominal malignancies ▶ duodenal perforation at ERCP ▶ colitis following a barium enema

RADIOLOGICAL FEATURES

- Gas radiates out from the hilum ▶ there is less marked gravity dependence than seen with aerobilia

US This is the most sensitive modality and can demonstrate moving gas bubbles ▶ there is a high-pitched random bubbling and squeaking sound with focal alias artefacts seen on spectral display (as the gas bubbles overload the system receivers)

XR/CT This can detect portal vein gas if large amounts are present ▶ air (−1000 HU) is seen within the main portal vein and its branches

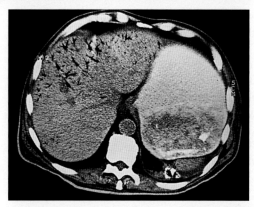

CT demonstrates air within the portal venous system of the liver in a postoperative patient unrelated to bowel necrosis.

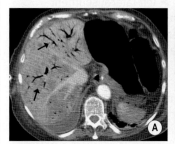
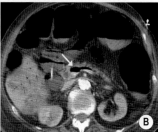
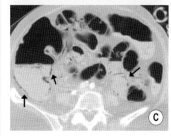

(A) Axial CECT showing extensive portal venous gas (arrows) within the liver in a patient with ischaemic bowel. (B) CECT in same patient showing gas within the main portal vein (arrow) and splenic vein. (C) Axial CECT on lung windows showing extensive pneumatosis in the bowel wall in the same patient.

PARENCHYMAL GAS

DEFINITION

- Intrahepatic parenchymal gas
- *Causes:* gas-forming organism within an abscess or infarct ▶ post-traumatic ▶ hepatic arterial thrombosis following liver transplantation ▶ following embolization or thermal ablation of liver tumours

RADIOLOGICAL FEATURES

US An echogenic area with posterior acoustic shadowing ▶ it may be difficult to define its extent when large ▶ it can be confused with adjacent bowel

CT This is the most sensitive for its delineation

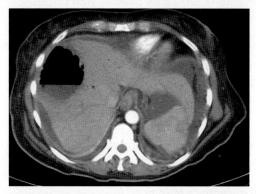

Large gas-forming abscess within the right lobe of the liver demonstrating a clear air-fluid level. A small amount of ascites and a small pleural effusion are also present.

343

ORTHOTOPIC LIVER TRANSPLANTATION

- This is an established treatment for end-stage liver disease (with ≥90% 1-year survival and ≥80% 5-year survival)
  - *Causes:* cirrhosis secondary to infective hepatitis (the most common cause) ▶ autoimmune disease ▶ alcohol abuse ▶ Alagille's syndrome
- The majority of donor livers are of cadaveric origin ▶ however, demand exceeds supply, leading to the development of:
  - *Split-graft procedures:* a single organ donation to benefit 2 or more patients ▶ typically the left lateral segment for a child and the right lobe for an adult recipient
  - *Living donors:* donation of the full right lobe (most common) ▶ full left lobe ▶ left lateral segment
  - *Auxiliary transplantation:* 'piggy-backing' a graft alongside the native liver as a temporary measure (e.g. in reversible liver failure)

Technique

- A 'piggy back technique' is now the standard procedure, preserving the retrohepatic IVC and anastomosing the donor IVC patch to the recipient hepatic veins (which are formed into a common cuff)
- The hepatectomy plane is 1 cm to either side of the middle hepatic vein and parallel to the 'principal plane'
- *Left lateral segment transplantation (paediatric):* donor segments II and III along with the left hepatic vein, left portal vein, left hepatic artery and left bile duct are removed ▶ the middle hepatic vein and middle hepatic artery (segment IV) are preserved in the donor
- *Right lobe transplantation (adult):* entire donor right lobe, right hepatic vein, right portal vein, right hepatic artery and right bile duct ▶ the middle hepatic artery (segment IV artery) and middle hepatic vein are preserved in the donor

Recipient assessment

- *Identify and characterize focal liver lesions:*
  - The Milan criteria is used for patients with cirrhosis and an increased risk of HCC: transplantation is performed if there is a single lesion (≤5 cm) or 3 lesions (≤3 cm)
  - 1–2 different imaging techniques are required to identify a HCC depending on lesion size (as this can be difficult to demonstrate within a cirrhotic liver) ▶ a biopsy is usually avoided due to the risk of tumour 'seeding'
  - Transplantation is rarely performed for a known cholangiocarcinoma (due to the poor prognosis)
- *Assess the patency of the portal vein and IVC:* this is usually with multiphase MRA or CTA
  - *Portal vein:* if this is occluded it is important to ascertain if the confluence of the SMV and splenic vein is involved as it will affect the surgical approach (vascular reconstructions can be used to 'jump' to this

confluence and allow successful grafting despite an occluded main portal vein)
  - *IVC:* the extent of the involvement is important with Budd–Chiari syndrome
- *Identify anatomical variants:* MRA and CTA can be used to assess variant hepatic arterial anatomy (variant portal vein anatomy is less of an issue)

Living donor assessment

- Usually the left lobe is resected ▶ increasingly the right lobe segments are removed (but there is a greater mortality)
- Cross-sectional and three-dimensional (3D) imaging techniques are used to detect variants of the arterial, portal venous, hepatic venous and biliary systems
  - Anomalies that cross the planned surgical division plane are the most important and may lead to complications for both the donor and recipient

Perioperative imaging

- *The detection of early complications:* haemorrhage ▶ haematoma and abscess formation ▶ anastomotic breakdown
  - It also allows image-guided drainage and aspiration
- *Surveillance imaging:* this is performed regularly for high-risk groups (e.g. paediatric transplants and complex vascular reconstructions) ▶ it detects sudden complications that may respond to an immediate intervention (e.g. hepatic arterial occlusion)

Graft failure

- **Causes of early graft failure:**
  - *Primary non-function:* hepatocyte function fails to recover in the newly perfused graft despite vascular patency and good perfusion at the time of surgery ▶ it is influenced by hepatic steatosis
  - *Hepatic artery thrombosis:* this occurs in 3–5% adults and 5–15% of children ▶ Doppler US is the initial mainstay of diagnosis ▶ it presents with:
    - Catastrophic liver failure with infarction and abscess formation ▶ Biliary complications (e.g. a leak or stricture formation) ▶ Silently with no obvious sequelae
  - *Portal vein thrombosis and IVC occlusions:* these are relatively rare
  - *Acute rejection:* this is infrequent due to improved immunosuppression
  - *Overwhelming sepsis*
- **Causes of late graft failure:**
  - *Causes:* chronic rejection ▶ chronic ischaemia ▶ biliary anastomotic failure ▶ diffuse biliary disease due to sepsis ▶ recurrence of the underlying disease (e.g. primary sclerosing cholangitis or hepatitis C infection)
  - The diagnosis is often made on biopsy

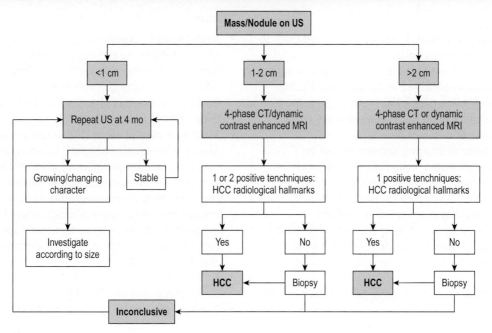

HCC diagnostic algorithm.

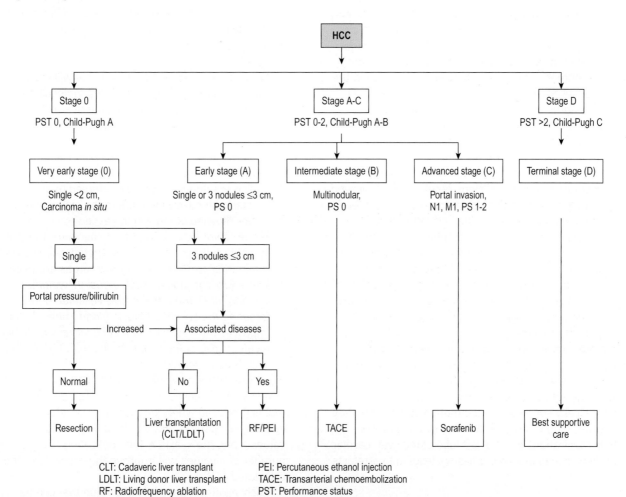

CLT: Cadaveric liver transplant   PEI: Percutaneous ethanol injection
LDLT: Living donor liver transplant   TACE: Transarterial chemoembolization
RF: Radiofrequency ablation   PST: Performance status

BCLC staging system and treatment strategy.

DIFFUSION WEIGHTED MR IMAGING OF THE LIVER

Technique

- DW MR imaging of the liver is usually performed prior to contrast material administration
- It uses a standard T2-weighted imaging sequence with application of a symmetric pair of diffusion sensitizing gradients on either side of the 180° refocusing pulse ▶ the use of parallel imaging techniques permits rapid imaging and reduction in motion artefact
- Although a number of imaging sequences can be applied, a single-shot spin-echo (SE) echo-planar technique is the most frequently used in combination with fat suppression (to reduce ghosting from respiratory motion and chemical shift artefact)
- Imaging may be performed during a breath hold, which attempts to freeze motion, or during free breathing with multiple signal acquisitions to reduce the effects of motion
  - *Breath-hold single-shot SE echo-planar imaging:* this is quick to perform
    - The whole liver can be evaluated in generally 1–2 breath holds of 20–30 s
    - *Disadvantages:* poorer signal-to-noise ratio (SNR) ▶ a greater sensitivity to distortion and ghosting artefacts ▶ a lower spatial resolution (with wider section thickness of 8–10 mm) ▶ a limitation on the number of *b* values that can be included in the measurement
  - *Free breathing:* this can also be combined with respiratory ± cardiac triggering ▶ high-quality diffusion images can be obtained as cyclical respiration is a coherent motion
    - The liver is typically evaluated in 3–6 min ▶ multiple signal acquisitions results in an improved SNR ▶ therefore thinner image sections can be obtained and more *b* values accommodated
    - *Disadvantages:* slight image blurring ▶ volume averaging with a longer measurement time may impair assessment of lesion heterogeneity ▶ respiratory triggering increases the acquisition time as the images are only acquired during part of the respiratory cycle (increasing the risk of patient movement)
- **The major limitations of diffusion-weighted MR imaging:** a low signal-to-noise ratio (SNR) inherent in the technique ▶ a susceptibility to motion artefact
  - As single-shot SE echo-planar sequences are intrinsically sensitized to the motion of diffusion, they are also highly sensitive to other kinds of motion (e.g. respiration) ▶ in the left lobe of the liver, cardiac motion results in spin dephasing, leading to artefacts

Theory

- **Static water protons:** these acquire an initial phase shift (the size of which is dependent upon the location along the sensitizing gradient) from the first diffusion-sensitizing gradient ▶ the second gradient will exactly reverse this phase shift as all protons remain in their original location
- **Moving water protons:** these acquire an initial phase shift (the size of which is dependent on the location along the sensitizing gradient) from the first diffusion-sensitizing gradient ▶ this is not exactly rephased by the second gradient (as the protons have moved from their original location and the second gradient is no longer a perfect match) ▶ this new reduced phase coherence results in attenuation of the measured signal intensity
  - Therefore the presence of water diffusion is observed as signal loss on DW MRI
- **b value:** this refers to the strength of the diffusion-sensitizing gradient, and is proportional to the gradient amplitude, the duration of the applied gradient and the time interval between paired gradients ▶ the sensitivity of the diffusion sequence is adjusted by varying the *b* value (most readily achieved by altering the gradient amplitude)
  - *Small b values* ($50–100$ s/mm²): this will result in signal loss in highly mobile water molecules ▶ the water molecules will have moved over relatively large distances by the time the rephasing gradient is applied ▶ consequently they will not regain their original phase information after application of the rephasing gradient.
    - The resulting images are referred to as 'black-blood' images due to the signal loss in the fast-flowing blood within vessels
  - *Higher b values* (≥ 200 s/mm²): as water movement in highly cellular tissues is restricted, such tissues retain their signal until higher *b* values are used
  - *Therefore applying a small diffusion-weighted gradient nulls the intrahepatic vascular signal (creating the so-called black-blood images) and improves the detection of focal liver lesions ▶ higher b values give diffusion information that helps focal liver lesion characterization*
- **Acquired diffusion coefficient (ADC):** for an individual voxel the ADC represents the slope (gradient) of a line that is produced when the logarithm of relative signal intensity of tissue is plotted along the y-axis versus *b* values along the x-axis ▶ the application of a greater number of *b* values will improve the accuracy of the calculated ADC
  - Each voxel will have an ADC value that can be combined visually as an ADC 'map'

- **T2 shine-through:** the signal intensity on diffusion-weighted images is dependent on water molecule diffusion and T2 relaxation time (it is based on a T2 sequence) ▶ therefore lesions with a high fluid content (e.g. cysts) can demonstrate high signal intensity even at high *b* values

- **DW MRI and tumour treatment:** effective tumour treatment results in an increase in the ADC value ▶ a transient reduction in ADC within 24–48 h after initiation of treatment has been observed (due to acute cell swelling) ▶ the ADC will subsequently decrease (due to tumour repopulation, fibrosis or tissue remodelling)

- **DW MRI imaging is a marker of cellularity,** therefore:
  - Benign solid lesions (e.g. FNH) may display restricted diffusion
  - Necrotic malignant lesions can demonstrate high ADC values
  - Therefore, DW MRI is most effectively interpreted in conjunction with other conventional MRI sequences.

b value	ADC	Cause
High	Low	Cellular tissue or tumour
Low	High	Cystic or necrotic tissue
High	High	T2 shine-through
Low	Low	Artefact or fat

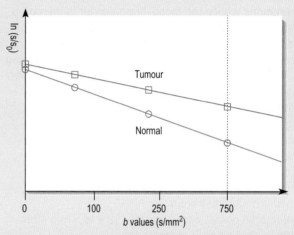

A graph showing the relationship of signal intensities (y-axis) vs *b* values (x-axis). The gradient of the line represents the ADC for a tissue, and the gradient of the line is steeper for normal tissue than tumour.

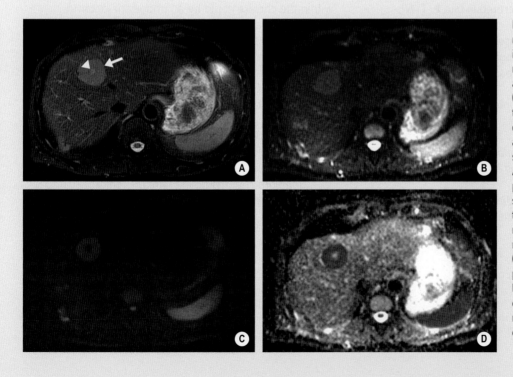

Diffusion imaging of a liver metastasis. (A) T2 fat-saturated image showing a high signal metastatic deposit (arrow) with a necrotic fluid filled centre (arrowhead). (B) At low *b* values, the metastasis is of high signal, demonstrating restricted diffusion, and the necrotic centre is also of high signal due to 'T2-shine through'. (C) At higher *b* values, the hypercellular periphery is of slightly reduced signal intensity (but still higher than the adjacent normal tissue). The necrotic centre loses proportionately more signal. (D) The hypercellular (restricted diffusion) nature of the periphery is confirmed by the signal loss on the ADC map, and the central high signal confirms the non restricted fluid nature of the necrotic centre.

MRI CONTRAST AGENTS

- MR imaging is an order of magnitude more sensitive to the effect of gadolinium than CT is to the effect of iodine – therefore a far lower dose of gadolinium is required for MR imaging
- Discontinue breast feeding for 24 hours following gadolinium ▶ only use gadolinium if absolutely necessary in pregnancy
- Extracellular MRI contrast agents do not cross the intact specialized vascular blood–brain barrier.
  - These agents accumulate in tissues with abnormal vascularity (malignant and inflammatory lesions) and in regions where the blood–brain barrier is disrupted
- Dynamic MR imaging of the liver is performed after bolus IV contrast injection ▶ fat-saturated three-dimensional (3D) volume interpolated MR imaging (e.g. VIBE, THRIVE, FAME) allows high spatial resolution imaging of the entire liver to be acquired in a 20-s breath hold
- Imaging is repeated in the arterial, portovenous and parenchymal phases of liver enhancement:
  - *Hepatic arterial phase:* typically 20–30 s after IV injection
  - *The portovenous phase:* 60–90 s after IV contrast medium administration
  - *Interstitial phase:* approximately 90 s to 5 min after administration of IV contrast agent
  - *Delayed hepatic enhancement phase:* this occurs at 15–30 min for Primovist and approximately 1–3 h for MultiHance
- **Hepatocyte selective gadolinium chelates:** paramagnetic compounds that are taken up by functioning hepatocytes and excreted in bile ▶ T1WI: increased SI
  - A major indication for their use is to characterize lesions as hepatocellular or non-hepatocellular:
    - *Hepatocyte-containing masses* (e.g. FNH): usually enhance
  - *Adenoma:* they appear hypointense as they do not contain normal biliary radicals
  - *FNH:* hyper- or isointense
  - *Metastases (non-hepatocellular) and hepatocellular carcinoma (poorly functioning hepatocytes):* frequently hypointense
- **Non-gadolinium contrast media:** unlike the gadolinium-based contrast media, dynamic imaging is not performed

- Teslascan is infused intravenously and its selective uptake by hepatocytes results in intense T1 liver signal enhancement at approximately 30 min, persisting for several hours
- **Reticuloendothelial system iron-based contrast media:** iron accumulates within Kupffer cells in the normal liver, resulting in reduction in signal intensity of the liver during T2*-weighted gradient-echo imaging ▶ lesions containing Kupffer cells demonstrate signal reduction, whereas lesions that are Kupffer cell depleted remain high signal
  - They are used most routinely to aid in HCC detection in high-risk patients ▶ HCC detection in cirrhosis with gadolinium may be difficult due to fibrosis, regenerating nodules and altered liver perfusion
  - NB: well-differentiated HCC may accumulate SPIO particles

Nephrogenic systemic fibrosis (NSF)

- The disease is characterized by scleroderma-like skin changes mainly affecting the limbs and trunk – this can progress to flexion contracture of joints ▶ the fibrotic changes may also affect other organs such as muscles, heart, liver and lungs
  - NSF is associated with gadolinium use and thus contraindicated with severe renal impairment (GFR <30 ml/min)
  - Use as low a dose as possible in moderate impairment (GFR 31-48 ml/min)
  - Immediate haemodialysis is not protective
- The stability of the binding of the gadolinium ion (Gd^{+++}) within the chelate could be an important factor in the pathogenesis ▶ the stability of the Gd chelates is influenced by the configuration of the molecule (whether linear or macrocyclic as well as its ionicity)
  - Macrocyclic chelates offer better protection and binding to Gd^{+++} (cf. linear molecules) ▶ therefore the least stable molecules are the non-ionic linear chelates
    - *High risk*: Omniscan (linear – non-ionic) ▶ OptiMARK (linear – non-ionic) ▶ Magnevist (linear – ionic)
    - *Medium risk*: Primovist (linear – ionic)
    - *Low risk*: ProHance (cyclic – non-ionic)

Classes	Non-specific extracellular gadolinium chelates	Hepatocyte selective gadolinium chelates	Non-gadolinium-based contrast media		
Examples	Magnevist ProHance Gadovist	MultiHance Primovist	Teslascan (manganese based)	Endorem (iron oxide based)	Resovist (iron oxide based)
Constituents	Low-molecular-weight gadolinium chelates	Low-molecular-weight gadolinium chelates: Gd-BOPTA, Gd-EOB-DTPA	Mangafodipir trisodium (MnDPDP)	Superparamagnetic iron oxide particles	Superparamagnetic iron oxide particles
Action	Distributes freely in the *extracellular* space	Initially distributes freely in *extracellular* space but undergoes *hepatic* excretion	Selective uptake by *hepatocytes* and excreted into bile ducts	Selective uptake by *Kupffer* cells	Selective uptake by *Kupffer* cells

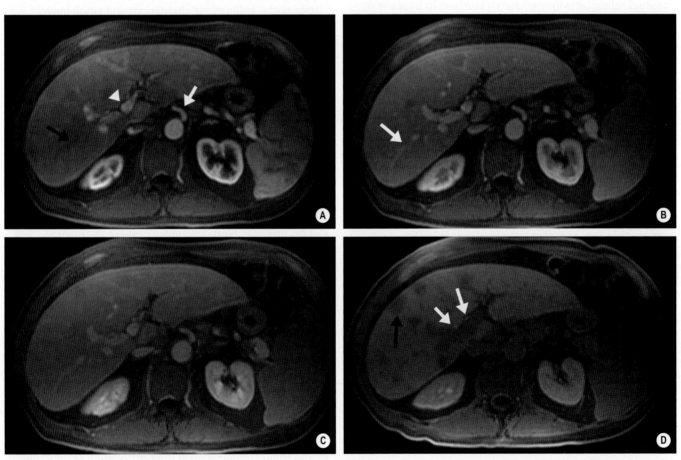

MR study of the liver with a hepatocyte specific gadolinium chelate. (A) Arterial phase. There is contrast within the hepatic artery (white arrow). Contrast within the portal vein (arrowhead) indicates that sufficient time has passed for arterial enhancement of any lesion, but the lack of contrast within the hepatic veins (black arrow) ensures that there has not been any significant washout of contrast from the liver parenchyma. (B) Contrast is now seen within the hepatic veins (white arrow), indicating that a true parenchymal phase of enhancement has been reached. (C) Interstitial phase at about 3 minutes. (D) Delayed imaging with a hepatocyte specific agent, as indicated by contrast excretion via the biliary tree (white arrows). The multiple liver metastases that are hepatocyte poor and do not take up contrast are now much more visible on delayed imaging.

3.7 BILIARY

MAGNETIC RESONANCE CHOLANGIOPANCREATOGRAPHY (MRCP)

Technique

- Heavily T2-weighted coronal oblique fast spin-echo sequence to obtain source data (aligned along the plane of the common bile duct [CBD])
  - Stationary water appears as areas of high SI and adjacent soft tissue is low SI (therefore it is not reliant on contrast excretion and can be used in jaundiced patients)
  - Fasting reduces any unwanted signal from the adjacent intestine
  - Breath-hold or non-breath-hold (respiratory triggered) imaging
- Source data allows MIP reformats to be generated (highlighting fluid-filled structures) – usually a number of coronal MIP reformats over 180°
- *Secretin:* this stimulates exocrine pancreatic secretion, distending the pancreatic duct and improving its visualization (acts immediately, returning to baseline at 10 min)
- *Functional MR cholangiography:* using delayed imaging at 30–60 min with the hepatobiliary excreted contrast agents Gd-EOB-DTPA (Primovist) or Gd-BOPTA (MultiHance)
  - *Uses:* liver donor transplant work-up ▶ the assessment of bile leaks and biliary communication with cysts ▶ the demonstration of segmental obstruction

Normal anatomy

- *Normal morphology:* only central intrahepatic ducts are normally seen (≤3 mm) ▶ extrahepatic ducts ≤7 mm (CBD up to 10 mm post cholecystectomy) ▶ pancreatic duct ≤3 mm ▶ accessory pancreatic duct in 45%
- *Right posterior hepatic duct* (segments VI/VII): almost horizontal course
- *Right anterior hepatic duct* (segments V/VIII): more vertical course
- *Left hepatic duct* (segments II–IV): joins the right to form the common hepatic duct ▶ separate drainage of segment I
- *Cystic duct insertion into common hepatic duct:* right lateral (50%) ▶ anterior (30%) ▶ posterior (20%)
- *Common variants:* an aberrant right posterior duct draining into the common hepatic duct or cystic duct ▶ drainage of the right anterior or posterior duct into the left hepatic duct ▶ a triple confluence at the hilum

Imaging pitfalls

- *Technique:* volume averaging artefacts in MIP reformats can obscure filling defects – source images must always be reviewed ▶ MIP reformats can also over- and underestimate strictures
- *Normal variants:* a long cystic duct running parallel to the CBD, stimulating a distended CBD ▶ a contracted sphincter mimicking an impacted stone
- *Intraductal factors mimicking filling defects:* aerobilia (non-dependent) ▶ flow phenomena (central signal void) ▶ debris ▶ haemorrhage
- *Extraductal factors:* pulsatile vascular compression from adjacent vessels mimicking a stricture (but no proximal dilatation) ▶ susceptibility artefact from surgical clips

HEPATOBILIARY SCINTIGRAPHY

- Hepatobiliary iminodiacetic acid (HIDA) scintigraphy: this is a bilirubin analogue labelled with ^{99m}Tc
  - It is injected intravenously with serial images obtained over 2–4 h (it requires near-normal bilirubin levels)
- There is normally accumulation of isotope within liver, bile ducts, gallbladder, duodenum and small bowel by 1 h
  - *Delayed hepatic activity:* hepatocellular disease (with corresponding elevated bilirubin levels)
  - *Non-demonstration of the gallbladder:* acute cholecystitis ▶ a contracted gallbladder (e.g. following a recent meal)
  - Drugs that may aid visualization:
    - *Cholecystokinin:* this contracts the gallbladder
    - *Morphine:* this causes spasm of the sphincter of Oddi, therefore distending the biliary tree

ENDOSCOPIC ULTRASOUND (EUS)

- This provides high-frequency grey-scale imaging (± colour Doppler) for the evaluation of the extrahepatic biliary tree, pancreas and duodenum ▶ it can also allow fine-needle aspiration cytology to be performed

ENDOSCOPIC RETROGRADE CHOLANGIOPANCREATOGRAPHY (ERCP)

- This allows direct bile and pancreatic duct opacification, as well as visual assessment of the duodenum and ampulla of Vater
  - *It also allows for:* biopsy ▶ brushings ▶ sphincterotomy ▶ stone extraction ▶ biliary stenting ▶ biliary stricture dilatation
- The main complication is the precipitation of pancreatitis
- The main pitfall is the presence of underfilled ducts above a stricture

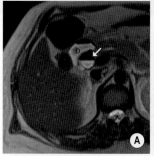
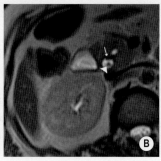
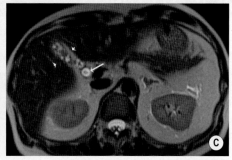

Example of intraductal factors causing potential pitfalls in interpretation. (A) Axial T2-weighted MRI shows an air-fluid level in a dilated proximal CBD in keeping with aerobilia (arrow), adjacent to the duodenum (D), which also shows an air-fluid level. (B) More distally in the same patient, the cause of the obstruction is seen with a dependent filling defect (arrowhead) in the distal CBD in keeping with a stone. This should not be confused with the non-dependent aerobilia also shown at this level (arrow). (C) Axial T2-weighted MRI in a different patient shows a central filling defect in a dilated CBD which is due to flow artefact (arrow). The patient also has chronic cholecystitis with a contracted gallbladder (arrowheads).

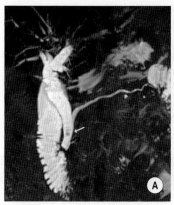
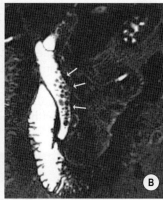

Example of a partial voluming artefact. (A) Coronal maximum intensity projection (MIP) reformat shows a possible filling defect (arrow) in the dilated distal CBD. (B) The thin section MRCP source image in fact demonstrates multiple filling defects (arrows) in the CBD, in keeping with stones.

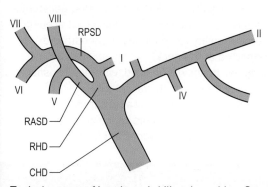

Typical pattern of intrahepatic biliary branching. Segments are numbered according to the system of Couinaud. CHD = common hepatic duct, RHD = right hepatic duct, LHD = left hepatic duct, RPSD = right posterior sectoral duct, RASD = right anterior sectoral duct.** (From Blumgart L H, Fong Y [eds] 2000 Surgery of the Liver and Biliary Tract, 3rd edn. WB Saunders, London, p 365, with permission.)

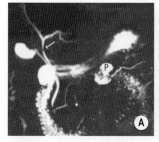
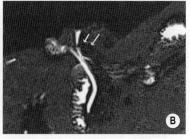

(A) Coronal MIP reformat suggests a stricture or possible filling defect in the common hepatic duct (arrow) but with no upstream dilatation. Incidental note is also made of a small pseudocyst (P) associated with the main pancreatic duct. (B) Thin-section MRCP image more clearly shows that this is due to extrinsic compression from the right hepatic artery, which appears as a subtle curvilinear signal void outside the duct and extending across it (arrows).

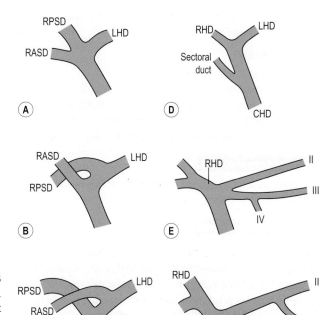

Variations of biliary branching patterns. The more common are A, B and C. Segments are numbered according to the system of Couinaud. CHD = common hepatic duct, RHD = right hepatic duct, LHD = left hepatic duct, RPSD = right posterior sectoral duct, RASD = right anterior sectoral duct.** (From Blumgart L H, Fong Y [eds] 2000 Surgery of the Liver and Biliary Tract, 3rd edn. WB Saunders, London, p 365, with permission.)

CHOLELITHIASIS (GALLSTONES)

Definition
- Stones present within the gallbladder – this affects 15% of the Western population (F>M) ▶ there is a small lifetime risk of developing a gallbladder carcinoma
- *Gallstone composition:* cholesterol (70%) ▶ pigment stones composed of calcium bilirubinate (up to 30%)

Clinical presentation
- Asymptomatic (80%) or presenting with biliary colic, acute or chronic cholecystitis, or obstructive jaundice

Radiological features

AXR Only 10–15% of calculi are visible (if they are calcified) ▶ larger stones tend to be laminated

US This has a sensitivity of > 95% for detecting gallstones ▶ gallstones appear as echogenic foci which cast acoustic shadows ▶ stone mobility is frequently demonstrated (unless it is impacted at the neck)
- NB: a gallbladder polyp will be fixed, with no acoustic shadow and may demonstrate vascularity
- 'Double-arc shadow' sign: two parallel curved echogenic lines separated by a thin anechoic space with dense acoustic shadowing in a gallbladder full of stones

CT Only a minority of gallstones are visible ▶ these are hypodense, hyperdense or of mixed density

Pearls
- **Reasons for non-visualization of the gallbladder:** a previous cholecystectomy ▶ a non-fasting state ▶ an abnormal gallbladder position ▶ emphysematous cholecystitis ▶ a gallbladder full of stones
- **Biliary sludge:** this is composed of calcium bilirubinate granules, cholesterol crystals and glycoproteins ▶ it is commonly seen with fasting states, critically ill patients, pregnancy and in those patients receiving total parenteral nutrition ▶ it resolves spontaneously in 50% of cases

US Fine, non-shadowing dependent echoes ▶ small gallstones can be difficult to detect if they lie within any sludge
- Sludge can be differentiated from a tumour by its mobility, lack of internal flow, and lack of an associated gallbladder wall abnormality
- Blood (haemobilia) and pus (empyema) can appear similar to sludge (the clinical setting aids the diagnosis)

CHOLEDOCHOLITHIASIS

Definition
Choledocholithiasis
- Stones within the bile duct
  - *Primary* (10%): arising within the bile duct (pigment stones)
  - *Secondary* (90%): stones that have passed from the gallbladder into the bile duct

Hepatolithiasis
- Intrahepatic stone formation
  - This may occur with common duct stones but is more often associated with other pathologies: benign strictures ▶ primary sclerosing cholangitis ▶ recurrent pyogenic cholangitis ▶ Caroli's disease

Clinical presentation
- Right upper quadrant pain ▶ obstructive jaundice ▶ pancreatitis

Radiological features

US An intraductal echogenic focus needs to be demonstrated in both the longitudinal and transverse planes (± duct dilatation) ▶ a duct diameter <4 mm carries a high negative predictive value for choledocholithiasis (regardless of the gallbladder status)
- Conditions mimicking a stone:
  - *Intraductal gas:* this has a linear nature and will be mobile

  - *Haemobilia and sludge:* this produces more diffuse echoes than a stone
  - *Surgical clips:* these will lie outside the duct lumen
  - *Parasites:* e.g. hydatid membranes

EUS This is more sensitive than standard US (with a sensitivity and specificity >90%)

NECT A ring density or soft tissue density within the bile duct and surrounded by bile (sensitivity 60–88% ▶ specificity >95%)

CT-IVC This has a high accuracy, with a reported sensitivity of up to 96% and a specificity of up to 98% ▶ it can diagnose stones that are <5 mm in diameter ▶ its main weakness is its reliance on a near-normal serum bilirubin

MRCP An intraluminal signal void visible in 2 thin-section orthogonal planes ▶ this has a high sensitivity (up to 94%) and specificity (99%) ▶ its quality is independent of the serum bilirubin levels
- False negative: stones <5 mm
- False positive: gas (gas will rise, stones are dependent) ▶ haemobilia ▶ flow voids

Pearl
- 8–15% of patients who are under the age of 60 years and who have undergone a cholecystectomy have duct stones

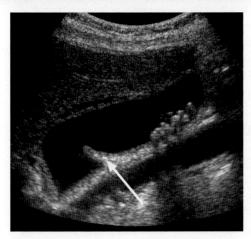

US shows multiple small shadowing stones. A normal fold (arrow) lies near the gallbladder neck.*

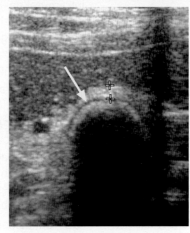

Gallbladder filled with stones producing the 'double-arc' sign ▶ hypoechoic line between two echogenic lines (arrow).*

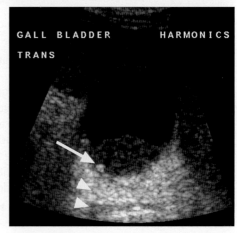

Sludge within which a small stone (arrow) casts a subtle acoustic shadow (arrowheads).*

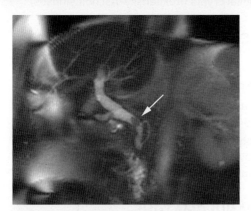

Choledocholithiasis. Single common duct stone (arrow) on thick-section, oblique, coronal MRCP.**

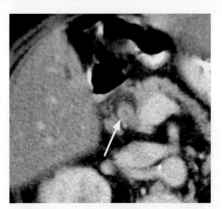

Choledocholithiasis. A distal common bile duct stone (arrow) is slightly dense compared with the surrounding low-density bile.*

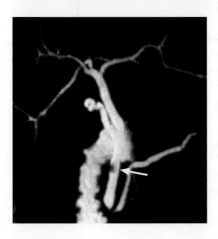

Choledocholithiasis. Single common duct stone (arrow) on thick-section, oblique, coronal MRCP. There has been a previous cholecystectomy.*

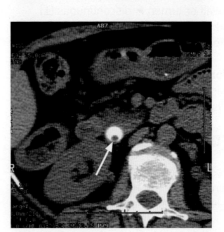

Choledocholithiasis. CT-IVC shows a small stone within the opacified distal common bile duct.*

ACUTE CALCULOUS CHOLECYSTITIS

Definition Gallbladder inflammation (which is secondary to gallstones in 90–95% of cases)

US This is the best initial imaging modality ▶ the signs include:

- A gallbladder wall thickness >3 mm ▶ gallbladder distension (>5 cm) ▶ pericholecystic fluid and gallbladder wall striations (± wall hyperaemia on Doppler) ▶ gallstones (common bile duct stones are suggested by abnormal liver function tests)
  - Fine echoes within the gallbladder may suggest the presence of sludge or pus (a gallbladder empyema)

CT Gallbladder wall thickening (>2 mm) ▶ subserosal oedema and gallbladder distension ▶ high-density bile ▶ pericholecystic fluid and inflammatory stranding within the pericholecystic fat ▶ variable enhancement of the gallbladder wall ▶ transient pericholecystic liver rim enhancement

- Gallstones are only seen in a minority (as they are often isoattenuating to biliary fluid)

Hepatobiliary scintigraphy There is non-visualization of the gallbladder at 2–4 h after isotope administration (secondary to inflammatory cystic duct obstruction)

- **Complications:** Gangrenous cholecystitis ▶ emphysematous cholecystitis ▶ empyema formation
- **Differential of gallbladder wall thickening:** a non-fasted or a generalized oedematous state ▶ hepatitis ▶ pancreatitis ▶ gallbladder wall varices ▶ adenomyomatosis ▶ gallbladder carcinoma

GANGRENOUS CHOLECYSTITIS

Definition Ischaemic necrosis of the gallbladder wall is a complication of acute cholecystitis

Radiological features

US Irregularity or asymmetrical thickening of the gallbladder wall ▶ internal membranous echoes resulting from sloughed mucosa ▶ pericholecystic fluid

CT Gas within the wall or lumen ▶ discontinuous (±) irregular mucosal enhancement ▶ internal membranes (representing sloughed mucosa) ▶ a pericholecystic abscess

- **Gallbladder perforation:** this is seen in 5–10% and is suggested by pericholecystic fluid and localized gallbladder wall disruption

EMPHYSEMATOUS CHOLECYSTITIS

Definition The presence of intramural (± intraluminal) gas due to gas-forming organisms ▶ it accounts for 1% of cases of acute cholecystitis, and has a relatively high mortality rate

- 50% of patients are diabetic (M>F) ▶ gallstones are only seen in <50% of patients

US Focal or diffuse bright echogenic lines (representing intramural gas) ▶ a curvilinear brightly echogenic band with acoustic shadowing seen within a non-dependent portion of the gallbladder (representing intraluminal gas)

- Small foci of intramural gas may cause ring-down artefacts and mimic adenomyomatosis

CT Intramural (± intraluminal) gas

ACUTE ACALCULOUS CHOLECYSTITIS

Definition Gallbladder inflammation in the absence of gallstones ▶ this is usually found in critically ill patients

- *Other causes:* prolonged fasting ▶ parenteral nutrition ▶ AIDS ▶ diabetes ▶ chemotherapy

US Gallbladder distension ▶ gallbladder wall thickening ▶ echogenic contents (± sloughed membranes or mucosa) ▶ pericholecystic fluid

- Gallbladder aspiration may aid the diagnosis ▶ localized gallbladder tenderness is a good predictive sign but it is difficult to assess

CHRONIC CALCULOUS CHOLECYSTITIS

Definition Chronic inflammation and thickening of the gallbladder wall which is secondary to gallstones

US/CT A contracted gallstone-containing gallbladder ▶ intramural epithelial crypts (Rokitansky–Aschoff sinuses)

CHRONIC ACALCULOUS CHOLECYSTITIS

Definition Unexplained biliary-type pain with no clear clinical, pathological or radiological criteria for diagnosis

US This may show gallbladder wall thickening (but no gallstones)

Cholescintigraphy This can assess the gallbladder contractility (following an IV infusion of cholecystokinin) ▶ an ejection fraction <35% indicates gallbladder dysfunction

XANTHOGRANULOMATOUS CHOLECYSTITIS

Definition A rare inflammatory disease of the gallbladder characterized by a focal, diffuse destructive inflammatory process with accumulation of lipid-laden macrophages ▶ it may simulate a malignancy radiologically and pathologically

Clinical presentation Cholecystitis or biliary obstruction (Mirizzi's syndrome)

Radiological features

US/CT Gallbladder wall thickening (focal or diffuse) ▶ the majority have gallstones (± perforation, abscess, or fistula formation)

- An associated gallbladder carcinoma is seen in a minority of patients

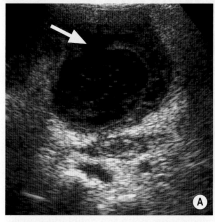
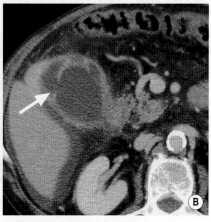

Acute cholecystitis with localized perforation on (A) US and (B) CT. The thickened gallbladder wall shows a local defect (arrow) and on CT there is small amount of intraperitoneal fluid and oedema of adjacent fat.*

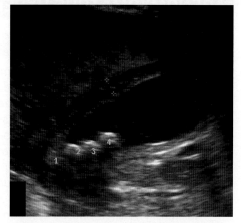

Acute cholecystitis. The gallbladder contains small stones in the neck (Nos 1–4) and its wall shows oedematous thickening (5 mm thickness).*

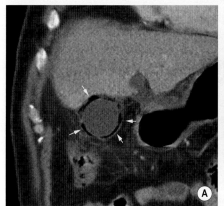
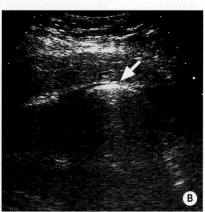

Emphysematous cholecystitis. (A) Coronal CT – intramural gas (arrows)** ▶ (B) US – intraluminal gas appears as a bright curvilinear echogenic band (arrow) with 'dirty' shadowing.*

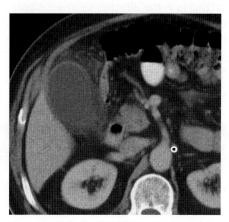

Acute cholecystitis on CT. The gallbladder wall is thickened with oedema in the adjacent fat.*

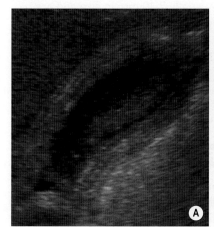
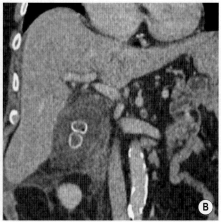

Acute cholecystitis. (A). US demonstrating a thickened inflamed gallbladder wall. (B) Coronal CT demonstrating marked pericholecystic inflammatory stranding with laminated calcified gallstones in situ.

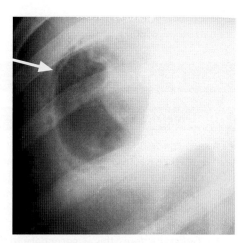

Emphysematous cholecystitis. Image showing intramural (arrow) as well as intraluminal gallbladder gas.*

ADENOMYOMATOUS HYPERPLASIA

DEFINITION

- This is otherwise known as adenomyomatosis or cholecystitis glandularis proliferans and is characterized by thickening of the gallbladder wall (resulting from epithelial and smooth muscle hyperplasia) ▶ it is associated with gallstones in 90% of cases
  - *Distribution:* fundal (the most common) ▶ segmental (usually within the mid-body) ▶ diffuse
  - The segmental form can lead to 'hourglass' deformity of the gallbladder
  - *Rokitansky–Aschoff sinuses:* cystic epithelial wall invaginations (which may contain small stones)

RADIOLOGICAL FEATURES

US Gallbladder wall thickening with secondary luminal narrowing ▶ the affected segment often contains wall bright echoes arising from the cystic spaces or from the small stones within them (and is often associated with 'comet-tail' ring-down artefacts)

CT Gallbladder wall thickening

MRI T2WI: intramural cystic spaces

CHOLESTEROLOSIS (STRAWBERRY GALLBLADDER)

DEFINITION

- This is due to cholesterol deposits within gallbladder wall macrophages ▶ it is associated with small polyps

RADIOLOGICAL FEATURES

US Echogenic foci within the gallbladder wall (with no acoustic shadowing)

GALLBLADDER FISTULAE

DEFINITION

- A rare condition due to either chronic stone disease (the majority) or neoplastic disease (the minority)
  - Cases due to chronic stone disease tend to fistulate with the duodenum ▶ cases due to neoplastic disease tend to fistulate with the colon
- *Cholecystoduodenal fistula:*
  - *'Gallstone ileus':* this is secondary to the antegrade passage of a gallstone and impaction within the terminal ileum
  - *Bouveret's syndrome:* this is secondary to the retrograde passage of a gallstone and obstruction within the stomach or duodenum

PORCELAIN GALLBLADDER

DEFINITION

- An asymptomatic and uncommon condition of mural wall calcification (focal or generalized) which is associated with chronic cholecystitis
  - Cholecystectomy is advocated as a carcinoma can occur in up to 30% of patients

RADIOLOGICAL FEATURES

US It may mimic an emphysematous cholecystitis

XR/CT Curvilinear calcification along the gallbladder wall

MILK OF CALCIUM BILE/LIMEY BILE

DEFINITION

Bile becomes very viscous, with a high concentration of calcium bilirubinate (due to stasis)

RADIOLOGICAL FEATURES

US Diffuse echoes similar to that seen with biliary sludge (but they are more echogenic with a tendency to layer out and produce an acoustic shadow)

CT/XR There may be layering of the high-density material

GALLBLADDER POLYPS

DEFINITION

- **Cholesterol polyps:** These account for the majority of polyps ▶ they are usually 2–10 mm in size and are often multiple ▶ they are not usually associated with gallstones
- **Adenomatous polyps:** These are usually up to 2 cm in size and are usually solitary ▶ they are often associated with gallstones
  - They are also associated with familial adenomatous polyposis and Peutz–Jeghers syndrome

RADIOLOGICAL FEATURES

US Both types appear as small echogenic non-shadowing foci adherent to the gallbladder wall (often the nondependent portion) ▶ they are usually non-mobile ▶ internal Doppler flow usually differentiates them from tumefactive sludge but this will not reliably distinguish between a benign and malignant polyp

- A diameter of >10 mm or local disruption of the adjacent gallbladder wall suggests malignancy

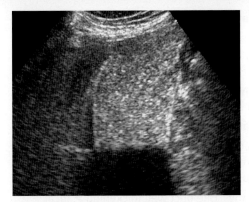

Milk of calcium bile producing fine echoes with a dependent layer that shadows.*

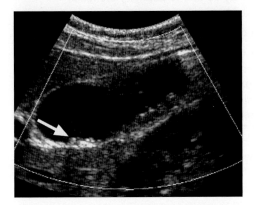

Adenomyomatous hyperplasia. Gallbladder wall thickening in the fundus is associated with small stones (arrow).*

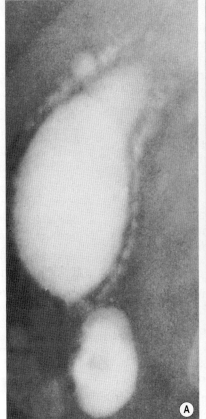
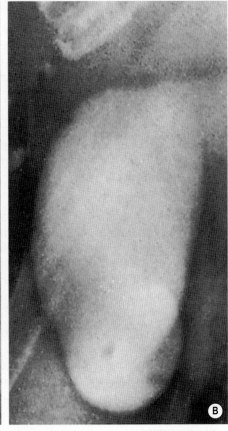

(A) Rokitansky–Aschoff sinuses shown on cholecystography. A stricture is also present. (B) Cholesterosis, showing fixed mural defects.†

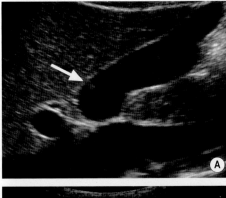
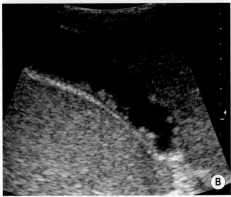

Gallbladder polyps. (A) Solitary, non-dependent and non-shadowing polyp (arrow). (B) Multiple, non-shadowing cholesterol polyps.*

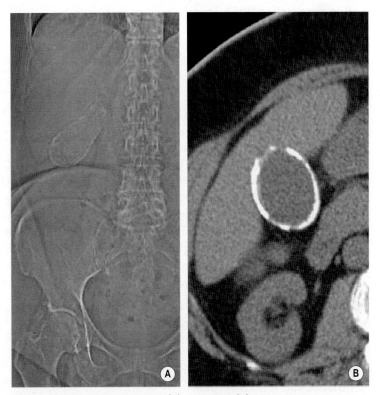

Porcelain gallbladder. Scout CT (A) and NECT (B).

Postoperative strictures

Definition A short (1–2 mm) stricture usually seen following cholecystectomy ▶ they usually involve the common duct (as well as the hepatic and aberrant ducts) ▶ stones may develop proximal to a stricture ▶ common following liver transplantation (anastomotic 9%, non-anastomotic 16%)

MRCP This can demonstrate the ducts above a complete stricture (unlike an ERCP)

- *Pitfall:* a common hepatic duct pseudostricture can be caused by the hepatic artery (or its right branch) crossing the duct

Sclerosing cholangitis

Definition Inflammation of the intrahepatic (20%) and extrahepatic (80%) ducts ▶ it has an unknown aetiology

- *Primary disease (primary sclerosing cholangitis):* this is idiopathic
- *Secondary disease:* this is the most common form ▶ 70% of patients have a background of inflammatory bowel disease (usually UC)

Cholangiography Characteristic diverticula-like out-pouchings alternating with strictures

- *'String of beads' appearance:* multiple segments of stricturing involving the intra- and extrahepatic ducts

US Bile duct wall thickening, which is most pronounced at the sites of stricturing ▶ outpouchings appear as local duct wall echogenic foci

CT/MRI Well-established disease is associated with areas of atrophy and hypertrophy within the liver

- **Bile duct stones (10%):** These appear as high-density lesions on CT
- **Cholangiocarcinoma (10%):** This should be suspected if there is progressive duct dilatation proximal to a stricture or if there is a nodule >1 cm

Mirizzi syndrome

Definition Chronic gallstone impaction within the gallbladder neck or cystic duct (or its remnant) leads to inflammation and fibrosis with associated common duct narrowing

- A fistula may develop between the gallbladder (or cystic duct) and the common duct – the stone may then partially or completely pass into the common duct

US Biliary dilatation down to a stone that is clearly not within the common duct

Cholangiography A smooth (2–3 cm in length) stricture most commonly seen in the upper and middle common duct ▶ it often has a concavity toward the right

IgG4-related sclerosing disease

- Immune-mediated multisystem disease most commonly presenting as autoimmune pancreatitis ▶ elevated serum IgG4 levels
- Extrapancreatic disease is common (hilar adenopathy in 80%/bile duct lesions in 75%)
  - Can mimic pancreatic cancer/cholangiocarcinoma/ PSC

Pancreatitis-related stricture

Definition Acute and chronic pancreatitis can produce biliary stricturing caused by fibrosis (± an inflammatory mass)

Cholangiography The strictures are smooth and tapering, extending over a few centimetres

HIV cholangiopathy

Definition This typically occurs in patients with an established diagnosis of HIV and is due to opportunistic infection (most commonly *Cryptosporidium*)

US/cholangiopathy Bile duct wall thickening ▶ focal strictures (intrahepatic ± extrahepatic) ▶ biliary duct dilatation (which may be due to papillary stenosis) ▶ gallbladder wall thickening is common

Acute bacterial cholangitis

Definition This is almost always caused by Gram-negative enteric organisms and is usually associated with at least partial bile duct obstruction (and is usually secondary to choledocholithiasis)

Clinical presentation Charcot's triad: fever + right upper quadrant pain + jaundice

Radiological features

US This can identify any duct stones as well as any bile duct wall thickening

Pearl Urgent imaging (US/CT/MRCP) is required to identify the cause and also for biliary tree drainage – this can be either endoscopic (ERCP and sphincterotomy) or transhepatic

Recurrent pyogenic cholangitis/oriental cholangiohepatitis

Definition Infection due to enteric bacteria or parasites (e.g. *Clonorchis sinensis*)

- This occurs mainly in South-East Asia or its emigrants ▶ it is characterized by recurrent episodes of cholangitis, biliary dilatation and strictures, together with bile duct stones (mostly intrahepatic)

US Duct dilatation ▶ stones that may not shadow ▶ gas is often present within the ducts

Cholangiography Duct dilatation and multiple duct stones (widespread or segmental) ▶ strictures ▶ ductal dilatation may be disproportionately prominent in the extrahepatic and central intrahepatic ducts (sparing the smaller peripheral ducts)

- *Clonorchis* is rarely identified as small filamentous wavy or elliptical filling defects

CT This identifies any associated hepatic abscesses and any lobar or segmental atrophy

- *Calcium bilirubinate stones:* these are seen within dilated ducts ▶ they are often intrahepatic and can be extensive

Complications Liver fibrosis ▶ portal hypertension ▶ cholangiocarcinoma

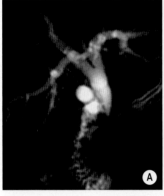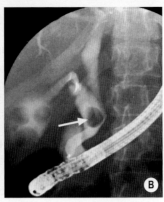

Mirizzi syndrome. MRCP (A) shows a stricture of the lower common duct caused by a stone (arrow) lying in an expanded cystic duct on ERCP (B). Multiple gallbladder stones are also seen.*

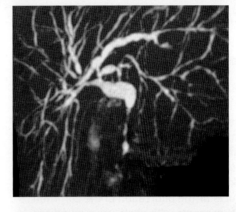

Primary sclerosing cholangitis. MRCP shows multiple intrahepatic and extrahepatic segments of stricturing + dilatation ('string of beads').*

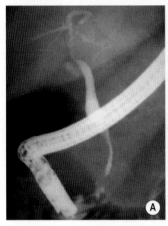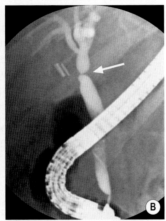

(A) Chronic pancreatitis. Typical smooth, elongated, incomplete stricture of the lower common bile duct. (B) ERCP shows a post-cholecystectomy stricture (arrow) which, characteristically, is very short.*

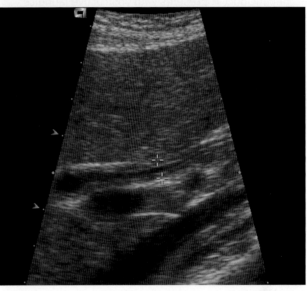

Primary sclerosing cholangitis. Typical bile duct wall thickening on US (calipers).**

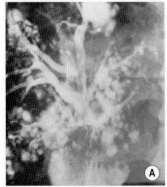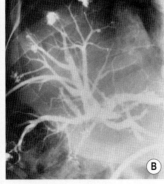

Acute suppurative cholangitis. (A) Abscess cavities communicate with dilated ducts. (B) After 5 days of external drainage most of the abscess cavities have healed and the ducts are less dilated.†

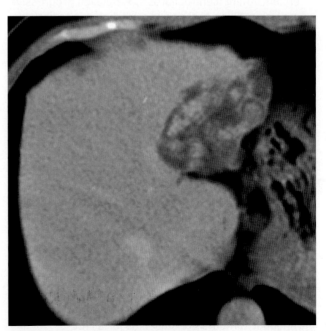

Recurrent pyogenic cholangitis. Multiple high-density stones lie in dilated ducts within an atrophic left lobe.**

CHOLANGIOCARCINOMA

Definition

- Adenocarcinomas originating from bile duct epithelium (>95%)
  - ▪ **Intrahepatic and peripheral to the liver hilum** (10%) ▶ peripheral to the secondary bifurcation of the left or right hepatic ducts ▶ <10% are diffuse or multifocal ▶ presents with abdominal pain/weight loss (obstructive jaundice is rare)
    - – *Treatment*: hepatectomy
  - ▪ **Hilar – Klatskin tumour** (25%) ▶ arising from one of the hepatic ducts or the bifurcation of the common hepatic duct ▶ presents with obstructive jaundice
    - – *Treatment*: bile duct resection + hepatectomy
  - ▪ **Extrahepatic** (65%): presents with obstructive jaundice
    - – *Treatment*: pancreatoduodenectomy
- Pathologically 3 types:
  - ▪ **Periductal infiltrating and stricture forming:** the most common ▶ concentric mural thickening with stricture formation (± fibrotic encasement of adjacent vascular structures)
  - ▪ **Mass forming (exophytic):** frequent central necrosis/fibrosis (± satellite nodules)
  - ▪ **Intraductal papillary growing:** often small but cause obstruction, can secrete mucin, which tends to produce duct expansion (± calcification)
- **Risk factors:** primary sclerosing cholangitis (> ulcerative colitis) ▶ Caroli's disease ▶ choledochal cyst ▶ previous *Clonorchis* exposure (Asia) ▶ exposure to benzene or toluene

Radiological features

- **Intrahepatic**
  - ▪ CT/MRI: initial irregular peripheral patchy enhancement (central fibrosis) ▶ delayed progressive central in-filling ▶ capsular retraction due to fibrosis ▶ T1WI: hypointense ▶ T2WI: hyperintense
- **Hilar**
  - ▪ CT/MRI: biliary dilatation with left and right duct disassociation ▶ hilar bile duct wall thickening (relatively hypervascular or with delayed enhancement) ▶ any mass is usually small ▶ T1WI: hypointense ▶ T2WI: hyperintense
- **Extraheptic (distal CHD or CBD)**
  - ▪ CT/MRI: short stricture or polypoid mass ▶ thickened enhancing wall

Pearls

- **Hilar unresectability due to involvement of:** the secondary confluence (bilateral) ▶ main portal vein ▶ both portal vein branches ▶ hepatic artery + portal vein ▶ vascular involvement on one side of the liver and extensive biliary disease on the other
- **Metastatic spread:** this is commonly to the hepatoduodenal and portocaval nodes ▶ haematogenous remote spread is uncommon
- Intrahepatic tumours are staged as for a HCC
- MRCP is better than US and CT at evaluating the proximal extent of any stricturing (which critically affects the treatment options)
- PET-CT is relatively insensitive

GALLBLADDER CARCINOMA

Definition
An uncommon tumour (adenocarcinoma in 90%)

Clinical presentation
There is usually a late presentation and consequently a very poor prognosis (unless it is detected incidentally at cholecystectomy) ▶ it presents during the 6th and 7th decades with RUQ pain (± biliary obstruction)

- *Risk factors:* cholelithiasis ▶ a porcelain gallbladder ▶ primary sclerosing cholangitis ▶ a choledochal cyst ▶ chronic infection
  - ▪ Any chronic inflammation will predispose to mucosal metaplasia

US/CT

- **Early (minority):** a polypoid intraluminal mass
- **Late (majority):** focal or diffuse irregular gallbladder wall thickening ▶ a large vascular mass within the gallbladder fossa with little or no gallbladder lumen identifiable (± central necrosis within larger lesions) ▶ biliary obstruction ▶ gallbladder stones are usually buried within the mass
  - ▪ There is early spread to the periportal lymph nodes (a nodal mass can extend down to the head of the pancreas) ▶ it can also spread to the adjacent liver (commonly involving segments IV and V)

MRI
T1WI: low SI ▶ T2WI: high SI ▶ T1WI + Gad: poor enhancement

Differential
Mirizzi syndrome ▶ gallbladder metastases ▶ adenomyomatosis ▶ xanthogranulomatous cholecystitis

Bismuth-Corlette classification of extrahepatic biliary strictures			
Type I	Below the confluence of left and right hepatic ducts	*Type IIIb*	Type II + left hepatic duct involvement
	Type I		Type IIIb
Type II	Extension to the confluence of left and right hepatic ducts	*Type IV*	Involving both hepatic ducts or multifocal involvement
	Type II		Type IV
Type IIIa	Type II + right hepatic duct involvement		
	Type IIIa		

Modified Bismuth classification of malignant hilar biliary obstruction based on proximal extent of tumour.**

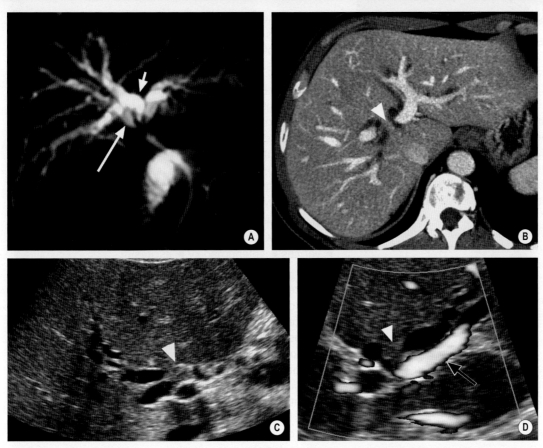

(A) Thick section oblique coronal MRCP. Small hilar cholangiocarcinoma (arrowhead) producing obstruction of the right posterior sectoral duct (short arrow), right anterior sectoral duct (long arrow) and left hepatic duct. (B) Axial portal phase CT. The small tumour is indicated by the arrowhead. (C) Longitudinal US. Again the tumour is indicated by the arrowhead. (D) Transverse colour Doppler US (black arrow: normal left portal vein).

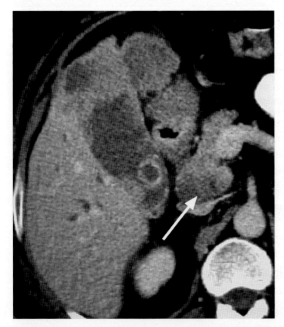

Gallbladder carcinoma. Advanced carcinoma extending outside the fundus, with a nodal metastasis posterior to the pancreatic head (arrow). An associated stone can be seen in the gallbladder neck.*

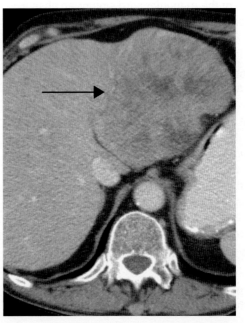

Portal venous phase CT demonstrating a large heterogeneous cholangiocarcinoma occupying the left lobe of the liver (arrow).

BILIARY ATRESIA

Definition A progressive obliterative inflammatory process, affecting the extrahepatic biliary tree and progressing centrally towards the intrahepatic interlobar ducts

- Type 1: CBD atresia
- Type 2: common hepatic duct atresia
- Type 3: intrahepatic duct atresia
- The aetiology is uncertain: perinatal and embryonic, environmental, infectious, immune and genetic aetiologies have been suggested
- Natural history of progressive fibrosis, cirrhosis and portal hypertension
- *Associated abnormalities occur in 10% of patients:* a preduodenal portal vein ▶ a choledochal cyst ▶ an absent IVC ▶ polysplenia and asplenia ▶ trisomy 13 ▶ situs inversus

Clinical presentation Persistent jaundice in the neonatal period (F>M) ▶ pale stools ▶ hepatomegaly

Radiological features

US The liver becomes large and coarse, with increased periportal reflectivity ▶ the biliary tree is not usually distended or dilated (due to the obliterative inflammatory process)

- The gallbladder is usually absent or rudimentary (it is seen in only 20%)
- *'Triangular cord' sign:* a highly reflective focus at the liver hilum cranial to the portal vein (representing the obliterated fibrosed biliary tree) ▶ if it persists after a Kasai procedure it may be a poor prognostic indicator
- The presence of the triangular cord sign or an absent or rudimentary gallbladder are high predictors of biliary atresia

99mTc-DISIDA This distinguishes biliary atresia from severe cholestasis

- 99mTc-DISIDA is extracted by the hepatocytes and secreted into the bile canaliculi and then into the bowel ▶ sequential imaging is performed during the first 60 min with delayed images taken at 2, 4, 6, and 24 h
- *Biliary atresia:* extraction is often normal with hepatic activity seen by 5 min ▶ failure to show excretion at 24 h (despite good parenchymal extraction) is suggestive of biliary atresia
  - The differential includes severe hepatocellular dysfunction

Preoperative PTC/PTTC and MRI These may play a role in difficult cases

Cholangiogram This is traditionally performed at laparotomy with a needle placed in the gallbladder or its remnant

Pearls The presence of a normal-sized gallbladder, which distends with fasting and contracts with feeding, suggests a diagnosis other than biliary atresia

- Percutaneous liver biopsy is required for a definitive diagnosis – this will show bile duct proliferation, periportal fibrosis, bile plugs and cholestasis

Treatment

- *Porto-enterostomy (Kasai procedure):* a jejunal loop is brought up as a Roux-en-Y up to the excavated porta hepatis to allow bile to drain through minute bile remnants or canaliculi into the bowel ▶ it is the primary treatment in patients who present before 60 days
- *Liver transplantation:* there is a significant morbidity and it requires long-term immunosuppression ▶ it is ultimately required in 70–80% of patients

Late complications These can occur even after a successful Kasai procedure: cirrhosis ▶ portal hypertension ▶ varices ▶ splenomegaly ▶ ascites

Other causes of neonatal jaundice Physiological jaundice of prematurity ▶ breast milk jaundice ▶ ABO incompatibility and other causes of haemolytic jaundice ▶ sepsis of any cause ▶ metabolic causes (e.g. galactosaemia, α_1-antitrypsin deficiency and cystic fibrosis)

- *Unconjugated hyperbilirubinaemia:* this is caused by prehepatic and hepatic forms of liver disease
- *Conjugated hyperbilirubinaemia* (which is almost always pathological): includes extrahepatic obstructive forms (e.g. biliary atresia, Alagille syndrome, biliary hypoplasia and choledocal cysts) and hepatic forms (e.g. TPN and cholestasis)

BILIARY HYPOPLASIA (ALAGILLE SYNDROME)

Definition A paucity in the number of intralobular bile ducts

- *'Non-syndromic':* this presents as an isolated finding
- *'Syndromic':* this was previously known as arteriohepatic dysplasia or Alagille syndrome

Clinical presentation Jaundice (presenting later than biliary atresia)

- *Syndromic form:* forehead bossing ▶ a pointed chin ▶ posterior embryotoxin of the eye ▶ butterfly vertebrae ▶ renal anomalies (hypoplastic or dysplastic kidneys and cystic disease) ▶ peripheral pulmonary branch stenoses

Radiological features

US A normal liver ▶ a normal or small gallbladder ▶ there is no triangular cord sign

99mTc-DISIDA No excretion into the bowel is seen in about 50% of biliary hypoplasias

Cholangiography Patent thin spidery ducts

Pearls The diagnosis is made on liver biopsy

- Management is conservative ▶ some complications may require liver transplantation
- *Late complications:* cirrhosis, portal hypertension and carcinoma

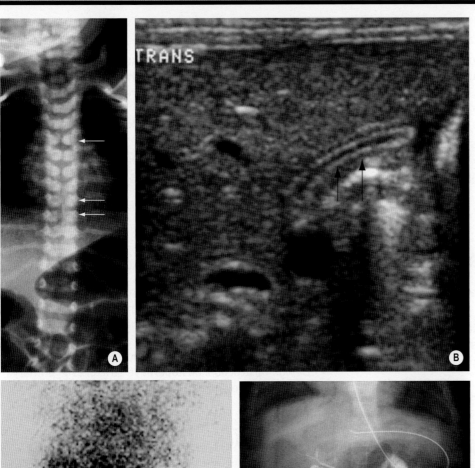

Alagille syndrome. Biliary hypoplasia. (A) Plain AP XR of the spine in a neonate with Alagille syndrome showing numerous hemivertebrae (arrows). (B) US of the liver in a 2-month-old boy with Alagille syndrome showing a small gallbladder (arrows). (C) Radionuclide scintigraphy in another child shows good extraction of the ^{99m}Tc-DISIDA by the liver, and excretion of some tracer into the bowel at 24 h. Both infants had biopsy-proven biliary hypoplasia. (D) Second image of a 2-month-old boy with prolonged neonatal jaundice. Preoperative cholangiogram shows a diminutive or hypoplastic but patent biliary tree consistent with biliary hypoplasia (non-syndromic). This was confirmed on biopsy.

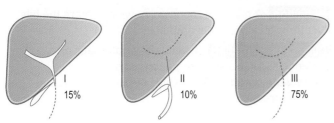

Types of biliary atresia. Type I (extrahepatic) ▶ Type II (intrahepatic) ▶ Type III (combined)

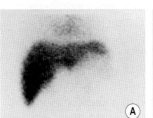
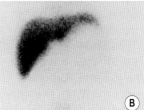

Biliary atresia. Radionuclide study of a 2-month-old baby boy. ^{99m}Tc-DISIDA scintigram. Following preparation with phenobarbital for 5 days, this radionuclide scintigram using ^{99m}Tc-DISIDA shows good extraction of the tracer by the liver at 2 min, and no excretion by the biliary tree into the bowel by 6 h (A) or 24 h (B). Biopsy confirmed biliary atresia. Ultrasound showed no gallbladder present.*

HAEMOBILIA

Definition Most cases of bleeding into the biliary tree result from a blunt or penetrating trauma, or an iatrogenic injury (e.g. following liver biopsy)

- *Other causes:* hepatic artery aneurysms ▶ tumours ▶ cholecystitis

US Haemobilia appears similar to sludge in either the gallbladder or bile ducts

CT Slightly hyperdense material within the gallbladder and bile ducts

Cholangiography A cast-like filling defect within the bile ducts

BILIARY LEAKS AND BILE DUCT INJURIES

Definition This usually occurs following either a cholecystectomy or trauma

US/CT/MRCP These can detect biliary *collections*

- MRCP cannot usually identify the source of a leak

HIDA scintigraphy/CT-IVC/ERCP These can detect biliary *leaks*

- HIDA scintigraphy is the most sensitive technique
- ERCP: allows the placement of a temporary stent

High-quality cholangiography This is the most important imaging investigation following a major bile duct injury

BILIARY CYSTIC DISEASE (CHOLEDOCHAL CYSTIC DISEASE)

Definition A rare condition that is associated with biliary tumours (a 20-fold increase in cholangiocarcinoma) ▶ the Todani classification:

- *Type I:* dilatation (saccular or fusiform) of the common bile duct ▶ this is the most common type
- *Type II:* a diverticulum of the extrahepatic biliary duct
- *Type III:* a choledochocoele
- *Type IV:* multiple dilatations of the intra- and extra-hepatic biliary tree ▶ this is the 2ⁿᵈ commonest type
  - Type 4a: fusiform dilation of the entire extrahepatic bile duct with extension of dilation into the intrahepatic bile ducts
  - Type 4b: Multiple cystic dilations involving only the extrahepatic bile duct
- *Type V:* Caroli's disease
- Types I and IV are characterized by a long common channel shared with the pancreatic duct ▶ there is a high incidence of stone development within the dilated ducts

Clinical presentation Type 1 cysts commonly present in childhood with pain, jaundice and a right upper-quadrant mass

- The presentation is otherwise similar to that seen with gallstone disease

ERCP, CT-IVC, PTC or contrast-enhanced MRCP These can be used ▶ cholangiography is the best test

CAROLI'S DISEASE

Definition A sporadic condition causing the formation of intrahepatic biliary cysts (with intrahepatic calculi) ▶ there is a risk of pyogenic cholangitis, intrahepatic abscess and cholangiocarcinoma formation

- *Associations:* medullary sponge kidney (80%) ▶ infantile polycystic kidney disease

US/CT A beaded appearance of the intrahepatic bile ducts with multiple cystic structures converging towards the porta in a branching pattern

- *'Central dot' sign:* a portal radical surrounded by a dilated bile duct

LIVER ATROPHY

Definition Lobar or segmental atrophy is frequently associated with contralateral lobar hypertrophy ▶ it may be associated with lobar or segmental bile duct obstruction due to malignant or benign causes

- *Malignant obstruction:* cholangiocarcinoma
- *Benign obstruction:* postoperative strictures ▶ primary sclerosing cholangitis

LOBAR OR SEGMENTAL DUCT OBSTRUCTION

Causes Stones ▶ postoperative strictures (which are usually right sided) ▶ primary sclerosing cholangitis ▶ cholangiocarcinoma

Clinical presentation

- A cholangitis or non-specific symptoms ▶ the serum bilirubin is usually normal but there is an elevated gammaglutamyl transferase and alkaline phosphatase

MRCP The best technique for evaluation

PARASITIC INFECTIONS: *ASCARIS LUMBRICOIDES*

Definition A parasitic roundworm which enters the bile duct through a duodenal ampulla

Clinical presentation It can be asymptomatic or result in cholangitis, cholecystitis, or pancreatitis

US/cholangiography A tube-like structure within the biliary tree

HYDATID DISEASE

Pearl Hepatic hydatid cysts may rupture into the biliary tree (potentially obstructing it) ▶ ruptured membranes are seen as curvilinear structures on US/cholangiography

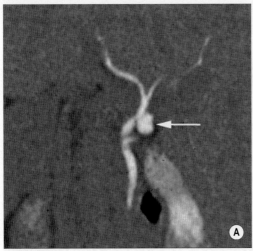

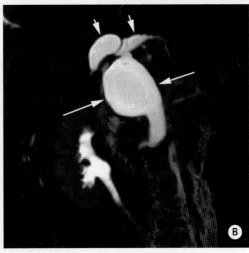

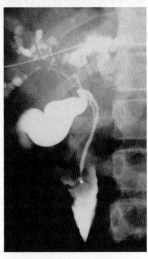

Choledochal cyst. (A) Curved CT-IVC reformat of a type II choledochal cyst (arrow). (B) Oblique coronal thick-slab MRCP of a type IV choledochal cyst demonstrating marked dilatation of the common hepatic duct (long arrows) and central intrahepatic ducts (short arrows) with no stricture or peripheral dilatation.**

Caroli's disease with characteristic strictures and segmental intrahepatic dilated ducts.†

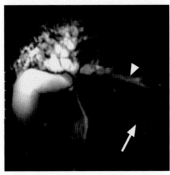

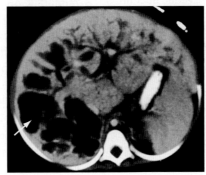

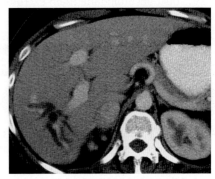

Hilar cholangiocarcinoma associated with marked right-lobe atrophy and left-lobe hypertrophy. MRCP shows a stricture with very dilated and crowded ducts in a small atrophic right lobe. Arrowhead = segment II ▶ long arrow = segment III (partially out of section).*

Caroli's disease. CT showing low attenuation areas surrounding the portal vein branches (arrow). The whole liver is involved, the right lobe more than the left.*

Right hepatic duct obstruction due to a postcholecystectomy stricture demonstrated on portal phase CT. The atrophic right lobe has rotated to lie in a characteristic posterior position. The left lobe is hypertrophic.*

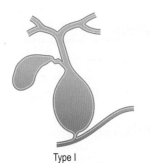

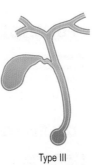

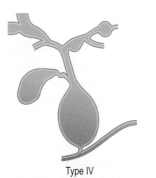

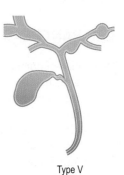

| Type I | Type II | Type III | Type IV | Type V |

Biliary cystic disease classification (after Todani).

3.8 PANCREAS

EMBRYOLOGY

- The pancreas develops in two parts from the endoderm of the primitive duodenum
- **Dorsal part:** this is the first part to appear, initially appearing as a diverticulum from the dorsal wall of the duodenum ▶ it forms the neck, body and tail of the gland and part of the head
- **Ventral part:** this develops more caudally and initially appears as a diverticulum from the developing bile duct ▶ it forms the remaining part of the head and uncinate process
  - ▪ The duodenum undergoes partial rotation and the 2 parts approximate each other and fuse
    - Before this occurs the dorsal duct (the duct of Santorini) opens into the duodenum proximal to the major papilla (the ampulla of Vater)
    - The ventral duct (the duct of Wirsung) opens into the major papilla with the CBD
  - ▪ Usually fusion of the two ducts occurs at the junction of the head and body of the gland, with the ventral duct becoming the main excretory pancreatic duct (in >90% of cases)

CONGENITAL ANOMALIES

PANCREAS DIVISUM

Definition This follows failure of fusion of the dorsal and ventral ducts (affecting 5–10% of the population) ▶ it is the commonest congenital pancreatic anomaly ▶ it may result in functional stenosis and pancreatitis and there is an increased incidence of pancreatic malignancies
- The duct of Wirsung drains the head and uncinate process of the pancreas (via the major papilla)
- The duct of Santorini drains the body and tail (via the more cranially positioned minor papilla)

ERCP/MRCP These allow visualization of the ducts ▶ secretin MRCP allows visualisation of functional stenoses at the minor papilla

ANNULAR PANCREAS

Definition Failure of normal rotation during development results in pancreatic tissue partially or completely encircling the duodenum ▶ this is the 2nd most common congenital anomaly
- It may cause proximal duodenal dilatation and symptomatic duodenal narrowing
- *Associations:* duodenal atresia and stenosis ▶ oesophageal atresia ▶ tracheo-oesophageal fistula ▶ Down's syndrome

Barium studies Narrowing of the duodenum at the level of the major papilla

CT Pancreatic tissue surrounding the duodenum

ERCP/MRCP These demonstrate a segment of pancreatic duct encircling the duodenum

PANCREATIC AGENESIS, HYPOPLASIA AND ECTOPIC PANCREAS

Definition Total pancreatic agenesis is rare – agenesis or hypoplasia of the dorsal part may occur
- Ectopic islands of pancreatic tissue may be found remote from the gland (e.g. within the gastric or duodenal wall)

Barium studies A smooth mural nodule, often with central umbilication (representing a rudimentary pancreatic duct)

MULTISYSTEM DISEASES WITH PANCREATIC INVOLVEMENT

CYSTIC FIBROSIS

Definition An autosomal recessive condition characterized by defects of serous and mucous secretion and involving multiple organs ▶ 85% of patients have severe exocrine pancreatic insufficiency and steatorrhoea
- Obstruction of the main pancreatic duct (and its side branches) by inspissated secretions results in acinar and ductal dilatation with subsequent atrophy of the acinar tissue

US/CT Marked fatty replacement of the normal pancreatic parenchyma ▶ dystrophic calcification ▶ pancreatic cysts

VON HIPPEL–LINDAU DISEASE

Definition An autosomal dominant condition characterized by renal cell carcinomas, phaeochromocytomas, retinal angiomatosis and cerebellar haemangioblastomas

Pearls The most common pancreatic lesions are simple pancreatic cysts ▶ serous cystic pancreatic neoplasms and pancreatic islet cell tumours may also occur

POLYCYSTIC KIDNEY DISEASE

Definition An autosomal dominant condition characterized by multiple renal cysts ▶ hepatic cysts may also occur and pancreatic cysts are seen in 10% of patients

OSLER–WEBER–RENDU DISEASE

Definition A vascular disorder characterized by telangiectasia of the skin, mucous membranes, GI and urinary tracts, liver and pancreas

Angiography Dilated pancreatic arteries supplying a racemose collection of vessels with early draining veins

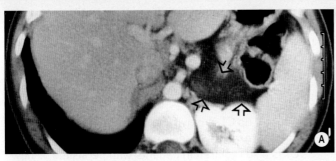
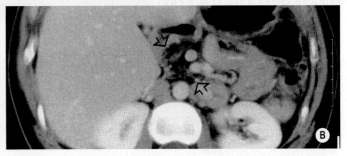

(A,B) Cystic fibrosis. CT through the level of the body and tail of the pancreas (arrows) shows fatty replacement of the gland.*

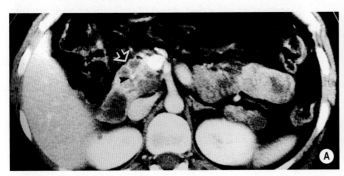
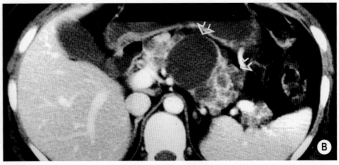

von Hippel–Lindau disease. (A) CT through the level of the head of the pancreas (open arrow) shows multiple small cysts and a central area of calcification (arrowhead) sited in a small serous cystadenoma. (B) Scan at the level of the body and tail of the pancreas (arrows) shows multiple cysts of different sizes. These were simple cysts, as distinct from the serous cystic neoplasm in the head of the pancreas.

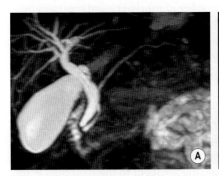
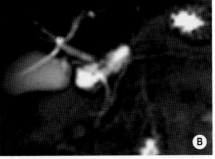
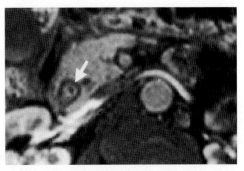

MRCP of normal pancreas and pancreas divisum. (A) Normal anatomy as demonstrated on MRCP. (B) Dorsal pancreatic duct drains into the minor papilla. The common bile duct drains separately into the major papilla.*

Annular pancreas. T1WI + Gad shows pancreatic tissue surrounding the second part of duodenum (arrow).†

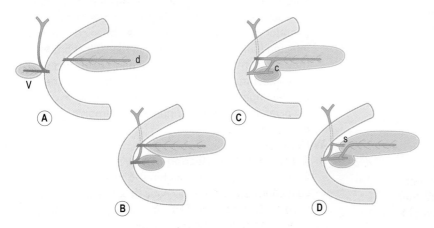

Embryological development of the pancreas. (A) Dorsal segment (d) draining through the duct of Santorini and minor papilla. Ventral segment (v) developing in association with the bile duct and draining through the duct of Wirsung and major papilla. (B) The ventral segment has rotated with the bile duct to occupy its definitive position. This is the arrested embryological position of the adult pancreas divisum. (C) A wide communication (c) has developed between the dorsal and ventral ducts. (D) The terminal portion of the dorsal duct or duct of Santorini (s) becomes relatively smaller and may disappear completely. This is the normal adult arrangement.

ACUTE PANCREATITIS

Definition Acute inflammation of the pancreas ▶ it may be caused by the reflux of bile and pancreatic enzymes into the pancreatic parenchyma

- *Causes:* cholelithiasis (50%) ▶ idiopathic (10–30% – possibly related to congenital duct anomalies such as pancreas divisum) ▶ alcohol (20–25%) ▶ trauma ▶ surgery ▶ metabolic (hyperlipidaemia and hypercalcaemia) ▶ viral infection (mumps, cytomegalovirus and AIDS) ▶ drugs (steroids and thiazide diuretics)

Atlanta classification of acute pancreatitis

- **Interstitial oedematous pancreatitis:** proteolytic enzymes injure the acinar cell, but not enough to cause necrosis
- **Necrotising pancreatitis:** peripancreatic necrosis alone carries a much better prognosis than parenchymal necrosis ▶ subdivided into:
  - Parenchymal necrosis alone
  - Peripancreatic necrosis alone (commonly within the retroperitoneum/lesser sac)
  - Combined type ± infection (the most common type)

Clinical presentation Epigastric pain ▶ nausea and vomiting ▶ raised serum amylase ▶ signs of haemorrhagic pancreatitis:

- *Cullen sign:* periumbilical bruising
- *Grey-Turner sign:* flank bruising

Radiological features

XR Left sided pleural effusion or atelectasis ▶ a gasless abdomen ▶ ascites ▶ intrapancreatic gas bubbles

- *'Colon cut off' sign:* a dilated transverse colon with an abrupt transition to a gasless descending colon
- *'Sentinel loop':* a localized segment of gas containing duodenum

Barium studies A widened duodenal sweep

- *'Frostberg inverted 3 sign:* this is due to segmental narrowing and fold thickening of the duodenum

US There is generalized (but less commonly focal) hypoechoic pancreatic enlargement ▶ ill defined pancreatic margins ▶ peripancreatic fluid ▶ hepatic steatosis (if there is an associated high alcohol intake)

- US can exclude cholelithiasis as cause, however it cannot reliably detect the presence of pancreatic necrosis

CECT

- *British Society of Gastroenterology Guidelines:* immediate CT is not indicated as the full extent of necrosis is only evident after 4 days (therefore the initial extent of necrosis may be underestimated) ▶

the contrast medium may also exacerbate any renal impairment

- An immediate CT should only be performed if the extent of necrosis dictates the management or if the diagnosis is unclear
- A follow up CT is only required if there is a failure to improve or a clinical deterioration
- CT is also required in patients with persisting or new organ failure continuing pain or sepsis
- **Interstitial oedematous pancreatitis** (70–80%)
  - A normal or enlarged gland of uniform enhancement (± peripancreatic fat stranding and thickening of the fascial planes) ▶ cuffs of fluid may be seen around the adjacent vessels ▶ CTSI for grading
- **Necrotising pancreatitis (a hallmark of severe acute pancreatitis)**
  - Heterogeneous areas of non-enhancement containing non-liquefied components ▶ if this involves >30% of the gland the mortality rate approaches 30% ▶ necrosis in more than 1 part (i.e. head and tail) ± distant fluid collections (i.e. paracolic gutter) are correlated with increased mortality
  - *Infected necrosis (20–70%):* this is suggested if there are gas bubbles within any necrotic tissue (this can also be caused by a fistula to the GI tract) ▶ it is a major determinant of morbidity and mortality (accounting for 80% of deaths from acute pancreatitis) ▶ if infection is confirmed by FNA then surgical intervention is required

Pearls Pancreatic and peripancreatic collections (sterile or infected)

- **Without necrosis**
  - *Acute peripancreatic fluid collections (APFC):* presents within 4 weeks and usually resorbed spontaneously without infection ▶ no non-liquefied components ▶ usually adjacent to the pancreas ▶ no discernible wall
  - *Pseudocyst:* after 4 weeks, an APFC may transition to a pseudocyst with a well-defined enhancing fibrous wall (containing no non-liquefied components – if solid internal material is present, the term pseudocyst should not be used) ▶ these can become infected (suggested by air within the collection) ▶ they can communicate with the pancreatic duct which may affect management ▶ rarely extend into the mediastinum ▶ 70% resolve spontaneously ▶ can be associated with rupture/infection/haemorrhage/pain/ biliary obstruction
- **With necrosis:**
  - *Acute necrotic collection (ANC):* presents within 4 weeks ▶ liquefaction within 2–6 weeks ▶ any collection replacing pancreatic tissue within 4 weeks is an ANC and not an APFC/pseudocyst ▶ an ANC may communicate with the pancreatic duct

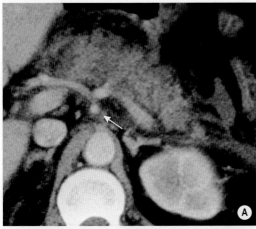

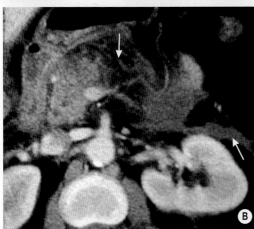

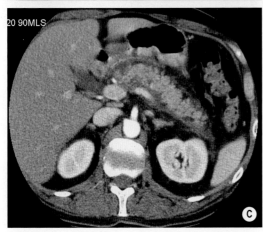

Mild acute pancreatitis. (A) Mild swelling of the gland that enhances uniformly but has indistinct margins because of peripancreatic oedema. There is inflammatory tissue around the coeliac axis (arrow). (B) Image at the level of the pancreatic head showing infiltration of the peripancreatic fat and fluid anterior to Gerota's fascia (arrows). (C) Different patient. Peripancreatic fluid with normally enhancing gland.*

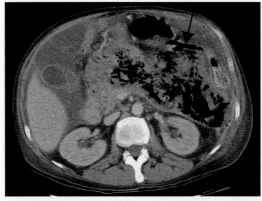

Infected pancreatic necrosis. CECT shows non-enhancement of pancreatic tissue with secondary gas formation (arrow).

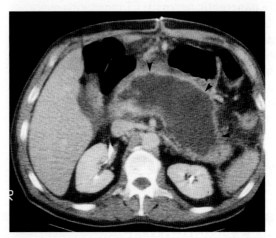

Walled-off necrosis containing necrotic debris. The more solid necrotic tissue contained within the abscess will not be adequately drained by percutaneous catheter drainage. The collection was successfully drained surgically.

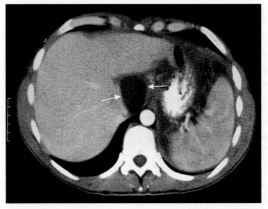

Pancreatic pseudocyst. A well-defined fluid collection with a thin wall (arrows) lies superior to the pancreas.**

ACUTE PANCREATITIS

- *Walled off necrosis (WON):* after 4 weeks an ANC may transition to a WON with a thickened non-epithelialized wall ▶ like ANC, a WON can involve the pancreas ± peripancreatic tissue, and any fluid collection occupying or replacing the pancreas after 4 weeks is a WON ▶ can be sterile or infected ▶ air bubbles within a WON are not always indicative of infection (if communication exists between the WON and GI tract)
- **Treatment**
  - **IEP/AFPC/pseudocyst:** usually self limiting and spontaneously resolves
  - **Necrotising pancreatitis:** if the clinical status allows, supportive treatment for 2 weeks followed by surgical/radiological drainage as required
  - **Sterile pancreatic necrosis:** CT monitoring every 7–10 days to exclude complication or infection ▶ percutaneous drainage and supportive measures as required
  - **Infected pancreatic necrosis:** percutaneous drainage/surgical debridement
- **Vascular involvement**
  - Intrapancreatic and peripancreatic arteries and veins may be eroded or thrombosed by pancreatic enzymes ▶ this may lead to pseudoaneurysm formation ▶ this can manifest as an episode of acute haemorrhage (due to vessel erosion, rupture of oesophageal, gastric, or mesenteric varices, or arterial pseuodaneurysm leakage)
  - This requires CECT (± angiography and vascular embolization) ▶ ideally all cases should be assessed with a post-contrast pancreatic protocol CT to enable vascular assessment ▶ splenic artery and vein are particularly at risk
- **GI involvement**
  - Direct extension of the inflammatory process can result in oedema, necrosis or perforation of the stomach or duodenal wall
  - Bowel involvement can occur due to pancreatic enzymes permeating through the mesenteric attachments (or secondary to vascular complications)
- **Bile duct involvement**
  - Oedema within the pancreatic head can cause a transient CBD obstruction
  - Severe or chronic pancreatitis can cause a persistent CBD obstruction or necrosis

CHRONIC PANCREATITIS

Definition

- Irreversible pancreatic inflammation with an increased risk of pancreatic carcinoma

Clinical presentation

- Chronic abdominal pain ▶ loss of exocrine and endocrine function (e.g. steatorrhoea and diabetes) ▶ weight loss
  - *Causes:* idiopathic ▶ alcohol abuse ▶ hyperparathyroidism ▶ hyperlidaemia ▶ hereditary ▶ following multiple attacks of acute pancreatitis

Radiological features

US/CT A heterogeneous pancreatic echotexture or attenuation ▶ parenchymal calcification (which may be seen on AXR) ▶ a dilated (>3mm) pancreatic duct (± CBD dilatation) ▶ atrophy or general pancreatic enlargement (differentiating between focal enlargement with ductal dilatation and a pancreatic carcinoma can be challenging – multiple biopsies may be required) ▶ splenic, mesenteric or portal vein thrombosis ▶ arterial stenosis or occlusion ▶ arterial pseudoaneurysm formation

ERCP/MRCP dilatation or multifocal stenoses of the main pancreatic duct and its lateral side-branches ▶ intraductal filling defects (representing protein plugs or calcification) ▶ narrowing of the intrapancreatic CBD
- *ERCP complications:* acute pancreatitis (in up to 10% of cases) ▶ haemorrhage ▶ cholangitis

Pearls

- **Groove pancreatitis**
  - A distinct form of CP affecting the groove between the pancreatic head, duodenum and CBD
  - CT: plate-like hypoattenuating poorly enhancing lesion between the pancreatic head and duodenum ± bile duct obstruction
  - EUS biopsy may be required
- **Autoimmune pancreatitis**
  - Affects patients without a history of biliary stones or alcohol abuse ▶ thought to be secondary to an immune mediated mechanism with abnormally elevated serum IgG4 levels
  - CT/MRI: diffuse or focal pancreatic enlargement ('sausage shaped' pancreas) with minimal peripancreatic stranding ▶ narrowed pancreatic duct (without dilatation) ▶ delayed enhancement ▶ focal AIP can be difficult to differentiate form pancreatic cancer
  - Responds well to steroid therapy

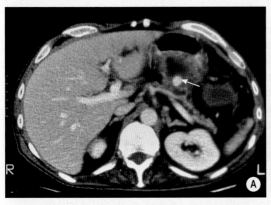

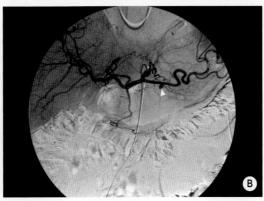

Pseudoaneurysm formation. (A) CECT shows high-density contrast collection (arrow) within a small retrogastric pseudocyst. (B) Coeliac axis angiogram confirms the presence of a pseudoaneurysm (arrowhead). This was embolized successfully.

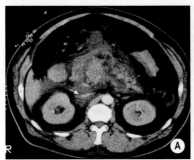

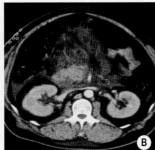

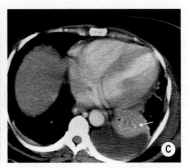

Moderately severe acute pancreatitis. (A) Inflammatory fluid is seen surrounding the inferior vena cava (arrow). (B) Extensive inflammatory changes involve the mesentery. (C) There is a left basal pleural effusion and collapse in the left lower lobe (arrow).*

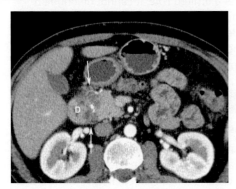

Groove pancreatitis: MDCT findings. There is a low-density mass (arrows) with some calcifications between the pancreatic head and duodenum (D).**

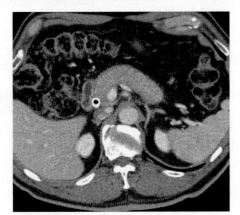

Autoimmune pancreatitis. MDCT shows uniform swelling of the gland in a patient without risk factors for pancreatitis.**

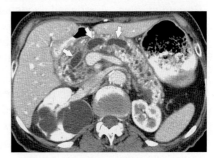

Chronic pancreatitis. Axial contrast-enhanced MDCT image shows diffuse calcifications in the pancreas with a dilated main pancreatic duct (arrows) measuring 9 mm and dilated side branches.©20

PANCREATIC DUCTAL ADENOCARCINOMA

DEFINITION

- An aggressive pancreatic malignancy arising from the ductal epithelium and causing a local desmoplastic response with a propensity to constrict or obstruct adjacent ducts or vessels ▶ there is early involvement of the adjacent structures by perivascular, perineural and lymphatic spread
- Only 10% of tumours are resectable at diagnosis with an overall 5-year survival rate of only 2–3%
  - *At presentation:* liver metastases (50%) ▶ lymph node involvement (40%) ▶ peritoneal deposits (35%)

CLINICAL PRESENTATION

- Weight loss ▶ anorexia ▶ abdominal pain (due to invasion of the coeliac plexus) ▶ obstructive jaundice
- It is commonly seen within the 7th to 8th decades (M>F) ▶ smoking is a significant risk factor

RADIOLOGICAL FEATURES

- Approximately 70% of adenocarcinomas arise within the head, neck or uncinate process – the remainder arise within the body or tail ▶ small masses may only be detectable by virtue of their differing imaging characteristics from normal tissue

US This differentiates obstructive from non-obstructive causes of jaundice ▶ a pancreatic tumour is a hypoechoic mass relative to the normal pancreas

Barium studies A widened duodenal loop ± mucosal irregularity (with spiculation and fold nodularity) ▶ a localized duodenal stricture or a double contour to the medial wall of the duodenal loop ▶ a 'reversed 3' sign of Frostberg

Cholangiography A pancreatic carcinoma produces a tight stricture that is often shouldered – this may have a blunt cut-off that is straight or convex upward or downward

CT Thin slices are used during the arterial phase and thicker slices during the portal phase acquisitions ▶ water is preferred to a positive oral contrast agent as the enhancement of the stomach and duodenal wall is more readily appreciated (allowing for the assessment of any invasion)

- Assessment with dual phase imaging:
  - *'Pancreatic' phase (late arterial enhancement):* as the tumour is hypovascular it will appear as a poorly enhancing focal area within densely enhancing normal pancreatic tissue
  - *Portal phase imaging:* this assesses for any vascular involvement and metastatic disease
- There is mass effect with alteration of the pancreatic contour ▶ the local desmoplastic response may mimic the appearances of a focal pancreatitis ▶ calcification is rare

- *'Double duct' sign:* this follows adjacent stricture formation within both the common bile and pancreatic ducts and is highly suggestive of a pancreatic carcinoma (less commonly a periampullary carcinoma) ▶ it leads to bile duct obstruction, upstream main pancreatic duct dilatation and pancreatic atrophy ▶ uncinate masses are often large before bile duct obstruction occurs (due to their location) and can encase the SMA before bile duct obstruction ▶ chronic pancreatitis may produce this sign but it will also demonstrate other distinguishing features (e.g. pancreatic calcification)
- *Courvoisier's sign:* an enlarged, non-tender and thin-walled gallbladder secondary to distal biliary obstruction (cf. cholecystitis with an enlarged, tender, thick-walled gallbladder)
- There is often retropancreatic extension with obliteration of the fat planes around the coeliac axis and SMA (indicating unresectable disease)

MRI This offers no significant advantage over CT ▶ T1WI (FS): tumour is of lower SI than the normal pancreas ▶ T2WI: there is often high SI (but this can be variable) ▶ T1WI + Gad: poor enhancement

ERCP This directly visualizes the duodenum and ampulla of Vater ▶ it also allows for cytological sampling and access for stent insertion

EUS and laparoscopic US This may be a helpful supplement in patients with potentially resectable disease ▶ although it can demonstrate a hypoechoic mass, there is poor visualization of the coeliac axis and splenic artery

FDG PET This has a limited role: it cannot distinguish between a malignant or inflammatory mass ▶ low sensitivity for the detection of liver metastases

- However it demonstrates high accuracy in the detection of local recurrence

PEARLS

Assessment of resectability (CT/MRI):

- In the absence of distant metastatic disease, perivascular invasion or vascular encasement are the most important criteria for unresectability ▶ tumours of the body and tail tend to be unresectable as these tend to have metastases at presentation
  - *CT findings indicating perivascular invasion:* soft tissue infiltration obscuring the vessel margin ▶ a vessel calibre change or contour deformity
    - >180° contact with tumour = vascular involvement ▶ ≤90° contact with tumour = low probability of vascular involvement
    - Complete arterial occlusion may result in splenic infarction
    - Tumours within the pancreatic head and uncinate process tend to affect the SMA ▶ tumours within the body and tail tend to affect the coeliac, hepatic or splenic arteries

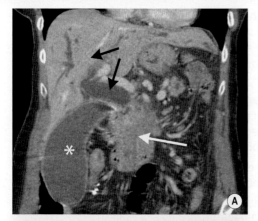

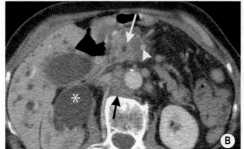

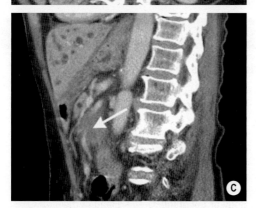

Pancreatic carcinoma. (A) Coronal CT demonstrating a mass within the pancreatic head (white arrow) with a significant associated desmoplastic response. There is associated common biliary and intrahepatic bile duct obstruction (black arrows), together with a distended thin-walled gallbladder (asterisk) (Courvoisier's sign). (B) Axial image demonstrating the pancreatic head mass within which can be seen the common bile duct (arrow). The mass is totally encasing the superior mesenteric vessels (arrowhead), making this unresectable disease. In addition, there is retroperitoneal spread that is encasing approximately 50% of the aortic circumference (black arrow). The right hydronephrosis (asterisk) is secondary to an obstructive tumour deposit within the pelvis. (C) Sagittal reformat demonstrating the tumour mass encasing the SMA (arrow).

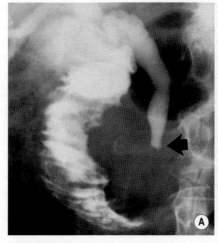
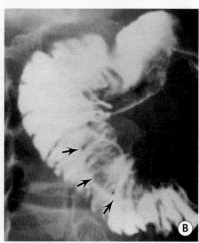

(A) Enlarged duodenal loop with a 'reversed 3' sign of Frostberg. Earlier PTC shows the characteristic 'gloved finger' obstruction of the intrapancreatic common bile duct pathognomonic of carcinoma of the pancreatic head. (B) Barium meal. A double contour (arrows) of the duodenal loop. Carcinoma of the pancreatic head.

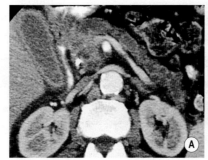
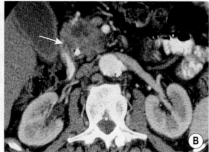

Pancreatic carcinoma. (A) Atrophy of the body and tail is seen, with a markedly dilated pancreatic duct. (B) The pancreatic head mass involves the duodenal wall (arrow).

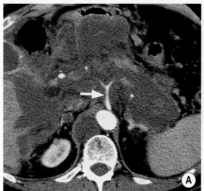
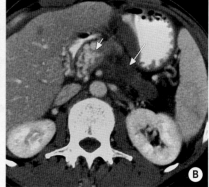

(A) Pancreatic carcinoma and adjacent adenopathy encasing the coeliac axis (arrow). (B) Venous occlusion. A tumour in the pancreatic body (long arrow) has occluded the splenic and portal veins, resulting in the development of multiple venous collaterals (small arrow). Note the presence of splenomegaly and a hepatic metastasis.

PANCREATIC DUCTAL ADENOCARCINOMA

PEARLS

- *Indirect CT findings of venous involvement* (often involving the superior mesenteric and splenic veins at the portal venous confluence): dilatation of small peripancreatic veins (± multiple venous collaterals) ▶ a 'tear drop' shape of the SMV
- *Unresectable disease:* vascular encasement (particularly if the tumour exceeds 50% of the vessel circumference) of the coeliac trunk/SMA
- SMV encasement (but a normal SMA) will not itself preclude resection as vein resection and interposition is an option
- *Invasion of adjacent structures (e.g. stomach, duodenum):* this will be shown by interruption of their normally enhancing wall ▶ duodenal involvement does not necessarily preclude curative surgery as the duodenum is removed as part of the procedure
- *There is early metastatic spread to the lymph nodes:* peripancreatic followed by coeliac, common hepatic, mesenteric and then para-aortic ▶ nodes may be involved without enlargement (nodes measuring >1 cm in short axis are suspicious for metastatic involvement)
- *Peritoneal spread:* this is commonly seen but the lesions are typically small and difficult to detect ▶ peritoneal involvement may be inferred if there is ascites
- *Distant metastases:* liver > lymph nodes > peritoneum > lung

Tumour markers (CA 19-9, CA 242, CEA) These are associated with pancreatic cancer but are not currently sensitive or specific enough for screening or the differentiation of benign from malignant pancreatic masses

Diagnosis This can be achieved with FNA biopsy ▶ this should be possibly avoided if the tumour is potentially resectable (due to the risk of cutaneous seeding)

Treatment Whipple's procedure: a radical pancreaticoduodenectomy with gallbladder removal ± distal gastric resection (a jejunal loop creates a gastrojejunal, choledochojejunal and pancreatojejunal anastamosis) ▶ alternatively can perform a PPPD (pylorus-preserving pancreatico-duodenectomy)
- This is associated with significant morbidity and mortality
- A radiologically guided coeliac axis block can help with pain relief

CYSTIC PANCREATIC TUMOURS

DEFINITION

- The commonest cystic mass within the pancreas is a pseudocyst (demonstrating a high amylase level following FNA) ▶ if there is a low amylase level then a cystic tumour has to be considered:

Intraductal papillary mucinous neoplasm (IPMN)

This is a rare cystic low-grade pancreatic tumour arising from the epithelial lining of the pancreatic ducts ▶ excessive mucin secretion results in duct dilatation and obstruction (it can involve the main or side ducts)
- *Location:* pancreatic head (58%) > body (23%) > tail (7%)
  - *Main duct IPMN:* high malignancy risk (invasive features in 50%)
    - Surgical removal usually advocated
  - *Branch duct IPMN:* lower malignancy risk (especially if < 3cm)
    - Close follow-up advocated if <3 cm and no signs of malignancy
  - *Mixed type IPMN:* dilatation of both the main and side branches
  - Predictors of malignancy: main pancreatic duct >9 mm ▶ mural enhancing nodules ▶ signs of invasion ▶ thick septa ▶ irregular wall

MRCP/MDCT/EUS/ERCP These can potentially detect a communication between the IPMN and pancreatic duct (no such communication exists with a mucinous cystic neoplasm)

Serous cystadenoma vs mucinous cystic tumour

	Mucinous cystic neoplasm (malignant potential)	Serous cystadenoma (benign potential)
Frequency	More common	Less common
Location	Body or tail of the pancreas	Head of the pancreas
Age	Younger patients	Older patients
Morphology	Fewer larger cysts (<6 cysts, >2 cm in diameter) ▶ solid enhancing nodules suggest a mucinous cystic neoplasm	Numerous tiny cysts (>6 cysts, <2 cm in diameter) ▶ they may appear solid on CT if the cysts cannot be resolved
Central scar	Absent	Present
Calcification	Amorphous peripheral mural calcification	Central stellate calcification ('sunburst')
Vascularity	Hypovascular	Hypervascular

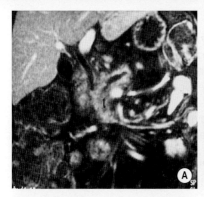

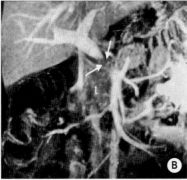

Unresectable carcinoma of the pancreas. (A) Coronal T1WI + Gad shows the ducts are obstructed by an ill-defined tumour (t), which is of slightly lower SI than adjacent pancreas ▶ maximum intensity projection (B) shows the lower end of the portal vein to be encircled (arrows) by extension of the tumour (t) from the head of the pancreas.

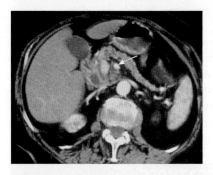

Unresectable pancreatic carcinoma. The uncinate process tumour encircles more than 50% of the circumference of the superior mesenteric artery (arrow).

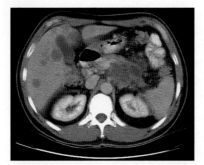

Pancreatic carcinoma with liver metastases. Portal venous phase CT shows poorly enhancing liver deposits secondary to a primary mass in the pancreatic body.

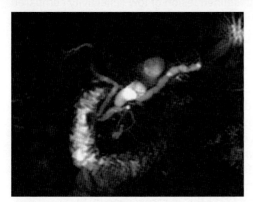

IPMN mixed type. MRCP shows, in a patient without history of pancreatitis, a dilated main duct with some cystic structures.**

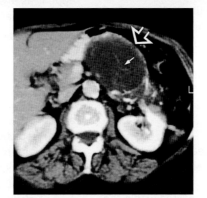

Mucinous cystadenocarcinoma. Contiguous CT images through the pancreas show a cystic mass (open arrow) replacing most of the body and tail of the gland. Areas of dystrophic calcification are noted within the wall of the cystic mass and small papillary excrescences and septa are also seen (small white arrows).*

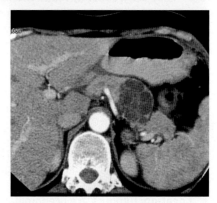

Benign serous cystadenoma. The tumour at the junction of the pancreatic body and tail shows the typical appearance of numerous small cysts.*

ENDOCRINE PANCREATIC TUMOURS AND ISLET CELL TUMOURS

DEFINITION

Functioning tumours

- Peptide hormone production produces a characteristic clinical syndrome

Insulinoma

- **Definition:** the commonest islet cell tumour (accounting for 50% of the total) presenting with hypoglycaemic episodes ▶ the diagnosis can be confirmed biochemically
- **Location:** there is no predilection for any particular part of the pancreas
- **Characteristics:** the tumour is usually solitary and small (<2 cm) ▶ 90% are benign
  - *'10% rule'*: 10% are associated with multiple endocrine neoplasia syndrome (MEN) type 1 (10%) ▶ 10% are multiple ▶ 10% are malignant

Gastrinoma

- **Definition:** the 2nd commonest islet cell tumour presenting with the Zollinger–Ellison syndrome (gastric hyperacidity with recurrent gastric and duodenal ulceration)
- **Location:** these can be ectopic (e.g. within the duodenal wall, stomach, or omentum)
  - *They are frequently found within the 'gastrinoma triangle':* formed by the junction of the cystic and the common hepatic duct superiorly, 2nd and 3rd parts of the duodenum inferiorly and the pancreatic duct medially
- **Characteristics:** they are often multiple, with a mean size of 3.5 cm ▶ 60% are malignant
  - $\frac{1}{3}$ are associated with MEN type 1

Glucagonoma

- **Definition:** this presents with diarrhoea, diabetes, necrolytic erythema migrans and glossitis (secondary to excessive glucagon secretion)
- **Location:** tumours are predominantly located within the pancreatic body and tail
- **Characteristics:** the average tumour size is 4–7 cm ▶ 60% are malignant

VIPoma

- **Definition:** this secretes vasoactive intestinal polypeptide leading to the WDHA syndrome (**w**atery **d**iarrhoea, **h**ypokalaemia, **a**chlorhydria) ▶ malignant transformation is seen in 60% of cases
- **Location:** tumours are predominantly located within the pancreatic body and tail ▶ 10% are ectopic (and found within the sympathetic chain and adrenal medulla)
- **Characteristics:** the average tumour size is 5–10 cm ▶ most tumours are benign, but 50% of intrapancreatic tumours are malignant

Somatostatinoma

- **Definition:** this presents with hyperglycaemia, gallstones and steatorrhoea (secondary to excessive somatostatin secretion)
- **Location:** tumours are located within the pancreatic head or duodenum
- **Characteristics:** the average tumour size is >4 cm ▶ >50% of tumours undergo malignant transformation

Non-functioning tumours

- **Definition:** these are the 3rd commonest islet cell tumour
- **Location:** they are commonly found within the pancreatic head
- **Characteristics:** they can be large at presentation (>5 cm), causing symptoms by mass effect (e.g. jaundice) ▶ they are nearly always malignant
- **Clinical presentation:** this is similar to a pancreatic adenocarcinoma – however there is a better prognosis as they can often be curatively resected or successfully treated with chemotherapy

RADIOLOGICAL FEATURES

US This detects >60% of solitary islet cell tumours ▶ they appear as a well-defined lesion of low reflectivity compared with the adjacent pancreas

Intraoperative US This is carried out if the preoperative location was unsuccessful ▶ it can visualize tumours as small as 3 mm (endoscopic and intraductal US is also available)

CT A tumour demonstrates early but transient enhancement (as it is hypervascular) ▶ there may be better depiction on portal phase imaging (there may be ring enhancement with an insulinoma)

- Radiological features suggesting a non-functioning endocrine tumour as opposed to an adenocarcinoma:
  - *Calcification (22%):* this is rarely seen in an adenocarcinoma
  - *Contrast enhancement:* this is not a feature of an adenocarcinoma

MRI T1WI (FS): low SI ▶ T2WI: high SI ▶ T1WI + Gad: solid or ring enhancement

Scintigraphy ^{111}In-pentetreotide and ^{123}I-MIBG can localize the appropriate cell type ▶ PET can be utilized using somatostatin receptor tracers (e.g. ^{68}Ga-dotatate)

Venous sampling This may localize a functioning tumour ▶ the hepatic vein is sampled after selective pancreatic arterial injection of a secretagogue (calcium for an insulinoma and secretin for a gastrinoma)

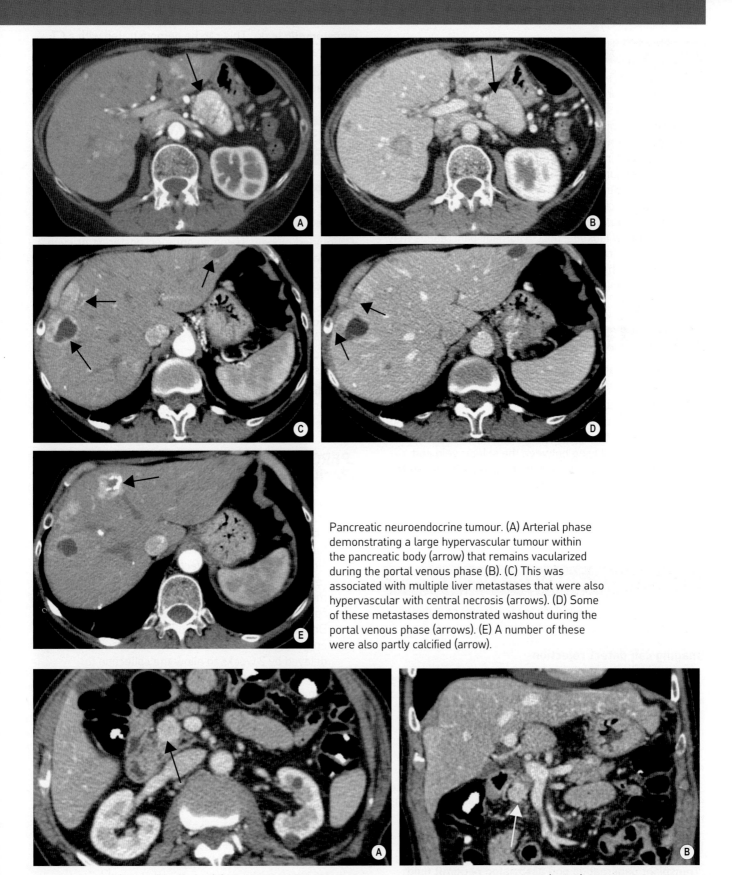

Pancreatic neuroendocrine tumour. (A) Arterial phase demonstrating a large hypervascular tumour within the pancreatic body (arrow) that remains vacularized during the portal venous phase (B). (C) This was associated with multiple liver metastases that were also hypervascular with central necrosis (arrows). (D) Some of these metastases demonstrated washout during the portal venous phase (arrows). (E) A number of these were also partly calcified (arrow).

Pancreatic neuroendocrine tumour. (A) A small hypervascular tumour is seen within the pancreatic head (arrow), which is also seen on the coronal view (B).

377

TRAUMA

DEFINITION

- Trauma may result in pancreatic contusion, laceration or a complete transection ▶ it is uncommon
- *Mechanism:* a severe direct impact or a forceful deceleration injury with midline compression of the pancreas against the vertebral column
  - Pancreatic injuries are often associated with other visceral injuries
- Blunt pancreatic injuries:
  - *Without ductal leakage:* these usually resolve spontaneously
  - *With ductal leakage:* post-traumatic pancreatitis may occur ▶ disruption of the main pancreatic duct is an important indicator of severity
  - *Other complications:* abscess, fistula or pseudocyst formation

RADIOLOGICAL FEATURES

US Peripancreatic fluid ▶ discontinuity of the normal pancreatic contour

CT This is the best investigation
- A pancreatic fracture line (± separation of the fragments) ▶ haematoma formation ▶ focal enlargement of the pancreas ▶ fluid lying between the splenic vein and pancreas ▶ increased peripancreatic fat attenuation ▶ thickening of the anterior renal fascia ▶ fluid within the lesser sac

ERCP/MRCP This is performed if a ductal injury is suspected

PANCREATIC TRANSPLANT IMAGING

- This is increasingly used for the treatment of diabetes (± a simultaneous renal transplant)

Imaging can detect rejection

US (acute rejection) Patchy or diffuse areas of decreased parenchymal echogenicity ▶ an enlarged graft

US (chronic rejection) Increased echogenicity ▶ a reduced graft size

Scintigraphy ^{99m}Tc-DTPA blood pool imaging: there is reduced graft perfusion

MRI This is the most sensitive technique ▶ T1WI: reduced SI (similar to skeletal muscle) ▶ T2WI: increased SI (similar to fluid)

Imaging can detect other complications

Transplant pancreatitis and associated perigraft fluid collections These are not uncommon and can be treated with percutaenous catheter drainage

Disruption of the cystoduodenostomy and an anastomotic leak This can be demonstrated with a CT cystogram

Other complications Abscess formation ▶ haemorrhage ▶ ischaemia ▶ graft-vessel thrombosis

INTERVENTIONAL RADIOLOGY IN THE PANCREAS

BIOPSY OF A PANCREATIC LESION

US-guided biopsy Using an anterior approach

CT-guided biopsy Using an anterior, posterior, or even a lateral approach
- It is usually necessary to pass the needle through normal abdominal tissue – most structures (except the spleen) can be traversed with a 20 or 22 G needle without significant morbidity
  - *FNA biopsy:* this provides a cytological aspirate
  - *Cutting needles (18–20 G):* these provide a core of tissue for histology

Complications Pancreatitis (the commonest complication –3%) ▶ a vasovagal reaction ▶ severe haemorrhage ▶ needle-track seeding (rarely seen)

PERCUTANEOUS DRAINAGE OF A PANCREATIC FLUID COLLECTION

- This usually follows acute pancreatitis with 2 main indications:
  - *To assess whether a fluid collection is infected:* a few millilitres are aspirated for microbiology
  - *Drainage of a known infected collection:* the best results are obtained using large catheters (≥12 F as most abscesses are viscous) ▶ drainage of separate collections is achieved with additional catheters
  - Drainage of a pancreatic collection following enzymatic destruction of pancreatic tissue is usually delayed by 2 weeks to allow the collection to sufficiently liquefy ▶ other peripancreatic collections can be drained immediately

OTHER INTERVENTIONAL RADIOLOGICAL PROCEDURES

Percutaneous access into dilated pancreatic ducts For either balloon dilation or stenting of benign pancreatic duct strictures

Percutaneous cystgastrostomy Creation of a communication between a pancreatic pseudocyst and the stomach (with the percutaneous insertion of a drainage catheter between the pseudocyst and stomach)

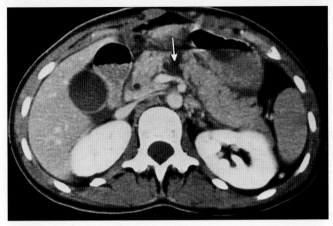

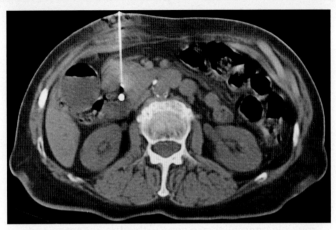

Pancreatic trauma. Following direct blunt trauma to the abdomen the pancreas is seen to be fractured (arrow). There was disruption of the main pancreatic duct.

CT-guided biopsy of the pancreas. A pancreatic mass is present and there is a plastic biliary stent in situ. Using an anterior approach, a 22-gauge needle has been inserted into the mass for biopsy. Fine-needle aspirate revealed adenocarcinoma.*

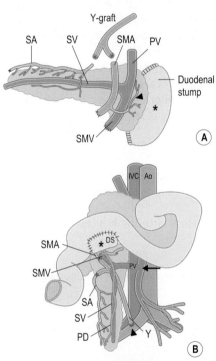

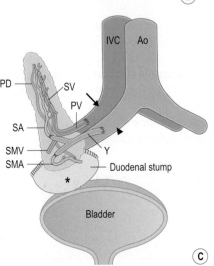

(A) Drawing of the donor pancreas (posterior view) demonstrates vascular reconstruction. The donor iliac Y-graft is attached to the donor splenic artery (SA) to supply the body of the pancreas, and to the donor superior mesenteric artery (SMA) to supply the head of the pancreas via the inferior pancreaticoduodenal artery (arrowhead). The donor portal vein (PV) functions as the main graft vein and drains the donor splenic vein (SV) and donor superior mesenteric vein (SMV). The donor duodenal stump (*) is harvested along with the pancreas. (B, C) Drawings (anterior view) illustrate the two types of pancreas transplants as seen through the overlying pancreas. (B) Portal venous and enteric exocrine drainage. The graft artery (Y) is attached to the common iliac artery (arrowhead) proximally ▶ the distal limbs are connected to the donor splenic artery (SA) and donor superior mesenteric artery (SMA). The graft vein (PV) is attached to the recipient superior mesenteric vein (arrow) for portal venous drainage. The donor splenic vein (SV) and donor superior mesenteric vein (SMV) are shown as well. Exocrine drainage is via the pancreatic duct (PD) to the duodenal stump (*), which is anastomosed to the jejunum. (C) Systemic venous and bladder exocrine drainage. The graft artery (Y) is attached to the common iliac artery (arrowhead) proximally ▶ the distal limbs are connected to the donor splenic artery (SA) and donor superior mesenteric artery (SMA). The graft vein (PV) is anastomosed to the recipient external iliac vein (arrow), providing systemic venous drainage of the donor splenic vein (SV) and donor superior mesenteric vein (SMV). Exocrine secretions are drained via the pancreatic duct (PD) to the duodenal stump (*), which is anastomosed to the bladder. Ao = aorta, IVC = inferior vena cava. ©21

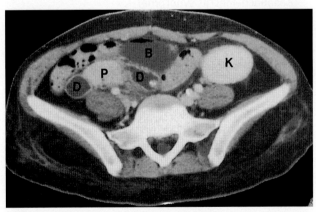

Post-pancreatic transplant CT study. Dynamic CT at the level of the head of the pancreatic allograft (P) shows an apparently normal gland. The attached duodenum (D) has been anastomosed to the urinary bladder (B). Contrast excretion by the transplanted kidney (K) has not yet reached the urinary bladder.**

3.9 SPLEEN

Normal variants and congenital anomalies

- **Splenunculus:** this represents ectopic splenic tissue of congenital origin ▶ they can be single or multiple and are usually found at the splenic hilum ▶ they have similar imaging (and enhancement) appearances to the spleen
- **Wandering spleen:** this follows laxity of the suspensory ligament ▶ torsion may occur
- **Polysplenia:** the spleen is divided into 2–16 masses ▶ this is a congenital syndrome associated with situs ambiguous, as well as cardiovascular and visceral anomalies
- **Asplenia (right isomerism):** an absent spleen and multiple anomalies are seen within the abdomen and thorax (e.g. situs ambiguous with right sidedness)
- **Splenogonadal fusion:** congenital fusion of splenic tissue and the gonad (usually left sided) ▶ it usually affects males

Splenosis

- Heterotopic autotransplantation of splenic tissue, which usually follows a traumatic rupture of the splenic capsule
  - **CT** Poorly marginated soft tissue nodules
- *Possible features:* subcapsular or intrasplenic haematoma ▶ laceration ▶ infarction ▶ haemoperitoneum ▶ pseuodoaneurysm formation

Benign mass lesions

- **Splenic cyst:** *True (primary) cyst:* this has a cellular lining ▶ it can be congenital (F>M) or secondary to echinococcal infection
- *False (secondary) cyst:* this does not have a cellular lining ▶ it is usually post-traumatic and probably represents an evolved haematoma
- **Haemangioma:** This is the commonest primary benign neoplasm of the spleen ▶ it may be part of the Klippel–Trénaunay–Weber syndrome
  - Large haemangiomas may lead to splenic rupture and anaemia, thrombocytopenia and coagulopathy (Kasabach–Merritt syndrome)
  - Enhancement following contrast
- **Lymphangioma:** These are multiple thin-walled, well-defined cysts ▶ they can be capillary, cavernous or cystic (the commonest type within the spleen) ▶ they are often subcapsular and can be single or multiple ▶ they are usually asymptomatic
  - **CT** They do not enhance
- **Hamartoma:** A rare benign lesion composed of an anomalous mixture of normal splenic elements ▶ they are usually single lesions
  - **US** A hyperechoic (± a cystic component) lesion
  - **NECT** An isodense or hypodense lesion

MRI T1WI: intermediate SI ▶ T2WI: high SI ▶ T1WI + Gad: slow enhancement with late filling in

Malignant mass lesions

- **Lymphoma and leukaemia:** Splenic lymphoma is usually part of a generalized lymphoma (usually NHL [non-Hodgkin's lymphoma]) ▶ there is splenomegaly (± multifocal deposits) – see separate section
- **Splenic angiosarcoma:** This is very rare but is the commonest non-lymphoid primary malignant tumour of the spleen ▶ there is a very poor prognosis ▶ CT: multiple nodules/solitary complex mass (cystic + solid)/haemorrhagic nodules/diffuse splenic involvement
- **Other primary tumours:** These are very rare (e.g. fibrosarcoma, leiomyosarcoma)
- **Metastatic disease:** This is rare and usually asymptomatic ▶ parenchymal lesions appear as hypodense nodules on CT
  - *Commonest primary sites:* breast ▶ lung ▶ colorectal ▶ ovary ▶ melanoma accounts for 50%
    - There may be cystic metastases from the ovary, breast, endometrium or skin
  - Calcification is uncommon (but can be seen with mucinous primary adenocarcinomas)
  - Ovarian, gastrointestinal or pancreatic tumours can lead to peritoneal splenic disease

Other splenic disorders

- **Splenic infarcts:**
  CT Low-density, wedge-shaped areas on CT – infarct of the whole spleen results in only rim enhancement of the capsule
  - *Causes:* embolic disease ▶ arteritis ▶ sickle cell disease ▶ pancreatitis
- **Splenic sarcoidosis:**
  CT Poorly enhancing 2–3 cm nodules ▶ splenomegaly ▶ adenopathy
- **Haemosiderosis:**
  MRI T1WI and T2WI: there is low SI due to the iron deposition
- **Amyloidosis:**
  CT Discrete low attenuation masses within an enlarged spleen ▶ diffuse low attenuation spleen with poor enhancement
- **Extramedullary haematopoiesis:** Splenomegaly ± focal masses of haematopoietic tissues (mimicking tumours)
- **Sickle cell anaemia:**
  XR/CT With chronic disease there is a small calcified spleen (due to repeated splenic infarction)

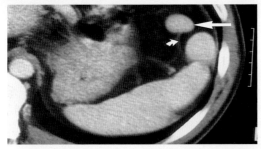

Accessory spleen. CECT shows a small accessory spleen (arrow) anterior to the spleen. Note the draining vein (curved arrow) from the accessory spleen can be seen to join the other veins draining the main spleen.*

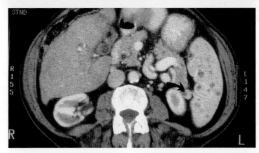

Splenic candidiasis. CECT shows multiple tiny hypodense lesions in the spleen from candidal microabscess. A small accessory spleen (curved arrow) at the splenic hilum is also involved.*

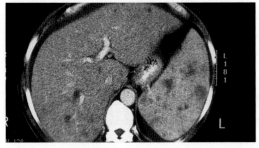

Lymphoma. CECT in a patient with NHL involving the liver and spleen. Multiple small poorly defined nodules can be seen in both the liver and spleen. A trace of ascites can also be seen anterior to the liver.*

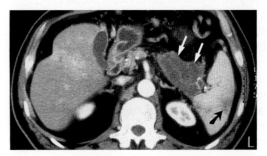

Splenic infarct. CECT shows a tumour mass (white arrows) in the tail of the pancreas causing occlusion to the splenic vein and a splenic infarct (black arrow).*

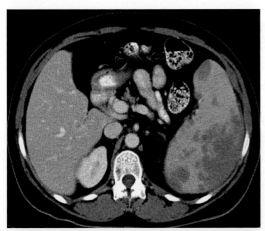

Splenic angiosarcoma. A heterogeneously enhancing mass expands the spleen on CT portal phase. FDG PET-CT demonstrates the associated increased metabolic activity.**

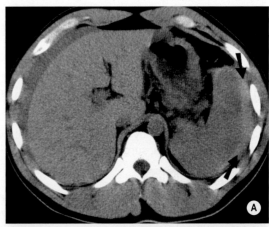

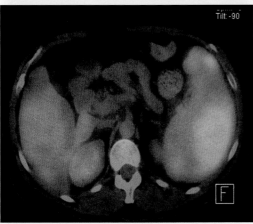

Splenic trauma. On the unenhanced CT (A) a rind of high-attenuation material (blood clot) is visible adjacent to the spleen (arrows), indicating the likely source of haemorrhage in this trauma patient. Only on the portal phase (B) is the splenic 'fracture' clearly visible (arrowheads).**

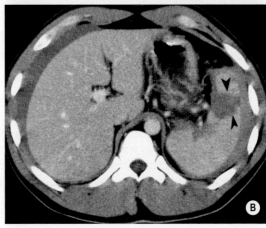

ASCITES

Definition

- >100 ml of free fluid within the peritoneal cavity due to benign or malignant causes
  - *Transudative fluid:* portal hypertension/cirrhosis/heart failure/nephrotic syndrome
  - *Exudative fluid:* infection/peritoneal carcinomatosis
  - *Blood:* trauma/tumour rupture/haemorrhagic diathesis
  - *Purulent fluid:* intestinal perforation
  - *Others:* bile (biliary leakage)/chyle (lymphatic obstruction)/pancreatitis fluid
- Exudates may be limited by peritoneal reaction/adhesions ▶ transudates diffuse freely
- Ascites usually seen in the pouch of Douglas (lowest most posterior space) ▶ upper abdominal ascites usually collects in Morison's pouch/hepatorenal space (most dependent area) ▶ fluid migrates to upper abdomen due to respiratory induced lower hydrostatic pressures ▶ fluid migrates along paracolic gutters – preferentially the right (as it is deeper and wider than the left and without an obstructing phrenicocolic ligament)

Radiological features

- **CT** Attenuation values range between 0 and +30 HU (>30 HU with increasing protein content or haemoperitoneum)
- *Loculated peritoneal fluid:* this is due to benign or malignant adhesions ▶ it appears as a cystic lesion with mass effect

INTRAPERITONEAL AIR

Definition

- This can be caused by a perforation of a hollow viscus, abdominal trauma, surgery or infection

Radiological features

- **CT** This is able to detect minute quantities of free air ▶ free air is most commonly seen anterior to the liver (if the patient is supine)

PERITONEAL INFECTION

Peritoneal abscess

- A localized collection of pus within the peritoneal cavity
- **CT** It initially appears as a mass of soft tissue attenuation – it then undergoes liquefactive necrosis with a mature abscess demonstrating wall enhancement and a near water attenuation centre (together with obliteration of the adjacent fat planes) ▶ gas within a loculated fluid collection is not pathognomonic for an abscess (a necrotic non-infected tumour or mass communicating with the bowel may contain air)

Peritonitis

- A generalized infective/inflammatory collection of intraperitoneal fluid occurring secondary to bacterial, granulomatous or chemical causes (bacterial peritonitis may be primary or secondary to an intraperitoneal abscess or due to rupture of a hollow viscus)
- **CT** Ascites ▶ peritoneal (± mesenteric) thickening

Tuberculous peritonitis

- This is rare and can be caused by rupture of a caseous lymph node or direct GI tract involvement by disease, lymphatic or haematogenous spread
- **CT** High attenuation proteinaceous ascites (20–45 HU) ▶ thickening and nodularity of the peritoneal surfaces ▶ enlarged low attenuation lymph nodes

SCLEROSING PERITONITIS

Definition Rare chronic peritoneal inflammation, common in patients undergoing continuous ambulatory peritoneal dialysis ▶ rare causes: long-term β blockers/sarcoidosis

CT Peritoneal thickening ▶ peritoneal calcification ▶ loculated fluid collections ▶ small bowel tethering

INFARCTION OF OMENTUM OR EPIPLOIC APPENDAGE (EPIPLOIC APPENDAGITIS)

Definition

- This occurs either as a result of torsion or from a spontaneous venous thrombosis ▶ it is a benign, self-limiting condition presenting with acute abdominal pain
  - *Epiploic appendages:* small pouches of peritoneum filled with fat and situated along the colon and upper part of the rectum

Radiological features

- **US** An ovoid non-compressible mass of high reflectivity situated under the abdominal wall
- **CT** A circumscribed fatty area with high attenuation streaks, often in the right lower quadrant
- In the case of epiploic appendagitis the lesion is seen in contact with the serosal surface of the colon (and usually exhibits a hyperattenuating rim and a central area of high attenuation corresponding to the thrombosed vessels)
- It is also associated with mild local bowel wall thickening

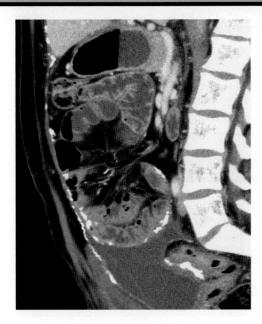

Sclerosing peritonitis. CECT shows a loculated fluid collection and extensive peritoneal calcification.*

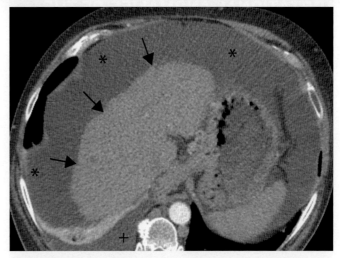

Ascites. The cirrhotic liver has an irregular edge (arrows) and is surrounded by ascites (*). A right pleural effusion with some collapsed lung is also evident (+).

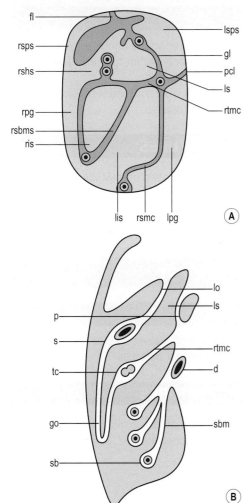

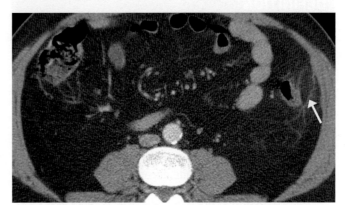

CECT showing an area of increased soft tissue attenuation and stranding of the pericolic fat (adjacent to the descending colon) in keeping with epiploic appendagitis.*

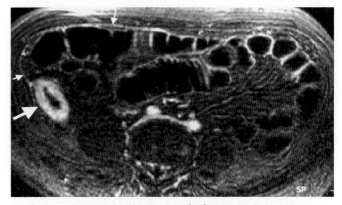

Peritoneal tuberculosis. T1WI + Gad (FS) depicting enhancement of the peritoneal lining (small arrows). There is involvement of the caecum characterized by homogeneous enhancement of the bowel wall (large arrow).*

(A) Coronal diagram showing division of the peritoneal cavity according to peritoneal attachments to the posterior abdominal wall. (B) Midsagittal diagram of the upper abdomen. Abbreviations: fl = falciform ligament; gl = gastrosplenic ligament; pcl = phrenicocolic ligament; ls = lesser sac; lsps = left subphrenic space; lpg = left paracolic gutter; lis = left infracolic space; rtmc = root of transverse mesocolon; rsbm = root of small bowel mesentery; ris = right infracolic space; rpg = right paracolic gutter; rshs = right subhepatic space; rsps = right subdiaphragmatic space; smb = small bowel mesentery; go = greater omentum; lo = lesser omentum; tc = transverse colon; sb = small bowel; s = stomach; p = pancreas; d = duodenum.**

ROTATIONAL ANOMALIES OF THE SMALL BOWEL MESENTERY

DEFINITION

- Rotational anomalies around the axis of the superior mesenteric artery occur when the normal process of fetal gut development is arrested
- It is characterized by the reversal of the normal relationship between the superior mesenteric artery and vein. The artery is now located to the right of vein ▶ there is twisting of the mesentery around the artery ▶ there is an absence of a normal horizontal duodenum
- It is usually asymptomatic in adults

DEVELOPMENTAL DEFECTS

DEFINITION

- Internal herniation occurs when the bowel and its mesentery can herniate into pouches or openings within the visceral peritoneum
  - *Paraduodenal hernia*: this is the commonest type and is caused by small bowel entrapment under the right or left mesocolon ▶ 3 times more common on the left
  - *Right-sided paraduodenal hernia*: bowel herniates through Waldeyer's fossa (behind the SMA and inferior to the third part of the duodenum) ▶ imaging findings include encapsulated small bowel loops within the right mid-abdomen with anterior displacement of the right colic vein, looping of the small intestine around the superior mesenteric vessels and an abnormal position of the superior mesenteric vein relative to the artery
  - *Left-sided paraduodenal hernia*: bowel herniates through Landzert's fossa located at the duodeno-jejunal junction ▶ the bowel becomes entrapped behind the descending mesocolon within the paraduodenal fossa with anterior displacement of the inferior mesenteric vein by the dilated encapsulated bowel loop ▶ CT shows a cluster of dilated bowel loops behind the stomach and pancreas, lateral to the duodeno-jejunal junction with anterior stomach displacement
  - *Transmesenteric hernias*: most common paediatric internal hernia, related to congenital mesenteric defects ▶ in adults usually related to previous surgery (e.g. Roux-en-Y anastamosis) ▶ more likely than other hernias to develop volvulus ▶ on CT appear as a cluster of dilated loops lying adjacent to the abdominal wall without overlying omental fat lateral to the colon which is displaced centrally – the mesenteric pedicle is engorged, stretched and crowded

LYMPHANGIOMA

DEFINITION

- The commonest subtype of a mesenteric cyst – it represents a congenital malformation of the bowel lymphatic vessels, frequently surrounding the loop of bowel from where it originates

RADIOLOGICAL FEATURES

US This can demonstrate internal septations

CT A large, thin-walled, single or multiloculated cystic mass ▶ its contents are of water-to-fat attenuation

MRI T2WI: high SI ± enhancement cyst wall and septa

ENTERIC DUPLICATION CYST

DEFINITION

- An uncommon congenital anomaly found anywhere along the GI tract (commonly within the ileum) and located on the mesenteric border
- It is lined with alimentary tract mucosa (occasionally gastric or pancreatic mucosa)

RADIOLOGICAL FEATURES

US Its wall is thick and composed of multiple layers, like those of the normal bowel wall

CT/MR A unilocular mass of predominantly water content and a thick wall that exhibits contrast enhancement

MESOTHELIAL CYST

DEFINITION

- This results from failure of coalescence of mesothelial-lined peritoneal surfaces

RADIOLOGICAL FEATURES

CT A fluid-filled mass with no discernible wall ▶ no internal septations are demonstrated (cf. a lymphangioma)

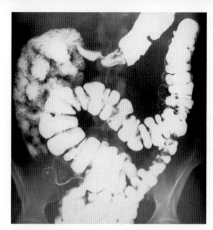

Small bowel loops are in the right upper quadrant in this patient with malrotation.••

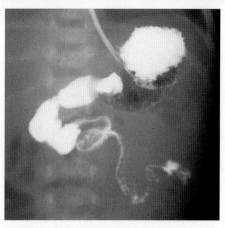

Typical corkscrew appearance of the duodenum and proximal jejunum associated with malrotation and midgut volvulus.©20

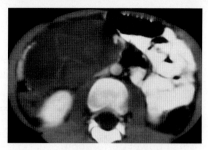

Cystic mesenteric lymphangioma. Enhanced CT depicting a multilocular cystic mass with thin internal septa, occupying the small bowel mesentery.*

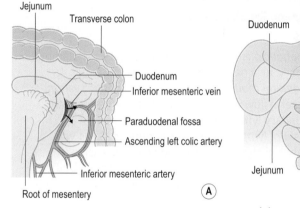

Development of a left-sided paraduodenal hernia. (A) Small bowel loops herniate into the descending mesocolon through the paraduodenal fossa posterior to the inferior mesenteric vein and ascending left colic artery. (B) Small bowel loops progressively herniate through an abnormal peritoneal pocket.

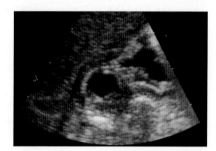

Duplication cyst of pylorus. Ultrasound showing echogenic mucosal layer and hypoechoic outer muscular layer.*

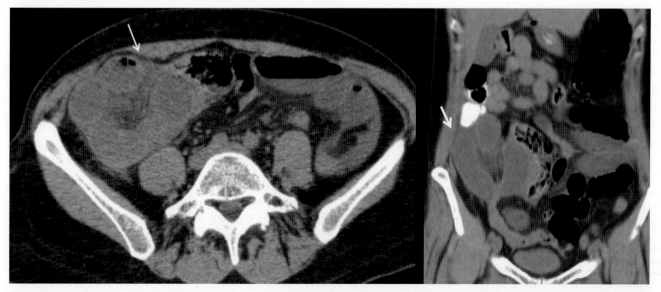

Transmesenteric internal hernia. Unenhanced axial and coronal reformatted CT show a cluster of dilated, fluid-filled loops of small bowel lateral to ascending colon (arrows) beneath anterior abdominal wall, displacing omental fat. Engorged vessels and adjacent mesenteric haziness are also evident, reflecting strangulating obstruction.**

Mesenteric lymphadenitis

Definition

- Benign lymph node inflammation within the ileal mesentery ▶ clinically it can mimic an appendicitis

US/CT Moderately enlarged mesenteric lymph nodes within the right lower quadrant (± ileal or ileocaecal wall thickening)

Small bowel perforation

Definition Perforation that is not associated with blunt trauma (e.g. a ruptured diverticulum or an intramural foreign body penetrating the wall)

CT Streaky mesenteric soft tissue densities associated with local extraluminal gas

Graft-vs-host disease

Definition A complication of heterotopic bone marrow transplantation

CT Focal or diffuse mural bowel thickening (usually within the ileum) ▶ it is associated with an increased size of any associated mesenteric vessels

Whipple's disease

Definition A systemic infectious disease primarily associated with malabsorption

CT Low attenuation mesenteric and retroperitoneal lymph nodes (due to the nodal deposition of fat and fatty acids) ▶ it is associated with diffuse intestinal wall thickening

Mesenteric panniculitis

Definition Chronic non-specific inflammation involving the small bowel mesenteric adipose tissue ▶ a rare, slowly progressive condition of unknown origin

- *Retractile or fibrosing mesenteritis:* a dominant fibrotic component is present

CT (mesenteric panniculitis) A well-delineated, inhomogeneous fatty mass located at the mesenteric root ▶ there is an absence of adjacent bowel loop involvement (or bowel displacement) ▶ there is mesenteric vascular envelopment (with a low attenuation halo surrounding the vessels)

MRI (mesenteric panniculitis) T2WI: hypointense capsule + contrast enhancement

CT (retractile mesenteritis) An infiltrative soft tissue mass with associated radiating linear strands of soft tissue attenuation (which may mimic a desmoid or carcinoid tumour) ▶ calcification may be present within the necrotic central portion of the mass

MRI (retractile mesenteritis) T1WI/T2WI: low SI

Non-inflammatory oedema

Definition A diffuse increase in mesenteric attenuation obscuring the mesenteric vessels

- *Causes:* hypoalbuminaemia ▶ cirrhosis ▶ nephrotic syndrome ▶ right-sided congestive heart failure ▶ mesenteric ischaemia ▶ vasculitis ▶ trauma

CT (mesenteric ischaemia) Mesenteric oedema can be focal or diffuse depending on the extent of vascular compromise

- Circumferential radially symmetric (<1.5 cm) bowel wall thickening ▶ increased mesenteric fat attenuation (secondary to oedema) ▶ decreased, delayed, or lack of small bowel enhancement ▶ intramural, mesenteric or portal venous gas with bowel infarction ▶ a low-density thrombus may be seen within the proximal mesenteric arteries

Radiation

Definition Radiation produces an endarteritis within the radiation port

CT Linear streaks of increased attenuation within the mesenteric fat (representing oedema) ▶ mesenteric retraction ▶ progressive small-vessel narrowing and vascular congestion ▶ bowel wall fibrosis ▶ thick-walled and straightened bowel loops

Mesenteric lymphoedema

Causes

- *Lymphatic obstruction:* this is secondary to inflammation, surgery, or a neoplasm
- *Congenital malformations of the lymphatic system:* collateral flow can occur via the mesenteries with secondary lymphoedema
- *Intestinal lymphangiectasia:* lymphatic stasis with mesenteric lymphoedema and chylous ascites
- *Metastatic disease:* lymph node involvement at the root of the small bowel mesentery may cause central lymphatic obstruction

Mesenteric and small bowel injuries

Definition An uncommon sequelae of blunt abdominal trauma

CT Free air and contrast extravasation (a highly specific sign – however their absence does not exclude a bowel wall injury) ▶ intestinal wall thickening (a non-specific sign) ▶ streaky densities within the mesenteric fat ▶ a mesenteric haematoma ▶ a triangle-shaped fluid collection within the mesentery

- *'Sentinel clot' sign:* the portion of blood closest to the source of bleeding may demonstrate the highest attenuation values (due to clot formation close to the bleeding source)

Intestinal obstruction

CT (strangulating obstruction) Engorgement of the mesenteric vessels ▶ haziness of the mesenteric fat ▶ blurring of the margins of the vessels and mesenteric fluid

CT (closed-loop obstruction) Any mesenteric involvement is less dramatic, with convergence of the dilated veins toward the point of obstruction

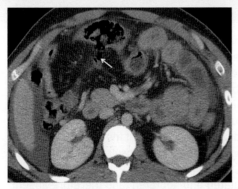

Small bowel perforation. CECT shows abnormally thickened loops of small bowel with adjacent free gas (arrow) in a patient with Crohn's disease.*

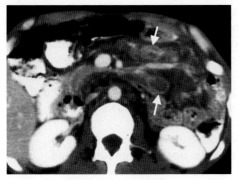

Whipple's disease. Non-enhancing low attenuation lymph nodes are seen within the small bowel mesentery (arrows).

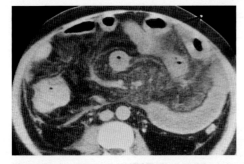

Mesenteric ischaemia. NECT shows diffuse haziness of the affected small bowel mesentery with effacement of the vascular markings, reflecting oedema, haemorrhage and venous congestion. Note also the thickened high attenuation bowel wall due to intramural haemorrhage.*

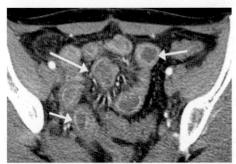

CECT showing multiple mildly thickened abnormally enhancing loops of small bowel (arrows) in a patient with previous pelvic radiotherapy for cervical cancer.*

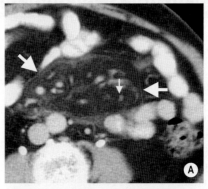

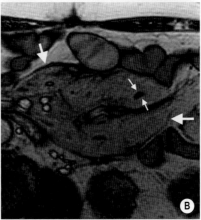

Mesenteric panniculitis. CECT (A) and true-FISP MRI (B) in a patient who presented with abdominal pain show a well-delineated fatty mass (large arrows) extending from the root of the small bowel mesentery toward the left abdomen, engulfing mesenteric vessels without distortion. Note the perivascular halo (small arrow).*

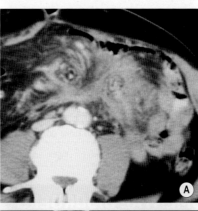

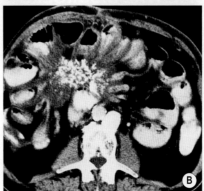

Fibrosing mesenteritis. (A) CECT in a patient who presented with fever of unknown origin demonstrates a fibrofatty mesenteric mass with irregular borders surrounding mesenteric vessels. Strands of soft tissue density are seen radiating from the mass to the adjacent mesenteric fat. (B) CT appearances. CECT demonstrating a large, ill-defined, soft tissue mesenteric mass with extensive calcification. Note retraction and thickening of the adjacent bowel loops.

NEOPLASTIC PERITONEAL DISORDERS

The majority of peritoneal neoplasms are malignant, and usually **secondary** to:

- **Direct invasion**
  - Malignant tumours (e.g. stomach/colon/pancreas/ovary) can spread directly along adjacent visceral peritoneal surfaces
  - Early peritoneal invasion: linear strands in the fat adjacent to the primary tumour
  - A mass contiguous with the primary reflects more advanced dissemination ▶ a mass may spread via ligamentous attachments to involve other structures
- **Intraperitoneal seeding (peritoneal carcinomatosis)**
  - **Definition:** malignant tumour seeding of the peritoneum ▶ malignant cells carried via peritoneal fluid
  - More aggressive tumours lead to peritoneal deposits close to the primary ▶ less aggressive tumours manifest deposits in remote areas
  - Anywhere where ascites pools will favour malignant growth, therefore the most common seeding sites are: the pouch of Douglas ▶ the distal small bowel mesentery (near the ileocaecal junction) ▶ the sigmoid mesocolon ▶ the greater omentum ▶ the right paracolic gutter
  - **CT** Sensitivity is reduced for tumour implants <1 cm in diameter

- Smooth nodular (or plaque-like) thickening and contrast enhancement of the parietal peritoneal surfaces of the diaphragm, liver and spleen (this can also be seen with tuberculosis, peritoneal mesothelioma and peritoneal lymphomatosis)
- Nodular tumour implants on the undersurface of the right diaphragm can indent the liver surface (mimicking capsular or subcapsular liver metastases)
- Ascites is not always present – if it is present it is often loculated and septated (and therefore absent from any dependent areas)
  - Calcified peritoneal implants seen pre-chemotherapy suggests that the primary site is usually a serous papillary cystadenocarcinoma of the ovary (or rarely a gastric carcinoma)
  - **Pseudomyxoma peritonei:** this follows rupture of a mucinous cystadenocarcinoma or cystadenoma of the ovary or appendix ▶ ascites (with septations representing mucinous nodules) and scalloping of the liver edge can be seen
    - **CT:** low attenuation masses
    - **MRI:** T2WI: moderately high SI masses
- **Lymphatic or embolic haematogenous spread**

Primary malignancy	Organ directly invaded	Route of invasion*
Stomach	Spleen	Gastrosplenic ligament
	Superior margin of the transverse colon	Gastrocolic ligament
Pancreas	Liver	Hepatoduodenal ligament
	Inferior margin of the transverse colon	Transverse mesocolon
	Spleen	Splenorenal ligament
Ovary	Diffuse spread through all adjacent peritoneal surfaces	

*Early peritoneal invasion is manifested as linear strands in the fat adjacent to the primary tumour

NEOPLASTIC OMENTAL DISORDERS

Definition **Primary neoplasms:** These are similar to those encountered within the mesentery

- Benign neoplasms are usually well circumscribed and localized within the omentum
- Malignant neoplasms frequently have indistinct margins and infiltrate any surrounding structures

Secondary neoplasms: These are more common than a primary neoplasm

- Tumours metastasizing to the omentum are similar to those responsible for peritoneal carcinomatosis (and usually an ovarian primary)
- Metastatic disease may involve the greater omentum by direct spread along the transverse mesocolon, gastrosplenic or gastrocolic ligaments (as well as by peritoneal or haematogenous spread)

Radiological features

CT

- *Early omental involvement:* irregular soft tissue permeation of the omental fat
- *Advanced omental involvement:* deposits range from discrete nodules to thick, confluent solid omental masses (omental 'cake') ▶ they may demonstrate enhancement

MRI T1WI: low SI areas within the high SI omental fat ▶ extensive involvement presents as an intermediate SI crescent-shaped mass ▶ T1WI + Gad: diffuse enhancement ▶ images are improved with fat suppression

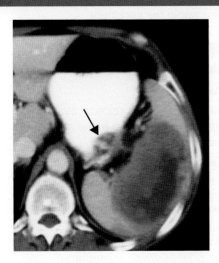

Direct spread of primary splenic lymphoma across the gastrosplenic ligament. The splenic lymphomatous mass has extended along the gastrosplenic ligament to invade the splenic hilar fat and produce mural thickening of the greater curvature of the stomach (arrow).*

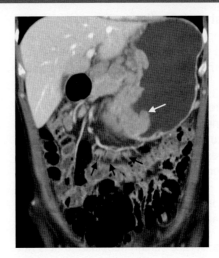

Direct extension of gastric carcinoma across the gastrocolic ligament. A greater curvature carcinoma (white arrow) has spread inferiorly along the gastrocolic ligament to the anterior surface of the transverse colon (black arrows).*

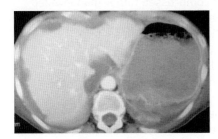

CT reveals the liver scalloping typical of pseudomyxoma peritonei.†

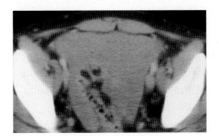

Peritoneal mesothelioma. CECT shows a soft tissue mass that obliterates the pelvic peritoneal spaces and engulfs the sigmoid colon.*

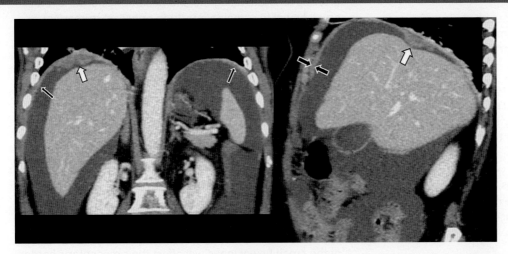

Coronal (left) and sagittal (right) reformations from axial MDCT images favour the visibility of peritoneal carcinomatosis. Irregular thickening and mild enhancement of the parietal peritoneum underneath both hemidiaphragms (long black arrows) and presence of masses (white arrows) corresponding to extensive peritoneal carcinomatosis. A small nodular deposit is barely seen at the left paracolic gutter (small thick black arrows), close to the phrenicocolic ligament.**

PRIMARY NEOPLASMS

Malignant peritoneal mesothelioma: The commonest primary peritoneal neoplasm (occurring in middle-aged men) ▶ it is associated with asbestos exposure (there is not always pleural involvement) ▶ it has a poor prognosis

CT Diffuse thickening or nodularity of the peritoneum ▶ it may diffusely infiltrate the mesentery, leading to omental and mesenteric thickening (with a 'stellate' configuration of the thickened perivascular bundles or 'pleated' thickening of the mesenteric leaves) ▶ peritoneal and omental masses (± local invasion into adjacent organs) ▶ nodular enhancement

- Any ascites is disproportionately small (cf. large-volume ascites with metastatic disease)

Cystic mesothelioma: A rare benign neoplasm that is not associated with asbestos exposure ▶ it is frequently seen within the pelvis and appears as a unilocular or complex cystic mass (stimulating a lymphangioma or ovarian carcinoma) ▶ cysts 1 mm to 6 cm

Fibromatosis: The commonest primary solid mesenteric tumour ▶ it can occur in an isolated form or can be associated with Gardner's syndrome ▶ it has a tendency to arise following either surgery or trauma ▶ often locally aggressive but do not metastasise

CT Highly collagenous: homogeneous ▶ myxoid: hypodense ▶ mixed: whorled appearance ▶ one or more usually large soft tissue attenuation masses (>10 cm) ▶ it often has irregular or ill-defined margins ▶ tethering, encasement or invasion of the adjacent bowel can be seen ▶ Can demonstrate greater enhancement than muscle

MRI T1WI: low to intermediate SI ▶ T2WI: variable SI

Lipoma: The 2nd commonest primary solid mesenteric tumour

CT A well-circumscribed homogeneous mass of fat attenuation

MRI T1WI/T2WI: high SI ▶ T1WI (FS): low SI ▶ internal septations are unusual

Liposarcoma: This is more commonly found within the retroperitoneum than within either the mesentery or peritoneum

CT/MRI A variable appearance reflecting its tissue composition – it can range from predominantly fat, fluid and soft tissue elements to an entirely soft tissue density mass ▶ fat is less likely in higher grade tumours

Pearl

- Primary mesenteric neoplasms are rare ▶ benign primary mesenteric tumours > malignant tumours ▶ secondary > primary malignancies
- Cystic > solid tumours

- Malignant tumours: often near the mesenteric root ▶ benign tumours: arise within the periphery

SECONDARY NEOPLASMS

Metastatic carcinoma

- The primary is usually the stomach, colon or ovary
- Most common malignancies spreading to the mesentery: metastatic carcinoma ▶ lymphoma

Intraperitoneal tumour dissemination The small bowel mesentery is frequently involved by intraperitoneally disseminated tumour with non-specific findings:

- Scattered nodules ▶ rounded, ill-defined soft tissue or cystic masses
- Any ascites can be loculated, and if large enough will tend to surround bowel loops which are tethered centrally by the rigid mesentery
- As metastatic deposits involve the mesentery surface, the mesenteric fat is compressed rather than invaded
- If ascites is extensive it surrounds bowel loops, which are tethered centrally by the rigid mesentery
- Involvement of small bowel mesentery is an independent survival prognostic factor
- Diffuse mesenteric infiltration may resemble mesenteric oedema
- Metastatic tumour nodules on the visceral peritoneal surfaces can become adherent to the serosa of the small bowel loops
- A severe desmoplastic response to the seeded metastases can cause marked fixation and angulation of the ileal loops (± obstruction)
- Fixation and thickening of the mesentery:
  - *Stellate form:* a radiating configuration of the mesenteric folds with thickened rigid perivascular bundles and encased, straightened vascular structures
  - *Pleated appearance:* sheets of soft tissue produce thickening of the mesenteric folds

Embolic metastases These spread via the mesenteric arteries to locate along the antimesenteric border of the small bowel (e.g. melanoma, lung or breast primaries)

CT Focal bowel wall thickening ▶ thickening of the mesenteric folds ▶ melanoma deposits may become large and ulcerated ▶ breast cancer deposits may cause multiple areas of small bowel luminal narrowing with prestenotic dilatations

Lymphatic dissemination This plays a minor role in the spread of metastatic carcinoma but it is the main pathway of dissemination of lymphoma to the mesenteric lymph nodes ▶ enlarged mesenteric lymph nodes occur at presentation in approximately 50% of patients with NHL

CT Confluent lymphomatous nodes may surround the superior mesenteric vessels producing a 'sandwich-like' appearance ▶ coexisting lymphomatous mural involvement of the small bowel loops will affect their mesenteric border

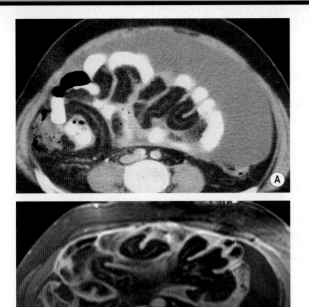

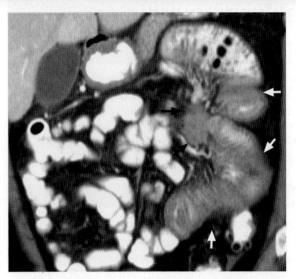

Mesenteric fibromatosis. CECT shows a soft tissue mass in the mesentery (black arrows) resulting in segmental jejunal ischaemia, manifested as symmetrical wall thickening (white arrows).*

Seeded gastric carcinoma along the small bowel mesentery. CECT (A) and post-gadolinium T1-weighted MR image (B) show thickening and enhancement of the mesentery together with ascites.*

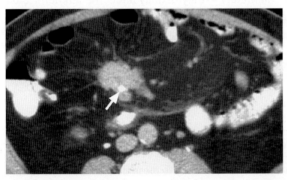

Carcinoid. CECT shows a mesenteric mass with radiating strands toward adjacent bowel loops. An area of dystrophic calcification is also evident (arrow).*

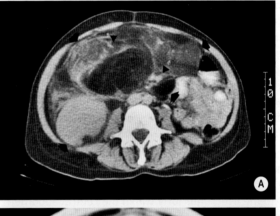

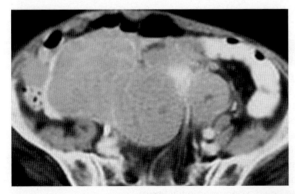

Mesenteric fibrosarcoma. CECT shows an enhancing soft tissue mass in the small bowel mesentery compressing a neighbouring small intestinal loop.*

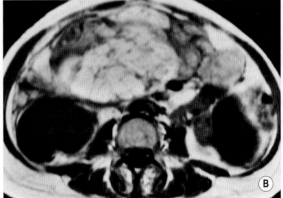

Liposarcoma: CT-MR pathological correlation. (A) CECT of the abdomen demonstrates a large mesenteric mass (arrows) with both fat and soft tissue densities, encasing large peripheral vessels (arrowheads). (B) T1WI demonstrating the multiple fibrous strands seen in this liposarcoma, as well as two components, one brighter centrally (corresponding to a fatty element) and a lower-intensity peripheral component (corresponding to an undifferentiated sarcomatous element).*

PNEUMOPERITONEUM

DEFINITION

- Free intra-abdominal gas – it usually indicates perforation of a viscus (it is often a peptic ulcer – a perforated appendix rarely demonstrates free gas)
  - *Other causes:* bowel obstruction ▶ appendicitis ▶ bowel ischaemia ▶ diverticular disease ▶ post colonoscopy

RADIOLOGICAL FEATURES

Erect CXR Gas is seen under the diaphragm (this can detect as little as 1 ml of free gas) ▶ do not confuse this appearance with Chilaiditi's syndrome (where intestine is seen between the liver and diaphragm) or a subphrenic abscess

Left lateral decubitus AXR Gas is seen between the liver and abdominal wall

Supine AXR Gas is seen within the RUQ – particularly within the subhepatic space and hepatorenal fossa (Morrison's pouch) ▶ triangular collections of air are seen within the abdomen (outlining the visceral contents) ▶ gas is seen on either side of the falciform ligament ▶ scrotal air can be seen in children

- *'Inverted V' sign:* gas is seen on either side of the umbilical ligaments
- *'Rigler's sign:* the outer and inner walls of a bowel loop are delineated by gas
- *'Football' or 'air dome' sign:* a central round air collection seen on a supine AXR in children (as air rises)

CT (lung window settings) This is the most sensitive technique for detecting small amounts of free gas (look anterior to the liver, anteriorly within the central abdomen and within the peritoneal recesses)

GAS WITHIN THE RETROPERITONEUM

DEFINITION

- Retroperitoneal gas can be seen particularly if the originating organ is retroperitoneal
  - *Causes:* a perforated posterior peptic ulcer ▶ a perforated sigmoid diverticular disease ▶ post colonoscopy

RADIOLOGICAL FEATURES

AXR/CT Gas is seen within the layers of the abdominal wall (flanks) or around the kidneys ▶ gas can track superiorly into the mediastinum and inferiorly into the buttock and thigh (classically gas is seen within the soft tissues of the left thigh from a diverticular perforation)

GAS WITHIN THE BOWEL WALL

Causes Intestinal infarction (following thrombosis or embolism of the superior mesenteric artery) ▶ pneumatosis cystoides intestinalis

Intestinal infarction

AXR/CT Linear gas streaks seen within the bowel wall ▶ non-specific dilated loops of small bowel ▶ thickening of the small bowel wall (due to submucosal haemorrhage or oedema) ▶ free gas (if there has been a perforation) ▶ mesenteric or portal venous gas (in advanced cases)

Pneumatosis cystoides intestinalis (pneumatosis coli)

Definition Cyst-like collections of gas within the submucosal or subserosal layers of the bowel wall (there is a normal overlying mucosa) ▶ the cysts can occasionally rupture, producing a pneumoperitoneum ▶ causes:

- *Pulmonary disease:* air tracks along the lung interstitium, via the mediastinum, to the retroperitoneum and mesentery (there is a known association with COPD)
- *Bowel necrosis:* this is seen with necrotizing enterocolitis and mesenteric thrombosis
- *Mucosal disruption:* this is seen with intestinal obstruction or trauma (e.g. endoscopy)

AXR/CT The cysts are well defined and closely packed (1–3 cm in diameter) ▶ they usually affect the left hemicolon

Treatment Prolonged high-dose oxygen therapy (the resultant altered diffusion gradients will collapse any cysts)

Gas within the wall of other organs	
Within the biliary tree	Following a gallstone ileus
Gallbladder	With emphysematous cholecystitis
Portal veins	Secondary to mesenteric infarction
Kidneys	Following emphysematous pyelonephritis
Pancreas	With infected necrosis or abscess
Urinary bladder	With infection or following catheter insertion

Causes of pneumoperitoneum without peritonitis*
Silent perforation of viscus that has sealed itself, in:
Patients on steroids
Unconscious patients
Patients being ventilated
The presence of other serious medical conditions
Postoperative
Peritoneal dialysis
Perforated cyst in pneumatosis cystoides intestinalis
Tracking down a pneumomediastinum
Stercoral ulceration
Leakage through a distended stomach (e.g. endoscopy)
Vaginal-tubal entry of air

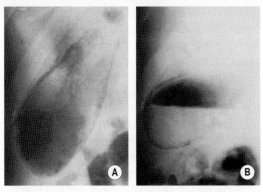

Emphysematous cholecystitis showing (A) gas in the lumen and wall of the gallbladder and (B) a gas–fluid level in the erect posture.†

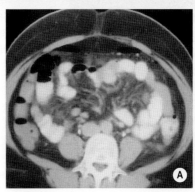

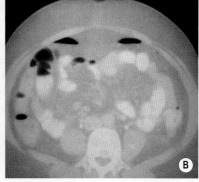

Free peritoneal gas due to perforated sigmoid diverticular disease. (A) CT viewed on abdominal window settings. (B) The same image viewed on broad window settings. The free gas deep to the anterior abdominal wall is more conspicuous in (B).*

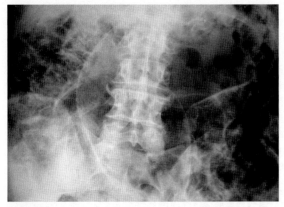

Pneumatosis coli. Multiple small gas-filled cysts are seen in association with the colon. There is also free peritoneal gas.*

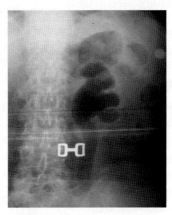

Emphysematous pyelonephritis. Patient with diabetes mellitus and sepsis. The left renal collecting system and ureter are distended and gas filled.*

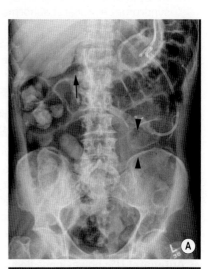

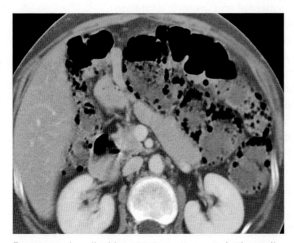

Pneumatosis coli with numerous gas cysts in the wall of the colon.*

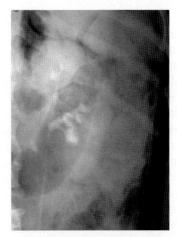

Retroperitoneal gas due to perforated sigmoid diverticular disease. Film from an IVU series. There is gas between the layers of the abdominal wall and around the upper pole of the left kidney.*

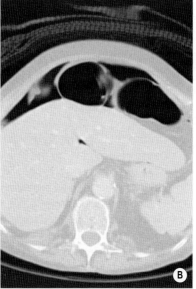

Rigler's sign. (A) Both sides of bowel wall are outlined due to gas being present internally and externally (arrowheads). In addition, triangular collections of air (arrow) are seen. (B) CT (lung windows) confirms a large amount of free intraperitoneal air.

393

OMPHALOCELE

- **Definition:** incomplete formation of the embryonic ventral abdominal wall leads to a congenital midline anterior abdominal wall defect around the umbilicus (the umbilical cord inserts at the tip of the defect)
  - *Larger omphaloceles (containing liver tissue):* these are due to failure of fusion of the lateral body folds
  - *Smaller omphaloceles (containing bowel only):* these are due to the persistence of the physiological herniation of the gut after the 10th week of fetal development
- Associated chromosomal abnormalities are common (50%): trisomy 13 and 18
  - *Beckwith–Wiedemann syndrome:* omphalocele (exomphalos) + macroglossia + gigantism (the 'EMG' syndrome) ▶ visceral abnormalities are seen in up to 70% of cases
- **Diagnosis:** this is made on antenatal ultrasound
- **Prognosis:** this depends upon the associated anomalies

GASTROSCHISIS (LITERALLY MEANING 'SPLIT STOMACH')

- **Definition:** a small defect in the ventral abdominal wall, classically to the right side of a normally positioned umbilicus ▶ it is thought to be due to a localized intrauterine vascular accident leading to full-thickness necrosis of a portion of the anterior abdominal wall
  - It typically occurs in the absence of any other anomalies
- **Antenatal US:** bowel loops floating freely in the amniotic fluid with no covering membrane
  - Exposure to the amniotic fluid damages the bowel and the extruded bowel loops are dilated and thickened (postnatally this can result in a thick, fibrous 'peel' covering the bowel loops)
- **Postnatal complications:** necrotizing enterocolitis (NEC) in up to 20% ▶ respiratory embarrassment following repair of the defect ▶ short bowel syndrome and intestinal dysmotility ▶ intestinal atresias and stenoses (secondary to the prenatal ischaemic insult)
  - The associated morbidity and mortality is mainly due to the associated GI problems (gastro-oesophageal reflux ▶ malrotation ▶ small bowel dilatation)
  - A markedly prolonged transit time (which can be >2 days) is compounded by the requirement for TPN (cholestatic liver disease is a major problem)
  - Approximately ⅓ of males have cryptorchidism, which may result in the testes passing through the defect

CLOACAL EXSTROPHY

- **Definition:** a rare midline infra-umbilical defect that arises due to an abnormality of the caudal body fold (M>F):

- Also known as OEIS complex (omphalocele/exstrophy/imperforate anus/spinal abnormalities) – representing different parts of the same spectrum
  - *Mild:* epispadias (urethral meatus opening on the penile dorsum) ▶ a cleft urethra in females
  - *Moderate:* bladder exstrophy: the bladder is exposed on the lower abdominal wall
  - *Severe:* cloacal exstrophy: abnormalities of the GU and GI tracts, CNS and MSK systems ▶ the cloaca opens onto the lower abdominal wall (open caecum and prolapsing terminal ileum between 2 hemi-bladders) ▶ omphalocele of varying size ▶ blind-ending short gut ▶ ambiguous external genitalia ▶ bilateral inguinal herniae ▶ spinal dysraphism ('open book' pelvis) ▶ renal/lower limb abnormalities
- **AXR:** the pubic bones are separated by >25 mm
- **USS:** antenatally the 'elephant's trunk' sign of the prolapsed terminal ileum is pathognomonic
- **Upper GI contrast study:** this can detect the presence of malrotation and also outlines the length of bowel present
- **MRI:** this can exclude an associated cord anomaly and delineate the pelvic organs and the pelvic floor musculature
- **Treatment:** the bladder and bowel are separated and repaired, with the abdominal wall defect closed

PRUNE BELLY (EAGLE–BARRET) SYNDROME

- **Definition:** a non-hereditary disorder consisting of:
  - *A congenital absence of the abdominal wall muscles:* giving a wrinkled and lax abdominal wall
  - *Urinary tract abnormalities:* renal dysplasia + gross pelvicalyceal and ureteric dilatation
  - *Cryptorchidism:* the bladder distension interferes with testicular descent
- **AXR:** a protuberant abdomen (resulting from the lack of abdominal musculature)
- **US/micturating cystourethrogram:** there are small kidneys with abnormal minimally dilated calyces and upper ureters – the lower ureters are tortuous and show disproportionate dilatation ▶ the bladder is thin walled, of a large capacity (without trabeculation) and has a wide neck ▶ there may be a patent urachus or a urachal diverticulum ▶ the posterior urethra is dilated proximally with typical conical narrowing (± dilatation of the anterior urethra)
  - **MCUG:** this is valuable for assessing the urethral anatomy but is dangerous if sepsis arises ▶ vesico-ureteral reflux is seen in ⅔ of patients
- **IVU:** this is rarely indicated
- **⁹⁹ᵐTc-DMSA:** this assesses the divided renal function
- **Dynamic renal scintigraphy:** this fails to show adequate drainage due to the gross dilatation
- **Long-term follow-up:** US and ⁹⁹ᵐTc-DMSA

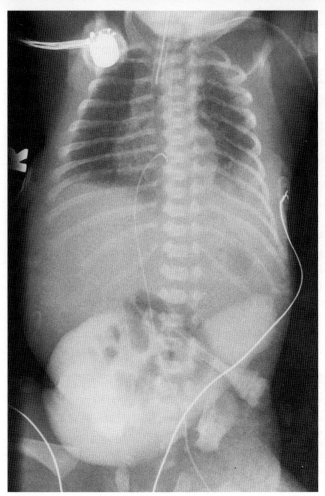

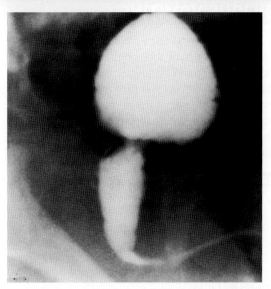

Prune belly syndrome. Image exposed near the end of micturition on a voiding cystourethrogram. The posterior urethra is dilated proximal to the membranous urethra and the calibre of the latter is normal. Posterior urethral valves are not present.*

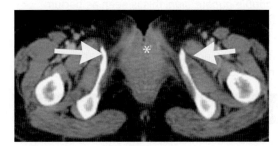

Gastroschisis. Several air-filled extra-abdominal loops of bowel are seen in this infant of 26 weeks' gestation. A small left congenital diaphragmatic hernia was also present.[†]

Cloacal exstrophy: axial CECT showing diastasis of the symphysis pubis (arrows) and midline defect in the lower anterior abdominal wall (*).

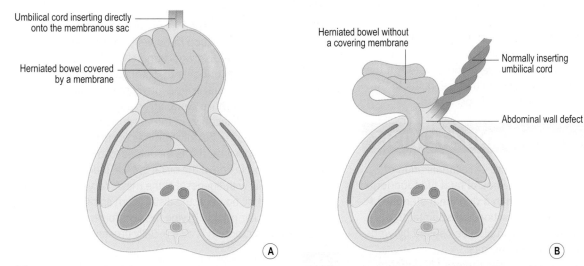

(A) Omphalocele. A midline abdominal wall defect with herniated bowel covered by a membrane. The umbilical cord inserts directly onto the herniated membranous sac. (B) Gastroschisis. The abdominal wall defect is adjacent to a normally inserted umbilical cord. The herniated bowel is not covered by a membrane.

NON-BILIOUS VOMITING

Definition Neonatal non-bilious vomiting due to a GI cause implies the presence of a lesion proximal to the ampulla of Vater and is most frequently due to GOR

- Congenital gastric obstruction is rare and is usually due to a web or diaphragm within the antrum and pylorus ▶ occasionally a true atresia is present with a fibrous cord uniting the two blind ends
- Other causes: enteric duplication cysts ▶ microgastria

Radiological findings

Prenatal

US Maternal polyhydramnios ▶ a large fetal gastric bubble

Postnatal

AXR With complete obstruction there will be a dilated stomach with no distal air

Upper GI series Vigorous gastric peristalsis and consistent filling defects within the antrum or pylorus at the site of the web

- *'Pseudo-double bubble' sign:* this is seen as barium outlines first the space between the antrum and pylorus, and then the duodenal bulb

US Persistent linear, echogenic structures arising from the antral or pyloric walls and extending centrally

BILIOUS VOMITING

Definition An obstruction distal to the ampulla of Vater – malrotation and a midgut volvulus constitute the greatest emergency

- *Other causes:* duodenal atresia and stenosis ▶ duodenal webs and diaphragms ▶ extrinsic duodenal compression (e.g. an annular pancreas or a preduodenal portal vein) ▶ small bowel atresia ▶ small bowel stenosis ▶ sepsis ▶ gastroenteritis
- If the AXR demonstrates a complete high intestinal obstruction then no further imaging is required (operative intervention irrespective of the cause) ▶ if the AXR shows a low intestinal obstruction (i.e. distal to the mid ileum) then a contrast enema is preferred

DUODENAL ATRESIA AND STENOSIS

Definition This is caused by failure of recanalization of the duodenal lumen after the 6th week of fetal life (duodenal atresia is much more common than a duodenal stenosis) ▶ in 80% of cases the level of obstruction is just distal to the ampulla of Vater ▶ obstruction can also be caused by webs and diaphragms or an annular pancreas

- *Associated anomalies occur in the majority of patients:* Down's syndrome (30%) ▶ malrotation (20–30%) ▶ congenital heart disease (20%) ▶ components of the VACTERL association may also be present

Clinical presentation Infants present early with bilious vomiting and upper abdominal distension (a preampullary obstruction presents with non-bilious vomiting)

Radiological features

Antenatal

US A dilated stomach and duodenal cap ▶ maternal polyhydramnios

Postnatal

AXR A gas-filled 'double bubble' of the stomach and duodenal cap ▶ distal gas will be present if the obstruction is partial (or rarely if there is a bifid pancreatic duct straddling the atretic segment)

Upper GI study A duodenal stenosis is seen as a narrowed area within the 2nd part of the duodenum ▶ a duodenal web may be seen as a thin, filling defect extending across the duodenal lumen

- *'Duodenal dimple' sign:* the pressure exerted by a NGT on the obstructing web can cause in-drawing of the duodenal wall at the site of the web's attachment

SMALL BOWEL ATRESIA AND STENOSIS

Definition These follow an intrauterine vascular insult (the vascular insult may be a primary or secondary event such as an antenatal volvulus or intussusception) ▶ an atresia is more common than a stenosis ▶ the proximal jejunum and distal ileum are the most frequently affected segments

Clinical presentation The majority of infants present with bilious vomiting in the immediate postnatal period ▶ abdominal distension is seen with more distal atresias

Radiological findings

AXR Dilated loops of small bowel are seen down to the level of the atresia (the loop of bowel immediately proximal to the atresia may be disproportionately dilated and have a bulbous contour) ▶ bubbles of distal gas are seen with a stenosis (cf. an atresia) ▶ fine intraluminal calcifications may be seen with a more distal atresia ▶ a meconium peritonitis (with calcification of the peritoneum) may be seen if an intrauterine perforation has occurred

- *'Apple peel' syndrome:* this is thought to follow an intrauterine occlusion of the distal SMA ▶ there is a proximal jejunal atresia, with agenesis of the mesentery and absence of the mid small bowel ▶ the distal ileum spirals around its narrow vascular pedicle (giving the syndrome its name) ▶ a malrotated microcolon is also usually present

Pearl

- Medical causes of bilious vomiting include functional immaturity of the colon and gastroenteritis

Causes of gastrointestinal obstruction[†]

Oesophagus
Oesophageal artesia ± tracheal-oesphageal fistula
Congenital oesophageal stenosis, web and diverticula
Extrinsic compression - vascular ring
                   - foregut duplication cyst
                   - neoplasm

Stomach
Gastric atresia
Antral web
Duplication cyst
Hypertrophic pyloric stenosis

Duodenum
Duodenal artesia
Duodenal web
Malrotation with midgut volvulus
Extrinsic compression - annular pancreas
                   - preduodenal portal vein

Small bowel
Jejunal and ileal atresia/stenosis
Meconium ileus ± meconium cyst, segmental volvulus
Midgut volvulus
Inguinal hernia
Necrotizing enterocolitis
Duplication cyst

Large bowel
Hirschsprung's disease
Functional immaturity/hypoplastic left colon syndrome
Colonic atresia/imperforate anus
Necrotizing enterocolitis
Duplication cyst

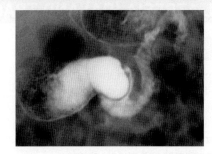

Duodenal web. Barium meal demonstrating a curvilinear filling defect or 'wind-sock diverticulum' in the second part of the duodenum with proximal dilatation.[†]

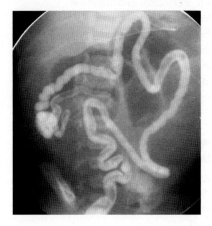

Ileal atresia. Contrast enema with microcolon and reflux into a non-dilated distal ileal segment with abrupt convex termination. A few meconium plugs are present.[†]

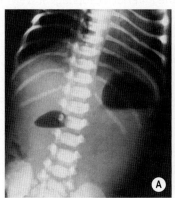 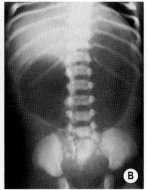

Duodenal atresia. Erect (A) and supine (B) AXR demonstrating the classic 'double bubble' sign.*

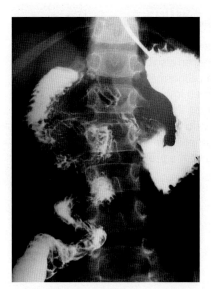

Malrotation and volvulus. Upper GI contrast medium study demonstrates the classical 'corkscrew' pattern of the duodenum and jejunum spiralling around the mesenteric vessels.*

OESOPHAGEAL ATRESIA (OA) AND TRACHEO-OESOPHAGEAL FISTULA (TOF)

DEFINITION

- This is due to abnormal partitioning of the laryngotracheal tube from the oesophagus by the tracheo-oesophageal septum during the 4th week of gestation ▶ it affects 1:3000–4500 live births
  - The atretic segment of the oesophagus tends to be at the junction of its proximal and middle thirds
  - A TOF (if present) is usually found proximal to the carina
  - Occasionally an isolated TOF can occur without an oesophageal atresia (the 'H'- or 'N'-type fistula)
- 50% of patients have associated congenital anomalies:
  - *VACTERL spectrum:* **V**ertebral anomalies ▶ an **A**norectal malformation ▶ **C**ardiovascular malformations (VSD, PDA, right aortic arch) ▶ **T**racheal anomalies ▶ an o**E**sophageal fistula ▶ **R**enal anomalies ▶ **L**imb anomalies
  - *Other anomalies:* duodenal atresia and stenosis ▶ an imperforate anus ▶ trisomy 18 and 21 ▶ Potter's syndrome

CLINICAL PRESENTATION

- **Antenatal (US):** maternal polyhydramnios
- **Postnatal:** an immediate presentation with choking, coughing, cyanosis and drooling (this is exacerbated during attempts to feed)
  - H-type fistulas generally present later in infancy or childhood with episodes of choking or apnoea during feeding, or recurrent respiratory tract infections

RADIOLOGICAL FEATURES

CXR An orogastric tube will curl up within the proximal oesophageal pouch (there can also be aspiration pneumonitis, vertebral anomalies or an abnormal cardiac silhouette)
- Gas within the abdomen implies a distal fistula (neonates with a H-type fistula commonly have a abdomen distended with gas)
- A gasless abdomen implies an isolated oesophageal atresia (or an atresia with a proximal fistula) ▶ there is

an absent fetal gastric bubble if there is an oesophageal atresia (but no TOF)
- *Isolated oesophageal atresia:* a long gap between the atretic segments is seen in association with 13 pairs of ribs

Upper GI study This can delineate an H-type fistula: the patient is placed prone and a horizontal X-ray is used ▶ contrast medium is injected under pressure (via a nasogastric tube with its tip in the distal oesophagus) and the tube is then slowly withdrawn under fluoroscopic guidance ('withdrawal oesophagram')
- The majority of these fistulas are seen at the level of the thoracic inlet
- *The gap between the oesophageal pouches can be assessed following the formation of a feeding gastrostomy:* under fluoroscopic guidance, a Heger dilator is inserted through the gastrostomy and retrogradely into the distal oesophagus ▶ a Repogle tube is simultaneously used to delineate the superior pouch ▶ as both tubes are radio-opaque, the degree of separation can be easily assessed
  - Alternatively CT can delineate the gap following the simultaneous injection of air into the upper pouch (via the Repogle tube) and via the gastrostomy

PEARLS

- The mortality rates are now no longer due to the oesophageal atresia itself, but due to the associated malformations
- A combined bronchoscopy and oesophagoscopy should be performed if there is a high clinical index of suspicion of an H-type fistula with negative imaging

Complications following surgical repair

- *Recurrent TOF (10%):* this should be suspected if the oesophagus is gas filled on CXR and if contrast medium studies show 'beaking' of the anterior oesophageal wall
- *Other complications:* anastomotic breakdown (10–20%) ▶ anastomotic strictures (up to 80%, more likely in long gap OA) ▶ disordered oesophageal and distal GI motility ▶ gastro-oesophageal reflux

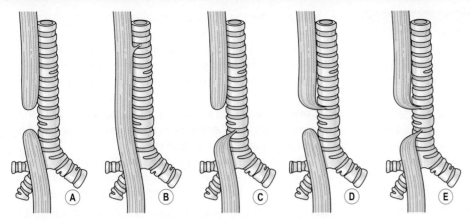

Oesophageal atresia and tracheo-oesophageal fistula. Diagrammatic representation of (A) isolated OA (9%), (B) H-type fistula (6%), (C) OA with distal TOF (82%), (D) OA with proximal TOF (1%) and (E) OA with TOF from both proximal and distal oesophageal remnants (2%).**

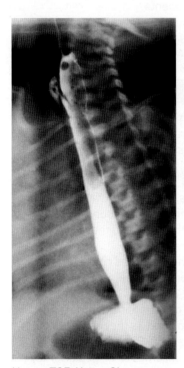

H-type TOF. Upper GI contrast study shows the fistula running obliquely at the level of the thoracic inlet.*

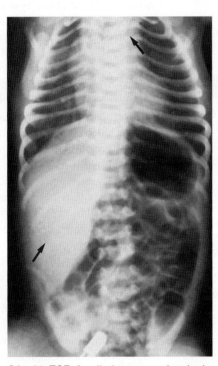

OA with TOF. A coiled nasogastric tube is seen in the dilated proximal oesophageal pouch (top arrow). The presence of distal air-filled bowel implies an associated TOF. Thirteen pairs of ribs are noted, compatible with VATER syndrome (lower arrow).

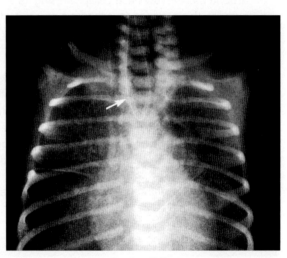

Oesophageal atresia. Supine CXR shows orogastric tube (arrow) curled in the proximal oesophageal pouch.*

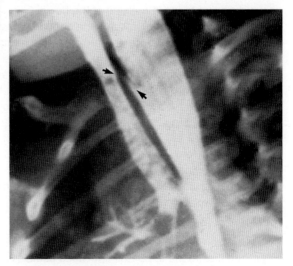

Contrast oesophagram demonstrating oblique track (arrows) of a TOF with contrast filling the tracheobronchial tree.†

399

MALROTATION

DEFINITION

- Malrotation is a generic term used to describe any variation in the intestinal position ▶ intestinal malfixation invariably accompanies malrotation in an attempt to fix the gut in place
  - *Peritoneal (Ladd) bands:* these stretch from the abnormally high-lying caecum, across the duodenum and to the region of the porta hepatis and the anterior and posterior abdominal walls ▶ Ladd bands can cause duodenal obstruction
- The abnormal positions of the duodenojejunal junction and caecum means that the base of the small bowel mesentery is short
  - *Midgut volvulus:* the midgut has a propensity to twist around this narrow base compromising its vascular supply – this can lead to ischaemic necrosis of the small bowel with an associated high mortality rate if undiagnosed

CLINICAL PRESENTATION

- This commonly presents within the 1st month of life with bilious vomiting ▶ older children may present with non-specific symptoms of chronic or intermittent abdominal pain, non-bilious emesis, diarrhoea, or a failure to thrive
- Symptoms of shock intervene if bowel ischaemia and necrosis have developed

RADIOLOGICAL FEATURES

AXR There are no specific features – it may be normal if a volvulus is intermittent or if there is incomplete duodenal obstruction due to loose twisting of the bowel
- A tight volvulus results in complete duodenal obstruction with a distended stomach and proximal duodenum (mimicking the 'double bubble' of duodenal atresia)
- *Closed loop obstruction:* this is a more ominous sign and is associated with distal small bowel obstruction ▶ the volvulus causes venous obstruction and small bowel necrosis – the small bowel loops will be thickened and oedematous (± pneumatosis) and any gas cannot be reabsorbed from the bowel lumen
- A gasless abdomen can be seen with prolonged vomiting, a closed loop obstruction with viable small bowel, or with a massive midgut necrosis

Upper GI study
- **Normal:** on a supine AXR the normal duodenojejunal junction lies to the left of the left-sided pedicles at the height of the duodenal bulb ▶ on a lateral view, the junction of the 2nd and 3rd parts of the duodenum is retroperitoneal

- **Malrotation:** the duodenojejunal junction is displaced inferiorly and to the right on a supine AXR ▶ the junction of the 2nd and 3rd parts of the duodenum turns sharply anterior ▶ the distal jejunal loops lie to the right of the midline ▶ the caecal pole may lie high and more to the left side
- **'Corkscrew' pattern:** this describes the duodenum and jejunum spiralling around the mesenteric vessels and is pathognomonic for a midgut volvulus
  - If Ladd bands are causing the duodenal obstruction rather than a volvulus the duodenojejunal course has been described as 'Z-shaped' rather than spiral

US A dilated, fluid-filled stomach and proximal duodenum if obstruction is present ▶ the superior mesenteric vein (SMV) lies ventral or to left of the superior mesenteric artery (SMA) in about $\frac{2}{3}$ of patients
- *'Whirlpool' sign:* the volvulus itself may be demonstrated (colour Doppler studies may show the SMV spiralling clockwise around the SMA)

PEARLS

- Normal fetal gut development:
  - The gut begins as a straight, midline tube, which, as it elongates and develops, herniates into the base of the umbilical cord
  - Between the 6th and 10th weeks of fetal development, the midgut loop rotates 90° anticlockwise around the axis of the SMA ▶ at this stage the duodenojejunal (proximal) loop lies to the right, and the caecocolic (distal) loop lies to the left
  - During the 10th week, the intestines return to the abdominal cavity (the proximal loop of bowel enters first)
  - Both the proximal and distal loops undergo a further 180° of anticlockwise rotation as they return to the abdominal cavity (a total of 270° of rotation)
  - The duodenojejunal loop comes to lie posterior to and the caecocolic loop anterior to the SMA ▶ the duodenojejunal junction (fixed by the ligament of Treitz) should lie in the left upper quadrant of the abdomen, and the ileocaecal junction within the right lower quadrant
- If there is complete duodenal obstruction on an AXR or clinical peritonitis, a neonate requires surgery rather than an upper GI study
- The majority of patients have an isolated bowel malrotation, but there is an increased association with: duodenal stenosis and atresia ▶ omphalocele ▶ gastroschisis ▶ congenital diaphragmatic hernia ▶ heterotaxy syndromes ▶ Hirschsprung's disease ▶ megacystis–microcolon–intestinal hypoperistalsis (Berdon) syndrome ▶ congenital short bowel without atresia

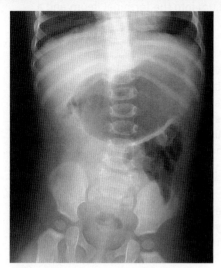

Malrotation and volvulus. AXR in a 12-month-old boy with bilious vomiting. The stomach is distended with a relative paucity of gas distally.[†]

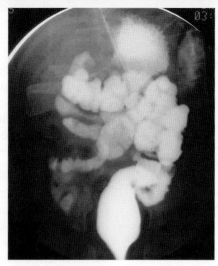

Follow-through examination demonstrating an abnormal high and medial caecal position. Malrotation confirmed at surgery.[†]

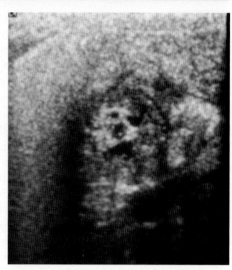

Ultrasound 'whirlpool' sign of midgut volvulus. Twisting mesenteric vessels with concentric rings of echogenic mesentery.[†]

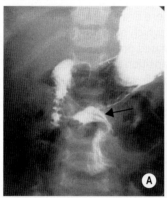

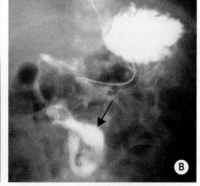

Malrotation. Contrast meal (A) demonstrating abnormally low position of the duodenojejunal junction (arrow). Further case (B) demonstrating both inferior and medial displacement of the duodenojejunal junction (arrow). The normal junction should lie to the left of the midline (over or lateral to the left vertebral pedicle) at the level of the pylorus.[†]

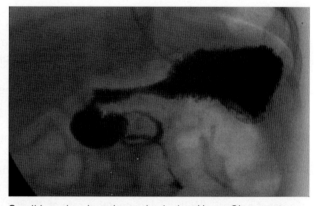

Small bowel malrotation and volvulus. Upper GI contrast study demonstrates the classical 'corkscrew' pattern of the duodenum and jejunum spiralling around the mesenteric vessels. Note the change in bowel calibre at the level of the duodenojejunal flexure.[**]

Transverse ultrasound images of the normal SMA:SMV relationship (A) and a malrotated child (B) in whom the SMV lies to the left of the SMA.[†]

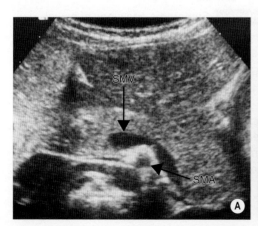

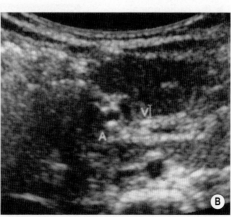

Hirschsprung's disease

Definition A form of functional low bowel obstruction due to failure of caudal migration of neuroblasts within developing bowel – this results in an absence of parasympathetic intrinsic ganglion cells in both Auerbach's and Meissner's plexi ▶ the distal large bowel from the point of neuronal arrest to the anus is *continuously* aganglionic ('skip lesions' are rare)

- *Short segment disease (75% of cases):* the aganglionic segment extends only to the rectosigmoid region ▶ short segment disease is sporadic (M > F)
- *Long segment disease:* this involves a portion of the colon proximal to the sigmoid colon ▶ long segment disease has a strong familial incidence (M = F)
- Variants of Hirschsprung's disease include *total aganglionosis coli* and *total intestinal Hirschsprung's disease* ▶ *ultrashort segment disease* is rare and involves only the anus at the level of the internal sphincter

Clinical presentation Neonatal abdominal distension ▶ vomiting ▶ failure to pass meconium (with a delay >48 h)

- It may unusually present later in childhood with chronic constipation and failure to thrive ▶ it can rarely present with an acute abdomen due to a colonic volvulus

AXR This typically shows a low bowel obstruction – commonly with colonic dilatation out of proportion to the small bowel ▶ absent rectal gas (a non-specific sign also seen with sepsis and NEC) ▶ retention of contrast medium above the sigmoid colon (>24 h – also non-specific)

- 5% of infants will have a pneumoperitoneum (occurring commonly within the ascending colon and which may be appendiceal)
- Intraluminal small bowel calcifications may be present with long segment disease
- A coexistent enterocolitis may lead to mucosal oedema, ulceration and spasm

Contrast enema (With a false-negative rate of 20–30%) ▶ a balloon catheter should not be used (the balloon can obscure the diagnostic features or even perforate the stiff aganglionic bowel)

- Lateral view:
  - *Short segment disease:* a narrow rectum with a cone-shaped transition zone to the more proximal, dilated and ganglionated bowel ▶ the radiological transition zone is commonly found distal to the pathological transition zone – in addition a transition zone may not be present in the neonate as it takes time for the proximal bowel to dilate
    - *Rectosigmoid ratio:* the rectum should always be the most distensible portion of the bowel with a rectosigmoid ratio >1 ▶ this ratio is reversed in short segment disease
  - *Total aganglionosis coli:* the findings are unreliable ▶ there is shortening of a normal-calibre colon (with loss of the normal redundancy of the flexures) ▶

muscle spasm, a pseudo-transition zone, easy reflux of contrast medium into the terminal ileum and a microcolon may also be seen

Pearls
- **Associations:** Down's syndrome (5%) ▶ ilial and colonic atresias ▶ cleft palate ▶ polydactyly ▶ craniofacial anomalies ▶ cardiac septal defects
- **Definitive diagnosis:** suction rectal biopsy
- **Treatment:** resection aganglionic bowel + 'pull through' + anastomosis to normal anal margin

Immature left colon (meconium plug syndrome or small left colon)

Definition A relatively common cause of neonatal bowel obstruction with delayed passage of meconium due to inspissated meconium ▶ it is possibly due to immaturity of the myenteric plexus

- It is *not* associated with cystic fibrosis

Clinical presentation Symptoms and signs of bowel obstruction (patients tend to be less ill than those with a mechanical obstruction)

AXR Distended small and large bowel loops to the level of the inspissated meconium plugs ▶ a few fluid levels are seen

Contrast enema Typically there is a microcolon distal to the splenic flexure, at which point there is an abrupt transition to a mildly dilated proximal colon (in Hirschsprung's disease the transition zone is more gradual and is uncommon at the splenic flexure) ▶ the rectosigmoid ratio is normal

- Discrete plugs of meconium are seen as filling defects within the dilated colon
- There is a therapeutic (as well as a diagnostic effect) if water-soluble contrast medium is used – meconium is typically passed soon after

Colonic atresia

Definition A rare condition due to an in utero vascular accident (the right colon is commonly affected) ▶ the atresia may take on the form of a diaphragm or web, fibrous cord or mesenteric gap defect

- It is associated with proximal atresias, gastroschisis and Hirschsprung's disease

Clinical presentation Symptoms and signs of bowel obstruction

AXR Features of a low intestinal obstruction

Contrast enema A distal microcolon, with obstruction to the retrograde flow of contrast medium at the point of the atresia

- *'Wind sock' configuration:* if a colonic diaphragm or web is present, the column of barium may cause the obstructing membrane to balloon into the proximal air-filled colon

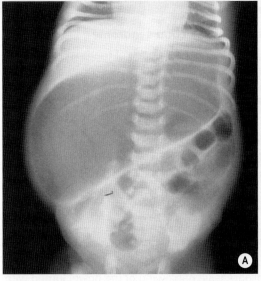
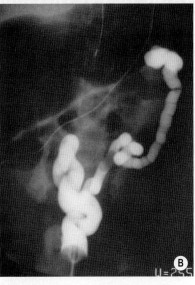

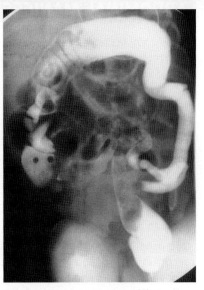

Colonic atresia. AXR (A) showing disproportionate dilatation of one bowel loop in a neonate with abdominal distension and failure to pass meconium. Contrast enema (B) showing a blind-ending colon with a convex distal border in the splenic flexure. The dilated air-filled proximal colonic segment can be seen. An isolated colonic atresia was confirmed at surgery.[†]

Small left colon syndrome. (A) Supine AXR shows a low obstruction with multiple dilated loops of bowel. (B) Contrast medium enema shows a microcolon distal to the splenic flexure. The transition point is abrupt.[†]

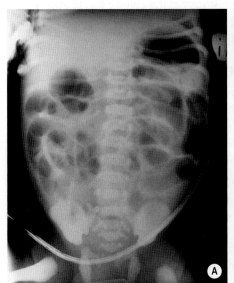
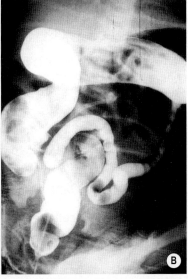

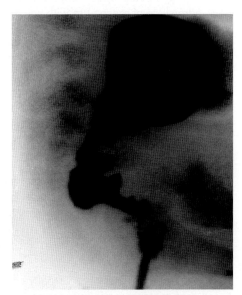

Functional immaturity (left colon syndrome). Contrast enema in a newborn term infant showing a relatively small left colon, transition zone at the splenic flexure and a large coiled meconium plug which was dislodged from the splenic flexure to the hepatic flexure during colonic filling.*

Rectosigmoid Hirschsprung's disease. Lateral view, contrast medium enema. The cone-shaped transition zone, abnormal rectosigmoid ratio and tertiary rectal contractions are demonstrated.*

ABDOMINAL MANIFESTATIONS OF CYSTIC FIBROSIS

The GI complications of cystic fibrosis result from abnormally viscous secretions within the hollow viscera and the ducts of the solid organs.

Meconium ileus

Definition This is a form of distal intestinal obstruction caused by inspissated pellets of meconium within the terminal ileum ▶ >90% of patients have cystic fibrosis (meconium ileus is the presenting feature of cystic fibrosis in 10–15%)

Clinical presentation Vomiting ▶ abdominal distension ▶ failure to pass meconium

Complications Intrauterine volvulus (due to a heavy, meconium-laden loop of bowel) ▶ a volvulus can lead to stenoses, atresias and perforation

- Perforation leads to a chemical meconium peritonitis with subsequent fibrosis and calcification
- Other causes of meconium peritonitis include a small bowel atresia or an intrauterine intussusception

AXR

- **Uncomplicated ileus:** small bowel dilatation ▶ fluid levels are scant
  - *A 'soap bubble' appearance:* this is due to an admixture of meconium with gas ▶ (classically seen within the right iliac fossa)
- **Complicated ileus:** intra-abdominal (bowel wall) or scrotal calcification ▶ prominent air-fluid levels
  - *A meconium pseudocyst:* this occurs due to a vascular compromise in association with an intrauterine volvulus ▶ the ischaemic bowel loops become adherent and necrotic, and a fibrous wall develops around them ▶ the wall may then calcify and the cyst can have a secondary mass effect

US

- **Uncomplicated ileus:** dilated bowel loops are filled with echogenic material (cf. echo-poor material with an ileal atresia)
- **Complicated ileus:** 'snow storm' ascites with a meconium peritonitis

Contrast enema There is a virtually empty microcolon ▶ reflux of contrast medium is seen into a small terminal ileum (with numerous pellets of meconium outlined) ▶ there are proximally dilated mid-ileal loops

Pearls A Gastrografin enema may be therapeutic in an uncomplicated case – Gastrografin is hypertonic and will draw water into the bowel lumen by osmosis, softening the meconium and allowing it to pass ▶ there is a risk of perforation (5%) or a fluid–electrolyte imbalance (therefore only use half-strength Gastrografin in a well-hydrated infant)

- Bowel obstruction in neonates with cystic fibrosis can be due to either meconium ileus or meconium plug syndrome

Distal intestinal obstruction syndrome

Definition Impaction of mucofeculent material within the terminal ileum and right colon (which is seen in 10–15% of older children with cystic fibrosis) ▶ it is potentially fatal

Clinical presentation Colicky abdominal pain and distension ▶ nausea and vomiting ▶ constipation ▶ a right iliac fossa mass

AXR Faecal loading of the colon with a 'bubbly' appearance ▶ right-sided abdominal mass ▶ dilated small bowel

Treatment Oral Gastrografin (± a Gastrografin enema) to soften and mobilize the stool

Fibrosing colonopathy

Definition A colonic stricture due to the irreversible and sometimes progressive narrowing of the bowel lumen with associated submucosal fibrosis and fatty infiltration ▶ it often involves the right side of the colon

- High-strength pancreatic enzyme supplements have been implicated in its aetiology

Clinical presentation Distal intestinal obstruction

AXR/MRI/US Thickened bowel wall

Contrast enema Shortening of the colon with narrowing of the colonic lumen ▶ loss of the colonic haustration ▶ nodular thickening of the colonic wall

Treatment Surgical resection

Pancreatic insufficiency

Definition This occurs in 80–85% of children with cystic fibrosis and manifests as malabsorption (chiefly of fat and proteins) ▶ 30–50% of patients have glucose intolerance (with 1–2% requiring insulin therapy)

AXR Punctate calcification within the pancreas

US A small echogenic pancreas

CT/MRI Fatty replacement of the pancreas

Miscellaneous

- **Liver cirrhosis:** this results from impaired biliary drainage with associated portal hypertension (there can be splenomegaly and gastric varices)
- **Chronic cholecystitis:** there is a small, thick-walled gallbladder (gallstones are seen in 10% of patients)
- **Intra-abdominal malignancy:** cystic fibrosis is associated with cancers of the oesophagus, stomach, small bowel, colon, liver, biliary tract, pancreas and rectum
- **Other bowel manifestations:** peptic ulcer disease ▶ GOR ▶ oesophagitis ▶ oesophageal stricture ▶ thickened nodular mucosal folds within the duodenum and small bowel
  - Intussusception: this occurs in 1% of patients (usually between the ages of 9–12 years) ▶ it is usually ileocolic)

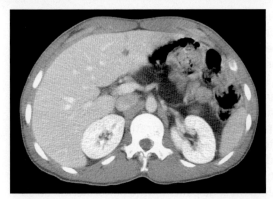

Fatty replacement of the pancreas in a patient with cystic fibrosis.••

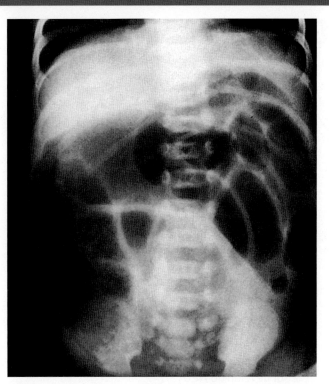

Meconium ileus. Supine AXR shows a low obstruction with multiple, dilated loops of bowel and a 'soap bubble' appearance in the right lower quadrant.*

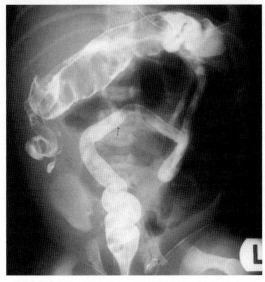

Meconium ileus. Contrast enema demonstrating a microcolon with reflux into dilated distal ileum. Multiple filling defects of inspissated meconium are seen within the distal ileum (superimposed over the transverse colon) and the colon.[†]

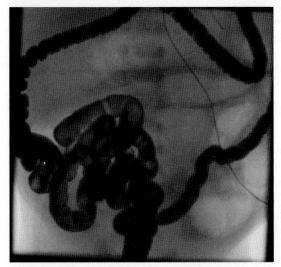

Meconium ileus. Contrast enema demonstrates the empty microcolon. Contrast medium refluxes into the narrow terminal ileum, where pellets of meconium are outlined.**

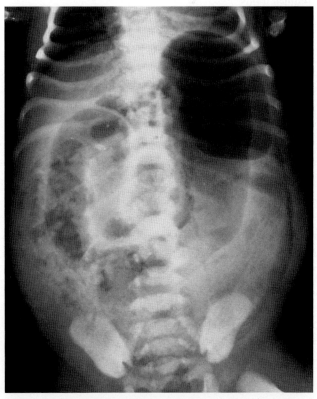

Meconium ileus. AXR showing loops of dilated bowel with a 'bubbly' appearance of meconium mixed with air in the right side of the abdomen. Free air is seen, indicating a perforation.[†]

405

NECROTIZING ENTEROCOLITIS

DEFINITION

- This is an often severe enterocolitis that affects primarily premature infants (with an increasing incidence due to the increased survival rates of very low birth weight infants of a younger gestational age)
  - NEC can also be seen in term infants (particularly those with polycythaemia, cyanotic congenital heart disease and gastroschisis)
- Initially superficial, the inflammatory process can extend to become transmural ▶ diffuse or discrete involvement of the bowel can occur ▶ the most commonly affected sites are the terminal ileum and colon (up to 50% of cases involve both the small and large bowel)
- The aetiology remains unknown, but immaturity of the gut mucosa and immune response (coupled with ischaemia and hypoxia) are felt to contribute ▶ there is also a possible infectious cause
  - *Additional risk factors:* sepsis ▶ early enteral feeding ▶ umbilical arterial and venous cannulation ▶ maternal cocaine abuse
    - Breastfeeding is associated with a decreased risk of developing NEC

CLINICAL PRESENTATION

- Usually presents in the 2nd week of life, following enteral feeds
- The initial clinical symptoms and signs are non-specific: lethargy ▶ hypoglycaemia ▶ temperature instability ▶ bradycardia ▶ feeding intolerance ▶ increased gastric aspirates ▶ gastric distension
  - Disease progression leads to vomiting and diarrhoea (often with the passage of blood or mucus in the stool), and eventually to shock
  - Severely affected infants may have visibly erythematous anterior abdominal walls, with palpable distended loops of bowel
- Perforation will occur in $\frac{1}{3}$ of children and occurs most commonly in the ileocaecal region (affecting 60% of cases)

RADIOLOGICAL FEATURES

AXR An early sign is diffuse gaseous distension of both the small and large bowel (or isolated gastric distension) ▶ serial XRs (taken every 6–12 h) will demonstrate fixed bowel loop dilatation and thickening (oedema) with loss of distinction of the bowel walls

- If the diameter of a bowel loop is greater than the width of the L1 vertebral body then it is likely to be dilated
- **Intramural gas (pneumatosis intestinalis):** this is a more specific sign, and an increasingly extensive pneumatosis correlates with an increased NEC severity
  - *Submucosal gas:* 'bubbly' lucencies in the bowel wall
  - *Subserosal gas:* linear bowel wall lucencies
- **Portal venous gas:** this is seen in approximately 10% of cases and is associated with severe NEC (its presence does not necessarily imply a fatal outcome) ▶ the disappearance of intramural or portal venous gas may herald imminent perforation rather than recovery
- **Indicators of imminent perforation:** free intraperitoneal fluid ▶ the 'persistent loop' sign: a solitary, dilated loop of bowel present over 24–36 h
- **Perforation:** $< \frac{2}{3}$ of patients will have free air visible on a plain XR (almost all patients who perforate will do so within 30 h of diagnosis) ▶ commonly ileocaecal region
  - *'Football' sign:* a large elliptical central abdominal lucency in the supine position (due to rising intra-abdominal air)
  - *'Telltale triangle' sign:* the collection of small amounts of free intraperitoneal air between loops of bowel seen with a supine, cross-table lateral or decubitus view

Contrast enema Its use in the acute situation (if the other signs are ambiguous) is controversial due to the risk of sepsis and perforation

US This is more sensitive than an AXR in the detection of ascites and portal venous gas

- **Portal venous gas:** echogenic particles flowing within the portal vein or focal areas of intrahepatic increased echogenicity
- **The 'circle sign':** this is indicative of bubbles of gas circumferentially within the bowel wall and is seen as a continuous, echogenic ring in cross-section
- **Perforation:** the presence of free intraperitoneal fluid may be an indicator of perforation (it is seen in only 20% of patients)

PEARLS

- The overall mortality rate from NEC is approximately 30%
- Perforation is not an absolute indication for surgical intervention – peritoneal drains are used in the initial resuscitation (delaying the need for surgery and allowing time for systemic recovery) ▶ in some instances a peritoneal drain may provide definitive treatment
- **Complications:** a late complication is stricturing, which can be single or multiple, and occurs in up to $\frac{1}{3}$ of patients ▶ the majority of strictures are short, are found in the colon and are diagnosed up to 3 months following the acute illness
  - *Other late complications:* an acquired intestinal atresia (rare) ▶ abscess formation ▶ enteric fistulas ▶ enterocyst formation ▶ obstruction secondary to adhesions ▶ malabsorption ▶ short bowel syndrome following surgical resection

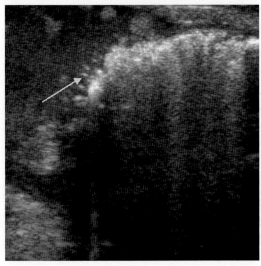

The use of ultrasound in the diagnosis of necrotising enterocolitis. Echogenic dots representing intramural gas bubbles of pneumatosis intestinalis (arrow) in the oedematous bowel wall.** (Image reproduced from Imaging in Medicine, August 2011;3[4]: 393–410. With the permission of Future Medicine Ltd.)

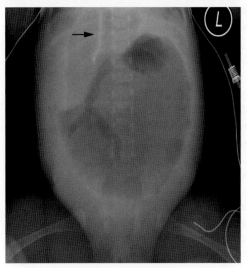

The 'football' sign: free intraperitoneal air has collected superiorly in this supine AXR, creating a central lucency. The free air is also outlining the falciform ligament (arrow).

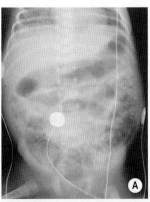
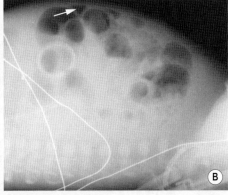

Necrotizing enterocolitis. Supine AXR (A) demonstrating extensive 'bubbly' pneumatosis in a 16-day-old premature infant born at 28 weeks' gestation. No definite free air seen. However, lateral shoot-through XR (B) shows a small triangle of free air beneath the anterior abdominal wall (arrow). A localized ileal perforation was found at laparotomy.[†]

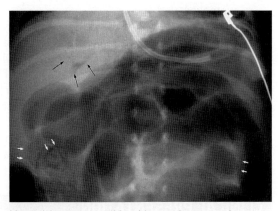

Necrotizing enterocolitis with portal venous air. Branching lucencies throughout the liver represent gas within the portal venous system (*black arrows*). Intramural air is also present (*white arrows*).©20

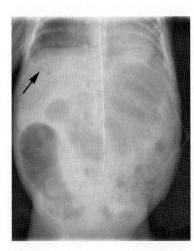

NEC. Supine AXR demonstrating gas within the hepatic portal veins (arrow), together with subserosal bowel wall gas (best seen in the left lower quadrant).

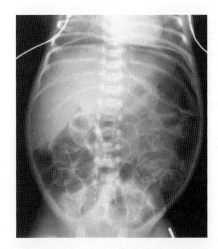

Free intraperitoneal air in perforated necrotizing enterocolitis demonstrated by lucency over the entire abdomen ('football' sign), subdiaphragmatic air and outlining of both sides of the bowel wall (Rigler's sign).[†]

ANORECTAL MALFORMATIONS

DEFINITION

- Anorectal malformations include anorectal atresia and an imperforate anus (± an anomalous connection between the atretic anorectum and the genitourinary tract) ▶ it results from the failure of descent and separation of the hindgut and the GU tract during the 2nd second trimester (affecting 1 in 1500–5000 live births)
  - *A high lesion:* the rectum ends above the puborectalis sling
  - *A low lesion:* the rectum ends below the puborectalis sling
- Classification gradually being accepted based upon the type of fistula present (important for surgical planning) ▶ perineal fistulas, also:
  - Males: fistula to prostatic/bulbar urethra or bladder neck
  - Females: fistula to vaginal vestibule
- It is associated with Down's syndrome (2–8%) as well as:
  - *The VACTERL sequence* (45% of patients)
  - *The OEIS complex* (5% of patients): **O**mphalocele + bladder **E**xstrophy + an **I**mperforate anus + **S**acral anomalies
  - *Currarino's triad:* an anorectal malformation (commonly anorectal stenosis) + bony sacral anomalies (classically a 'scimitar sacrum' with unilateral hypoplasia of the lateral aspect of the vertebral bodies) + a presacral mass lesion (e.g. an enteric cyst, teratoma, anterior meningocele or dermoid)
  - The cloacal malformation only occurs in females, with a single perineal opening for the urethra, vagina and rectum

CLINICAL PRESENTATION

- **Low lesions:** usually there is a visible perineal opening ▶ the orifice may be located more anteriorly than normal (an ectopic anus) and it may be stenotic or covered with a membrane ▶ there is no communication with the GU tract ▶ low lesions also include an isolated rectal atresia or stenosis
  - Female patients with low lesions will have separate urethral and vaginal orifices with an intact hymen
- **High lesions:** there is no visible perineal fistula ▶ rarely the rectum ends blindly
  - Male patients will usually have a fistulous tract between the atretic anorectum and the posterior urethra (less commonly a fistula to the bladder or anterior urethra)
    - Female patients usually have fistulas from the atretic anorectum to the vagina or vestibule

RADIOLOGICAL FEATURES

Inverted lateral XR   A radio-opaque marker is placed over the anal dimple and the distance between the pouch of rectal gas and the marker is measured ▶ distance <1 cm implies a more distal atresia
- *False positives:* if a patient is imaged during the 1st 24 h of life (as any gas may not have yet reached the rectum)
  - ▶ if the infant has not been held prone for long enough
  - ▶ if meconium has impacted within the distal rectum
- If an infant is crying or straining, the rectal pouch can descend through the levator sling and a high lesion may be misinterpreted as a low one

Supine AXR   This can detect any associated bony anomalies of the spine
- *Intravesical air:* this implies a high lesion (with a rectovesical fistula or a rectourethral fistula in a boy)
- *Calcified intraluminal meconium:* this implies a high lesion in a boy (meconium calcifies when it comes into contact with urine)

Transperineal US   This measures the distance of the rectal pouch from the perineum ▶ there are problems with interpretation as for an inverted lateral XR

Augmented pressure colostogram   This is performed in infants with high lesions following the initial formation of a colostomy ▶ a Foley catheter is inserted into the distal segment of colon and a balloon is inflated to 5 ml ▶ water-soluble contrast is then hand injected to distend the distal colon and define the fistulous tract

PEARLS

- Renal US is mandatory in all infants with anorectal atresia ▶ a spinal US will exclude any associated spinal cord lesions (e.g. cord tethering) as these are not uncommon associations
  - Alternatively a pre- and postoperative MRI can study the pelvic floor and reveal any associated renal or spinal anomalies
- **Low lesions:** these are treated with an anoplasty or dilatation soon after birth
- **High lesions:** these are treated with a colostomy and then definitive repair

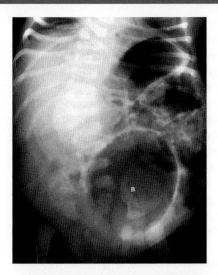

Colovesical fistula. Supine AXR shows intravesical air and vertebral segmentation anomalies in a male infant with a high anorectal malformation. B = bladder.*

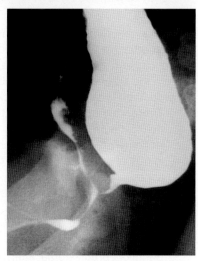

Recto-urethral fistula. Augmented pressure colostogram in a male infant with a high anorectal malformation.*

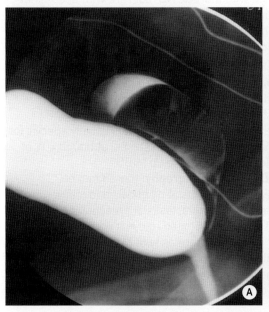

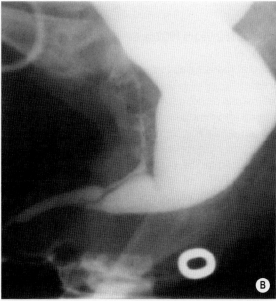

Anorectal atresia with urethral fistula. Micturating cystogram (A) demonstrating fistula from the distal rectal pouch to the posterior urethra and distal loopogram. (B) showing a fistula to the anterior urethra.†

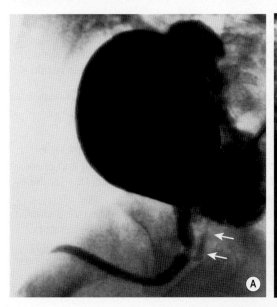

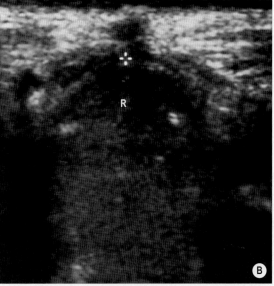

Imperforate anus. (A) Communication between the posterior urethra and the rectum (arrows). (B) Transperineal US scan illustrates the distance from the pouch (R) to the anal dimple (marker) as well as calcific densities within the meconium within the rectal pouch.§

NEUROBLASTOMA (NB)

Definition

- A malignant tumour arising from primordial neural crest cells (these normally develop into the adrenal medulla and sympathetic ganglia) ▶ tumours can arise from the adrenal glands or usually anywhere along the sympathetic chain within the neck, thorax and abdomen
  - *Thorax*: tumours arise within the posterior mediastinum
  - *Abdomen:* tumours arise within the retroperitoneum in 60% of cases, and of these, 40% occur within the adrenal glands
  - It is the 2nd commonest paediatric abdominal cancer (after Wilms' tumour)
- Classification of neural crest tumours
  - Neuroblastoma: malignant
  - Ganglioneuroblastoma: intermediate features
  - Ganglioneuroma: well differentiated and benign

Clinical presentation

- The median age at diagnosis is 2 years (90% are diagnosed at <5 years of age)
- It presents with an incidental mass or abdominal pain ▶ other presenting features:
  - *Symptoms due to metastatic disease* (metastases frequently present): bone and joint pain ▶ proptosis (orbital metastases) ▶ anaemia ▶ weight loss ▶ fever
  - *Excess hormone production:* hypertension (elevated catecholamines are produced in 95% of patients) ▶ intractable watery diarrhea (VIP)
  - *Horner's syndrome:* this follows involvement of the stellate ganglion

Radiological features

CXR A calcified mass ▶ paravertebral widening within the lower chest (due to any retrocrural spread)

AXR A non-specific soft tissue mass with calcification seen in up to 50% of cases

Long bones Metastases can appear as ill defined areas of bone destruction ▶ a solitary lesion may appear as a lytic, moth eaten or permeating destructive area interspersed with sclerotic trabeculae ▶ there may be a laminar periosteal reaction
- Common sites are the skull and long bone metaphyses ▶ they are not seen within the hands, feet, or clavicles

US A heterogenous and hypervascular mass of varying echogenicity ▶ hypoechoic areas are secondary to haemorrhage and necrosis

US/cross-sectional imaging *This determines the local disease extent*
- An aggressive large and heterogenous mass which invades the adjacent structures and readily crosses the midline ▶ it tends to surround and engulf (rather than displace) large vessels ▶ there will be external compression on the kidney ▶ the tumour may invade the spinal canal, kidney or liver

- *Skull metastases:* usually located spheno-orbital region ▶ these appear as an infiltrating mass causing permeative bone destruction and spiculated bone changes – these may extend into the scalp soft tissues or push through the skull inner table
- **CT:** calcification is seen in up to 85% of cases (diffuse, mottled, finely stippled or coalescent) ▶ erosion of the pedicles is suggestive of intraspinal extension ▶ low attenuation areas represent areas of haemorrhage and necrosis ▶ mild heterogeneous enhancement reflects areas of vascularity alternating with areas of necrosis, haemorrhage and cystic change
- **MRI:** T1WI: a low SI mass (high SI with haemorrhage) ▶ T2WI: a high SI mass ▶ T1WI (FS) + Gad: heterogenous enhancement
  - *Extradural extension (dumb-bell syndrome):* this is common with thoracic NB, but rare with abdominal tumours
  - *Bone metastases:* T1WI: low SI ▶ T2WI: high SI
- **Whole body MRI:** limited experience ▶ excellent sensitivity in detecting disease, but low specificity

Scintigraphy *This determines the distal disease extent*
- **mIBG** (^{131}I- or ^{123}I-labelled): an analogue of the catecholamine precursors taken up by catecholamine-producing cells ▶ it is usually specific for NB (primary tumour and metastases) although 20% of primary lesions do not take up MIBG
- **^{99m}Tc-MDP bone scintigraphy:** this should be performed in all patients at diagnosis and follow-up as $^2/_3$ of patients have metastases at presentation
- **FDG PET:** this has a limited role ▶ it demonstrates a similar imaging pattern as with MIBG (diffuse abnormal skeletal uptake with extensive bone marrow involvement) ▶ it cannot visualize lesions in the cranium because of the high physiological activity within the brain

Pearls

- Neuroblastoma tends to regress in size with treatment but the regression is frequently incomplete (leaving a small residual soft tissue mass which is often calcified) ▶ MIBG is required to determine whether this residual tissue is fibrosis or viable tumour
- **Staging (see appendix):**
  - $^2/_3$ of patients have metastatic bone disease at diagnosis
    - *Involved sites:* the skeleton ▶ bone marrow ▶ lymph nodes ▶ liver ▶ rarely the lung and brain
- **Stage IV–S:** this has a better prognosis with a tendency to spontaneously regress
  - The hepatomegaly may be massive despite a small primary lesion (and may cause severe respiratory complications in very young patients) ▶ there may be bone marrow lesions and palpable subcutaneous nodules

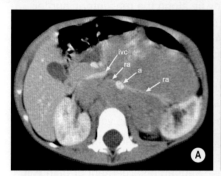

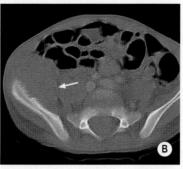

Abdominal neuroblastoma. CECT. (A) A prevertebral tumour extends across the midline in the retroperitoneum, displaces and encases the aorta (a) anteriorly and encases the renal arteries (ra). The inferior vena cava (ivc), partially encased, is displaced anterolaterally and compressed by the tumour and nodes. The mass extends to both the renal hili. (B) Infiltrative lesion to the right iliac bone with a large soft tissue component (arrow) that projects inwards as a space-occupying mass.*

International neuroblastoma risk group staging system	
Stage	
L1	Localised tumour not involving vital structures as defined by the list of image-defined risk factors and confined to one body compartment
L2	Locoregional tumour with presence of one or more image-defined risk factors
M	Distant metastatic disease (except stage MS)
MS	Metastatic disease in children younger than 18 months with metastases confined to skin, liver and/or bone marrow
Adapted from Monclair et al.	

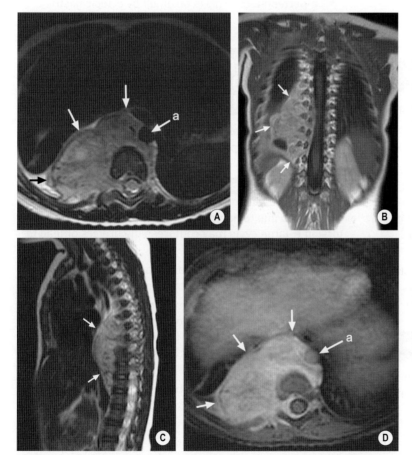

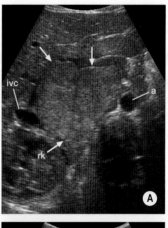

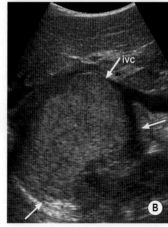

Thoracic neuroblastoma with intraspinal extension. MRI. (A,B) Axial and coronal T1WI + Gad. (C) Sagittal T1WI + Gad. (D) Axial T2WI. Large posterior mediastinal mass (arrows) with anterior and lateral displacement of the aorta (a), which is encased. There is massive tumour extension into the canal through the right neural foramina to displace the spinal cord to the left. Extension into the right paraspinal soft tissues is evident.*

Abdominal neuroblastoma. (A) Transverse US through the right abdomen shows a solid paraspinal mass (arrows) anterior to the right kidney (rk). The aorta (a) and inferior vena cava (ivc) are displaced by the mass. (B) Longitudinal image through the right flank shows the mass (lower arrows) and the stretched inferior vena cava (ivc).*

MESENTERIC LYMPHADENITIS

- Definition: A common cause of abdominal pain in childhood ▶ can present as an acute abdomen ▶ symptoms are caused by swelling of mesenteric lymph nodes in reaction to a trivial, often asymptomatic viral infection
  - A diagnosis of exclusion

USS Multiple enlarged nodes at the root of the mesentery ▶ the hyperechoic fatty hilum is preserved ▶ normal Doppler signal within the nodes

CHRONIC INTESTINAL PSEUDO-OBSTRUCTION

Definition Definition: this represents a spectrum of diseases that have common clinical manifestations consisting of recurrent symptoms mimicking bowel obstruction over weeks or years ▶ due to visceral neuropathy or myopathy (familial or non-familial) resulting in non-coordinated intestinal motility

- Rare ▶ presents from newborn to adulthood

AXR bowel loops with pronounced dilatation

Diagnosis Intestinal manometry and biopsy

HENOCH–SCHÖNLEIN PURPURA

- Definition: Acute small vessel vasculitis occurring almost exclusively in childhood
- Manifestations: purpuric skin lesions (without thrombocytopaenia) ▶ arthritis ▶ nephritis
  - GI manifestations: oedema ▶ bleeding ▶ ulceration ▶ intussusception of the intestine (usually ileoileal, but ileocolic can occur)
- HSP is usually completely reversible with healing in 3–4 weeks

USS Uni- or multifocal bowel wall thickening accompanied by reduced peristalsis with normal or slightly dilated bowel loops between the thickened segments ▶ there can be a small amount of intra-peritoneal fluid

ENTERIC DUPLICATION CYSTS

Definition Uncommon congenital anomalies due to abnormal canalisation of the GI tract ▶ they can occur anywhere along the length of the gut but are most frequent in the ileum where they lie along the mesenteric border and share a common muscle wall blood supply ▶ they have a mucosal lining and 43% contain gastric mucosa ▶ the majority do not communicate with the GI tract

- Gastric duplication cysts: <5% ▶ usually found on the greater curve ▶ when located in the antropyloric region they may cause gastric outlet obstruction and present in the neo-natal period with non-bilious vomiting

Clinical presentation Usually present in the first year of life with vomiting or abdominal pain ▶ infection or haemorrhage can cause sudden enlargement or pain ▶ it can act as a lead point for intussusception

AXR Can assess for bowel obstruction ▶ displacement of bowel loops ▶ soft tissue mass

USS Often a spherical large cyst (echoic contents if bleeding into the cyst)

- Classical feature: 'double layer' sign: bowel wall lining the cyst with an inner echogenic mucosal layer and an outer hypoechoic muscular layer

^{99m}Tc-pertechnate This is taken up by ectopic gastric mucosa

MESENTERIC CYSTS (INTRA-ABDOMINAL LYMPHANGIOMA)

Definition A lack of communication of small bowel or retroperitoneal lymphatic tissue with the main lymphatic vessels, resulting in the formation of a cystic mass

Clinical presentation Often present in childhood, with an acute presentation of pain, abdominal distension, fever or anorexia due to haemorrhage into the cyst, infection or torsion ▶ large cysts may compress the ureters or lead to bowel obstruction

AXR Soft tissue mass displacing bowel loops (occasionally the cyst wall is calcified)

USS A thin walled, uni- or multilocular cystic mass that may be adherent to the solid organs and bowel ▶ the cyst wall consists of a single layer (cf. enteric duplication cysts) ▶ echogenic debris if the cyst is haemorrhagic, chylous or infected

MRI This can characterize the cyst contents

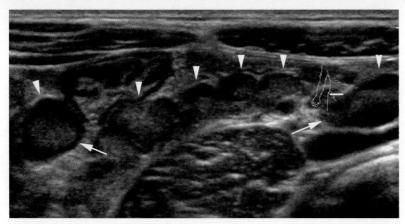

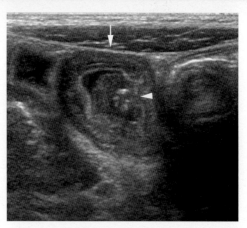

Sonographic appearance of mesenteric lymphadenitis. Multiple, unremarkable mesenteric lymph nodes (arrowheads) with preserved hyperechoic fatty hilum (arrows).**

Henoch–Schönlein purpura. Sonographic features of bowel wall thickening (arrow) due to intramural haemorrhage (arrowhead) in a child with Henoch–Schönlein purpura.**

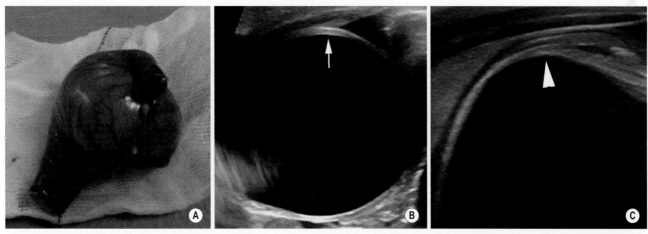

Intestinal duplication cyst. (A) Pathological specimen of a resected duplication cyst. (B) Sonographic features of the duplication cyst showing an anechoic cyst with a 'double layer' sign of the cyst wall. (C) Magnified image of the cyst wall revealing multiple layers in keeping with an intestinal duplication cyst.**

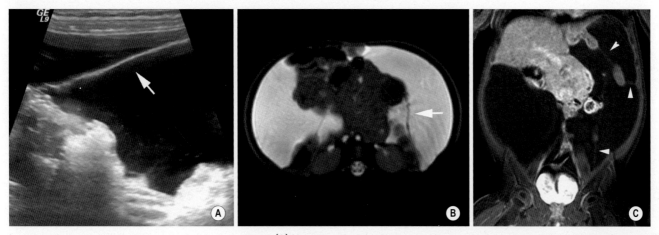

Imaging characteristics of mesenteric lymphangioma. (A) Ultrasound of the abdomen shows a large, septated fluid-filled structure with debris. (B) T2W MRI shows a large, septated cystic mass, displacing the bowel cranially and towards the midabdomen. (C) T1W fat-saturated MRI after administration of intravenous contrast shows subtle enhancement of the intracystic septae.**

GENITOURINARY

4.1 KIDNEYS

Glomerulonephritis

Definition A proliferative and necrotizing abnormality of the glomeruli ▶ it is usually primarily renal but may be part of a systemic vasculitis (e.g. SLE, PAN, Goodpasture's or Wegener's)

US/CT/MRI

- **Acute:** symmetrically swollen kidneys ▶ no papillary or calyceal abnormality
- **Chronic:** small kidneys ▶ smooth, normal pelvicalyceal systems ▶ prominent renal sinus fat

Acute tubular necrosis (ATN)

Definition Deposition of cellular debris within the tubules causing a *reversible* acute oliguric renal failure ▶ it usually follows an episode of severe ischaemia associated with hypotension, dehydration, or nephrotoxin exposure

US Swollen kidneys ▶ increased echogenicity within the cortex and pyramids

IVU (oliguric phase) A persistent nephrogram ▶ little or no filling of the pelvicalyceal system

Acute cortical necrosis

Definition Ischaemic necrosis of the cortex (with sparing of the medulla and medullary pyramids) causing *irreversible* renal damage ▶ the insult is more severe than that seen with ATN and is usually due to obstetric shock

AXR Patchy or linear renal calcification (with a 'pencil line' or 'double tramline' appearance)

US *Acute:* a hypoechoic renal cortex ▶ *chronic:* cortical calcification

CECT There may be opacification of the spared subcapsular cortex (its blood supply is from capsular vessels)

Papillary necrosis

Definition Ischaemic necrosis involving the renal medullary pyramids and papillae (these regions are particularly sensitive to hypoxia)

- *Causes:* analgesic abuse ▶ diabetes ▶ sickle-cell disease or trait ▶ obstruction complicated by infection ▶ acute infection ▶ haemophilia ▶ renal vein thrombosis ▶ acute renal failure in infancy

CT/IVU

- There is usually bilateral symmetrical involvement – unilateral involvement can occur with ascending infection or renal vein thrombosis ▶ the papillary and calyceal changes are rarely uniform
  - *Acute:* enlarged affected kidneys
  - *Chronic:* renal atrophy with a regular type of surface scarring (due to atrophy of the cortex overlying the damaged papillae and hypertrophy of the intervening columns of Bertin)
- **Calyces:**
  - *'Lobster claw deformity':* initially the necrotic areas erode the papilla tip and excavate from the fornices into the pyramids

- *'Egg in cup' appearance:* with progression contrast curves around the papilla from both fornices
- **Papillae:** the papilla initially swells and may eventually slough into the pelvicalyceal system causing colic, haematuria or hydronephrosis (as it appears as a filling defect it can mimic tumour, calculus or a blood clot) ▶ if the papillae fail to separate (necrosis in situ) the calyces may appear normal ▶ the papillae may calcify (with spotty calcification in a ring or triangle around a translucent centre)
- **Remaining defect:** calyceal clubbing resulting from a flattened or concave pyramidal tip

Medullary sponge kidney

Definition A common benign collecting duct ectasia occurring within the renal pyramids ▶ it is usually bilateral (but can be unilateral or segmental)

AXR Medullary nephrocalcinosis: punctate medullary calcification (representing small calculi within ectatic tubules)

IVU A striated nephrogram: multiple linear or saccular contrast collections within the medulla (do not confuse with a normal papillary blush)

- **Associations:** Wilms' tumour ▶ phaeochromocytoma ▶ horseshoe kidney ▶ Caroli's disease ▶ hemihypertrophy

Megacalycosis/polycalycosis

Definition An increased number of calyces (polycalycosis) or calyces with an abnormal rounded shape (megacalycosis)

Focal reflux nephropathy (chronic atrophic pyelonephritis)

Definition Focal parenchymal loss with clubbing of the underlying calyces – it usually follows a childhood infection associated with reflux

IVU/CT Small kidneys ▶ cortical scarring (representing parenchymal loss) with underlying clubbed calyces ▶ localized scars are more common within the upper pole (R>L)

- It can be unilateral or bilateral with part or all of the kidney involved (± a dilated renal pelvis and ureters)

Nephrocalcinosis

Definition Deposition of calcium within the renal parenchyma and outside of the pelvicalyceal system

CT/IVU

- *Medullary nephrocalcinosis (95%):* this is usually the product of a metabolic disorder (e.g. hyperparathyroidism/renal tubular acidosis) resulting in a raised serum calcium or a tubular defect resulting in hypercalciuria ▶ calcification is usually bilateral and diffuse
- *Cortical nephrocalcinosis (5%):* this is seen in acute cortical necrosis of any cause ▶ calcification is usually punctate and patchy (classically with a 'tramline' appearance)

Renal parenchymal disease

Glomerulonephritis ▶ *acute tubular necrosis* ▶ *acute cortical necrosis*	No papillary or calyceal abnormality ▶ no focal cortical loss
Papillary necrosis ▶ *medullary sponge kidney* ▶ *megacalycosis/polycalycosis*	Papillary or calyceal abnormality ▶ no focal cortical loss
Obstructive nephropathy ▶ *focal reflux nephropathy*	Papillary or calyceal abnormality ▶ focal cortical loss

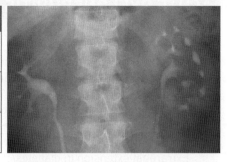

Left megacalycosis with numerous calyces showing poorly developed flattened papillae.[†]

Causes of nephrocalcinosis

Site	Cause
Cortical	Acute cortical necrosis
Medullary	**Associated with a metabolic disorder** Hyperparathyroidism Sarcoidosis Drug related (e.g. hypervitaminosis D, milk–alkali syndrome) Myelomatosis Primary or secondary hyperoxaluria Hyperhyroidism Osteoporosis
	Associated with renal tubular defects Idiopathic hypercalciuria Medullary sponge kidney Renal tubular acidosis
Focal	**Linear or rim calcification** Renal artery aneurysm Real cyst
	Amorphous calcification Calcified haematoma Tuberculosis Renal cell carcinoma (in 10%) Calcified renal papilla

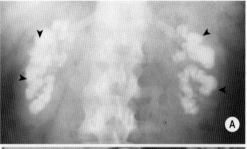

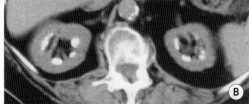

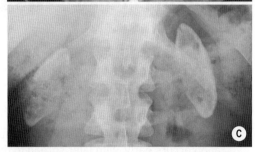

(A) Medullary nephrocalcinosis (arrowheads) with the corresponding CT appearances (B). (C) Cortical nephrocalcinosis.[∫]

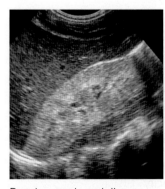

Renal parenchymal disease. Longitudinal US of the right kidney shows increased reflectivity compared to the adjacent liver.*

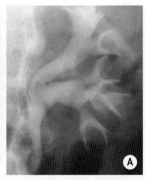

Papillary necrosis. (A) Lobster claw deformity. (B) Focal papillary contrast collections (arrows) associated with abnormal calyces (arrowheads).[∫]

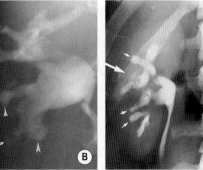

Analgesic nephropathy. Characteristic 'egg in cup' cavities (short arrows) and a 'horn' (long arrow).*

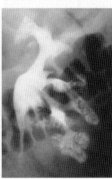

Medullary sponge kidney. The collecting system and renal pelvis appear normal. However, there are striated and saccular collections of contrast material within the renal papilla of the medulla.[∫]

ACUTE PYELONEPHRITIS

Definition

- Bacteriuria, pyrexia and flank pain due to an ascending infection in 85% (usually *E. coli*), or haematogenous seeding in 15% (*S. aureus*)
  - *Risk factors:* diabetes ▶ vesicoureteric reflux (VUR) ▶ urinary obstruction ▶ pregnancy ▶ instrumentation ▶ immune deficiency
  - Extrarenal extension in diabetes/immunocompromised patients

Radiological features

- This is a clinical diagnosis – imaging is rarely required during uncomplicated adult disease ▶ it can however be useful if the diagnosis is in doubt or to exclude obstruction or abscess development

IVU Focal or diffuse renal swelling ▶ delayed and poor pelvicalyceal system filling ▶ a dense, persistent or striated nephrogram (with severe disease)

US Normal in 80% ▶ focal (lobar) renal swelling or diffuse renal swelling with severe disease ▶ the affected segments are hypoechoic (they can be hyperechoic with haemorrhage) ▶ reduced corticomedullary differentiation (due to oedema) ▶ focal or diffuse reduced perfusion

NECT Reduced renal attenuation (which can be increased with haemorrhage) ▶ renal swelling with acute disease

CECT During the nephrographic phase there can be areas of patchy enhancement or band/wedge-shaped areas of decreased enhancement extending from the papillae to the renal margin ▶ delayed persistent enhancement ▶ any abnormal parenchymal enhancement may persist for >2 months and may develop into a scar ▶ extrarenal extension

MRI Similar features as for CT

DMSA Can demonstrate areas of chronic scarring

Pearls

- **Complications:** abscess formation ▶ emphysematous pyelonephritis ▶ xanthogranulomatous pyelonephritis ▶ cortical atrophy and renal failure
- **Causes of a sterile pyuria:** TB ▶ fungal infections ▶ glomerulonephritis ▶ interstitial nephritis
- Renal abscess: usually due to ascending infection (*E. coli*) ▶ haematogeneous spread due to *S. aureus*
- CT: non-enhancing fluid centre ± gas ▶ thick irregular wall ± enhancement ▶ inflammatory changes in the perinephric space

RENAL TUBERCULOSIS (TB)

Definition

- The kidneys are the 2nd commonest site of TB involvement after the lung (even though the CXR is normal in 35–50% of cases it usually follows haematogenous spread from the lung)
  - Lesions spread via the tubular lumen to the papilla and hence to the collecting system ▶ papillary ulceration occurs early, with later spread to the collecting system leading to fibrosis and stricture formation

Clinical presentation

- Lower tract symptoms ▶ haematuria ▶ sterile pyuria

Radiological features

IVU/CT Although both kidneys are seeded, clinical manifestations are usually unilateral (>70% of cases)

- **Early:** *an enlarged kidney* ▶ irregularity and destruction of ≥1 papillae (resembling papillary necrosis)
- **Late:** *an atrophic kidney*
  - **Renal calcification (30%):** this appears as punctate or curvilinear renal parenchymal calcification or as calcification within a caseous pyonephrosis (with a characteristic cloudy appearance in the distribution of the dilated calyces)
    - *'Tuberculous autonephrectomy':* this may progress to homogeneous calcification within a dilated pelvicalyceal system so that the kidney appears as a lobulated calcified mass

  - *Ureteric calcification:* this is the 2nd commonest site of calcification with a typical beaded appearance ▶ calcification of the bladder, vas deferens and seminal vesicles is rarely seen
  - *Cavitations:* these are usually irregular and communicate with the collecting system ▶ widespread cavitations may mimic hydronephrosis (but the pelvis and infundibula of the calyces are not dilated unless there is an associated obstruction)
  - *Fibrotic strictures:* these can occur anywhere within the renal tract
    - *Hydrocalycosis:* a local calyceal dilatation due to a partial stricture of a major infundibulum (the infundibulum appears 'cut off' with a complete stricture) creating a 'phantom calyx'
    - *Ureter:* a 'corkscrew' appearance (due to multiple stenoses) ▶ a 'pipestem' appearance (due to a rigid and aperistaltic ureter)
    - *Renal pelvis:* a 'purse string' stenosis
  - *Bladder:*
    - *Early:* trabeculation ▶ bladder wall irregularity ▶ a slight decrease in capacity
    - *Late:* a thick-walled small-capacity bladder demonstrating calcification ▶ bladder TB is almost always associated with renal TB ▶ often there is VUR into a widely dilated upper tract

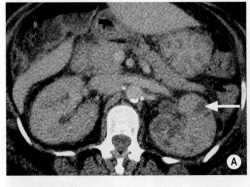

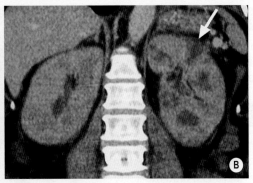

Diffuse unilateral acute pyelonephritis. (A) Axial and (B) coronal enhanced CT shows wedge- and band-shaped areas of reduced enhancement in the left kidney (arrow). There is associated perinephric inflammatory change.*

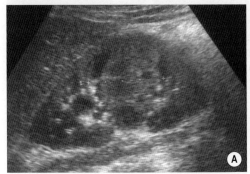

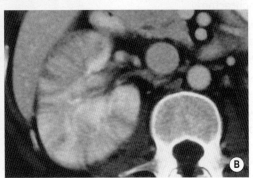

(A) Focal severe pyelonephritis appearing on US as a slightly heterogeneous mass.[†]
(B) Acute pyelonephritis. CECT demonstrating reniform enlargement of the right kidney with numerous striations due to parenchymal oedema and urine stasis within the renal tubules.[∫]

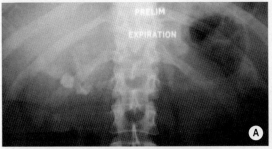

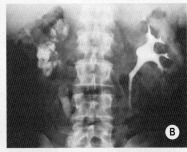

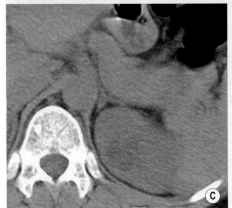

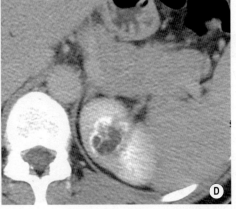

Urinary tract tuberculosis. The plain film (A) demonstrates calcification within distended upper pole calyces. Classical end-stage upper tract tuberculosis is the autonephrectomy (B) in which the chronically obstructed pelvicalyceal system is filled with calcifying caseous pus associated with complete renal parenchymal destruction. In this case there is also similar calcifying pus in an obstructed dilated upper ureter.[†]
(C) Unenhanced axial CT demonstrates hypodense area at the upper pole of the left kidney medially with marginal enhancement at contrast-enhanced axial CT (D).**

EMPHYSEMATOUS PYELONEPHRITIS

DEFINITION

- A rare fulminating form of acute necrotic pyelonephritis due to a gas-producing organism (usually *E. coli*) ▶ it is associated with diabetes and obstruction

RADIOLOGICAL FEATURES

Emphysematous pyelonephritis Gas within the renal parenchyma (which can be focal or diffuse) + the collecting system ± the perinephric space ▶ there is a high mortality rate (>60%) and it may require nephrectomy

Emphysematous pyelitis Gas within the pelvicalyceal system and ureter only ▶ it has a lower mortality rate, and percutaneous drainage and antibiotics may be sufficient

Perinephric emphysema Gas within the perinephric space

Emphysematous cystitis Gas within the bladder and bladder wall (due to *E. coli* or *C. albicans*) ▶ the patient is usually diabetic

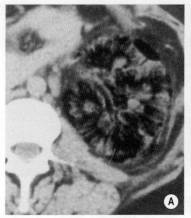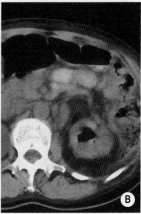

(A) CT demonstrating diffuse emphysematous pyelonephritis. (B) Emphysematous pyelitis. CT demonstrating gas within the collecting system.[†]

XANTHOGRANULOMATOUS PYELONEPHRITIS (XGP)

DEFINITION

- Chronic renal parenchymal inflammation with replacement of the normal renal parenchyma with lipid-laden histiocytes ▶ it is secondary to chronic urinary infection (e.g. *E coli* or *Proteus mirabilis*) and obstructing calculus disease ▶ it is associated with diabetes ▶ renal pelvis initially affected, later corticomedullary areas are affected (± peri-renal extension)
  - There are diffuse (common) or focal (uncommon) forms ▶ the focal form can mimic a tumour

RADIOLOGICAL FEATURES

IVU/US/CT A renal staghorn calculi (70%) ▶ an enlarged (global or focal) non-excreting kidney ▶ dilated affected calyces with internal echoes or debris ▶ a heterogeneous kidney with multiple non- or rim-enhancing low attenuation areas (-15 to -20 HU) representing dilated calyces and xanthomas ▶ perinephric extension (± a thickened Gerota's fascia) is common ▶ hilar/para-aortic adenopathy

MRI Necrotic areas are hyperintense on T2WI ▶ T1WI: intermediate SI (high protein content within cavities)

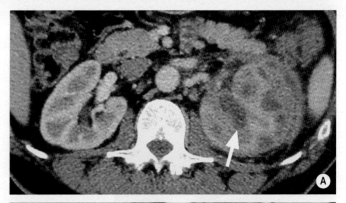
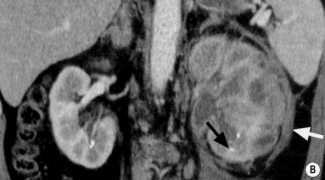

Diffuse left xanthogranulomatous pyelonephritis. (A) CT shows dilated calyces (arrow) with a thinned parenchyma. (B) Note the perinephric inflammatory change (white arrow) and calcification (black arrow).*

RENAL ABSCESS

DEFINITION

- A renal parenchymal collection secondary to acute pyelonephritis (Gram-negative or anaerobic bacilli) or haematogenous spread of infection (*S. aureus*)

RADIOLOGICAL FEATURES

US A heterogeneous renal mass with areas of cystic necrosis (± shadowing due to gas)

CT There is a heterogeneous central portion of near-fluid density (with no enhancement) ▶ there are enhancing thick irregular walls (± perinephric inflammatory change) ▶ gas within the lesion is diagnostic

MRI T1WI: low SI rounded thick walled lesion ▶ T2WI: high SI depending on fluid/debris content ▶ T1WI+Gad: rim enhancement

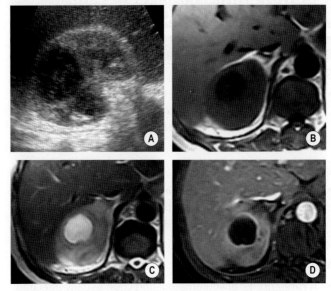

Renal abscess. (A) Ultrasound shows a hypoechoic right renal lesion with internal echoes. (B) Axial T1-weighted MRI shows a hypointense parenchymal lesion. (C) Axial T2-weighted MRI demonstrates hyperintensity relative to the surrounding renal parenchyma with a thick margin. (D) There is marginal enhancement on Gd-enhanced GRE T1-weighted axial image.**

PERINEPHRIC ABSCESS

DEFINITION

- An extension of renal infection into the perinephric space with subsequent abscess formation

RADIOLOGICAL FEATURES

IVU Loss of the renal outline (± psoas shadow) ▶ absent renal function

CT A perinephric rim-enhancing fluid collection (± debris, septations and gas) ▶ this may extend in any direction

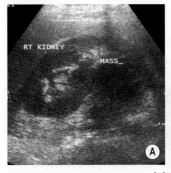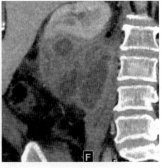

Perirenal and psoas abscess. (A) Ultrasound shows a hypoechoic lesion which appears to lie within and posterior to the lower pole of the right kidney. (B) Contrast medium-enhanced coronal CT demonstrates a multilocular cystic lesion with marginal and septal enhancement extending to the right psoas muscle.**

SQUAMOUS METAPLASIA, LEUKOPLAKIA, MALACOPLAKIA, AND CHOLESTEATOMA

DEFINITION

Squamous metaplasia

- Replacement of the normal transitional epithelium by squamous epithelium (which may become keratinized) ▶ it is associated with recurrent urinary tract infections and calculi

Leukoplakia

- Areas of squamous metaplasia seen as sharply defined white patches on the renal pelvic mucosal surface ▶ it appears as thickened folds and irregularity of the renal pelvis

Malacoplakia

- A rare chronic granulomatous infection usually affecting women (secondary to *E. coli* infection) and which is more common in immunosuppressed patients ▶ small plaques are visible on the mucosal surfaces (bladder > upper urinary tract)

  IVU Multiple small filling defects within the renal pelvis and ureter (they are too small to be seen within the bladder)

  US Focal hypoechoic renal masses – these may become large enough to mimic a tumour ▶ there may be impaired renal function if the parenchyma is involved

Urinary cholesteatoma

- A mass of desquamated keratin lying free within the lumen and demonstrating a typical whorled appearance

PYELOURETERITIS CYSTICA

DEFINITION

- Small benign submucosal cysts of the renal pelvis and ureter ▶ it is associated with urinary tract infection and chronic obstruction

RADIOLOGICAL FEATURES

IVU Multiple small filling defects indenting the renal pelvis and ureter

BILHARZIA (URINARY SCHISTOSOMIASIS)

DEFINITION

- This is due to a fluke infestation (*Schistosoma haematobium*) ▶ the worm enters the skin and matures

within the liver (via the portal vein) ▶ ova are then deposited within the bladder or ureteric submucosa (via the perivesical plexus) ▶ the ova produce an inflammatory reaction, leading to granuloma and stricture formation

RADIOLOGICAL FEATURES

Ureters These are grossly dilated and tortuous (± strictures) ▶ there can be multiple filling defects (representing granulomas or ureteritis cystica) ▶ parallel lines of ureteric calcification can be seen

Bladder This is small and fibrosed with wall calcification (which can be fine, granular, linear or irregular)

Complications

- Bladder squamous cell carcinoma (with chronic infection)

FUNGAL INFECTIONS

DEFINITION

- An opportunistic infection (often *C. albicans*) due to the increased use of antibiotics, immunosuppressive agents and steroids ▶ diabetics are at increased risk

RADIOLOGICAL FEATURES

US/CT A round, shaggy (sometimes laminated) fungus ball within the renal pelvis or bladder (it may extend into the ureter as a cylindrical filling defect) ▶ it is highly echogenic on US, and it may demonstrate air within the collecting system and bladder

PYONEPHROSIS

DEFINITION

- Pus within the renal pelvis and calyces following an ascending infection in an obstructed kidney (e.g. secondary to a calculus or PUJ obstruction) ▶ there is a risk of septicaemia and endotoxic shock (especially with attempted drainage)

RADIOLOGICAL FEATURES

US An obstructed kidney ▶ debris or gas (dense shadowing) within the renal pelvis ▶ cortical loss or a perinephric abscess if long-standing

CT High-density material (± layering) within a dilated pelvicalyceal system ▶ there may be a renal or perinephric abscess ▶ thickening of the renal pelvis (>2 mm)

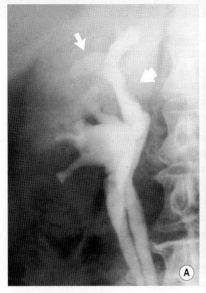
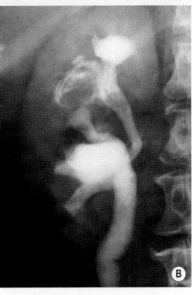

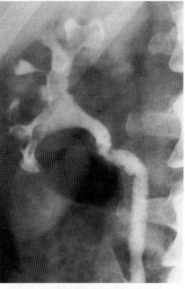

Cholesteatoma of the kidney. Recurrent urinary tract infection for many years. (A) IVU 1975. Filling defect in upper pole calyx (arrow). Also there is a flat defect in the infundibulum (broad arrow). The latter is consistent with leukoplakia. (B) IVU 1979. Extensive irregular filling defects with typical whorled pattern in the upper pole.*

Pyeloureteritis cystica. A staghorn calculus occupies much of the collecting system.*

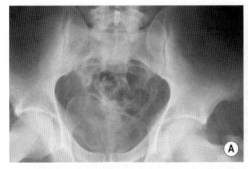
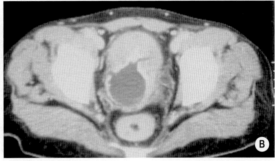

Schistosomiasis. Plain XR (A) showing linear calcification along the bladder wall and distal left ureter. CT (B) demonstrating bladder wall calcification and thickening – this may be gross and (as here) associated with rectal wall thickening.[†]

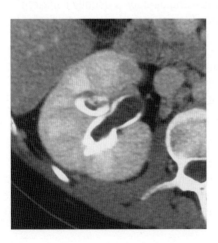

Calyceal fungus debris. CECT demonstrating radiolucent material forming a cast of the calyces. The material was fungal debris in this immunosuppressed patient.[ſ]

Chronic pyonephrosis. There is marked cortical loss and modest collecting system dilatation. The CT also demonstrates the pelvic calculus responsible and a multiloculated perinephric abscess, which has extended laterally into the abdominal wall and posteriorly into the psoas muscle.[†]

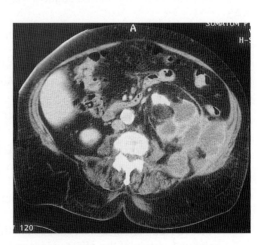

RENAL ARTERY STENOSIS (RAS)

Definition

- Narrowing of the renal artery accounts for 1–5% of all causes of hypertension
  - *Mechanism:* decreased glomerular perfusion results in renin release via the juxtaglomerular baroreceptors ▶ the resultant increased renin (and angiotensin II) levels leads to vasoconstriction

Atheromatous RAS

- This is the commonest cause of RAS (70–80%) and is most commonly seen in men over 50 years old ▶ atheroma involves the origin (ostial) or proximal ⅓ of the renal artery ▶ there can be post-stenotic dilatation
  - Ostial lesions are caused by aortic plaques ▶ renal arterial lesions are caused by eccentric atheromatous plaques of the proximal renal artery

Fibromuscular dysplasia (FMD)

- This is the most common cause of a non-atheromatous RAS and is the 2nd most common cause of an RAS (15–20%) ▶ it typically occurs in young women
- Medial fibroplasia is the commonest form, causing multiple short stenoses (with a 'string of beads' appearance on angiography)
- It involves the distal main renal artery (and its major branches) ▶ it can also affect the external iliac and carotid arteries
- It dilates easily with excellent angioplasty results

Takayasu's disease

- This is a rare disease affecting the aorta and its branches ▶ aortic disease may consist of diffuse or focal stenoses, occlusion, or a fusiform AAA ▶ can be resistant to dilatation

Radiological features

US In the absence of any other renal disease, a significant discrepancy in renal size should suggest the presence of RAS

Duplex US This is a limited technique, as up to 42% of renal arteries are not visualized

- *RAS:* a renal artery peak systolic velocity >100 cm/s ▶ a renal artery to aortic velocity ratio (RAR) >3.5 ▶ a 'parvus and tardus' effect within the intrarenal vessels (due to velocity reduction and slowing of the acceleration of the systolic upstroke)

Angiotensin-coverting enzyme (ACE) renography

- Baseline dynamic renal imaging is performed using either ^{99m}Tc-DTPA or ^{99m}Tc-MAG3
- Imaging is repeated after the administration of an ACE inhibitor
  - *Positive ACE renogram:* a reduction in the total and relative function of the affected kidney (>5–10%) and/or a delayed time to peak maximum activity and prolonged intrarenal parenchymal transit

CTA Multidetector CT provides excellent spatial resolution (superior to MRA)

- Post-processing of data includes curved multiplanar reformats (MPRs), maximum intensity projections (MIPs) and volume rendering
- Stenoses may be overestimated if there is low soft tissue contrast (e.g. with inadequate opacification or a slice thickness greater than the vessel diameter)

MRA This uses gadolinium-enhanced 3D spoiled gradient echo imaging during a single breath-hold (+ bolus tracking)

- Smaller fields of view increase the spatial resolution ▶ it has a sensitivity (97%) and specificity (92%) comparable with intra-arterial angiography for detecting stenoses within the main and segmental arteries
- Dynamic imaging may also provide functional imaging similar to scintigraphy

DSA Formally the gold standard ▶ it is increasingly being replaced by non-invasive methods

- An aortogram is essential to demonstrate the number and location of the renal arteries and also the presence of any aortic or proximal renal vascular abnormalities
- Selective arteriography should not be performed in RAS (except as a prelude to renal angioplasty) as it may cause renal artery dissection or occlusion
  - Consider angioplasty or stenting if a gradient is greater than 15 mmHg (or 10% of the systolic pressure)

Pearls

- Screening is indicated in high-risk patients:
  - With an abrupt onset of hypertension (<30 or >50 years)
  - With hypertension unresponsive to drug therapy
  - With a unilateral small kidney or abdominal bruits

Renal angioplasty and stenting

- High restenosis rates following percutaneous transluminal angioplasty (PTA) led to renal stenting with metallic stents becoming the dominant strategy for atheromatous lesions – angioplasty is usually sufficient for non-atheromatous lesions
- No clear benefit in most cases over medical treatment alone
- The kidney must be salvageable (e.g. a renal length >8 cm and a satisfactory GFR)
- *Indications:* resistant hypertension ▶ rapidly developing renal failure ▶ flash pulmonary oedema ▶ critical stenosis in a single kidney
- *Complications* (with a greater potential than seen in peripheral vascular disease): renal artery rupture and perforation ▶ branch occlusion ▶ occlusion of the main renal artery ▶ cholesterol emboli ▶ a short-term deterioration in renal function (due to the contrast medium given)

Middle aortic syndrome A rare condition whereby renal artery stenoses are associated with abdominal aortic coarctation (± visceral artery stenoses) ▶ it may be associated with Williams' syndrome or neurofibromatosis

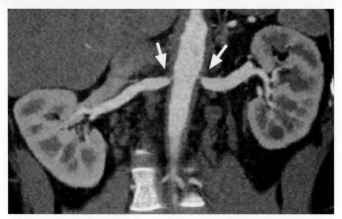

Takayasu's disease. Curved multiplanar coronal reformat CT demonstrating the bilateral renal artery stenosis (arrows) and diffuse aortic wall thickening.*

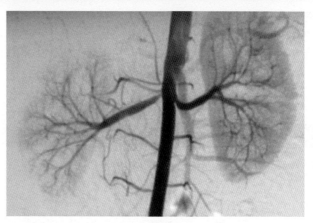

DSA demonstrating a right renal artery stenosis.*

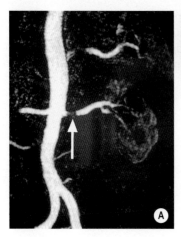
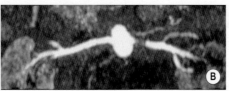

MRA. (A) Coronal MIP of a patient with significant left renal artery stenosis (white arrow). (B) Axial MIP of the same patient.*

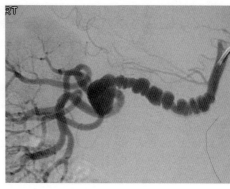

Fibromuscular dysplasia. On a selective right anterior oblique (RAO) DSA the characteristic saccular dilatations and the web-like stenoses are clearly evident.*

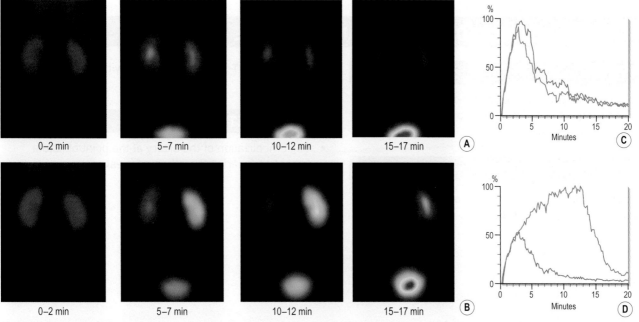

(A) MAG3 dynamic scintigram before captopril, showing a relatively normal dynamic study. (B) The same patient following captopril time–activity and measured parameters. (C) The pre-captopril time–activity and (D) the time–activity curves and measured parameters after captopril on the abnormal right kidney (red line, right kidney ▶ blue line, left kidney).*

RENAL ARTERY ANEURYSMS

DEFINITION

- A focal renal arterial dilatation is rare
  - *Causes:* congenital ▶ mycotic ▶ post-traumatic ▶ atherosclerotic ▶ vasculitic ▶ fibromuscular hyperplasia

RADIOLOGICAL FEATURES

US A cystic mass demonstrating arterial flow

CT/MR angiography Characteristic curvilinear aneurysmal calcification may not be seen with MRI ▶ both will demonstrate aneurysmal dilatation

PEARL

Treatment Embolization coils or stents can be used if there is hypertension or if there is a risk of rupture
- *Increased rupture risk:* an aneurysm >2.5 cm ▶ absent wall calcification ▶ occurring during pregnancy

POLYARTERITIS NODOSA

DEFINITION

- An autoimmune arteritis affecting medium and small-sized arteries

RADIOLOGICAL FEATURES

CT/MR angiography 2–3 mm aneurysms (± areas of arterial narrowing) ▶ aneurysms tend to be more peripheral than with FMD

- CTA and MRA cannot demonstrate changes within the smaller vessels – this requires DSA
- A *'moth-eaten' nephrographic appearance:* thromboses can result in small renal infarcts

ARTERIOVENOUS MALFORMATIONS AND FISTULAE

DEFINITION

- These are usually iatrogenic or post-traumatic (but can rarely be congenital) ▶ it may lead to impaired renal function due to a 'steal' effect

RADIOLOGICAL FEATURES

Doppler US High-velocity turbulent flow within an abnormal vascular communication

Angiography/CT Enlarged vessels with early filling of the renal veins

TREATMENT

- Coil embolization of the artery at the point of fistula formation (sparing the other arteries)

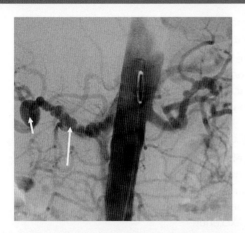

Renal artery aneurysm. On this AP aortogram the pigtail catheter is positioned just above the renal arteries. There is fibromuscular disease involving the distal right renal artery (long arrow) with an aneurysm (short arrow).*

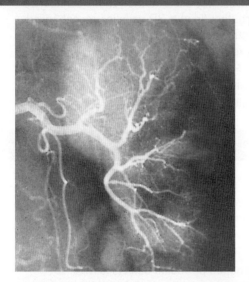

Polyarteritis nodosa. Renal angiogram showing multiple microaneurysms.†

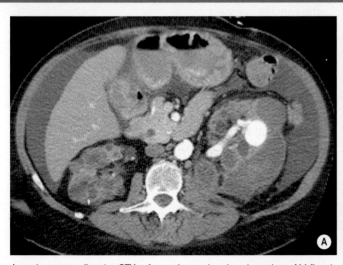

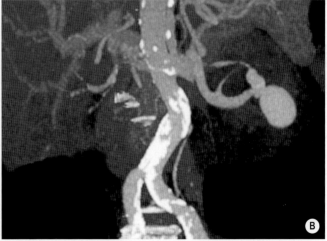

Arteriovenous fistula. CTA of a patient who developed an AV fistula following a renal biopsy. (A) Axial CT. (B) MIP of the CTA.*

RENAL VEIN THROMBOSIS

DEFINITION

- Renal vein occlusion by thrombus can be caused by: membranous glomerulonephritis (the commonest adult cause) ▶ nephrotic syndrome ▶ dehydration ▶ hypercoagulable states ▶ renal or left adrenal tumours

CLINICAL PRESENTATION

- Acute loin pain or haematuria ▶ with chronicity venous collaterals can open with only slightly impaired renal function

RADIOLOGICAL FEATURES

IVU

- *Acute:* an enlarged kidney ▶ a faint or absent nephrogram ▶ absent pelvicalyceal filling (which may also be stretched and compressed by an oedematous renal parenchyma) ▶ rarely there may be an increasingly dense nephrogram (± striations)

- *Chronic:* a normal or atrophic kidney ▶ retroperitoneal venous collaterals can indent the PC system

US Acutely there may be a large oedematous kidney with loss of corticomedullary differentiation ▶ renal vein thrombus and a lack of flow within the main veins (± reversed end diastolic flow within the parenchymal veins)

- A normal study does not exclude the diagnosis

CECT A filling defect within the renal vein (which can be enlarged or of normal calibre) ▶ prolonged irregular parenchymal enhancement ▶ prolonged corticomedullary differentiation ▶ the 'cortical rim' sign ▶ delayed or absent contrast medium excretion

- *Chronic changes:* the renal vein may be atrophic with curvilinear calcification and collateral vessel formation

MRI False positives may occur at the venous confluence (due to fast or turbulent flow) ▶ 3D gadolinium-enhanced MRA may differentiate benign from tumour thrombus

- *Spin-echo sequences:* high SI thrombus
- *Gradient-echo sequences:* low SI thrombus

DSA This is rarely used ▶ selective renal venography may identify any filling defects

RENAL INFARCTION

DEFINITION

- Thromboembolic occlusion of a renal artery usually leads to a focal renal infarction (less commonly total infarction) ▶ over time the infarcted area decreases in size with scar formation and tissue retraction
  - *Causes:* atrial fibrillation ▶ aortic aneurysm ▶ trauma ▶ thrombosis (due to atheroma or vasculitis)

CLINICAL PRESENTATION

- Pain and haematuria (it can be confused with renal colic)

RADIOLOGICAL FEATURES

IVU A renal cortical scar (± deformity of the underlying calyces) ▶ this can progress to a shrunken end-stage kidney

Dynamic DTPA imaging Reduced or absent blood flow within the affected area during the initial flow phase of the study ▶ there is failure of tracer uptake on later images

Doppler US

- *Complete occlusion:* the kidney appears normal but demonstrates no flow
- *Segmental or focal infarction:* a wedge-shaped mass (with a similar appearance to pyelonephritis)

CECT Wedge-shaped perfusion defects (similar to the appearance of acute pyelonephritis) with later scar formation

- *'Cortical rim' sign:* a rim of cortical enhancement from the capsular vessels

MRI Reduced corticomedullary differentiation

- T1WI and T2WI: a low SI infarct (unless there is associated haemorrhage) ▶ T1WI + Gad: no enhancement

DSA This defines the site of any arterial block

- *Early:* an absent nephrogram or wedge-shaped defect
- *Late:* typical scar formation

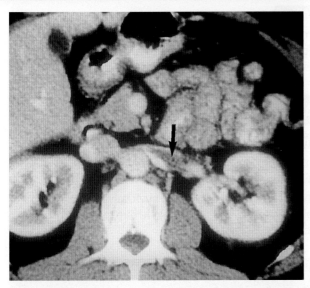

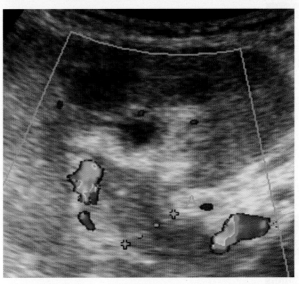

Renal vein thrombus in a patient with nephrotic syndrome. CECT at the level of the renal veins shows thrombus in the left renal vein (arrow).*

Oblique US view of a renal transplant demonstrating an expanded thrombosed renal vein (blue cursor) full of echogenic thrombus. Patent renal arteries are seen adjacent to it.

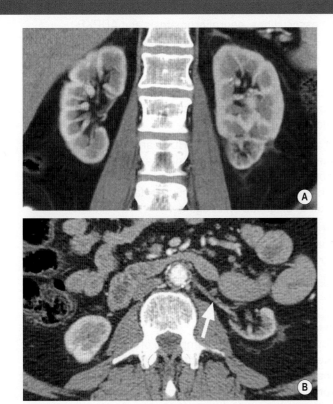

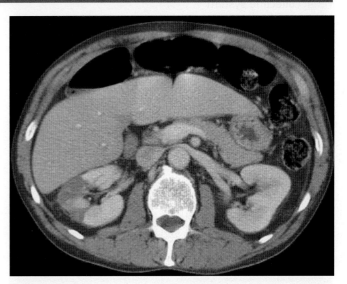

Axial CECT demonstrating multiple wedge-shaped low attenuation infarcts within the right kidney. There is also reduced attenuation of the right liver lobe (relative to the left), also caused by the same underlying embolic phenomena.

Focal infarction. (A) CT demonstrating focal infarction of the lower pole of the left kidney due to (B) occlusion of an accessory lower pole renal artery (arrow).*

SEROUS RENAL CYST

Definition

- This is the commonest form of renal cystic disease and there are often multiple cysts present (affecting up to 50% of the population)

  US An anechoic well-defined thin-walled mass (with posterior acoustic enhancement)

  CT A well-defined rounded mass (0–20 HU) with an imperceptible wall ▶ a 'beak sign' can be seen with large lesions

  MRI T1WI: low SI ▶ T2WI: high SI ▶ T1WI + Gad: no enhancement

PARAPELVIC AND PERIPELVIC CYSTS

Definition

Parapelvic cyst A renal serous cyst arising from the renal parenchyma and expanding into the renal sinus

Peripelvic cyst A cyst of lymphatic origin which may track along the renal infundibula ▶ it can be confused with hydronephrosis (but it will not demonstrate a connection with the dilated renal pelvis)

US Simple cysts distorting (but rarely obstructing) the renal collecting system

ACQUIRED CYSTIC KIDNEY DISEASE (ACKD)

Definition

- This occurs in 13% of patients with chronic renal disease (prior to dialysis) and in 90% of patients after 5 years of haemo- or peritoneal dialysis ▶ there is an increased risk of developing renal cell carcinoma – following transplantation any ACKD (and the increased RCC risk) persist

US This is distinguished from ADPKD as the kidneys are small or normal in size, and demonstrate fewer and smaller cysts

HYDATID (ECHINOCOCCAL) CYSTS OF THE KIDNEY

Definition

- Renal cystic disease due to echinococcal infection ▶ this is rarely seen (even in endemic areas)
  - The cysts may rupture into the collecting system, giving rise to acute flank pain followed by the voiding of hydatid scolices (± haematuria)

US A mainly intrarenal multicystic structure with thick walls (± calcification)

ADENOMA

Definition

- Small renal tumours (<3 cm) have historically been regarded as adenomas rather than carcinomas ▶ however an adenoma may still rarely metastasize

HAEMANGIOMA

Definition

- A rare benign vascular tumour that is generally cavernous rather than capillary

US/IVD/CT A renal mass with pyelocalyceal distortion ▶ a pyelocalyceal filling defect may be due to the tumour or associated blood clot

ANGIOMYOLIPOMA

Definition

- A benign lesion composed of fat, smooth muscle and abnormal blood vessels – the imaging appearances depend upon the various proportions of these tissue components that are present
  - It mainly affects females (during the 5th decade) but is also associated with tuberous sclerosis (affecting a younger age group with multiple lesions) ▶ other associations: neurofibromatosis and ADPKD

US A circumscribed, highly reflective mass (it may not be echogenic if there is a greater proportion of muscle, or if it has undergone haemorrhage or necrosis) ▶ it can be confused with a small hyperechoic RCC (although an angiomyolipoma may demonstrate posterior acoustic shadowing)

CT A fatty mass (–15 to –20 HU) ± areas of increased tissue density ▶ fat within a renal mass is diagnostic of an angiomyolipoma (but ensure that it is not perinephric fat that has been engulfed by tumour) ▶ fat poor AMLs can be difficult to diagnose on imaging

MRI Fatty regions will demonstrate signal loss on out of phase imaging ▶ NECT is the definitive technique for confirming the presence of fat

Angiography Can demonstrate multiple small aneurysms and an 'onion layer' appearance

Pearl

- Angiomyolipomas are composed of thick-walled, inelastic blood vessels with a risk of haemorrhage if the lesion is >4 cm ▶ embolization can control bleeding tumours and can reduce the risk of haemorrhage within enlarging lesions ▶ large vascular tumours are embolized to reduce bleeding risk (especially if future pregnancy is likely)

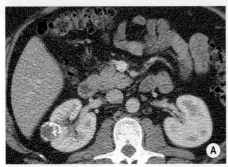
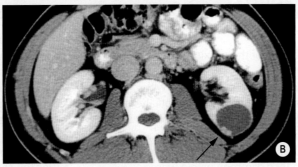

Bosniak IIF renal cyst. CT demonstrates heavy calcification in a small cyst which was difficult to evaluate at US. Despite the absence of enhancement on CT, the lesion was considered too atypical to be a Bosniak II lesion, and was classified as a 2F cyst for observation.** (B) Cystic renal cell carcinoma. CECT demonstrates a small peripheral nodule of enhancing tumour (arrow) in the wall of the cyst (Bosniak class IV).*

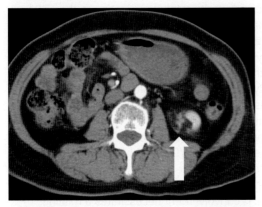

Non-contrast CT of 44-year-old woman with angiomyolipoma. There is a left renal mass (arrow) that has hypoattenuating components consistent with fat, which is virtually diagnostic of angiomyolipoma.**

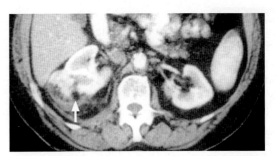

Bleeding angiomyolipoma. Axial CT shows perirenal blood and inflammatory change surrounding the right kidney following a spontaneous bleed. The central fat density (arrow) suggests an angiomyolipoma.*

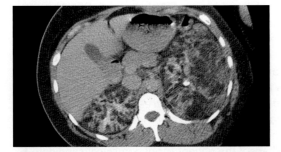

Axial CT demonstrating multiple angiomyolipomas in a patient with tuberous sclerosis.

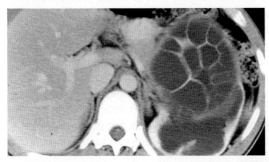

Hydatid disease of the kidney. There is a cystic mass in the left kidney with a multiloculated internal appearance from the presence of many daughter cysts. The mass is causing marked pelvicalyceal dilatation.*

Bosniak classification (based upon CT findings) for complicated renal cysts		
Class	**Behaviour**	**Imaging features**
Class I	Benign	A simple benign cyst
Class II	Benign	One or more (<1 mm) septa ▶ thin mural calcification ▶ fluid contents of increased attenuation (due to haemorrhage or infection) ▶ no enhancement (unlike a malignant lesion)
Class IIF	Benign (requires follow-up) for up to 5 years	Lesions with multiple class II features ▶ >3 cm hyperdense cysts ▶ totally intrarenal hyperdense cysts
Class III	Possibly malignant	Thickened septae ▶ nodular calcification ▶ solid non-enhancing areas *This needs biopsy or surgery to exclude malignancy*
Class IV	Malignant	Cystic masses which are clearly malignant (with solid enhancing) nodules or irregular walls

RENAL CELL CARCINOMA

Definition
- Thought to arise from the cells of the proximal convoluted tubule
- It usually occurs spontaneously but is associated with von Hippel–Lindau disease and long-term haemodialysis
  - *Clear cell carcinoma* (85%): seen in 36% of patients with von Hippel–Lindau disease
  - *Papillary tumour* (10–15%): often multiple ▶ type 1 and type 2 (the latter is less common with a worse prognosis) ▶ common in failing kidneys
  - *Chromophobe tumour* (5%)
  - *Collecting duct tumour (rare)*: poor prognosis

Clinical presentation
- The classic clinical triad of a palpable mass, flank pain and haematuria is only seen in about 10% of cases ▶ it can also present with fever (PUO), weight loss, anorexia, paraneoplastic syndromes and polycythaemia
- It usually presents during the 5th–7th decades (2M:1F) ▶ it is bilateral in 5% of cases

Radiological features

US Small tumours are usually hyperechoic ▶ larger tumours can be isoechoic (± central necrosis) ▶ cystic tumours have thick or irregular walls with variably sized intracystic tumour nodules

CT

Preferred method for staging
- *NECT:* a solid mass of heterogeneous attenuation (>20 HU) with low density central areas ▶ calcification can be present (5–10%)
- *CECT:* increased attenuation (>10 HU) suggests a solid mass ▶ increased attenuation >20 HU between NECT and nephrogenic phases is suggestive of malignancy (as is >10 HU between the corticomedullary and nephrogenic phases) ▶ lesser values can be due to pseudoenhancement ▶ there is a significantly increased risk of metastases with tumours >3 cm
  - *Clear cell carcinoma:* significant (heterogeneous) enhancement
  - *Papillary tumour:* poor enhancement
  - *Chromophobe tumour:* similar appearance to an oncocytoma
- *Signs suggestive of renal capsule invasion:* an indistinct renal outline ▶ perirenal fascial thickening ▶ strands of tissue (or a discrete mass) extending into the perirenal fat
- *Renal vein or IVC thrombus:* a filling defect present within an expanded vein ▶ enhancing vessels can be seen within a tumour thrombus
  - It can be difficult to distinguish between direct tumour invasion of the vein (which may enhance) from a bland thrombus ▶ flow related artefacts may also complicate the assessment
  - Isolated renal vein enlargement is an unreliable sign as it can be caused by increased blood flow secondary to tumour hypervascularity

MRI This is used for staging if a CECT is contraindicated or if frequent follow-up is required in high-risk patients
- T1WI: low to intermediate SI ▶ T2WI: slightly high SI ▶ T1WI + Gad: immediate heterogeneous enhancement which decreases on delayed images ▶ homogeneous enhancement is more likely in small, low-grade tumours
  - *Venous invasion:* MRI is superior to CT in differentiating benign from malignant thrombus in either the renal vein or IVC ▶ T1WI: normal flow voids are replaced by relatively high tumour SI

Pearls
- **Lymphatic drainage:** renal lymphatics drain to the para-aortic nodes, ultimately terminating in the cisterna chyli (drainage directly to the mediastinum can occur)
- **Distant metastases:**
  - *Liver:* hypervascular lesions
  - *Lungs:* the most common site of metastatic disease
  - *Bones:* lytic and expansile lesions
  - It can also metastasize to the adrenals, brain and contralateral kidney
- **Venous invasion:** this usually represents intraluminal tumour (the wall of the IVC is rarely invaded) ▶ its presence reduces disease survival
  - Assessing the degree of invasion aids surgical planning: IVC involvement necessitates a midline laparotomy approach ▶ extension above the level of the hepatic veins requires a thoracic surgical approach
- **CT-guided radiofrequency (heat)/cryo (cold) ablation:** these are noninvasive options for treating smaller peripheral lesions (T1a lesions) ▶ RENAL nephrometry/PADUA score aids assessment for ablation (see appendix) ▶ cryoablation allows real-time image-guided assessment of ablation zone (cf. RFA), but is more prone to bleeding (no coagulant effect) ▶ care has to be taken to avoid damage to renal pelvis/surrounding non-renal structures
- **Embolization:** preoperative embolization is less popular than in the past ▶ can be used to control symptomatic haemorrhage if the patient is not a surgical candidate ▶ distal embolizations are preferred as parasitic supplies from other vessels (e.g. lumbar arteries) is common ▶ can use polyvinyl alcohol/glue/Onyx
- **CT limitations:**
  - It has a limited accuracy in differentiating T2 from early T3a disease (this is only important clinically if nephron-sparing surgery is being considered)
  - CT is limited at predicting nodal involvement (with an accuracy of 83–89%): using 1 cm as an upper limit of normal, nodal micrometastases are missed in 4% of patients ▶ false-positive nodes can be due to reactive hyperplasia
  - Perinephric stranding is seen in T3 disease (tumour) but can also be seen with T1 and T2 disease (due to any associated oedema, vascular engorgement or fibrosis)

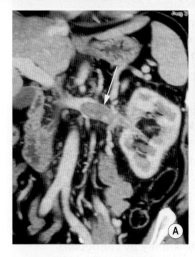

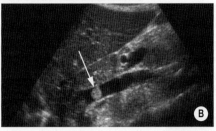

Advanced renal cell carcinoma. (A) Coronal CECT demonstrates tumour thrombus extending into the left renal vein but not into the cava (arrow). (B) US in a different patient shows tumour as a soft tissue nodule of intermediate echogenicity within the IVC (arrow).[†]

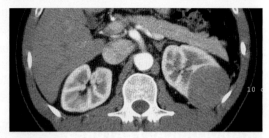

Papillary carcinoma. CECT demonstrates a large poorly enhancing homogeneous mass seen in the left kidney.*

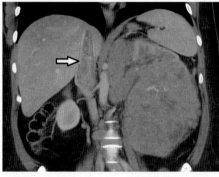

T3b Renal cell carcinoma. Coronal post-contrast CT demonstrates tumour thrombus extending into the right renal vein and the cava (see arrow) (radiological stage T3b).**

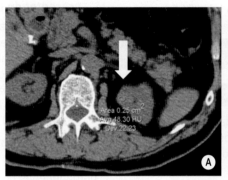

Renal cell carcinoma on CT in a 71-year-old man. (A) There is a cortical-based left upper pole renal mass (arrow) which has attenuation of 48 HU on unenhanced CT within a region of interest placed over the lesion. This alone is suspicious for a solid lesion. (B) Following intravenous contrast administration, the lesion (arrow) measures 75 HU, indicating definitive enhancement and suggesting renal neoplasm.**

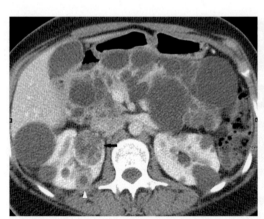

Von Hippel–Lindau and renal tumours. Single-phase post-contrast CT demonstrates multiple renal and pancreatic cysts in a patient with known von Hippel–Lindau. There is a cystic RCC in the mid pole of the right kidney (see arrow), which was subsequently removed at open partial nephrectomy. There is a further smaller mass in the posterior aspect of the right kidney (see arrowhead).**

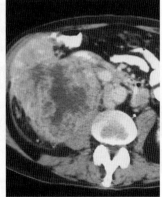

Right renal cell carcinoma invading the psoas muscle and anterior abdominal wall.[†]

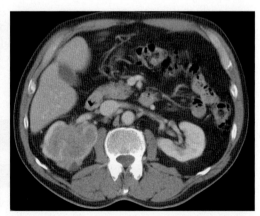

Chromophobe tumour. Post-contrast CT demonstrates a large enhancing right renal mass which was confirmed following nephrectomy as a chromophobe renal cancer. The appearances are indistinguishable from that of a clear cell cancer. Chromophobe tumours have a better prognosis than clear cell carcinoma.**

ONCOCYTOMA

DEFINITION

- This arises from the epithelial cells of the proximal tubule (the oncocyte) ▶ It was previously considered benign, but it is now known that it can metastasize ▶ as they can mimic a RCC they require surgical resection

RADIOLOGICAL FEATURES

US Usually a solitary and unilateral solid isoechoic mass (1–20 cm) internal echoes ▶ a stellate hypoechoic centre (due to a necrotic centre with tumours >5 cm)

CT A well-defined solid mass (± a low attenuation central scar) ▶ an apparent pseudocapsule (compression of adjacent renal tissue) ▶ it may extend into and engulf perinephric fat ▶ good enhancement (except the central scar) ▶ CT cannot accurately distinguish from RCC

SARCOMA

DEFINITION

- A rare, solid, malignant tumour originating from mesenchymal cells (usually a leiomyosarcoma)
- It tends to metastasize haematogenously – lymphadenopathy is uncommon

RADIOLOGICAL FEATURES

- Non-specific imaging features make distinction from a renal cell carcinoma difficult:
  - A large renal mass invading the renal vein and IVC ▶ early metastases are common
  - *Its location may give a diagnostic clue:* close to the renal capsule, the wall of intrarenal blood vessels, or the renal pelvis
- It tends to metastasize haematogenously – lymphadenopathy is uncommon

LYMPHOMA

DEFINITION

- *Primary lymphoma of the kidney:* this is very rare (no lymphatic tissue is present within the kidneys)
- *Secondary lymphoma:* due to haematogenous spread or contiguous invasion from adjacent retroperitoneal lymphadenopathy ▶ the kidneys are much more frequently involved in non-Hodgkin's lymphoma (particularly if the disease has relapsed)

RADIOLOGICAL FEATURES

- *The commonest pattern (60%) is multiple masses (a solitary renal mass is only seen in 15% and may be indistinguishable from an RCC)*

US Hypoechoic renal deposits without posterior acoustic enhancement

NECT Well-defined homogeneous iso- or hypo-attenuating masses ▶ significant regional adenopathy is usually seen (± associated hydronephrosis)

CECT A 'density reversal pattern': a lesion is more dense than the surrounding renal parenchyma before contrast medium administration and less dense thereafter

MRI T1WI: intermediate SI ▶ T2WI: intermediate-to-low SI ▶ STIR: high SI

- *Direct infiltration of the kidney by contiguous retroperitoneal nodal masses is the 2nd commonest presentation (25%)*

CT/MRI Associated encasement of renal vessels and extension into the renal hilum and sinus (it may resemble a TCC) ▶ occasionally soft tissue mass(es) can be seen within the perirenal space (which may encase the kidney without any evidence of parenchymal invasion)

- *Diffuse renal infiltration (resulting in global enlargement) is the least common presentation*

US Diffuse renal enlargement (uniformly hypoechoic)

CT The normal parenchymal enhancement is replaced by homogeneous non-enhancing tissue

PEARL

- **Leukaemia:** diffuse bilateral symmetrical renal enlargement ▶ loss of the normal renal architecture

TUMOURS METASTATIC TO THE KIDNEY

DEFINITION

- Metastases are due to haematogenous (most common), direct or lymphatic spread
  - *Commonest primary tumours:* melanoma ▶ bronchus ▶ colorectal ▶ breast ▶ testicular ▶ gynaecological

RADIOLOGICAL FEATURES

- Haematogenous metastases are usually small (<3 cm), multiple and confined to the renal cortex ▶ hypovascular ▶ renal vein invasion is atypical ▶ usually more infiltrative and less exophytic than an RCC
- Diffuse infiltration can be seen with bronchial SCC

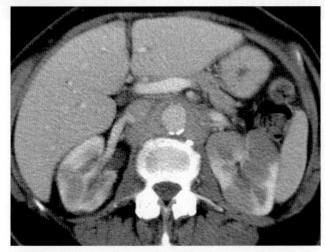

Lymphoma of the kidney. Post-contrast CT demonstrates multifocal solid masses in both kidneys with para-aortic nodal disease highly suggestive of lymphoma. Biopsy of the renal mass is required to confirm and characterize before treatment, which will not be surgical.**

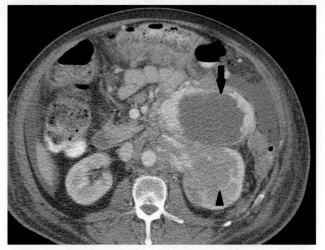

RCC and lymphoma. Post-contrast CT demonstrates a complex left renal mass. There is an irregular hypervascular mass in the upper pole of the left kidney (see arrow), as well as a poorly enhancing soft-tissue mass in the lower pole (see arrowhead). Incidental para-aortic nodes were seen. Biopsy of both components was performed, confirming the presence of a clear cell carcinoma in the upper pole and a lymphoma of the lower pole. There was no previous history of lymphoma. Following chemotherapy, the lower pole renal mass responded, as did the nodal disease. Nephrectomy was performed for the clear cell carcinoma of the upper pole.**

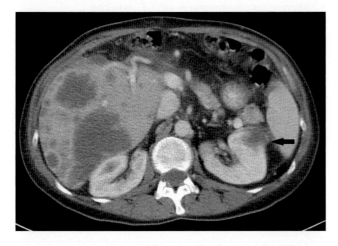

Metastatic disease to the kidney. Post-contrast CT in a patient with advanced metastatic cholangiocarcinoma demonstrates multiple metastases to the liver with a similar metastatic deposit in the left kidney (see arrow). Renal metastases in advanced metastatic disease are not uncommon, but are rarely clinically significant.**

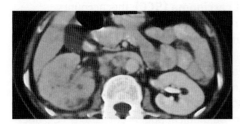

Renal sarcoma. CECT showing an expanded kidney with areas of tumour enhancing to a lesser degree than normal renal tissue

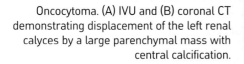

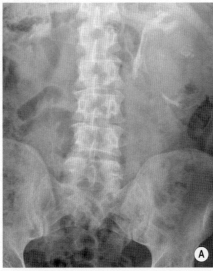

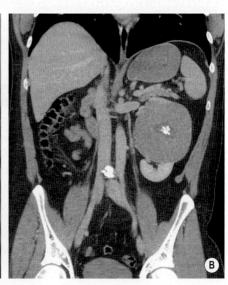

Oncocytoma. (A) IVU and (B) coronal CT demonstrating displacement of the left renal calyces by a large parenchymal mass with central calcification.

TRANSITIONAL CELL CARCINOMA OF THE UPPER URINARY TRACT

DEFINITION

- Transitional cell carcinoma (TCC) originates from the transitional epithelium of the renal pelvis and ureter
- Urothelial carcinoma (90%)
  - *Other types:* squamous cell ▶ adenocarcinoma ▶ carcinocarcinoma ▶ small cell carcinoma ▶ papilloma
- Similar tumours arise from the transitional epithelium of the bladder
  - *Location:* upper tracts: 10% ▶ bladder: 90%
  - *Usual grade at diagnosis:* upper tracts: high ▶ bladder: low
  - *Invasive at diagnosis:* upper tracts: 60% ▶ bladder: 15%
- Similar risk factors exist for all TCCs (smoking or exposure to chemicals containing aromatic hydrocarbons)
- It accounts for 90% of renal pelvic tumours, although overall they are much less commonly seen than a renal cell carcinoma (accounting for <10% of all renal tumours) ▶ synchronous and metachronus TCCs are common
- The extrarenal pelvis is the commonest location (cf. the infundibulocalyceal region) ▶ ureteric tumours are most commonly seen in the lower $\frac{1}{3}$ of the ureter and are least commonly seen within the upper $\frac{1}{3}$ of the ureter
- Early tumours are confined to the collecting system, but with disease progression they can extend into the renal parenchyma and the retroperitoneum ▶ IVC and renal vein invasion is uncommon ▶ haematogenous metastases are rare but lymph node spread is common:
  - *Regional nodes for the renal pelvis:* renal hilar, paracaval, aortic and retroperitoneal nodes
  - *Regional nodes for the ureter:* renal hilar, iliac, paracaval, periureteral and pelvic nodes
  - *Distant metastases:* liver, lung and bone

CLINICAL PRESENTATION

- It is commonly seen during the 6th and 7th decades (3M:1F) ▶ frank haematuria ▶ abdominal pain ▶ abnormal urine cytology

RADIOLOGICAL FEATURES OF TCC

- **Ureteric TCC:** 75% are unilateral
  - **IVU/CTU:** a sessile or polypoidal intraluminal filling defect with surrounding ureteric dilatation ▶ cupping of the contrast medium around the upper or lower convex margin of a lesion ▶ contiguity of the lesion with the ureteric wall ▶ a stippled appearance caused by contrast material entering the interstices of the tumour ▶ strictures (± proximal obstruction)
- **TCC within a calyx:** it may obstruct only a portion of the kidney

- **CT:** an iso- or hypodense ill-defined tumour mass or wall thickening visible against the low inherent urine density ▶ invasion of the renal sinus or parenchyma (± an associated hydrocalyx, oncocalyx, PUJ obstruction or hydronephrosis) ▶ if large enough a TCC can obliterate the renal sinus fat (which is not seen with an RCC) ▶ calcification within a tumour is rare ▶ there is poor enhancement
- **CTU:** opacification of the collecting system improves the conspicuity of a TCC (and is seen as a filling defect)
- *Differential:* thrombus (denser than renal parenchyma with no enhancement) ▶ calculi (most are >200 HU) ▶ fungus ball or sloughed papilla (which may be dependent) ▶ pyeloureteritis cystica

PEARLS

- **Suggested imaging protocol:**
  - *Microscopic haematuria:* no CT required
  - *Macroscopic haematuria, <45 years:* USS first, if negative then CTKUB. If this is also negative for stone disease as a cause for haematuria, then proceed to CTIVU
  - *Macroscopic haematuria, >45 years:* CTIVU
  - *Upper tract surveillance for TCC:* CTIVU
- **Treatment:** open or laparoscopic nephroureterectomy (if resectable) ± bladder cuff – due to the risk of tumour recurrence within the remaining tissues
  - *Endoscopic management:* solitary kidney ▶ bilateral synchronous tumours ▶ renal insufficiency ▶ comorbid disease
  - *Regional lymphadenectomy:* inconclusive evidence at present
  - *Chemotherapy:* no proven effect
- **TNM staging:** see Section 9
- **Squamous cell carcinoma (SCC):** this accounts for 5–10% of all renal pelvic tumours (and a smaller percentage of ureteric tumours) ▶ it tends to occur in older patients and carries a poor prognosis
  - It is associated with chronic irritation of the urothelium (metaplasia), as seen with leukoplakia, calculi and schistosomiasis infection
  - It has similar radiological appearances to a TCC but is more aggressive in nature – often involving the renal parenchyma and perinephric tissues with metastases at presentation
  - **Hereditary nonpolyposis colon cancer (HNPCC) syndrome:** an autosomal dominant condition that is associated with a high incidence of tumours of the renal pelvis, ovaries and small bowel (together with colorectal cancer)

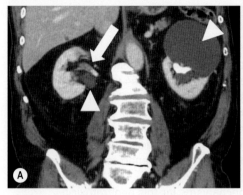

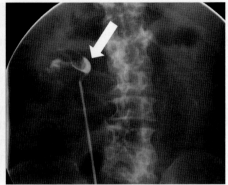

Transitional cell carcinoma of renal collecting system. (A) There is a hypoenhancing mass (arrow) in the upper pole collecting system of the right kidney on CT urography obtained in the nephropyelographic phase by split bolus technique. There are parapelvic cysts in both kidneys (arrowheads). (B) There is a smooth filling defect (arrow) in the upper pole collecting system producing a phantom calyx appearance on retrograde pyelography.**

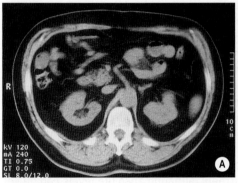

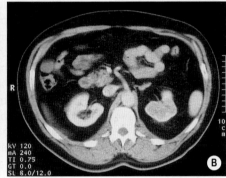

Infiltrating left upper pole TCC with similar density to normal renal tissue and obliterating the sinus fat (A) and enhancing less than normal renal tissue (B).†

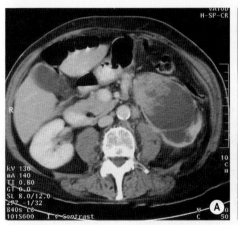

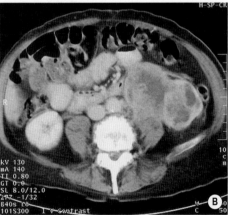

Squamous cell carcinoma developing within a chronic hydronephrosis (A). The tumour has extended out of the collecting system and is invading the psoas muscle (B).†

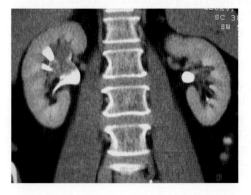

Transitional cell tumour seen on a coronal reformat CT urogram.*

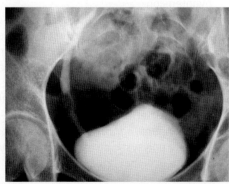

Transitional cell tumour seen on an IVU as a filling defect in the distal ureter.*

437

RENAL FAILURE

DEFINITION

- Acute or chronic renal impairment due to many causes:
  - Renal tract obstruction
  - Autosomal dominant polycystic kidney disease (ADPKD)
  - Tuberous sclerosis (there are multiple renal cysts indistinguishable from autosomal dominant polycystic kidney disease)
  - Acquired cystic kidney disease (ACKD)
  - Renovascular disease
  - Contrast medium nephrotoxicity

RADIOLOGICAL FEATURES

US/NECT/MRI This can demonstrate any underlying cause (e.g. obstruction or ADPKD)
- **US:** this is the first-line investigation, demonstrating increased parenchymal reflectivity and an increased intrarenal arterial resistive index
  - *Chronic renal failure:* small kidneys with cortical thinning

99mTc-MAG3 dynamic radionuclide renography This is the simplest and safest way to assess renal perfusion in patients with renal failure, helping to differentiate reversible causes (e.g. ATN) from other conditions with a poorer prognosis (e.g. cortical necrosis)
- *ATN:* relatively good renal perfusion is maintained, even in the presence of anuria or severe oliguria ▶ however little or no excretion is seen
- *Obstruction:* renal perfusion is maintained
- *Acute renal failure due to intrinsic parencyhmal disease or major vessel obstruction:* perfusion is severely impaired or absent

High-dose IVU This is not often performed (having been replaced by other imaging modalities)
- *Immediate faint persistent nephrogram:* proliferative or necrotizing disorders (e.g. acute glomerulonephritis) ▶ renal vein thrombosis ▶ chronic severe ischaemia
- *Immediate distinct persistent nephrogram:* acute tubular necrosis ▶ acute-on-chronic renal failure ▶ acute hypotension
- *Increasingly dense nephrogram:* acute obstruction ▶ acute hypotension ▶ acute tubular necrosis ▶ acute pyelonephritis ▶ renal vein thrombosis ▶ acute glomerulonephritis ▶ acute papillary necrosis
- *Rim nephrogram:* severe hydronephrosis ▶ acute complete arterial occlusion (due to cortical perfusion by capsular arteries)
- *Striated nephrogram:* acute ureteric obstruction ▶ infantile polycystic disease ▶ medullary sponge kidney ▶ acute pyelonephritis.

PEARLS

Contrast medium nephrotoxicity

- This is defined as a rise (which is usually reversible) in the serum creatinine by >25% or 44 μmol/L during the first 3 days following the administration of IV contrast medium (for which there is no other explanation)
  - Although there are a number of risk factors for contrast medium nephrotoxicity, there is no evidence that IV contrast media are nephrotoxic to patients with normal renal function
- There are 2 mechanisms for this nephrotoxicity:
  - The vasoactive substances endothelin and adenosine lead to a decreased renal blood flow
  - High osmolality contrast media cause a marked diuresis with excretion of increased amounts of sodium – this activates the tubuloglomerular feedback mechanism, leading to vasoconstriction of the afferent arterioles and a reduction of the GFR
- A recent estimated glomerular filtration rate (eGFR) level should be available for all patients with a history of renal disease or diabetes, and for all patients undergoing an angiographic procedure
  - Generally an eGFR < 60 ml/min/1.73 m^2 indicates renal impairment, although absolute levels can be set locally
- Try and avoid using iodinated contrast media with impaired renal function ▶ if it is necessary use the following steps:
  - Ensure the smallest dose possible is used
  - Ensure the patient is well hydrated pre- and post-procedure
  - Consider using an iso-osmolar non-ionic dimeric contrast agent (e.g. iodixanol – 'Visipaque')
- There is insufficient evidence to suggest that any pharmacological treatment will reduce the incidence of contrast-induced nephropathy
- **Metformin:** if the serum creatinine is normal (or eGFR 60 ml/min/1.73 m^2) there is no need to stop metformin following contrast administration ▶ if the serum creatinine is elevated (or eGFR <60 ml/min/1.73 m^2) then metformin may need to be discontinued for 48 hours post-contrast administration
- **Pregnancy:** iodinated contrast may be used in exceptional circumstances ▶ no special precautions are required regarding breastfeeding

Nephrogenic systemic fibrosis
- Gadolinium administration in renal failure can lead to nephrogenic systemic fibrosis – a systemic condition primarily affecting the skin (skin thickening/flexion contractures/parasthesia/pruritus)

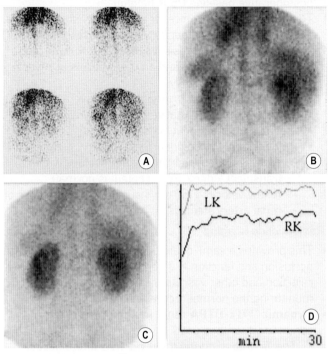

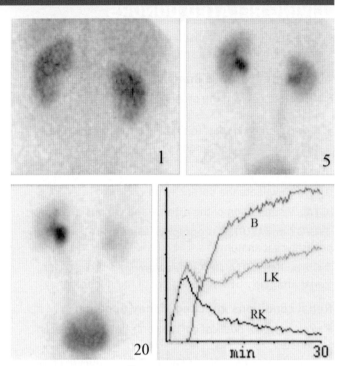

Acute tubular necrosis. ^{99m}Tc-MAG3 study shows perfusion of both kidneys is reduced (A) and excretion images at 1 min (B) and 20 min (C) show persistent retention of the tracer in the kidney with no excretion. Renogram curves (D) show immediate uptake but no clearance. LK, left kidney ▶ RK, right kidney.[†]

Low-grade obstruction. ^{99m}Tc-MAG3 diuretic study images at 1, 5 and 20 min show normal uptake and clearance on the right ▶ normal uptake on the left but incomplete clearance. Renogram curves (bottom right) show normal right side and normal uptake on the left but after an initial fall the excretion curve rises again. B, bladder ▶ LK, left kidney ▶ RK, right kidney.[†]

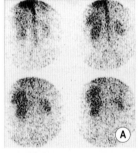

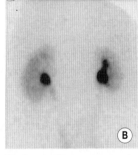

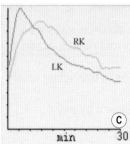

Right renal artery stenosis. ^{99m}Tc-MAG3 dynamic study shows reduced blood flow to the smaller right kidney on the perfusion series (A), delayed excretion on the 15-min image (B), and the renogram curve (C) shows reduced uptake, delayed Tmax, and slower clearance from the right kidney. LK, left kidney ▶ RK, right kidney.[†]

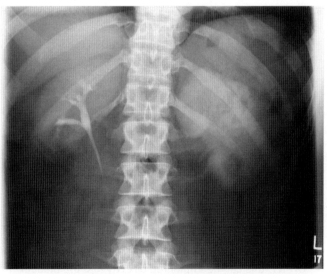

Dense nephrogram with delay in appearance of contrast in the left collecting system characteristic of high-grade obstruction.[†]

PREOPERATIVE INVESTIGATION OF LIVING RELATED DONORS

- Live-related renal transplantation accounts for a minority of UK renal transplants

Aims of preoperative imaging

- *Donor:* to confirm the presence of a normal contralateral kidney
- *Transplanted kidney:* to exclude a major abnormality and outline its vascular anatomy

Investigations

US To evaluate the parenchyma

CTA Visualization of the arterial and venous anatomy

IVU/CT and IVU/MR urography Demonstration of the pelvicalyceal anatomy

^{51}Chromium-EDTA GFR measurement + ^{99m}Tc-DMSA renal imaging GFR assessment of the donor kidney

Renal conditions affecting kidney donation

- *Pelvicalyceal duplication:* the contralateral kidney is donated
- *A solitary renal cyst or unilateral mild reflux nephropathy (with only one scar):* the ipsilateral kidney is donated
- *Accessory renal arteries (20%):* these are technically more difficult to transplant and vascular complications more likely ▶ a single renal artery with very proximal branching is also difficult to transplant

Surgical technique

- The transplant kidney is placed extraperitoneally within the recipient's iliac fossa
  - Usually a right kidney is placed within the left iliac fossa (and vice versa) as these permit easier vascular anastomoses ▶ this results in the renal pelvis lying anteriorly and the vessels posteriorly
- *Renal artery:*
  - *Cadaveric kidney:* an aortic patch (Carrel patch) is removed together with the renal artery and anastomosed to the external iliac artery
  - *Live donor kidney:* the renal artery is anastomosed (end-to-side) to the external iliac artery ▶ it is occasionally anastomosed to the internal iliac artery (end-to-end)
- *Renal vein:* this is anastomosed (end-to-side) to the external iliac vein
- *Ureter:* this can be implanted directly into the bladder – a submucosal tunnel will reduce the incidence of vesicoureteric reflux ▶ rarely a uretero-ureteric anastomosis is performed

POSTOPERATIVE INVESTIGATION OF THE TRANSPLANTED KIDNEY

US

- This will assess any pelvicalyceal system dilatation ▶ the pelvicalyceal system is normally mildly dilated during the early postoperative period (therefore an early postoperative baseline US is helpful)
- The investigation of choice for renal artery stenosis
  - *Power and colour Doppler:* permits assessment of the vascularity and resistive index (RI) ▶ it can also assess the interlobar and arcuate vessels at several levels within the kidney
  - *A normal transplant artery:* this will have a similar spectral pattern to a native renal artery with flow maintained throughout diastole
  - *An abnormal transplant artery:*
    - RI >0.8 (although slightly high RI values within a transplant kidney are accepted as normal)
    - A flow velocity >150 cm/s suggests the presence of renal artery stenosis

Radionuclide imaging

- This provides a semi-quantitative evaluation of the graft perfusion and function ▶ it permits early detection of rejection and other vascular complications as well as monitoring the normal recovery from ATN
- **Dynamic ^{99m}Tc-DTPA renal imaging:** this is the commonest method used
  - *The 'first pass' during the initial 30 s after injection:* multiple dynamic 5 s images will demonstrate the renal perfusion and allow the construction of a renal perfusion index from the renal and iliac vessel time–activity curves
  - *Between 80 and 180 s after injection:* as tracer is filtered into the glomeruli, the uptake is an index of renal function
  - *Up to 20 min after injection:* tracer concentration should decrease within the renal parenchyma, appearing within the collecting system at 5 min and subsequently draining into the bladder ▶ a normal examination will exclude obstruction or the extravasation of urine

CT

- This can guide interventional procedures

DSA

- Indications:
  - *Renal artery stenosis:* this may occur as early as 6 weeks, and presents with abnormal renal function and hypertension
  - *Primary non-function:* this is due to transplant artery occlusion
  - *Severe haematuria:* this can follow a biopsy

MRI

- T1WI + Gad: this will evaluate parenchymal perfusion
- MRA: this will evaluate any renal artery stenosis
- MR-IVU: these heavily T2-weighted sequences can evaluate the collecting system

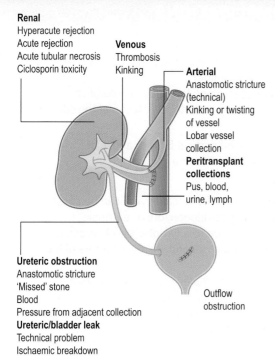

Renal
Hyperacute rejection
Acute rejection
Acute tubular necrosis
Ciclosporin toxicity

Venous
Thrombosis
Kinking

Arterial
Anastomotic stricture
(technical)
Kinking or twisting
of vessel
Lobar vessel
collection

**Peritransplant
collections**
Pus, blood,
urine, lymph

Ureteric obstruction
Anastomotic stricture
'Missed' stone
Blood
Pressure from adjacent collection

Ureteric/bladder leak
Technical problem
Ischaemic breakdown

Outflow
obstruction

Possible postoperative problems encountered
with a renal transplant.[†]

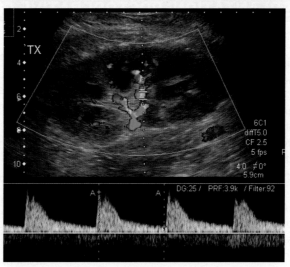

24D Normal spectrum from the interlobar renal artery
within a transplanted kidney, demonstrating good end
diastolic flow (EDF) with a vertical systolic upstroke.©28

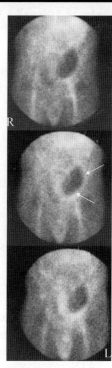

Acute oliguria after renal transplantation. Anterior
view dynamic images 2, 5 and 10 min after injection
of ⁹⁹ᵐTc-DTPA show a photon-deficient area (arrows)
which represents the totally ischaemic graft in the
left iliac fossa. Diagnosis: renal vein thrombosis.[†]

Imaging findings in primary non-function*			
Imaging technique	**ATN**	**RVT**	**RAT**
US	Good arterial and venous flow	No venous flow	No venous flow, no arterial flow
US Doppler	Normal arterial and venous flow due to a swollen kidney	Damped systolic peak with reverse arterial flow in diastole	Very late – no flow
⁹⁹ᵐTc-DTPA blood flow	Good	Photon-deficient area	Photon-deficient area
⁹⁹ᵐTc-DTPA filtration	Moderate	Very poor	Nil
⁹⁹ᵐTc-DTPA transit	Very slow and progressive	Often normal	Nil
ATN, acute tubular necrosis ▶ RVT, renal vein thrombosis ▶ RAT, renal artery thrombosis.			

Imaging findings with a rising creatinine in renal transplants*			
Imaging technique	**Rejection**	**Ciclosporin toxicity**	**Obstruction**
US	Good arterial and venous flow	Good arterial and venous flow	Dilatation of the calyces, pelvis and ureter
⁹⁹ᵐTc-DTPA blood flow	Reduced markedly	Moderate reduction	Normal
⁹⁹ᵐTc-DTPA filtration	Moderate reduction	Reduced markedly	Normal or reduced
⁹⁹ᵐTc-DTPA transit	Slow, but isotope seen	Slow with retention	Slow and progressively rising in bladder and parenchyma

RENAL TRANSPLANTATION: POSTOPERATIVE COMPLICATIONS

Rejection

- **Hyperacute rejection:** This is due to circulating antibodies within the recipient at the time of transplantation ▶ it results in immediate graft failure that is evident at surgery and requires immediate removal (imaging plays no role)
- **Acute rejection:** This is mediated through cellular immunity (mismatched HLA) ▶ it usually begins 1 week after transplantation (as the T cells must differentiate prior to rejection)
- **Chronic rejection:** A chronic inflammatory and immune response leading to long-term loss of function and subsequent fibrosis

US

- **Acute rejection:** non-specific graft swelling ▶ loss of corticomedullary differentiation ▶ decreased renal sinus fat echogenicity with a hyperechoic cortex (producing conspicuous pyramids) ▶ reduced diastolic flow within the intrarenal arteries (which is also seen with ATN, ciclosporin toxicity, renal vein thrombosis, acute pyelonephritis and obstruction) ▶ possible flow reversal
- **Chronic rejection:** a small kidney with diffuse parenchymal thinning (often with increased parenchymal reflectivity and loss of corticomedullary differentiation) ▶ reduced patchy cortical perfusion
- An increased RI (>0.8) and loss of corticomedullary differentiation are sensitive but non-specific indicators of graft dysfunction

MRI

- **Acute rejection:** T1WI: increased renal cortical SI (with a resultant loss of corticomedullary differentiation which can also occur with ATN and ciclosporin toxicity)

Radionuclide imaging   Decreased perfusion (± graft swelling)

Acute tubular necrosis (ATN)

- ATN is the commonest cause of early graft failure following almost exclusively cadaveric transplantation (it occurs as a result of graft ischaemia)
  - It is difficult to distinguish from acute rejection (and therefore requires biopsy) ▶ the main role of imaging is the exclusion of any treatable causes

US   Non-specific swelling of the kidney ▶ enlargement of the pyramids and reduced amplitude of the sinus echoes

- **Doppler US:** there is usually normal perfusion, but there can be globally reduced perfusion with severe cases (± reduced intrarenal arterial diastolic flow) ▶ an increased RI (>0.8) and loss of corticomedullary differentiation

Radionuclide imaging   There is an almost normal first-pass perfusion phase, with uptake at 80–180 s

(consisting of a blood pool only with no selective uptake or excretion) ▶ rejection may be identified by a decrease in perfusion (± renal swelling)

- *An acute vascular event:* this may be identified by absent perfusion producing a photopenic focus at the site of the graft

MRI   T1WI: increased cortical SI with a loss of corticomedullary differentiation

Obstruction

- This is seen in up to 10% of cases and can be caused by ureteric strictures, blood clots or extrinsic compression (e.g. due to a lymphocele) ▶ ureteric strictures are usually secondary to ischaemia of the distal ureter
  - Some ureteric strictures can be treated with percutaneous balloon dilatation
  - An RI >0.75 may indicate the presence of obstructive pelvicalyceal dilatation

Urine Leak

- This occurs in up to 5% of transplants (± urinoma) and usually within the first two postoperative weeks
- It commonly involves the distal ureter (which may be subject to early vascular compromise) and the bladder (with a leak from the anterior cystotomy site)

Fluid collections

- *Haematoma or abscess:* this occurs during the early postoperative period
- *Lymphocele:* this occurs 4–8 weeks post surgery

Vascular complications

- **Renal artery occlusion (1%):** This usually occurs within the early postoperative period and is associated with severe acute rejection
- **Renal artery stenosis (≤10%):** This usually affects the anastomosis or proximal donor artery ▶ a late complication
- Signs: renal artery velocity >2.5 m/s ▶ gradient of 2:1 between stenotic and pre-stenotic segment ▶ spectral broadening ▶ downstream turbulence
- **Arteriovenous fistula or pseudoaneurysm formation:** This is usually a complication following a biopsy, antegrade pyelography, or percutaneous nephrostomy
- It is often small and self-limiting, but can give rise to gross haematuria with clot retention or renal ischaemia
- *Diagnosis:* Doppler US ▶ DSA (± embolization)
- **Renal vein thrombosis:** Doppler US will demonstrate absent venous signals and arterial waveform changes (with sharp systolic peaks and retrograde flow during diastole due to the reduced venous outflow)

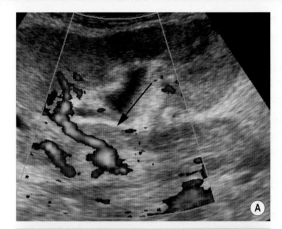

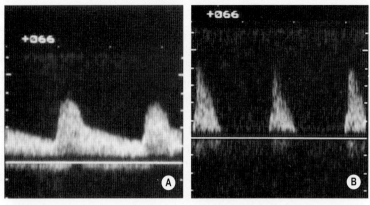

Duplex Doppler US. Spectra obtained from the interlobar arteries in (A) a normal transplant kidney and (B) a transplant kidney undergoing rejection. Note the absent diastolic flow.*

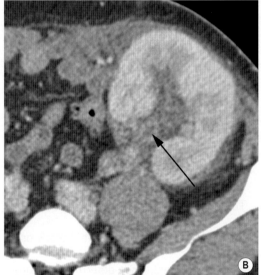

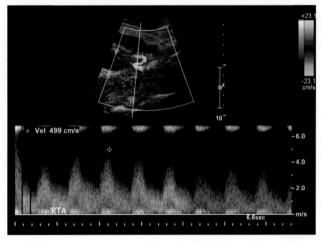

Renal artery stenosis. Doppler US demonstrates abnormality of colour flow, elevated systolic velocities and spectral broadening in the renal transplant artery consistent with a significant artery stenosis.**

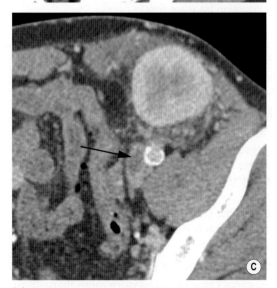

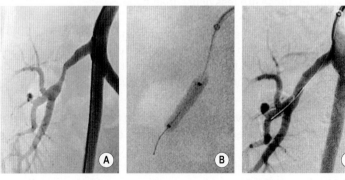

(A) US demonstrating the renal vein travelling from the transplant which is full of echogenic thrombus. This partially extends into the iliac vein. CT images confirming the renal vein thrombosis (B) extending into the iliac vein (C) (arrows).*

Renal transplant stenosis and balloon angioplasty procedure. (A) Injection through a long sheath with the tip in the common iliac artery and the guidewire in the external iliac artery. Note the normal-appearing internal iliac artery to the right and the transplant artery to the left on this left anterior oblique (LAO) 45° view. The ostium of the transplant artery appears normal and there is a severe tubular stenosis in the distal artery just before the renal hilum. (B) After the transplant artery was catheterized and a wire passed through the stenosis, the catheter was exchanged for the balloon catheter. (C) With the guidewire across the stenosis, a post-ballooning injection into the long sheath demonstrates a very satisfactory postangioplasty appearance.*

UROLITHIASIS

Definition

- Stones form when the concentration of two ions in solution exceeds the saturation point
- *Risk factors:* race (with a higher risk for the Caucasian and Asian populations) ▶ diet ▶ occupation ▶ water hardness ▶ a urological anatomical abnormality ▶ urinary stasis
- *Calculi commonly lodge at natural points of narrowing:* the ureteropelvic junction ▶ where the iliac vessels cross the ureter ▶ the ureterovesical junction
- *Bladder calculi:* these occur as a result of stasis (most commonly), infection or the presence of a foreign body ▶ they can also descend from the upper urinary tract
  - *Composition:* a mixture of magnesium, ammonium and phosphate apatite ▶ uric acid mixed with urate

Clinical presentation

- Classically there is acute severe ipsilateral loin-to-groin pain (± nausea and vomiting) ▶ there can also be renal angle tenderness and microscopic haematuria
- Renal impairment at presentation suggests the presence of a complicating factor (e.g. underlying renal disease or septicaemia) ▶ rarely renal failure may be secondary to bilateral obstructing calculi or a calculus within a single functioning kidney
- A delayed presentation is often complicated by infection proximal to an obstructing calculus ▶ matrix calculi are often infected (e.g. *E. coli, Proteus* and *Candida*)

Radiological features

KUB The majority of calcium-containing stones are radio-opaque

- *Oxalate stones:* these are denser than bone
- *Cysteine stones:* these are less dense than bone
- *Uric acid stones:* these are radiolucent
- It has a poor sensitivity due to overlying bowel gas and extrarenal calcification (e.g. pelvic phleboliths) ▶ tomography may improve the detection rate ▶ it is useful for monitoring the progress of stone fragments following ESWL

IVU A dense nephrogram with delayed excretion ▶ a column of contrast may be seen down to the point of obstruction

- The degree of ureteric dilatation is not related to the stone size
- *'Steinstrasse':* this describes a number of calculi that are bunched up in a linear fashion within a ureter (commonly following ESWL)

US An echogenic focus (± acoustic shadowing) ▶ there can be pelvicalyceal or ureteric dilatation

- Stones within the pelvicalyceal system can only be reliably identified if they are greater than 5 mm in size (as small stones are less likely to cast an acoustic shadow) ▶ ureteric stones are poorly visualized unless they are located within the proximal ureter or VUJ
- USS can miss acute obstruction in 30% (it can take hours for hydronephrosis to develop) ▶ physiological hydronephrosis can be seen in pregnancy (R>L)

NECT This is the investigation of choice

- It detects greater than 99% of stones ▶ exceptions include pure matrix stones and stones made of indinavir sulphate
- *Secondary CT signs:* ureteric and collecting system dilatation ▶ nephromegaly ▶ perinephric and periureteric stranding ▶ 'soft tissue rim' sign: pelvic phleboliths will not have a surrounding rim of soft tissue (ureteric wall)
- *Factors influencing the choice between ESWL and PCNL:* stone size ▶ dependency of the relevant calyx and its draining infundibulum
  - Stones that are denser than 1000 HU respond less well to ESWL

Magnetic resonance urography (MRU)

- This is used if other investigations are contraindicated
- It can identify the site of obstruction, but the definitive identification of a stone (seen as a signal void) may be difficult

Scintigraphy This can determine the divided renal function:

- It helps decide between minimally invasive therapy or nephrectomy
- If bilateral stones are present, it can determine the side with better function (to treat first)

Pearls

Treatment

- Spontaneous stone passage: 2–4 mm (76%) ▶ 5–7 mm (60%) ▶ 7–9 mm (48%) ▶ >9 mm (<25%)

Extracorporeal shock wave lithotripsy (ESWL)

- The best results are obtained with renal calculi measuring less than 2.5 cm and composed of calcium oxalate or uric acid ▶ it is also used for upper ureteric stones (cf. ureteroscopy for lower ureteric stones)
- *Contraindications:* clotting anomalies ▶ a high BMI ▶ urinary tract infection ▶ distal obstruction ▶ stenosis of the relevant calyceal neck

Percutaneous nephrolithotomy (PCNL)

- *Indications:* renal calculi that measure more than 2.5 cm ▶ calculi that have not responded to ESWL (or other factors making ESWL technically impossible) ▶ a large calculus (e.g. a staghorn calculus) requiring initial debulking

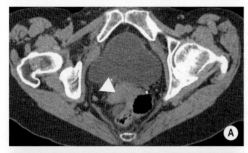

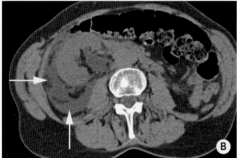

(A) A small calculus is seen at the right VUJ (arrowhead). (B) This has caused proximal obstruction. As a result of the increased pressures, the right pelvicalyceal system has spontaneously ruptured and decompressed the system. A large amount of perinephric urine is now demonstrated (arrows). This does not usually require any further treatment and will resolve spontaneously.

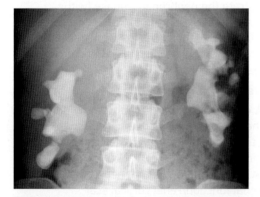

Bilateral staghorn calculi are seen on the control image of an IVU series.*

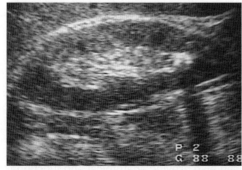

US demonstrating a small solitary renal calculus which is seen as an echogenic focus with marked posterior acoustic shadowing.†

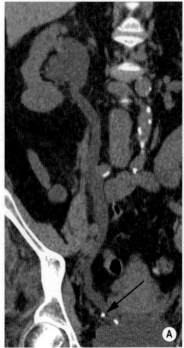

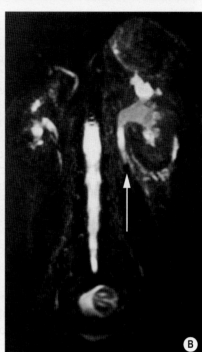

(A) Coronal NECT demonstrating right-sided hydronephrosis and hydroureter. This has been caused by a small calculus (arrow) near the right VUJ. Note the right pelvic phlebolith near the calculus (arrowhead) which could be easily mistaken for a calculus but which in this instance is clearly outside the line of the right ureter. (B) Maximum intensity image from a heavily T2WI (MRU) demonstrates a stone in the proximal left ureter represented as a focus of signal void (arrow). There is associated obstruction and perinephric high SI in keeping with oedema.*

Types of urinary tract stones and their aetiology		
Composition	**Aetiological factors**	**Percentage of all stones**
Calcium oxalate/ calcium oxalate mixed with calcium phosphate	An underlying metabolic disorder (e.g. idiopathic hypercalciuria or hyperoxaluria) ▶ in 25% no metabolic abnormality is identified	75
Struvite or matrix calculi (composed of magnesium ammonium phosphate)	Renal infection	10–15
Uric acid	Hyperuricaemia or hyperuricosuria ▶ it is idiopathic in 50%	6
Cysteine	A renal tubular defect	1–2
Other stones (e.g. xanthine stones, which may be related to a metabolic abnormality, or indinavir stones, which are drug related) are uncommon and account for <5% of all renal stones.		

METHODS OF IMAGING IN OBSTRUCTION

Pathophysiology

- *Acute obstruction:* there is initially a paradoxical increase in renal blood flow (due to afferent arteriolar dilatation mediated by prostaglandin release) ▶ 3–5 h later there is afferent arteriolar vasoconstriction (with reduced renal blood flow)
  - Permanent renal damage commences 4–7 days later (which is complete and unrecoverable by 6 weeks)
- *Chronic obstruction:* a reduction or increase in the renal size ▶ dilatation of the collecting system ▶ a normal or reduced nephrogenic phase ▶ parenchymal loss

Radiological features

IVU *Obstructive nephrogram:* an increasingly dense nephrogram (lasting up to 24 h with a peak density at 6 h) ▶ this is seen with acute obstruction and only in kidneys with normal renal blood flow, GFR and tubular function

- *Delayed contrast excretion:* the delay in contrast excretion depends on the degree of obstruction
- *Ureteric or pelvicalyceal dilatation:* this may be minimal during the first few days
- *Heterotopic excretion:* this is due to vicarious excretion of contrast media into the gallbladder
- *Spontaneous pyelosinus extravasation:* it may produce symptom relief

US This is an excellent method of detecting obstruction – however is does not provide functional information and it can be difficult to distinguish a prominent extrarenal pelvis from mild hydronephrosis ▶ false-negative results may arise if there is a large staghorn calculus

- There may not be hydronephrosis visible in very early obstruction
- Dilatation of the pelvicalyceal system is a poor indicator of the severity of obstruction (the absence of dilatation does not exclude obstruction)
  - Grade I: minimal calyceal dilatation
  - Grade II: mild hydronephrosis
  - Grade III: moderate hydronephrosis
  - Grade IV: severe hydronephrosis
- **Doppler US:**
  - *Colour Doppler:* an absent vesicoureteric jet is seen with acute obstruction
  - *An elevated resistive index (>0.7):* this can be seen with obstruction ▶ the RI can help differentiate between pregnancy-related ureteric dilatation and mechanical obstruction

CT

- **NECT:** hydronephrosis and hydroureter to the level of the obstruction
- **CECT:**
  - *Acute obstruction:* prolongation of the usually transient, early corticomedullary nephrogram ▶ contrast medium will eventually opacify the medullary pyramids (causing a homogeneously dense nephrogram)
    - *A reverse corticomedullary nephrogram:* if obstruction is unrelieved for several days the medullary pyramids may actually become more densely opacified than the cortex
  - *Chronic obstruction:* hydronephrosis ▶ parenchymal thinning (± a shell or rim nephrogram)
- **CT urography (CTU)**
  - Consider oral hydration ± frusemide infusion ± prone imaging
  - *NECT:* this will demonstrate any calcification within the renal tract
  - Nephrographic phase: 80–100 s delay ▶ highest sensitivity for renal parenchymal masses
  - Excretory phase: 5–15 min after contrast injection
  - *'Split dose' imaging:* 'split dose imaging' can reduce dose
    - Approximately 50% of the IV contrast medium load is administered ▶ imaging is then performed at approximately 5–15 min after injection (this demonstrates the urographic phase with opacification of the pelvicalyceal systems and ureters)
    - Just prior to imaging (approximately 100 s) the remaining contrast bolus is administered ▶ therefore these images will also concurrently demonstrate the nephrogenic phase (with enhancement of the parenchyma)
    - a disadvantage of this technique is that ureteric contrast may obscure subtle iso-attenuating tumours not seen on NECT

Radionuclide radiology

- **⁹⁹ᵐTc-DTPA or MAG-3 diuresis renography:** this will usually help to distinguish obstructive from non-obstructive dilatation, and will localize the site of any obstruction
- **⁹⁹ᵐTc-DMSA renography:** this can measure the differential renal function/renal cortical scar detection
  - Measurement of individual renal function while the kidney is obstructed may underestimate the amount of recoverable function

MR urography (MRU) Consider oral hydration ± frusemide infusion ± prone imaging

- **A heavily weighted T2 sequence:** this is akin to an MRCP and can demonstrate the urine-filled ureter (adequate distension can be achieved with IV hydration and the use of a diuretic) ▶ it can be used in poorly functioning hydronephrotic kidneys
- **An excretory MR:** this uses a gadolinium contrast agent and T1WI ▶ it can also provide anatomical and functional information about the kidney

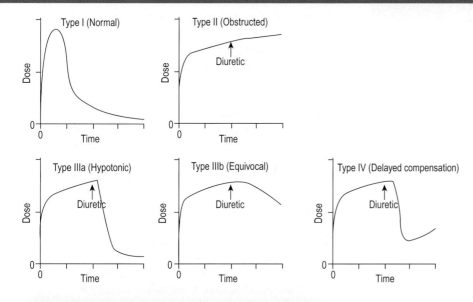

Type I (Normal)
Type II (Obstructed) — Diuretic
Type IIIa (Hypotonic) — Diuretic
Type IIIb (Equivocal) — Diuretic
Type IV (Delayed compensation) — Diuretic

Type I – Normal Normal uptake with prompt washout. Rapid rise in curve, peaks at 2–5 min, with a normal rapid washout (curve falls quickly). **Type II – Obstructed** Rising uptake curve, no response to diuretic (i.e. curve continues to rise [obstruction]). Anything but an exponentially falling curve could be considered evidence of obstruction. Beware false positive – dehydration, poor renal function, massive dilatation, bladder effect. **Type IIIa – Hypotonic** An initially rising curve which falls rapidly in response to diuretic (non-obstructive dilatation). Dilatation result of stasis rather than obstruction. **Type IIIb – Equivocal** An initially rising curve which neither falls promptly following injection of diuretic nor continues to rise. **Type IV – Delayed compensation (Homsy)** Delayed double peak. The initial washout due to the diuretic is good but the curve flattens or even rises. Flow rate too high for system and obstructs. (Intermittent obstruction).

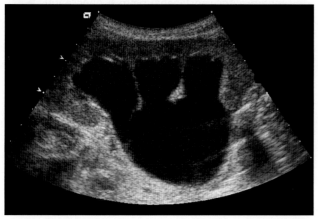

Ultrasound of the kidneys showing hydronephrosis and cortical atrophy.*

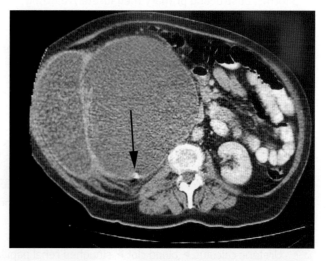

CT of long-standing hydronephrosis of the right kidney with the appearance of a shell nephrogram. The appearance was diagnosed as a PUJ obstruction although nephroureterectomy demonstrated tumour obstructing the distal ureter. An incidental small calculus is also noted in the calyceal system (arrow).*

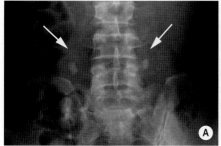
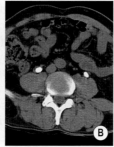
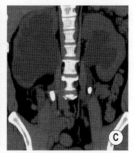

(A) Plain abdominal XR. Bilateral large ureteric calculi (arrows). (B) Unenhanced axial CT at the level of the stones. (C) Coronal multiplanar reformation (MPR) sections demonstrating the same bilateral ureteric calculi with bilateral hydronephrosis and renal atrophy.*

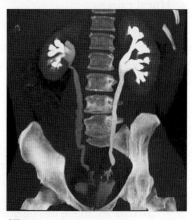

CT urography for ureteric leaks and fistulas. Bilateral lower ureteric leaks following laparoscopic myomectomy.*

447

NON-OBSTRUCTIVE DILATATION OF THE UPPER URINARY TRACT

Vesicoureteric reflux (VUR)   Congenital or acquired incompetence of the VUJ

- Severe reflux may cause massive hydronephrosis ▶ upper tract distension peaks during reflux and is better assessed with a micturating cystogram than an IVU

Postobstructive dilatation   The collecting system often fails to return to its normal calibre after the relief of obstruction

Megacalyces   A congenital non-obstructive dilatation of the calyces, associated with hypoplasia of the medullary pyramids (the renal pelvis and ureter are normal)

- Usually unilateral (and more common in males) ▶ renal *cortical* thickness and function remain normal (cf. postobstructive atrophy)

Polycalycosis   A congenital increase in the number of calyces ▶ renal function remains normal

Primary megaureter   Ureteric dilatation (>7 mm) in the absence of a *mechanical* obstruction and due to deficient musculature (VUR is present in a minority) ▶ a functional obstruction is present

- 3 forms: obstructing primary megaureter/refluxing primary megaureter/non-obstructing non-refluxing primary megaureter
- The consistent abnormality is a relatively normal calibre but non-distensible juxtavesical ureteric segment that fails to transmit peristalsis ▶ absence of a fixed anatomical obstruction is confirmed by unimpeded retrograde passage of a ureteric catheter

MECHANICAL URINARY TRACT OBSTRUCTION

Congenital ureteric obstruction (e.g. ureteric duplication)

Acquired ureteric obstruction

- **Intraluminal causes**
  - Ureteric calculus ▶ blood clot ▶ sloughed renal papilla
- **Mural causes**
  - Urothelial neoplasms ▶ tuberculous ureteritis ▶ schistosomiasis
  - *Radiation ureteritis:*
    - *IVU:* mucosal irregularity ▶ short or long distal ureteric strictures
    - *CT:* IVU findings + thickening and stranding of the ureteric wall
  - *Endometriosis:*
    - This uncommonly affects the urinary tract (bladder > ureter) ▶ ureteric disease is usually extrinsic
    - *MRI:* high T1 and T2 signal seen within the haemorrhagic lesion
  - *Strictures:* these can be postoperative, traumatic or idiopathic

Extrinsic causes

- *Large pelvic tumours:* cervix ▶ ovary ▶ prostate ▶ rectosigmoid ▶ colon
- *Retroperitoneal tumours:* sarcoma ▶ desmoid ▶ metastases ▶ lymphoma (this characteristically displaces and narrows the ureters over lengthy segments)
- *Metastases:* carcinoma of the ovary, cervix, uterus, colon, bladder and prostate may invade the ureters by direct extension or by spread to periureteric lymph nodes ▶ lung, breast, stomach, pancreas and gallbladder metastases tend to cause a marked retroperitoneal desmoplastic reaction (resembling retroperitoneal fibrosis)
- *Strictures:* post surgical ▶ radiotherapy ▶ trauma ▶ ureteric infection
- *Retroperitoneal fibrosis (periaortitis)*
  - A retroperitoneal inflammatory and fibrotic reaction leading to trapping of one or both ureters
    - Causes: idiopathic ▶ aortoiliac surgery ▶ inflammatory aortic aneurysm ▶ pancreatitis ▶ extravasated urine ▶ trauma ▶ radiotherapy ▶ methysergide therapy
  - *CT:* a plaque-like mass surrounding the aorta or iliac arteries (± loss of the fat plane between the mass and psoas muscle) ▶ the mass tends not to displace the aorta anteriorly (cf. lymphoma) ▶ the ureters tend to be displaced medially with narrowing at the L4–5 level
- *Hydronephrosis of pregnancy:*
  - This affects 90% of pregnant women with unilateral or bilateral dilatation of the renal pelvis and ureter by the 3rd trimester ▶ there is usually right-sided ureteric dilatation down to the pelvic brim ▶ it usually resolves postpartum
    - Causes: it is usually due to an enlarging uterus compressing the ureters against the iliac arteries as they enter the pelvis ▶ there may also be decreased ureteric tone (due to maternal hormones)
  - *MR urography:* the investigation of choice for pregnant patients with loin pain
- *Retroperitoneal infection or inflammation:* tuberculosis ▶ fungal adenitis ▶ sarcoidosis ▶ malacoplakia ▶ chronic granulomatous disease
- *Retroperitoneal vasculitis:* Wegener's polyarteritis ▶ Churg–Strauss syndrome
- *Pelvic lipomatosis* (pushing distal ureters medially)
- *Gynaecological causes:* endometriosis ▶ pelvic inflammatory disease ▶ uterine prolapse ▶ hydrocolpos
- *Gastrointestinal causes:* Crohn's disease ▶ diverticulitis ▶ appendicitis ▶ pancreatitis ▶ GI malignancy

Bladder causes of ureteric obstruction

- *Secondary to a scarred contracted bladder:* tuberculosis ▶ schistosomiasis ▶ radiotherapy ▶ interstitial cystitis
- *Benign prostatic hypertrophy*
- *Prostate cancer:* due to local invasion of the bladder base or ureters

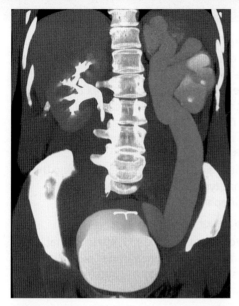

A megaureter predisposes to recurrent urinary tract infections.*

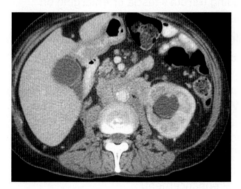

Retroperitoneal fibrosis (periaortitis). There is a concentric soft tissue abnormality surrounding the aorta with obstruction of the left ureter. Differential diagnosis includes lymphoma and retroperitoneal metastases.*

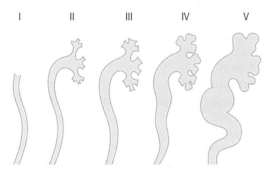

Radiographic grades of reflux. (I) Ureter and upper collecting system without dilatation ▶ (II) mild or (III) moderate dilatation of the ureter and mild or moderate dilatation of the renal pelvis, but no, or only slight, blunting of the fornices ▶ (IV) moderate dilatation and/or tortuosity of the ureter with moderate dilatation of the renal pelvis and calyces and complete obliteration of the sharp angle of the fornices but maintenance of papillary impression in the majority of calyces ▶ (V) gross dilatation and tortuosity of ureters, renal pelvis and calyces ▶ papillary impressions are not visible in the majority of calyces.

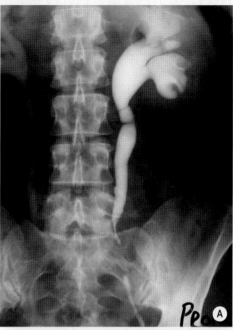

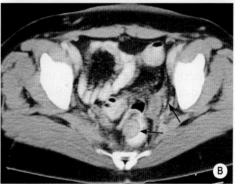

Ureteric endometriosis. (A) IVU demonstrates extrinsic compression in the distal left ureter with proximal ureteric dilatation. (B) CT demonstrates an abnormal soft tissue mass on the left side of the pelvis which is causing ureteric dilatation. There is a similar soft tissue mass of endometriotic tissue surrounding the sigmoid colon.*

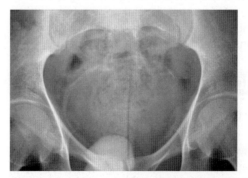

Urinary tract schistosomiasis. The characteristic curvilinear calcification in the bladder wall is seen on the control film of an IVU series.*

449

UPPER URINARY TRACT TRAUMA

DEFINITION

- Renal injury occurs in 8–10% of cases of abdominal trauma
  - Blunt force (90%); penetrating trauma (10%)
- *Segmental renal infarct:* these are relatively common in blunt trauma and result from stretching and subsequent occlusion of a branch of the renal artery, an accessory renal artery, or a capsular artery ▶ as an isolated renal injury they should be considered a non-surgical lesion (Grade 1)
- *Subcapsular renal haematoma:* these are rare (particularly in older adults) as the renal capsule is not easily separated from the cortex ▶ usually this injury will resolve without specific treatment but a large haematoma compressing the kidney to near systolic level pressures may require surgical release of the renal tamponade
  - *Page kidney:* localized ischaemia within the compressed cortex may lead to non-function or the onset of late hypertension
- *Renal lacerations:* these are usually self-limiting injuries, and are typically accompanied by small amounts of perinephric haemorrhage
- *Main renal artery occlusion:* in blunt trauma the kidneys are displaced outward towards the lateral retroperitoneum with consequent stretching of the intima beyond its elastic limit and subsequent dissection ▶ later clot begins to form on and around the disrupted intima leading to partial or complete occlusion (usually between the proximal and middle $\frac{1}{3}$ of the vessel)
- *Renal vein disruption:* this is less common than an arterial injury but it can produce extensive perinephric bleeding (but as the venous pressure is low this is usually limited to the retroperitoneum)
- *Renal pelvis disruption:* this occurs following hyperextension and secondary overstretching of the pelvis ▶ there is gross contrast and urine extravasation near the pelviureteric junction ▶ usually the involved kidney remains intact with limited parenchymal dysfunction

RADIOLOGICAL FEATURES

US A negative examination does not exclude a renal injury

Renal angiography This is not recommended (introduced delay may prevent kidney salvage)

CT of minor renal injury (grades I, II)

- *Contusions:* ill-defined low attenuation areas ▶ a striated nephrographic pattern within the affected area (due to the differential flow through the contused parenchyma)
  - *Delayed imaging:* focal renal parenchymal extravasation

- *Segmental renal infarct:* they appear as sharply demarcated wedge-shaped areas of low attenuation and typically involve the renal pole(s)
- *Subcapsular renal haematoma:* a convex or lenticular blood collection (limited by the renal capsule) which may indent the renal parenchyma ▶ some delay in renal perfusion may be seen secondary to an increased resistance to arterial perfusion
- *Lacerations:* these are superficial (only involving the cortex) ▶ they are typically accompanied by small amounts of perinephric haemorrhage

CT of major renal injury (grade III)

- *Deep renal fractures:* these extend into the renal collecting system with a contained urine leak (urinoma) ▶ urine leaks resolve spontaneously in the majority of cases (particularly if there is unimpeded antegrade urine flow)
- *Large perinephric haematoma:* a high attenuation collection distending Gerota's fascia or enlarging on serial CT studies

CT of catastrophic renal injury (grade IV and V)

- *Renal arterial occlusion:* this can be partial or complete ▶ there will be a lack of renal opacification (cf. the aorta) but there may be peripheral enhancement from collateral vessel perfusion (the 'rim' sign) ▶ there may be a diminished renal size
  - As there is no arterial perfusion, contrast medium within the IVC may retrogradely flow into the renal veins (leading to collecting system opacification without cortical enhancement)
- *Renal pedicle disruption:* there can be extensive perinephric bleeding, which is usually limited to the retroperitoneum
  - Ongoing bleeding into the kidney or surrounding tissue appears as patchy dense contrast material surrounded by less dense clotted blood ▶ typically the attenuation values of extravasated arterial contrast medium is >80 HU (but within <15 HU of an adjacent artery)
- *Renal vein occlusion:* this leads to a delayed and progressively dense nephrogram ▶ venous thrombus/increased renal size
- *Injury to the renal pelvis:* contrast or urine extravasation occurs near the pelviureteric junction ▶ delayed images will show the collection of high density contrast adjacent to the injury ▶ partial disruption of the renal pelvis is suggested if there is opacification of the distal ureter
- *Renal fragmentation:* this may result in a completely fragmented kidney
- *Other features:* an extensive or enlarging perinephric haematoma ▶ a renal pseudoaneurysm ▶ a major arteriovenous communication

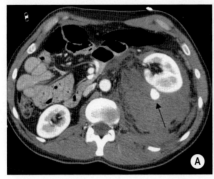
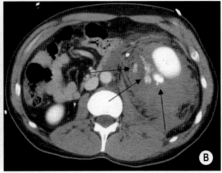

A 22-year-old male victim of motor vehicle collision. Arterial phase MDCT image (A) demonstrates a large left perinephric haemorrhage with an oval focus of high density adjacent to the posterior aspect of the mid-kidney (arrow). Portal venous phase image at the level of the lower pole (B) shows the focus has remained dense and increased in size (arrows), diagnostic of active bleeding.**

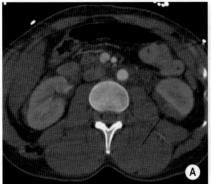
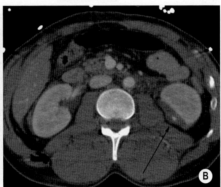

Arterial phase image of contrast-enhanced MDCT of patient who fell demonstrates subcapsular haematoma flattening the posteromedial aspect of left kidney (A). There is a small focus of hyperdensity within the subcapsular haematoma (arrow). Portal venous phase image (B) shows increase in size of focus of hyperdensity (arrow), indicating active bleeding. Note small amount of right perinephric haemorrhage.**

Indications for renal imaging in acute trauma	
Indication	**Imaging study**
Penetrating flank and back trauma	CT chest/abdomen/pelvis with IV and oral contrast medium
Gross haematuria	CT abdomen/pelvis with oral and IV contrast medium if haemodynamically stable or resuscitated
Haemodynamically unstable requiring emergency surgery	Intraoperative IVU when stabilized
Haemodynamically stable with microscopic haematuria, but no other indication for abdominal-pelvic CT	Observation until resolution of haematuria
Haemodynamically stable with microscopic haematuria, but other indications for abdominal-pelvic CT (+abdominal examination, decreasing haematocrit, indeterminate result of peritoneal lavage or abdominal ultrasound, unreliable physical examination)	CT abdomen/pelvis with oral and IV contrast medium
Haemodynamically stable with or without microscopic haematuria with evidence of major flank impact (e.g. a lower posterior rib or lumbar transverse process fracture ▶ major contusion of flank soft tissues)	CT abdomen/pelvis with oral and IV contrast medium

UPPER URINARY TRACT TRAUMA

Pearls

- Microscopic haematuria without hypotension is unlikely to be associated with a major renal injury in adult blunt trauma – however there is some evidence that in the paediatric population microscopic haematuria without hypotension can be associated with a significant renal injury
  - CT is therefore recommended for both gross and microscopic haematuria in children

Suggested CT technique for renal trauma

- Thin section (0.75/1.5 mm) MDCT ▶ images are obtained during the arterial phase with injection triggered at a threshold density of 100 HU within the ascending aorta ▶ this allows for the assessment of renal parenchymal integrity and function, the extent of any perinephric haematoma and if there is any active bleeding
- A delayed CT can be performed at 2–3 min to evaluate for any parenchymal, collecting system, ureteral or bladder injuries

Management

- *Grades I and II (minor) injuries:* these are usually managed conservatively
- *Grade III (major) injuries:*
  - *An infected urinoma:* this can be percutaneously drained under radiological guidance ▶ persistent collecting system leaks are treated with a nephrostomy or a double-J ureteral catheter ▶ surgery may be required if a leak is extensive and is not responding to non-surgical techniques
  - *A perinephric haematoma:* haemorrhage is most likely to occur from a renal arterial branch ▶ if the patient is haemodynamically stable and there are no other injuries then distal embolization of the bleeding site(s) can be performed ▶ if the patient is haemodynamically unstable, then surgery is required
- *Grade IV and V injuries:*
  - *Renal arterial occlusion:* this requires renal revascularization and usually has to be performed within <2 h following the injury (longer delays may be successful if there are adequate collateral vessels or there is only a partial occlusion) ▶ options include immediate nephrectomy/ non-operative management/endovascular or surgical revascularization
  - *Renal pedical disruption:* if the patient is stable, active bleeding sites and post-traumatic pseudoaneurysms, arteriovenous fistulae or arteriocalcyeal communications can be confirmed by selective renal angiography and selectively embolized with Gelfoam pledgets (followed by coils)
  - *Disruption to the ureter or pelviureteric junction:* partial disruptions can be treated with a ureteric stent ▶ complete disruptions require surgery
  - *Renal fragmentation:* this usually requires a nephrectomy

URETERAL INJURY

Definition

- A ureteral injury may involve contusion, a partial tear, or complete disruption
- *Blunt trauma:* injury typically occurs at the pelviureteric junction and is caused by hyperextension with overstretching of the ureter, or compression of the ureter against a lumbar transverse process
- *Penetrating trauma:* these involve the upper ureter in 70% and the distal ureter in 22% ▶ they account for <1% of all penetrating urinary system injuries
- *Iatrogenic injury:* these occur in ≤2.5% of patients undergoing gynaecological surgery for non-malignant conditions ▶ the risk is increased with haemorrhage, endometriosis, uterine enlargement and adhesions
  - *Recognized at surgery:* immediate repair
  - *Delayed presentation:* patients can present with fever, loin pain, fistula formation, infection or obstruction

Radiological features

CT urogram Mild fat stranding or a small amount of adjacent low density fluid around the injury ▶ progressing to contrast accumulating in the peri-ureteric tissues on delayed imaging ▶ a partial (cf. complete) tear is suggested if the distal ureter opacifies

Retrograde pyelography This can document the site and extent peaks and retrograde flow during diastole due to

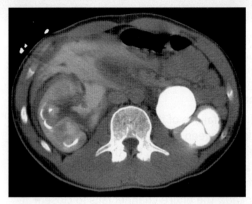

A 24-year-old man involved in motor vehicle collision with bilateral UPJ obstruction. A 10-min delayed image of contrast-enhanced MDCT demonstrates extensive iodinated urine extravasation from injured right collecting system. The left collecting system shows UPJ obstruction without injury.**

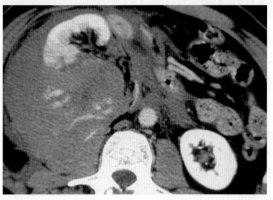

CT of active renal haemorrhage. Multiple foci of active bleeding are seen in the centre of a large perinephric haematoma displacing the kidney markedly anteriorly. There is haemorrhage in both the anterior and posterior pararenal spaces. The posterior part of the kidney is lacerated.*

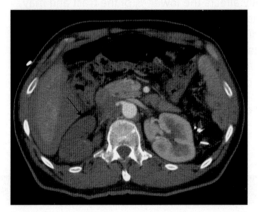

Arterial phase MDCT image of patient involved in motor vehicle collision demonstrates characteristic findings of main renal artery injury. There is abrupt cut-off of the proximal right renal artery with small amount of surrounding haemorrhage, small renal size and lack of perfusion to most of the kidney. Note minimal peripheral renal enhancement (arrow) due to intact collateral capsular vessels (rim sign).**

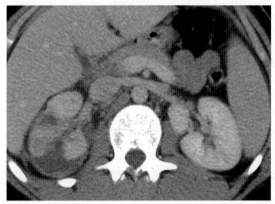

Renal fracture shown on CT. This contrast-enhanced CT of the kidneys in a patient who was in a motor vehicle collision shows a fractured right kidney. There are two lacerations in the right kidney. The fracture more anterior is only a partial-thickness laceration while the more posterior laceration extends through the full thickness of the renal parenchyma, and is therefore a renal fracture.ʃ

Contrast-enhanced spiral CT grading of blunt renal injury	
Injury grade	**Description or CT finding**
I	Superficial laceration(s) involving cortex Renal contusion(s) <1 cm subcapsular haematoma Perinephric haematoma not filling Gerota's space and no active bleeding Segmental renal infarction
II	Deeper renal laceration extending to medulla, with intact collecting system >1 cm subcapsular haematoma with intact renal function Perinephric haematoma limited to and not distending the perinephric space; no active bleeding
III	Laceration extending into collecting system with urine extravasation limited to retroperitoneum Perinephric haematoma distending perinephric space or extending into pararenal spaces; no active bleeding
IV	Fragmentation (three or more segments) of the kidney (usually partially devitalized with large perinephric haematoma) Devascularization >50% of parenchyma Main renal pedicle injury Active bleeding by CT Extravasation of urine into peritoneal cavity or extensive extravasation Subcapsular haematoma compromising renal perfusion

4.2 BLADDER

CONGENITAL ANOMALIES

Bladder agenesis

- A rare condition which is usually associated with absence of the urethra and other congenital abnormalities ▶ there is marked upper tract dilatation and renal dysplasia which is incompatible with life

Bladder hypoplasia (dwarf bladder)

- This is extremely rare and is usually associated with other urinary tract anomalies

Bladder duplication

- Each bladder receives the drainage from an ipsilateral ureter and bladder drainage is via two separate urethras
  - *Incomplete duplication:* the bladders are fused caudally with one draining urethra (associated urinary tract anomalies are less common)
  - *'Hourglass' bladder:* partial or complete bladder division from a sagittal or transverse septum

Bladder diverticula

- *Hutch diverticulum:* a congenital weakness of the bladder wall located near the VUJ (it is usually associated with reflux)
- *Bladder ear:* a diverticulum descending into the internal inguinal ring

- *Acquired diverticula:* these are the result of bladder outlet obstruction (± infection) ▶ they are usually multiple and may contain calculi (25%) or tumour (<5%)

Urachal anomalies

- These result from failure of the normal closure of the communication between the bladder urachus and allantois (which normally forms the median umbilical ligament) ▶ an adenocarcinoma can arise within the urachal remnant
  - *Patent urachus:* the entire channel fails to close ▶ it presents with urine leakage at the umbilicus
    - US/CT/MRI: a fluid-filled tubular structure
  - *Urachal cyst:* the umbilical and bladder ends of the channel are closed but a mid portion remains patent ▶ it usually affects the lower $\frac{1}{3}$ of the tract and may present as a cystic mass on imaging
  - *Urachal diverticulum:* urachal dilatation only involving the bladder component
  - *Urachal sinus:* urachal dilatation only involving the umbilical component

Bladder exstrophy/prune-belly syndrome

- See Section 3 Chapter 12, Paediatric gastrointestinal disorders

INFLAMMATORY DISEASE

Chronic cystitis

- This follows repeated bacterial infections (usually with *E. coli*)
  - *Predisposing factors:* reflux ▶ bladder outlet obstruction ▶ bladder diverticulae

AXR/CT Bladder wall thickening ▶ bladder wall irregularity associated with trabeculation ▶ a diminished bladder capacity

- *Cystitis cystica:* hyperplastic submucosal urothelial cells occurring in response to chronic infection (central necrosis can give a pseudocystic appearance) ▶ it is characterized by granulomatous nodular cystic cavities
- *Cystitis glandularis:* glandular proliferation within the mucosa and lamina propria
  - *'Cobblestone' appearance:* multiple rounded defects seen on the lateral or posterior bladder walls
- *Leukoplakia:* developing squamous metaplasia in response to chronic inflammation ▶ white patches are commonly seen on the trigone and bladder base

Cystitis emphysematosa

- An inflammatory lesion associated with gas vesicles within the bladder wall

AXR/CT

- *'Cobblestone' effect:* small gas-filled vesicles usually seen unilaterally

- Gas within the bladder lumen ▶ gas within the bladder wall and appearing as a 'ring' within the pelvis

Causes of gas within the bladder wall and pneumaturia

- *Instrumentation of the GU tract*
- *Fistula formation between the GI and GU tracts*
- *Emphysematous cystitis:* infection (commonly *E. coli*) in association with diabetes

Fungus ball

- This follows infection with *Candida albicans* and may occur following prolonged antibiotic therapy, protracted use of steroids, immunosuppression, severe debilitating disease, or diabetes

US Echogenic luminal masses (without posterior acoustic shadowing)

NECT High attenuation masses containing internal gas locules (with occasionally gas around them)

CTU Bladder filling defects with contrast occasionally entering the fungus balls

Differential diagnosis Neoplasia ▶ blood clot ▶ cellular debris

Tuberculosis/malacoplakia/schistosomiasis

- See Section 4 Chapter 1, Renal tract infection/inflammation

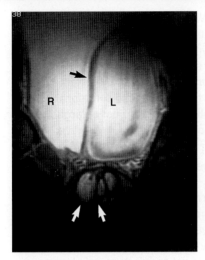

Congenital bladder duplication in a patient with multiple genitourinary anomalies including penis didelphys (white arrows): T2WI. Both right (R) and left (L) urinary bladders are fully distended. The bladder septum (black arrow) is well visualized.*

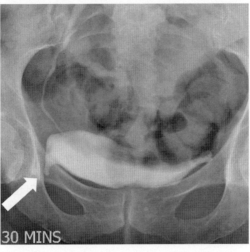

Bladder ear at intravenous urogram in a 61-year-old woman. Pelvic radiograph 30 min following intravenous contrast medium administration demonstrates a bladder ear (arrow).**

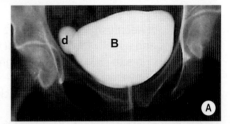

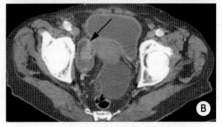

Acquired bladder diverticulum. (A) Voiding cystourethrogram – oblique projection. The urinary bladder (B) has a smooth outline. There is a narrow-necked bladder diverticulum (d). (B) In a different patient a CT demonstrates a large right-sided Hutch diverticulum containing a large tumour (arrow).*

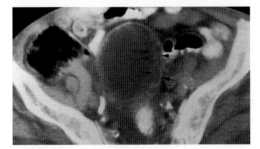

Cystitis cystica. Cystic lesions (arrows) are seen within the thickened bladder wall.*

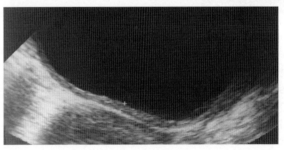

Bladder US shows diffuse thickening of the bladder wall in a patient with dysuria and pyuria.∫

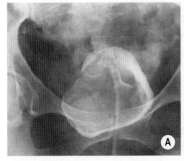

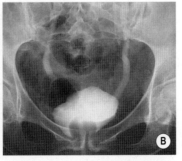

Fulminant haemorrhagic cystitis in a patient with gross haematuria and dysuria. (A) A cystogram demonstrates a large filling defect consistent with a blood clot. (B) An IVU performed 4 weeks later shows nodular thickening of the bladder that has a reduced capacity.∫

BLADDER TUMOURS

Definition

- *Superficial neoplasms* (70–80%) – 70% are papillary tumours and usually low grade ▶ *flat neoplasms* or carcinoma in situ (30%) – typically higher grade and likely to become invasive if untreated
- 20–30% of bladder tumours are muscle invasive at diagnosis
- 70% recur within 3 years (10–20% of these are more aggressive)
  - *Transitional cell carcinoma* (TCC): 90% of all epithelial tumours ▶ 40% will have areas of atypical histology with a worse prognosis
  - *Squamous cell carcinoma* (SCC): 6–10% of all epithelial tumours ▶ it is associated with chronic infection (e.g. schistosomiasis) and bladder calculi ▶ usually high grade at presentation
  - *Adenocarcinoma*: 1% of all epithelial tumours ▶ it is associated with bladder exstrophy and urachal remnants ▶ mucus found in the urine
- **Papillary neoplasm grading:** (1) papillomas ▶ (2) papillary neoplasms of low malignant potential ▶ (3) low-grade tumours ▶ (4) high-grade tumours

Clinical presentation

- Haematuria ▶ dysuria ▶ pelvic pain ▶ hydronephrosis
- Peak incidence: 6th and 7th decades (M>F) ▶ $\frac{1}{3}$ of patients have multifocal disease at presentation
- Urine cytology is not sensitive for superficial tumours

Radiological features

- *Location:* commonly around the region of the trigone or along the lateral bladder walls ▶ bladder diverticula: increased TCC risk (urine stasis), and worse prognosis (not all wall layers are present and earlier spread)

US A sessile or pedunculated mixed echogenicity mass projecting into the bladder lumen (± vascularity)

CT This is useful for showing distant metastases and detecting perivesical fat invasion (T3b) ▶ it cannot distinguish between lesions limited to the lamina propria (T1) and those invading the superficial (T2a) and deep (T2b) muscle

- A sessile or pedunculated soft tissue mass projecting into the bladder lumen (± overlying calcification or associated blood clots) ▶ localized bladder wall thickening ▶ increased tumour enhancement
- *Perivesical fat invasion (T3b):* poor external bladder wall definition ▶ increased perivesical fat density
- *Adjacent visceral invasion (T4a):* no distinct fat plane is present between the bladder and rectum, uterus, prostate or vagina
  - T2WI: high SI material within the affected organ and contiguous with the bladder tumour
- *Pelvic side wall invasion (T4b):* soft tissue extending into the obturator internus muscle ▶ strands of soft tissue extending from the main tumour mass to the pelvic side wall

- *Pelvic lymph nodes (N1–N3):* malignant involvement if >7 mm ▶ rare in superficial tumours (<T2b) but the incidence increases with deep muscular involvement and then extravesical spread
  - *Pattern of nodal spread:* obturator and external iliac nodes, followed by the internal and common iliac nodes ▶ often involved nodes are not enlarged
- *Distant metastases:* bone ▶ lungs ▶ brain ▶ liver

MRI It is better than CT for the evaluation of tumours at the bladder base or dome and for differentiation between T3a and T4 disease

- T1WI: similar SI to normal wall ▶ higher SI to urine
- T2WI: higher SI to normal wall ▶ lower SI to urine ▶ it may distinguish between superficial (T2a) and deep (T2b) muscle invasion by the integrity of the bladder wall 'black line' between the superficial and deep muscle layers
- T1WI + Gad: a higher SI relative to normal bladder wall (with similar enhancement characteristics with CT)
  - Bladder wall tumour or perivesical extension demonstrates earlier enhancement than simple inflammatory post-biopsy change
  - Metastatic lymph nodes demonstrate earlier enhancement than non-metastatic nodes
- DWI: ↑ signal ▶ ADC: ↓ signal (mirroring tumour grade)

CT/MRI Imaging shortly after transurethral resection (<6 weeks) means any perivesical abnormality may be neoplastic (T3b) or reactive/inflammatory ▶ upper tract obstruction is associated with more aggressive tumours

Pearls

Risk factors Carcinogens present within cigarette smoke (the most important factor) ▶ aromatic amines ▶ cyclophosphamides

Treatment

- *Tumour confined to the bladder wall or if there is minimal extravesical spread:* surgical resection (TURBT or cystectomy)
- *Superficial tumours:* intravesical chemotherapy (BCG)
- *Extensive extravesical spread:* systemic chemotherapy or palliative radiotherapy

Monitoring response to therapy

- Biopsy is usually required as imaging cannot alone confidently distinguish between granulation tissue and recurrence
- *IVU/cystoscopy:* this evaluates the upper tracts and bladder for metastatic lesions (every 1–2 years)
- *Radiotherapy changes on MRI:* T2WI: thickened and high SI within the outer muscle layer ▶ T1WI + Gad: enhancement (but this cannot distinguish from recurrent tumour)
- *Dynamic contrast-enhanced MRI:* delayed tumour enhancement in patients responding to chemotherapy (early enhancement in non-responders)

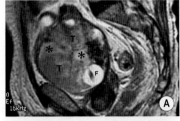
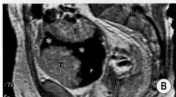

MRI of TCC. (A) Sagittal T2WI and (B) sagittal T1WI + Gad show a large bladder tumour (T) as well as blood clot (*). The use of contrast allows differentiation between the two by showing enhancement of the tumour and not the blood clot. F, Foley balloon catheter.*

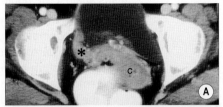
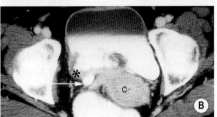

Stage T4 bladder TCC with invasion of the cervix: CECT (A) 60 s and (B) 5 min post injection. The intraluminal tumour (*) extension is seen better on the early post-contrast images, but recognition of the invasion of the ureter (long arrow) and cervix (c) is easier when both images are analysed.*

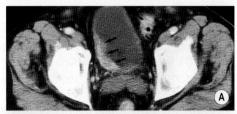
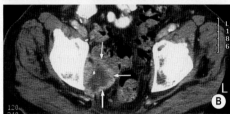

Bladder TCC with local recurrence. CT images before (A) and after (B) radical cystectomy. The tumour (black arrows) involves the right lateral and posterior bladder. Local recurrence to the cystectomy site and right pelvic side wall is seen 1 year later (B white arrows).*

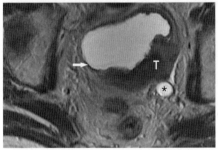

Stage T3b TCC. Axial T2WI: large tumour (T) at the left lateral bladder extending into the perivesical fat. Left hydroureter (*) is present. Normal bladder wall (arrow) shows low signal intensity.*

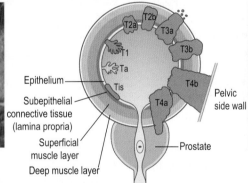

Schematic depiction of local staging of bladder carcinoma.*

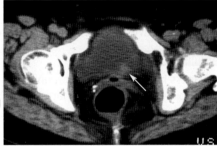

Bladder phaeochromocytoma. An unenhanced CT image in a woman with a history of hypertension shows small rounded mass along the left posterolateral aspect of the bladder (arrow).**

Other bladder tumours	
Malignant	
Lymphoma	Bladder usually secondarily involved (primary disease rare) ▶ focal mural mass or diffuse bladder thickening
Leiomyosarcoma/ rhabdomyosarcoma	Large heterogeneous ulcerated and necrotic mass
Metastases	Usually secondary to direct local spread (haematogeneous seeding is rare)
Benign	
Leiomyoma	Usually in females ▶ soft tissue masses with smooth margins ▶ low SI on T2WI
Paragangliomas	Arise from chromaffin cells in sympathetic nerves near the bladder ▶ hypertension ▶ anxiety or syncope on voiding (catecholamine release) ▶ occasionally malignant ▶ smoothly marginated masses
Nephrogenic adenoma	Benign ▶ secondary to chronic inflammation ▶ bladder wall thickening or lobulated masses
Inflammatory pseudotumour	

BLADDER INJURY

Definition

- Trauma to the bladder can be due to:
  - *Blunt abdominal trauma:* the most common cause (90% follow a motor vehicle accident)
  - *External penetrating agents:* stab wounds ▶ bone fragments
  - *Internal penetrating agents:* cystoscopes ▶ resectoscopes
- Classification of traumatic bladder injuries: bladder contusion ▶ intramural (partial-thickness) laceration ▶ full-thickness laceration with intra- or extraperitoneal rupture
  - *Intraperitoneal bladder rupture* (10–20%): this follows blunt trauma and usually occurs at the bladder dome ▶ it requires surgical repair
  - *Extraperitoneal bladder rupture* (80–90%): this is due to perforation of the bladder by bone spicules or by pulling of the fascial connections between the bladder and pelvis ▶ it usually involves the anterolateral wall near the bladder base ▶ it is associated with disruption of the urogenital diaphragm (and posterior urethra)
  - 60–90% of patients with a traumatic bladder rupture have associated pelvic fractures ▶ 2–11% of patients with pelvic fractures have a ruptured bladder

Clinical presentation

- Gross haematuria ▶ suprapubic pain ▶ ascites ▶ an inability to void ▶ abnormal urea and electrolytes

CT cystography This is more accurate than standard cystography for the detection of bladder injuries ▶ performed after a urethral injury has been excluded and catheterization is deemed safe ▶ at least 300 ml needs to be instilled

- **Intraperitoneal bladder rupture:** free intraperitoneal contrast medium is seen outlining the peritoneal recesses and bowel loops
- **Extraperitoneal bladder rupture:** contrast extravasates into the surrounding extraperitoneal space, often spreading in an irregular and often streaky manner along the fascial planes (with a 'flame-shaped' appearance)
  - *Urine can dissect into the following:* the anterior prevesical space of Retzius ▶ the anterior abdominal wall ▶ the inguinal region(s) and upper thigh(s) ▶ the lateral paravesical and presacral spaces ▶ the perineum, scrotum and rarely the retroperitoneum
- **Subserosal rupture:** this is rare and is characterized by elliptical extravasation adjacent to the bladder

SCROTAL INJURY

Definition Scrotal injury can be due to: penetrating wounds ▶ following the direct impact of a high-velocity object against the testis ▶ following compression of the testis against the pubic arch and impacting object

US This is the imaging technique of choice

- *Scrotal haematoma:* an echogenic collection between the tunica dartos and tunica vaginalis or within the scrotal septum ▶ this will become sonolucent with time
- *Haematocele:* a complex collection between the leaves of the tunica vaginalis
- *Testicular contusion:* a focal region of heterogeneous echotexture
- *Hydrocele:* a liquefied haematoma or serous collection between the layers of the tunica vaginalis ▶ an echolucent fluid collection around the testis
- *Testicular rupture:* a poorly defined testicular margin (due to the tearing of the tunica albuginea) with extrusion of the testicular parenchyma into the scrotal sac ▶ it is associated with testicular laceration, fragmentation, infarction and intratesticular haematoma formation
- *Testicular dislocation:* this is typically into the inguinal canal ▶ testicular torsion can also occur

URETHRAL TRAUMA

Definition Injuries commonly involve the male membranous urethra (which is relatively fixed within the urogenital diaphragm and subjected to shearing forces) ▶ injuries occur in 10% of pelvic fractures (M>F)

- *Type I injury:* a stretched and narrowed urethra secondary to a haematoma elevating the bladder ▶ no tear is present
- *Type II injury:* a urethral tear above the urogenital diaphragm
- *Type III injury:* a urethral tear below the urogenital diaphragm ▶ these are virtually always complete tears
- *Complete tears:* these require surgical repair
- *Partial tears:* these are usually treated conservatively with catheterization

Clinical presentation Gross haematuria ▶ meatal blood ▶ a non-palpable prostate ▶ an inability to void

- Anterior urethral injury ▶ Buck's fascia intact: limited to corporal bodies ▶ Buck's fascia disrupted: haematoma within the scrotum/perineum/anterior abdominal wall

Retrograde urethrography Contrast extravasates from the urethra into the retropubic space (type II injury) or into the perineum (type III injury)

- *Partial tear:* contrast medium fills the bladder
- *Complete tear:* no bladder opacification

MRI This defines the pelvic floor anatomy and can guide the surgical reparative approach ▶ it can assess the degree of fibrosis and any injuries to the periurethral tissues

- T1WI: this is useful for haematoma identification
- T2WI: this evaluates the direction of displacement of a urethral tear and the distance between the torn ends

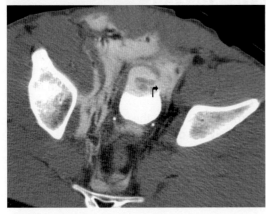

CT of extraperitoneal bladder rupture. Delayed CECT across the pelvis reveals urine extravasation into the extraperitoneal fascial planes around the bladder and tracking to the presacral space. The bladder wall defect is directly observed (curved arrow).

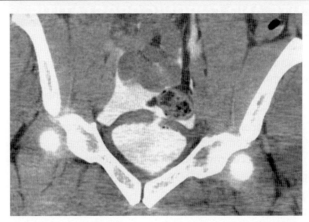

CT cystogram (coronal reformat) of a patient with intraperitoneal bladder injury demonstrating high-density fluid surrounding bowel loops and the precise site of injury at the dome.**

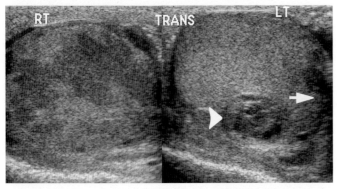

US of testicular contusion and haematoma. The right testicle shows areas of lower echogenicity in an irregular pattern, suggesting contused parenchyma. The left testicle shows a linear fracture (arrow) and a rounded focus of mixed echo texture, indicating haematoma (arrowhead).

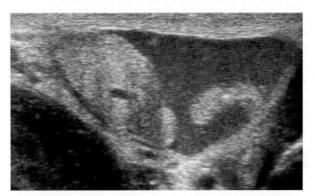

US of a ruptured testis. The testicular parenchyma is fragmented and an echogenic haematocele fills the hemiscrotum.*

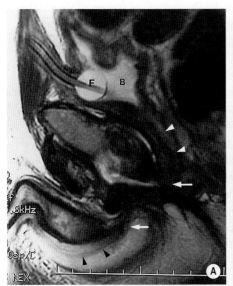

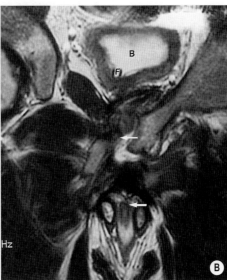

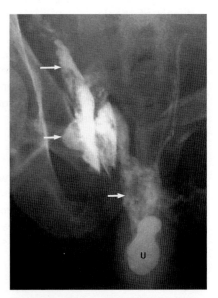

Traumatic urethral tear. (A) Sagittal and (B) coronal T2WI show a membranous urethral tear (arrows) with a superior–inferior gap of 2.5 cm between the two ends of the urethra. White arrowheads, prostatic urethra ▶ black arrowheads, bulbar urethra ▶ B, bladder ▶ F, Foley catheter.

Traumatic urethral injury. Retrograde urethrogram shows opacification of the anterior urethra (u) and extravasation of contrast medium (arrows) from the urethra.*

4.3 PROSTATE

ACUTE AND CHRONIC PROSTATITIS

Definition

- The same organisms that produce acute prostatitis can cause chronic prostatitis
  - *Healthy adults:* E. coli and staphylococci are the predominant causative organisms
  - *Immunocompromised patients:* unusual organisms are more commonly seen (e.g. a gonococcal, streptococcal, mycotic or viral aetiology)

Voiding cystourethrogram A narrowed, elongated or straightened prostatic urethra

- If chronic prostatitis is associated with a urethral stricture, the increased voiding pressure results in reflux of contrast into the prostatic ducts

TRUS

- Periprostatic inflammation within the periurethral glands: mass effect and heterogenous echogenicity
- Peripheral zone: ill-defined hypoechoic areas (which can mimic malignancy)

MRI Variable reported experiences:

- T2WI: multiple small areas of high SI with acute and chronic prostatitis ▶ areas of low SI due to chronic prostatitis and scarring
- *Chronic prostatitis:* heterogeneous SI

Pearls

Granulomatous prostatitis

- *Non-specific:* this is more common and results from the escape of prostatic contents, bacterial products or urine into the prostatic tissue
- *Specific:* this is produced by a known aetiological agent (e.g. *Mycobacterium*, schistosomiasis, malacoplakia or fungal infection)

Prostatic TB

- This is almost always secondary to TB elsewhere (e.g. within the GU tract) ▶ abscess formation (with caseation, cavitation and fibrosis) ▶ rupture into the periprostatic space, urethra or rectum may occur ▶ rarely fistulas may form within the perineum

KUB Prostatic calcification

Cystourethrogram

- *Early:* filling of the prostatic ducts without cavitation
- *Late:* greatly dilated prostatic ducts ▶ varying degrees of prostatic parenchymal destruction (sloughing may produce irregular cavities – in advanced cases the entire prostate seemingly occupied by a smooth-walled cavity)

PROSTATIC ABSCESS

Definition

- This usually begins within the peripheral zone but may spread to other areas ▶ it usually follows a urinary tract infection with E. coli or *Proteus* ▶ it is rarely seen in infants and children
- The abscess may rupture into the urethra, rectum or perineum (or rarely the peritoneum)

Antegrade/retrograde cystourethrogram Smooth prostatic cavitation (up to several cm) ▶ a radiographic diagnosis can only be made when the abscess has penetrated the urethra (allowing contrast medium into the cavity)

TRUS An echo-poor liquid abscess

MRI Discrete rounded foci: T1WI: intermediate-to-low SI ▶ T2WI: high SI ▶ T1WI + Gad: no enhancement

- It can be treated with percutaneous CT- or TRUS-guided drainage

BENIGN PROSTATIC HYPERTROPHY (BPH)

Definition

- Benign nodular enlargement of the prostate gland involving the transitional and periurethral zones (carcinoma typically affects the peripheral zone)

Cystourethrography An elongated and compressed urethra

IVU/retrograde cystogram Bladder outlet obstruction producing bladder trabeculation, diverticulae or calculi formation (± hydroureters and hydronephrosis)

- *J-shaped or 'fish-hook' ureters:* as the prostate enlarges, the bladder floor is elevated and the trigone pushed upwards

TRUS A prostate volume >30 ml ▶ an enlarged central gland with well-defined or poorly demarcated hypoechoic or mixed echogenicity nodules (± hyperechoic foci) ▶ a thick surgical pseudocapsule may be seen interposed between an enlarged central and normal peripheral gland

CT A prostate gland seen ≥2–3 cm above the symphysis pubis is unequivocal evidence of enlargement

MRI T2WI: nodular hyperplasia demonstrates heterogeneous SI ▶ stromal hyperplasia demonstrates homogeneous low-to-medium SI ▶ a surgical pseudocapsule appears as a low SI margin between the adenoma and peripheral zone

Pearl

- Prostatic artery embolization has potential for controlling the symptoms of BPH ▶ embolisation of the prostatic arteries with an embolic agent (e.g. PVA particles)

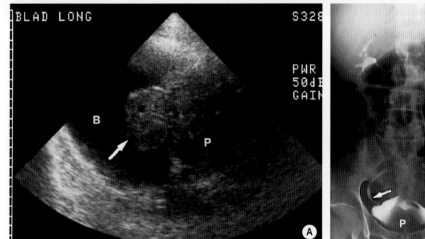
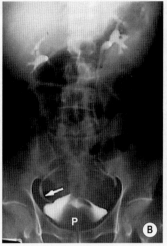
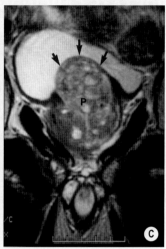

Benign nodular hyperplasia demonstrated on a (A) suprapubic US scan: markedly enlarged prostate gland (P) with enlargement of the intravesical portion (arrow) which protrudes into the urinary bladder (B). Benign nodular hyperplasia on (B) IVU and (C) coronal plane T2WI. On the IVU study the enlarged prostate gland (P) elevates the bladder floor and causes a J-hooking (fish-hooking) deformity of the distal ureters (arrow). No obstruction is seen. The MRI provides direct visualization of the prostate (P) and its impression upon the bladder floor (arrows).*

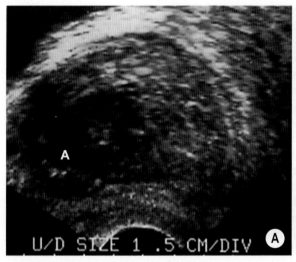
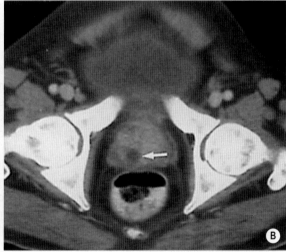

Prostatic abscess as seen by (A) TRUS and (B) CT. On US, the area of the abscess (A) is seen as an ill-defined hypoechoic pattern. On CT, liquefaction within the abscess (arrow) is even better appreciated.*

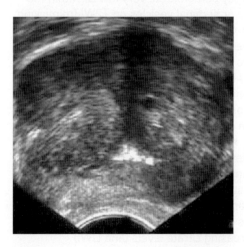

TRUS (transverse images) in a patient with clinical prostatitis. There is some benign prostatic enlargement. There is calcification at the junction of the peripheral and central gland and a slightly moth-eaten appearance to the central gland.†

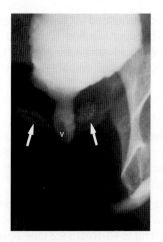

Reflux into the prostatic duct and visualization of prostatic acini (arrows) during a voiding cystourethrogram. The reflux was secondary to chronic prostatitis and was associated with a previous urethral stricture. v, verumontanum.*

PROSTATE CARCINOMA

DEFINITION

- This is predominantly a latent tumour but it demonstrates malignant potential that correlates with the histological grade, tumour volume and stage
- **Histology:** adenocarcinoma (>95%) ▶ it is rarely a squamous or transitional cell carcinoma (very rarely a sarcoma in 0.1–0.2%)
  - Prostatic intraepithelial neoplasia (PIN) is the precursor to an invasive carcinoma
- **Site:** peripheral zone (70%) > transitional zone (20%) > central zone (10%)
  - NB: BPH tends to arise from the transitional zone

CLINICAL PRESENTATION

- Lower urinary tract symptoms ▶ haematuria ▶ bone pain ▶ uraemia (following ureteric infiltration and obstruction) ▶ rectal bleeding
  - A general haemorrhagic state can exist due to prostatic fibrinolysin activity
- There is an increasing incidence with age (it is seen in 90% of men at 90 years) ▶ it is rare before the age of 50 years

RADIOLOGICAL FEATURES

TRUS Its main role is for performing guided needle biopsies (targeted and systematic sampling)
- *Tumour:* a hypoechoic region usually within the peripheral zone (it may be difficult to appreciate if it involves the entire zone) ▶ there is improved detection with colour and power Doppler
- *Extracapsular extension:* contour deformity and irregularity of the capsule ▶ direct tumour extension into the periprostatic fat
- It demonstrates a poor sensitivity for seminal vesicle or bladder neck invasion, as well as for lymph node metastases

CT This is not recommended for routine staging (it cannot distinguish between various T2 stages) ▶ however it is useful for detecting advanced adenopathy (>1 cm in size) – however microinvasion within normal nodes cannot be assessed
- If no pelvic adenopathy is demonstrated, imaging only up to the aortic bifurcation is sufficient

Radionuclide bone scintigraphy This is a screening tool for detecting bony metastases ▶ metastatic disease is uncommon in T1 or T2 tumours with a Gleason score <7 and a PSA <20 ng/ml

MRI This is used for local staging ▶ an endorectal coil (eMRI) is preferred
- Reported according to PI-RADS v.2 (see Appendix)
- **T1WI:** Detection of haemorrhage

- **T2WI:** a non-specific low SI area within the peripheral zone (which can also be caused by radiotherapy, hormone therapy or prostatitis) ▶ wedge-shaped areas tend to be benign ▶ a normal peripheral zone does not exclude the presence of a carcinoma ▶ tumour detection within the central and transitional zones is hampered by their inherent benign hypertrophic heterogeneity ▶ transitional features of concern: ill-defined nodule/spiculated margin/anteriorly located lesion with a lenticular or fusiform shape
- **DWI:** high SI
- **ADC map:** lower values than normal peripheral glandular tissue ▶ values can correlate with Gleason score ▶ prostatitis can give intermediate values
- **DEC MR imaging:** tumour angiogenesis results in an earlier and higher enhancement peak than normal tissue, as well as earlier and more pronounced washout ▶ prostatitis and BPN can show moderate enhancement
- **Extracapsular invasion (T3a):** T2WI: an irregular capsular bulge or irregular capsular margin ▶ an obliterated rectoprostatic angle ▶ neurovascular bundle asymmetry ▶ angulation or a step-off appearance of the prostate contour ▶ focal capsular retraction and thickening ▶ broad (>12 mm) capsular tumour contact ▶ breech of the capsule with evidence of direct tumour extension
- **Seminal vesicle invasion (T3b):** T2WI: direct tumour extension into and around the seminal vesicles ▶ low SI seminal vesicles ▶ tumour extension along the ejaculatory ducts ▶ seminal vesicle dilatation distal to the tumour ▶ non-visualization of the ejaculatory duct
- **Bladder base invasion (T4):** sagittal plane T2WI: tumour interruption of the low SI bladder wall
- **Nodal metastases (M1a):** T1WI: pelvic lymph nodes >8 mm (stage N1)
- **Bone metastases (M1b):** T1WI and T2WI: well-defined low SI lesions (due to their sclerotic nature)
- **Imaging post-prostatic biopsy:** post-biopsy haemorrhage may demonstrate very low SI within the peripheral zone or seminal vesicles on T2WI (mimicking a carcinoma) ▶ this has to be correlated with the T1WI (which will have a corresponding region of high SI if this is indeed due to haemorrhage) ▶ ideally post-biopsy imaging should be performed no less than 3 weeks after biopsy to minimize these effects

3D ^{1}H MR spectroscopic imaging (MRSI): this provides a 3D metabolic map of the prostate gland (normal prostate: high citrate levels ▶ prostate cancer: reduced citrate levels and high choline levels)
- It significantly improves evaluation of any extracapsular extension and staging ▶ can direct biopsies
- There is a linear correlation of increasing tumour aggressiveness (Gleason grade) with increasing choline levels and decreasing citrate levels (and DWI)

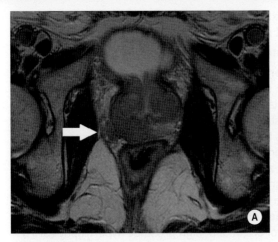

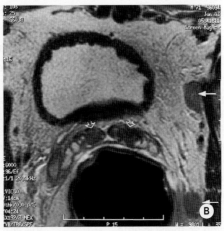

Prostate carcinoma. (A) Axial T2WI demonstrating a low signal focus within the right peripheral lobe with extracapsular tumour extension (arrow). (B) Low SI within the medial aspects of both seminal vesicles representing invasion (open arrows). There is involvement of local pelvic lymph nodes (arrow).*

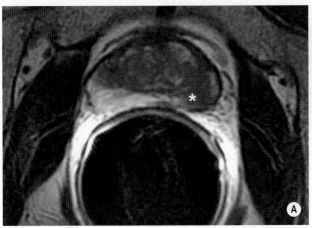

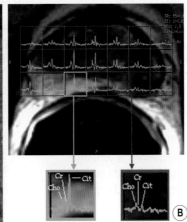

MRI and 3D ¹H MR spectroscopy of prostate carcinoma. (A) Axial T2WI (endorectal coil), with (B) superimposed MR spectroscopic grid and corresponding spectral array to the superimposed grid. The tumour (*) is seen as a low SI in the left peripheral gland. The corresponding MR spectroscopic grid shows concordant results with abnormal metabolism in this area: green box, healthy tissue ▶ red box, cancer ▶ Cho, choline ▶ Cr, creatine ▶ Cit, citrate.*

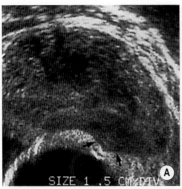

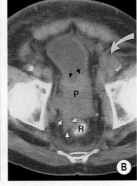

(A) Stage T3 prostate carcinoma. TRUS demonstrating an ill-defined hypoechoic area (arrows) within the peripheral zone. The tumour is causing a localized bulge of the prostatic outline beyond the expected contour of the gland. This is the most reliable finding in diagnosing transcapular invasion. (B) CT demonstration of prostatic carcinoma with regional lymph node metastasis. The prostate gland (P) is markedly enlarged and there is direct tumour extension into the perirectal region (small white arrows), rectum (R) and the bladder base (small black arrows). Pronounced left external iliac adenopathy is present (curved arrow).*

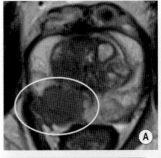

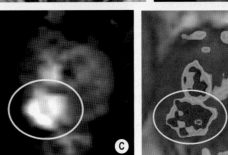

Multi-parametric MR images of a 64 year old man with a PSA level of 13 ng/mL and 1 negative TRUS biopsy session, showing a typical case of a peripheral zone tumour. With MR-guided biopsy a GS 4 + 4 = 8 was found. (A) Axial T2-weighted image. (B) Axial ADC map. (C) Axial DWI with b = 1400. (D) Axial DCE image.**

PROSTATE CARCINOMA PEARLS

Screening Digital rectal examination and serum PSA is more sensitive than TRUS alone
- **Normal PSA:** ≤4 ng/ml ▶ PSA density and PSA velocity can also be assessed

Diagnosis TRUS-guided needle biopsy

Gleason score The Gleason score is the sum of the microscopic pattern most commonly observed (1–5) + the 2nd most common pattern (1–5)
- Gleason score ≤5: well differentiated
- Gleason score 6–7: moderately differentiated
- Gleason score ≥8: poorly differentiated

Pattern of tumour spread Local direct extension through the prostatic capsule (apical tumours are more likely to demonstrate extracapsular extension as there is little capsule present at this level) ▶ rectal involvement is uncommon as Denonvillier's fascia is an effective barrier
- *Nodes:* obturator ▶ presacral, internal and common iliac ▶ para-aortic
- *Haematogenous spread:* this is commonly seen with advanced disease ▶ metastases commonly appear as sclerotic bone lesions within the axial skeleton (vertebral column and ribs) as there is direct communication between the periprostatic and vertebral venous plexi ▶ metastasizes to the lungs and liver (less common)

Treatment The key treatment determinant is whether the disease is organ confined (T2 and potentially curative) or has spread beyond the prostate margins (T3+ and not curative)
- *Organ-confined (T1 or T2) disease:* watchful waiting ▶ radical prostatectomy ▶ radiotherapy (external or brachytherapy) ▶radiation therapy causes atrophy and fibrosis (resulting in a small diffusely low T2 signal prostate)
- *Non-organ-confined (T3+ or metastatic) disease:* hormone (anti-androgen) therapy ▶ localized radiotherapy (e.g. for bone metastases)

Monitoring patients after therapy *PSA levels:* this is the primary method of following up patients
- *Local recurrence:* TRUS and MRI only provides a limited assessment and requires biopsy confirmation
- *Local recurrence:* T2WI: hyperintense ▶ ADC map: low ▶ DCE MRI: early enhancement ▶ MRSI: usually suffers from susceptibility artefact (surgical clips)
- *Typical recurrence locations:* around the anastomosis ▶ retrovesical ▶ within the bladder wall/seminal vesicles ▶ lateral surgical margins of the prostatectomy bed

Prostate anatomy and imaging

Normal anatomy
- **Base:** extends from the bladder floor and seminal vesicle/ejaculatory duct junction to a level just above the greatest transverse dimension of the gland
- **Mid-gland:** greatest transverse gland diameter to the level of the ejaculatory duct orifices (at the verumontanum)

- **Apex:** extends from just below the verumontanum to the external urethral sphincter/urogenital diaphragm

Zonal anatomy
- **Peripheral zone (PZ) (70%):** this is the predominant site of origin of a prostatic carcinoma
- Posterolateral to the peripheral zone, and within the periprostatic fat, lie the neurovascular bundles (NVB) ▶ this is the commonest initial site of extracapsular extension in prostatic carcinoma
- **Central zone (CZ) (25%):** this atrophies with age ▶ on transrectal ultrasound it is not easy to distinguish between the central and transition zones
- **Transition zone (TZ) (5%):** this enlarges with age ▶ it is the site of origin of benign prostatic hypertrophy (BPH)

Radiological investigations

Transrectal US (TRUS) This demonstrates the zonal anatomy well
- **Peripheral zone:** homogeneous medium echogenicity
- **Transition zone:** lower heterogenous echogenicity
- **Corpora amylacea:** dense echogenic foci seen at the margin between peripheral and transition zones
- **Capsule:** this is not visualized, but lies at the junction of the peripheral zone and the periprostatic fat
- **Seminal vesicles:** 'bow-tie' configuration (transaxial)
- **Vas deferens:** a rounded area toward its insertion at the medial aspect of the seminal vesicles (transverse plane) ▶ anterior to the vesicles (sagittal plane)
- **Volume measurement:** use the ellipsoid formula: $V = \frac{1}{2}(L \times AP \times W)$

MRI 1.5T vs 3T: imaging at 3T gives a higher signal to noise ratio, reduces imaging time ▶ drawbacks of 3T imaging are increased susceptibility artefacts and dielectric effects
- **T1WI:** homogeneous intermediate SI throughout
- **T2WI:**
- **Peripheral zone:** of higher SI than either central or transition zones (which demonstrate similar lower SI)
  - *Prostate base:* the peripheral zone surrounds the posterolateral aspect of the central zone
  - *Prostate apex:* the peripheral zone is nearly concentric around the urethra
- **Transition zone:** this demonstrates more heterogeneous SI with age (due to BPH)
- **Surgical pseudocapsule:** seen in older subjects at the interface between the transition and peripheral zones
- **True prostate capsule:** a thin low SI rim surrounding the peripheral zone
- **Neurovascular bundles:** punctate signal voids posterolateral to the capsule (at 5 and 7 o'clock)
- **Seminal vesicles:** a 'grape-like' configuration – with high SI fluid and a low SI seminal vesicle walls
- **Periprostatic venous plexus (PVP):** this is located at the anterolateral aspect of the prostate gland

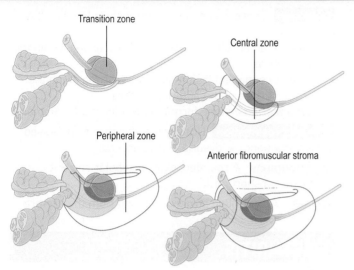

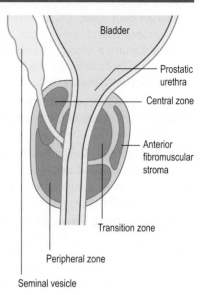

Zonal anatomy of the prostate as described by J. E. McNeal (Am J Surg Pathol 1988: 12;619–633). The transition zone surrounds the urethra proximal to the ejaculatory ducts. The central zone surrounds the ejaculatory ducts and projects under the bladder base. The peripheral zone constitutes the bulk of the apical, posterior and lateral aspects of the prostate. The anterior fibromuscular stroma extends from the bladder neck to the striated urethral sphincter.

Sagittal cross-section through the prostate.

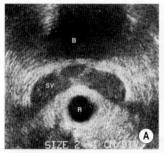

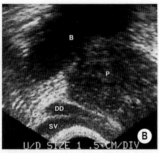

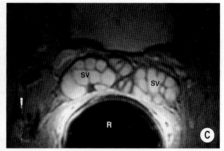

Normal seminal vesicles. (A) Transaxial and (B) sagittal plane TRUS. On the transaxial plane the seminal vesicles (SV) seen between the rectum (R) and bladder (B) demonstrate a 'bow-tie' configuration. On the sagittal image the seminal vesicles (SV) are seen posteriorly and above the prostate gland (P) ▶ B, urinary bladder. The ductus deferens (DD) is seen anterior to the seminal vesicles in the sagittal plane. (C) Axial T2WI of normal seminal vesicles.

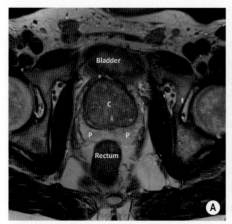

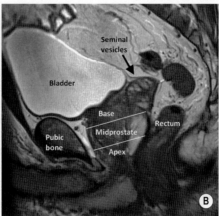

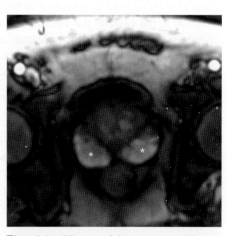

(A) Axial T2-weighted MR image showing the prostate and its zonal anatomy. The peripheral zone (P) is shown as a crescent-shaped hyperintense structure; the central gland (C) is depicted as a structure with heterogeneous signal intensity. (B) Sagittal T2-weighted image showing the craniocaudal segmentation of the prostate and its relation to the adjacent structures.**

T1-weighted image of the prostate with hyperintense signal (*) in the peripheral zone caused by haemorrhage.**

4.4 URETHRA

CONGENITAL ANOMALIES

Müllerian duct cysts Usually the caudal Müllerian duct is obliterated apart from its distal tip (which forms the verumontanum) ▶ incomplete obliteration may lead to the formation of cysts between the bladder and rectum which can present with urinary frequency or obstructive symptoms

MRI/US Midline cystic structures which are located within the posterior portion of the prostate gland (superior to the verumontanum)

Prostatic utricle This is a cavity communicating with the posterior urethra and derived from the caudal Müllerian duct (the male homologue of the uterus) ▶ it is often associated with maldevelopment of the genitalia

Posterior urethral valves (PUV) These are thickened mucosal folds within the posterior urethra which commonly extend inferiorly ▶ they are located near the distal verumontanum and result from the abnormal migration of mucosal folds (Wolffian duct remnants) from the verumontanum to the membranous urethra

- This only affects males and is usually diagnosed during fetal development or early infancy

Clinical presentation Bilateral hydronephrosis ▶ progressive oligohydramnios during pregnancy (± pulmonary hypoplasia) ▶ obstructive symptoms ▶ infection ▶ haematuria

- Up to 4 types have been described:
  - *Type 1* (the most common): two mucosal folds at the level of the verumontanum with a ventral central slit-like orifice
  - *Type 3:* this has a pin-point, eccentric orifice which results in forward ballooning of the valve, giving a 'wind in the sail' appearance on an oblique MCUG projection ▶ there is a high association with renal dysplasia and minimal upper tract dilatation

MCUG or prenatal US These can visualize the PUV as well as any bladder neck hypertrophy (which is a constant feature) ▶ there may be dilatation of the posterior urethra proximal to the valve ▶ the valve is visualized as an acute-calibre transition on the oblique/lateral urethral projection at micturition ▶ vesicoureteric reflux may be present (and is associated with poor renal function on the affected side) ▶ DMSA scanning to evaluate renal function, with MAG-3 and USS follow-up

Other urethral anomalies

- *Recto-urethral fistula:* this rare abnormality is usually associated with an imperforate anus ▶ air within the bladder confirms the diagnosis
- *Urethral duplication:* there is usually complete duplication with one of the urethras ending as a hypospadias
- *Hypospadias:* absence of the ventral aspect of the distal urethra
- *Epispadias:* absence of the dorsal aspect of the distal urethra

URETHRAL DIVERTICULUM

Definition These occur more commonly in females than males

- *Females:* an acquired lesion usually occurring within the mid urethra
- *Males:* a congenital lesion usually occurring along the ventral surface of the anterior urethra
- **Complications:** stone formation ▶ infection ▶ carcinoma

Clinical presentation Urinary incontinence ▶ increased urinary frequency ▶ dysuria ▶ dyspareunia

Urethrography A rounded, oval, or tubular sac ▶ it usually has a short neck

CT/MRI A fluid-filled structure arising from the urethra

URETHRITIS

Definition

- *Gonococcal:* an ascending gonorrhoeal infection involving the anterior urethra and extending into the glands of Littre
- *Non-gonococcal: Chlamydia trachomatis* ▶ *Ureaplasma urealyticum* ▶ tuberculosis ▶ schistosomiasis

Clinical presentation Dysuria and urethral discharge

Urethrography Luminal irregularity with filling defects representing sloughed mucosa ▶ strictures ▶ reflux into the glands of Littre, Cowper's gland ducts, prostatic ducts and seminal vesicles ▶ pseudodiverticulae

- *'Watering-can' perineum:* multiple fistulas may involve the cutaneous perineum

STRICTURES

- *Inflammatory:* these usually involve the proximal bulbar urethra (which is the site of the periurethral glands) ▶ there is proximal dilatation and it classically follows a gonococcal urethritis
- *Traumatic:* these usually involve the bulbomembranous area and tend to form more quickly than inflammatory strictures ▶ they tend to affect solitary, short segments
- *Iatrogenic:* these occur at fixed and narrowed sites of the urethra (e.g. the membranous and penoscrotal junction) as a result of pressure necrosis
  - *TURP resectoscope:* smooth, short-segment strictures
  - *Indwelling catheter:* long strictures with superimposed infection
- *Neoplastic:* this is a rare cause of stricture formation

Diagnosis Urethrography or US

Treatment Balloon dilatation ▶ ureteroscopy ▶ surgery

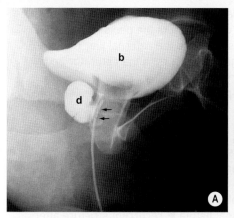 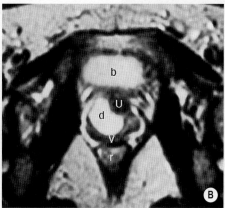 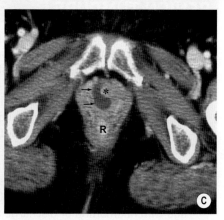

Urethral diverticulum. (A) Voiding cystourethrogram and (B) axial T2WI of urethral diverticulum (d) posterolateral to the urethra (U) in a female patient. There is also posterior displacement of the vagina (V). Arrows, catheter in urethra ▶ b, bladder ▶ r, rectum. (C) Axial CT image of a urethral diverticulum (arrows) in another female patient seen arising from the right wall of the urethra (*). R, Rectum.*

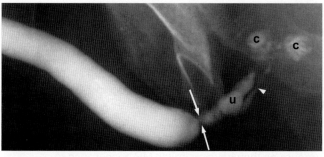 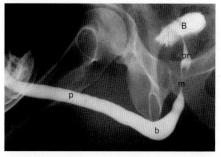

Urethral stricture with reflux into Cowper's glands. Retrograde urethrogram shows a tight bulbar stricture (arrows) with reflux on contrast seen into the Cowper's gland duct (arrowhead) and into Cowper's glands (c). u, Urethra.*

Normal retrograde urethrogram. Retrograde injection of contrast medium showing normal opacification of the male urethra. b, Bulbar urethra ▶ m, membranous urethra ▶ p, penile urethra ▶ pr, prostatic urethra ▶ B, bladder.*

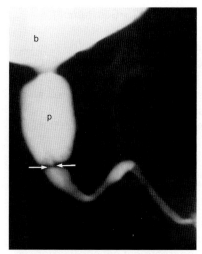 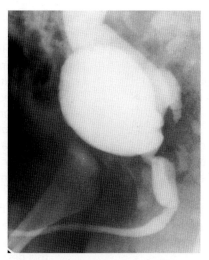 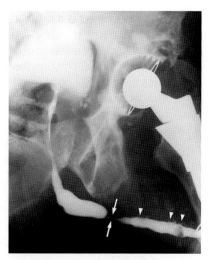

Posterior urethral valves. Voiding cystourethrogram demonstrating posterior urethral valves (arrows) with proximal dilatation of the posterior urethra (p). b, Bladder.*

Posterior urethral valves. MCUG done on the first day of life reveals bladder neck hypertrophy with a dilated posterior urethra. There is an abrupt change in calibre of the urethra, although the exact outline of the posterior urethral valve cannot be seen. Reflux into a ureter was also clearly seen.*

Urethral stricture with reflux into the glands of Littre. Retrograde urethrogram shows a tight stricture along the penile urethra (arrows). Reflux of contrast medium into the glands of Littre (arrowheads) is also demonstrated.*

BENIGN TUMOURS

- These tumours are rare and include: papillary adenoma ▶ squamous cell papilloma ▶ transitional cell papilloma ▶ nephrogenic adenoma ▶ inflammatory and fibrous polyps
  - *Inflammatory and fibrous polyps:* finger-like processes (1–2 cm long) originating near the verumontanum and presenting with intermittent obstruction
  - *Urethral caruncle:* transitional and squamous cell papillomas are found within the distal ⅓ of the urethra ▶ they present between 20 and 40 years of age with haematuria or discharge and are seen as smooth solitary or multiple filling defects

URETHRAL CARCINOMAS

Definition These are rare tumours (2F:1M)
- **Females:**
  - Squamous cell carcinoma (60%) > transitional cell carcinoma (20%) > adenocarcinoma (10%) > undifferentiated carcinoma and sarcoma (8%) > melanoma (2%)
  - *Anterior urethral tumours:* these arise from the distal ⅓ of the urethra ▶ they are usually low-grade tumours with an early presentation and a good prognosis
    - Tumours involving the external meatus spread to the superficial and deep inguinal lymph nodes
  - *Posterior or 'entire' urethral tumours:* these arise from the proximal ⅔ of the urethra ▶ they present later with an advanced grade and a poorer prognosis
    - Lymphatic spread is to the hypogastric, external iliac and sacral nodes
  - Lymph node metastases occur before blood-borne spread ▶ at presentation there can be pelvic nodal metastases (20%) and distant metastases (10–15%)
  - *Risk factors:* previous urethral trauma ▶ infection ▶ caruncle formation
- **Males:**
  - This can be regarded as two different conditions:
    - The commonest type is carcinoma of the prostatic urethra which is usually a TCC and has a strong association with bladder TCC
    - Carcinoma within the remainder of the urethra is strongly associated with chronic urethral inflammation: 75% of these are squamous cell carcinomas
      - Adenocarcinomas of the mid urethra are rare ▶ they may arise from the glands or ducts of Cowper's or Littre
  - Spread is by direct invasion as well as lymphatic spread (distant blood-borne metastases are rare)
    - *Penile urethra:* this drains along its ventral surface to the bulbar region and the superficial and deep inguinal lymph nodes
    - *Bulbar/membranous urethra:* this drains initially along the dorsal vein of the penis (behind the symphysis pubis) to the external iliac nodes ▶ drainage then occurs to the obturator and hypogastric nodes
  - *Risk factors:* previous urethral strictures (up to 75% of cases)

Clinical features

- **Females:** non-specific features: haematuria ▶ dysuria ▶ increased urinary frequency ▶ perineal pain ▶ palpable inguinal nodes
- **Males:** penile bleeding ▶ outlet obstruction ▶ a palpable mass ▶ a perineal fistula ▶ recurrent stricture after urethroplasty and excess bleeding after stricture dilatation

Radiological features

Urethrography This only assesses any luminal abnormalities and not the extent of tumour invasion into the periurethral tissues ▶ carcinoma appears as multiple serial irregular filling defects or as an irregular stricture

CT This is limited by poor soft tissue contrast (the tumour and surrounding corporeal bodies are poorly differentiated) ▶ it is the most common method for evaluating nodal metastases

MRI This is limited in the detection of small malignant tumours as they have a similar MR appearance to benign disease – however the strength of MRI lies in the localization and staging of a diagnosed urethral carcinoma
- **Women:** T1WI: a low SI mass which cannot be differentiated from the periurethral muscular layer ▶ T2WI: a high SI mass with disruption of the 'target-like' appearance of the urethra ▶ T1WI + Gad: tumour enhancement
- **Men:** T1WI: a low-to-intermediate SI mass (relative to the surrounding corporeal body) ▶ T2WI: a low SI mass
  - Tumour extension (with stage):
    - *Corporeal tissue (T2):* T2WI: a low SI mass within the corporeal tissue
    - *Tunica albuginea (T2):* T2WI: disruption of the low SI tunica
    - *Anterior vagina (T3):* T2WI: loss of the normal low SI and involvement of the vaginal mucosa
    - *Bladder neck (T3):* a mass infiltrating the bladder wall (and associated with wall thickening) ▶ T2WI: increased bladder neck SI
    - *Extension across the urogenital diaphragm (T3):* this determines the treatment options (surgery vs radiation)

URETHRAL METASTASES

- **Females:** invasion from tumours of the bladder, uterus, cervix and bowel
- **Males:** invasion from tumours of the bladder, prostate and testes

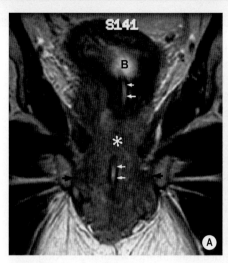
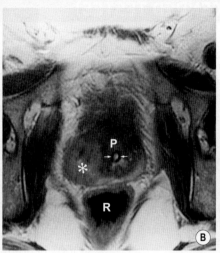
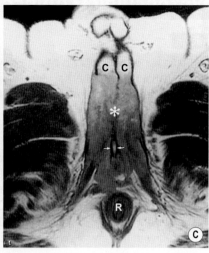

MR of urethral carcinoma in a male patient. (A) Coronal and (B, C) axial MR images show a large mass (*) arising from the urethra, encasing the Foley catheter (white arrows), invading the corpora cavernosa (c) and extending beyond the genitourinary diaphragm (black arrows) invading the prostate (P). B, Bladder ▶ R, rectum.*

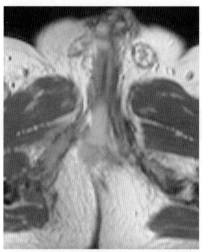

Transverse T1WI + Gad showing invasion of the penile bulb and muscles of the right side of the pelvic floor by a urethral carcinoma.†

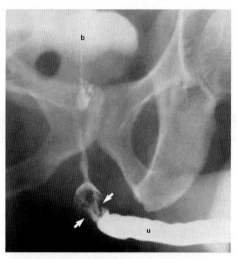

Urethral carcinoma. Retrograde urethrogram shows an irregular stricture (arrows) at the membranous–bulbar junction associated with mass-like filling defects. u, Urethra ▶ b, bladder.*

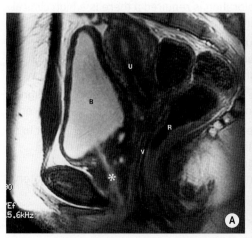
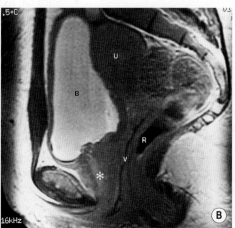

MR of urethral carcinoma in a female patient. (A) Sagittal T2WI and (B) sagittal T1WI + Gad show irregular urethral thickening and enhancement representing tumour (*). B, Bladder ▶ R, rectum ▶ V, vagina ▶ U, uterus.*

4.5 MALE REPRODUCTIVE SYSTEM

CRYPTORCHIDISM (UNDESCENDED TESTES)

Definition

- The testis is normally drawn caudad towards the inguinal canal by the gubernaculum, which is attached to its lower pole – differential growth between the gubernaculum and abdominal wall may account for this migration
  - An undescended testis may be found anywhere along its normal course of descent from the retroperitoneum to the inguinal canal
- 80% are found within the inguinal region and are usually palpable ▶ the condition is bilateral in 10–25% of cases ▶ usually right sided ▶ unilateral testicular agenesis is associated with ipsilateral renal agenesis

Radiological features

- The role of imaging for the work-up of cryptorchidism is controversial – it has been suggested that imaging does not influence the subsequent surgical planning

US This can detect an undescended testis within the inguinal region with a high-resolution linear array transducer (it is best demonstrated in the transverse plane) ▶ the testis may be atrophic and difficult to locate

CT/MRI This can image the entire retroperitoneum ▶ it is useful if an inguinal testis has not been demonstrated with US ▶ superior to *USS* in detecting near normal non-palpable testes
- **MRI:** T1WI: the testes are of low SI ▶ T2WI and STIR: the testes are of high SI

Pearls

- It can be an isolated abnormality or in association with other abnormalities (e.g. prune-belly syndrome, Beckwith–Wiedemann syndrome, congenital rubella, renal agenesis)
- Its prevalence parallels the gestational age: it is found in 100% of premature male infants weighing < 900g, 3–4% of infants > 2.5 kg, < 1% of infants by 1 year (as most testes spontaneously descend)
- It is a risk factor for subfertility (even if unilateral) and subsequent testicular tumour development (usually a seminoma)
- *Orchidopexy:* this does not reduce the risk of malignancy within the ipsilateral or contralateral testis (however it does allow for earlier detection)

TESTICULAR TORSION

Definition

- An abnormal twist of the spermatic cord as a result of testicular rotation
  - Normally the tunica vaginalis converges posteriorly, fixing the testis to the scrotal wall ▶ this attachment may be deficient or patulous, allowing the testis to rotate (a 'bell-clapper' deformity)
  - It can be complete (at least 360° of rotation) or incomplete ▶ the degree of torsion determines the severity of testicular ischaemia and the rapidity of any irreversible changes
  - *Acute:* lasting between 24 h and 10 days ▶ *subacute or chronic:* > 10 days
- It is commonly seen during the 1st year of life or during adolescence (when the testicle is rapidly enlarging)
  - *Intravaginal:* this affects an older age group and is common
  - *Extravaginal:* this affects infants and is rare (the testis and tunica vaginalis twist at the external ring)

Radiological features

- Imaging should not delay surgical exploration – imaging studies are the exception rather than the rule

US Non-specific appearances: a swollen hypoechoic testis is usually not salvageable (a normal testis often is)

- *Acute:* an enlarged heterogeneous testis and epididymis
- *Chronic:* a reactive hydrocele

Colour Doppler US Absent or markedly reduced testicular blood flow ▶ the demonstration of normal blood flow does not exclude torsion (which can be intermittent)

99mTc scintigraphy An infarcted testis appears as a photon-deficient area ▶ it is often surrounded by a rim of increased activity (representing hyperaemia)

Pearls

- Surgical exploration is required if there is a high clinical suspicion but normal imaging

Missed testicular torsion Salvage rates are closely related to the time to diagnosis (80% during the first 6 h, falling to 20% after 24 h)

Torsion of the testicular appendix (hydatid of Morgagni) The most common cause of acute scrotal pain in children

US A focal heterogeneous soft tissue mass adjacent to the upper epididymal pole ▶ it demonstrates a central hypoechoic region and an associated hydrocele ▶ its appearances may be misleading, suggesting inflammatory change only

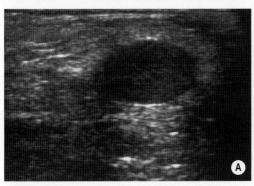 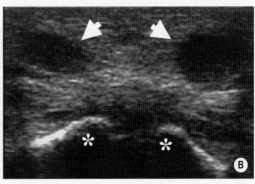

(A) US of an undescended infantile testis. The testis lies within the inguinal canal surrounded by suprapubic fat. (B) Bilateral undescended testes, transverse US view. The testes (arrows) are demonstrated at the level of the superior pubic rami (asterisks).*.†

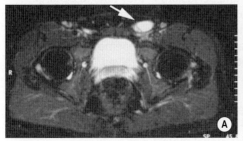 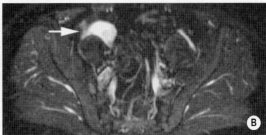

Transverse STIR MRI images demonstrating undescended testis (arrows) within the suprapubic pouch (A) and pelvis (B).†

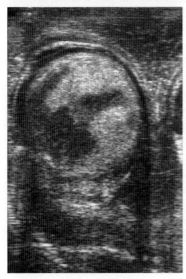 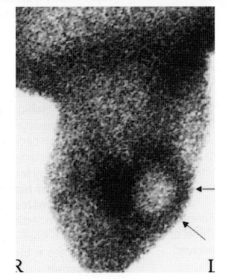 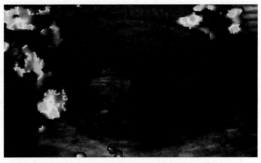

Infarcted testicle. There are extensive areas of reduced echogenicity within the testicle and the adjacent epididymis is also markedly swollen.†

Testicular torsion – anterior view. 99mTc-pertechnenate study demonstrates an intensely hyperaemic rim of tissue surrounding a photon-deficient infarcted left testis (arrows).†

Doppler of an enlarged testis showing no Doppler flow within the infarcted testis and only in the surrounding epididymis. ©27

PRIMARY TESTICULAR MALIGNANCIES

Definition

- **Germ cell origin (95%):**
  - *Seminoma (40%):* a peak incidence during the 4th and 5th decades
  - *Non-seminomatous germ cell tumour* (NSGCT) (60%): a peak incidence during the 3rd and 4th decades
    - *Adults:* embryonal tumour > yolk sac tumour > teratoma
    - *Children:* although testicular tumours are rare they are usually a yolk sac tumour (which is more common than a teratoma)
- **Gonadal stromal tumours (non-germ cell) (1%):** these are of Leydig, Sertoli or theca cell origin: they are usually benign but endocrinologically active ▶ there can be premature virilization (Leydig tumours secreting androgens) or gynaecomastia (Sertoli tumours secreting oestrogens)
- **Lymphoma (4%):** this is common in older males

Clinical features

- A painless unilateral scrotal mass ▶ acute pain due to haemorrhage (10% of cases)

Radiological features

US This cannot reliably distinguish between tumour types ▶ the approximate appearances:

- *Seminoma:* a well-defined and homogeneous mass, which is hypoechoic relative to the surrounding parenchyma ▶ it may be multifocal
- *Embryonal cell tumour:* this is less homogeneous and well defined
- *Teratoma:* a mixed reflectivity mass (± cystic spaces and calcification)

Doppler US Increased tumour flow is common but this cannot differentiate a benign from a malignant tumour

CT This is used for staging

- Nodes are considered abnormal if they are > 1 cm in size (however the usual issues regarding false-negative examinations and enlarged nodes due to reactive hyperplasia remain)
- *Testicular tumours typically spread via the lymphatics:* this is initially to the para-aortic nodes (up to the level of the renal hila) ▶ inguinal nodes are not usually involved unless there is scrotal wall invasion
  - *Left-sided lesions:* these involve the upper left para-aortic chain, and are situated closer to the left renal vein than the aortic bifurcation
  - *Right-sided lesions:* these involve the anterior inter-aorticocaval recess and paracaval nodes ▶ deposits tend to be more caudad than left-sided metastases ▶ they may potentially be located posterior to the 3rd part of the duodenum with an impact on surgical management

- *Distant nodal spread:* para-aortic nodes ▶ retrocrural nodes ▶ supraclavicular nodes (via the thoracic duct) ▶ posterior mediastinal or subcarinal nodes (via direct spread through the diaphragm)
- Contralateral nodal disease and inferior spread to the inguinal nodes only occurs following well-established ipsilateral disease (e.g. nodes > 2 cm) ▶ isolated pelvic adenopathy may occur (but is more often seen with testicular maldescent or scrotal involvement)
- *Distant metastases:*
  - Haematogenous spread (via the thoracic duct) is predominantly to the lungs ▶ these are frequently subpleural and basal (representing areas of maximal ventilation and perfusion) ▶ they tend to be large lesions (up to a few cm) ▶ mediastinal adenopathy is less common than with lung metastases
  - Brain metastases are usually haemorrhagic ▶ the liver and bones can also be involved

Pearls

- **Stages:** stage I: no metastases ▶ stage II: abdominal metastases ▶ stage III: supradiaphragmatic metastases ▶ stage IV: extranodal metastases
- **Risk factors:**
  - *Cryptorchidism* (10%): the risk persists after orchidopexy with an increased risk in a normal contralateral testis
  - *A previously treated testicular cancer:* there is an increased risk of developing a malignancy in the contralateral testis
  - *Others:* mumps orchitis ▶ testicular microlithiasis ▶ infective orchitis ▶ infertility
- **Treatment:**
  - *Seminoma:* orchidectomy + para-aortic radiotherapy (stage I) ▶ orchidectomy + chemotherapy for advanced disease ▶ extremely radiosensitive
  - *NSGCT:* orchidectomy + retroperitoneal lymphadenectomy (stage I) ▶ orchidectomy + chemotherapy for advanced disease
- **Other testicular tumours:**
  - *Testicular metastases:* suspect in a patient > 50 years with a testicular mass
    - *Primary sites:* prostate ▶ kidney ▶ bronchus ▶ pancreas ▶ bladder ▶ thyroid
  - *Leukaemia*
    - Testicular involvement is seen in acute leukaemia (50%) and chronic leukaemia (25%) ▶ overt clinical involvement is rare
    - It is a common site of relapse following treatment (due to limited testicular penetration by chemotherapeutic agents)
    - **US:** non-specific appearances ▶ diffuse multifocal infiltrating lesions ▶ possibly hyperechoic
  - *Hodgkin's disease/non-Hodgkin's lymphoma:* see separate section

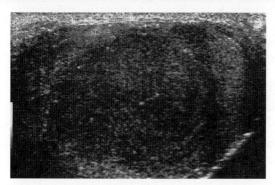

Seminoma: longitudinal US view. The slightly hypoechoic lesion is almost replacing the entire testis. Microcalcifications are seen in the normal and abnormal parenchyma.*

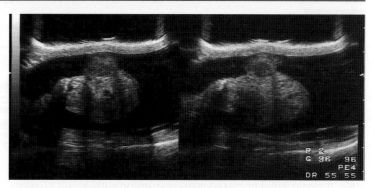

Testicular US showing virtually complete replacement of normal testicular tissue by metastatic prostate cancer. An associated hydrocele is also present.[†]

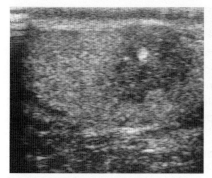

US of an NSGCT which is hypoechoic but relatively well defined and containing at least one area of calcification.[†]

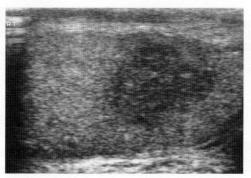

US of a seminoma showing homogeneous reduction in echogenicity.[†]

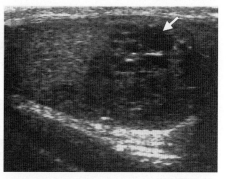

Teratoma of the testis (US). The cystic areas (arrow) within the lesion are characteristic.*

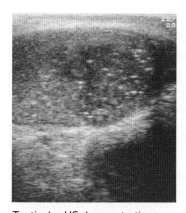

Testicular US demonstrating microlithiasis and the development of a seminoma.[†]

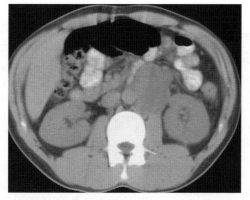

CT demonstrating a large left-sided metastatic para-aortic mass partly encasing the aorta.[†]

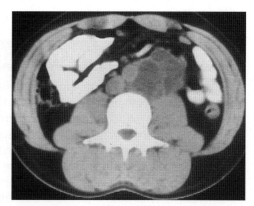

CT demonstrating a substantial cystic lymph node mass due to a testicular NSGCT.[†]

	Seminoma	**Teratoma**
Alpha-fetoprotein (AFP)	Elevated	Elevated
Human chorionic gonadotrophin (hCG)	Less commonly elevated	Elevated
Adjuvant treatment	Radiosensitive	Chemosensitive

CYSTS

Definition These can be unicameral or multiseptate (up to 10% of testicular US studies) ▶ it needs to be distinguished from a cystic tumour

- **Causes:** previous trauma ▶ inflammation ▶ embryonal remnants

EPIDERMOID CYST

Definition An uncommon benign tumour consisting of layers of keratin within a fibrous capsule

US A cystic, solid or mixed avascular lesion with a characteristic whorled appearance

MRI T2WI: alternating high SI and low SI layers ▶ no enhancement

TESTICULAR ABSCESS

- **Acute:** associated with an epididymitis ▶ **chronic:** includes tuberculosis

US A low or mixed reflectivity region (± calcification if chronic)

TUBULAR ECTASIA

Definition Benign cystic dilatation of the rete testis which affects older men ▶ possibly secondary to epididymal obstruction ▶ epididymal cysts in 85%

MRI T1WI/PD: reduced SI compared with normal testis ▶ T2WI: the lesion is undetectable

TESTICULAR MICROLITHIASIS

Definition Multiple (> 5) sub mm highly reflective foci present in one or both testes ▶ it is thought to result from degenerating cells within the seminiferous tubules

- It is found in normal men (2.4%) and debate exists as to whether it represents a premalignant condition
- Annual US follow-up (to 50 years) may be advisable
- *Other associations:* cryptorchidism ▶ infertility ▶ Klinefelter's syndrome ▶ testicular infarction ▶ alveolar microlithiasis

US Small hyperechoic foci that are too small to cast an acoustic shadow

HYDROCELE

Definition A small amount of fluid surrounding the testicle is normal – excessive fluid is the commonest cause of a scrotal mass and can be:

- *Congenital:* occurring during infancy and due to a patent processus vaginalis ▶ it usually resolves spontaneously
- *Acquired:* trauma ▶ tumour ▶ infection

US A fluid collection surrounding the anterior and lateral aspects of the testis ▶ anechoic or multiple low reflectivity echoes (representing cholesterol crystals) ▶ it may be multiloculated and indistinguishable from an organizing haematoma

SPERMATOCELE/EPIDIDYMAL CYST

Definition These are related lesions caused by dilated epididymal tubules

- *Spermatocele:* a retention cyst of the head of the epididymis ▶ it contains sperm
- *Epididymal cyst:* these are found anywhere within the epididymis ▶ they do not contain sperm ▶ they can be single or multiple well-defined anechoic cysts

VARICOCELE

Definition Dilated tortuous veins of the pampiniform plexus ▶ it is associated with male infertility

- *Causes:* idiopathic (invariably left sided due to more indirect drainage of left testis into left renal vein) ▶ secondary to incompetent valves within the spermatic vein

US Multiple serpiginous tubules > 2 mm in diameter superior and posterior to the testis (they may extend to the inferior pole of the testis) ▶ there is increased prominence on standing

- Spontaneous flow may not be seen – flow may be demonstrated with coughing, rapid inspiration or the Valsalva manoeuvre

ACUTE EPIDIDYMITIS

Causes E. coli ▶ Pseudomonas ▶ Aerobacter ▶ Neisseria gonorrhoeae ▶ Chlamydia

- *Tuberculous epididymitis:* this is secondary to prostatic tuberculosis ▶ the testis may be involved by direct extension ▶ it may be difficult to distinguish from tumour

US An enlarged entire epididymis (occasionally only involving the head) ▶ a hypoechoic or heterogeneous echotexture ▶ increased colour Doppler flow (cf. torsion)

ORCHITIS

Definition This is seen in association with a systemic viral illness (e.g. mumps) or in association with a bacterial epididymitis

US Testicular swelling (with reduced echogenicity) ▶ possible long-term testicular atrophy

- *Colour Doppler:* increased vascularity ▶ there may be reduced vascularity if there is associated ischaemia or infarction

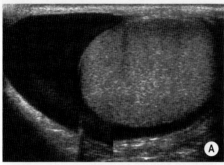 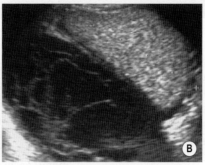

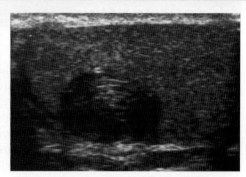

Longitudinal US view of normal testis and moderately sized hydrocele (A). Longitudinal US views of organizing scrotal haematoma following trauma (B). The adjacent testis is compressed but otherwise normal. A septated hydrocele may present a similar appearance.*

US of epidermoid cyst of testis in a young adult.*

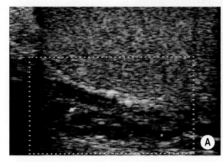 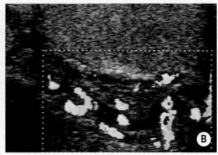

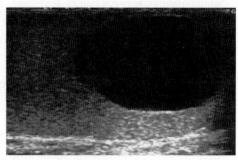

US of an asymptomatic left varicocele. At rest (A), there is little detectable flow on colour Doppler. During Valsalva manoeuvre the flow is enhanced (B).*

US of intratesticular cyst of unknown aetiology in a man referred with clinical diagnosis of epididymal cyst.*

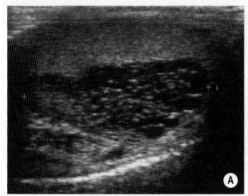 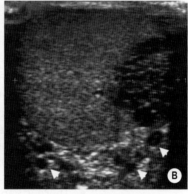

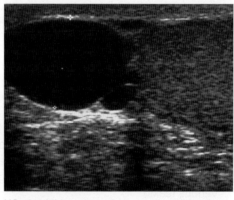

Tubular ectasia of the rete testis. Longitudinal (A) and transverse (B) US views. There is a superficial resemblance to testicular teratoma. Typical cystic lesions of the epidydimis are demonstrated (arrowheads).*

US of epididymal cyst in head of epididymis.

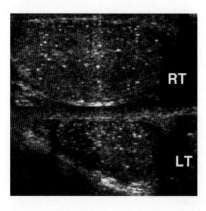

Microlithiasis of the testes. Longitudinal US views demonstrate unilateral atrophy. The cause was unknown. Microlithiasis involves both the normal and atrophic testis.*

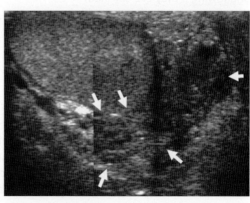

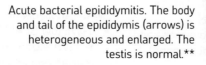

Acute bacterial epididymitis. The body and tail of the epididymis (arrows) is heterogeneous and enlarged. The testis is normal.**

ERECTILE FAILURE

Definition

- In normal males the response to humoral and neurogenic stimuli is reduced vasoconstriction resulting in increased flow to the cavernosal arteries ▶ this compresses the subtunical venules against the tunica albuginea and results in a rise in intracavernosal pressure (approximating systolic pressure).
  - Erectile failure is seen in 5% of men aged 40 years (15% aged 70 years)
- *Causes:* Peyronie's disease ▶ vasogenic causes (due to failure of the veno-occlusive mechanism to provide adequate venous resistance during erection) ▶ endocrine abnormalities ▶ renal failure ▶ chronic liver disease ▶ neurological disorders (e.g. Parkinson's disease and multiple sclerosis) ▶ smoking ▶ depression ▶ AIDS

Radiological features

- The aim is to demonstrate adequate arterial inflow and a normal reduction in venous outflow

Dynamic infusion cavernosometry

- Following the insertion of a needle into the corpus cavernosum, the amount of saline flow required to maintain an erection can be measured

  - *Normal:* 120 ml/min (without using smooth muscle relaxants)
- An alternative method utilizes an intracavernosal injection of papaverine, followed by monitoring of the intracavernosal pressure
  - *Normal:* intracavernosal pressure should approach mean arterial blood pressure within 5–10 min ▶ failure to achieve this may be due to either impaired inflow or an inability to reduce outflow
  - *Abnormal:* with arteriogenic impotence but normal veno-occlusive function, there is a slow rise in pressure that never reaches systemic blood pressure

Iodinated contrast cavernosogram

- This is performed after cavernosometry
  - *Normal:* no venous drainage occurs
  - *Abnormal:* there is leakage from the dorsal, crural or cavernosal veins

Doppler US Cavernosal arteries with a peak systolic velocity < 35 cm/s are associated with angiographic arterial disease

OTHER PENILE CONDITIONS

Peyronie's disease

Definition Palpable fibrotic plaques within the tunica albuginea of the corpora cavernosa (following a vasculitis of the subtunica connective tissue) ▶ the penis is characteristically curved

- Erectile dysfunction can result from the fibrotic penile deformity impairing sexual intercourse or due to a vasogenic erectile failure (the plaques can obstruct distal corpora cavernosal flow as well as being associated with venous leaks)

US The method of choice ▶ hyper- or hyporeflective peripheral lesions within the corpora cavernosa (± acoustic shadowing if they are calcified)

Contrast cavernosography The plaques appear as filling defects or as a deformity of the normal contour of the corpus

MRI This is better at demonstrating plaques at the penis base ▶ post-gadolinium plaque enhancement suggests inflammatory change

Penile trauma

Definition This can follow a penetrating or blunt injury (the latter is associated with sexual intercourse)

- *'Fractured penis':* disruption to the corpora cavernosa and penile tunica albuginea may occur (± urethral damage)

US/MRI These can demonstrate a tunical tear in men with a penile fracture (which may guide surgery) ▶ the diagnosis is essentially clinical

Penile carcinoma

Definition A keratinized squamous cell carcinoma which almost always starts within the sulcus and proceeds with local invasion into the glans and along the shaft ▶ advanced disease may invade the urethra, prostate and perineum

- There is early lymph node spread but late haematogenous spread

Staging There is a TNM classification in addition to the flowing staging:

- *Stage I:* confined to the glans or foreskin
- *Stage II:* shaft invasion
- *Stage III:* regional lymph nodes
- *Stage IV:* distant metastases

US This can demonstrate the tumour margins ▶ it is not able to differentiate between invasion of the subepithelial tissue and invasion into the spongiosum (it can demonstrate invasion into the tunica albuginea)

MRI An ill-defined, infiltrating lesion

- T1WI: low SI ▶ T2WI: low SI (cf. the corpora cavernosa) ▶ T1WI + Gad: this is ideal for evaluating the tumour margin and any extension

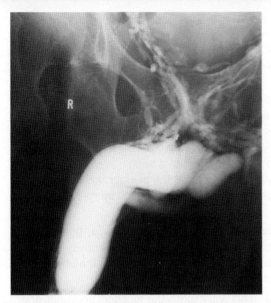

One cause of erectile dysfunction. Cavernosogram showing opacification of the cavernosa and marked venous leakage.†

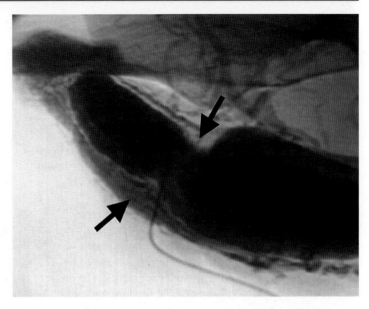

Peyronie's disease. Cavernosogram in a patient with erectile failure confined to the distal penis. There is a circumferential stricture (arrows) of the mid-shaft of both corpora cavernosa.*

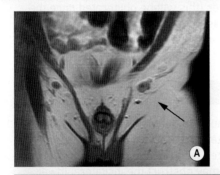

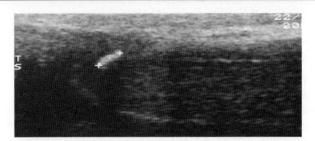

Longitudinal US of a penis in Peyronie's disease showing a small calcified echogenic plaque with distal acoustic shadowing.†

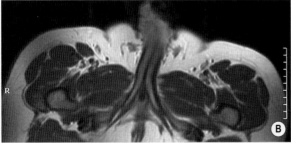

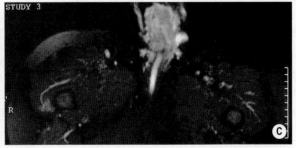

MRI scan of extensive penile carcinoma. Axial T1WI + Gad (B) shows destruction of the normal anatomy of the glans and shaft by the irregular enhancing mass of tumour. This is seen on the axial STIR (C), which also demonstrates upstream dilatation of the urethra, a finding generally only seen with advanced tumours. The coronal T1WI + Gad (A) demonstrates the presence of inguinal lymph nodes. These are not particularly enlarged but the node on the left (arrow) shows central necrosis characteristic of squamous cell carcinoma metastasis.†

4.6 PAEDIATRIC GENITOURINARY DISORDERS

DUPLEX KIDNEY

DEFINITION

- A congenital abnormality where drainage of the kidney is via two collecting systems (occurring in 3% of individuals)
  - Partial < complete
  - Bilateral > unilateral
- **Complete duplication**
  - The ureters draining the two moieties never join
  - Classically the upper moiety ureter obstructs (its ectopic ureteral orifice is often stenotic) and the lower moiety ureter tends to demonstrate vesicoureteric reflux (due to an incompetent valve)
    - The upper moiety ureter usually enters the bladder as a ureterocele ▶ such ectopic drainage is almost always associated with dysplastic function of the upper moiety of the kidney
  - **Weigert–Meyer rule:** the upper moiety ureter inserts into the bladder *inferomedial* to the lower moiety ureter
    - *Other ectopic insertions of the upper ureteric moiety:* bladder neck ▶ posterior urethra ▶ seminal vesicle or ejaculatory duct ▶ vagina
- **Incomplete duplication**
  - The two ureters join at any level above the bladder
  - 'Yo-yo' reflux: this may occur if urine refluxes from one ureteric moiety into the other (rather than draining into the bladder) if there is ureteric duplication above the bladder – a septated renal pelvis is the mildest variant of this condition

CLINICAL PRESENTATION

- Asymptomatic ▶ the development of a UTI
- *Pain:* secondary to intermittent obstruction at the PUJ level of the lower moiety or due to 'yo–yo' reflux with incomplete duplication
- *Continuous wetting in a girl:* due to an ectopic insertion of the upper moiety into the vagina
- *Vaginal prolapse:* the ureterocele prolapses out of the bladder
- *Bladder neck obstruction:* following prolapse of a ureterocele

RADIOLOGICAL FEATURES

- One of the cardinal signs of a duplex system is a change in the axis of the lower moiety
  - The lower moiety calyces are medial to the upper moiety calyces (giving the lower moiety of the kidney a longitudinal axis which points to the ipsilateral shoulder)

US A duplex kidney is longer than normal in bipolar length (for an uncomplicated duplex) ▶ the kidney may simply show two distinct renal pelves

- *Upper moiety:* this is usually dilated ▶ this may be normal, small, or dysplastic ▶ it may be anechoic and resemble a 'cyst' (which is an obstructed ureterocele) ▶ these findings are generally associated with a dilated ureter
- *Lower moiety:* in complete duplication the lower moiety may be normal and difficult to recognize ▶ the calyces and pelvis of a lower moiety may be dilated with no ureteric dilatation (suggesting a PUJ stenosis) ▶ reflux is likely when a dilated ureter is seen
- *Ureterocele:* this is seen at the bladder base if it is intravesical ▶ it can be so large as to be mistaken for a bladder

IVU *'Drooping lily' sign:* an obstructed upper pole moiety will not opacify – the opacifying lower pole moiety will be displaced inferiorly by the mass effect from the obstructed and enlarged upper pole moiety

99mTc-MAG3 This will assess the function, drainage, and the presence of any reflux (especially with late images) ▶ if a moiety is non-functional it will not be visualized (this is important to recognise when there is a small severely dysplastic upper moiety) ▶ with incomplete duplication the upper and lower moieties may be normal or there may be reduced function of either element

- 'Yo-yo' reflux is seen with an incomplete duplication

Micturating cystourethrography A ureterocele appears as a filling defect along the posterolateral wall of the bladder on early images (this will be obliterated once the bladder is full of contrast medium)

- VUR may be detected (usually into the lower moiety) ▶ reflux into the upper moiety is rarely detected

PEARLS

Ureterocele A submucosal dilatation of the intramural distal ureter, which often projects into the bladder lumen ▶ it is usually associated with the upper moiety ureter of a duplex system (and may obstruct the ipsilateral lower moiety ureter)

- It may also prolapse into the urethra (causing bladder outlet obstruction) or present as a labial and interlabial mass
- Ureteroceles that are not associated with a duplex system tend to be small and are not associated with significant obstruction (unless complicated by calculi)

IVU *A 'cobra's head' appearance:* a contrast-filled structure (the ureterocele cavity) with a thin radiolucent wall (the ureterocele wall) surrounded by contrast within the bladder

US A thin-walled cystic structure projecting into the bladder lumen

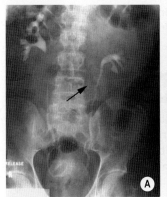
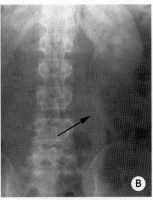

The classical 'drooping lily' sign on IVU (A). The lower pole moiety has been displaced inferolaterally by an upper pole hydronephrosis. This usually occurs due to obstruction of the upper pole moiety ureter at its orifice associated with an ectopic insertion or a ureterocele. (B) In this case it is due to a calculus in the upper pole moiety ureter (arrow).[†]

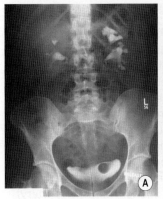
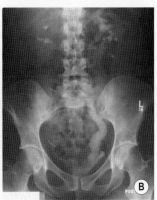

Full-length film from an IVU series showing a non-opacified partly obstructing ureterocele surrounded by opacified urine in the bladder (A). A later full-length film shows opacification of the distended upper moiety ureter running down to the opacified ureterocele (B).[†]

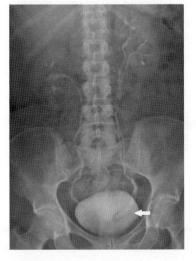

IVU demonstrating a duplex left kidney with complete ureteric duplication. The upper moiety ureter is seen entering the bladder as a ureterocele with a typical 'cobra's head' appearance (arrow).

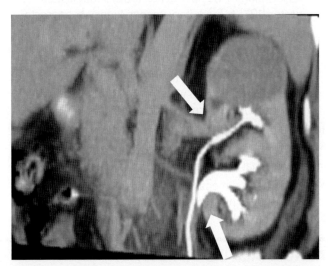

Partial duplication of the left renal collecting system on CT in a 61-year-old woman. Coronal CT reformation shows separate drainage systems for the upper and lower moieties of the left kidney (arrows).[**]

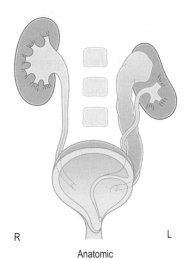
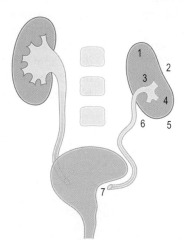

R   L

Anatomic   Urographic

Ectopic ureterocele. Diagrammatic representation of the anatomical and urographic appearances of an ectopic ureterocele of the left upper moiety without function. Diagnosis of this entity on IVU depends on recognition of indirect signs: 1, increased distance from the top of the visualized collecting system to the upper border of the nephrogram ▶ 2, abnormal axis of the collecting system ▶ 3, impression upon the upper border of the renal pelvis ▶ 4, decreased number of calyces compared to the contralateral kidney ▶ 5, lateral displacement of the kidney and ureter ▶ 6, lateral course of the visualized ureter ▶ 7, filling defect in the bladder.

479

ABNORMALITIES OF FUSION

HORSESHOE KIDNEY

Definition A common renal anomaly (affecting 1:400 live births and M > F) whereby in utero contact between the metanephric tissue of the developing kidneys results in a midline connection (isthmus) between the lower poles ▶ the isthmus may be anything from a fibrous band, to more commonly a block of renal tissue

- The ascent of the fused kidney is arrested by the inferior mesenteric artery during development, resulting in a low abdominal position (the isthmus lies anterior to the aorta and IVC but posterior to the inferior mesenteric artery) ▶ its abnormal position makes it more susceptible to injury
- It is always associated with malrotation so that the pelves and ureters pass anteriorly over the fused lower poles
  - *Associations:* PUJ obstruction (30%) ▶ duplicated ureter (10%) ▶ medullary sponge kidney ▶ anorectal and musculoskeletal anomalies
  - *Complications:* renal pelvic dilatation (± PUJ obstruction) ▶ renal calculi or infection ▶ there is an increased risk of renal tumours (e.g. a Wilms' tumour) ▶ may be associated with trisomy 18 (Edwards' syndrome) and Turner's syndrome

US This may not detect the abnormal axes of the kidney

⁹⁹ᵐTc-DMSA An anterior view is useful to show all functioning renal tissue (especially over the spine)

CT/MRI These can easily demonstrate a horseshoe kidney (the upper poles point superolaterally, the lower poles inferomedially)

Pancake kidney A rare fusion anomaly whereby both kidneys have failed to ascend from the pelvis and have fused

CROSS-FUSED RENAL ECTOPIA

Definition One kidney is displaced across the midline and is fused inferiorly to the other relatively normally positioned kidney (both ureters enter the bladder in a normal position) ▶ there is an increased incidence of VUR into the crossed kidney

Clinical presentation It may present as an abdominal mass or as an obstructive uropathy with a PUJ obstruction ▶ it is more common on the right (M>F) – the left kidney is more commonly the ectopic kidney

US An unusually large kidney on the affected side and an absent kidney on the opposite side

⁹⁹ᵐTc-MAG3 study This is performed if surgery is being considered for a PUJ obstruction

⁹⁹ᵐTc-DMSA scintigram Patchy uptake of the isotope owing to the anatomical abnormality and dysplasia that exists to some degree

MCUG This may provide further anatomical information

PANCAKE KIDNEY

- Occurs when bilateral pelvic kidneys fuse

ABNORMALITIES OF POSITION

MALROTATED KIDNEY

- The upper pole of the kidney is located more laterally than the lower pole (the upper pole calyces are therefore lateral to the lower pole calyces) ▶ a malrotated kidney may develop urological complications, be more susceptible to trauma, or indicate that pathology in an adjacent organ is displacing the kidney

ECTOPIC KIDNEY

- *Failure of complete ascent:* this results in a pelvic kidney (the majority) ▶ there is an increased risk of trauma, VUR and calculus formation (due to urinary stasis)
- *Overascent:* this is almost always limited by the diaphragm but if there is eventration of the diaphragm or a Bochdalek hernia an intrathoracic kidney may result ▶ this can resemble a posterior mediastinal mass

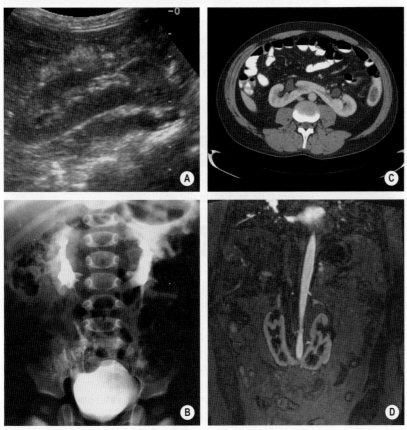

Horseshoe kidney. (A) Longitudinal US. (B) Axial CT image. (C) IVU demonstrating lower renal poles merging inferomedially. (D) T2WI MR urogram.§,†

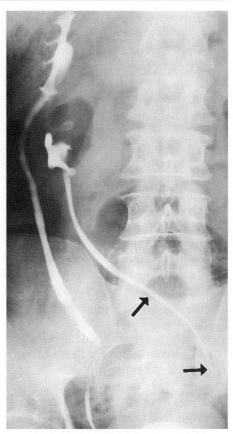

Cross-fused ectopia demonstrated on IVU. The abnormally positioned left kidney still drains into the left VUJ (arrows).ʃ

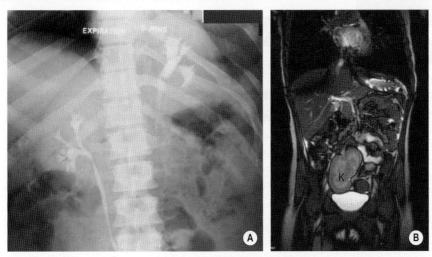

Ectopic kidneys. An intrathoracic kidney seen on IVU (A). (B) Coronal T2WI demonstrating a pelvic kidney (K).†,§

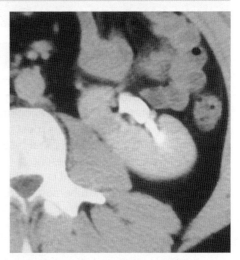

Renal malrotation. CT demonstrating a malrotated kidney with the renal pelvis draining the kidney anteriorly rather than the normal medial position.ʃ

UNILATERAL RENAL AGENESIS

DEFINITION

- This follows failure of the ureteric bud to reach the metanephros (affecting 1 in 1250 live births) ▶ the ipsilateral ureter and hemitrigone fail to develop but occasionally a ureteric stump may remain ▶ as an antenatal diagnosis is uncommon this suggests that agenesis may represent an involuted multicystic kidney ▶ bilateral renal agenesis is incompatible with life
  - It can be difficult to differentiate between unilateral agenesis and a small non-functioning kidney (especially if it is ectopically located)

ASSOCIATIONS

- Ipsilateral urogenital abnormalities are common (absence of the vas deferens or absence of the seminal vesicle) ▶ cardiovascular, gastrointestinal and musculoskeletal anomalies ▶ the VATER syndrome
- Females with renal agenesis have a 70% incidence of Müllerian anomalies (vaginal/uterine agenesis, or unicornuate uterus which are part of Mayer–Rokitansky–Küster–Hauser syndrome)
- Bilateral renal agenesis results in Potter's syndrome consisting of oligohydramnios, pulmonary hypoplasia and facial abnormalities (low set ears/broad flat nose/prominent infraorbital skin folds)

RADIOLOGICAL FEATURES

US/CT/MRI There is compensatory hypertrophy of the normal contralateral kidney

99mTc-DMSA This can exclude a small ectopic kidney

TUBEROUS SCLEROSIS

DEFINITION

- An autosomal dominant condition characterized by multiple hamartomas in the brain, skin, kidneys, liver, lungs and heart (e.g. a cardiac rhabdomyosarcoma)
  - *Renal manifestations:* this is most commonly an angiomyolipoma (AML) ▶ renal cysts or a renal carcinoma can also be present
    - If renal cysts are found in a child < 5 years with no family history, tuberous sclerosis must be excluded

RADIOLOGICAL FEATURES

US Multiple cysts (similar to ADPKD) ▶ during later childhood there may be multiple small rounded echogenic foci throughout the renal parenchyma representing multiple AMLs (with an increased risk of haemorrhage if an AML is > 4 cm)

CT Multiple fat-containing renal masses

SUPERNUMERARY KIDNEYS

- This is extremely rare ▶ it is usually left sided, hypoplastic and caudally positioned

SEPTUM OF BERTIN

- This represents a prominent column of Bertin (cortical tissue that separates the pyramids) ▶ it is usually located at the junction of the upper and middle ⅓ of the kidney ▶ it may be mistaken for a renal mass and is associated with a bifid renal pelvis consisting of two pelvices joined proximal to the ureteropelvic junction – the upper calyces drain into the upper pelvis, while the mid and lower calyces drain into the lower pelvis ▶ the ureters may also join distal to the ureteropelvic junction with a Y configuration (which is usually asymptomatic unless there is 'yo-yo' reflux precipitating recurrent infections)

DROMEDARY HUMP

- This represents a prominent superolateral border of the left kidney (due to compression by the adjacent spleen) ▶ it may be mistaken for a renal mass

SINUS LIPOMATOSIS

- There is increased renal sinus fat

PERSISTENT FETAL LOBULATION

- Renal tissue develops as a series of 8–16 lobules and the lobulated structure persists at birth – this feature normally disappears over the first 5 years of life as the kidney grows

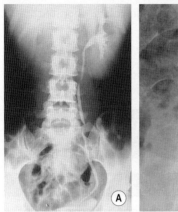
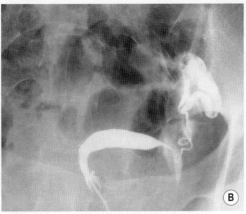

Unicornuate uterus associated with unilateral renal agenesis. (A) IVU demonstrating agenesis and compensatory hypertrophy of the remaining kidney. (B) Hysterosalpinography demonstrates a left-sided unicornuate uterus.[f]

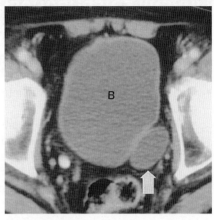

A seminal vesicle cyst (arrow) adjacent to the bladder (B) in a patient with unilateral renal agenesis.[f]

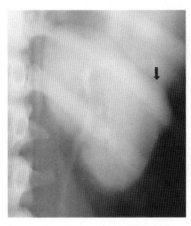

Dromedary hump. A nephrogram demonstrates a focal convex bulge (arrow) along the lateral margin of the left kidney, thought to be due to splenic impression on the kidney.[f]

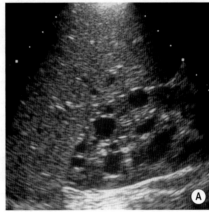

Tuberous sclerosis. (A) Longitudinal US of the right kidney. The left kidney had similar appearances. Both kidneys contain multiple cysts of varying sizes. The appearances on US are indistinguishable from autosomal dominant polycystic kidney disease. This child had the skin stigmata of tuberous sclerosis. (B) Longitudinal US of the right kidney of another patient. There were similar appearances in the left kidney. This shows the more usual appearances of tuberous sclerosis in the kidney with the small echogenic foci of angiomyolipomas.*

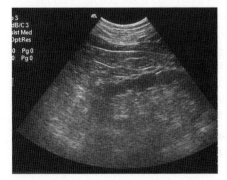

Renal US demonstrating the characteristic pattern of persistent fetal lobulation.

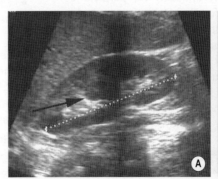
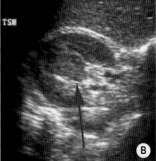

Septum of Bertin. Longitudinal (A) and transverse (B) scans (arrows).[†]

JUVENILE NEPHRONOPHTHISIS/ MEDULLARY CYSTIC DISEASE

DEFINITION

- Medullary cysts associated with interstitial fibrosis and tubular atrophy
  - *Juvenile nephronophthisis:* juvenile-onset (autosomal recessive) ▶ there is a prolonged course with an average disease duration of 10 years
  - *Medullary cystic disease:* adult-onset (autosomal dominant) ▶ there is a rapidly progressive course with death occurring within approximately 2 years

CLINICAL PRESENTATION

- An early urine concentrating defect, with a salt wasting polyuria, polydipsia, growth retardation and anaemia

RADIOLOGICAL FEATURES

US Hyper-reflective kidneys (which are small or normal in size) ▶ loss of corticomedullary differentiation ▶ the late development of corticomedullary cysts

DMSA scintigram During the early stages (when the tubules are affected to a greater degree than the glomeruli) the kidneys may not be visible – yet a ^{99m}Tc-DTPA scintigram may be almost normal

PEARLS

- It is associated with skeletal abnormalities, congenital hepatic fibrosis and mental retardation
- *Diagnosis:* renal biopsy

DYSPLASIA/CYSTIC DYSPLASIA

DEFINITION

- Abnormal metanephric differentiation with persistence of fetal renal tissue in the form of nests of metaplastic cartilage associated with primitive ducts
  - If it is bilateral then renal failure will develop (possibly not until the 2nd decade)
  - *Associations:* a duplex kidney ▶ posterior urethral valves ▶ malpositioned kidneys (e.g. cross-fused renal ectopia, a horseshoe or a pelvic kidney) ▶ various syndromes (e.g. Beckwith?Wiedemann)

RADIOLOGICAL FEATURES

US A small kidney with loss of the normal corticomedullary differentiation and hyper-reflectivity ▶ a variable number and size of cysts ▶ dilatation is uncommon (unless it is associated with VUR)

^{99m}Tc-DMSA scintigraphy Focal defects ▶ poor function (to a varying degree)

MCUG Blunted calyces which are few in number ▶ a dilated and rather perpendicular renal pelvis with a tortuous and dilated ureter

MULTICYSTIC DYSPLASTIC KIDNEY (MCDK)

DEFINITION

- Ureteral obstruction or atresia during the metanephric stage inhibits nephron development (and failure of union of renal mesenchyme and ureteric bud) – as a result the collecting tubules enlarge into cysts with the formation of immature glomeruli and tubules
- MCDK is always non-functioning with an atretic ureter ▶ usually contralateral VUR

CLINICAL PRESENTATION

- Asymptomatic ▶ an abdominal mass (it is the 2nd most common neonatal abdominal mass after hydronephrosis) ▶ recurrent UTIs
  - It is usually unilateral ▶ there is a natural tendency towards involution (M>F)

RADIOLOGICAL FEATURES

- The appearance is related to:
  - The time of onset
    - *Early:* a small renal pelvis with multiple cysts
    - *Late:* a large central dilated pelvis, mimicking hydronephrosis, which may communicate with the associated cysts
  - The location of the obstruction or atresia
    - *Proximal ureter:* multiple enlarged cysts within an enlarged kidney
    - *Distal ureter:* a few cysts within an atrophic kidney
- Differentiating MCDK from PUJ obstruction: residual parenchyma is central (MCDK) or peripheral (PUJO)

US Variable appearances: a large kidney with multiple large cysts or a hypoplastic and echogenic atophic kidney ▶ there is little identifiable renal parenchyma

- *'Cluster of grapes' appearance:* visible cysts are usually anechoic and of variable sizes (often with a dominant large cyst sited peripherally)

Indications for surgery A large mass impeding breathing or feeding ▶ an enlarging mass ▶ a mass that is > 5 cm by 1 year of age

Prognosis This depends upon the function of the contralateral kidney (bilateral MCDK is incompatible with life) ▶ the contralateral kidney is associated with PUJ obstruction or ureteric stenosis (30%)

Comparison of renal cystic diseases

	ADPKD	Tuberous sclerosis	ARPKD	MCDK	Simple cyst
Inheritance	AD	AD	AR	None	None
Distribution	Bilateral unequal	Bilateral	Bilateral equal	Uni- or bilateral	Unilateral
Kidney size	Normal or large	Normal or large	Very large (>90th centile)	Small or large	Normal
Extrarenal manifestations	Cysts in the liver, spleen, pancreas	Cardiac rhabdomyomas, intracranial tubers	Congenital hepatic fibrosis	None	None
Age at presentation	3rd decade	Often < 18 months	Neonate and childhood	Antenatal, rare in childhood	Onset in adult life
Cyst size	Visible cysts of variable size	Similar to ADPKD, ± angiomyolipomas	Generally small	Large then often involute	Variable
Diagnosis	US, genetic	US, cardiac echo, cranial MRI	US, IVU, liver biopsy	US, MAG3	US, IVU
Malignancy risk	No	Yes	No	Rare	No

ADPKD, autosomal dominant polycystic kidney disease ▶ ARPKD, autosomal recessive polycystic kidney disease ▶ MCDK, multicystic dysplastic kidney ▶ AR, autosomal recessive ▶ AD, autosomal dominant.*

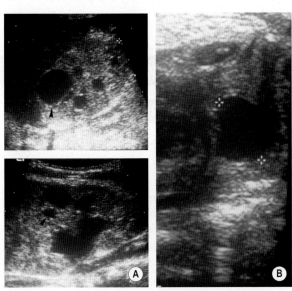

Cystic dysplasia. (A) Longitudinal US of the right (top) and left (bottom) kidneys. Both kidneys are hyperechoic and contain small cysts (arrowheads) with some dilatation of the collecting system on the left. This male infant also had dilated ureters. (B) Longitudinal US of the posterior urethra during voiding shows the dilatation of the posterior urethra. This infant had posterior urethral valves.*

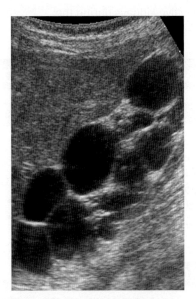

Multicystic dysplastic kidney. Longitudinal US of the right renal area. This shows the right renal fossa filled with multiple cysts of varying sizes and no normal renal parenchyma.*

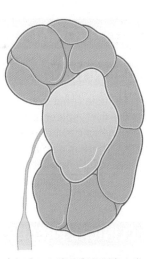

A hydronephrotic multicystic dysplastic kidney. The renal parenchyma is dysplastic and replaced by numerous cystic areas. The upper ureter is atretic. There is a dominant central cyst within the area where the renal pelvis would be expected, and surrounded by radially arranged similar cysts.

AUTOSOMAL RECESSIVE POLYCYSTIC KIDNEY DISEASE (ARPKD)

DEFINITION

- A rare genetic disorder (involving chromosome 6) where the renal parenchyma is replaced by numerous tiny (1–8 mm) cysts
  - *4 subtypes:* perinatal ▶ neonatal ▶ infantile ▶ juvenile
  - There is an association with periportal hepatic fibrosis and subsequent liver failure – this increases in frequency with the age of presentation until the juvenile subtype where the liver disease predominates
    - *Younger children:* renal disease predominates
    - *Older children:* liver disease predominates

CLINICAL PRESENTATION

- Most cases present during the neonatal period with oligohydramnios and Potter's syndrome

RADIOLOGICAL FEATURES

US

- *Prenatal:* bilateral highly reflective kidneys during the fetal period (a non-specific sign)

- *Infant:* symmetrically and markedly enlarged kidneys (the kidneys appear relatively less enlarged as the infant grows) ▶ a characteristic hyper-reflective cortex and medulla ▶ small 1–2 mm cysts may be seen within the medulla ('pepper and salt' kidney) ▶ there can occasionally be large cysts of different sizes seen in later childhood (mimicking ADPKD)
  - *Liver:* hepatosplenomegaly is usually seen in most children after the 1st year of life ▶ increased echogenicity within the periportal regions (due to bile duct proliferation and fibrosis) ▶ single or multiple cysts communicating and closely related to the biliary tree (± biliary ectasia) ▶ splenomegaly, portal hypertension and varices

IVU A streaky nephrogram (as contrast medium pools within ectatic collecting ducts) ▶ distorted calyces with full collecting systems

99mTc-DMSA scintigraphy Bilateral focal defects within enlarged kidneys on a background of high activity

HIDA scintigram An enlarged left lobe of the liver (in children > 1 year of age) ▶ delayed passage of isotope through the liver with areas of pooling and prominence of the duct system

AUTOSOMAL DOMINANT POLYCYSTIC KIDNEY DISEASE (ADPKD)

DEFINITION

- Multiple renal cysts seen in association with cysts in the liver, spleen and pancreas ▶ although it has 100% penetrance, it demonstrates a variable expression
  - There is also an association with intracranial aneurysms within the circle of Willis ▶ it is rarely associated with congenital hepatic fibrosis (cf. ARPKD)

CLINICAL PRESENTATION

- Hypertension ▶ renal insufficiency ▶ cyst complications (e.g. haematuria or pain) ▶ an abdominal mass
  - It commonly presents after the 3rd decade of life (but may present in childhood or antenatally) ▶ 64% of presenting children (< 10 years) will have renal cysts – this increases to 90% between 10 and 19 years

RADIOLOGICAL FEATURES

IVU Enlarged kidneys with classically stretched calyces ▶ occasional cyst calcification

US

- *Prenatal:* highly reflective kidneys (similar to ARPKD)
- *Infancy/adult:* variable appearances from a normal kidney, to a few cysts, to multiple cysts involving the cortex and medulla of an enlarged kidney ▶ typically there is unequal but bilateral involvement

CT As the cysts are prone to haemorrhage and infection, they may become thick walled, septated, calcified, or contain internal debris

MRI This can be a useful technique in differentiating between simple cysts, haemorrhagic cysts and neoplasms

PEARL

- A renal neoplasm may coexist with adult polycystic renal disease (the diagnosis can become difficult in these cases)

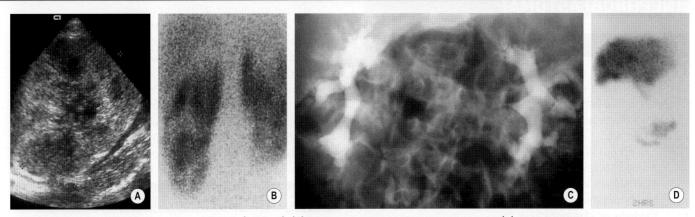

Autosomal recessive polycystic kidney disease (ARPKD). (A) Longitudinal US of the right kidney and (B) DMSA scintigram on a patient with ARPKD. US shows the typical appearances of a large hyperechoic kidney. The left kidney appeared similar. The DMSA scintigram shows photon-deficient areas in both the kidneys, particularly in the polar regions. These defects do not correspond to visible cysts on US. The child had no history of urinary tract infection. (C) IVU on a patient with ARPKD showing the streaky radiation of contrast medium as it passes through the ectatic tubules. (D) HIDA scintigram: delayed image after 2 h showing retention of tracer within the liver, an enlarged left lobe, and a 'patchy' appearance as the tracer has accumulated in the ducts. Similar appearances have been reported in Caroli's syndrome with congenital hepatic fibrosis.*

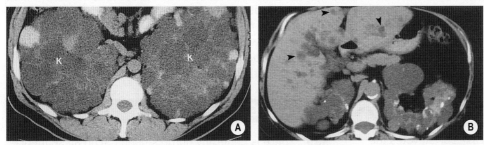

Autosomal dominant polycystic kidney disease. (A) NECT demonstrates massive kidney (K) enlargement with the normal renal parenchyma replaced with renal cysts. Some of these cysts are high attenuation, indicating previous haemorrhage. (B) Extensive bilateral cysts are noted. Some of these cysts contain calcifications. As is common, numerous simple cysts (arrowheads) of the liver are also present.ʃ

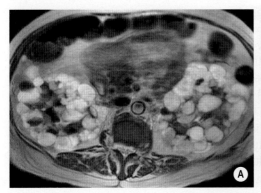

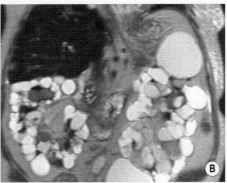

Autosomal dominant polycystic kidney disease. (A) Axial T2WI demonstrating the renal parenchyma replaced by multiple cysts. (B) Coronal T2WI in the same patient.

WILMS' TUMOUR (NEPHROBLASTOMA)

DEFINITION

- A renal tumour arising from metanephric blastema cells (the primitive embryonic renal parenchyma) ▶ a solid lesion with a fibrous pseudocapsule ▶ variable areas of haemorrhage and necrosis ▶ it may invade the renal vein and IVC
  - *Extrarenal Wilms' tumours are rare:* retroperitoneum ▶ inguinal region ▶ pelvis
  - *Metastases:* local para-aortic nodes ▶ haematogenous spread to the lungs (less commonly the liver or skeleton)

CLINICAL PRESENTATION

- It most commonly presents as an asymptomatic abdominal mass ▶ haematuria ▶ less commonly pain, fever or hypertension
- Peak incidence at 3 years (M = F)
- It is the 3rd most common childhood malignancy after leukaemia and brain tumours
- 10% are bilateral ▶ ⅔ are synchronous tumours ▶ ⅓ are metachronous tumours

RADIOLOGICAL FEATURES

US A solid hyperechoic mass (± cystic areas)

CT Typically a large heterogeneously enhancing exophytic renal mass (enhancing less than normal kidney) ▶ a pseudocapsule may be visible ▶ calcification is unusual (< 10%) ▶ variable haemorrhage/necrosis

- *'Claw' sign:* normal renal tissue is typically stretched at the periphery of the lesion
- *Tumour spread:* typically by direct extension with displacement of any adjacent structures (cf. a neuroblastoma where tumour encases or elevates the aorta)
- *Vascular invasion:* this is seen in 5–10% (involving the renal vein, IVC and right atrium) ▶ it can also invade the renal pelvis and ureter

MRI T1WI: low SI ▶ T2WI: high SI ▶ T1WI + Gad: heterogeneous enhancement (often poor)

PEARLS

- **Treatment:**
  - *North America:* surgical excision is followed by adjuvant chemotherapy (per surgical staging)
  - *Europe:* initial chemotherapy (after biopsy confirmation) with subsequent resection
- **Prognosis:** 4-year overall survival rates: stages I–II (86–96%) ▶ stage IV (up to 83%) ▶ stage V (70%)

- There is a poorer outcome for the much less common diffuse anaplastic Wilms' tumours
- **Associated congenital anomalies (15%):** cryptorchidism ▶ horseshoe kidney
- **Associated syndromes:** Beckwith–Wiedemann (macroglossia + exophthalmos + gigantism) ▶ hemihypertrophy ▶ Denys–Drash (pseudohermaphroditism) ▶ Soto's (cerebral gigantism) ▶ Bloom's (immunodeficiency and facial telangiectasia) ▶ WAGR (Wilms' tumour + Aniridia + Genitourinary abnormalities + mental Retardation)

NEPHROBLASTOMATOSIS

DEFINITION

- Persistence of the metanephric blastema beyond 36 weeks' gestation, with multiple and diffuse nephrogenic rests ▶ these rests have the potential to form a nephroblastoma or Wilms' tumour
  - It is seen in 1% of normal infant kidneys, in 41% of patients with a unilateral Wilms' tumour, in 94% of metachronous bilateral Wilms' tumours, and in 99% of multicentric or bilateral Wilms' tumours
- Nephroblastomatosis may be unifocal, multifocal or diffuse
- **Perilobar nephrogenic rest:** these are located at the periphery of a renal lobe
  - *Associations:* Beckwith–Weidemann syndrome ▶ hemihypertrophy ▶ trisomy 18
- **Intralobar nephrogenic rest:** these are located anywhere within a renal lobe
  - *Associations:* DRASH syndrome ▶ WAGR syndrome ▶ sporadic aniridia

RADIOLOGICAL FEATURES

MRI There is generally homogeneous SI on all sequences (including T1WI + Gad) – this is in contrast to a Wilms' tumour which is heterogeneous

- **Multifocal (juvenile) nephroblastomatosis:** this is the most common form

  US/CT/MRI The nephrogenic rests resemble normal renal cortex and are scattered throughout the kidneys ▶ they may be nodular or plaque-like ▶ after contrast administration they may become hypodense (CT) or hypointense (MRI) due to their relatively poor perfusion
- **Superficial diffuse nephroblastomatosis:** a superficial continuous rind of rest tissue around the renal medulla

  US This demonstrates a thick band of reduced echogenicity around the medulla ▶ there is reduced corticomedullary differentiation

  CT/MRI Abnormal tissue surrounding the renal periphery which is non-enhancing

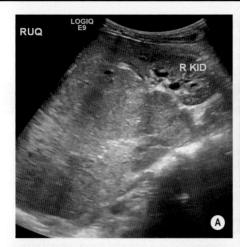

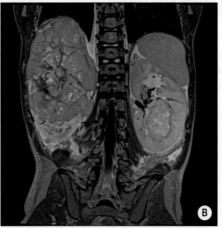

(A) Wilms' tumour. Large heterogeneous mass on US arising from the upper right kidney with inferior displacement of the lower renal pole. (B) Bilateral Wilms' tumour. MRI is now the gold standard for assessment of bilateral disease. Here, a small mass in the left kidney may be overlooked by the large right-sided mass.**

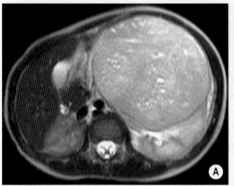

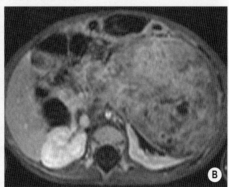

Wilms' tumours. MRI. (A) Axial T2WI and (B) axial T1WI + Gad show a large tumour growing exophytically anterior to the left kidney.*

Distinguishing features between a Wilms' tumour and a neuroblastoma		
	Wilms' tumour	**Neuroblastoma**
Age at presentation	Peak incidence between 2 and 3 years	< 2 years
Renal mass effect	Intrinsic mass effect (the CT 'claw sign' helps confirm the renal origin of the tumour)	Extrinsic mass effect (as the originating cells are from the retroperitoneal neural crest cells)
Calcification	Affects a minority of tumours	Seen in 85%
Effect on the aorta	Displacement	Encasement and elevation
Extension across the midline	Less common	Common

Wilms' tumour staging	
Stage I	Tumour is confined to the kidney (with no capsular or vascular invasion)
Stage II	Tumour extends beyond the renal capsule into the perinephric space ▶ vessel infiltration
Stage III	Positive lymph nodes within the abdomen or pelvis ▶ peritoneal invasion ▶ residual tumour at the surgical margin
Stage IV	Metastatic disease outside the abdomen or pelvis
Stage V	Bilateral tumours at original diagnosis

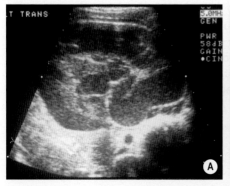

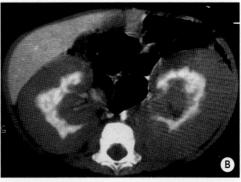

Nephroblastomatosis. (A) US demonstrating uniformly hypoechoic lesions surrounding the periphery of an enlarged kidney in a diffuse type of nephroblastomatosis. (B) Delayed CECT sections demonstrate these lesions, typically showing reduced vascularity in a fairly homogeneous pattern. Dense contrast medium is seen within the normal renal parenchyma.*

RHABDOID TUMOUR OF THE KIDNEY

Definition

- The most aggressive malignant renal tumour in childhood (it originates from the renal sinus) ▶ renal vein invasion is common and it can also metastasize to the lungs, liver and brain
- It accounts for 2% of all paediatric renal neoplasms and presents during the 1st year of life
- It is associated with a paraneoplastic hypercalcaemia (a non-specific finding as it is also found with a mesoblastic nephroma) ▶ it is also associated with simultaneous primitive neuroectodermal tumours (usually occurring within the posterior fossa)

CT The mass is indistinguishable from a Wilms' tumour

- *'Peripheral fluid crescent' sign:* this has been described but it is not pathognomonic

CLEAR CELL SARCOMA OF THE KIDNEY

Definition

- A highly malignant childhood renal tumour (accounting for 4% of all childhood renal neoplasms) ▶ there are no known genetic associations and no reports of bilateral tumours ▶ M >> F
  - It has a particular predilection for skeletal metastases (> 20%) ▶ it can also metastasize to the lungs

Clinical presentation

- A palpable abdominal mass ▶ haematuria ▶ lethargy
  - There is a marked male preponderance with a peak age of incidence similar to a Wilms' tumour (2–3 years of age)

US A heterogeneous mass of soft tissue echogenicity

CT There are no specific radiological features allowing a distinction to be made from a Wilms' tumour

Bone scintigraphy Bone metastases (with no lung deposits) suggests a clear cell sarcoma rather than a Wilms' tumour

LYMPHOMA AND LEUKAEMIA

Definition

- Renal involvement (± retroperitoneal adenopathy) is seen in 12% of children with non-Hodgkin's lymphoma ▶ it is most commonly a B-cell Burkitt's lymphoma

US Renal enlargement with an altered echotexture is typical for lymphoma and leukaemia

CT Multiple, and usually bilateral, nodules are typical ▶ diffuse infiltration may be seen ▶ there is usually widespread disease elsewhere

MESOBLASTIC NEPHROMA

Definition

- A renal tumour derived from early renal mesenchyme typically involving the renal sinus (usually there is no herniation into the renal pelvis, unlike a MLCN) ▶ it does not invade the vascular pedicle nor does it metastasize

Clinical presentation

- It is the most common solid neonatal renal neoplasm, presenting as an abdominal mass ▶ it almost exclusively occurs within the first 6 months of life (90% are diagnosed at < 1 year of age) ▶ M>F

US A solid non-calcified renal mass demonstrating heterogeneous reflectivity (heterogeneity suggests cystic change or necrosis) ▶ hypoechoic areas represent cystic change or necrosis ▶ there is no invasion of the vascular pedicle (complete excision carries an excellent prognosis)

US and CT These cannot reliably distinguish this from a Wilms' tumour

99mTc-DMSA The tumour will demonstrate uptake (cf. no uptake with a Wilms' tumour)

MULTILOCULAR CYSTIC NEPHROMA (MLCN)

Definition

- An uncommon cystic renal mass which is derived from the metanephric blastema (with a sporadic association with other anomalies)
- Nephrectomy is curative (this is recommended because of the malignant potential)

Clinical presentation

- It has a bimodal distribution: it is seen more commonly in boys < 4 years of age and in women in the 5th or 6th decades

US A multilocular renal mass with multiple cysts and septations ▶ a thick fibrous capsule is present

CECT A multilocular cystic mass with the cystic component usually of water attenuation ▶ it is typically unilateral and found within the lower pole ▶ there may be curvilinear calcification and moderate septal enhancement

- It characteristically herniates into the renal hilum

Isotope imaging A non-functioning mass

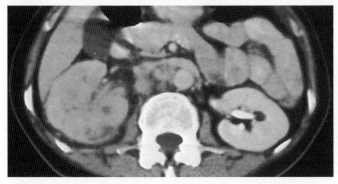
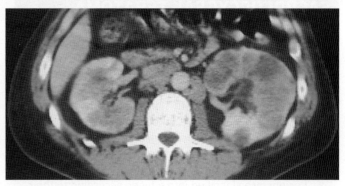

CECT of a renal sarcoma showing a generally expanded kidney with areas of tumour enhancing less well than normal renal tissue.[†]

CECT demonstrating renal lymphoma. There are bilateral relatively well-defined intermediate-to-low-density deposits of lymphoma.[†]

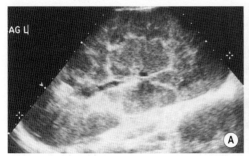
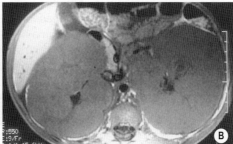

Non-Hodgkin's lymphoma of the kidneys. Longitudinal renal US (A) in a 5-year-old boy showing multiple isoechoic masses within a 17 cm kidney. Axial T1WI (B) and coronal STIR (C) confirming gross enlargement of both kidneys with complete loss of the normal renal architecture. Differential diagnoses include lymphoma, leukaemia and nephroblastomatosis.[†]

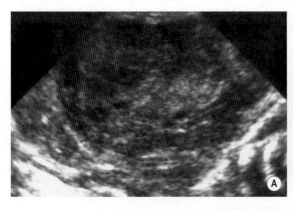
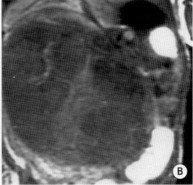

Mesoblastic nephroma. (A) US demonstrating a inhomogeneous renal mass. (B) An MRI confirms the extent and character of the lesion.[§]

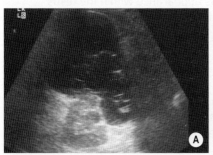
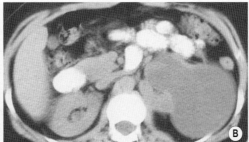
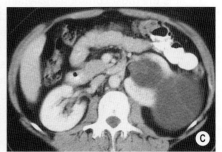

Multilocular cystic nephroma on ultrasound (A) and CT before (B) and after (C) contrast. Note the lesion typically bulging into the renal pelvis.[†]

SACROCOCCYGEAL TERATOMA

Definition

- This is the most common presacral tumour and is a congenital lesion containing derivatives of the three germinal layers arising from the ventral surface of the coccyx ▶ lesions are mostly non-familial and occur more frequently in girls ▶ although almost all lesions are benign at birth, sacrococcygeal teratomas have the potential for later malignant transformation and hence require surgical removal
  - Lesions are classified into 4 types according to their location
    - *Type I:* predominantly external
    - *Type II:* external and intrapelvic
    - *Type III:* superior extension into the abdomen
    - *Type IV:* entirely presacral with no external component
  - Lesions may be evident at birth or present later (type IV)
  - The tumour marker for sacrococcygeal teratoma is α-fetoprotein

Radiological features

MRI A solid lesion attached to the sacrum (cf. an anterior sacral meningocele which is cystic)
- *Benign:* this is usually a cystic mass (± calcification and fat)
- *Malignant:* a predominantly solid lesion, which may invade adjacent structures or metastasize to the chest

OTHER PRESACRAL LESIONS

- Anterior myelomeningocele ▶ neuroenteric cyst ▶ spinal dysraphism associated with a sacral defect
  - Less commonly a neuroblastoma or lymphoma

RHABDOMYOSARCOMA

Definition

- Although the term suggests a mesenchymal tumour derived from striated muscle, the tumour frequently arises in sites lacking striated muscle
  - It is the most common malignant neoplasm of the pelvis in children (the GU tract is the 2nd most common site for a paediatric rhabdomyosarcoma after a head and neck location)
    - *Boys:* most arise from the prostate or bladder base
    - *Girls:* most arise from the bladder, vagina or uterus
  - *Histological types:* embryonal and alveolar (embryonal is the more common and has a better prognosis)

Clinical presentation

- Pelvic tumours may be very large at presentation and present as an abdominal mass ▶ prostate tumours may cause urinary obstruction and manifest with marked bladder distension or acute retention

Radiological features

US A typically solid but heterogeneous mass ▶ the vascularity can be quite variable

MRI Oedema and later non-specific soft tissue thickening after radiotherapy may suggest an increase in tumour size or persisting tumour, which can lead to discrepancies between the MRI findings and surgical or biopsy results
- Prostate tumours commonly infiltrate locally into the perivesical tissues and into the bladder base with anterosuperior spread into the space of Retzius
- T1WI + Gad: a solid heterogeneous enhancing mass (± adenopathy)

Pearls

- Rhabdomyosarcomas in favourable sites such as the vagina have up to 94% 3-year survival
- Tumours in the prostate and bladder have a worse prognosis, with a 3-year survival of approximately 70%

PAEDIATRIC SCROTAL MASSES

Definition

- Intratesticular benign and malignant tumours are relatively common neoplasms in children
  - *Primary testicular neoplasms:* germ cell tumours (the most common and often with calcifications) ▶ endodermal sinus tumour and embryonal carcinomas ▶ paratesticular rhabdomyosarcomas (including tumours arising within the spermatic cord, epididymis and penis and accounting for 12% of scrotal tumours in boys)
  - *Secondary sites of disease:* leukaemia ▶ lymphoma ▶ neuroblastoma (although it is seen much less frequently than in adults)

Clinical presentation

- A palpable scrotal mass

Radiological features

US A heterogeneous appearance within the testis ▶ increased Doppler flow ▶ it may mimic infection

CT/MRI This allows evaluation of the regional lymph nodes

Pearl

- A paratesticular rhabdomyosarcoma has a good outlook in children younger than 10 years, with a greater than 90% 5-year survival

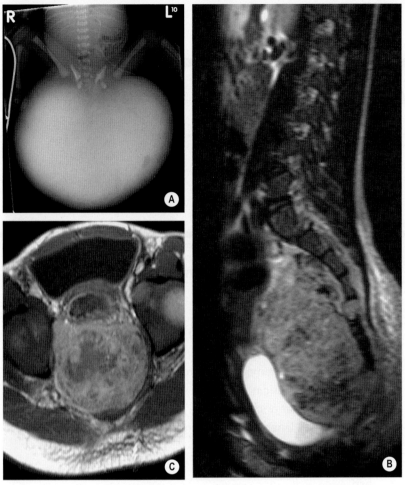

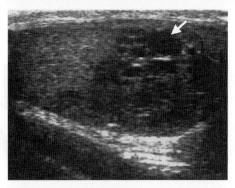

Teratoma of testis. US. The cystic areas (arrow) within the lesion are characteristic.*

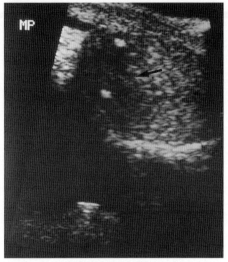

Sacrococcygeal teratomas. (A) Plain AXR showing a very large external component to a sacrococcygeal teratoma in a newborn. (B) Sagittal T2WI in another infant showing a large intrapelvic component to the sacrococcygeal teratoma. Note the teratoma, posterior to the uniformly high SI bladder, is of intermediate heterogeneous signal, and is invading the sacrum. (C) Axial T1WI in the same patient showing the heterogeneous mass in a presacral location.*

Embyonal cell carcinoma of testis. Longitudinal US shows a testicular mass (arrow) containing 2 echogenic foci, consistent with calcifications. The interface between tumour and normal parenchyma is poorly defined.ʃ

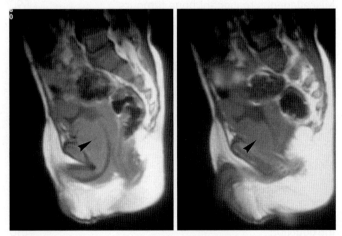

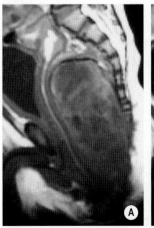

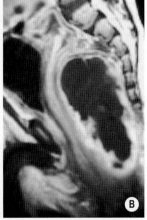

Prostatic rhabdomyosarcoma. MRI sagittal T1WI through the pelvis showing a large mass of intermediate SI centred on the prostate (arrowheads). A catheter is seen to traverse the urethra with the balloon in a collapsed bladder. The appearances are those of the bladder/prostate rhabdomyosarcoma.*

Rhabdomyosarcoma. (A) Sagittal T1WI. (B) Sagittal T1WI + Gad showing a large cystic mass lesion due to an embryonal rhabdomyosarcoma in the presacral region extending to the perineum. The mass demonstrates vivid peripheral enhancement after contrast medium administration, but no obvious central enhancement was seen. Note that the bladder and bowel are displaced anteriorly. No intraspinal extension was evident.*

5.1 SKELETAL TRAUMA

GENERAL CONSIDERATIONS

XR Two orthogonal views are required ▶ it is poor at soft tissue assessment

- Displacement and obliteration of the normal fat pads can be a clue to an acute fracture haematoma or joint distension ▶ a lipohaemarthrosis (fat and blood within the joint space) is evidence of an intra-articular fracture

Scintigraphy Uptake is related to any osteoblastic activity ▶ it is much more sensitive than XR

CT Small fractures may not be detected due to volume averaging

MRI This is ideal for assessing the ligaments, tendons, cartilage and muscle ▶ it is very sensitive for the detection of bone oedema (T1WI: low SI ▶ T2WI: high SI)

- Normal tendons and ligaments are devoid of signal on all routine pulse sequences ▶ sprains and tears increase their water content (T2WI: high SI) ▶ fat-suppressed sequences increase the conspicuity of any increased signal
- **Tendinitis:** this leads to tendon enlargement and increased intratendinous signal intensity
  - *Partial tear:* this may be seen as an irregularity within the tendon shape with associated high SI (T2WI)
  - *Complete tear:* the tendon is discontinuous, absent or unrecognizable
- **Ligamentous injury**
  - *Grade I injury* (mild sprain): abnormally increased SI around an otherwise normal-appearing ligament
  - *Grade II injury* (severe sprain): abnormal thickening ± abnormal SI within the ligament
  - *Grade III injury* (complete disruption of the ligament): a disrupted ligament

US High-resolution transducers are ideal for assessing tendon, ligament and muscle injuries

- Normal tendons appear as hyperechoic parallel lines within the longitudinal plane ▶ artefactual areas of hypoechogenicity may result from incorrect transducer placement
- *Tendinitis:* this is seen as an increased tendon thickness with altered echogenicity (focal or diffuse)
- *Tear:* this appears as a hypoechoic gap within the tendon (often fluid is seen within the tendon sheath)
- **Pathological fracture:** this occurs where substantially less force is required to cause a fracture in a weakened bone
  - *'Banana fracture':* pathological fractures tend to be oriented transversely within long bones
  - *Causes:* metastatic disease ▶ benign tumours (e.g. an enchondroma or a solitary bone cyst) ▶ Paget's disease ▶ renal osteodystrophy ▶ osteogenesis imperfecta
- **Stress fracture (fatigue fracture):** this occurs due to chronic repetitive trauma on normal bone ▶ a subtle periosteal reaction or a transverse band of linear

sclerosis may develop 1–2 weeks after the onset of symptoms
  - *Common sites:* metatarsal shafts ('march fractures') ▶ pubic rami ▶ femoral neck ▶ tibial and fibular shafts ▶ calcaneal tuberosity
- **Insufficiency fracture:** this is caused by normal activity on abnormal bone (e.g. osteopenic bone in the elderly)
- **Joint prosthetic loosening:** a widened radiolucency at either the bone–cement or prosthesis–bone interface (> 2 mm) ▶ prosthetic migration ▶ periosteal reaction

FRACTURE DESCRIPTION

- **Location:** e.g. proximal, middle or distal shaft
- An **open** (disruption of the overlying skin, suggested by gas within the adjacent soft tissues) vs a **closed** fracture (with intact overlying skin)
- A **complete** (a fracture extending across the full width of the bone) vs an **incomplete** fracture (e.g. a paediatric greenstick fracture)
- A **transverse** vs an **oblique** vs a **spiral** (due to significant torsional force) fracture
- **Distraction** (separation) vs **impaction** vs **overriding** (overlapping without impaction) of the fracture fragments
- Joint **dislocation** (the articular surfaces are completely separated) vs **subluxation** (there is partial contact between the articular surfaces)
- An **avulsion** fracture: there is separation of the bone fragment at the ligament or tendinous attachment site (it is usually a transverse fracture)
- An **osteochondral** fracture: there is disruption of the articular cartilage and underlying subchondral bone ▶ a fracture fragment can become a joint loose body
  - *Common sites:* femoral condyles ▶ patella ▶ talar dome
- **Comminuted** fracture: > 2 separate bone fragments
- **Butterfly fragment:** a large triangular fragment usually orientated along the long axis of the bone
- The proximal fragment is considered the point of reference when describing the displacement of a distal fragment:
  - Anterior, posterior, medial or lateral (e.g. one shaft width medial displacement)
  - Angulation of the long axis of the distal fragment relative to the proximal fragment (varus vs valgus)
- Associated soft tissue injuries:
  - **Joint effusion:** elevation of the elbow anterior fat pad is suggestive of a fracture
  - **Lipohaemarthrosis:** a fat-fluid level within a joint (commonly from trauma-induced release of bone marrow fat) ▶ this can be seen on a horizontal lateral view of the knee ▶ it can also be seen within the shoulder

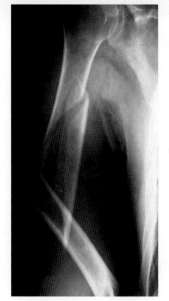

A comminuted fracture of the midshaft of the right humerus demonstrates a medial butterfly fragment (large arrow). There is marked lateral angulation at the fracture line between the major fracture fragments.*

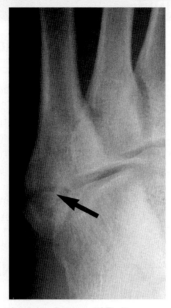

Avulsion fracture. AP views of the foot demonstrate a horizontal lucency at the base of the fifth metatarsal (arrow), representing an avulsion injury at the insertion site of the peroneus brevis tendon.*

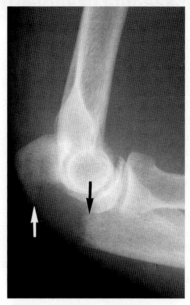

Distracted fracture of the olecranon. Lateral view of the elbow in a patient who was struck by a bus, causing fracture of the olecranon process of the ulna (arrows). Note the wide distraction of the fragments, caused by retraction of the triceps brachii inserting on the proximal fragment.*

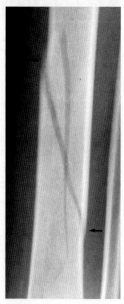

Spiral fracture. AP projection of the leg demonstrates a spiral fracture of the tibia. Note the sharp ends of the fracture fragments (arrows), which may cause significant soft tissue injury.*

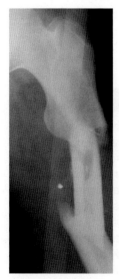

Segmental fracture. AP view of the left hip demonstrates a three-part fracture of the proximal femoral shaft, due to massive trauma in a motor vehicle accident.*

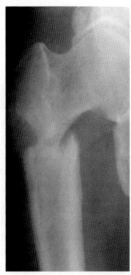

Pathological 'banana fracture'. A transverse subtrochanteric fracture of the right femur with varus angulation. A transverse fracture in a long bone (particularly the subtrochanteric region of the femur) is almost always due to an underlying abnormality (in this case a metastatic lesion within the lateral cortex).*

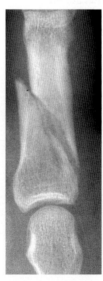

An oblique fracture of the proximal phalanx of the fourth digit. There is minimal override of the fracture fragments.*

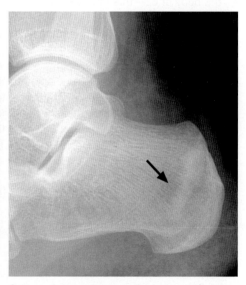

Calcaneal stress fracture. A lateral view of the calcaneus demonstrates linear sclerosis within the tuberosity (arrow) of a stress fracture.*

ASSESSMENT OF CERVICAL SPINE INJURIES

NORMAL RADIOLOGICAL ANATOMY (LATERAL XR)

- The cervical spine is normally lordotic – this may be absent due to patient positioning, the presence of a hard collar or muscular spasm
- Minimum imaging requirement: AP view, AP odontoid peg view, and lateral view
  - Lateral view: all seven cervical vertebrae (including the C7/T1 junction) must be visualised ▶ this may require a swimmer's view if they are not demonstrated on the lateral view
- 4 imaginary continuous curves should be present, and appear smooth without interruption:
  1. *Anterior spinal line* (passing along the anterior borders of the vertebral bodies and anterior odontoid peg)
  2. *Posterior spinal line* (passing along the posterior borders of the vertebral bodies)
  3. *Spinolaminar line* (the junction of the laminae with the spinous processes) ▶ in children the spinolaminar line may have an offset of 2 to 3 mm at the C2–C3 and C3–C4 levels with flexion and extension
  4. *Facet joint line* (posterior aspect of the facet joints – superimposed on a lateral view) ▶ a double fact joint line ('bow-tie' sign) indicates a rotational abnormality, usually a fracture dislocation of the facet joints
- The odontoid process is usually tilted posteriorly on the body of C2 – this may otherwise may indicate an odontoid fracture
- Slight anterior subluxation of C2 on C3 is a common appearance in children
- Kyphotic angulation of the spine associated with widening of the gap between 2 spinous processes implies rupture of the posterior ligamentous structures
- The atlantoaxial distance measured at the base of the dens between the anterior cortex of the dens and posterior cortex of the anterior arch of C1:
  - *Adults:* <3 mm
  - *Children:* <5 mm
- Assessment of the prevertebral tissues (to exclude a retropharyngeal haematoma):
  - *Adults:* <5 mm (at the level of C3 and C4) ▶ <22 mm (at the level of C6)
  - *Children:* no more than $\frac{2}{3}$ of the width of the C2 body (at the level of C3 and C4 ▶ <14 mm (at the level of C6)

NORMAL RADIOLOGICAL ANATOMY (AP VIEW)

- The spinous processes should form a continuous (although often slightly irregular) line ▶ they may appear bifid (a normal finding) – the central point is midway between the 2 tubercles of the spinous process
- The C2–7 vertebrae should be of a similar height

NORMAL RADIOLOGICAL ANATOMY (OPEN MOUTH VIEW)

- This is used to detect an odontoid process fracture and confirm integrity of the C1 ring
  - *Neutral position:* the lateral margins of the lateral masses of C1 should align with C2
- With rotation the atlas normally moves as a unit with lateral facet offset on one side and medial offset on the opposite side
  - *Adults:* bilateral offset indicates a C1 ring fracture
  - *Children:* bilateral offset is a normal variant (due to discrepant growth of C1 and C2)

RADIOGRAPHIC SIGNS OF INSTABILITY

- The cervical spine is divided into 3 columns:
  - *Anterior column:* the anterior longitudinal ligament and the anterior $\frac{1}{2}$ of the vertebral body
  - *Middle column:* the posterior $\frac{1}{2}$ of the vertebral body and the posterior longitudinal ligament
  - *Posterior column:* the posterior ligamentous complex
- Instability is suggested if there is: abnormal spinous process fanning ▶ a widened disc space ▶ horizontal displacement of one body on another (> 3.5 mm) ▶ angulation > 11° ▶ disrupted facets or multiple fractures
- Instability is more likely if more than 1 column is disrupted
  - *Stable:* fractures limited to the vertebral or posterior elements
  - *Unstable:* fractures involving both the vertebral body and posterior elements

PEARLS

- Fractures and dislocations are most common within the lower cervical spine (C4–C7), the thoracolumbar junction (T10–L2), and the craniocervical junction (C1–C2) – these are relatively mobile areas ▶ the thoracic spine is relatively rigid (restricted by the thoracic cage)
  - Usually the upper vertebral body is displaced anteriorly relative to the lower vertebral body
  - There is often an anterior wedge compression fracture of the lower vertebral body and fractures involving the laminae, facets, or spinous processes
  - Alternatively, there may be a disruption of the joint capsule of the facet joints and interspinous ligament without associated fractures
  - At times there may be no significant fracture associated with a dislocation, since the injury is limited to the intervertebral disc, facet joint capsules and intervening ligaments
- Paraspinal haematomas (e.g. a retropharyngeal mass) may point to an otherwise obscure fracture or dislocation

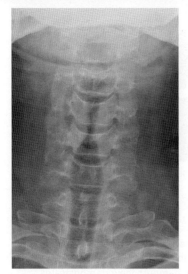

C-spine XR. AP view of the cervical spine showing normal alignment of the vertebral bodies with no loss in vertebral body height. Posterior elements are intact.

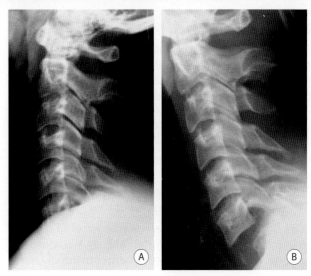

We must demonstrate all seven cervical vertebrae. (A) Initial cross-table lateral XR examination of the spine reveals only six cervical vertebrae. (B) A repeat examination was obtained while pulling down on the shoulder, which demonstrates a fracture-dislocation at C6–7 not apparent on the initial XR.*

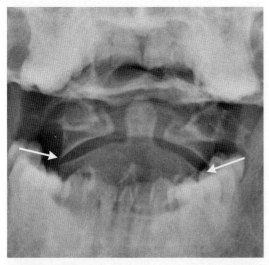

C-spine XR. Open-mouth view of the cervical spine shows the normal alignment of the lateral masses of C1 with C2 (arrows).

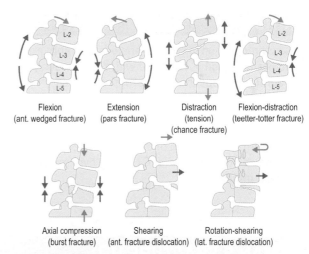

Pathomechanics of spinal injury. Each force produces a characteristic injury as visualized on the lateral XR. **Flexion** creates an anterior wedged deformity of the vertebral body. **Extension** results in a small triangular fragment separated from the anterior inferior margin of the vertebral body. **Distraction** creates horizontal fractures in the posterior element and little or no wedging of the vertebral body. **Flexion-distraction** creates a horizontal fracture of the posterior elements and anterior wedging of the vertebral body. **Axial compression** is characterized by anterior wedging of the vertebral body and retropulsion of the posterior superior margin of the vertebral body as in burst fractures. **Shearing** results in fracture–dislocations manifested by anterior displacement of the vertebra above the level of dislocation carrying with it a triangular avulsed fragment from the anterior superior margin of the vertebral body below. Fractures of the laminae and superior facets are commonly encountered. **Rotational** forces are combined with shearing to produce an anterior lateral dislocation of the spine.

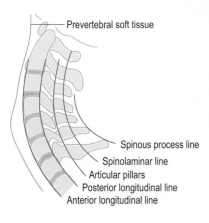

- Prevertebral soft tissue
- Spinous process line
- Spinolaminar line
- Articular pillars
- Posterior longitudinal line
- Anterior longitudinal line

On the lateral XR 4 imaginary continuous curves should be present: (1) anterior vertebral body line (2) posterior vertebral body line (3) spinolaminar line (4) posterior spinous process line.

JEFFERSON FRACTURE (C1)

DEFINITION

- The oblique superior articulating surfaces of the lateral masses of the atlas are driven down and laterally – this disrupts the anterior and posterior arches of the atlas (there can be a single disruption of each arch)

MECHANISM

- An axial compression injury to the top of the skull ▶ it is an uncommon injury
  - **STABLE injury** (unless there is associated disruption of the tranverse atlantal ligaments)

AP XR Bilateral offset of the lateral masses of C1 relative to the lateral margin of the C2 vertebral body ▶ a widened space between the dens and medial border of the C1 lateral masses

Lateral XR It may be impossible to distinguish this from an isolated fracture of the posterior arch of the atlas

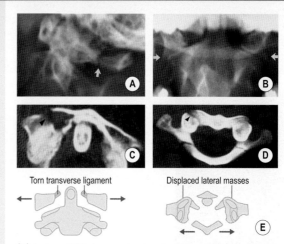

Torn transverse ligament

Displaced lateral masses

(A) Lateral XR demonstrates fracture of the posterior arch of atlas (arrow) – indistinguishable from an isolated fracture of the C1 posterior arch. (B) Open-mouth view demonstrates bilateral displacement of the C1 lateral masses (arrows). (C,D) CT demonstrates a single fracture in the right portion of the anterior arch (arrowhead) and bilateral fractures of the posterior arch.

POSTERIOR ARCH FRACTURE (C1)

DEFINITION

- This is commonly non-displaced and bilateral and neurologically benign ▶ take care with differentiating it from neural arch gaps that are normal variations

MECHANISM

- It results from compression of the arch between the occiput and spinous process of C2 during hyperextension
  - **STABLE injury**

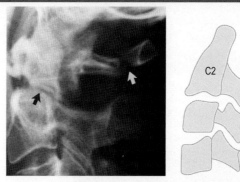

Fracture of the posterior arch of C1 (white arrow) combined with fracture at the base of the dens. Note the posterior dislocation (black arrow).*

HANGMAN'S FRACTURE (C2)

DEFINITION

- Traumatic spondylolisthesis of C2 with a fracture through both pedicles, separating the posterior elements from the vertebral body ▶ fracture lines tend to be oblique and symmetrical ▶ there may be an associated avulsion fracture of the anteroinferior C2 margin
- The C2 vertebral body subluxes anteriorly relative to C3 but the posterior elements remain normally aligned – as the spinal canal effectively widens in AP diameter there is often little neurological injury

MECHANISM

500
- A hyperextension injury
  - **UNSTABLE injury**

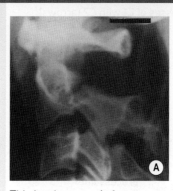

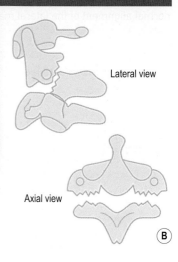

Lateral view

Axial view

This is a hangman's fracture with subluxation of C2 upon C3 and a widely displaced fracture in the neural arch.

ODONTOID (DENS) FRACTURE (C2)

DEFINITION

- This can be mistaken for an os odontoideum (either congenital or post traumatic)
- *Type 1 (high):* an avulsion fracture of the superolateral portion of the tip of the dens by the intact alar ligament – **STABLE injury**
- *Type 2 (high):* a transverse fracture at the base of the dens (the commonest type) – **UNSTABLE injury**
- *Type 3 (low):* a fracture of the superior portion of the axis body with extension through one or both of its superior articular facets (it is not technically a dens fracture) – **UNSTABLE injury**

MECHANISM

- A hyperflexion or hyperextension injury

AP XR The Mach effect (due to the inferior cortical margin of the posterior arch of the atlas crossing the base of the dens) may mimic a dens fracture

Lateral XR Anterior tilt of the odontoid ▶ prevertebral soft tissue swelling

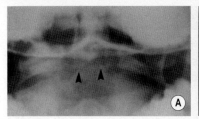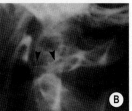

High (Type 2) dens fracture in frontal (A) and lateral (B) projections. The fracture lines (arrowheads) are confined entirely to the base of the dens.*

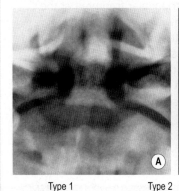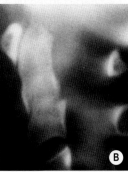

Type 1   Type 2   Type 3

Low (Type 3) dens fracture. (A) No fracture line is apparent. This is frequently the case in this type of fracture. (B) A lateral tomogram clearly demonstrates the fracture line and the tilting of the dens.*

EXTENSION TEARDROP FRACTURE (C2)

DEFINITION

- A fracture of the anteroinferior corner of body of C2 (which is avulsed by an intact anterior longitudinal ligament) ▶ it is not associated with a neurological deficit
- It may occur in isolation or be associated with a hangman's fracture ▶ it may occasionally involve the lower cervical vertebral bodies

MECHANISM

- An extension injury
  - **UNSTABLE injury**

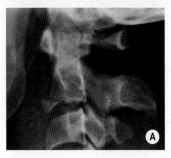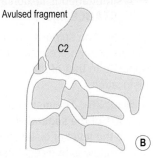

C2 extension teardrop fracture. Note the triangular fragment arising from the anteroinferior vertebral body margin and the marked swelling in the retropharyngeal tissue (haematoma). There is slight posterior subluxation of C2 upon C3 (hyperextension mechanism and disruption of the intervertebral disc).*

FLEXION TEARDROP FRACTURE (C3–C7)

DEFINITION

- A fracture–dislocation that is usually associated with a spinal cord injury (associated with significant spinal displacement at time of injury)

MECHANISM

- Hyperflexion and axial compression
  - **UNSTABLE injury**

XR It is characterized by a triangular fragment at the anteroinferior aspect of the involved vertebral body (the 'teardrop') ▶ the anterior vertebral body height is reduced with associated prevertebral soft tissue swelling
- Posterior displacement of the fractured vertebra and diastasis of the interfacetal joints indicates longitudinal ligament, intervertebral disc and posterior ligament complex disruption

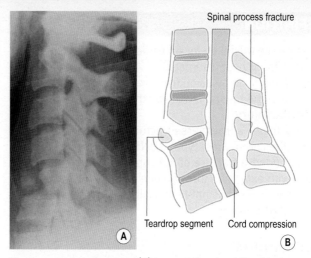

Flexion teardrop fracture. (A) Lateral C-spine XR with the cervical spine in the flexed attitude. A single large fragment (anteroinferior corner of the C5 body) is present. The 5th vertebral body is posteriorly displaced. Widened interfacetal and interspinous spaces between C5 and C6 indicate complete disruption of the posterior ligament complex and bilateral interfacetal dislocation.*

UNILATERAL LOCKED FACETS/UNLATERAL INTERFACETAL DISLOCATION (C3–C7)

DEFINITION

- Dislocation of the interfacetal joint on the side opposite to the direction of rotation (the dislocated facet comes to rest anterior to the subjacent facet and is thus 'locked')

MECHANISM

- A simultaneous flexion and rotation injury
  - **STABLE injury**

AP XR The spinous processes cephalad to the level of the dislocation are rotated off the midline (in the direction opposite to that of the rotation) and point to the side of the dislocation

Lateral XR The dislocated vertebra is anteriorly displaced by <50% of the sagittal vertebral body diameter ▶ the spine above the level of dislocation is obliquely oriented (the spine below is in direct lateral orientation)
- 'Bow tie' or 'butterfly' appearance: the appearance of the articular masses on an oblique projection

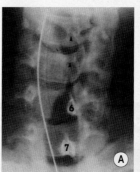
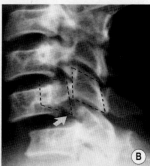

Unilateral locked facets. (A) Frontal XR – the spinous processes from C6 and above (arrowheads) are rotated off the midline. (B) Unilateral locked facets (C5–6). The 'bow tie' or 'butterfly' configuration of the facet is characteristic of this lesion (dashed lines). Note that at the level of dislocation, the vertebrae above are in the oblique projection and those below are in the lateral projection. One can see that the inferior facet of one side (arrow) lies anterior to the vertebra below.*

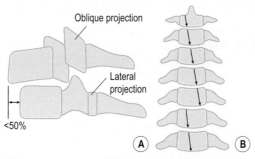

(A) Lateral diagram. (B) AP diagram. The spinous processes above the injury are rotated off the midline.

BILATERAL LOCKED FACETS/BILATERAL INTERFACETAL DISLOCATION (C3–C7)

DEFINITION

- Both facet joints at the level of injury are dislocated and all the interosseous ligaments (including the intervertebral disc) are disrupted
- It is usually associated with a neurological deficit

MECHANISM

- Extreme neck flexion
  - **UNSTABLE injury**

Lateral XR Anterior displacement of the involved vertebra for at least 50% of the sagittal vertebral body diameter ▶ the articular masses of the superior vertebrae lie anterior to the articular masses of inferior vertebrae (thus 'locking' the facets) ▶ there are often associated bilateral laminar fractures of the superior vertebrae

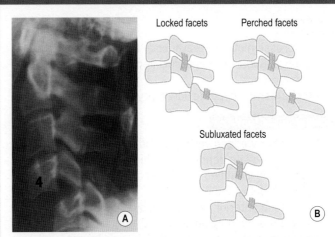

Bilateral locked facets at C4–5 (interfacetal dislocation). Note that the lateral mass of the inferior facet of C4 is locked anteriorly to the superior facet of C5.*

CLAY SHOVELLER'S FRACTURE (C6–T1)

DEFINITION

- A spinous process avulsion (C6–T1)

MECHANISM

- It is usually caused by rotation of the upper trunk with a fixed cervical spine (occasionally as the result of a direct blow)
  - **STABLE injury** (isolated fractures of the other indent posterior elements are rare)

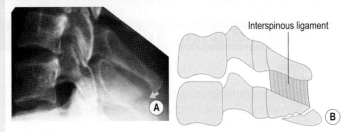

Clay shoveller's fracture (arrow) of the spinous process of C6–7.*

HYPERFLEXION SPRAIN (C3–C7)

DEFINITION

- A pure soft tissue and posterior ligamentous injury

MECHANISM

- Acute flexion without axial compression
  - **STABLE injury**

Lateral XR Localized kyphotic angulation ▶ widening of the interspinous and interlaminar space ('fanning') ▶ interfacetal joint subluxation ▶ posterior widening and anterior narrowing of the intervertebral disc (± 1–3 mm of vertebral anterior displacement)
- It is accentuated by flexion views (but must be supervised by a radiologist) ▶ the injury is associated with delayed instability

PEARL

Spinal cord injury without radiological abnormality (SCIWORA)
- Hyperextension dislocation at the time of injury, with the spine relatively normally aligned subsequently ▶ MRI will demonstrate any cord injury

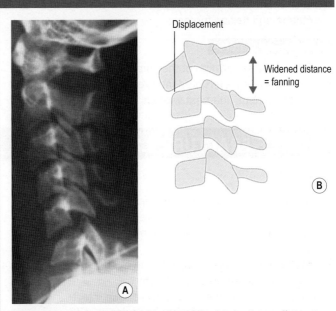

Hyperflexion sprain. Note widening of the interspinous distance at C5–6 with additional widening of the facet joints, and superior subluxation of the facets of C4 on C5 and posterior intervertebral joint. This picture indicates severe ligamentous disruption.†

SIMPLE WEDGE (COMPRESSION) FRACTURE (T1–L5)

Definition

- Compression of a vertebral body between adjacent vertebral bodies ▶ it is associated with a paraspinous haematoma
- **Mechanism:** a hyperflexion injury

Radiological features

XR Anterior wedged vertebral body deformity and vertebral end-plate depression (which is usually superior) ▶ impaction is identified by a faint sclerotic band just beneath the deformed end-plate

- Decreased anterior vertebral body height (the anterior cortical margin may be disrupted, angulated or impacted) ▶ the posterior height is maintained (as the posterior elements remain intact)
- *Lumbar spine:* a fracture is usually limited to the superior end plate and subjacent vertebral body
- *Paraspinous haematoma:* a localized lateral bulge of the mediastinal stripe

Pearls

Lesions that may mimic a compression fracture

- A non-united vertebral ring epiphysis ▶ Schmorl's nodes (an irregular lucent defect at the end-plate with irregular sclerotic margins) ▶ a limbus vertebra (a distant separate ossicle found on the anterosuperior margin of the vertebral body and representing a developmental abnormality of the ring apophysis)

Burst fracture

- This is common at the thoracolumbar junction (resulting from an axial compression force) ▶ a fragment from the superoposterior vertebral body may be displaced into the spinal canal with the potential for neurological injury
- Unlike a simple compression fracture the vertebral body posterior cortex is disrupted
- **STABLE injury** (it may become an **UNSTABLE injury** if there is a neurological deficit or retropulsed fragments)

FRACTURE–DISLOCATION (T10–L2)

Definition

- This most commonly occurs at the T10–L2 level (at the junction of mobile and relatively immobile segments) ▶ neurological injury is common
  - *Stable:* limited to a vertebral body or the posterior elements only
  - *Unstable:* involving both the vertebral bodies and the posterior elements
- **Mechanism:** it is due to a combination of shearing, rotation and flexion forces

Radiological features

AP XR Wide separation of the spinous processes
- There may be a disrupted intervertebral disc, facet joint or interspinous ligament without an associated fracture

- *Vertebral body above the injury level:* anterior dislocation
- *Vertebral body below the injury level:* an anterior wedge compression fracture with a triangular bony fragment avulsed from its anterosuperior surface

Pearls

- Isolated posterior element fractures do not commonly occur without an associated vertebral body fracture
- It can be associated with a paraspinal haematoma (a retropharyngeal or paraspinal mass)

XR This is difficult to identify within the lumbar spine as it is the same density as paraspinal muscle

CHANCE FRACTURE (L1–L5)

Definition

- Horizontal splitting of the vertebral body with little compression (a 'seatbelt' fracture)
- It is commonly associated with intra-abdominal and neurological injuries
- **Mechanism:** anterior hyperflexion over an object (e.g. a seatbelt) that serves as a fulcrum
- The posterior ligaments usually remain intact ▶ ligament rupture: ligament irregularity, with haemorrhage into the epidural fat ('dirty fat' sign)
- Soft tissue chance injury: posterior ligamentous injury without posterior bony injury

Radiological features

AP XR A transverse fracture of the spinous processes (± the pedicles)

Lateral XR A horizontal fracture involving the spinous processes, laminae, articular masses and vertebral body
- The vertebral body is tilted (with a widened interspinous space) at the injury site with little anterior wedging
- There may be disruption of the ligaments and intervertebral discs without an associated fracture

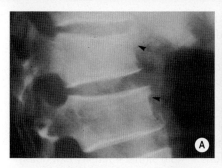
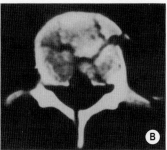

(A) Simple wedge (compression) fracture of the T11–12 bodies. The posterior vertebral body walls are maintained and the posterior elements are intact without evidence of dislocation. (B) Burst fracture of L3. CT reveals severe comminution and a fracture at the junction of the lamina and spinous process on the right, with posterior fragment displacement into the neural canal.*

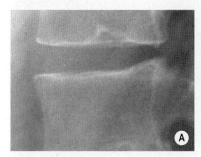
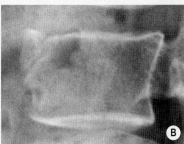

(A) Schmorl's nodes. Note the sharply defined dome-like densities arising from the end-plate in these two adjacent vertebrae. (B) Limbus vertebra. There is a well-marginated ossicle at the anterosuperior vertebral body margin. The underlying vertebral body margin is well defined.*

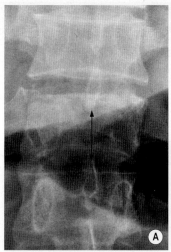
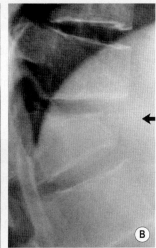

Fracture–dislocation of T11–12. AP projection (A) showing wide separation of the spinous processes of T11–12 (arrows) and obliteration of the T12–L1 vertebral disc space. There is also a fracture of the right T12 vertebral body (anterosuperior margin). (B) A dislocation is demonstrated, with displacement of a small bone fragment from the anterosuperior margin of the vertebra below the level of dislocation (arrow). There is characteristic wedging of the vertebral body below the level of dislocation.*

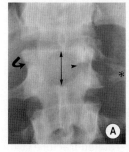
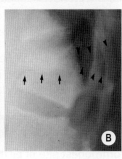

Chance fracture

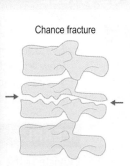

Chance fracture of L1. The frontal projection (A) shows a comminuted fracture of the left transverse process (*), transverse fracture of the left pedicle (arrowhead), separation of the T12 and L1 laminae and spinous processes (double arrow) and a fracture of the right superolateral cortex of L1 (curved arrow). (B) Lateral projection indicating a distracted transverse fracture of the spinous process and laminae (arrowheads). Arrows indicate the horizontal fracture of the body with anterior wedging.*

ANTERIOR SHOULDER DISLOCATION

DEFINITION

- This is due to an indirect force from abduction, external rotation and extension
- It account for 95% of all shoulder dislocations
- The glenohumeral joint is inherently unstable - injury or abnormality of the static stabilisers makes the joint prone to recurrent dislocation

RADIOLOGICAL FEATURES

XR There is medial and inferior displacement of the humeral head beneath the corocoid process (the humerus is externally rotated) ▶ it is associated with an avulsion fracture of the greater tuberosity

CLINICAL PRESENTATION

Hill–Sachs fracture

- A V-shaped deformity of the humeral head caused by the impaction of the anterior glenoid rim on the posterosuperior humeral head ▶ there is an increased risk for recurrent dislocations ▶ once the humeral head is relocated, the signs of a Hill–Sachs lesion are a notch in the superolateral humeral head and a sclerotic vertical line of impacted bone

Bankart lesion

- A fracture of the anteroinferior glenoid rim ▶ the labrum can become displaced ▶ there is an increased risk for recurrent dislocations ▶ fluid signal intensity extending between the glenoid and labrum is the primary sign of a labral tear ▶ more severe injury can be associated with a bony injury of the glenoid rim (bony Bankart lesion)

'Pseudodislocation'

- Inferolateral displacement of the humeral head relative to the glenoid ▶ it is due to a large haemarthrosis

Luxatio erecta

- An unusual inferior dislocation caused by severe arm hyperabduction ▶ the humeral head impinges upon the acromion, which acts as a fulcrum ▶ the arm is 'locked' in abduction

POSTERIOR SHOULDER DISLOCATION

DEFINITION

- This is related to seizures, electrocutions or a direct blow to the humeral head ▶ it accounts for 5% of all shoulder dislocations

RADIOLOGICAL FEATURES

XR The craniocaudal relationship between the humerus and glenoid is undisturbed ▶ the congruity of the humeral head with the glenoid often appears maintained on the AP view ▶ there is subtle widening of the joint (> 6 mm) or the bones overlap on a Grashey view (a Y or axillary view can confirm this)

- *'Electric light bulb' sign:* the humerus is in fixed internal rotation, causing the head and neck of the humerus to appear like an electric light bulb
- *'Trough sign':* a corresponding impaction fracture of the medial humeral head

PEARL

- Acute trauma is also associated with rotator cuff tears
- The location of any labral and humeral injury is opposite to an anterior dislocation (reverse Bankart lesion/reverse Hill–Sachs defect)

FRACTURES OF THE SCAPULA AND CLAVICLE

DEFINITION

Scapula

- Fractures are usually due to falls or a crush injury ▶ they are usually located within the scapular neck or body
- *Associations:* ipsilateral upper rib and clavicle fractures ▶ pulmonary contusions and pleural effusions

Clavicle

- Evaluation requires a straight and a cranially angled AP view ▶ fractures of the mid-third are the most common ▶ distal fractures may disrupt the coracoclavicular ligaments (± involve the acromioclavicular joint)

PEARL

Clavicle is the commonest site of birth-related fracture (± shoulder dystocia and obstetric brachial plexus palsy)

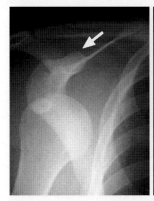
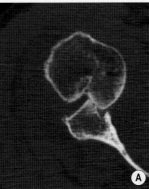
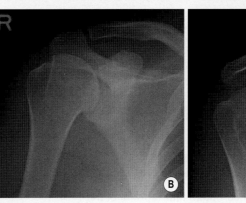

Anterior (subcoracoid) shoulder dislocation. AP XR demonstrates the humeral head located inferomedial to the glenoid, beneath the coracoid process (arrow).*

(A) Anterior dislocation with axial oblique view on CT scan shows the effect of impaction of the glenoid on the humeral head, resulting in a V-shaped bony defect in the humeral head referred to as a Hill–Sachs lesion. (B) The humeral head is now back in joint. Note the defect in the superior contour and the vertical sclerotic line of impacted bone.**

AP view showing fracture of the inferior glenoid margin known as a Bankart lesion.**

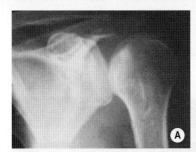
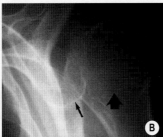
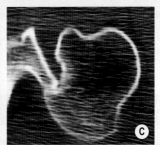
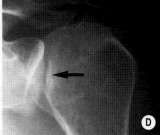

Posterior shoulder dislocation. (A) Note the circular appearance of the humeral head. (B) Trans-scapular XR shows posterior dislocation of the humeral head (large arrow) relative to the glenoid (small arrow). (C) CT shows impaction of the anterior humeral head on the posterior glenoid, which is seen as the 'trough sign' on an AP XR (arrow) (D).*

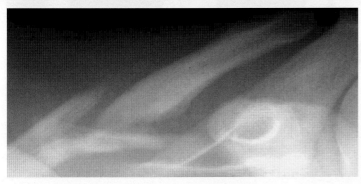
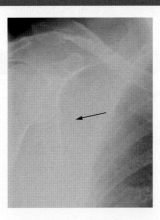

Fractured right scapular neck (arrow) seen on a CXR.

Clavicular injuries. The middle third of the clavicle is the most common location for clavicle fractures.*

ACROMIOCLAVICULAR JOINT INJURY

ANATOMY

- The AC joint normally measures < 5 mm and the undersurface of the acromion aligns with the distal clavicle (AP view) ▶ the coracoclavicular distance is 11–12 mm
- Weight-bearing views will emphasize any ligamentous disruption

CLINICAL PRESENTATION

Grade I injuries An incomplete tear (sprain) of the acromio-clavicular ligaments with a widened AC joint ▶ minor separation (if any) at the AC joint

Grade II injuries A complete tear of the AC ligaments and a partial tear of the coracoclavicular ligaments ▶ ACJ widening with <50% superior displacement of the lateral clavicle

Grade III injuries A complete disruption of the AC and coracoclavicular ligaments ▶ >100% superior displacement of the lateral clavicle (increased coracoclavicular distance)

Grade IV injuries Posterior displacement of the lateral clavicle

PEARL

- Grade I + II injuries usually resolve spontaneously
- Grade III + IV injuries are treated surgically

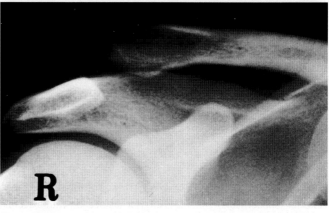

First-degree separation of the right acromioclavicular joint on weight bearing.*

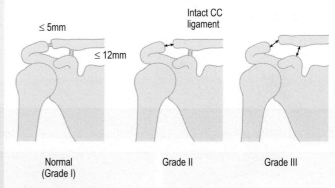

Different grades of acromioclavicular joint injury.

STERNOCLAVICULAR DISLOCATION

DEFINITION

Anterior dislocation

- This is the most common injury (with superior displacement of the clavicle)

Posterior dislocation

- This is more serious (there is a risk of injury to the great vessels at the thoracic inlet as well as tracheal compression)

RADIOLOGICAL FEATURES

XR This is difficult to diagnose with a routine XR (CT is preferred)

- There may be widening of the joint or overlap of the medial clavicle and manubrium

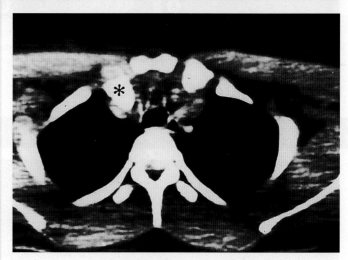

Posterior sternoclavicular joint dislocation. CT image demonstrates posterior displacement of the medial right clavicle (*) relative to the manubrium.*

PROXIMAL HUMERAL FRACTURES

DEFINITION

- Fractures tend to be spiral (they can also be angulated and overriding due to muscular contraction on the individual fragments)
- They are most commonly seen in the elderly ▶ they usually involve the surgical neck and are associated with separation of the greater tuberosity
- Children: the normal proximal growth plate has an irregular contour and can be mistaken for a fracture ▶ fractures can be significant as the physis accounts for 80% of longitudinal growth of the humerus

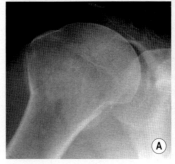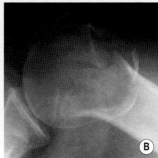

Fracture of the humeral neck. AP (A) and axillary (B) views of the left shoulder demonstrate an acute comminuted fracture of the surgical neck of the humerus. Note the separation of the greater and lesser tuberosities.*

Neer classification	
1 part	There is no displacement of the fracture fragments
2 part	There is displacement of 1 fragment
3 part	There is displacement of 2 fragments (1 tuberosity remains in contact)
4 part	There is displacement of 3 fragments

SLAP LESIONS

DEFINITION

- Tears affecting the anterosuperior labrum, with biceps tendon involvement ▶ common in overhead throwing athletes
- **SLAP: S**uperior **L**abrum from **A**nterior to **P**osterior (in relation to the biceps tendon insertion)

MECHANISM

- These occur after a forced extension injury, during rapid arm abduction during a fall, and during the deceleration phase of throwing
  - *Type I:* degenerative fraying or a tear of the superior labrum
  - *Type II:* detachment of the labral–bicipital complex from the superior glenoid
  - *Type III:* a bucket handle tear of the superior labrum
  - *Type IV:* type III with extension into the biceps tendon

PEARL

- Most important features to describe:
  - Extent of labral tear (clockface terminology)
  - Involvement of biceps anchor and tendon
  - Presence of associated rotator cuff tears

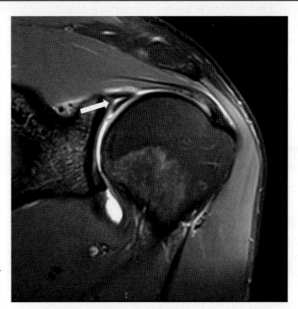

Coronal FS T2W MR arthrogram image. There is high SI contrast medium extending into the substance of the superior labrum, indicating a superior labrum anterior to posterior (SLAP) tear.**

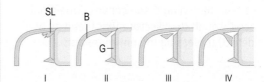

Types of SLAP lesions. Coronal section at the level of the labral–bicipital complex, SL: superior labrum ▶ B: biceps tendon ▶ G: glenoid cartilage.

SHOULDER IMPINGEMENT SYNDROME/ROTATOR CUFF TEARS

ANATOMY

- There is a restrictive space between the acromion, coracoacromial arch and acromioclavicular joint (superiorly) and the humeral head and greater tuberosity (inferiorly) ▶ the rotator cuff tendons (supraspinatus, infraspinatus, teres minor and subscapularis) pass through this space

MECHANISM

- There is potential 'pinching' of the distal centimetre of the supraspinatus tendon (representing a vascular watershed region) between the coracoacromial arch and humeral head on abduction and external rotation ▶ variations in the shape of the anteroinferior acromion, together with osteoarthritic change, can exacerbate any impingement ▶ initially there is reversible oedema and haemorrhage in the tendon, leading to tendinopathy (inflammatory and thickened tendon) leading to eventual tendon failure ▶ calcific tendinopathy is characterized by intrasubstance deposition of calcium hydroxyapatite crystals
  - *Type I damage:* myxoid degeneration (tendinosis) within the tendon ▶ there is no surface defect
  - *Type II damage:* a partial thickness tear ▶ can involve the articular surface (commonest) or bursal surface (less common)
  - *Type III damage:* a full thickness tear with communication between the shoulder joint and the subacromial–subdeltoid bursa ▶ supraspinatus is most commonly affected

RADIOLOGICAL FEATURES

XR Narrowing of the subacromial space (specific but non-sensitive sign of a full thickness tear) ▶ tendon calcification

US Using high-frequency linear array probes ▶ calcific tendinopathy seen as echogenic deposits (± acoustic shadowing)
- *Normal:* an echogenic fibrillar structure
- *Tendinosis:* swelling with diffuse or focally reduced echogenicity
- *Partial tear:* a focal anechoic structure or a fissure within the tendon
- *Full thickness tear:* flattening of the convex superficial tendon surface through to a discrete tear (seen as a hypoechoic defect) traversing the entire tendon

MRI In addition this allows assessment of the acromion, ACJ and subacromial–subdeltoid bursa
- **Normal tendon:** a hypointense structure on all sequences
- **Cuff degeneration:** T1WI and PD: intermediate SI ▶ T1WI: similar changes can be seen within a normal distal supraspinatus tendon due to the 'magic angle' effect:
  - This occurs where the tendon is at 55° to the magnetic field (B_0) ▶ at this particular angle the parallel cartilaginous fibres constrain proton movement – the resultant shortening of T1 relaxation results in an increased SI on T1WI (this effect is not seen with T2WI)
- **Partial tear:** this can be difficult to differentiate from tendinosis (until the tear is visible)
- **Full thickness tear:** T1WI/T2WI/PD: high SI which can be seen to cross the full tendon thickness (± tendon retraction) ▶ fluid within the subacromial-subdeltoid bursa (as there is no longer a barrier to fluid movement previously provided by an intact tendon) ▶ fatty atrophy of the rotator cuff muscles ▶ the tendon defect allows upward subluxation of the humeral head ▶ flattening or concavity of the subacromial fat plane
- *MRI is also able to assess any additional causes of impingement:* ACJ degenerative change ▶ acromial and lateral calvicular spurs ▶ a laterally downward sloping acromion
- *Os acromiale (an unfused epiphysis):* this must be recognized preoperatively to avoid rendering the acromion unstable

Arthrography/MR arthrography Contrast can pass from the glenohumeral joint through the rotator cuff defect (the rotator cuff is normally a barrier) to opacify the subacromial–subdeltoid bursae

ADHESIVE CAPSULITIS (FROZEN SHOULDER)

DEFINITION

- A clinical syndrome of pain associated with severely restricted shoulder joint movement ▶ the diagnosis is often clinical

RADIOLOGICAL FEATURES

Arthrography Joint capsule contraction ▶ irregularity of the capsular insertion ▶ a reduction in joint volume

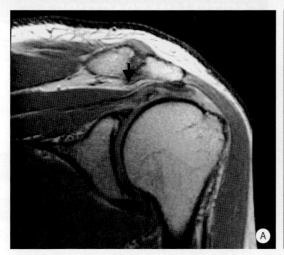
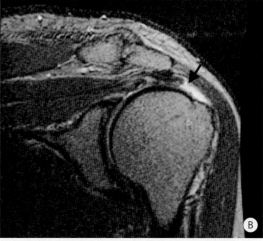

Supraspinatus tear. (A) Extensive degenerative change is present in the ACJ with fibrous tissue extending inferiorly to impinge upon the supraspinatus tendon (arrow). (B) The full thickness supraspinatus tear is indicated by termination of the tendon fibres abruptly with fluid within the empty space (arrow).

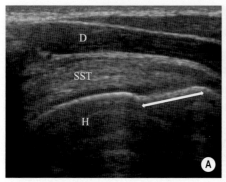
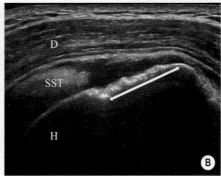
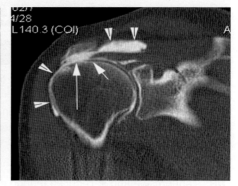

Normal longitudinal US image of the supraspinatus tendon (A). The echogenic tendon inserts across the footprint of the greater tuberosity (double arrow). A full thickness tear of supraspinatus (B) is demonstrated as a focal deficiency of the tendon which is filled by low reflective joint fluid. D, deltoid muscle; H, humeral head; SST, supraspinatus tendon.**

Oblique coronal reformatted CT arthrogram images of the shoulder in two different patients. Single-contrast arthrogram demonstrates a full-thickness supraspinatus tendon tear. There is a large gap (long arrow) with extension of contrast material from the glenohumeral joint into the subacromial/subdeltoid bursa (arrowheads). Note the tendon retraction to the level of the humeral head (short arrow).©35

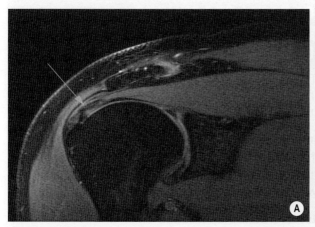
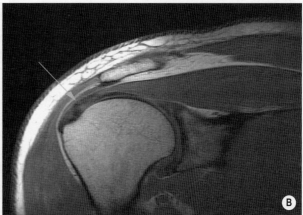

Oblique coronal PD (FS) (A) and oblique coronal PD image (B). MR images demonstrate mild thickening and heterogeneously increased signal intensity in the supraspinatus tendon consistent with tendinosis (arrows).©35

SUPRACONDYLAR FRACTURE

DEFINITION

- The commonest paediatric elbow injury
- Due to a fall on an outstretched hand
- Associated neurovascular damage (brachial artery/median + ulnar nerves) may lead to Volkmann's ischaemia of the forearm ▶ malunion may lead to a cubitus varus deformity

Lateral XR Elevated anterior and posterior fat pads ▶ $< \frac{1}{3}$ of the humeral capitellum resides anterior to the anterior humeral line

- An anterior fat pad may be visible normally – a posterior fat pad is always abnormal ▶ absence of the fat pad sign does not exclude a fracture (effusions are not always present)

EPICONDYLITIS OF THE ELBOW

DEFINITION

- *'Tennis elbow'*: tearing of the extensor tendons attaching to the lateral epicondyle
- *'Golfer's elbow'*: injuries to the common flexor and pronator muscle group that are attached to the medial epicondyle

XR This is usually normal

US Tendon swelling ▶ reduced tendon echogencity ▶ focal hypoechoic areas representing a tear

MRI Inflammatory changes within the tendinous attachment ▶ a visible tendon defect ▶ haemorrhage and haematoma formation

ELBOW DISLOCATION

DEFINITION

- This invariably involves a posterolateral dislocation of the radius and ulna (in relation to the humerus) ▶ a fracture of the ulnar coronoid process is frequently present
- An isolated radial head dislocation is extremely rare in adults – a synchronous ulna fracture should be excluded
- Myositis ossificans is a complication

RADIAL HEAD DISLOCATION

- Radio-capitellar line: a line drawn along the mid shaft of the radius proximal to the tuberosity which should pass through the capitellum – if not, the radial head is dislocated

CAPITELLUM FRACTURE

DEFINITION

- This is usually an osteochondral injury
- It is due to a valgus impaction force
- It may be difficult to diagnose on XR (MRI is very sensitive)

OLECRANON FRACTURE

DEFINITION

- The fracture fragments are often distracted (secondary to muscular contraction)
- It is due to a direct blow to the elbow or an avulsion injury (due to triceps contraction)

PROXIMAL RADIAL FRACTURE

DEFINITION

- A radial head fracture is usually oriented vertically ▶ a radial neck fracture tends to be impacted and slightly angulated

XR It is commonly difficult to identify on an AP or lateral view (an oblique projection may be required)

Positive fat pad sign This is a secondary non-specific sign of an intra-articular fracture (due to an elbow effusion or haemarthrosis)

- *'Sail' sign:* displacement of a normally visible anterior fat pad away from the anterior humerus
- Visualization of a posterior fat pad (which is not usually visible)
  - NB: if the capsule has ruptured the fat pads may not be visible

FOREARM FRACTURES

DEFINITION

- The radius and ulna are fixed along their length by an interosseous membrane ▶ a displaced fracture of one bone necessitates fracture or displacement of the other

Monteggia fracture dislocation

- This is rare (due to a fall on a flexed arm)
- It is an anteriorly angulated fracture of the proximal ulna with an associated anterior dislocation of the radial head

Galeazzi fracture dislocation

- This is rare (due to a fall on a flexed arm)
- It is a dorsally angulated distal radial fracture associated with a disruption of the distal radioulnar joint

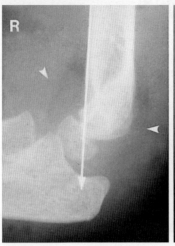
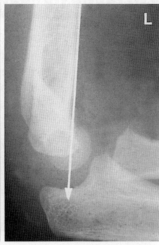

Supracondylar fracture. The left humerus is normal ▶ the line extending from the anterior cortex of the shaft passes through the middle ⅓ of the capitellum. A similar line on the right cuts the posterior ⅓ of the capitellum indicating anterior fragment displacement (and vice versa for posterior displacement). A haemarthrosis displaces both fat pads (arrowheads).[†]

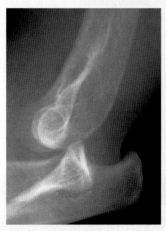
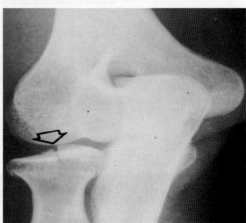

Complete dislocation of the elbow. Lateral XR demonstrating posterior dislocation of the radius and ulna relative to the humerus. Ulnar coronoid process fractures are often associated with this injury.*

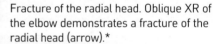

Fracture of the radial head. Oblique XR of the elbow demonstrates a fracture of the radial head (arrow).*

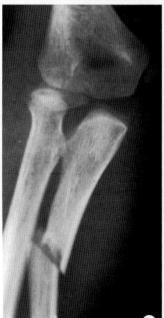
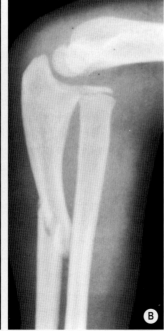
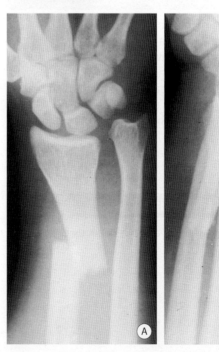

Monteggia fracture–dislocation of the proximal forearm. AP (A) and lateral (B) views demonstrate an anteriorly angulated fracture of the proximal ulna and anterior dislocation of the radius relative to the capitellum.*

Galeazzi fracture–dislocation of the distal forearm. AP (A) and lateral (B) views of the distal arm demonstrate a displaced fracture of the radius and diastasis of the distal radioulnar joint, with ulnar dislocation.*

SCAPHOID FRACTURE AND AVASCULAR NECROSIS

DEFINITION

- Most are non-displaced transverse fractures through the middle (or 'waist') of the scaphoid (70%) and account for 75% of all carpal fractures
- The scaphoid blood supply is via an artery entering the bone at its waist – non-union of fracture fragments interrupts the blood supply to the *proximal* fragment (leading to osteonecrosis)

CLINICAL PRESENTATION

- Pain within the anatomical snuffbox

TECHNIQUE

- Multiple views are required for accurate evaluation (especially an AP view in maximum ulnar deviation) ▶ it may not be seen on the initial film – if there is clinical or radiological suspicion perform a repeat film at 7–10 days (± scintigraphy or an immediate MRI)

XR/CT Sclerosis, resorption and collapse of the proximal pole of the scaphoid ▶ these can detect late osteonecrosis – a dense necrotic fragment is due to a combination of disuse osteoporosis of the surrounding bone and fat necrosis of the avascular segment

MR

- *Early:* bone marrow oedema commonly on both sides of the fracture (T2WI and STIR: high SI)
- *Late:* an avascular *proximal* pole (T1WI: low SI, T2WI: intermediate or low SI)

TREATMENT

- **Before avascularity is established:** surgical screw fixation of the proximal pole
- **Once avascularity is established:** corticocancellous graft or prosthesis

KIENBÖCKS DISEASE (LUNATOMALACIA)

DEFINITION

- Avascular necrosis of the lunate which is usually secondary to a trivial trauma
- It is associated with a negative ulnar variance:
  - *Normal:* the distal articular surfaces of the radius and ulna are within 2 mm of each other (with the forearm and carpus in the neutral position)
  - *Negative ulna variance:* the ulna is shorter than the radius
  - *Positive ulna variance:* the ulna is longer than the radius

CLINICAL PRESENTATION

- It presents between the 3rd and 5th decades (M:F 2:1)

RADIOLOGICAL FEATURES

XR This is normal during the early stages

MR staging

- *Stage I:* bone oedema ▶ the bone shape is preserved
- *Stage II:* sclerosis (which is low SI on all sequences) ▶ normal bone morphology
- *Stage III:* the bone collapses craniocaudally (with resultant proximal capitate migration)
- *Stage IV:* the end stage with well-defined collapse ▶ there is widespread adjacent degenerative change ▶ bone oedema is not a feature

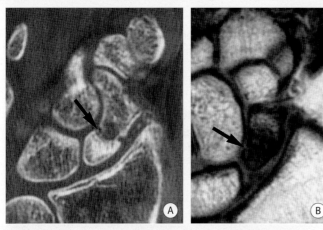

Osteonecrosis of the proximal scaphoid pole. Direct coronal CT (A) demonstrates the unhealed fracture through the scaphoid waist (arrow). The proximal pole is dense, indicating ischaemia or osteonecrosis. Coronal T1WI image (B) demonstrates abnormal low SI in the proximal fragment (arrow).*

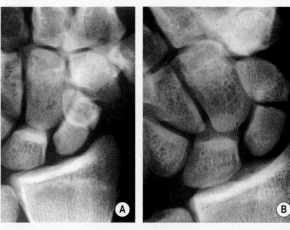

Fracture of the scaphoid. In the PA projection (A), the scaphoid is somewhat rotated, and a fracture is difficult to see. The navicular view with the wrist in ulnar deviation (B) demonstrates a lucent band traversing the waist of the scaphoid, representing a fracture. Such fractures can be difficult to detect in the acute setting ▶ occasionally, reimaging the patient 7?10 days after injury may demonstrate the fracture due to hyperaemia of the surrounding bone.*

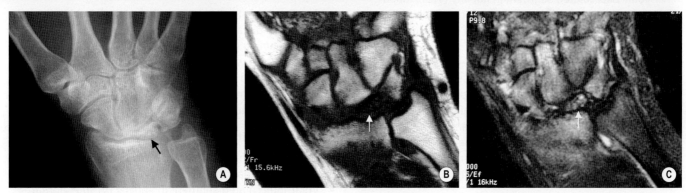

Kienböck's disease. (A) The lunate is collapsed and sclerotic, indicating avascular necrosis (arrow). (B) T1-weighted MR image. The normal fatty marrow is replaced by low-signal material, indicating that the bone is avascular (arrow). (C) Fat-saturated FSE T2-weighted sequence shows a paucity of inflammatory change.*

CARPAL FRACTURES

DEFINITION

Triquetral fracture

- The second most common carpal fracture (15%)
- There is usually a small avulsion fragment on the dorsal surface of the bone at the dorsal radiocarpal ligament attachment – this is best seen on a lateral XR

Hamate fracture

- This may involve the hook or it may involve the dorsal surface (it is not uncommonly seen in golfers or baseball players)

Trapezium fracture

- This occurs secondary to abduction and hyperextension of the thumb ▶ it manifests as a vertical fracture within the lateral aspect of the bone

CARPAL DISLOCATIONS

DEFINITION

- Disruption of the intrinsic wrist ligaments results in intercalated segment instability (dissociative carpal instability)
  - Dorsal intercalated segment instability (DISI): scapholunate ligament involvement ▶ scapholunate diastasis (>3 mm) ▶ increased scapholunate angle (>60°) with dorsal rotation of the lunate (lateral view) and volar rotation of the scaphoid
  - volar intercalated segment instability (VISI): lunotriquetral ligament disruption ▶ volar rotation of the lunate (lateral view) ▶ reduction of scapholunate angle (<30°)
- There is a sequence of increasingly severe injuries:
  - *Scapholunate dissociation:* rotary subluxation of the scaphoid and disruption of the scapholunate ligament
  - *Perilunate dislocation:* disruption of the scapholunate, lunocapitate and lunotriquetral ligaments
  - *Lunate dislocation:* disruption of the volar radiocarpal ligaments in addition to the ligamentous disruptions described for a perilunate dislocation

Scapholunate dissociation (the most common)

- *'Terry Thomas' or 'Madonna' sign:* a widened scapholunate space seen on an AP XR (> 4 mm – the normal is 2 mm)
- The scaphoid may rotate on its axis with volar movement of its distal pole (due to a disrupted scapholunate ligament) ▶ on a lateral view the resultant angle between the lunate short axis and the scaphoid long axis is > 60° (the normal is 30–40°) ▶ rotatory subluxation results in apparent scaphoid foreshortening on an AP view with projection of the distal pole cortex over the waist ('signet ring' sign)

Perilunate dislocation

- The lunate maintains its normal relationship to the radius – the remainder of the carpus and hand shifts dorsally (lateral view) ▶ it is associated with a scaphoid fracture (and less commonly the capitate)
- The lunate loses its normal trapezoidal configuration and takes on the appearance of a triangular wedge of pie (AP view)
- On a lateral XR a vertical line through the centre of the lunate should inferiorly pass through the radial articular surface and superiorly through the centre of the capitate – if not a carpal dislocation is certain

Lunate dislocation

- The lunate dislocates anteriorly (volarly) and tilts so that its distal articular surface faces the palm ▶ the remaining carpal bones maintain their normal relationships with each other and with the radius
- A lunate and a perilunate dislocation can appear identical on an AP XR ▶ differentiation of lunate versus perilunate dislocation is best made on a lateral XR

Carpal instability

- This is commonly due to a ligamentous injury of the proximal carpal row
- Volar intercalated segment instability (VISI) ▶ dorsal intercalated segment instability (DISI)

PEARL

- Triangular fibrocartilage (TFC) complex
  - The TFC is composed of fibrocartilage, and is formed by the triangular fibrocartilage discus, radioulnar ligaments, and ulnocarpal ligaments
  - Tears can present as ulnar wrist pain
    - Degenerative: central TFC perforation, associated with positive ulnar variance (long ulna), which can lead to ulnar abutment on the triquetrum
    - Traumatic: often affecting the ulnar attachments, and associated with ulnar styloid fractures ▶ any also involve the dorsal and radial radio-ulnar ligaments and lead to DRUJ instability

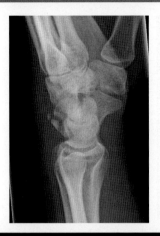

Small bone fragments are visible on the dorsum of the wrist. These indicate a triquetral fracture; there was no abnormality on the AP view.**

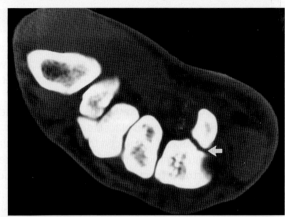

Fracture of the hook of the hamate. Axial CT demonstrates separation of the hook of the hamate (arrow), indicating an acute fracture.*

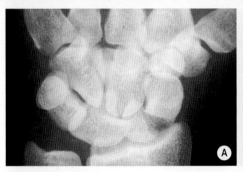

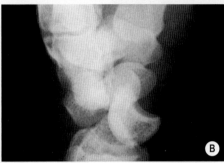

Posterior trans-scaphoid perilunate fracture–dislocation. The AP view (A) demonstrates overlap of the lunate and capitate, with a 'wedge of pie' appearance of the lunate. There is a fracture of the scaphoid. The lateral view (B) demonstrates slight volar tilt of the lunate, with the remainder of the carpus and hand posteriorly dislocated.*

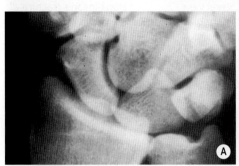

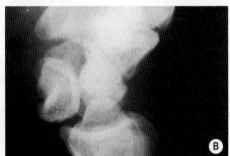

Anterior lunate dislocation. AP view (A) can be indistinguishable from a perilunate dislocation. The lateral view (B) shows volar displacement, dislocation and tilt of the lunate. The remainder of the carpus is normally aligned with the radius.*

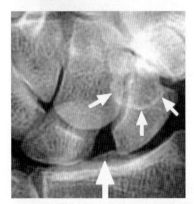

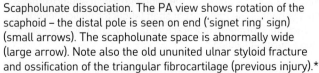

Scapholunate dissociation. The PA view shows rotation of the scaphoid – the distal pole is seen on end ('signet ring' sign) (small arrows). The scapholunate space is abnormally wide (large arrow). Note also the old ununited ulnar styloid fracture and ossification of the triangular fibrocartilage (previous injury).*

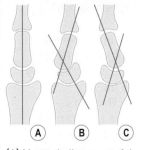

(A) Normal alignment of the wrist allows a continuous line to be drawn through the radius, lunate and capitate. (B) Abnormal alignment: palmar flexion instability (VISI). The lunate is rotated towards the palmar surface of the wrist, with the capitate rotated towards the dorsal surface. (C) Dorsiflexion instability (DISI) – the converse of B.

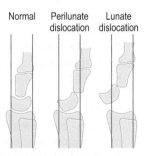

Diagram showing the lateral alignment of the lunate in relation to the carpus and distal radius in normal circumstances, perilunate dislocation and lunate dislocation.

517

COLLES' AND RELATED FRACTURES

DEFINITION

- **Colles' fracture:** Colles' original description specifically describes *only* an impacted distal radial fracture with dorsal displacement of the distal fracture fragment ▶ it can be associated with ulnar styloid avulsion
- **Smith's fracture (reverse Colles'):** A distal radial fracture with a *volarly* displaced distal fragment
- **Barton's fracture:** A displaced fracture of the volar lip of the distal radius (without involvement of the dorsal lip)
- **Reverse Barton's fracture:** The opposite condition (with a fracture of the dorsal lip)
- **Hutchinson's fracture (chauffeur's fracture):** An isolated fracture of the radial styloid process

RADIOLOGICAL FEATURES

XR ■ **Colles' fracture:** neutralization or reversal of the normal slight (10°) volar tilt of the distal radial articular surface implies an impacted fracture
- An indirect sign of an acute distal forearm fracture: displacement or obliteration of the pronator quadratus fat plane (which is normally seen adjacent to the anterior surface of the distal radius)

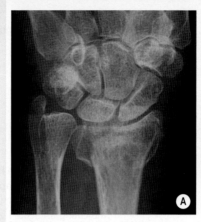
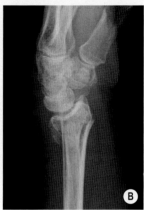

(A, B) A fracture of the distal radius, which on the lateral is displaced dorsally. There is an associated fracture of the ulnar styloid. There is no intra-articular involvement. This is a Colles' fracture.**

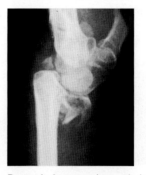

Barton's fracture. Lateral view of a comminuted fracture of the volar rim of the distal radius.*

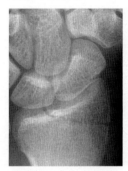

Hutchinson's fracture of the radial styloid, usually due to a direct blow.*

METACARPAL FRACTURES

DEFINITION

- **Fractures of the 4th and 5th metacarpals:** These are common and usually result from punching a hard object (a 'boxer's' fracture) ▶ they may involve the midshaft or distal end of the bone (the distal fragment is usually volarly angulated)
- **Bennett's fracture:** An oblique fracture at the base of the 1st metacarpal involving the 1st carpometacarpal joint ▶ it is often unstable (the distal fragment is distracted by the unopposed abductor pollicis longus muscle)
- **Rolando's fracture:** This is similar to a Bennett's fracture – but there is comminution of the base of the 1st metacarpal ▶ this injury is less prone to displacement of the distal fragment (due to comminution at the thumb base)

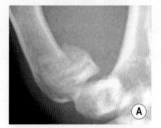
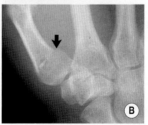
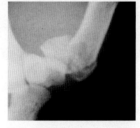

Rolando's fracture of the thumb. Comminution of this intra-articular fracture prevents abduction and retraction of the metacarpal shaft (less likely to require surgical fixation than a Bennett's fracture).*

(A) Bennett's fracture–dislocation of the thumb base. The oblique fracture extends into the joint with radial and proximal displacement of the metacarpal shaft (abductor pollicis longus contraction). Extra-articular fracture (arrow, B) generally does not require surgical fixation.*

GAMEKEEPER'S/SKIER'S THUMB

DEFINITION

- This follows a forced abduction of the thumb – it results in disruption of the ulnar collateral ligament of the 1st MCP joint ▶ displaced tears require surgery
- Stener lesion: in a displaced tear the ligament is torn from the distal insertion and retracts proximally around the aponeurosis of adductor pollicis

RADIOLOGICAL FEATURES

XR It is radiographically occult unless it is associated with a small avulsion fragment arising from the base of the proximal phalanx ▶ radial stress placed on the thumb will demonstrate radial deviation at the MCP joint

US/MR This may demonstrate the completely torn ligament

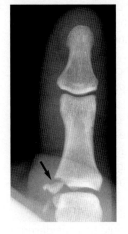

Gamekeeper's, or ski-pole, fracture. An AP view of the thumb demonstrates a bony fragment adjacent to the medial aspect of the base of the proximal phalanx of the thumb (arrow) representing an avulsion of the MCP joint ulnar collateral ligament (leading to significant thumb instability).*

VOLAR PLATE FRACTURE

DEFINITION

- This occurs at either the PIP or DIP joint as a result of forced hyperextension (± dislocation)

RADIOLOGICAL FEATURES

Lateral XR A subtle flake of bone arising (but separate) from the volar aspect of the base of the more distally involved phalanx

- The bone fragment represents an avulsion of the volar plate (the palmar ligamentous stabilizer of the IP joint)

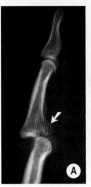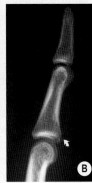

Volar plate avulsion. The patient in (A) demonstrates dorsal subluxation of the middle phalanx, with a volarly displaced avulsion fracture of the volar plate (arrow). In a different patient (B), there is no displacement – the fracture fragment is very subtle (arrow).*

MALLET (DROP) FINGER/BOUTONNIÈRE INJURY

DEFINITION

- **Mallet finger:** A direct blow to the fingertip causes DIP hyperflexion with disruption of the deep component of the extensor tendon
- **Boutonnière injury:** Avulsion of the middle extensor slip ▶ this occurs at the base of the middle phalanx

RADIOLOGICAL FEATURES

XR

- **Mallet finger:** An avulsion fragment may be seen adjacent to the dorsal aspect of the base of the distal phalanx ▶ it can result in a flexion deformity ▶ it may occur without an associated fracture
- **Boutonnière deformity:** PIP flexion ▶ DIP extension

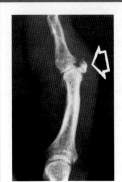

Mallet finger. There is a fracture fragment dorsal to the base of the distal phalanx, indicating avulsion of the extensor tendon. The fixed flexion deformity at the DIP joint is due to the unopposed action of the flexor tendon.*

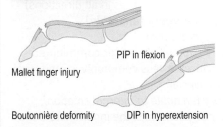

Mallet finger injury

PIP in flexion

Boutonnière deformity   DIP in hyperextension

519

PELVIC INJURIES

- The pelvis acts as a bony ring – any disruption of one part of the ring necessitates a matching disruption elsewhere within the ring (similar rings exist around the obturator foramen)
- **Stable injuries:** the pelvic rim is fractured in one place or there is a peripheral fracture ▶ *causes:* a direct blow, avulsion or stress injuries
  - *Straddle injury (stable)*
    - *Straddle injury:* fractures of the ischial and pubic rami (which are often bilateral) with superior displacement of the medial fragments ▶ it is caused by landing on a hard object whilst in a straddle position (e.g. a bicycle accident)
      - Often an associated urethral injury – a retro-grade cystourethrogram should be considered
  - *Avulsion injury (stable)*
    - This follows the action of associated muscles on the pelvis ▶ it is common in athletes ▶ as avulsed apophyses continue to form bone, this can lead to bizarre mass like appearances
  - *Insufficiency fracture (stable)*
    - This is common in elderly patients ▶ it usually involves the sacral alae (usually accompanied by insufficiency fractures of the body of the pubis)
      - **XR**: it is difficult to identify
      - **Scintigraphy**: increased activity (sacral alae)
        - *'Honda' sign:* increased activity ('H' shape)
  - *Iliac wing injury (stable)*
    - *Duverney's fracture:* an isolated iliac wing fracture following a direct blow to the pelvis ▶ associated with internal iliac artery haemorrhage
- **Unstable injuries:** these are fractures or dislocations within the anterior and posterior aspects of the pelvic ring ▶ they are associated with a significant pelvic injury
  - *4 main patterns of fracture:* lateral compression/AP compression/vertical shearing forces/complex hybrid
  - *AP compression injury (unstable)*
    - Commonly occurring during a head on collision
    - *AP type 1 injury:* symphyseal diastasis (<2.5 cm) and vertical pubic rami fractures ▶ no significant ligamentous injury (pelvis is essentially stable)
    - *AP type 2 injury ('open-book' fracture):* progressive widening of the symphysis (>2.5 cm), or fracture lines consequent upon disruption of the sacroiliac, sacrotuberous and anterior sacroiliac ligaments ▶ intact posterior sacroiliac ligaments ▶ unstable to external rotation/stable to internal rotation
    - *AP type 3 injury:* additional posterior sacroiliac disruption (unstable to all forces in all directions)
  - *Lateral compression injury (unstable)*
    - Commonest injury pattern
    - *LC type 1 injury (stable):* oblique or comminuted pubic rami fractures ▶ less commonly symphyseal disruption and overlap
    - *LC type 2 injury (unstable to internal rotation):* after the anterior pelvis fails, the innominate bone

internally rotates, pivoting on the anterior margin of the sacroiliac joint, disrupting the posterior sacroiliac ligament (type 2a) or fracturing the iliac blade (type 2b)
    - *LC type 3 injury (unstable):* 'roll-over' injury – type 2 pattenr on the side of impact, but the contralateral hemipelvis is externally rotated
    - *'Bucket handle' fracture:* a sacroiliac fracture with contralateral ischiopubic rami fractures of the superior and inferior pubic bones ▶ displacement is uncommon
  - *Vertical shear injury (unstable)*
    - Unilateral impact (fall from a height) ▶ 1 injury type only (complete ligamentous disruption with multidirectional instability ▶ vertical pubic rami fractures with cephalad displacement on the side of impact
    - *Malgaigne's complex:* a fracture of the medial ilium or sacrum seen in conjunction with fractures of the superior and inferior rami on the ipsilateral side ▶ superior displacement of the affected hemipelvis
- **Acetabular fracture (stable or unstable)**
  - *Anterior wall fractures:* rare ▶ rarely displaced ▶ managed conservatively
  - *Posterior wall fractures*: force along a femur when seated is directed through the posterior wall (RTA) ▶ in children any involvement of the tri-radiate cartilage potentially affects future growth ▶ fractures >40% of posterior wall depth require internal fixation (as do impacted fragments)
  - *Anterior/posterior column fractures:* coronal fracture plane cleaving the acetabulum into anterior and posterior segments (both extending through obturator ring) – anterior column injury disrupts the iliopectineal line – posterior column injury disrupts the ilioischial line
  - *Transverse fractures*: these split the acetabulum into upper and lower halves (ilioischial and iliopectineal lines are disrupted, intact obturator ring)
  - *Complex fractures*

EXTRA-ARTICULAR HIP PAIN

- *Snapping iliotibial band* (external type)
  - Guteus maximus lies over the greater trochanter before abruptly moving posteriorly to bring the iliotibial band into contact with the greater trochanter
- *Snapping iliopsoas tendon* (internal type)
  - The iliopsoas tendon rotates abnormally before abruptly reversing and forcefully striking the superior pubic ramus
- *Ischiofemoral impingement*
  - Predominantly affects females ▶ impingement of quadratus femoris as it passes through a narrowed space between the ischial tuberosity and lesser trochanter of the femur

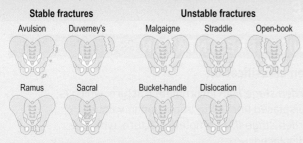

Stable fractures   Unstable fractures

Avulsion   Duverney's   Malgaigne   Straddle   Open-book

Ramus   Sacral   Bucket-handle   Dislocation

Schematic diagram showing types of stable and unstable fractures of the pelvis (see text).

Site of avulsion	Muscle (group) involved
Anterior superior iliac spine	Sartorius
Anterior inferior iliac spine	Rectus femoris
Ischial tuberosity	Hamstrings
Inferior pubic ramus	Adductors
Greater femoral trochnater	Hip rotators
Lesser femoral trochanter	Iliopsoas

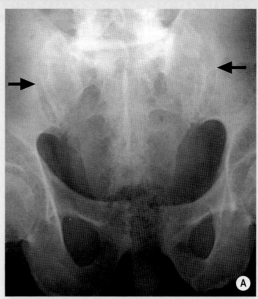

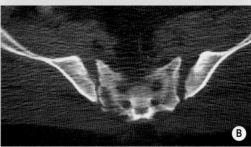

Open-book pelvic injury. AP pelvic XR (A) demonstrating widened sacroiliac joints (arrows) and pubic symphysis diastasis. CT (B) shows widened sacroiliac joints and external angulation of the iliac wings.*

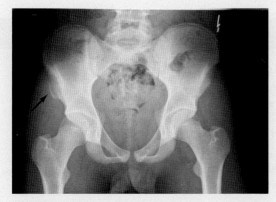

Avulsed anterior superior iliac spine as a result of the action of sartorius (arrow).*

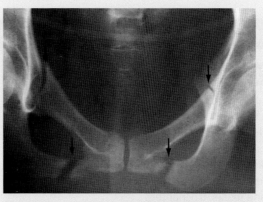

Straddle injury. There are slightly displaced fractures of the superior and inferior pubic rami bilaterally (arrows), due to a direct blow to the perineum.*

521

INTRACAPSULAR NECK OF FEMUR FRACTURE

DEFINITION

- These are commonly seen in the elderly following minor trauma (due to the background osteoporosis)
  - Hip fractures in younger adults are usually due to severe trauma (e.g. RTA)
- *Fracture types:* capital ▶ subcapital ▶ transcervical ▶ basicervical ▶ intertrochanteric ▶ subtrochanteric
- Displaced fracture fragments significantly increase the complication rate (e.g. poor union, arthritis, avascular necrosis)
- Fractures of the pubic rami and greater trochanter can mimic the signs of a hip fracture

RADIOLOGICAL FEATURES

XR A non-displaced impacted femoral neck fracture may only be represented by a sclerotic band traversing the femoral neck, or subtle disruption of the normal trabecular pattern (with valgus angulation of the primary compressive trabeculae)

- Subtle non-displaced fractures may be missed, presenting only when displacement has occurred

CT Allows accurate surgical planning and assessment of fracture fragments

MRI T1WI: low SI fracture line ▶ T2WI: high SI marrow oedema, low SI fracture line

Bone scintigraphy Increased uptake at the fracture site

CLINICAL PRESENTATION

Garden classification

- *Garden stage I:* an incomplete fracture, which is undisplaced (including impaction in valgus)
- *Garden stage II:* a complete fracture, which is undisplaced
- *Garden stage III:* a complete fracture, which is incompletely displaced (with contact between the fracture fragments)
- *Garden stage IV:* a complete fracture, which is completely displaced (with no contact between the fracture fragments)

Occult fracture

- This can be detected on MRI (immediately) and bone scintigraphy (24–72 h later)

PEARLS

- The blood supply to the adult femoral head is principally via recurrent arteries entering the hip from the lateral aspect of the femoral neck – fractures proximal to this can disrupt the blood flow resulting in AVN (avascular necrosis) ▶ the risk is directly related to the proximity of the fracture (unfortunately most are subcapital and therefore at high risk for AVN)
- There is a reduced risk with impacted fractures (and therefore these are usually stabilized with compression screws and allowed to heal) ▶ displaced fractures (which are high risk) require pre-emptive prosthetic implantation

EXTRACAPSULAR NECK OF FEMUR FRACTURE

DEFINITION

- This includes intertrochanteric and subtrochanteric fractures ▶ these do not interrupt the blood supply and there is therefore no significant AVN risk (a compression screw or a plate combination allows fragment impaction and stabilization)
- They are often comminuted with separation of the greater and lesser trochanters

CLINICAL PRESENTATION

Isolated greater trochanter fracture

- These are common (due to elderly falls)

Isolated lesser trochanter fracture

- This is often pathological (e.g. due to a metastatic deposit) ▶ uncommon in the elderly

Subtrochanteric fractures

- These are often pathological (they are seen with metastatic disease, myeloma and Paget's disease)
- They are usually transversely orientated fractures

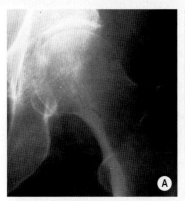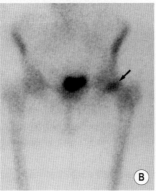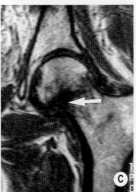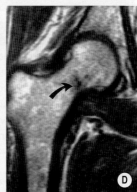

Occult hip fracture. AP XR of the left hip (A) demonstrates no fracture. Bone scintigram (B) demonstrates increased radionuclide activity in the left subcapital region (arrow). Coronal T1WI (C) clearly shows a well-demarcated line of decreased SI in the subcapital region of the left femoral neck consistent with a non-displaced fracture (arrow). MRI on the left hip (D) shows a subtle medial femoral neck fracture (curved arrow) not demonstrated on the scintigram or on the conventional radiograph.*

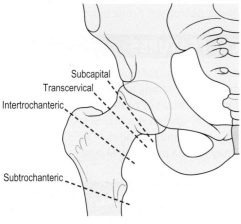
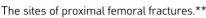

The sites of proximal femoral fractures.**

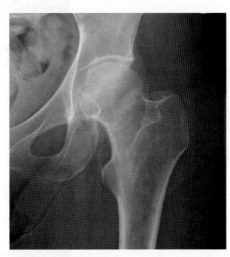

Subtle interruption of the trabecular lines of the femoral neck. There is ill-defined sclerosis extending across the neck. These signs suggest an impacted fracture.**

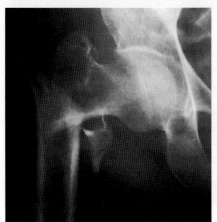

Intertrochanteric fracture. There is varus deformity and separation of the trochanters.*

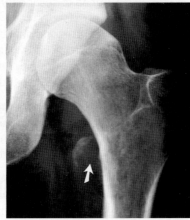

Avulsion fracture of the lesser trochanter. Note the separation of the lesser trochanter (arrow) in an area of permeative bone destruction. Such fractures are almost always pathological when seen in adults ▶ this patient had multiple myeloma.*

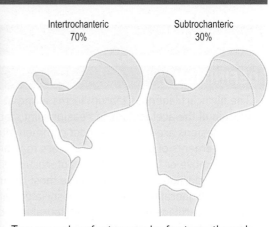

Two examples of extracapsular fractures through the neck of femur.

POSTERIOR DISLOCATION OF THE HIP

DEFINITION

- This is the most common type and usually due to a motor vehicle accident where the femur is driven posteriorly after hitting the dashboard
- It is often associated with a fracture through the posterior wall of the acetabulum with small fragments present inside and outside the joint (these may prevent reduction)

RADIOLOGICAL FEATURES

CT This is often required for assessment

CLINICAL PRESENTATION

Anterior dislocation
- This tends to result in displacement of the femoral head into the obturator foramen ▶ this is rarely seen

ILIOPSOAS BURSITIS

DEFINITION

- The iliopsoas bursa is interposed between the iliopsoas muscle and the anterior hip capsule (lateral to the femoral vessels) ▶ it communicates with the joint in 15% of cases
- It may become enlarged with increases in intra-articular fluid pressure (e.g. secondary to rheumatoid arthritis or osteoarthritis)

CLINICAL PRESENTATION

- Pain, swelling or a femoral neuropathy

LABRAL TEARS

DEFINITION

- The fibrocartilagenous labrum forms a ring at the margin of the acetabulum, increasing joint stability ▶ labral lesions are one of the most common internal derangements of the hip ▶ labral tears may be degenerative or traumatic ▶ the anterosuperior and superior portions of the labrum are most commonly affected ▶ labral tears are often associated with adjacent articular cartilage damage – and a labral tear can be a precursor to osteoarthritis
- *Femoroacetabular impingement:* traumatic tears may arise from impingement between the femoral head and neck, and acetabular rim
  - ▪ *'Cam' impingement:* caused by the presence of an abnormal osseous 'bump' found on the anterior or lateral aspect of the femoral head–neck junction ▶ this produces abnormal contact between the femur and acetabular rim (typically presenting in athletic young men) ▶ repeated contact between the osseous bump and anterior acetabulum during hip flexion results in a labral tear ▶ acetabular delamination ('carpet lesion') is common ▶ an α angle > 50° is abnormal
  - ▪ *'Pincer' impingement:* this results from over-coverage of the femoral head by the acetabulum ▶ on hip flexion there is impingement between the acetabular rim and femoral neck leading to labral and cartilage damage ▶ a centre-edge angle > 40° is abnormal ▶ coxa profunda and protrusion acetabula predispose to this condition ▶ it is common in middle-aged women

CLINICAL PRESENTATION

- Pain, clicking and a decreased range of motion

RADIOLOGICAL FEATURES

MRI Gold standard imaging technique is MR arthrography – a torn labrum may appear small, irregular, absent or demonstrate linear penetration of contrast into the tear ▶ T1WI / T2WI: a normal labrum is a low SI triangular structure on coronal and sagittal images ▶ fluid tracking through the tear may form a para-labral cyst

SLIPPED UPPER FEMORAL EPIPHYSIS (SUFE)

DEFINITION

- This is a Salter–Harris type I fracture through the epiphysis ▶ the slip is usually posteromedial and can lead to secondary AVN or premature closure of the physis
- *Causes:* increased shear forces (adolescent growth spurt) ▶ obesity (increased shear forces) ▶ there may be an intrinsic cartilagenous weakness ▶ there is a hormonal role (during adolescence)

CLINICAL PRESENTATION

- An acute or chronic presentation in adolescents and young children (M>F) ▶ it is bilateral in up to $\frac{1}{3}$ of cases

RADIOLOGICAL FEATURES

XR A line drawn along the superior border of the proximal femoral metaphysis (Klein line) does not intersect part of the proximal femoral epiphysis ▶ this is best demonstrated on a frog leg lateral view

MRI This can demonstrate early oedema (T2WI and STIR)

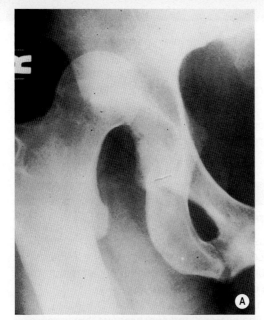

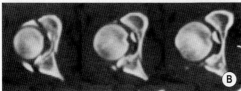

Fracture–dislocation of the right hip. AP XR (A) before relocation shows the femur dislocated posterosuperiorly. No bony fragments are seen. CT images (B) after relocation. Multiple fragments are seen, including a large intra-articular fragment. There is a fracture of the posterior acetabular wall.*

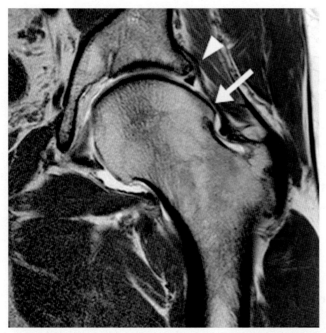

Cam deformity and labral tear. Coronal T1-weighted MR arthrographic image. High signal intra-articular contrast medium is shown penetrating between the labrum and acetabulum (arrowhead) indicating a labral tear. There is an osseous bump, or cam deformity of the lateral femoral head (arrow).**

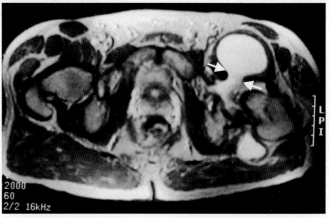

Iliopsoas bursa. A fluid-containing structure is seen to arise anterior to the left hip on a T2W image in this patients with a hip effusion. This communicates with the underlying joint via a neck lateral to the iliopsoas tendon (arrows).*

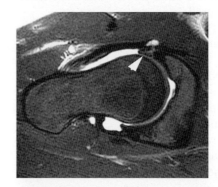

Oblique axial T2WI (FS) showing a complex labral tear with intrasubstance tearing (white arrow) and detachment that underwent intrasubstance suture banding and reattachment.©35

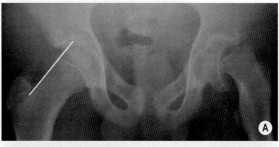

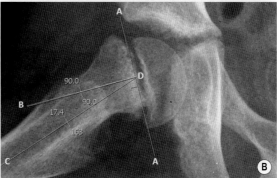

Slipped capital femoral epiphysis. (A) Left slipped capital femoral epiphysis. Klein's line is shown on the right. This line should normally intersect approximately the lateral sixth of the capital femoral epiphysis in the AP projection. (B) The slip angle—between (1) a line [BD] perpendicular to the plane of the growth plate [AA] and (2) a line [CD] parallel to the longitudinal axis of the femoral shaft in the frog lateral projection—is 17.4°.**

AVASCULAR NECROSIS OF THE HIP

DEFINITION

- This describes a segment of dead trabecular bone and marrow involving the femoral head and extending to the subchondral plate ▶ it is also called osteonecrosis or ischaemic necrosis

MECHANISM

- Interruption of the arterial inflow (traumatic or compressive) or impaired venous drainage (e.g. increased marrow pressure or intraluminal vascular obstruction)
- **Elderly patients:** the commonest cause is a subcapital femoral neck fracture
- **Younger patients:** this is usually a non-traumatic cause (and commonly bilateral)
- *Causes:* steroids ▶ radiation
  - *Sickle cell anaemia:* due to trapping of abnormal RBCs
  - *Alcohol abuse and pancreatitis:* due to fat embolization
  - *Gaucher's disease:* due to marrow infiltration and subsequent vascular compromise
  - *Caisson disease:* rapid decompression after breathing pressurized air causes microbubbles of nitrogen to precipitate out and occlude small vessels

RADIOLOGICAL FEATURES

MRI This is more sensitive than CT or scintigraphy in the early detection of AVN
- *Stage 0:* asymptomatic
  - **XR:** this is normal
  - **MRI:** there may be non-specific bone marrow oedema within the femoral head (fat-suppressed T2WI or STIR is needed for optimal sensitivity)
- *Stage I:* clinical symptoms
  - **XR:** there are normal trabeculae ▶ there is minor osteoporosis
- *Stage II:* there is more diffuse osteoporosis with osteosclerosis ▶ an infarct is distinguished from normal bone by a shell of reactive bone
  - **XR:** the findings lag behind the pathology (weeks to months)
  - **MRI:** a *'double line' sign* (80%): a serpiginous low SI line (on T1WI and T2WI) with an adjacent rim of high SI (T2WI) oedema ▶ this describes a low signal sclerotic line next to a high signal hypervascular line demarcating the extent of the lesion
- *Stage III:* the femoral head loses its spherical shape
  - **MRI:** a *'crescent sign'*: a low SI line (on all sequences) paralleling the subarticular cortex and representing a subchondral fracture ▶ this precedes overt collapse

of the femoral head, and the joint space remains normal
- *Stage IV:* further collapse with cartilage destruction, joint space reduction and secondary osteoarthritis

Scintigraphy This detects AVN earlier than XR ▶ there is initially a photopenic region followed by increased activity (representing revascularization, repair and secondary osteoarthritis)

PEARLS

Legg–Calvé–Perthes disease

- Spontaneous AVN occurring without a known insult in children (it commonly occurs between 4 and 9 years) ▶ patients present with a painful limp (it can mimic an irritable hip or infective arthritis)
- It is usually unilateral (but bilateral in 15%) ▶ it can occasionally be bilateral and synchronous, but is more usually metachronous (and therefore asymmetrical) – synchronous disease should raise the possibility of an epiphyseal dysplasia
- There are 4 stages of disease: (1) devascularization ▶ (2) collapse and fragmentation ▶ (3) re-ossification ▶ (4) remodelling

XR A loss of height, fragmentation and sclerosis of the femoral head with disease progression ▶ there can be a coxa magna deformity with lateral uncovering of the capital femoral epiphysis (± irregularity of the epiphysis)
- *'Crescent' sign':* a radiolucent subchondral fissure

US A hip effusion lasting > 6 weeks is associated with the development of Legg–Calvé–Perthes disease (± capital femoral epiphyseal fragmentation and poor coverage of the femoral head)

MRI Signal abnormalities may be detected less than 3 months following the disease onset
- T1WI: typically low SI ▶ T2WI/STIR (fat suppressed): high SI ▶ T1WI + Gad: this identifies any viable bone ▶ complete loss of SI (on all sequences) represents dead bone

Other examples of AVN (and the affected region)

- Kienböck's disease (lunate)
- Köhler's disease (navicular)
- Freiberg's disease (2nd or 3rd metatarsal heads)
- Kümmell's disease (spine)
- Proximal scaphoid pole and talar dome (post-traumatic)

Transient osteoporosis of the hip (top)

- Self-limiting painful condition of uncertain aetiology ▶ may go on to involve other parts of the skeleton (regional migratory osteoporosis)

MRI Extensive bone marrow oedema involving the femoral head ± neck

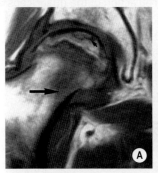
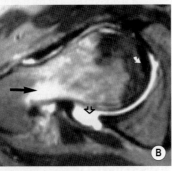

Coronal T1WI MRI (A) demonstrates a well-defined lesion in the subcortical bone demarcated by a line of low signal, consistent with AVN of the femoral head (small arrow). An ill-defined zone of reduced SI in the medial femoral neck (arrow) represents a subcapital fracture. (B) An oblique axial STIR image oriented along the long axis of the femoral neck shows low signal in the region of AVN (small arrow) and high signal in the posterior femoral neck fracture (arrow). There is a small joint effusion (open arrow).*

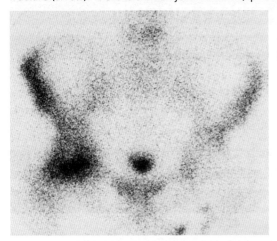

Radioisotope bone scan in avascular necrosis. Increase in uptake is demonstrated around the infarcted area, indicating healing at the margins of the infarct.†

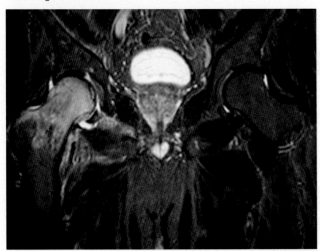

Transient osteoporosis of the right hip. Coronal T2-weighted fat-saturated image shows extensive bone marrow oedema in the right femoral head and neck.

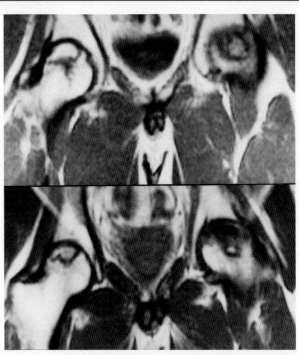

Avascular necrosis. Coronal T1WI of the hip showing a serpiginous zone of low signal around the avascular areas.†

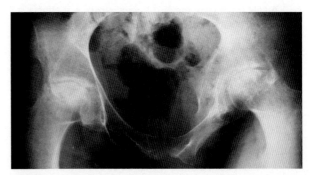

Avascular necrosis. Structural failure with fractures of both femoral heads. There is subarticular cyst formation and sclerosis resulting from trabecular compression.†

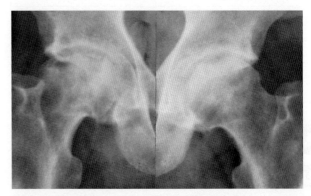

Avascular necrosis of the hips. Note mixed sclerosis and lucency of the femoral heads, with collapse of the weight-bearing surface but maintenance of the joint spaces, indicating intact articular cartilage.†

TIBIAL PLATEAU FRACTURE

DEFINITION

- Lateral tibial plateau fractures are the most common (90%) and often due to a 'bumper' injury (lateral side of the knee is struck forcing the knee into valgus)
- Fragments that are depressed > 8–10 mm are usually surgically lifted (a non-displaced tibial plateau fracture can be difficult to detect)
- Small bone fragments around the knee usually signify a significant avulsion injury

RADIOLOGICAL FEATURES

`CT/MRI` These are useful for defining the position and size of any comminuted fragments
- Subtle injuries can be detected via:
  1) Loss of clarity of the normal lateral plateau cortex
  2) Impaction of the subcortical trabeculae resulting in sclerosis
  3) Lateral displacement of the tibial margin beyond a vertical line inferiorly from the lateral femoral condyle

Schatzker classification		
	Description	**Injury mechanism**
Type I	A split fracture of the lateral tibial plateau ▶ no depression	Valgus stress ▶ it affects younger patients with strong bones
Type II	A split depression of the lateral tibial plateau	Valgus and axial stress ▶ it affects older patients with osteoporosis
Type III	Depression of the lateral tibial plateau	Often following a fall ▶ it affects older patient with osteoporosis
Type IV	A medial tibial plateau fracture (split or split depression types)	Varus stress ▶ it often follows a severe trauma
Type V	Split medial and lateral tibial plateaus	Pure axial stress ▶ it often follows a severe trauma
Type VI	A metaphyseal fracture that separates the articular surface from the diaphysis ▶ this may involve the medial or lateral tibial plateaus	It often follows a severe trauma

PATELLAR FRACTURE

DEFINITION

- This may be due to a direct blow or an indirect forced contraction of the quadriceps mechanism (with the knee fixed in flexion)
  - *Direct force:* this results in a linear fracture (or a stellate pattern if a greater force is involved)

- *Indirect force* (more common): this usually results in a transverse fracture and retraction of the quadriceps muscle
- It must be distinguished from a *bipartite patella*:
  - This is a normal variant representing a separate ossification centre within the superolateral patella (it is bilateral in 80%) ▶ a bipartite fragment will have a smooth well-corticated edge (unlike a fracture)

SEGOND FRACTURE

DEFINITION

- An avulsion fracture involving the posterolateral margin of the tibial plateau (representing an avulsion of the ilotibial band)
- It is associated with an accompanying disruption of the anterior cruciate ligament and a meniscal injury

TIBIAL STRESS FRACTURE

RADIOLOGICAL FEATURES

`XR` This may be normal ▶ there can be slight cortical thickening (± a subtle periosteal reaction)

`Scintigraphy/MR` These may be necessary to make a correct diagnosis

BUMPER FRACTURE

DEFINITION

- A proximal fibula fracture (often occurring in a pedestrian struck by an automobile bumper)
- The peroneal nerve is anatomically close to the proximal fibula and may be damaged

OSTEOCHONDRAL FRACTURE

DEFINITION

- A type of fracture in which the articular cartilage at the end of a joint also becomes torn – this usually occurs along the articular surfaces of the patella or femoral condyles
- The commonest location is within the lateral aspect of the medial femoral condyle

RADIOLOGICAL FEATURES

`MRI` This can demonstrate the size and location of the lesion, and help to determine the integrity of the overlying cartilage ▶ if the cartilage is disrupted, fluid from the joint can track into the space between the fragment and the remainder of the bone
- T2WI: high SI extending between the two areas of bone

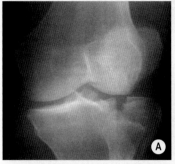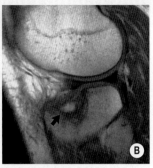

Lateral tibial plateau fracture. (A) XR demonstrating a fracture without significant depression. (B) Sagittal MRI in a different patient illustrating fragment depression (arrow).

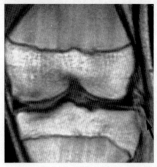

Segond fracture of the knee. Coronal PD MRI demonstrates avulsion of the bony insertion of the iliotibial band (arrow) – there is a close association with an ACL injury.*

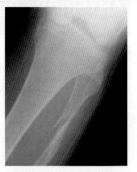

Bumper fracture: fractured proximal fibula.

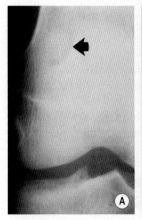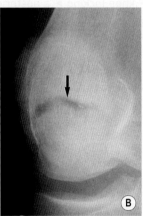

A bipartite patella (A) is usually superolateral in location – the fragment is often smaller than the 'defect' in the patella. The edges are smooth and sclerotic (arrow). An acute fracture of the patella (B) demonstrates fragments that fit together like puzzle pieces – the edges are indistinct (arrow).*

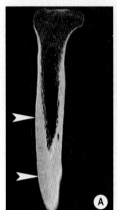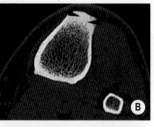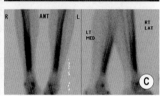

Tibial stress fractures. (A) Sagittal CT reformat demonstrates multiple perpendicular lucencies (arrowheads) in the anterior tibial cortex. (B) CT scan reveals a radiolucent fracture line (arrowhead) and cortical thickening (arrow). (C) 99mTc MDP bone scan shows increased focal radiotracer uptake anteriorly (R>L).©35

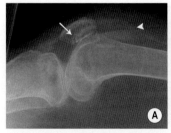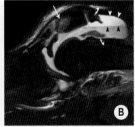

(A) Cross-table lateral radiograph of the knee shows a layering fat-fluid level parallel to the floor typical of a lipohemarthrosis (arrowhead), essentially diagnostic of an intra-articular fracture. If not for the lipohemarthrosis, the subchondral fracture at the patellar undersurface (arrow) might be overlooked. (B) On a sagittal T2WI (FS) a lipohemarthrosis is easy to identify. Remember, the patient is supine during imaging on most MR systems, so cellular blood products, with higher specific gravity, layer posteriorly (black arrowheads) while the serum component (white arrowheads) layers anteriorly. Intra-articular fat is often entrapped and can take on a more globular configuration within the effusion (curved arrows). A lipohemarthrosis indicates the presence of an intracapsular fracture, and MRI with fat suppression can often clue the imager in to the location of a nondisplaced fracture by demonstrating bone marrow edema (arrow).©35

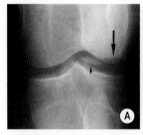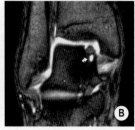

Osteochondral fracture. (A) AP view demonstrating a curvilinear defect in the lateral femoral condyle (arrow) representing an osteochondral injury and the displaced fragment (small arrow) located in the knee joint. (B) Coronal T2WI of an ankle demonstrates high SI between a fracture fragment in the talar dome and the native talus (arrow). Fluid can track between the fragment and the talus only if the overlying cartilage is disrupted.*

ANTERIOR CRUCIATE LIGAMENT (ACL) INJURY

Definition

- Disruption of the ACL is commonly due to rotation of the femur on the tibia at the time of a varus or valgus stress ▶ the ACL is particularly vulnerable after the collateral ligaments have already been torn – therefore it is unusual for an ACL injury to exist in isolation (associated meniscal injuries are seen in 68% of acute injuries)
- The mid substance of the ligament is injured more frequently than the proximal or distal portions

Clinical presentation

- An audible click at the time of injury ▶ a painful knee (± a haemarthrosis) ▶ a positive draw sign (implying disruption of the anteromedial band of the ACL)

Radiological features

MRI

- *A normal ACL (oblique sagittal images):* an elongated ovoid signal void from the medial aspect of the lateral femoral condyle to the anterior tibial spine
- *Sprain:* T2WI: high SI within the tendon
- *Partial tear:* attenuation of some fascicles (which may appear indistinct due to amorphous intermediate SI representing oedema and haemorrhage)
- *Complete tear:* a discontinuity within the low signal band ▶ no ACL is identified ▶ there is oedema and haemorrhage
- *Chronic injury:* a thickened or thinned ACL with no acute oedema
- *Secondary signs:* bunching up of the posterior cruciate ligament ▶ anterior translation of the femur on the tibial condyles ▶ a wavy patellar ligament ▶ 'pivot shift' injury: bone contusions within the posterolateral tibia and articular surface of the lateral femoral condyle ▶ an avulsion fracture of the anterior aspect of the tibial spine ▶ 'lateral notch' sign: abnormally deep indentation of the condylopatellar sulcus of the lateral femoral condyle on a lateral XR

Pearls

- **Treatment:** conservative, primary repair or reconstruction
  - *Repair:* this is suitable for a tear at either the tibial or femoral attachment (avulsion of an associated bone fragment is associated with a good prognosis)
  - *Reconstruction:* mid substance interstitial tears are not good candidates for repair
- Associated with Segond fractures (avulsion of a fracture fragment from the lateral margin of the lateral tibial condyle at the joint capsule attachment)
- Associated with O'Donaghue's triad (tears of the ACL, MCL and medial meniscus)
- Children: anterior tibial spine fractures > ACL rupture (tensile ACL strength > bone)

POSTERIOR CRUCIATE LIGAMENT (PCL) INJURY

Definition

- Disruption of the PCL usually occurs following a forced posterior displacement of the tibia ▶ it is less common than an ACL injury, and is usually associated with ACL, meniscal or collateral ligament damage
- Partial tears are more common than complete tears or avulsions
- Associated soft tissue injury is common (tears of the ACL, medial collateral ligament, and posterolateral corner)

Clinical presentation

- Pain ▶ knee locking ▶ a posterior draw sign

Radiological features

MRI

- *A normal PCL:* a thick, curved signal void extending from the medial femoral condyle to the mid-portion of the posterior tibial plateau
- *PCL injury:* abnormal internal tendon signal ▶ thickening, disruption, haemorrhage and discontinuity of the tendon

PATELLOFEMORAL DISLOCATION

Definition

- This is the most common dislocation involving the knee ▶ it is due to a valgus stress with internal rotation (and often combined with a medial blow to the patella) ▶ it causes lateral dislocation of the patella relative to the trochlear groove of the femur
- It is associated with disruption of the medial patellar retinaculum and matching osteochondral fractures or contusions in the medial aspect of the patella and lateral femoral condyle

Clinical presentation

- It is clinically undiagnosed during the initial presentation in the majority of patients (as it often reduces spontaneously or is reduced by the patient)

TRUE KNEE DISLOCATION

Definition

- Dislocation at the tibiofemoral joint ▶ this is an unusual injury following a strong force ▶ the tibia may dislocate anteriorly or posteriorly
- There is a close association with an intimal injury or disruption of the popliteal artery (angiography is generally performed with a knee dislocation and a reduced dorsal pedal pulse)

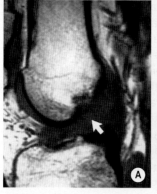
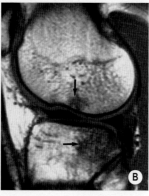

MRI appearance of acute ACL rupture. Sagittal T1WI of the knee (A) demonstrates a mass of intermediate SI in the expected location of the ACL (arrow), consistent with a complete tear. Further laterally (B), low SI in the posterior tibia and lateral femoral condyle represents typical contusions seen in association with ACL injury (small arrows).*

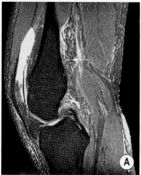
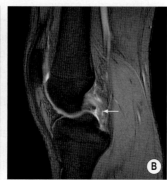

(A) Sagittal PD (FS) MR image shows a tear of the femoral attachment of the PCL (arrowhead) with associated rupture of the posterior capsule and fluid within the popliteal fossa (arrow). (B) Sagittal gradient-echo T2WI shows a complete disruption of the PCL (arrow).©35

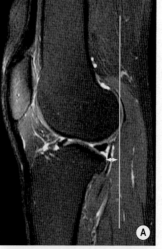
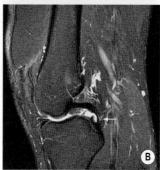

(A) Sagittal PD (FS) MR image through the lateral femoral condyle. A tear of the ACL has resulted in anterior tibial translation. There is an increased distance (arrows) between the posterior tibia margin and a tangent drawn to the lateral femoral condyle (white line). (B) Sagittal PD (FS) MR image shows a partial tear of the PCL that is markedly thinned close to its tibial insertion (arrow).©35

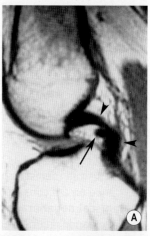
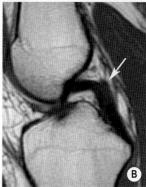

Meniscofemoral ligaments. (A) Sagittal PD image: the ligament of Humphrey (arrow) anterior to the PCL. (B) Sagittal T1WI: the ligament of Wrisberg (arrow) posterior to the PCL.

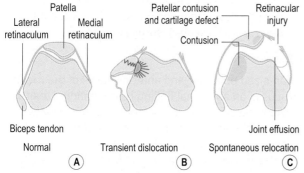

Transient patellar dislocation. (A) Normal relationship of the patella and retinacula. (B) Transient lateral patellar dislocation results in disruption of the medial retinaculum. Contractile force of the vastus medialis causes the medial facet of the patella to strike the lateral femoral condyle. (C) The resultant MRI findings: disruption of the medial patellar retinaculum / patellar and femoral contusions / joint effusion.

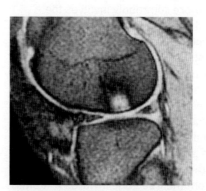

Bone 'bruising' of the femoral condyle, following knee dislocation. MRI gradient-echo image, showing the typical appearances of a focal area of increased signal.†

531

Meniscal injury

- **Normal meniscus:** a triangular area of homogeneous signal void (on all sequences) ▶ sagittal MRI images show a bow-tie configuration at the periphery, appearing as two triangles representing the anterior and posterior horns as you progress towards the intercondylar fossa
- **Discoid meniscus:** this is a normal developmental variant as a result of failure of resorption of its central portion ▶ it usually affects the lateral meniscus ▶ it can cause knee locking as well as being more prone to injury (tears)
  - A discoid meniscus has a continuous body appearance on ≥ 3 consecutive sagittal 4–5 mm images
- **Meniscal degeneration:** this is equivalent to meniscal grade I and II injuries ▶ it is usually asymptomatic ▶ it is most commonly seen affecting the posterior horn of the medial meniscus
  - T1WI/T2WI/PD: focal or globular intrasubstance areas of high SI representing 'myxoid' or 'hyaline' degeneration due to imbibed synovial fluid
    - These changes do not extend to the articular surface
- **Meniscal cyst:** a cyst extending from a meniscal tear (usually horizontal) ▶ it commonly affects the anterior horn of the lateral meniscus or the posterior horn of the medial meniscus
- **Meniscocapsular separation:** this commonly involves the posterior medial meniscus ▶ it results from damage to the supporting meniscotibial (coronary) or meniscofemoral ligaments, typically at their meniscal attachment (± a meniscal tear) ▶ it commonly affects the posterior horn of the medial meniscus ▶ it is associated with medial collateral ligament injuries
  - Sagittal MRI: > 5 mm of posterior articular tibial cartilage is 'uncovered' due to the anterior displacement of the medial meniscus
  - T2WI: increased SI within the meniscotibial or meniscofemoral ligaments, with high SI fluid seen between the posterior horn of the medial meniscus and the joint capsule
- **Torn meniscus:** this is represented by high intrameniscal SI extending to the superior or inferior articular surface ▶ it more commonly involves the medial meniscus (as this is tethered by the coronary ligaments) ▶ it presents with pain (± knee locking) ▶ a tear may be horizontal or vertical (longitudinal or radial) depending upon whether it reaches one meniscal surface or two ▶ it is a complex tear if two or more tear configurations are present
  - *T1WI/T2WI/PD:* linear increased vertical or horizontal SI extended to the articular surface
  - *Vertical tear:* this is commonly traumatic
  - *Horizontal tear:* this is commonly degenerative ▶ it usually extends from the free edge inwards ▶ it often involves the posterior horn of the medial meniscus
  - *Longitudinal tear:* a vertical tear occurring along the longitudinal axis of the outer ⅓ of the meniscus, beginning in the peripheral posterior horn and propagating circumferentially (the anterior horn is usually spared) ▶ may heal spontaneously as the peripheral meniscus has a better blood supply
  - **Radial tear:** a radially orientated vertical tear (perpendicular to the meniscal free edge) ▶ it is most commonly seen affecting the junction of the anterior horn and body of the lateral meniscus ▶ associated with acute fractures and ACL tears if the posterior horn of the lateral meniscus is affected
    - 'Parrot beak' tear: a small oblique tear
    - 'Ghost meniscus': a tear traversing the full meniscal width, splitting the meniscus into two parts ▶ a 'ghost meniscus' appearance where the image slice passes through the split
  - **Meniscal flap tear:** a meniscal tear on both a longitudinal and radial orientation can generate a flap of meniscal tissue that may become displaced into the joint space ▶ it often affects the posterior horn/body of the medial meniscus
  - **'Bucket-handle' tear:** a vertical peripheral meniscal tear extending circumferentially but remaining attached at its anterior and posterior attachments to the meniscal horns – these attachments may become broken, allowing displacement of the free fragment into (commonly) the intercondylar notch ▶ medial > lateral meniscus
    - *Coronal images:* meniscal fragments at the notch with a small meniscal body
      - 'Double delta' sign: a flipped meniscal fragment adjacent to the anterior horn of the originating meniscus appears as 2 triangular shapes adjacent to each other
    - *Sagittal images:*
      - 'Double posterior cruciate ligament' sign: this represents a displaced fragment beneath the PCL
    - Tears > 1 cm require surgical intervention
  - **General treatment principles:**
    - *Inner ⅓* (avascular): debridement
    - *Middle ⅓* (avascular/vascular): debridement vs surgical repair (depending upon the vascularity)
    - *Lateral ⅓* (vascular): surgical repair

Pearls

- Similar-sized posterior and anterior horns of the medial meniscus is an abnormal finding representing a tear or a previous resection, as the posterior horn is usually larger than the anterior horn (the horns of the lateral meniscus are usually similarly sized)
- T2WI: this is less sensitive than T1W or PD imaging for tears – however it is more specific
- **Pitfalls:** a normal transverse meniscal ligament (connecting the medial and lateral anterior horns) can be mistaken for an anterior horn tear ▶ the popliteus tendon can be mistaken for a tear of the posterior horn of the lateral meniscus ▶ the meniscofemoral ligaments can be mistaken for a posterior horn tear
  - *Ligament of Humphrey:* this runs anterior to the PCL
  - *Ligament of Wrisberg:* this runs posterior to the PCL

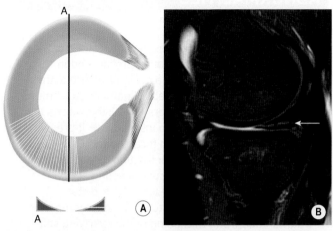

(A) Horizontal/oblique tear. This schematic shows the appearance of a horizontal meniscal tear 'A' seen on a sagittal image through the meniscus. The tear can extend to the articular surfaces or the free apical edge of the meniscus. (B) Sagittal T2WI (FS) image through the knee demonstrating a horizontal tear (arrow) with extension to the free apical margin of the body and posterior horn of the meniscus.©35

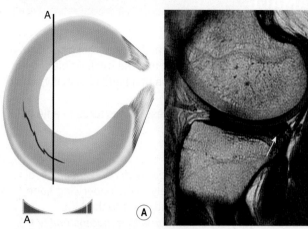

(A) Vertical tear. This schematic shows the appearance of a vertical meniscal tear 'A' seen on a sagittal image through the meniscus. The tear can extend to both the superior and inferior articular surfaces of the meniscus. (B) Sagittal PD image showing a vertical tear through the posterior horn of the lateral meniscus (arrow).©35

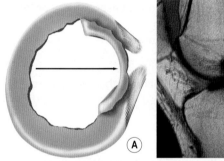

(A) Bucket handle tear. This schematic shows a centrally displaced fragment of meniscal tissue due to an extensive vertical longitudinal tear. (B) Sagittal PD image through the knee demonstrating a bucket handle tear and 'double PCL' sign. A displaced medial meniscal bucket handle tear is seen with the displaced fragment located centrally in the intercondylar notch below the posterior cruciate ligament (arrow) causing the appearance of a 'double PCL'.©35

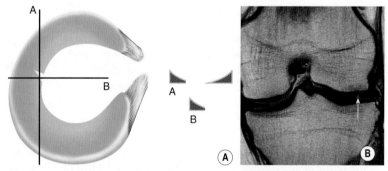

(A) Radial tear. This schematic shows a radial tear along the free edge of the meniscal body. This causes a blunted appearance on the sagittal 'A' and coronal 'B' images. (B) Coronal PD image through the knee showing a blunted appearance to the normal triangular configuration at the free apical margin of the meniscal body consistent with a radial tear.©35

Historical grading of meniscal tears (T1WI/PD)		Association with tear	Clinical significance
Grade I	Focal or globular areas of high SI within the central meniscus ('myxoid degeneration') ▶this does not extend to the articular surface	None	None
Grade II	Horizontal clefts of high SI ▶ this extends to the capsule periphery but not the meniscal articular surface (a 'meniscal fissure')	Low	It predisposes to a tear (particularly if it involves the posterior ⅓ of the medial meniscus)
Grade III	High SI within the meniscus that comes into contact with either the superior or inferior articular surface	A tear is present	Pain ± knee locking

MEDIAL COLLATERAL LIGAMENT DAMAGE

Definition

- The MCL extends from the medial femoral epicondyle and attaches below the joint into the medial tibial metaphysis ▶ it appears as a thin band of signal void (on coronal images)
- The MCL is injured with excess valgus force to a flexed knee

Radiological features

- **Grade I injury:** *a minimal tear with no instability* ▶ a normal MCL is applied closely to the underlying bone
  - T2WI: high SI in tissues adjacent to the MCL
- **Grade II injury:** *a partial tear with minor instability* ▶ displacement away from the bone
  - T2WI: MCL oedema and haemorrhage (also within the adjacent soft tissues)
- **Grade III injury:** *a complete tear with gross instability:* loss of ligament continuity ± interposed fluid and fibrosis
  - T2WI: disruption of the MCL fibres with interposed fluid
- **Chronic tear:** a thickened MCL with normal SI

Pearls

- **Associations:** medial and posterior capsular tears (with a complete rupture) ▶ a lateral tibial plateau bone contusion (± a non-displaced compression fracture)
- **Treatment:** isolated MCL tears are commonly treated non-surgically
- **O'Donoghue's triad:** MCL injury + ACL injury + medial meniscus damage
- **Pellegrini–Stieda lesion:** post-traumatic ossification of the femoral attachment of the medial collateral ligament

LATERAL COLLATERAL LIGAMENT COMPLEX AND POSTEROLATERAL CORNER INJURY

Definition

- These are associated with medial tibial compression fractures and bone contusions (in keeping with a forced varus strain on the knee)
- It can lead to iliotibial band disruption with severe injuries (a Segond injury heralds the presence of an associated ACL injury)
- Posterolateral corner injuries may lead to posterolateral instability

Radiological features

MRI Similar imaging features as for an MCL injury

Pearl

- Treatment is usually conservative (surgical repair may be needed if there is associated ACL injury or an unstable knee)

EXTENSOR MECHANISM ABNORMALITIES

Definition

- Extensor mechanism injuries include trauma to the quadriceps muscle, patella and patellar tendon
- **Sinding–Larsen injury:** an avulsion fracture of the lower patellar pole (the patellar ligament attachment)
- **Patellar tendinosis** ('jumpers knee'): this affects the superior and inferior tendon insertions ▶ it presents with anterior knee pain with focal tenderness
- **Osgood–Schlatter disease:** traction osteochondritis of the tibial tubercle ▶ it occurs in young active patients (and is usually self-limiting) ▶ distal patellar tendinopathy/tibial tubercle enlargement or fragmentation, and thickening of the overlying soft tissues

Radiological features

MRI Abnormal signal or size of the musculotendinous unit (MTU) suggests an intrasubstance injury or partial tear ▶ complete disruption is usually manifested as discontinuity of the normal black

- **Patellar tendinosis**
  US Tendon swelling with reduced echogenicity or loss of the internal fibrillar pattern
  MRI T2WI: high SI ▶ T1WI: low SI

Osgood–Schlatter disease

MRI Hypertrophy ± fragmentation of the tibial tubercle ▶ soft tissue swelling ▶ increased T2 SI in and around the distal patellar tendon

Pearls

- **The normal patella craniocaudal position:** the patellar tendon length = the patella height (± 20%) (Insall–Salvati ratio)
  - *Patella alta* (a high patella): this is associated with chondromalacia patellae, subluxation and cerebral palsy
  - *Patella baja* (low patella): this is associated with polio, juvenile chronic arthritis and achondroplasia

Patellar dislocation Prone to dislocate laterally (valgus force of the quadriceps) ▶ usually transient and relocates spontaneously

MRI subcortical bone marrow oedema of the medial patella and lateral femoral condyle ('kissing' contusions) ▶ usually an associated tear of the medial patellar retinaculum ± osteochondral patellar fracture

'Housemaid's knee' Bursitis of the superficial infrapatellar/deep infrapatellar/prepatellar bursae

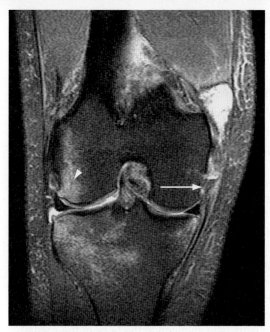

Coronal PD (FS) MR image. Valgus injury with bony avulsion of the femoral attachment of the MCL (arrow) and lateral compartment microfracture (arrowhead).©35

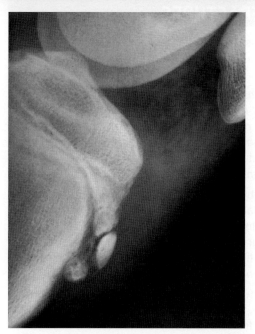

Osgood–Schlatter disease. Fragmentation may be seen and a portion of the tibial tubercle ossification centre is elevated.†

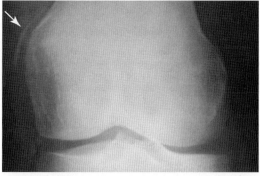

Pellegrini–Steida lesion. Post-traumatic calcification in relation to the medial femoral condyle (arrow).†

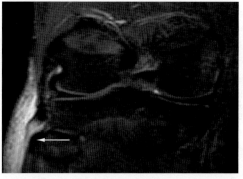

Coronal STIR MR image. There is an avulsion of the fibular collateral ligament (arrow) with the small fragment of periosteum from the fibular head.©35

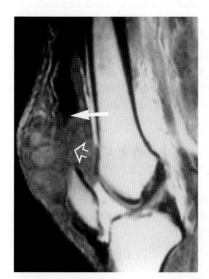

Complete rupture of the quadriceps tendon in a dialysis patient. Sagittal T1WI of the knee demonstrates quadriceps tendon rupture with a large amorphous area of haemorrhage (open arrow) just above the inferiorly retracted patella. Note the retracted quadriceps tendon (long arrow).*

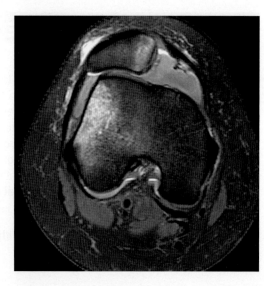

Acute patellar dislocation–relocation. Axial proton density fat-saturated image shows typical bone marrow oedema reflecting 'kissing contusions' of the medial patella and lateral femoral condyle. Note the shallow trochlea sulcus and lateral patella tilt which predispose to dislocation.**

ANKLE FRACTURES

- **Weber classification:** this is based upon the location of the distal fibular fracture relative to the distal fibula joint mortise

Weber A fracture A transverse fracture of the distal fibula *below the joint mortise* (an avulsion injury) + an oblique fracture of the medial malleolus (an impaction injury) ▶ there is a preserved tibiofibular complex ▶ it can be treated with closed reduction and casting
- *Following ankle supination*

Weber B fracture (the most common) An oblique, spiral lateral malleolar fracture *at the level of the joint mortise* (an impaction injury) + avulsion of the deltoid ligament (± avulsion fracture of the medial malleolus) ▶ there is partial rupture of the tibiofibular complex ▶ it may require surgery
- *Following ankle supination with external rotation*

Weber C fracture A proximal fibula fracture *above the joint mortise* ▶ there is avulsion of the deltoid ligament (± an avulsion fracture of the medial malleolus) ▶ there is a ruptured tibiofibular complex ▶ this usually requires surgery
- *Following ankle pronation with external rotation*

Pilon fracture A comminuted supramalleolar distal tibial fracture extending into the tibial plafond ▶ it is caused by axial loading and impaction of the talar dome against the tibial plafond (driving the fragments apart) ▶ it is associated with distal fibular fractures

Tillaux and triplanar fractures See paediatric fracture section

Trimalleolar fracture A fractured posterior lip of the distal tibia + a fractured medial and lateral malleoli

Maisonneuve fracture An avulsion fracture of the medial malleolus – the force is dissipated superiorly causing disruption of the interosseous ligament (joining the fibula and tibia) with an associated proximal fibula fracture ▶ it usually requires surgery

ACHILLES TENDON RUPTURE

Definition
- This is most common in middle-aged men (following sporting activity) ▶ it is an injury following a low-impact condition, which implies the presence of previous chronic degeneration (e.g. diabetes) ▶ the tendon insertion can be affected by impingement from a prominent posterior calcaneal process (Haglund's bump)
- Tears usually occur within 3 cm of the distal calcaneal insertion point (a relatively avascular 'critical' zone)

Normal tendon

MRI The tendon appears as a signal void (with a semilunar shape on axial images)

Achilles tendinosis Chronic degeneration can precede a tear (as there is no inflammation it is not a 'tendinitis')
MRI Diffuse tendon swelling and thickening ▶ T2WI/STIR: high SI

Achilles tendon tear

Lateral XR Soft tissue swelling and obliteration of the pre-Achilles fat pad
MRI/US Diffuse swelling and thickening ▶ T2WI/STIR: high SI
- *Partial tear:* T2WI: linear focal regions of high SI
- *Complete tear:* T2WI: tendon disruption with high SI between the ends of the torn ligament ▶ retraction of the proximal tendon ▶ T1WI: high SI (representing acute haemorrhage)

Posterior tibialis tendon injury The 2nd most common ankle tendon injury ▶ usually maintains the medial arch of the foot ▶ it commonly affects females without a history of trauma (usually during the 5th and 6th decades) ▶ the tendon is usually involved at the level of the medial malleolus (avulsion of the tendon from the navicular is typical in young patients)
- *Normal posterior tibialis tendon:* this is approximately 2 times as large as the adjacent flexor digitorum longus tendon

MRI Increased SI and tendon enlargement with injury

ANKLE LIGAMENT INJURIES

Definition
- Stretching and distraction (sprain) of the ankle ligaments following a medial or lateral ankle distraction ▶ inversion > eversion injury

XR of a mid-ligament rupture Soft tissue swelling only
XR of a rupture at a bone insertion This may cause an avulsion fracture (which is usually proximal – e.g. involving the malleoli) ▶ fracture fragments can be confused with well-corticated normal accessory ossification centres (some may represent old traumatic avulsions)

MRI It usually evaluates the lateral ligaments but can also evaluate the medial ankle ligaments (deltoid/tibio-spring/spring ligaments)▶ lateral ligaments: anterior talofibular ligament is the weakest and the 1st to be injured (if this is intact then the remaining lateral collateral ligaments are almost always intact)
- *Grade I:* anterior talofibular stretching or tearing
- *Grade II:* anterior talofibular tearing with calcaneofibular ligament stretching
- *Grade III:* disruption to the anterior and posterior talofibular ligaments as well as the calcaneofibular ligament (an unstable ankle)

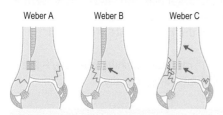

Diagram showing the Weber classification for ankle fractures.

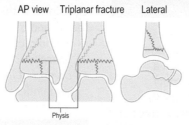

Diagram showing the fracture configuration in a triplanar fracture.

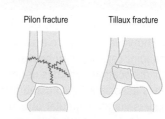

Diagram showing the fracture configuration in a Pilon fracture and Tillaux fracture.

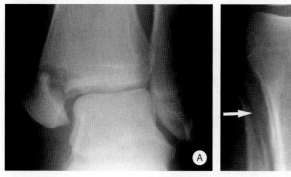

Maisonneuve fracture. AP XR of the ankle (A) demonstrates a transverse fracture of the medial malleolus. More cranially (B) there is a fracture of the proximal fibula (arrow), indicating extension of the injury plane along the interosseous membrane.*

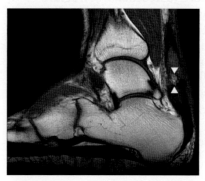

Complete tear of the Achilles tendon. Sagittal T1WI shows high signal at the site of a complete tear of the Achilles tendon. Arrowheads demarcate the length of fiber discontinuity. The tendon is thickened.©35

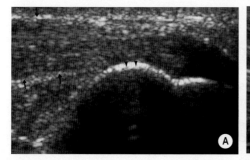
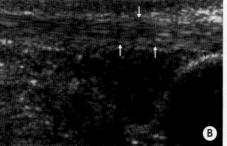
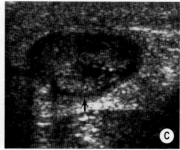

Partial tear/strain of the Achilles tendon. Longitudinal US (A) demonstrates thickening of the tendon (arrows) proximal to its calcaneal attachment (arrowheads). (B) Normal Achilles tendon (arrows). (C) Axial US in the mid-substance of the abnormal right tendon reveals a rounded anterior margin (arrow) and focal areas of decreased echogenicity.*

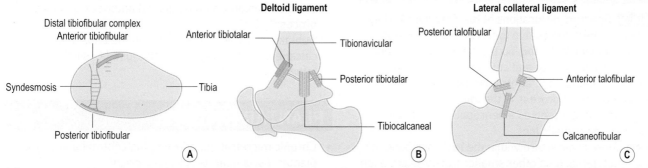

(A) Diagram showing the anatomy of the ligaments around the ankle when viewed from above. (B,C) Diagrams showing the components of the deltoid and lateral collateral ligaments of the ankle. The distal tibiofibular complex (including the anterior and posterior tibiofibular ligaments and syndesmosis) is an important ankle stabilizer.

TALAR FRACTURE

Definition The talus has no muscular or tendinous attachments – however in severe trauma the adjacent ligaments and joint capsule may be disrupted with a resultant talar dislocation (which is usually anterior)

- Dislocation is associated with osteonecrosis (as the blood supply is via the capsular attachments) ▶ most of the blood supply to the talar dome enters via the distal talus – therefore a talar neck fracture can result in talar dome osteonecrosis
- **Transchondral fracture (osteochondral fracture of the talar dome/osteochondritis dissecans/osteochondral fracture)**
  - This follows an impaction injury (with impingement of the talar dome against the posteromedial tibia and fibular styloid) ▶ the osteochondral fragment lies either within a bone crater (with fluid deep to the fragment) or it is detached and migrates into the joint space
    - **XR** It can be difficult to diagnose (MRI is often necessary)

CALCANEAL FRACTURE

Definition A comminuted impaction fracture within the body of the calcaneus with flattening of the subtalar portion of bone ▶ it is usually due to a compressive force (e.g. a fall from a height) ▶ it is commonly associated with lumbar spinal compression fractures or pilon fractures

- *Boehler's angle:* the normal angle is between 20 and 40° ▶ an impacted fracture will reduce or reverse this angle (a normal angle does not exclude a fracture) ▶ unreliable in children
- **Calcaneal stress fractures:** These have a vertical linear sclerotic appearance

XR A fracture is well seen on an axial heel (Harris) view

CT This is ideal for evaluating complex calcaneal fractures (including any extension into the subtalar joint)

LISFRANC FRACTURE DISLOCATION

Definition Fracture–dislocations at the TMT joint ▶ they follow severe shear forces due to forced plantar flexion

- Anterior impingement: this occurs between bony spurs on the dorsal talar neck and anterior tibial plafond
- Posterior impingement: associated with a large os trigonum or stieda process of the talus

▶ they are frequently seen as a neuropathic fracture–dislocation in the diabetic foot

- Usually there is a fracture within the recessed base of the 2nd metatarsal (and other smaller fractures are seen along the margins of the TMT joints)

Normal anatomy The 1st metatarsal is aligned with the medial cuneiform ▶ the 2nd metatarsal with the middle

cuneiform ▶ the 3rd metatarsal with the lateral cuneiform ▶ the 4th and 5th metatarsals with the cuboid

- *Homolateral injury:* all the metatarsals are shifted laterally
- *Divergent injury:* the 1st metatarsal shifts medially – the remainder of the forefoot shifts laterally

METATARSAL STRESS FRACTURE

Definition This is commonly seen with overuse – the classic is the 'march fracture' seen in military recruits and runners

XR Periosteal new bone formation is seen along the shafts of the 2nd, 3rd and 4th metatarsals

5TH METATARSAL AVULSION FRACTURE

Definition This follows forced inversion of the foot with associated rupture of the peroneus brevis attachment to the base of the 5th metatarsal

- **Jones (dancer's) fracture:** An extra-articular fracture of the proximal 5th metatarsal

XR The fracture line will invariably be transverse (as opposed to a normal accessory ossification centre at the base of the 5th metatarsal which appears as a longitudinal lucency along its lateral aspect)

FREIBERG'S INFRACTION

Definition An osteochondritis resulting from repetitive trauma which commonly affects the 2nd metatarsal head

XR Sclerosis, flattening and collapse of the 2nd metatarsal head (it may affect other metatarsals)

TARSAL COALITION

- Developmental fusion of ≥2 hind foot bones ▶ osseous or non-osseous ▶ most common is calcaneonavicular coalition (fusion via an elongated anterior calcaneal process
- Subtalar coalition: fusion between the talus and calcaneus at the middle subtalar joint ('C-sign' on a lateral radiograph)

PLANTAR FASCIITIS

- Chronic microtrauma affecting the central band of the plantar fascia near its calcaneal origin

US/MRI Fascial thickening (>5 mm) and loss of normal fibrillar structure

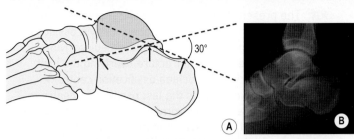

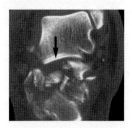

(A) Line drawing showing how Bohler's angle is constructed and measured. (B) The calcaneus is abnormal with flattening of Bohler's angle as the highest point in the middle is depressed so that joining the three points results in an almost straight line. A posterior fracture is evident.**

CT of a comminuted fracture of the calcaneus demonstrates complete disruption of the posterior subtalar joint (arrow).*

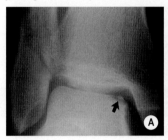

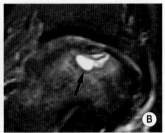

Osteochondral fracture of the medial talar dome. Oblique XR (A) demonstrates a lucency separating a small bony fragment from the talar dome (arrow) – also note the fractured lateral malleolus. Sagittal STIR image (B) demonstrates an osteochondral fragment of the talar dome separated from the talus by high signal fluid (arrow).*

Transchondral fracture classification		
Stage	**Description**	**Treatment**
Stage I	Compression fracture (with a normal XR, and bone marrow oedema on MRI)	Immobilization
Stage II	A partially detached osteochondral fragment*	Surgery (curettage, drilling, pinning)
Stage III	A detached osteochondral defect remains within an underlying crater	Surgery (curettage, drilling, pinning)
Stage IV	A detached osteochondral defect has migrated	The defect is excised to prevent early joint degeneration

*Fluid seen deep to the fragment, or a fissure within the overlying cartilage indicates that the fragment is at risk of loosening

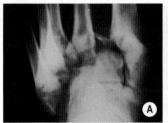

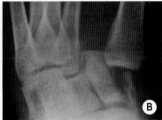

(A) Homolateral Lisfranc fracture–dislocation. All five metatarsals are displaced laterally. Oblique (B) projection of a divergent Lisfranc fracture–dislocation.*

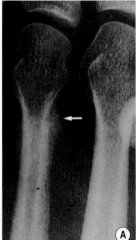

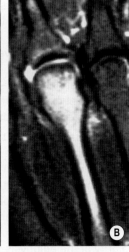

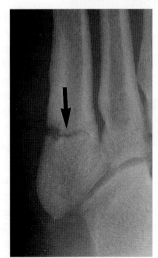

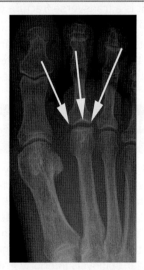

Stress fracture of the metatarsal ('march fracture'). AP radiograph (A) demonstrates fluffy periosteal new bone along the distal shaft of the 3rd metatarsal (arrow). (B) Coronal STIR image demonstrates increased SI within the distal 2nd metatarsal.*

Fracture of the proximal shaft of the 5th metatarsal ('true Jones fracture') (arrow).*

Anteroposterior radiograph of the forefoot showing evidence of Freiberg's disease with squaring off and flattening of the subchondral plate of the second metatarsal head (arrows).

5.2 PAEDIATRIC FRACTURES

GREENSTICK/TORUS FRACTURE/ PLASTIC BOWING

Definition In the paediatric skeleton the soft bone tends to bend and partially break (greater elasticity)

- **Greenstick fracture:** the bone cortex and periosteum break on the convex side of a long bone only
- **Torus fracture:** the bone cortex buckles on the concave side
- **Plastic bowing:** a long bone bends, rather than breaks (multiple oblique microfractures are present) ▶ in the forearm, a non-bowed bone may fracture or dislocate

EPIPHYSEAL INJURIES

Definition Injuries are graded according to the Salter–Harris classification (types I–V) ▶ injuries become more serious as the grade rises, with an associated risk of growth disturbance or avascular necrosis ▶ there is a worse prognosis within the lower limb than the upper limb

- *Types I and II:* the epiphysis remains intact ▶ good prognosis
- *Types III and IV:* the epiphysis is fractured ▶ poorer prognosis
- *Type V:* a very rare crushing injury of the physeal cartilage ▶ it is usually associated with types 1–IV injuries

CT This is useful in planning complex fracture treatment

MRI This visualizes the non-ossified growth plate cartilage, soft tissue or ligamentous injury (as well as the non-ossified epiphyses in very young children)

SUPRACONDYLAR FRACTURE

Definition This is the most common elbow fracture in children ▶ it is a transverse fracture of the distal humerus (proximal to the humeral condyles)

XR A joint effusion (with elevated anterior and posterior fat pads) ▶ the mid-third of the capitellum is displaced posterior to the anterior humeral line

MEDIAL CONDYLAR/EPICONDYLAR FRACTURE

Definition This is an avulsion injury (due to contraction of the forearm flexor muscles during a fall on an outstretched arm or an impaction injury from a fall onto the olecranon)

- A medial condylar fracture extends to the trochlear articular surface (an epicondylar injury is extra-articular)
- Valgus stress causes displacement of the medial epicondylar epiphysis inferiorly ▶ it may be associated with ulnar nerve injury

XR The presence of a trochlea ossification centre in the absence of a normally sited medial epicondyle ossification centre suggests that there is a displaced epicondylar fracture (with the displaced fracture overlying the joint space and mimicking a trochlea ossification centre) ▶ as the lateral epicondyle is the last ossification centre to appear, if there is a bone fragment adjacent to the lateral aspect of the distal humerus and it is not possible to identify the 5 other centres, a fracture must be present

- **Ossification order at the elbow** (CRITOL): **C**apitellum, **R**adial head, **I**nternal (medial) epicondyle, **T**rochlea, **O**lecranon, **L**ateral epicondyle

Pearl 'Little leaguer's elbow': chronic apophysitis around the medial epicondyle due to low energy repetitive traction forces

TODDLER'S FRACTURE

Definition An undisplaced oblique fracture of the middle/ distal tibial diaphysis in young children ▶ it may not be seen on an initial XR (perform delayed XR or scintigraphy – periosteal reaction + sclerosis)

- This is not suspicious for NAI (in isolation) if the toddler is ambulant

ANKLE FRACTURES

Definition

- Children's physes are more likely to fail than the ankle ligaments ▶ those of the distal tibia and fibula fuse at the same time (if only one is fused suspect an epiphyseal injury)
- Triplane and Tillaux fractures tend to occur in adolescence around the time of distal tibial epiphyseal fusion ▶ CT is used for assessment prior to reduction

Triplane fracture A Salter–Harris type IV epiphyseal injury: an oblique coronal fracture through the distal tibial metaphysis extending horizontally through the lateral part of the physis before running vertically through the epiphysis in the sagittal plane

- *Lateral XR:* it appears as Salter–Harris type II fracture (due to metaphyseal extension)
- *AP XR:* it appears as type III injury

Tillaux fracture A Salter–Harris type III injury due to avulsion of the anterior tibiofibular ligament: the fracture line runs through the anterolateral aspect of the distal tibial physis until it reaches the part that has fused, and then passes downwards through the epiphysis and into the joint ▶ no fracture component in the coronal plane (cf. triplane fracture)

- As the majority of the epiphysis has already fused there is no growth arrest (but the fracture must be reduced to restore joint congruity)

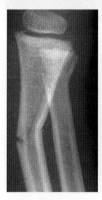
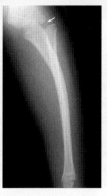
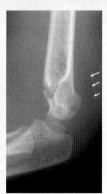

Supracondylar fracture of the distal humerus with elevation of the posterior fat pad (arrows). The mid ⅓ of the capitellum is also displaced posterior to the anterior humeral line.*

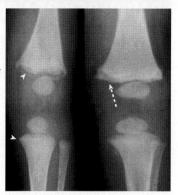

Classic metaphyseal lesions with different appearances. 'Corner fracture' (a thick rim only, arrowhead), 'bucket handle' (a thick rim projected away from the shaft, arrow) and a thin disk with a thick rim (stippled arrow).**

Greenstick fractures of the distal radius and ulna.*

Plastic bowing of the ulna with dislocation of the radial head (arrow).*

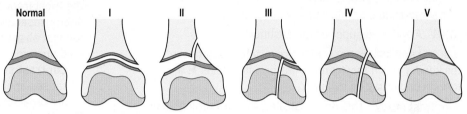

Illustration of the Salter–Harris classification of fractures. (Type I) The fracture is isolated to the growth plate and causes epiphyseal separation, without adjacent bone fracture. The fracture line passes through the hypertrophic layer of the physis. (Type II) This is the most common growth plate fracture and is usually seen in children between the ages of 10 and 16. As a result of shearing or avulsive force, the fracture splits the growth plate and then passes into the metaphysis, separating a small fragment of bone. (Type III) The fracture line passes through the epiphysis, and then horizontally across the growth plate. This is most commonly seen at the distal tibia in children aged 10–15. (Type IV) This is a vertically orientated fracture, involving both the epiphysis and metaphysis, and crossing the growth plate. This is most commonly seen in the distal humerus and tibia. (Type V) This fracture, results from a compressive force, crushing the growth plate. Damage to the growth plate can cause subsequent deformity. The diagnosis is often made retrospectively when growth arrest is discovered at a later date.**

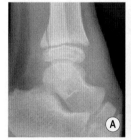
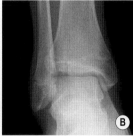
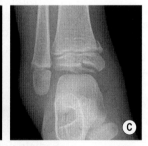
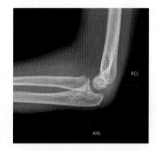

Various Salter–Harris fractures. (A) Salter–Harris II fracture of the distal left tibia. (B) Salter–Harris III fracture of the distal right tibia. (C) Salter–Harris fracture of the distal left tibia.**

Normal lateral film of the elbow. The two lines drawn on the radiograph are used to assess the elbow joint. Anterior humeral line (AHL): one-third of the capitellum should lie anterior to this line. In the young child where there is only partial ossification of the capitellum, this measurement is less valid. RCL—on a lateral film, a line drawn along the shaft of the proximal radius should pass through the capitellum.**

Clinical impact guidelines: the I in CRITOL

The ossification centre for the internal (i.e. medial) epicondyle is the point of attachment of the forearm flexor muscles. Vigorous muscle contraction may avulse this centre. The most common injury mechanism is a fall on an outstretched hand. Avulsions also occur in children who are involved in throwing sports, hence the term "little leaguer's elbow". When a major displacement of the internal epicondyle occurs the bone can become trapped within the elbow joint. This is a well recognised complication of a dislocated elbow, occurring in 50% of cases following an elbow subluxation or dislocation. A major avulsion is easy to overlook when an elbow has been transiently dislocated and then reduces spontaneously because the detached epicondyle may, on the AP radiograph, be mistaken for the normally positioned trochlear ossification centre. I before T. Though the CRITOL sequence may vary slightly there is a constant: the trochlear (T) centre always ossifies after the internal epicondyle. Therefore apply this rule: if the trochlear centre (T) is visible then there must be an ossified internal epicondyle (I) visible somewhere on the radiograph. If the internal epicondyle is not seen in its normal position then suspect that it is trapped within the joint.

RADIOLOGY OF NON-ACCIDENTAL INJURY (NAI)

DEFINITION

- **NAI**: a spectrum of injuries due to child abuse ▶ this includes physical, sexual and emotional abuse

Clinical presentation

- This ranges from vague minor symptoms to life-threatening shock

Specific injuries

- **Oropharyngeal injuries**: pharyngeal perforation may lead to a retropharyngeal abscess, mediastinitis, haemorrhage, or interstitial emphysema

  CXR A widened superior mediastinum

  Lateral soft tissue neck XR Preverterbral soft tissue thickening which may contain gas or a fluid level ▶ a foreign body may be evident

  Contrast study This demonstrates an extraluminal leak

  CT / MRI This detects soft tissue abnormalities

- **Abdominal injuries:**
  - These are secondary to a direct blunt trauma or to a sudden deceleration after the child is thrown ▶ CT is the investigation of choice ▶ US is portable and readily available
  - Abdominal injuries demonstrate a lower incidence in NAI than either skeletal or brain injuries (skeletal or brain injuries predominate with increasing age)
    - There is a significant associated morbidity and mortality (up to 50%) ▶ the average age for abuse related fatal visceral injury is 2 years
  - **Solid organs:** in NAI the liver is injured more frequently than the spleen or kidneys (the reverse is true for accidental trauma)
  - **Bladder:** rupture in the absence of a pelvic fracture (following a direct blow against a full bladder)
  - **Urethra:** following sexual abuse (with associated rectal, perineal and genital injuries)
  - **Pancreas:** trauma commonly results from a direct midline blow where the pancreas crosses the midline (resulting in an injury at the junction of the body and tail) – this is the most common cause of childhood acute pancreatitis ▶ acute haemorrhagic pancreatitis is highly suggestive of NAI
    - Due to its retroperitoneal location, associated injuries often mask what may already be slowly evolving clinical signs
  - **Adrenals:** injuries can be isolated or in association with other visceral injuries ▶ unilateral haemorrhage tends to be right sided (and often clinically silent)
    - **CT:** low attenuation homogenous masses within the gland (± thickening of the ipsilateral crus and free intraperitoneal blood)

- **GI tract**: bowel injuries are rare in accidental trauma but more often seen with NAI (due to blows across the abdomen) ▶ the mesenteric side of the bowel is more prone to vascular tears and the antimesenteric side to perforation ▶ intense bowel wall enhancement is seen with the 'shock bowel' syndrome
- **Duodenum:** the 2nd and 3rd parts are the most commonly injured (following direct compression against the vertebral column) ▶ intramural haematomas of the duodenum and jejunum are the most frequent bowel trauma finding in NAI ▶ submucosal and subserosal bleeding may cause luminal obstruction ▶ a haematoma may act as a lead point for intussusception
  - **Contrast study:** acute duodenal haematoma causes an intramural mass with thickened proximal folds (a 'coiled spring' appearance)
- **Bowel rupture and perforation:** this commonly affects the 2nd and 3rd parts of the duodenum (just distal to the ligament of Treitz), and the ileocaecal junction ▶ colonic injuries are rare (due to protection from the bony pelvis and its peripheral location)
- **Mesenteric injuries:** severe injuries result from SMA avulsion with mesenteric ischaemia ▶ ischaemic strictures are late complications

- **Thoracic injury**
  - Direct contusion of lungs and pleura is rare even in the presence of rib fractures ▶ pneumothoraces and effusions are uncommon (cf. accidental trauma) ▶ diaphragmatic rupture may occur

Dating fractures: radiographic changes in childhood fractures			
Radiological feature	**Early**	**Peak**	**Late**
Soft tissue resolution	2–5 days	4–10 days	10–21 days
Periosteal new bone	4–10 days	10–14 days	14–21 days
Loss of fracture line definition	10–14 days	14–21 days	42–90 days
Soft callus	10–14 days	14–21 days	2 years to physeal closure
Hard callus	14–21 days	21–42 days	
Remodelling	3 months	1 year	
©10			

SKELETAL INJURIES IN NON-ACCIDENTAL INJURY

General features No fracture is pathognomonic on its own ▶ mid-clavicular and humeral fractures are well known birth injuries

Features associated with possible NAI Multiple fractures ▶ rib fractures (regardless of type) ▶ femoral fractures in non-ambulant children ▶ mid shaft humeral fractures ▶ skull fractures ▶ metaphyseal injuries ▶ uncommon sites (e.g. scapula) ▶ any fracture with a delayed presentation

RCR Referral Guidelines Skeletal survey (+ skull radiographs) in children < 2yrs with a suspicion of abuse ▶ CT brain for any infant < 1 yr with evidence of physical abuse or any child presenting with physical abuse + encephalopathic features, neurological signs of haemorrhagic retinpathy ▶ MRI brain may be helpful ▶ bone scintigraphy if the skeletal survey is equivocal ▶ CT if chest or abdominal injury suspected

Fractures that occur infrequently with a high specificity for abuse Metaphyseal, rib and scapular (esp. acromial) fractures ▶ fractures of the outer ⅓ of the clavicle ▶ sternal fractures ▶ spinous process fractures

Fractures with moderate specificity for abuse Multiple fractures ▶ bilateral fractures and fractures of differing ages ▶ vertebral fractures or subluxation ▶ digital injuries in non-mobile children ▶ spiral fractures of the humerus ▶ epiphyseal separations ▶ complex skull fractures (i.e. those that are wider than 5 mm, depressed, occipital and growing fractures)

Fractures that occur frequently but have a low specificity for abuse Mid-clavicular fractures ▶ simple linear skull fractures of the parietal bone ▶ single diaphyseal fractures (with the exception of spiral fractures of the humerus) ▶ greenstick fractures

Radiological features

Skeletal survey This is usually performed in children <2 years old (with the highest yield) ▶ repeat XR's after 10–14 days enhances occult fracture detection (especially the ribs) ▶ precise dating of a fracture is not possible (estimates are based on the pattern of healing)

Skeletal scintigraphy This becomes positive within hours of injury ▶ it is the most sensitive in detecting rib, scapular, spinal, diaphyseal and pelvic fractures (as well as periosteal trauma) ▶ it has a low sensitivity for fractures of the skull or flat bones, or healed and metaphyseal fractures ▶ the epiphyses normally show high uptake (do not confuse with a fracture) ▶ physiological periosteal new bone and the periosteal prominence accompanying rapid growth do not demonstrate uptake

MRI Not routinely indicated for bony assessment in NAI

US This is not routinely performed ▶ it can demonstrate subperiosteal haemorrhage, fracture separation of the epiphysis, costochondral injuries and occult long bone fractures before they become evident radiographically

Differential diagnosis of non-accidental injury in children			
Disease	**Shaft fracture**	**Periosteal reaction**	**Metaphyseal abnormality**
Normal bone density			
Non-accidental injury	+	+	+
Birth trauma	+		±
Congenital indifference to pain	+	+	+
Myelodysplasia	+	+	+
Osteomyelitis	-	+	+
Congenital syphilis	-	+	-
Vitamin A intoxication	-	++	-
Caffey's disease	-	+	-
Prostaglandin E therapy	-		
Metaphyseal and spondylometaphyseal dysplasias	-	-	+
Osteopenic bones			
Osteogenesis imperfecta	+	-	+
Rickets	+	+	+
Scurvy	-	+	+
Leukaemia	-	+	-
Methotrexate therapy	+	-	±
Menkes' kinky hair syndrome	-	+	+

Skeletal survey*
AP and lateral chest – lateral to include sternum
Upper limbs – AP both forearms, AP both humeri, PA both hands and wrists
Lower limbs – AP both femora done individually
AP both tibiae and fibulae
AP both ankles, coned, with ankle joints flexed at 90°
Dorsiplantar both feet
AP abdomen and pelvis
Lateral of thoracolumbar spine
Lateral cervical spine
AP and lateral skull – add a Townes' view if there is occipital injury
Additional views at radiologist's discretion
All films to be checked by a radiologist
It is essential to have the following: – metal markers on all films – correct patient identification labelling – radiographs should ideally be done on high-resolution film but there is increasing use of modern digital equipment

©11

543

METAPHYSEAL FRACTURES ('CORNER' OR 'BUCKET HANDLE' FRACTURES)

Definition These are highly characteristic of and specific for NAI ▶ a series of microfractures across the metaphysis following 'shearing forces' sustained during violent shaking

Mechanism of injury They occur during shaking (acceleration and deceleration forces applied directly to a limb) or following direct wrenching or twisting of the limb using the extremities as 'handles' (in children >2 years old metaphyseal trauma results in diaphyseal and epiphyseal fracture separation)

Clinical presentation They are most commonly seen in non-mobile abused infants (<18 months of age) ▶ they are usually asymptomatic and found incidentally

Location They are most frequently seen around the knees and ankles but also occurs at the shoulder, elbow, wrists and hips

XR Corner fractures ▶ metaphyseal subperiosteal reaction (the loosely attached periosteum is frequently stripped by shearing forces leading to subperiosteal bleeding) ▶ a metaphyseal lucent line immediately adjacent to the epiphyseal plate (a subtle sign) ▶ repeated trauma leads to an irregular fluffy appearance to the metaphyses

- Repeat XR after 2 weeks may show healing, and a repeat XR after 5–6 weeks may clarify whether a metaphyseal irregularity represents a normal variant (most fractures will have healed by then)

LONG BONE DIAPHYSEAL FRACTURES

Definition The most common fracture in NAI (it is 4 times as common as a metaphyseal fracture)

- *There should be increased suspicion if:* they are multiple, bilateral, or found in a state of healing ▶ if they are of differing ages or when there is a fracture through callus ▶ if a femoral fracture occurs in non mobile children ▶ if they are associated with fractures that have a high specificity for abuse

Location The femur, humerus and tibia are the most frequently injured bones

XR Transverse fractures (direct trauma) ▶ spiral fractures (twisting or a pulling force and always suspicious for abuse – particularly in the humerus)

Pearl Common accidental injuries that can also occur in NAI: a 'toddlers' fracture' (only in mobile children) ▶ supracondylar and metaphyseal torus fractures

IMPACTION FRACTURES

Definition These are most common at the metadiaphyseal junction of the distal femur and proximal tibia (due to

impaction forces when a child is forcibly thumped down onto their legs)

XR The bone cortex buckles anteriorly and there is an incomplete crush fracture of the bone shaft

PERIOSTEAL NEW BONE

Definition Physiological subperiosteal new bone formation (SPNBF) is seen as a normal physiological phenomenon between 6 weeks and 6 months of age and should be differentiated from periosteal new bone formation as a result of occult fracture or a gripping injury

- *SPNBF:* it always has an organized lamellar appearance ▶ it is symmetrical and more common within the lower limbs ▶ it is confined to the diaphysis (and never extends to the metaphysis) ▶ it demonstrates normal uptake on bone scintigraphy (there is increased uptake with trauma)
  - Outside this age range periosteal reaction is abnormal – it is usually seen with a fracture repair, or as a consequence of a gripping or twisting force

XR Periosteal reaction is evident about 7 days post injury (as the periosteum is only loosely attached and readily separates) ▶ it may be florid in repetitive or severe twisting injuries

VERTEBRAL INJURIES

- These are relatively rare in NAI
- Vertebral body compression fractures commonly occur in the thoracolumbar region ▶ babies are susceptible to cervical injuries (as there are flexible supporting ligaments)

CERVICAL SPINE INJURIES

- Injuries typically affect the 1st and 2nd cervical bodies (disproportionate head size and under-developed neck muscles)
- 'Spinal Cord Injury Without Radiographic Abnormality' (SCIWORA) ▶ spinal cord injury without fracture as the spinal column has more flexibility than the spinal cord in children
- Normal anatomical variants misinterpreted as injuries:
  - Pseudo-subluxation at C2/3 and C3/4 (up to 4 mm is allowed)
  - Open-mouth view: a pseudo-Jefferson fracture may be seen due to ossification of the C1 lateral mass exceeding that of C2
  - Pseudo anterior vertebral wedging of up to 3 mm can be normal (especially C3)

RIB FRACTURES

Definition Rib fractures are usually rare due to the elasticity of the thoracic cage in children ▶ solitary or multiple rib fractures are considered synonymous for NAI once other causative factors (e.g. osteogenesis imperfecta) have been excluded

Clinical presentation 80% are clinically occult ▶ the majority occur at <2 years of age ▶ they commonly follow violent shaking with thoracic compression ▶ not usually associated with chest wall bruising ▶ typically multiple (positioned immediately above each other in a line) ▶ unilateral in 50% ▶ may be solitary ▶ they are not usually seen with paediatric cardiopulmonary resuscitation

XR Multiple fractures of varying ages ▶ they occur particularly medial to the costotransverse articulation ▶ fractures can occur anywhere along the rib, but fractures to the posterior rib arches are particularly associated with NAI ▶ they are rarely accompanied by associated lung contusions

- *Subtle signs:* expansion and widening of the ribs

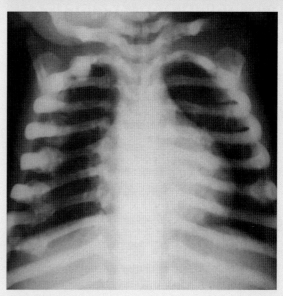

NAI. CXR demonstrating multiple rib fractures at different stages of healing.†

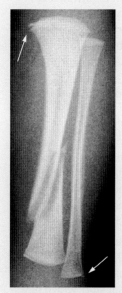

Diaphyseal fracture. XR of the left lower leg demonstrating a mildly diastatic oblique fracture of the distal tibia. There are also metaphyseal corner fractures of the proximal tibia and distal fibula (arrows).*

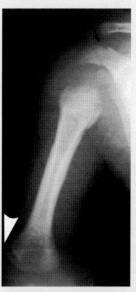

Fracture of the acromion (black arrow). There is also a metaphyseal fracture of the distal humerus (white arrowhead). A thick pathological periosteal reaction of the proximal humerus extending into the metaphysis is evident.*

BRAIN INJURY IN NON-ACCIDENTAL INJURY (NAI)

- NAI is the leading cause of serious head injury and death in infants <2 years of age

MECHANISMS

- Direct trauma with skull fractures ± underlying brain injury ▶ repeated trauma, shaking or strangulation ▶ impact injuries (including acceleration and deceleration injuries) ▶ whiplash shaking injuries

TYPES OF INJURY

- *Primary injury:* SDH or EDH ▶ subarachnoid haemorrhage ▶ cortical contusion ▶ diffuse axonal shearing injury ▶ intracerebral and intraventricular haemorrhage
- *Secondary injury:* hypoxic ischaemic damage resulting from: cerebral oedema ▶ reduced cerebral blood flow ▶ shock or vasospasm

'Whiplash shaken baby syndrome'

- The association of a SDH (± SAH), massive cerebral oedema, retinal haemorrhages, fractured ribs and metaphyseal injuries in the absence of any external signs of cranial trauma
- The child is often held by the rib cage and squeezed (resulting in fractured ribs and a raised CVP)
- A young infant is particularly prone to this as there is a relatively large head in relation to the body size (in association with poor head support and control) ▶ the brain is also relatively small in relation to the cranium, generating shearing forces ± ruptured cortical veins ▶ axonal injuries due to the differing density between white and grey matter ▶ midbrain injures due to limited upper brainstem mobility (set by the tentorium)
- *Other possible sequelae:* hypoxia secondary to respiratory embarrassment (following squeezing of the chest during shaking) ▶ carotid occlusion secondary to a violent neck motion

Complications of brain injury

- Arachnoiditis leading to obstructive hydrocephalus ▶ a communicating hydrocephalus from alteration in the CSF dynamics ▶ cerebral atrophy ▶ cerebral arterial and venous infarction ▶ multicystic encephalomalacia

Parenchymal brain injuries

- *Intraparenchymal haemorrhagic contusions:* visible at the white matter/cortex junction
  - CT: spontaneously hyperdense (acute), hypodense (chronic)
  - MRI: better seen with MRI ▶ T1WI: increased SI (intermediate phase) ▶ T2*WI: low SI (late phase) ▶ SWI: low SI (late phase)

- *Shearing diffuse axonal injuries:* seen in the subcortical region, centrum ovale, corpus callosum, cerebral peduncles
  - CT: initially visible if haemorrhagic
  - MRI: demonstrated if non-haemorrhagic ▶ DWI is useful for changes in anisotrophy

Subdural haematoma

- This is the most common intracranial finding in NAI with a high specificity for abuse (as it requires the application of severe forces) ▶ it results from trauma associated with rotation between the brain and dura – this leads to shearing of the bridging veins within the subdural space
- There is an increased suspicion of NAI if there is:
  - The presence of SDH without a skull fracture (implying a shaking injury)
  - Bilateral SDH's
  - SDH's of different ages (the density of blood on CT and MRI varies with its age)
  - SDH in the presence of retinal haemorrhages (implying an acceleration–deceleration force)
  - An acute interhemispheric fissure SDH or closely related to the falx and layering over the tentorium (evident as a bright and irregularly thickened falx)
    - This must be distinguished from a normal falx (which may appear bright against the background of an abnormally low density brain)
    - In accidental trauma subdural bleeds do not usually extend into the falx (localised over the cerebral convexities)
  - NB: a non abuse subdural collection can be seen in 'benign macrocrania'

Diffuse hypoxic-ischaemic lesions

- Focal ischaemic lesions in multiple locations, either in the MCA territory, with a subarachnoid haemorrhage is highly suggestive of abuse ▶ ischaemic lesions preferentially involve the basal ganglia ▶ lesions are more diffuse preserving only the posterior fossa

CT Loss of the grey-white matter differentiation ▶ parenchymal hypoattenuation (oedema) ▶ relative preservation in density of the thalami, basal ganglia and cerebellum (hence the term 'reversal sign' which is associated with a poor prognosis – it may also occur with drowning, fits, status asthmaticus, and cardiac arrest)

- An acute interhemispheric fissure subdural haemorrhage together with the acute reversal sign is highly suggestive of a shaking NAI

MRI + DWI is very sensitive in demonstrating early hypoxic-ischaemic change ▶ MR spectroscopy: high concentration of lactate compared with creatine and NAA

Radiological investigations

SXR This is not a reliable predictor of intracranial injury
- It should be performed in all children <2 years of age with a suspected injury
- Bilateral, stellar or depressed fractures or fractures through the midline are suspicious ▶ a growing fracture with a leptomeningeal cyst is more common with NAI than in accidental injury

Transfontanellar US Imaging via a patent fontanelle in neonates and small babies may detect a subdural haematoma (peripheral anechoic collection) ▶ parenchymal contusions (hypoechoic or cystic lesions, particularly at the grey white matter junction)

CT This is performed in an obtunded or neurologically unstable child, or if there is a skull fracture ▶ the oedema is usually massive and worse within the parieto-occipital region ▶ it appears as diffusely decreased grey and white matter density with decreased or lost grey-white matter differentiation ▶ relative preservation in density of the thalami, basal ganglia and cerebellum
- An acute interhemispheric fissure subdural haemorrhage together with the acute reversal sign is highly suggestive of a shaking NAI

MRI Indicated if a CT is equivocal ▶ gradient echo T2* to detect blood products – susceptibility weighted imaging (SWI) is more sensitive for small haemorrhages ▶ FLAIR is useful for demonstrating an extra axial acute bleed (can be difficult to interpret in the first months of life) ▶ DWI to assess for hypoxic-ischaemic change and axonal injuries

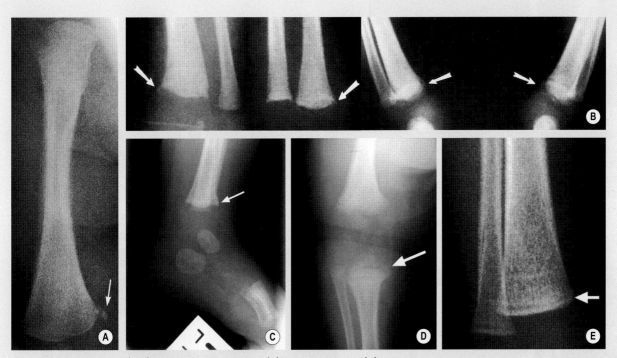

Metaphyseal fractures. (A,B) XRs of the right femur (A) and both ankles (B) demonstrating metaphyseal corner fractures of the distal femur and both distal tibia (arrows). The angled tangential view reveals the 'bucket-handle' appearance of the fracture. (C) XR of the left ankle demonstrates a metaphyseal corner fracture of the distal tibia (arrow). (D) Angled tangential view of the right lower limb demonstrates the 'bucket-handle' appearance (arrow). (E) XR of the right ankle demonstrates subtle metaphyseal fractures evident as a metaphyseal lucent line (arrow).*

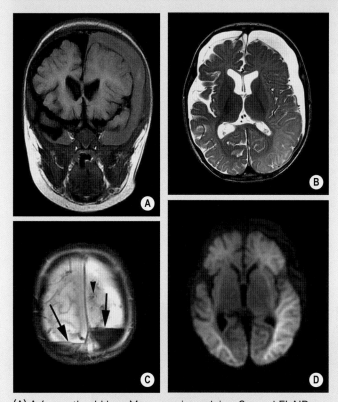

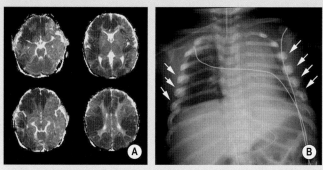

(A) A 3-month-old girl. Sudden pallor, loss of consciousness, then seizures; blood found with lumbar puncture. DWI with ADC maps reveals multiple ischaemic lesions. (B) Continuing, chest radiographs after resuscitation in the intensive care unit: multiple rib fractures with callus (arrows). Shaken baby.**

(A) A 4-month-old boy. Macrocrania, malaise. Coronal FLAIR image demonstrates circumferential bilateral subdural collections. (B) Continuing, T2 axial slice confirms subdural collections, with hyperintensity of the posterior regions of the brain. (C) Continuing, susceptibity-weighted image shows punctiform parenchyma bleeding (arrowhead) and fluid–fluid levels within the surrounding subdural collections.
(D) Continuing, diffusion-weighted image better demonstrates bilateral cortico-subcortical ischaemic lesions.**

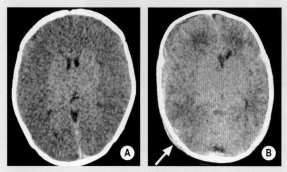

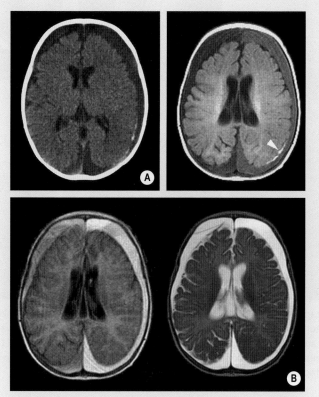

Reversal sign in hypoxic–ischaemic encephalopathy.
(A) NECT of an abused baby who was shaken, demonstrating the 'reversal sign'. The brain is oedematous with loss of grey–white matter differentiation and reduced density. There is relative preservation in density of the thalami and basal ganglia. (B) NECT demonstrating an oedematous, swollen brain with reduced grey–white matter differentiation and mass effect. Small bilateral hyperdense subdural bleeds are present. A right posterior parietal skull vault fracture is present and is associated with an overlying scalp haematoma (arrow).*

(A) A 4-month-old boy, somnolent, presenting with a right periorbital haematoma. CT demonstrated subacute, subdural collections bilaterally, with recent bleeding on the left side.
(B) Continuing, MRI performed 3 days later. Axial T1, flair and T2-weighted images. Right and left subdural collections exhibit different signal intensities, maybe in relation to different bleeding but also to blood concentration in each collection. Note also subarachnoid bleeding on the left side, better seen on T1 (arrowhead). Skeletal survey revealed multiple rib fractures.**

5.3 SOFT TISSUE IMAGING

LOCALIZED CALCIFICATION AND OSSIFICATION

Definition Deposition of calcium pyrophosphate dihydrate or calcium hydroxyapatite within soft tissues is called mineralization or calcification
- *Metastatic:* the result of abnormal calcium metabolism
- *Calcinosis:* occurring with a normal calcium metabolism
- *Dystrophic:* related to tissue damage
- *Ossification:* bony trabeculae are discernible (either ectopic or heterotropic) ▶ calcium deposits tend to be more densely sclerotic than in normal bone
- The differential diagnosis is divided into:
  - Generalized calcification (see separate section)
  - Localized calcification
  - Ossification

LOCALIZED CALCIFICATION – TRAUMA

Definition Any cause of focal soft tissue necrosis (e.g. injection sites, radiation damage, thermal injuries) can predispose to calcification
- Blunt trauma can cause fat necrosis within the subcutaneous tissues and areas of dystrophic calcification
  - Any haematoma (particularly subperiosteal) may calcify
- **Calcific myonecrosis:** calcification of atrophic muscles occurring 1–2 months after a severe crush injury

LOCALIZED CALCIFICATION – TUMOURS

Definition Widespread soft tissue calcification is a rare manifestation of disseminated malignancy where there is hypercalcaemia associated with extensive bone destruction (e.g. metastases, leukaemia and myeloma)
- Localized intratumoral calcification may occur within any soft tissue tumour due to haemorrhage or necrosis
- **Benign mineralizing tumours:** soft tissue chondroma (punctuate or 'ring and arc' calcification) ▶ lipoma (ossification can occur, especially if it is parosteal) ▶ haemangiomas (phleboliths)
- **Malignant mineralizing tumours:** extraskeletal osteosarcoma ▶ extraskeletal chondrosarcoma ▶ synovial sarcoma (with a central rather than peripheral distribution)

HETEROTOPIC OSSIFICATION

Definition This follows inappropriate differentiation of fibroblasts into osteoblasts in response to local inflammation
- Developmental causes include fibrodysplasia ossificans progressiva, melorheostosis and progressive osseous heteroplasia
- **Post-surgical:** this particularly occurs following a total hip arthroplasty (± pain and restricted movement)
- **Post-traumatic:**
  - *Pellegrini–Stieda lesion:* ossification of the medial collateral knee ligament
  - *Neurogenic heterotropic ossification:* soft tissue ossification associated with CNS injuries (with prolonged unconsciousness and spinal trauma) ▶ there is a periarticular distribution (commonly affecting the hips) ▶ surgery is associated with recurrence
  - *Avulsion of an ossification centre:* in the skeletally immature an avulsed ossification centre may continue to grow ▶ this may present later as a large ossified soft tissue mass (commonly affecting the pelvic and hamstring pelvic origins)

MYOSITIS OSSIFICANS

Definition Heterotopic bone formation within muscles, tendons and fascia following trauma ▶ it is possibly due to haematoma ossification or displacement of periosteal elements into the soft tissues
- Haemorrhage is followed by mineralization ▶ this is first seen in the periphery with a gradual reduction in the size of the mass (which are both helpful in distinguishing from a mineralizing soft tissue sarcoma)
- Early biopsy should be avoided (as it can resemble a soft tissue osteosarcoma)
- It is associated with burns and paraplegia ▶ it is commonly seen around the elbow and in the thigh

Angiography A hypervascular lesion

Scintigraphy Increased activity

MRI T2WI/STIR: florid perilesional oedema involving the whole affected muscle compartment
- **Pseudomalignant myositis ossificans:** this is similar radiographically and pathologically to myositis ossificans (but there is no history of trauma)

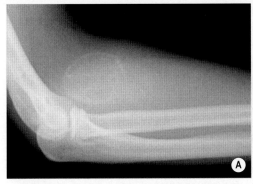
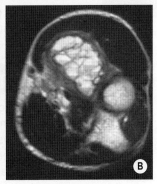

Antecubital myositis ossificans. (A) The plain XR shows the characteristic peripheral ossification and multiple high SI fluid levels (haemorrhage) on the axial MR image (B).[†]

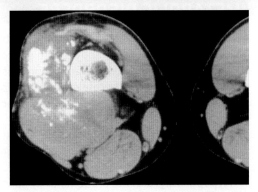

Synovial sarcoma. Axial CT demonstrating a soft tissue mass lateral and posterior to the femur containing calcifications.*

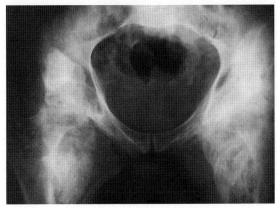

Myositis ossificans associated with paraplegia. Very extensive ossification is seen around both hips.[†]

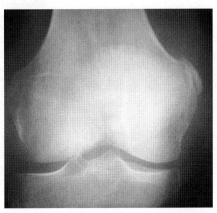

Pellegrini–Stieda lesion of the medial femoral condyle.[†]

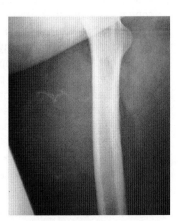

Calcified liposarcoma.[†]

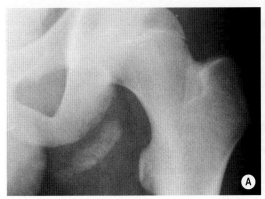
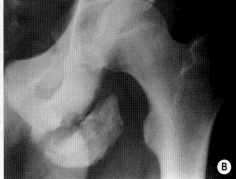

Ischial avulsion. (A) XR at presentation shows the avulsed ischial apophysis. (B) Three years later the apophysis has continued to grow to form a large ossified mass.*

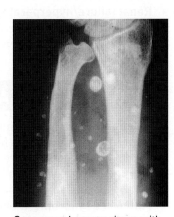

Cavernous haemangioma with multiple phleboliths.[†]

METABOLIC DISORDERS

- This results from prolonged elevation of the serum calcium (or more importantly serum phosphate) ▶ many causes, but chronic renal failure is the most common
- **Primary hyperparathyroidism**: calcification is typically seen involving arteries, cartilage (chondrocalcinosis), and periarticular tissues
- **Secondary hyperparathyroidism**: soft tissue and vascular calcification is more common than in primary disease ▶ chondrocalcinosis is infrequent
- **Hypoparathyroidism**: predominantly subcutaneous calcification (also with basal ganglia calcification) ▶ osteosclerosis ▶ premature epiphyseal closure ▶ band-like paraspinal calcification (mimicking DISH)
- **Pseudohypoparathyroidism**: there are similar features to hypoparathyroidism but it is associated with growth deformities (rounded facies, broad bones, cone epiphyses, short metacarpals and metatarsals – especially the 1st, 4th and 5th)
- **Pseudopseudohypoparathyroidism**: XR features are identical to pseudohypoparathyrodism (but with a normal serum calcium and phosphate)
- **Hypervitaminosis D**: smooth lobulated amorphous calcium hydroxyapatite masses within the periarticular regions, bursae, tendon sheaths and the joint capsule ▶ dense metaphyseal bands and cortical thickening (± osteosclerosis) in children ▶ most of these features are absent in adults (osteosclerosis may be the only manifestation)

ARTERIAL CALCIFICATION

- **Monkeberg's arteriosclerosis**: finer 'pipe-stem' calcification seen with medial degeneration
- **Diabetes**: calcification of the small vessels of the feet
- **Renal failure/hyperparathyroidism**: a fine more generalized pattern of arterial calcification
- **Aneurysms**: rounded, curvilinear and crescentic calcification

VENOUS CALCIFICATION

- **Phleboliths**: these are common and represent a calcified venous thrombus (leading to a small circular calcified density) ▶ they are often seen within pelvic veins ▶ they are also seen in chronic varicosities and cavernous haemangiomas
- **Maffucci's syndrome**: multiple phleboliths (haemangiomas) and enchondromas
- **Venous incompetence**: subcutaneous calcification and organized periosteal new bone formation
- Pearl Venous mural calcification is rare

BACTERIAL INFECTION

• Dystrophic calcification may occur within resolving abscesses (e.g. spine TB)

- **Extensive calcified lymphadenitis**: old TB infection ▶ histoplasmosis ▶ coccidioidomycosis
- Leprosy is a rare cause of nerve calcification

PARASITIC INFECTION

- **Echinococcosis** (hydatid): liver and lung calcifications
- **Schistosomiasis**: urinary tract calcifications
- **Cystercicosis** (pork tapeworm: Taenia solium): larvae show a predilection for muscle, subcutaneous tissues and the brain ▶ calcified dead cysts are oval with a lucent centre and are orientated in the direction of the muscle fibres

FIBRODYSPLASIA OSSIFICANS PROGRESSIVA (MYOSITIS OSSIFICANS PROGRESSIVA)

Definition A congenital connective tissue disorder with an autosomal inheritance and variable penetrance ▶ it is unrelated to myositis ossificans

Clinical presentation There is progressive swelling and ossification of the fascia, aponeuroses, ligaments, tendons and skeletal muscle connective tissues

- It usually affects the neck and shoulder girdle first (before the onset of multifocal calcification which ultimately progresses to ossification)

Radiological features Progressive ossification produces large masses that can bridge bones (and can also cause respiratory compromise within the thorax)

- *Associated skeletal abnormalities*: short 1st metacarpals and metatarsals ▶ small cervical vertebral bodies with relative prominence of the pedicles

CONNECTIVE TISSUE DISORDERS (ACQUIRED)

- Crystal deposition diseases
- Dermatomyositis
- Scleroderma (progressive systemic sclerosis)
- Calcium pyrophosphate dehydrate deposition disease (CPPD)

TUMORAL CALCINOSIS

Definition this is an autosomal dominant condition leading to a defect of phosphorus metabolism (with a normal serum calcium)

Radiological features Large multilocular juxta-articular cystic lesions filled with calcific fluid (calcium hydroxyapatite) ▶ these can demonstrate fluid-fluid levels ▶ the joints are normal

- Their large size can lead to restricted joint motion, bone erosions, superficial ulceration and secondary infection

Pearl Surgery is often associated with recurrence of the mass

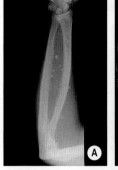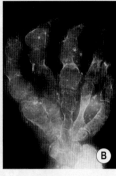

Haemangiomas (two different cases). (A) Extensive cavernous haemangioma of the forearm indicated by the numerous phleboliths. (B) Maffucci's syndrome with multiple enchondromas and soft tissue haemangiomas.*

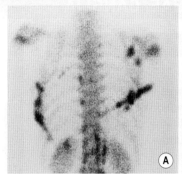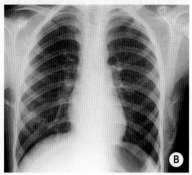

Fibrodysplasia ossificans progressiva. (A) Posterior 3-h skeletal scintigram of the trunk showing linear foci of increased activity corresponding to the soft tissue ossification. (B) Chest radiograph showing bilateral chest wall ossification.*

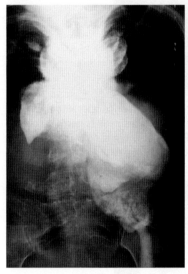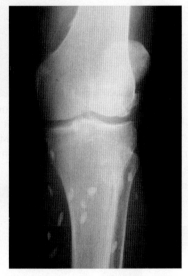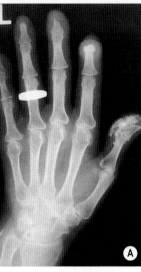

Old tuberculosis (Pott's disease) of the spine. The resultant spinal deformity is obscured by the massive calcified paravertebral abscesses.*

Cysticercosis. AP radiograph of the knee showing multiple calcified oval cysts aligned along muscle planes.*

Scleroderma. (A) Acro-osteolysis and (B) calcinosis circumscripta.†

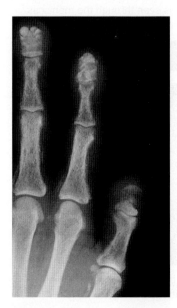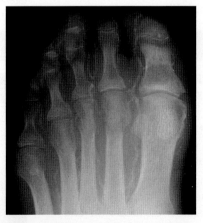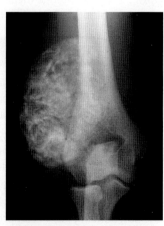

Chronic renal failure. PA hand radiograph showing the florid features of secondary hyperparathyroidism including terminal phalangeal resorption, soft tissue calcification, subperiosteal resorption, vascular calcification and osteopenia.*

Arterial calcification. Heavy vascular calcification in a diabetic patient. Resorption of the 1st and 2nd terminal phalanges due to repeated infection.*

Tumoral calcinosis with heavy periarticular calcification.*

SYNOVIAL CYST, BURSAE, GANGLIA

DEFINITION

Synovial 'cysts'

- Benign uni- or multilocular periarticular soft tissue masses ▶ they represent a herniation of synovial tissue through a weakened joint capsule (therefore they are fluid-filled and lined with synovium)

Bursae

- Open or closed synovium-lined sacs which are usually found over bony prominences or between muscles and tendons (e.g. subacromial, olecranon, iliopsoas and prepatellar regions)
- **Baker's cyst:** fluid accumulation within the semimembranosus–gastrocnemius bursa and located posterior to the knee

Ganglia

- This contains myxoid matrix ▶ it does not communicate with the joint cavity or tendon sheath – therefore it is not lined with synovium (cf. synovial cysts and bursae) ▶ it is the commonest cause of a mass in the hand and wrist
- **Meniscal cyst:** this is a variant of a ganglion cyst seen in association with knee meniscal degeneration and tears (joint fluid is forced through the meniscal tear into the surrounding tissues) ▶ meniscal surgery is required in addition to addressing the cystic component

RADIOLOGICAL FEATURES

- All these lesions have similar imaging characteristics:

US A well-defined hypoechoic mass (with posterior acoustic enhancement)

CT It is hypodense with respect to muscle ▶ there is peripheral enhancement

MRI T1WI: isointense (hyperintense if there is a high protein content) ▶ T2WI/STIR: high SI

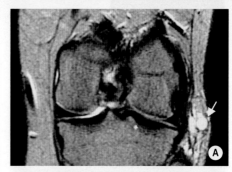

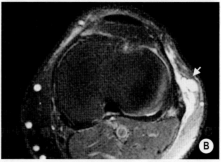

Ganglion. (A) A cystic structure is seen to arise lateral to the lateral meniscus (arrow) but the meniscus itself is normal. (B) Axial FSE T2-weighted MR image. There is no evidence of extension of the cystic lesion (arrow) deep to the lateral collateral ligament.*

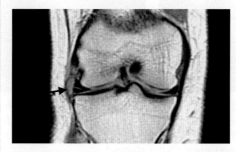

Meniscal cyst. A cystic structure is seen arising deep to the lateral collateral ligament (arrow), intimately related to the lateral meniscus. An oblique tear is seen through the meniscus confirming that this represents a meniscal cyst.*

LIPOMA

Definition A superficial or deep well-defined mass composed of mature fat (adipocytes) ▶ it is the most common mesenchymal tumour in adults (rare in children)

XR Areas of relative lucency ▶ calcification is seen with chronic lesions ▶ larger lesions may cause pressure erosion of the underlying cortical bone

US Variable appearances (ranging from a focus of increased reflectivity to the same echo characteristics as the surrounding fat) ▶ compressible ▶ elliptical with long axis parallel to skin surface

CT A mass of fat attenuation (−65 to −120HU)

MRI T1WI/T2WI: isointense to fat ▶ shows fat suppression ▶ fine septa can be seen ▶ can have fibrosis/necrosis in deep tumours

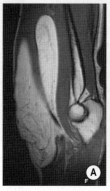
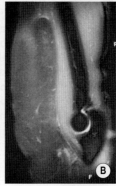

Inter- and intramuscular lipoma between biceps brachii and deeper brachialis muscle on sagittal (A) T1WI and (B) fat-suppressed PD imaging.†

LIPOSARCOMA

Definition This is the 2nd most common adult malignant soft tissue tumour after malignant fibrous histiocytoma ▶ it usually arises within the buttock, thigh, leg or retroperitoneum
- Low-grade and well-differentiated liposarcomas are also known as an atypical lipoma ▶ local recurrence is common (but it does not tend to metastasize)

Radiological features A high-grade liposarcoma is indistiguishable from any other soft tissue sarcomas (it may be so cellular that no fat is detectable) ▶ it may appear biphasic (with intermingled atypical lipoma and intermediate or high-grade sarcoma)
- Suspicion should be aroused if incomplete fat suppression ▶ thick nodular septa ▶ focal non-lipomatous areas

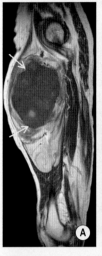
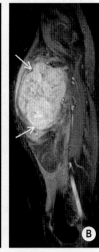

Dedifferentiated liposarcoma. Sagittal T1 (A) and STIR (B) MR images showing a lipomatous mass. At the superior aspect of the mass there is a well-defined non-fatty tumour, corresponding to the dedifferentiated component (arrows).**

VASCULAR TUMOURS

Definition
- **Haemangioma:** benign vascular tumours of infancy – rapid initial growth followed by slow involution ▶
  - In adults usually a low flow venous vascular malformation (dysplastic thin walled post capillary vessels) ▶ variable thrombosis and dystrophic calcification ▶ multiple tissue planes can be affected
- **Malformations:** congenital dysplastic vascular channels – enlarge with the patient and do not regress
  - *High flow:* arteriovenous malformations/ arteriovenous fistulas
  - *Low flow:* venous/lymphatic/capillary/mixed

Clinical presentation
- **High flow malformation:** pain ▶ tissue overgrowth ▶ bleeding ▶ high output cardiac failure ▶ pulsatile skin abnormality (thrill and bruit)
- **Low flow venous malformation:** blue skin discoloration (soft and compressible) ▶ possibly pain and infiltration of local structures with reduced mobility and skeletal remodeling

XR Phleboliths are a specific sign

USS Phleboliths (echogenic foci with acoustic shadowing) ▶ compressibility
- *Low flow:* Doppler will often show no flow within a mass (monophasic and low velocity if seen)
- *High flow:* High USS flow rates

MRI Usually well defined despite any local infiltration ▶ classified into high flow (by the presence of flow voids and arterial feeding vessels) or low flow
- T1WI: mildly hyperintense to muscle ▶ possible focal hyperintensity if small amounts of fat
- T2WI: serpigenous channels between solid soft tissue matrix ▶ fluid–fluid levels with areas of static blood
- T1WI + Gad: enhancement on delayed images but no arterial or early venous filling

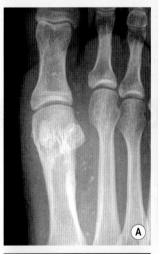
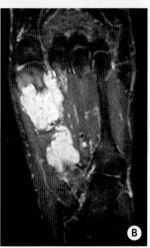
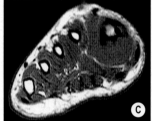

Venous malformation. Dorsoplantar radiograph of the great toe (A) shows soft tissue swelling and phleboliths. Cortical thickening and subtle remodelling of the metatarsal is noted. Axial STIR MR image (B) shows a lobular, hyperintense mass with faint low-signal septation. Coronal T1W imaging (C) shows pressure erosion and cortical thickening of the plantar aspect of the metatarsal by a circumferential mass, which in this case is isointense to muscle.**

Pearl
- Clinical syndromes associated with vascular malformations: Kasabach–Merritt, Maffucci, Osler–Weber–Rendu, Klippel–Trenaunay–Weber, Gorham and Proteus syndromes

555

DESMOID TYPE FIBROMATOSIS (AGGRESSIVE FIBROMATOSIS/EXTRA-ABDOMINAL DESMOID)

Definition

- Tumours composed of fibroblasts with varying amounts of collagen ▶ they may remain relatively dormant for many years (usually painless) ▶ occurs in deep soft tissues ▶ typically locally invasive but does not metastasize ▶ young adults commonly affected ▶ common sites: shoulder/chest wall/back/thigh/head + neck ▶ symptoms arise due to infiltration or mass effect on adjacent structures

Radiological features

USS Heterogeneous solid mass, mimicking a sarcoma

MRI T1WI: low signal bands representing dense collagen bundles
- T2WI (fat suppressed): it may be difficult to see
- T1WI + Gad: there is limited enhancement (as it is hypovascular)

Pearl

- The mainstay of treatment is surgery ▶ local recurrence is common ▶ radiotherapy and chemotherapy have been used with variable success

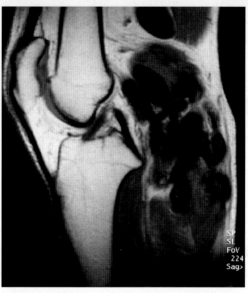

Aggressive fibromatosis (extra-abdominal desmoid). Sagittal T1WI MRI showing an extensive low signal intensity mass behind the knee.*

SOFT TISSUE SARCOMA

Definition

- A rare tumour arising from mesenchymal tissue ▶ most common tumour of late adult life is the 'pleomorphic undifferentiated sarcoma' (formerly malignant fibrous histiocytoma) – commonly occurring in the extremities and retroperitoenum

Radiological features

- Poorly characterized by imaging
- Most tumours are well defined (associated pseudocapsule) ▶ ill defined lesions can be benign (e.g. aggressive fibromatosis or post traumatic) and therefore not predictive of malignant potential
- *Features suspicious of malignancy:* deep seated large mass (a significant minority arise superficially in skin and subcutaneous fat) ▶ heterogenous appearances on MRI ▶ tumour necrosis ▶ size >5 cm

Pearl

Synovial sarcoma

- Usually a slow growing mass located at the extremities (commonly the lower limb) and close to a joint ▶ <10% are intra-articular
- Frequently a large, deep, multilobular septated mass ▶ calcification (30%) ▶ haemorrhage (40%) ▶ fluid–fluid levels (18%) ▶ bone erosion/invasion (21%)
  - 'Triple signal': areas of high, low and isointensity c/w fat on T2WI

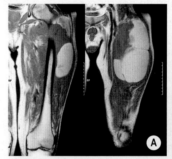
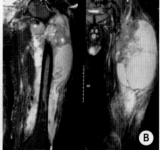
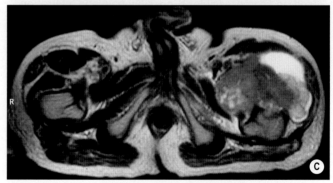

Necrotic soft tissue sarcoma of the thigh. (A) Coronal T1WI MRI showing a large soft tissue mass with invasion of the proximal femoral diaphysis. The mass shows hyperintense areas either due to subacute haemorrhage or fat. (B) Coronal STIR image. The hyperintense areas in (A) do not fat suppress, indicating that this represents haemorrhage and not a lipomatous tumour. (C) Axial T2WI image showing the solid and cystic/necrotic components of the tumour as well as the invasion of the anterior femur.*

BENIGN NERVE SHEATH TUMOURS

- A nerve seen entering and exiting a lesion is patho-gnomonic for either a schwannoma or neurofibroma

Schwannoma

- This arises from the Schwann cells surrounding a nerve – therefore it results in eccentric nerve displacement ▶ typically small and slow growing ▶ multiple tumours with NF-2

MRI A small fusiform mass with tapering margins

Neurofibroma

- *Localized NF:* slow growing mass arising from a peripheral nerve or larger central nerve ▶ usually solitary (multiple in NF1)
- *Diffuse NF:* diffuse skin thickening
- *Plexiform NF:* infiltration of a large nerve or plexus ▶ extension into adjacent tissues (lobulated mass) ▶ bone/soft tissue overgrowth

Benign nerve sheath tumour imaging features

- Mass arising from a nerve (entering or leaving)
- Fusiform morphology
- *'Split fat' sign:* mass splitting fat within the intermuscular space and displacing muscle
- *'Target' sign:* T2WI: low SI centrally with a high peripheral SI ring peripherally
- *'Fascicular' sign:* T2WI: T2WI/PD: ring-like low SI areas within a mass (representing fascicular bundles)
- *Schwannoma:* heterogeneous mass ▶ cystic change ▶ fluid–fluid levels ▶ haemorrhage ▶ calcification
- *Diffuse neurofibroma:* infiltrative thickened skin ▶ T1WI + GAD: enhancement

Morton's neuroma

- Perineural fibrosis of a plantar digital nerve (this is not a tumour) ▶ it typically occurs level with the metatarsal heads (often the 3rd or 4th metatarsals)

US A hypoechoic intermetatarsal mass ▶ compression helps distinguish it from an associated bursa

MRI A small well-demarcated teardrop-shaped mass ▶ it is easily seen on T1WI and fat-suppressed contrast-enhanced sequences (due to its fibrotic nature)

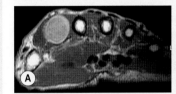
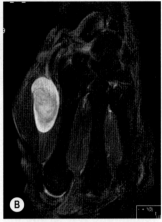

Schwannoma. Axial proton-density (A) and coronal T2W imaging with fat saturation (B) show a well defined, fusiform mass in the dorsum of the hand, between the thumb and index metacarpals. A fascicular sign is seen in (A) and a target sign in (B).**

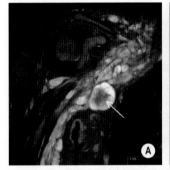
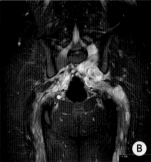

Plexiform neurofibromas of the right brachial plexus (A) and sciatic nerves (B). Coronal STIR images showing marked lobular enlargement of major central nerves in a patient with neurofibromatosis type 1. A target sign is seen in the brachial plexus mass (arrow).**

MALIGNANT PERIPHERAL NERVE SHEATH TUMOUR (MPNST)

Definition This is also called a neurofibrosarcoma or malignant schwannoma ▶ it is an aggressive, locally invasive large lesion (distant metastases to the lung are common) ▶ rapid enlargement ± pain

- It is frequently associated with NF-1 ▶ it occasionally arises from a pre-existing neurofibroma

MRI It usually involves the major nerve trunks (e.g. the sciatic nerve, brachial and sacral plexus) ▶ large heterogeneous lobular mass with no target sign (± haemorrhage) ▶ it appears as a fusiform shape with a longitudinal orientation in the direction of the nerve ▶ it can demonstrate irregular margins and heterogeneous SI ▶ peripheral rather than central enhancement

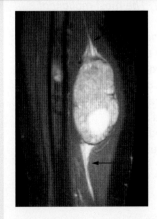

Malignant peripheral nerve sheath tumour (MPNST) in the posterior compartment of the thigh on a sagittal fat-suppressed T2-weighted TSE image showing the sciatic nerve (arrow) entering and exiting the heterogeneous mass.†

5.4 GENERAL CHARACTERISTICS OF BONE TUMOURS

AGE AT PRESENTATION

- Metastases are the commonest malignant bone tumours in patients that are > 45 years of age (an atypical metastasis is more common in this age group than a classical primary malignant tumour)
  - Primary malignant bone tumours are rare before 5 years of age
  - *1st decade:* these are commonly disseminated bone lesions of leukaemia and neuroblastoma
  - *2nd decade:* it is usually an osteosarcoma or Ewing's sarcoma

RATE OF GROWTH

Benign and low-grade malignant neoplasms

- These tend to remain within the intramedullary cavity (until late) ▶ there is slow erosion of the endosteal cortex (leading to endosteal scalloping) ▶ periosteal new bone formation can lead to bone expansion and a well-defined sclerotic rim

High-grade malignant tumours

- These commonly extend through the cortex at presentation with associated cortical destruction, a non-sclerotic rim and an adjacent extraosseous mass

Lodwick pattern I (geographical) *Benign and low-grade malignant neoplasms*
- There is a narrow zone of transition (a few mm) ▶ the most actively growing lesions (e.g. a GCT) have a non-sclerotic margin ▶ the least aggressive lesions show a sclerotic rim of varying thickness
- Type 1A: a rim of sclerosis between the lesion and the host bone
- Type 1B: a very well-defined lytic lesion but no marginal sclerosis
- Type 1C: slightly less sharp, non-sclerotic margin

Lodwick pattern II (moth-eaten) *The next most aggressive pattern*
- The zone of destruction is made up of multiple ill-defined coalescing lucent areas (2–5 mm) and implies cortical involvement (purely medullary lesions are not visible)

Lodwick pattern III (permeative) *The most malignant pattern*
- This is composed of multiple coalescing small ill-defined lesions (≤ 1 mm) with a zone of transition of several cm ▶ XR can underestimate the extent of involvement
  - *'Saucerization' of the outer cortical margin:* tumour that is temporarily restrained by the periosteum erodes back through cortical bone
    - *Example:* malignant round cell tumours ▶ osteosarcoma ▶ most metastases ▶ certain stages of osteomyelitis ▶ Langerhans cell histiocytosis

PERIOSTEAL REACTION

- No type of periosteal reaction is pathognomonic – however it does help indicate the aggressiveness of a lesion

Thick well-formed (solid) periosteal reaction This indicates a slow rate of growth (it is not necessarily a benign tumour, as it may be seen with a low-grade chondrosarcoma)

Laminated ('onion peel') periosteal reaction This indicates subperiosteal extension of tumour, infection or a haematoma ▶ lesions demonstrating periodic growth (e.g. Ewing's sarcoma) may show a multilaminated pattern

Codman's triangle This indicates the limit of subperiosteal tumour in a longitudinal direction ▶ bone formation only occurs at the tumour margins

Spiculated, vertical or 'hair-on-end' periosteal reaction This is seen with the most aggressive tumours (e.g. osteosarcoma or Ewing's sarcoma) ▶ the most rapidly growing lesions may not be associated with any radiographically visible periosteal reaction (as mineralization of periosteum can take weeks)

MATRIX MINERALIZATION

- **Chondral calcifications:** linear, curvilinear, ring-like, punctuate or nodular
- **Osseous mineralization:** cloud-like and poorly defined, whereas diffuse matrix mineralization in benign fibrous tumours produces the characteristic 'ground-glass' appearance (e.g. fibrous dysplasia)
- **Chondroid or osteoid matrix mineralization:** this is often central ▶ it is often peripheral in benign lesions such as a bone infarct or myositis ossificans

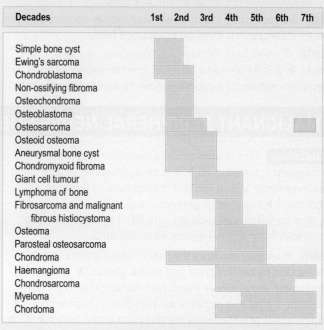

Decades	1st	2nd	3rd	4th	5th	6th	7th
Simple bone cyst							
Ewing's sarcoma							
Chondroblastoma							
Non-ossifying fibroma							
Osteochondroma							
Osteoblastoma							
Osteosarcoma							
Osteoid osteoma							
Aneurysmal bone cyst							
Chondromyxoid fibroma							
Giant cell tumour							
Lymphoma of bone							
Fibrosarcoma and malignant fibrous histiocystoma							
Osteoma							
Parosteal osteosarcoma							
Chondroma							
Haemangioma							
Chondrosarcoma							
Myeloma							
Chordoma							

Peak age incidence of bone tumours.

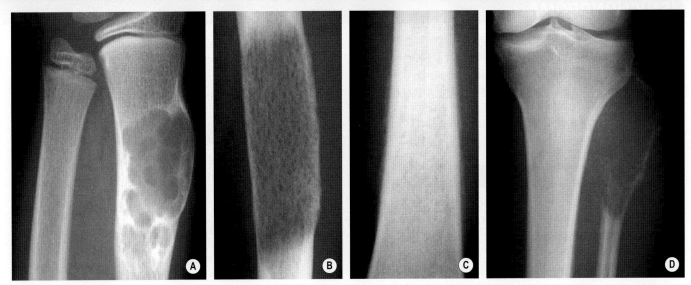

Patterns of bone destruction. AP XRs. (A) A non-ossifying fibroma (NOF) demonstrating features of slow growth: a sharp, 'geographic' margin, endosteal scalloping and bone expansion with an intact overlying cortex. (B) A renal carcinoma metastasis with a 'moth-eaten' appearance. (C) A primary bone lymphoma showing a 'permeative' pattern of bone destruction. (D) A lytic lesion with expansion and destruction of the cortex, indicating an aggressive growth pattern.*

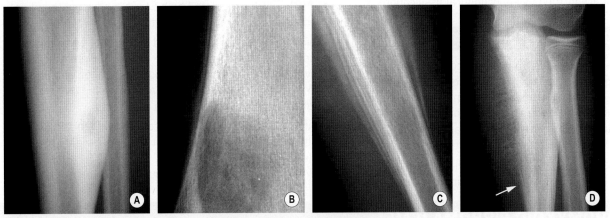

Patterns of periosteal reaction. (A) A solid periosteal reaction due to osteoid osteoma. (B) A single, laminated periosteal reaction associated with a Brodie's abscess. (C) A multilaminated periosteal reaction associated with Ewing's sarcoma. (D) A 'hair-on-end' type vertical periosteal reaction associated with Ewing's sarcoma. Note also the Codman's triangle (arrow).*

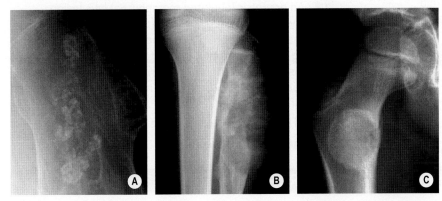

Patterns of matrix mineralization. (A) Metachondromatosis showing typical chondroid calcification. (B) Osteosarcoma showing typical osseous mineralization. (C) Fibrous dysplasia showing typical ground-glass mineralization.*

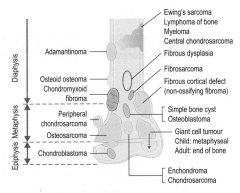

Site of origin of bone tumours.

5.5 BENIGN BONE TUMOURS

(EN)CHONDROMA

DEFINITION

- Chondroma: a benign intramedullary neoplasm consisting of mature hyaline cartilage ▶ it is commonly centrally located (and then referred to as an enchondroma)
- It is the 2nd commonest benign chondral lesion (after an osteochondroma)

CLINICAL PRESENTATION

- An incidental finding ▶ a pathological fracture (60%) ▶ pain in the absence of a fracture or a rapid size increase is potentially malignant
- Age: 10–80 years (M = F)

Location The tubular bones of the hands (40–65%): proximal phalanges > metacarpals or middle phalanges ▶ femur, tibia and humerus (25%) ▶ small bones of the feet (7%)

- A metaphyseal or diaphyseal location (rarely located within the epiphysis) ▶ often eccentric
- It is not found within the skull (it is only found within bones that are formed by endochondral ossification)

RADIOLOGICAL FEATURES

XR A well-defined oval or lobulated eccentric lytic lesion ▶ cortical expansion and chondral (popcorn) type calcification ▶ the overlying cortex may be thin and scalloped ▶ a narrow or sclerotic zone of transition ▶ no periosteal reaction (unless fractured) ▶ a solitary lesion in 75%

- 'Reverse Madelung' deformity: a short distal ulna

MRI Lobular margin ▶ T1WI: intermediate SI ▶ T2WI: high SI (due to the water content of hyaline cartilage) ▶ punctate areas of signal void (matrix mineralization) ▶ there is a hypointense rim with septations ▶ T1WI + Gad: septal enhancement

Scintigraphy No increased uptake

PEARLS

- Differentiation between a large enchondroma + grade 1 chondrosarcoma can be difficult ▶ lesion size >5–6 cm and deep endosteal scalloping are suggestive of chondrosarcoma

Periosteal chondroma Rare and occurs in children and young adults ▶ it affects the long bone metaphyses (proximal humerus ▶ femur, tibia and the tubular bones of the hands and feet) ▶ no malignant potential ▶ the differential includes a periosteal chondrosarcoma/periosteal osteosarcoma

- **XR:** a 1–3 cm well-defined area of cortical erosion ▶ a mature periosteal reaction ▶ chondral-type calcification (50%) ▶ rarely a thin external shell of bone is present
- **MRI:** T2WI: a lobulated high SI mass adjacent to but not infiltrating the underlying cortex

Ollier's disease Characterized by multiple enchondromas ▶ sporadic (and not inherited) ▶ usually unilateral ▶ bone growth may be impeded (with bowing or angulation)

- Malignant change (5–30%) ▶ an associated risk of a glioma, pancreatic or ovarian carcinoma

Maffucci's syndrome A rare condition characterized by multiple enchondromas and soft tissue haemangiomas (phleboliths) ▶ unilateral in 50%

- Malignant change (20%) ▶ usually > 40 years

CHONDROMYXOID FIBROMA (CMF)

DEFINITION

A benign tumour composed of immature myxoid mesenchymal tissue with early cartilagenous differentiation

CLINICAL PRESENTATION

- Pain and swelling (it can be asymptomatic)
- 75% of patients present between 10 and 30 years of age (75%) ▶ (M:F, 2:1)

Location 60% are found within the long bones (25% are within the upper ⅓ of the tibia) ▶ 40% are found within the flat bones (10% within the ilium) ▶ 17% are found within the small tubular bones of the hands and feet ▶ metaphyseal and eccentric in the medulla

RADIOLOGICAL FEATURES

XR An eccentric lobulated metaphyseal lytic lesion arising within the medulla ▶ it can cross into the epiphysis ▶ an associated well-circumscribed sclerotic border with thinning and expansion of the cortex ▶ the lesion long axis parallels the bone long axis ▶ periosteal reaction or soft tissue extension is uncommon ▶ matrix calcification in seen in 12% of cases

MRI There are no characteristic features

Scintigraphy Increased uptake

PEARL

Differential: chondrosarcoma ▶ adamantinoma ▶ fibrous dysplasia ▶ ABC

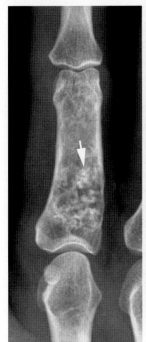

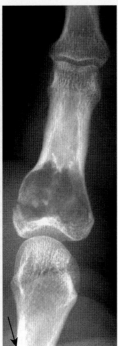

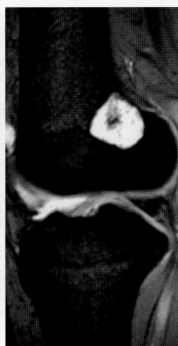

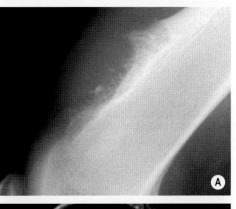

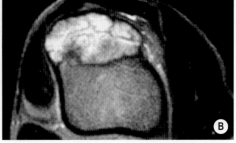

Enchondroma. AP radiograph of the index finger showing a lobular, mildly expansile lesion with typical chondral matrix mineralisation (arrow).**

AP XR of a proximal phalangeal enchondroma with associated pathological fracture (arrow).*

Sagittal T2WI MRI of a distal femoral chondroma – calcification is manifest as focal areas of signal void.*

Periosteal chondroma. (A) Lateral XR showing a calcified surface lesion. (B) Axial fat-suppressed T2WI showing a hyperintense lobulated lesion, without medullary infiltration.*

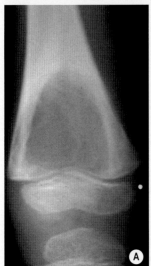

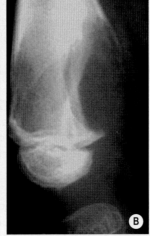

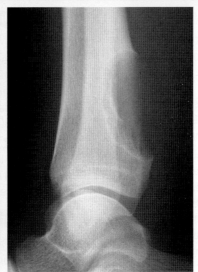

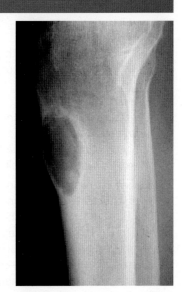

Chondromyxoid fibroma of the distal femoral metaphysis. (A,B) Large osteolytic defect bulging outward.*

Chondromyxoid fibroma. Lateral radiograph of ankle shows a well-defined, eccentric lytic lesion arising eccentrically within the distal tibial metaphysis.©35

Chondromyxoid fibroma. Lateral XR showing expansion of the anterior cortex.*

OSTEOCHONDROMA

Definition

- A cartilage-capped exostosis (representing a bony outgrowth) ▶ usually a developmental anomaly ▶ it possesses its own growth plate and will stop growing with skeletal maturity
- The most common benign bone lesion

Clinical presentation

- It presents between 2 and 60 years (M:F, 2:1)
- It can present with mechanical problems: an enlarging mass ▶ pressure on any adjoining structures (e.g. nerves or blood vessels) ▶ bursa formation (due to irritation of local soft tissues)
  - Rarely the stem can fracture

Location The long bones – especially around the knee (35%) ▶ the proximal humerus or femur ▶ the flat bones (e.g. the ilium or scapula)

- Lesions are initially metaphyseal but migration to the diaphysis occurs over time (classically pointing away from the joint)

Radiological features

XR A continuous bony outgrowth from a normal cortex ▶ it can have a long slim neck (pedunculated) or be broad based (sessile) ▶ the marrow cavity extends into the exostosis (essential feature for diagnosis) ▶ the cartilage cap develops punctuate calcification with age

US/CT/MRI These allow assessment of the cartilage cap – it should be < 5 mm (T2WI: high SI)

Scintigraphy There will be variable activity

Pearls

- *Differential:* periosteal chondroma ▶ parosteal osteosarcoma

- Chondrosarcomatous change within the cartilage cap (occurring in <1% of cases) should be suspected if:
  - There is an increase in pain or size (particularly after skeletal maturation)
  - If the cartilage cap measures >1 cm (CT) or >2 cm (MRI)
  - The development of ill-defined margins

Diaphyseal aclasia (multiple hereditary exostosis) A rare autosomal disorder with multiple osteochondromas occurring particularly at the ends of the long bones, ribs, scapulae and iliac bones (they may be larger than in the solitary form) ▶ this may lead to shortened or deformed limbs (e.g. a reverse Madelung deformity with a short distal ulna) ▶ the metaphyses can be widened and dysplastic

- Vertebral involvement is rare ▶ the cranial vault is spared ▶ malignant degeneration in 3–5%

Bizarre parosteal osteochondromatous proliferation (BPOP)

- A rare, tumour-like disorder
- Calcified masses arise adjacent to the cortex of the small bones of the hands and feet – there is no continuity between the lesion and the underlying bone ▶ there is no cartilaginous cap but it can resemble an osteochondroma
- *Differential:* soft tissue chondroma ▶ florid reactive periostitis

Dysplasia epiphysealis hemimelica (Trevor's disease) Irregular overgrowth of part of an epiphysis which lies on one side of a single limb (resembling an osteochondroma) ▶ the leg is commonly affected

CHONDROBLASTOMA

Definition

A benign cartilage tumour with proliferation of immature cartilage cells (1% of all bone tumours)

Clinical presentation

- 80–90% occur between 5 and 25 years (M:F, 3:1)
- It presents with joint pain (± a synovial reaction) ▶ commonly presents as a monoarthropathy (typically located in the epiphyses and provoking a synovial reaction)

Location It is usually seen in skeletally immature patients, affecting the long bone epiphyses (40% are seen around the knee, and 33% within the proximal femur)

- Also found within apophyses and sesamoid bones (epiphyseal equivalents) such as the femoral greater trochanter and patella (the commonest patella tumour)
- It usually affects the calcaneus or talus in the foot
- The flat bones are mostly affected if >30 years old

Radiological features

XR An eccentric spherical or lobular lytic lesion with a fine sclerotic margin centred within the epiphysis (40%) ▶ it extends into the metaphysis (55%) with partial closure of the growth plate

- Matrix mineralization (30%) ▶ linear periosteal reaction (30–50%)

MRI T1WI: intermediate SI ▶ T2WI: variable SI including fluid levels due to secondary aneurysmal bone cyst change (15%) ▶ there is associated marrow and soft tissue oedema ▶ there may be a reactive joint effusion

Pearl

An 'aggressive' (atypical) chondroblastoma A rare variant associated with cortical destruction and soft tissue involvement ▶ rarely associated with lung metastases

- Differential of a lytic epiphyseal lesion:
  - *Children:* Brodie's abscess
  - *Adults:* subchondral cyst ▶ clear cell chondrosarcoma

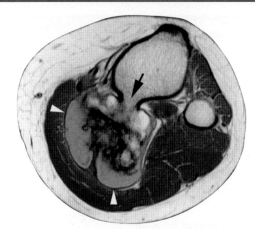

Osteochondroma. MRI features. (A) Axial PDW FSE MRI through the proximal tibia showing medullary continuity (arrow) between the osteochondroma and host bone. The cartilage cap is mildly hyperintense and surrounded by a thin, hypointense perichondrium (arrowheads).**

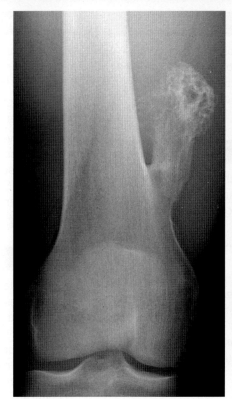

Osteochondroma. AP XR showing a typical pedunculated osteochondroma.*

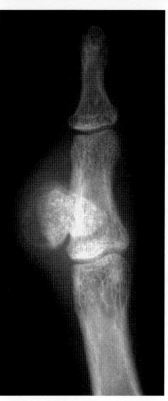

BPOP. AP XR showing a bizarre parosteal osteochondromatous proliferation adjacent to the middle phalanx.*

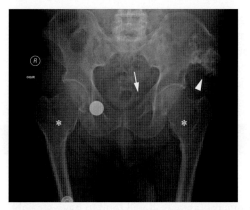

Diaphyseal aclasia demonstrating the typical femoral neck modelling deformity (asterisks), a small osteochondroma arising from the left superior pubic ramus (arrow) and malignant transformation of a left iliac wing osteochondroma (arrowhead). A coin was left in the right pocket.

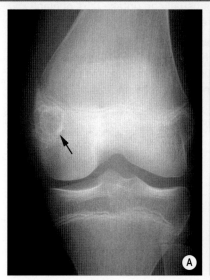

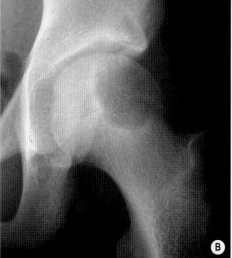

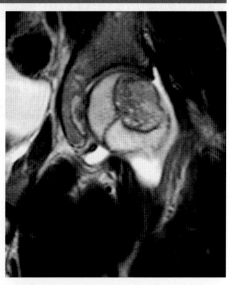

Chondroblastoma in the immature and mature skeleton. (A) AP XR showing a lobulated, lytic lesion (arrow) adjacent to the open growth plate and limited to the epiphysis. (B) AP XR showing extension of the lesion across the fused growth plate.*

Chondroblastoma of the left femoral head. Coronal fat-suppressed T2WI showing the hypointense lesion with surrounding marrow oedema and reactive joint effusion.*

563

OSTEOBLASTOMA

DEFINITION

- A benign bone tumour producing osteoid and woven bone ▶ it is histologically similar to an osteoid osteoma, but is differentiated by its size (> 1.5–2 cm) ▶ tends to show a more aggressive growth pattern ▶ does not resolve spontaneously

CLINICAL PRESENTATION

- Any pain is usually more chronic and less severe than with an osteoid osteoma (and is rarely relieved by aspirin) ▶ there can be a painful scoliosis (with tumour at the concavity apex)
  - 80% of cases present at < 30 years of age (M:F, 2–3:1)

Location 40–50% are within the spine and sacrum – 90% are eccentrically located within the neural arch with a painful scoliosis (± expansion or absence of the pedicle) ▶ potential extraosseous extension

- Other major sites: the diaphyses or metaphyses of the long bones (commonly the humerus)

RADIOLOGICAL FEATURES

XR A predominantly lytic lesion (>2 cm) ▶ larger lesions have greater matrix mineralization and may expand the bone with surrounding reactive sclerosis

CT This often reveals occult calcification (punctate/nodular/generalized)

MRI Reactive marrow and soft tissue changes (which may extend across several vertebrae) dominate ▶ there may also be secondary ABC changes ▶ T1WI: low or intermediate SI ▶ T2WI: intermediate or high SI ▶ T1WI + Gad: enhancement

Scintigraphy This is always positive

PEARLS

- An osteoblastoma may produce an extracortical mass causing spinal cord compression with a soft tissue component
- *'Aggressive osteoblastoma'*: a locally aggressive lesion which is commonly within the sacrum and capable of producing metastases
- *Differential (long bones)*: Brodie's abscess ▶ chondromyxoid fibroma ▶ Langerhans' cell histiocytosis

BONE ISLAND (ENOSTOSIS)

DEFINITION

- A congenital developmental focus of medullary cortical bone

CLINICAL PRESENTATION

- An asymptomatic incidental finding

Location It is commonly seen within the pelvis, femur and other long bones

RADIOLOGICAL FEATURES

XR A dense sclerotic focus with a spiculated margin blending with the trabeculae of adjacent bone

MRI It is hypointense on all sequences (equivalent to cortical bone)

- Unlike a sclerotic metastasis, it will tend to have straight edges and the very dense bone can cause adjacent susceptibility artefacts

Scintigraphy There is usually no uptake (25% of giant bone islands show increased uptake)

Osteopoikilosis and osteopathia striata An autosomal dominant condition with multiple bone islands located in a periarticular distribution ▶ they can appear either round (osteopoikilosis) or elongated (osteopathia striata) in shape

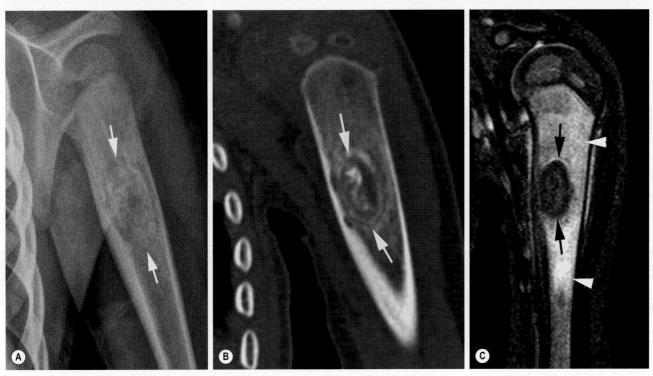

Osteoblastoma. (A) AP radiograph of the left proximal humerus showing a large mixed lytic-sclerotic lesion (arrows) in the medullary cavity with associated periosteal thickening. (B) Coronal CT MPR shows the oval, mineralised lesion (arrows). (C) Coronal STIR MRI demonstrates a hypointense tumour (arrows) with extensive reactive oedema-like marrow changes (arrowheads).**

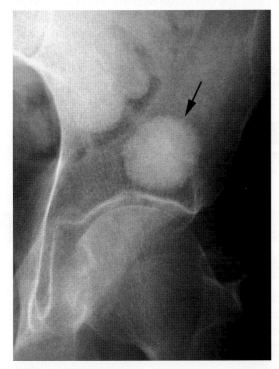

Giant bone island. AP XR showing a uniformly sclerotic bone island (arrow) in the supra-acetabular region of the ilium.*

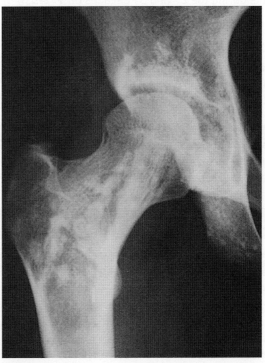

Osteopoikilosis.†

OSTEOMA

DEFINITION

- A slow-growing tumour consisting of predominantly cortical or, less often, cancellous bone ▶ it represents a dysplastic developmental anomaly

CLINICAL PRESENTATION

- It is usually asymptomatic, although it can affect sinus drainage (leading to mucocoele formation) ▶ it can also cause CSF rhinorrhoea, pneumocephalus or meningitis

Location Cortical (ivory) osteomas commonly affect the paranasal sinuses (frontal and ethmoid > sphenoid sinuses)

▶ it is less often found within the mandible, long bones or spine (causing backache)

RADIOLOGICAL FEATURES

XR/CT A homogeneous smooth dense lesion with a well-defined spherical margin ▶ it is attached to underlying bone ▶ it rarely exceeds 2–3 cm diameter

PEARL

- Multiple osteomas occur in Gardner's syndrome

OSTEOID OSTEOMA

DEFINITION

- A benign hamartoma affecting the cortex (80%), medullary cavity or subperiosteum ▶ it produces osteoid and woven bone

CLINICAL PRESENTATION

- Night pain relieved by aspirin (as it secretes prosta-glandins) ▶ it may result in disuse osteoporosis, muscle wasting or limb overgrowth in children ▶ a painful scoliosis can be caused by spinal lesions (on the concave side)
- It presents during the 2nd and 3rd decades (M:F, 2–3:1)

Location It can affect any site: appendicular skeleton > spine
- 50% are within the metaphysis or diaphysis of the tibia or femur ▶ 15% are intra-articular (causing synovitis)
- 90% of spinal lesions are within the neural arch (with associated dense vertebral pedicles)

RADIOLOGICAL FEATURES

XR/CT The characteristic feature is the nidus (which can be of a lucent, sclerotic or mixed density) ▶ the osteoma

is < 1.5 cm in diameter (cf. an osteoblastoma) ▶ there is surrounding reactive medullary sclerosis and periosteal reaction (which is greater in younger patients with subperiosteal lesions)
- 'Vascular groove': thin serpentine channels in the thickened bone around the nidus
- A periosteal reaction is absent if the lesion is intra-articular, within the terminal phalanges, deep within medullary bone, or at tendon or ligament insertions
- CT is the study of choice

MRI It can be mistaken for an aggressive lesion due to the reactive bone and soft tissue oedema and an associated soft tissue mass ▶ T1WI: low SI ▶ T2WI: high SI ▶ T1WI + Gad: arterial enhancement, early washout, and delayed enhancement within the peripheral bone

Scintigraphy The 'double density' sign: focal intense activity (at the nidus) with surrounding lesser activity (due to reactive sclerosis)

PEARL

- **Treatment:** spontaneous resolution ▶ surgical curettage ▶ CT-guided radiofrequency ablation

TUMOURS OF NEURAL TISSUE

DEFINITION

- This includes schwannomas and neurofibromas
- Tumours can cause pressure erosion when they arise in close proximity to bone (especially if they are intraspinal)
- Intraosseous benign nerve sheath tumours are very rare and usually affect the mandible ▶ lesions within the appendicular skeleton are extremely rare, with no diagnostic XR features

PEARL

Neurofibromatosis Skeletal lesions (such as the classical tibial pseudoarthrosis or spinal deformity) are rarely due to intraosseous neural tissue but are related to an overall mesenchymal disturbance

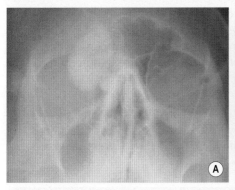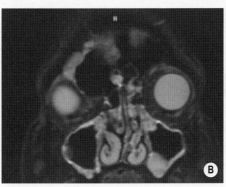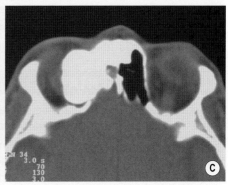

Osteoma. (A) Plain XR. (B) Coronal STIR images underestimate the lesion since bone and air are both black. (C) Axial CT shows extension into the orbit.*

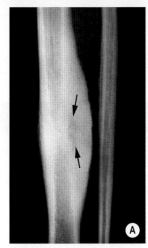

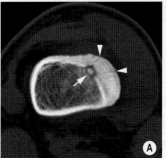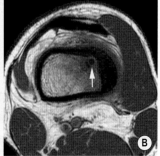

Osteoid osteoma. (A) Axial CT shows a densely mineralised intracortical nidus (arrow), with solid adjacent periosteal thickening containing multiple vascular channels (arrowheads). (B) Axial T1W SE MRI clearly demonstrates the hypointense nidus (arrow) and the cortical thickening.**

Osteoid osteoma. (A) AP XR shows solid thickening of the anterolateral tibial cortex containing a small nidus (arrows). (B) Lateral 99mTc-MDP scintigram showing the 'double-density' sign.

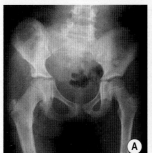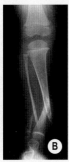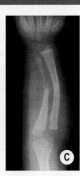

(A) Hemihypertrophy in a 7-year-old girl with neurofibromatosis. Anteroposterior view of the pelvis shows hypertrophied right hemipelvis, right hip, and right femur. (B) A 1-year-old girl with neurofibromatosis and congenital pseudarthrosis of the right tibia and fibula. Anteroposterior view of the right leg shows the pseudarthrosis in the distal diaphysis of the tibia and fibula. There is tapering, overriding, and angulation of the fragments. (C) A 2.5-year-old boy with neurofibromatosis and congenital pseudarthrosis of the left ulna. Anteroposterior radiograph of the forearm shows interruption of the continuity of the ulna, with significant tapering, and underdevelopment of the distal ulnar fragment. There also is mild lateral bowing of the radius.©34

SIMPLE BONE CYST (UNICAMERAL BONE CYST)

DEFINITION

- A solitary uni- or multilocular cyst ▶ unknown aetiology

CLINICAL PRESENTATION

- It often presents with a pathological fracture
- It presents between 5 and 15 years of age (M : F, 2.5 : 1)

Location It extends from the proximal metaphysis into the diaphysis with growth, and has usually healed by the time it reaches the mid diaphysis (and respects the physis) ▶ proximal humerus (60%) > proximal femur (30%) ▶ occasionally the cyst adheres to the growth plate and extension into the epiphysis/apophysis is reported (2%)

RADIOLOGICAL FEATURES

XR A *central* lytic lesion with cortical thinning (cf. an eccentric ABC) ▶ symmetrical bone expansion ▶ a periosteal reaction only if there is a pathological fracture ▶ it typically measures 6–8 cm with its long axis parallel to the bone ▶ apparent trabeculation is common

- *'Falling fragment' sign* (5%): a fracture fragment penetrating the cyst and falling with gravity (this is pathognomonic)

MRI T1WI: low to intermediate SI ▶ T2WI: high SI – there can be fluid-fluid levels (representing haemorrhage) and pericystic oedema if it has fractured ▶ T1WI + Gad: no enhancement

PEARL

- *Differential:* ABC ▶ fibrous dysplasia

ANEURYSMAL BONE CYST (ABC)

DEFINITION

- A true neoplasm: it is an expansile cavity composed of thin-walled blood-filled cystic cavities (accounting for 1–2% of primary bone lesions)
- It represents a reparative process and can be induced by trauma or tumour

CLINICAL PRESENTATION

- It usually presents during the 2nd decade, with the majority occurring before growth plate fusion, unlike a GCT (M = F)
- Scoliosis or neurological symptoms (if it occurs within a neural arch)

Location Long bones (> 50%) ▶ spine (20%) ▶ the pelvis is the commonest site of flat bone involvement (5–10%) ▶ it can also be intracortical or subperiosteal

- *Spine:* it usually occurs within a neural arch with vertebral body extension (unilateral collapse can result in a structural scoliosis)

RADIOLOGICAL FEATURES

XR An eccentric purely lytic expansile intramedullary lesion within long bone metaphysis (it is occasionally central) ▶ it extends to the growth plate (but respects it with rare extension to the articular surface)

CT An egg shell thin cortex ▶ marginal periosteal reaction ▶ fine septal ossification ▶ apparent trabeculation due to ridging of the endosteal cortex ▶ marginal periosteal reaction

MRI T1WI: cysts of different SI (representing temporal haemorrhage) ▶ a thin sclerotic margin with internal hypointense internal septa ▶ T2WI: fluid-fluid levels ▶ reactive medullary oedema ▶ T1WI + Gad: enhancing internal septa

Scintigraphy *'Doughnut' sign:* a photopenic centre with increased peripheral uptake

PEARLS

- Secondary ABC change can be seen in a variety of preceding lesions: NOF ▶ chondroblastoma ▶ GCT ▶ fibrous dysplasia ▶ osteoblastoma ▶ osteosarcoma
- The absence of fluid levels may indicate a 'solid' variant of ABC (commonly reported in the long bones)
- *Treatment:* surgical curettage or radiotherapy
- *Differential:* telangiectatic osteosarcoma

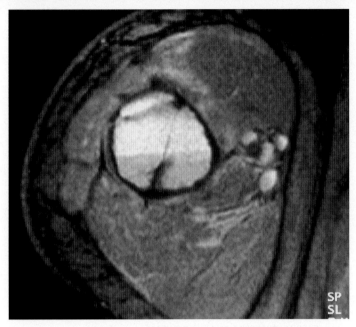

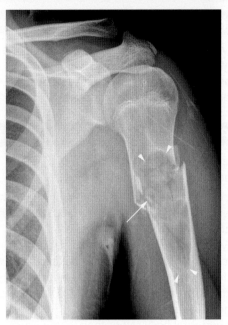

Simple bone cyst of the proximal humerus. Axial T2WI shows fluid levels indicative of previous fracture.*

Simple bone cyst. AP left humerus demonstrating a well-defined osteolytic lesion within the diaphysis (arrowheads), with a pathological fracture and internal fragments (arrow).**

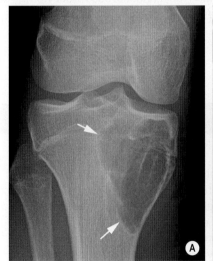

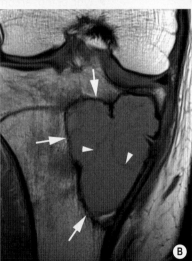

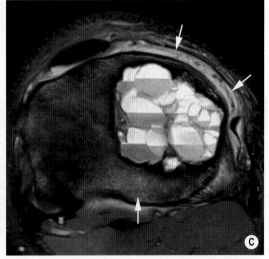

Aneurysmal bone cyst. (A) AP radiograph showing a mildly expansile lytic lesion with a thin sclerotic margin (arrows) located eccentrically within the proximal tibial metaphysis. (B) Coronal T1W SE MRI showing an intermediate SI lesion (arrows) with thin internal septae (arrowheads). (C) Axial fat-suppressed T2W FSE MRI demonstrates multiple fluid–fluid levels fi lling the lesion with mild surrounding reactive medullary and soft-tissue oedema (arrows).**

GIANT CELL TUMOUR (GCT) (OSTEOCLASTOMA)

DEFINITION

- An aggressive benign neoplasm arising from osteoclasts – it represents 5% of all primary bone tumours
- It is richly vascular with numerous giant cells, with tumour forming neither bone nor cartilage

CLINICAL PRESENTATION

- Localized pain and swelling
- It presents at 20–45 years of age (M:F, 2:3)

Location It originates within the metaphyseal side of the growth plate (with epiphyseal extension) ▶ it is seen in the skeletally mature patient

- Nearly always occurs in a subarticular or subcortical region (adjacent to a fused apophysis) of a long bone ▶ knee (distal femur or proximal tibia: 55%) ▶ distal radius (10%) ▶ proximal humerus (6%) ▶ sacrum (7%) – this is the commonest site in the spine
- It affects the vertebral body rather than the neural arch (unlike most benign spinal tumours)

RADIOLOGICAL FEATURES

XR A subarticular eccentric lytic lesion with a well-defined non-sclerotic margin (a poorly defined margin indicates an aggressive lesion) ▶ almost 100% involve subchondral or apophyseal bone at presentation

(it involves the metaphysis adjacent to the growth plate in the immature skeleton) ▶ apparent trabeculation or cortical expansion is common ▶ periosteal reaction is seen with a pathological fracture (15%) ▶ there can be cortical destruction or extraosseous extension (50%) ▶ 5–7 cm in size

- Sacral lesions appear as a lytic destructive lesion extending to the SI joint

MRI T1WI: low–intermediate SI (high SI indicates haemorrhage) ▶ STIR: heterogeneous high SI ▶ T2WI: fluid–fluid levels – profound low SI (haemosiderin) indicates chronic haemorrhage ▶ marrow oedema

Scintigraphy *'Doughnut' sign:* a photopenic centre with increased peripheral uptake

PEARLS

- A GCT can complicate Paget's disease
- Malignant change is recognized (benign lesions can rarely metastasize to the lungs)
- Multifocal metachronous GCT can occur (often within the hands) ▶ associated with hyperparathyroidism
- **Treatment:** surgical curettage (there is a tendency to recur)
- **Differential:** ABC ▶ chondroblastoma ▶ brown tumour ▶ lytic osteosarcoma ▶ malignant fibrous histiocytoma ▶ lytic metastasis (especially renal)

LIPOMATOUS BONE LESIONS

True intraosseous lipoma

- This arises within the medulla, producing expansion (sometimes with endosteal scalloping and trabeculation) ▶ calcification may be present (particularly centrally) ▶ it can resemble a cyst or even fibrous dysplasia ▶ it usually affects the lower limb (especially the calcaneus)

CT/MRI It can demonstrate fatty matrix tissue

Parosteal lipoma

- This may cause benign pressure erosion of bone and formation of circumferential periosteal new bone ▶ a combination of peripheral ossification with a tumour composed of a fatty matrix establishes the diagnosis ▶ rare ▶ frequently encountered around the proximal radius, where it may cause posterior interosseous nerve palsy

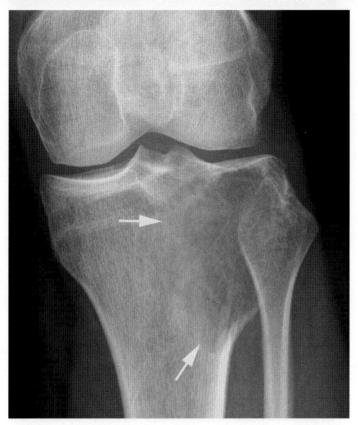

Giant cell tumour. AP radiograph of the knee showing an eccentric, subarticular lytic lesion of the proximal tibia with a poorly defined margin (arrows) and destruction of the lateral cortex.**

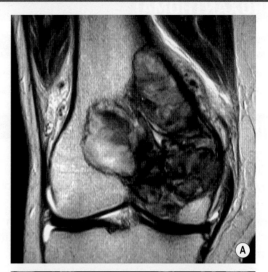

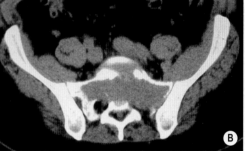

(A) Coronal T2WI showing a distal femoral GCT with predominantly low SI due to haemosiderin deposition from chronic haemorrhage. (B) CT of the sacrum showing a GCT. Note the extension to the left sacroiliac joint.*

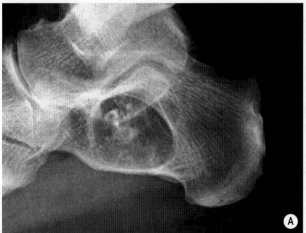

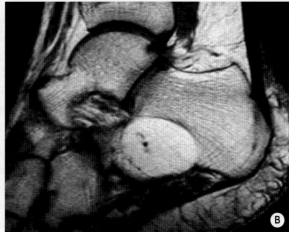

Intraosseous lipoma of the calcaneus. (A) Lateral XR showing a geographic, calcified lytic lesion. (B) Sagittal T1WI showing the hyperintense fatty nature of the lesion.*

NON-OSSIFYING FIBROMA (NOF) (FIBROXANTHOMA)

DEFINITION

- A benign hamartomatous lesion ▶ it represents a developmental defect arising within tubular bone trabeculae

CLINICAL PRESENTATION

- Asymptomatic ▶ pain with a pathological fracture ▶ usually seen during the 2nd decade of life
- It may be multiple or familial ▶ there is an association with neurofibromatosis (5%)

Location Long bone metaphyses (close to the growth plate) ▶ essentially intracortical ▶ the majority involve the lower limbs (the distal femur or tibia)

RADIOLOGICAL FEATURES

XR An intracortical lobulated lesion with a soap bubble appearance ▶ an oval shape with its long axis parallel to the bone ▶ it enlarges into the medullary cavity ▶ a narrow zone of transition with a sclerotic margin ▶ no matrix calcification ▶ periosteal reaction if a pathological fracture occurs

MRI T1WI: intermediate SI ▶ T2WI: 80% demonstrate low SI (but with marginal and septal high SI) ▶ T1WI + Gad: enhancement

- Marginal sclerosis appears as a low SI rim

Scintigraphy Increased uptake with active lesions ▶ decreased uptake with involution

PEARLS

- Spontaneous involution can occur with bone replacing fibrous tissue ▶ a healed NOF may demostrate homogeneous sclerosis

Fibrous cortical defect Histologically and radiologically identical to a NOF (but < 2 cm in size) ▶ common in children (regarded as a normal variant) ▶ commonly located within the distal femoral or proximal tibial metaphysis

Jaffe–Campanacci syndrome Multiple (usually unilateral) NOFs with café au lait spots

Benign fibrous histiocytoma This has the same histology as a NOF but occurs during the 3rd to 5th decade ▶ it resembles a GCT on XR but with a well-defined sclerotic margin (representing slower growth) ▶ $\frac{1}{3}$ occur about the knee

DESMOID (DESMOPLASTIC FIBROMA)

DEFINITION

- A rare, locally aggressive benign neoplasm which is histologically similar to soft tissue fibromatosis

CLINICAL PRESENTATION

- Usually between 10 and 30 years (M = F)

Location Long bone metaphyses (56%) ▶ mandible (26%) ▶ ilium (14%)

RADIOLOGICAL FEATURES

XR Subperiosteal or intraosseous tumours which can be large at presentation (>5 cm) ▶ a permeative or moth-eaten lesion, or an expanding trabeculated lesion

MRI T1WI: heterogeneous intermediate SI ▶ T2WI: high SI ▶ T1WI + Gad: irregular enhancement

PEARLS

- Although considered benign, metastases have been reported ▶ recurrence is common ▶ rarely associated with fibrous dysplasia
- *Differential:* a well-differentiated fibrosarcoma

LIPOSCLEROSING MYXOFIBROUS TUMOUR

DEFINITION

- A benign fibro-osseous bone lesion – histologically it is composed of immature bone and fibrous tissue (xanthomatous and myxoid elements are frequently present) ▶ ischaemic ossification may be found within altered fat
- It may be related to fibrous dysplasia or represent end-stage degeneration of an intraosseous fibrous lesion or lipoma ▶ it rarely undergoes malignant transformation

CLINICAL PRESENTATION

- Asymptomatic (but can present with pain)
- There is a wide age range at presentation (usually during the 4th–6th decades)

Location 90% occur within the central metadiaphysis of the proximal femur

RADIOLOGICAL FEATURES

XR A lytic or ground-glass geographic lesion ▶ there is often a markedly sclerotic border ▶ amorphous mineralization is usually present ▶ the matrix is globular and irregular

MRI Non-specific appearances (T1WI: homogeneous ▶ T2WI: heterogeneous high SI)

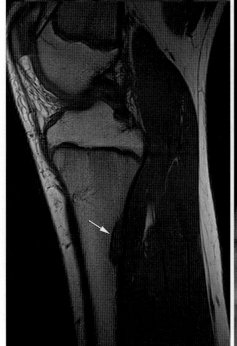

Non-ossifying fibroma: MRI. Sagittal pre-gadolinium T1-weighted MRI with fat saturation, depicting a well-defined cortical lesion with a sclerotic low signal rim (arrow).**

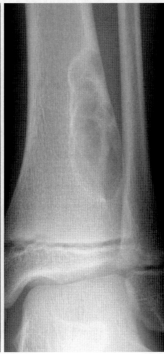

AP XR of the ankle showing a classical distal tibial NOF.*

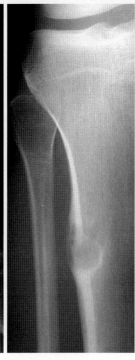

AP XR showing a diaphyseal fibrous cortical defect of the proximal tibia.*

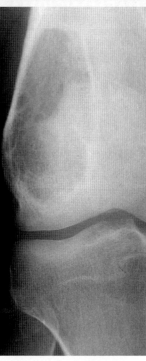

AP XR of the distal femur showing a benign fibrous histiocytoma.*

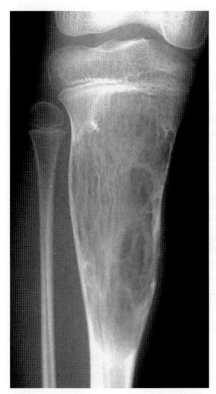

AP XR of the proximal tibia showing a desmoplastic fibroma.*

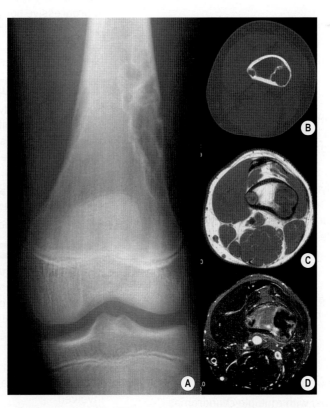

Non-ossifying fibroma/ fibrous cortical defect. Anteroposterior radiograph (A), axial CT scan (B), and axial T1WI (C) and T2WI (FS) (D) MR images show a fibrous cortical defect arising medially and a non-ossifying fibroma arising laterally in the distal femoral diaphysis. The CT scan confirms the cortical origin of both lesions, and the low signal intensity on the MR images indicates the predominantly fibrous nature of the matrix.©35

HAEMANGIOMA

Definition

- A congenital vascular malformation (formed from newly formed blood vessels)
  - *Capillary:* these most commonly arise within the vertebral bodies
  - *Cavernous:* these are most commonly seen within the skull vault
- Bone expansion and extraosseous extension are recognized features

Clinical presentation

- This is usually asymptomatic – although complications include vertebral collapse and neurological symptoms ▶ it can present at any age

Location The spine (the commonest site, with an 11% autopsy incidence) ▶ the calvarium (the 2nd commonest site) ▶ the long bones

Radiological features
Spine

- Vertical trabeculation within a vertebral body – this may extend into the neural arch ▶ there are normal-sized vertebral bodies (cf. Paget's disease)

XR/sagittal CT Coarse vertical trabeculations (secondary to hypertrophy of the primary and erosion of the secondary trabeculae)

Axial CT Dense 'dots' within a fatty matrix

MRI T1WI/T2WI: high SI (fat content) ▶ vascular lesions may have reduced signal intensity (T1WI) ▶ T1WI + Gad: enhancement

Long bones

- Striated lesions are found within the epiphyses and metaphyses of the long bones ▶ the direction of the linear striations is along the long axis of the bone

Flat bones

- Multiple, well-defined lytic lesions producing a soap-bubble effect
  - Skull: radiating mature spiculation can produce a sunburst appearance (with expansion of the outer > the inner table)

Pearls

Aggressive haemangiomata These can have extraosseous extension (which is associated with spinal neurological symptoms)

Lymphangioma Another type of vascular malformation that can occur in bone

Maffucci's syndrome Soft tissue cavernous haemangiomas (phleboliths) with multiple chondromas

CYSTIC ANGIOMATOSIS

Definition

- A multifocal condition of either blood or lymphatic vessels

Clinical presentation

- It usually presents with pain and swelling due to visceromegaly (spleen) ▶ pathological fractures can occur
- 50% present before the age of 20 years

Location The commonest sites: ribs and pelvis ▶ there is a centripetal distribution (few lesions are distal to the elbow or knee)

Radiological features

XR Numerous lytic lesions ▶ these are round or oval with a fine sclerotic rim

Pearls

- Chylous pleural effusions may develop
- The prognosis is worse with visceral involvement (which is unrelated to bone involvement)

MASSIVE OSTEOLYSIS

Definition

- Extensive cystic angiomatosis – a non-malignant proliferation of bony vascular or lymphatic structures ▶ it results in progressive bony destruction (± soft tissue extension)
- A rare, non-hereditary disorder (also known as Gorham's disease, vanishing bone disease, or haemangiomatosis)

Clinical presentation

- Pain is not an early feature ▶ there is progressive weakness and limitation of movement of the affected area (with a useless or flail limb months later)
- It is seen in children and young adults

Location The common sites include the shoulder, mandible and pelvis ▶ there is progressive resorption of a single bone (paired bones, several contiguous ribs or segments of the spine can also been affected)

Radiological features

CT/MRI Lytic destruction of the metaphysis or diaphysis of a long bone with associated cortical erosion ▶ there is tapering of the bone ends

- There can be a pathological fracture with little callus formation and no attempt at healing

Pearls

- It may be life threatening if the spine or thorax is involved
- Only complete excision of the affected bone can halt the disease progress ▶ spontaneous arrest has been rarely reported

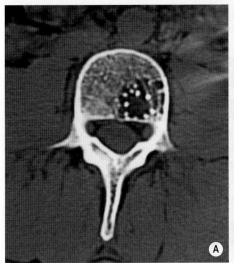
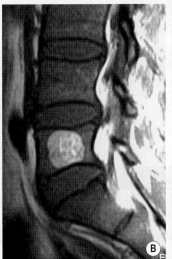
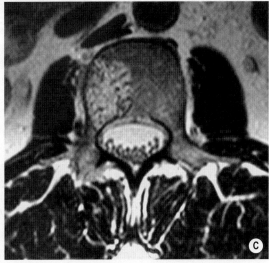

Haemangioma of bone. (A) Axial CT showing a vertebral body haemangioma with fatty matrix and thickened primary trabeculae. (B) Sagittal T1WI showing a haemangioma of L5 with high SI due to fat. (C) Axial T2WI showing a vertebral haemangioma in the right side of L2.*

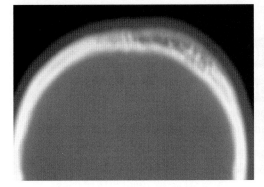

Coronal CT multiplanar reconstruction showing a haemangioma of the skull vault.*

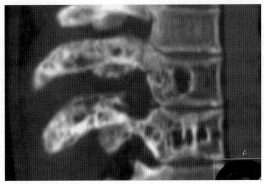

Coronal oblique CT multiplanar reconstruction showing angiomatosis affecting the vertebrae and adjacent ribs.*

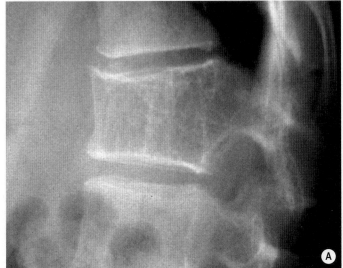
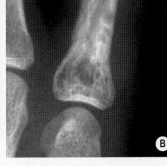

Haemangioma of bone. (A) Coned lateral XR showing a diffuse haemangioma of the T12 vertebral body. (B) AP XR showing a haemangioma with multiple intraosseous vascular channels.*

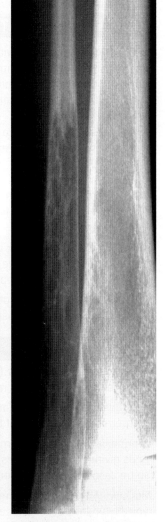

Gorham's disease. AP XR showing extensive lytic destruction of the fibular metaphysis and diaphysis.*

FIBROUS DYSPLASIA (LICHTENSTEIN–JAFFE DISEASE)

DEFINITION

- A developmental disorder of the bone (which ceases growth with maturity)
- Medullary bone is replaced with well-defined areas of fibrous tissue which can then ossify (but which are unable to produce mature lamellar bone)

CLINICAL PRESENTATION

- Painless (unless there is an associated fracture) ▶ limb or growth deformity ▶ usually < 30 years old (M = F)

Location Typically within long bone metadiaphyses

Monostotic (70–85%) Commonest sites: ribs (30%), proximal femur (20%), craniofacial bones (20%)

Polyostotic It may involve up to 75% of the skeleton (>50% are within the skull and facial bones) ▶ café au lait spots (30–50%) ▶ asymmetrical or unilateral distribution

RADIOLOGICAL FEATURES

XR A geographic lesion with bone expansion, deformity and endosteal scalloping with diffuse ground-glass matrix mineralization ▶ a thick sclerotic margin ('rind' sign) is characteristic ▶ a periosteal reaction only with an associated fracture
- Skull base lesions tend to be sclerotic (cf. lucent lesions elsewhere) ▶ there is greater involvement of the outer table of the calvarium
- Pseudoarthrosis of the tibia
- 'Shepherd's crook deformity': a varus deformity of the proximal femur is a late finding (due to bone softening and expansion)

MRI T1WI: low SI ▶ T2WI: low or high SI ▶ internal septations and cystic change with associated fluid levels ▶ T1WI + Gad: uniform and septal enhancement

Scintigraphy Increased uptake ▶ best technique for identifying polyostotic disease

PEARLS

- Malignant change is rare (0.5%) and more common in the polyostotic form ▶ it may follow radiotherapy

Cherubism An inherited (autosomal dominant) symmetrical involvement of the mandible and maxilla

Leontiasis ossea Involvement of the facial and frontal bones giving a leonine facies (resembling a lion) ▶ there can be associated cranial nerve palsies

McCune–Albright syndrome Polyostotic fibrous dysplasia (typically unilateral) + ipsilateral café au lait spots (coast of Maine) + endocrine disturbances (most commonly precocious puberty in girls)

Mazabraud's syndrome Fibrous dysplasia (most commonly polyostotic) + soft tissue myxomata

IMPLANTATION EPIDERMOID

DEFINITION

- A cyst lined by epidermis and containing exfoliated squames ▶ associated with a history of a penetrating injury (resulting in epithelial cells being carried into the underlying bone)

Location Usually within the terminal phalanx of the hand

RADIOLOGICAL FEATURES

XR A well-defined, slightly expansile, round lytic lesion

PEARL

- *Differential:* enchondroma (although rarely found within the terminal phalanx)

OSTEOFIBROUS DYSPLASIA

DEFINITION

- This histologically resembles fibrous dysplasia and the stroma of adamantinoma

CLINICAL PRESENTATION

- It is seen from birth to 40 years, with 50% of cases presenting at < 10 years of age (M = F)

Location The tibia is affected in > 90% (with the anterior mid-diaphyseal cortex affected in $\frac{2}{3}$) ▶ the ipsilateral fibula is affected in 20% ▶ multiple lesions can occur in the same bone ▶ bilateral involvement can occur

RADIOLOGICAL FEATURES

XR
- *Early infancy:* tibial expansion and bowing with a sclerotic rim
- *3 months of age:* multilocular ground-glass matrix mineralization similar to fibrous dysplasia (with an eccentric location) ▶ may be purely lytic

MRI No characteristic features

Scintigraphy Increased uptake

PEARL

- It can resolve spontaneously – but may be a precursor of an adamantinoma

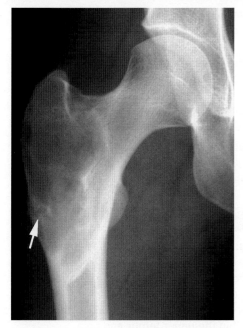

Fibrous dysplasia. AP XR showing a well-defined expanded lesion with typical ground-glass matrix mineralization and a thick, sclerotic margin (rind sign). A stress fracture is present in the lateral cortex (arrow).*

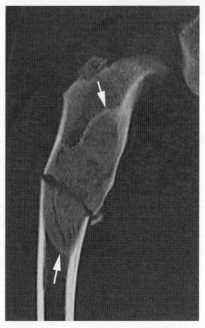

Fibrous dysplasia. Coronal CT MPR of the proximal femur showing a well-defined lesion with a 'ground-glass' matrix (arrows), through which there has been a pathological fracture.**

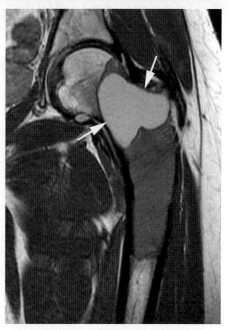

Fibrous dysplasia. Coronal T1W SE MRI showing a lesion in the left femoral neck with combined intermediate and increased SI (arrows), the latter due to haemorrhage.**

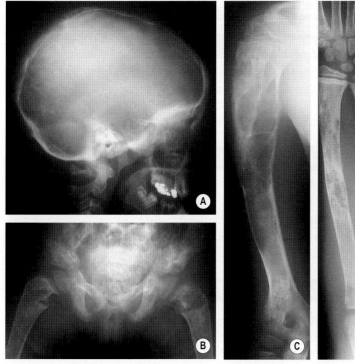

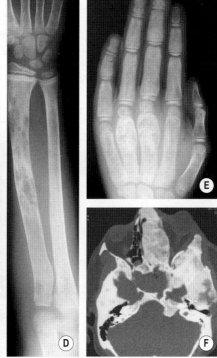

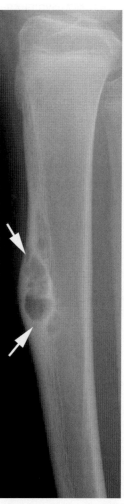

Fibrous dysplasia. (A) Patchy sclerosis affecting the vault and the base of the skull. (B) Radiolucent areas in the femoral necks and pelvic bones. Bilateral coxa vara. This is an early ?shepherd?s crook? deformity. Widening of the upper femoral epiphyseal plates, due to associated hypophosphataemic rickets. (C) Multiple radiolucent areas causing expansion. The margins are sclerotic and extend over several millimetres (a ?rind? appearance). Scalloping of the cortex. (D) The radiolucent areas predominantly affect the radius in a ray distribution. (E) The metacarpals and phalanges of the second to fifth fingers show expansion and deformity. Multiple radiolucent clearly defined lesions with relative sparing of the thumb and carpus. (F) CT demonstrating expanded and abnormally mineralized bone occupying the skull base.

Osteofibrous dysplasia. Lateral radiograph of the proximal tibia showing a lobular lesion (arrows) within the anterior cortex.**

PAGET'S DISEASE (OSTEITIS DEFORMANS)

DEFINITION

- A metabolic osteoclastic disorder characterized by abnormal osseous remodelling ▶ it is commonly polyostotic and asymmetrical
- It has an unknown aetiology but it may be caused by a viral infection (possibly paramyxovirus)
  - *Initial lytic (hot) phase:* increased osteoclastic activity results in bone resorption (with osteoblastic activity lagging behind) ▶ this is not commonly seen radiographically
  - *Intermediate (mixed) phase:* increased bone resorption is followed by increased formation of abnormally coarsened trabeculae ▶ corticomedullary differentiation is lost
  - *Late sclerotic (cold) phase:* osteoblastic activity predominates, generating disorganized bone of increased density

CLINICAL PRESENTATION

- It is predominantly found in the elderly (2M:1F) ▶ it is usually asymptomatic and found incidentally
- *Other presentations:* pain ▶ deafness (due to cranial nerve compression) ▶ insufficiency fractures ▶ high-output cardiac failure

Location   Apart from the skull, the weight bearing and persisting red marrow areas are the most commonly involved areas (sacrum and lumbar spine > skull, pelvis and femur) ▶ no bone is exempt although lesions of the fibula are rare

RADIOLOGICAL FEATURES

XR

- **Skull:** basilar invagination can be seen:
  - *Osteoporosis circumscripta:* the initial lytic phase (sparing the inner table) may persist within the skull (predominantly affecting the frontal and occipital bones)
  - *'Cotton wool' appearance:* osteoporosis circumscripta progressing to a mixed pattern
- **Pelvis:** a thickened ileopectineal line (an early sign) ▶ protrusio acetabuli
- **Long bones:** disease usually starts at the end of a bone (except for the tibia where it begins in the tuberosity) ▶ as it extends into the diaphysis it is demarcated from normal bone by a V-shaped zone of transition ('flame-shaped' lysis) ▶ there is an increased cortical width ▶ weakened bones can bow under the stress of weight bearing

- **Vertebrae:** enlargement of the vertebral body, neural arch and pedicle involvement distinguishes it from metastatic disease
  - *'Picture frame' appearance:* condensed thickened end plates and vertebral margins enclosing a cystic spongiosa
  - *'Ivory' vertebrae:* sclerotic vertebral bodies ▶ there can be collapse (± cord compression)

Scintigraphy   Very hot lesions are seen during the lytic phase ▶ it is able to detect polyostotic disease

MRI   This is better used for assessing any complications

PEARLS

- **Complications:** secondary osteoarthritis ▶ cranial nerve palsies ▶ high-output cardiac failure
  - *'Banana' fractures:* insufficiency fractures involving the convex cortical surface
  - *Pathological fractures:* these are usually transverse and seen within the upper femur and tibia
  - *Malignant degeneration* (<1%): osteosarcoma > MFH > chondrosarcoma

POST-TRAUMATIC CORTICAL DESMOID

DEFINITION

- This is a benign lesion resulting from a chronic avulsive stress at the femoral origin of the medial head of gastocnemius ▶ it is regarded as a normal variant (but can be confused with an aggressive tumour)

CLINICAL PRESENTATION

- Asymptomatic or with mild pain (affecting the adolescent age group)

Location   The characteristic site is the posterior aspect of the supracondylar ridge of the medial femoral condyle ▶ it is twice as common within the left femur ($\frac{1}{3}$ are bilateral)

RADIOLOGICAL FEATURES

XR/MRI   A poorly defined lytic lesion ▶ there is no soft tissue extension ▶ it can appear concave or convex ▶ there is periosteal reaction

PEARLS

- It heals without treatment
- Similar lesions can be seen at the pectoralis major and deltoid insertions

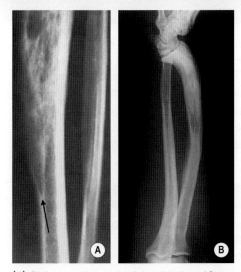

(A) Oblique radiograph of the tibia in a 60-year-old man with Paget's disease shows sharply demarcated lysis along the distal anterior cortex (arrow) of the tibia ('blade of grass' appearance). The proximal tibia shows bony expansion and has a mixed sclerotic and lytic appearance, indicating more advanced disease. (B) Radiograph of the forearm shows cortical expansion, sclerosis, and bowing of the radius characteristic of Paget's disease.©34

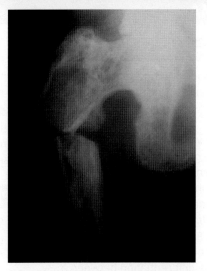

Complete transverse fracture in the upper femur in established Paget's disease. Sharply defined and at right angles across the shaft of the bowed bone. The clarity of the margin militates against a malignant pathology underlying this typical pathologic fracture.©35

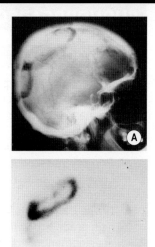

Osteoporosis circumscripta. Two circular focal areas of active osteolysis in Paget's disease (A) are reflected as areas of increased uptake on scintigraphy (B).[†]

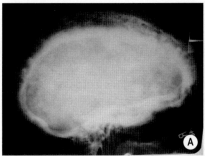

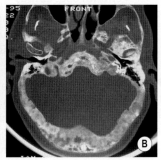

(A) Gross Paget's disease of the skull. Note the marked thickening of the vault, the multiple 'cotton wool' opacities, and the extensive involvement of the base of the skull. (B) Compression and distortion of the internal auditory meatuses and middle ears is shown on CT secondary to Paget's disease of the skull.©35

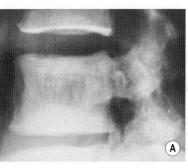

Paget's disease. (A) 'Picture frame' appearance in a vertebral body. The pedicles are also enlarged. (B) The bone scan demonstrates increased uptake.[†]

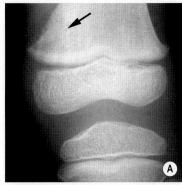

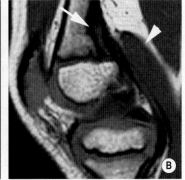

Cortical desmoid (Bufkin lesion). (A) AP XR showing a distal femoral metaphyseal cortical desmoid (arrow) appearing as a poorly defined lytic lesion. (B) Sagittal T1WI showing the lesion (arrow) at the site of origin of the medial head of gastrocnemius (arrowhead).*

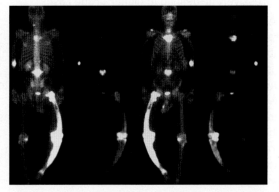

A whole-body radionuclide scintiscan (late phase using 99mTc-labeled diphosphonate) shows a predominantly right-sided distribution of disease but also the apparently random sites of involvement. Note, however, the area of photon deficiency in the right femur. This should raise the possibility of a sarcoma, which was confirmed histologically.©35

5.6 MALIGNANT BONE TUMOURS

CHONDROSARCOMA

DEFINITION

- A malignant cartilage-producing tumour – it generally has a better prognosis than an osteosarcoma (due to late metastases)
- **Classification:**
  - *Central* (intramedullary) vs *peripheral*
  - *Primary* vs *secondary* (e.g. arising in a pre-existing bone lesion such as a central enchondroma or a peripheral osteochondroma)
  - *Grade I:* low grade ▶ *Grade II:* myxoid ▶ *Grade III:* high grade ▶ *dedifferentiated:* this refers to the development of an adjacent non-chondroid tumour (e.g. an osteosarcoma, fibrosarcoma, or MFH)
- A major consideration is the differentiation between a chondroma and a low-grade chondrosarcoma

CLINICAL PRESENTATION

- This is rare in children with > 50% of patients over 40 years of age (M:F, 1.5:1) ▶ secondary chondrosarcoma tends to present at a slightly younger age (4th + 5th decades)
- Most are low-grade tumours found incidentally ▶ it can present with insidious pain, a palpable mass or a pathological fracture

Location It usually affects the pelvis, proximal femur and proximal humerus (it is rare distal to the elbow or knee) ▶ it is found within the metaphysis (± epiphyseal extension) ▶ 9% of chondrosarcomas occur in the ribs, making this the most common rib primary (other than myeloma) ▶ rare in the hands and feet (c/w enchondroma)

RADIOLOGICAL FEATURES

- General features of central chondrosarcoma are those of a lytic lesion, well-defined in low grade cases and progressively ill-defined in higher grade cases

XR A well-defined lytic lesion with chondroid matrix mineralization (chondroid calcification visible in 75%, described as ring-and-arc, punctate, stippled or popcorn) ▶ there is a narrow zone of transition
- *Slow growth:* this allows reactive change with periosteal new bone + bone expansion + endosteal resorption (endosteal scalloping > ⅔ of the cortical width suggests a chondrosarcoma rather than a chondroma) ▶ an increased cortical thickness (if the periosteal reaction outweighs the cortical scalloping)
- *More aggressive tumours:* cortical destruction ▶ one should consider dedifferentiation to a more malignant type

CT/MRI This can demonstrate a large extraosseous mass which is commonly seen with pelvic lesions (which are often radiographically and clinically occult)

- T1WI: hypointense to muscle ▶ T2WI: multilobulated high SI lesion ▶ matrix mineralization appears as foci of signal void ▶ T1WI + Gad: minimal peripheral or septal enhancement (as it is poorly vascularized)

Scintigraphy A chondrosarcoma will demonstrate greater activity than that seen within the anterior iliac crest ▶ cannot reliably distinguish between benign and malignant lesions

PEARLS

- Suspect the development of a chondrosarcoma within a pre-existing osteochondroma if:
  - There is increased pain or continued growth after skeletal maturity
  - There is destruction of part of the calcified cap or ossified stem
  - **US/CT/MRI:** these can assess the cartilage cap – it should be < 5 mm with an osteochondroma (but is often > 20 mm with malignant change)

Periosteal chondrosarcoma (juxtacortical chondrosarcoma)

- This is rare (and more common in men) ▶ it involves the outer long bones (usually the distal femoral or proximal humeral metaphyses) ▶ there is a good prognosis after resection

XR A calcified juxtacortical cartilagenous mass (>5 cm in length) with cortical thickening and periosteal reaction ▶ distinguished from the other surface form of chondrosarcoma (peripheral chondrosarcoma) by a lack of continuity with underlying medullary bone

Mesenchymal chondrosarcoma

- This is rare, affecting a younger age group than with a conventional chondrosarcoma (3rd and 4th decades) ▶ it has a very much more cellular malignant matrix than a normal chondrosarcoma (high grade malignancy)

XR It is indistinguishable from a central chondrosarcoma ▶ there is often chondroid calcification ▶ there is a predilection for the ribs and mandible
- Local recurrence and metastases occur early (and more commonly than with a conventional chondrosarcoma)

Clear cell chondrosarcoma

- This is rare ▶ it is a low-grade tumour with a better prognosis and slow growth ▶ can be mistaken for a subchondral cyst/intraosseous ganglion

XR It resembles a chondroblastoma or chondromyxoid fibroma – except it almost always involves the ends of the long bones after closure of the growth plate (esp. the proximal femur or humerus) ▶ it has a lytic appearance (± a loculated or 'soap bubble' appearance)

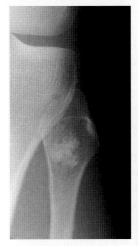

Chondrosarcoma. AP XR showing a mineralized lesion of the fibula due to low-grade chondrosarcoma. The lesion cannot be radiologically differentiated from a chondroma.*

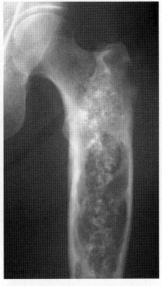

AP radiograph of the femur showing an extensive central chondrosarcoma with typical chondroid matrix, cortical expansion and thickening with endosteal scalloping.**

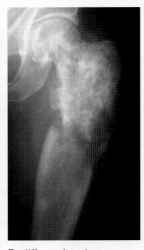

Dedifferentiated chondrosarcoma. AP XR showing a proximal femoral chondrosarcoma with an adjacent area of lytic destruction and a pathological fracture.*

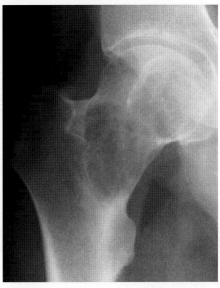

AP radiograph of the hip showing a clear-cell chondrosarcoma as a well-defined lytic lesion extending up to the articular margin.**

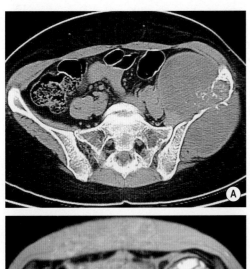

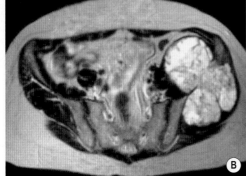

Chondrosarcoma of the left ilium. Axial CT (A) and T2WI (B) show a large extraosseous mass.*

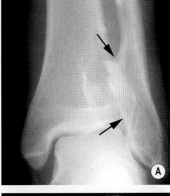

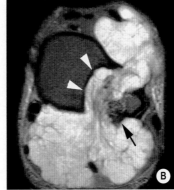

Peripheral chondrosarcoma. (A) AP XR showing an osteochondroma of the distal fibula (arrows). (B) Axial fat-suppressed T2WI shows a large malignant cartilage cap surrounding the osteochondroma (arrow) and causing pressure erosion of the adjacent tibia (arrowheads).*

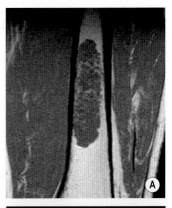

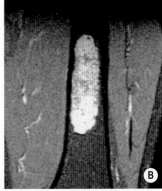

Chondrosarcoma of the femur. (A) Coronal T1WI and (B) STIR image show a large lobulated intramedullary lesion, which is particularly hyperintense on STIR.*

581

CONVENTIONAL CENTRAL OSTEOSARCOMA

DEFINITION

- Commonest non-haematological primary bone malignancy ▶ a malignant osteoid producing tumour
- It is usually a primary central osteosarcoma (75%) – the remainder are made up of other variants distinguished by site and histological grade ▶ it can occur secondary to Paget's disease, post radiotherapy or as a dedifferentiated chondrosarcoma
- *Classification:*
  - Central (conventional high or low grade)
  - Intracortical
  - Surface (parosteal, periosteal or high grade)

CLINICAL PRESENTATION

- Pain or a palpable mass (usually > 6cm at presentation) ▶ pathological fracture
- 80% of cases present between 10 – 30 years ▶ uncommon under 10 years of age ▶ rare under 5 years of age ▶ there is a 2nd smaller peak occurring above the age of 40 years which is seen commonly within the flat bones and vertebrae and usually secondary to a pre-existing disorder (e.g. Paget's)

RADIOLOGICAL FEATURES

`Location` it commonly affects the metaphyseal region of a growing long bone (50-75% are seen around the knee, and within the distal femur or proximal tibia) ▶ other common sites include the proximal humerus and femur ▶ it can cross the growth plate with epiphyseal extension seen in 75% of cases

`XR` moth-eaten or permeative lytic bone destruction arising eccentrically within the medullary cavity – there can be associated medullary sclerosis due to mineralised tumour osteoid (which has been described as 'solid', 'amorphous', 'cloud-like' and 'ivory-like') ▶ there is a wide zone of transition ▶ there can be cortical destruction with an extra-osseous mass and cloudlike matrix mineralization ▶ a spectrum of appearances from purely lytic (13%) to purely sclerotic

- *Periosteal reaction:* a 'sunburst' appearance perpendicular to the cortex ▶ a lamellated / onion skin appearance with reactive Codman's triangles seen at the margins of the lesion
- A solely lytic lesion (13% of cases) may mimic an ABC

`MRI` this adds little to the diagnosis but is invaluable for local staging and assessing any extension (it can demonstrate any intramedullary and extraosseous extension as well as extension into the adjacent joint or across an open growth plate)

`FDG PET` established role in the evaluation of treatment response and for recurrent disease

PEARLS

- It is a highly vascular tumour with early haematogenous metastases to the lung (with a subpleural location, possible calcification, and potential pneumothorax formation) ▶ occasionally there are lymphatic metastases
  - *'Skip metastases':* metastasis within the same bone as the primary (5-8% of cases)

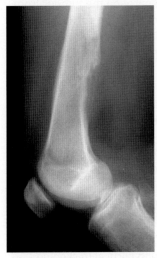

Lytic osteosarcoma. Lateral XR of the distal femur showing a lytic osteosarcoma.*

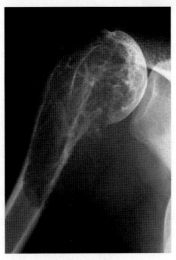

Low-grade central osteosarcoma. AP XR of the proximal humerus showing the lytic, trabeculated pattern.*

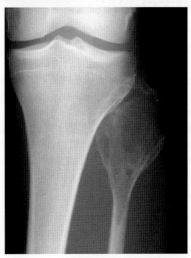

Pseudocystic osteosarcoma. AP XR of the proximal fibula showing an expanded, lytic lesion mimicking an aneurysmal bone cyst.*

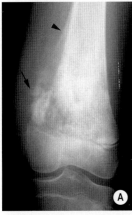
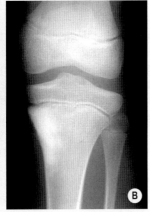

Conventional central osteosarcoma. (A) AP XR of the distal femur showing a classical osteosarcoma with mixed lytic and sclerotic areas, tumour bone formation in the extraosseous mass (arrow), and a proximal Codman's triangle (arrowhead). (B) AP XR of the proximal tibia showing dense metaphyseal sclerosis due to an osteoblastic osteosarcoma.*

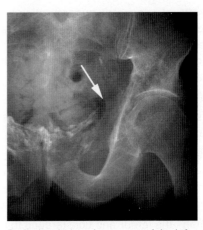

Radiation-induced sarcoma of the left superior pubic ramus manifest as a region of lytic bone destruction (arrow) with underlying radiation osteitis.*

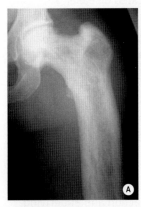
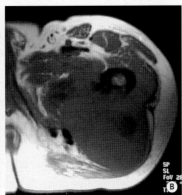
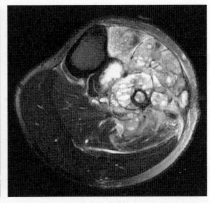

Paget's sarcoma. (A) AP XR of the proximal femur showing Paget's disease. (B) Axial T1WI shows an associated large soft tissue mass due to sarcomatous change.*

OTHER VARIETIES OF CENTRAL OSTEOSARCOMA

Primary multicentric osteosarcoma

- Multiple intramedullary osteosarcomas in the absence of pulmonary metastases
- **Synchronous:** multiple osteoblastic metaphyseal lesions occurring in children or adolescents ▶ it has a poor prognosis
- **Metachronous:** this affects older patients presenting with a solitary lytic or sclerotic lesion within a long or flat bone ▶ multiple lesions are seen after more than 5 months ▶ this has a better prognosis than a synchronous lesion

Telangiectatic osteosarcoma

- This is composed of septated blood-filled cavities (and can mimic an ABC) ▶ it accounts for 4-11% of all osteo-sarcomas with a mean age of presentation at 24 years (M:F 2:1) ▶ it is very malignant with a poor prognosis

Location femur, tibia and humerus

XR predominantly lytic lesions ± bone expansion

CT / MRI subtle matrix mineralisation ▶ extensive haemorrhage with fluid-fluid levels ▶ extra-osseous extension

- Thick peripheral, septal and nodular enhancement helps differentiate from an ABC

Small cell osteosarcoma

- This accounts for <1% of cases ▶ it has similar features to a conventional central osteosarcoma

Low-grade intramedullary osteosarcoma

- This well differentiated indolent lesion accounts for <1% of cases ▶ there is a mean age of presentation at 34 years, with a slight female preponderance

Location the femur and tibia (around the knee)

XR / CT 4 patterns: 1) lytic with varying degrees of coarse trabeculation ▶ 2) lytic with little trabeculation ▶ 3) densely sclerotic ▶ 4) mixed lytic and sclerotic

- It has a relatively benign appearance that can be mistaken for fibrous dysplasia, osteoblastoma or a low grade chondroid tumour ▶ extraosseous extension aids in the differentiation

SURFACE OSTEOSARCOMA

Definition A group of tumours that arise form the surface of bone – includes parosteal, periosteal and high grade surface osteosarcomas ▶ all types account for < 10% of osteosarcomas

Parosteal Commonest surface osteosarcoma; affects an older age group (the 3rd and 4th decades) ▶ it is slow growing with an excellent prognosis (unless it dedifferentiates to a high grade osteosarcoma in 20%) ▶ it has an equal sex incidence

Location posterior distal femoral metaphysis (60%), proximal humerus or tibia

XR a dense bony mass enveloping the metaphysis with a well defined radiolucent line separating the tumour from the normal cortex (it is only attached to the cortex at its origin) ▶ medullary invasion in 15% ▶ it may wrap around the bone ▶ satellite bony masses can be seen in the adjacent soft tissue

MRI T1WI: low SI ▶ T2WI ▶ low SI - high SI at the periphery may indicate higher grade or dedifferentiation

Differential osteochondroma ▶ juxtacortical myositis ossificans

- There is peripheral ossification in myositis ossificans, and central ossification in an osteosarcoma

Periosteal Intermediate grade chondroblastic tumour, with a mean age of presentation of 20 years ▶ there is a slight male preponderance

Location the proximal tibial or distal femoral diaphysis

XR 2 patterns: surface lesion with cortical thickening / erosion and perpendicular 'hair-on-end' periosteal reaction ▶ thin peripheral shell simulating a periosteal chondroma

MRI T2WI: lobulated high SI lesion (due to the chondroblastic nature of the lesion) ▶ marrow invasion is rarely demonstrated

High-grade Histologically this is the same as a conventional central osteosarcoma (but with a poorer prognosis) ▶ it is radiologically similar to the periosteal type but more aggressive in nature – it is usually larger with a greater degree of cortical destruction

Paget's sarcoma 50% of bone sarcomas arising after 50 years of age are secondary to Paget's disease (remainder are spindle cell / pleomorphic sarcomas or chondrosarcomas) ▶ malignant change is reported in up to 14% of cases of Paget's disease (M:F 2:1) ▶ it should be suspected if there is a change in pain or a pathological fracture ▶ it has a very poor prognosis

Location it is commonly seen within the pelvis, femur or humerus ▶ the spine is usually spared

XR / CT permeative bone destruction with a wide transition zone and a large soft tissue mass ▶ preservation of medullary fat signal in uncomplicated disease

Post radiation sarcoma

- this is common in treated breast cancer, lymphoma, head and neck cancers and gynaecological tumours ▶ it is usually an osteosarcoma ▶ it commonly occurs within the pelvis and shoulder girdle and has a poor prognosis
- **Criteria for diagnosis:** a history of radiotherapy or tumour arising within a radiation field ▶ a >3 - 4 year latency (mean latency of 15 years) ▶ a histology different from the original tumour
  - Usually > 30Gy is required

XR / CT permeative bone destruction, a soft tissue mass, matrix mineralisation, periosteal reaction and underlying radiation change (osteopaenia / radionecrosis) within the underlying bone

MRI aggressive tumour destroying bone with soft tissue extension

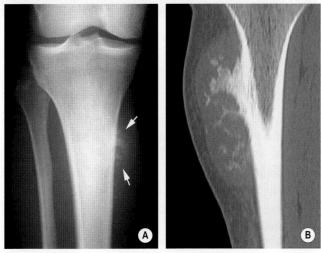

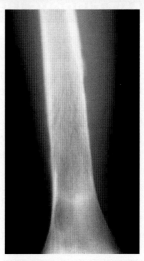

High-grade surface osteosarcoma of the proximal tibia. (A) AP XR shows a vertical periosteal reaction (arrows) arising from the medial metaphysis. (B) Sagittal CT multiplanar reconstruction shows the large associated soft tissue component. The features are similar to periosteal osteosarcoma, but more aggressive.*

Telangiectatic osteosarcoma. AP XR of the distal femur showing the classical 'iron-filing'-type destruction of the cortex.*

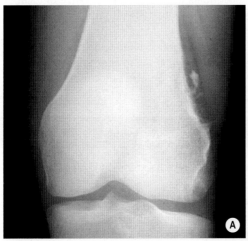

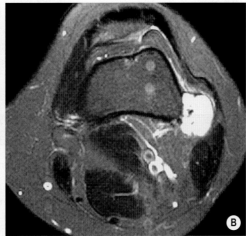

Periosteal osteosarcoma. (A) AP XR showing a spiculated periosteal reaction from the lateral femoral condyle and nodular matrix mineralization. (B) Axial fat-suppressed T2WI shows a lobular, hyperintense surface lesion consistent with a chondroblastic tumour.*

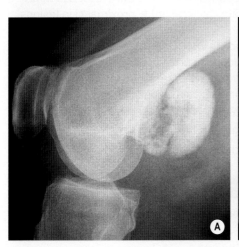

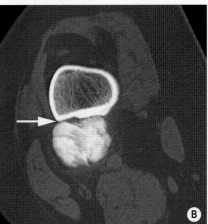

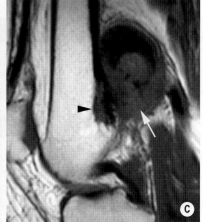

Parosteal osteosarcoma. (A) Lateral XR showing a dense, lobulated mass of bone arising from the posterior distal femur. (B) Axial CT shows a lucent line (arrow) separating the lesion from the underlying cortex. (C) Sagittal T1WI shows the low SI mass with central intermediate SI (arrow) indicating a region of dedifferentiation to high-grade tumour. Note also the intramedullary extension (arrowhead).*

MALIGNANT FIBROUS HISTIOCYSTOMA (MFH)

DEFINITION

- The most common primary malignant tumour of fibrous origin affecting bone – it originates from the bone marrow histiocytes
- Approximately 25% arise within a pre-existing lesion (especially Paget's disease, post radiotherapy, bone infarction or in relation to a dedifferentiated chondrosarcoma)
  - *Rare associations:* fibrous dysplasia ▶ non-ossifying fibroma ▶ chronic oteomyelitis ▶ total hip replacement
- It has a tendency to recur and metastasize

CLINICAL PRESENTATION

- It presents between 6 and 80 years, with a peak incidence during the 4th decade (M:F, 1.5:1)
- It has a non-specific presentation with insidious pain and swelling (pathological fractures are seen in 20%)

RADIOLOGICAL FEATURES

Location Predominantly the central metaphyses of the long bones (75%), and particularly found around the knee

▶ the humerus, pelvis, spine and ribs are less commonly involved

XR A lytic destructive lesion (resembling a metastasis) ▶ an extraosseous mass may be evident ▶ central mineralization and sclerotic margins are uncommon ▶ periosteal reaction is limited (unless a pathological fracture is present) ▶ it may extend to a subarticular surface (mimicking a giant cell tumour)

Scintigraphy Central photon-poor regions are sometimes seen (occasionally related to a pre-existing bone infarct)

MRI T1WI: intermediate-to-low SI ▶ T2WI: heterogeneous high SI: T1WI + Gad: variable enhancement ▶ it may show skip metastases

PEARLS

- Multicentric MFH is also recognized
- It may be indistinguishable from a fibrosarcoma
- It has a poor prognosis due to a high incidence of local recurrence and distant metastases (to the lungs, liver and brain)
- **Treatment:** Surgical resection (with wide margins) if there has been a good response to chemotherapy

FIBROSARCOMA

DEFINITION

- A malignant tumour of fibrous origin
- It can occur secondary to Paget's disease, a dedifferentiated chondrosarcoma, bone infarction post irradiation, or within a chronic sinus tract of osteomyelitis

CLINICAL PRESENTATION

- It presents between 20 and 50 years (M = F)
- It can present with insidious pain and swelling, or a pathological fracture

RADIOLOGICAL FEATURES

Location The long bones (70%): 50% arise within the lower limb (particularly around the knee) ▶ it is less commonly seen within the pelvis, humerus or jaw ▶ it is usually metaphyseal and arising eccentrically within the

medulla – often with epiphyseal extension (7% are purely diaphyseal)

XR A 'moth-eaten' destruction of bone with a wide zone of transition in the more malignant tumours ▶ cortical destruction (with little periosteal reaction) ▶ a loculated 'soap bubble' appearance ▶ a small extra-osseous mass (rarely with punctate calcification) ▶ proximal skip lesions can be seen

- *Low-grade lesion:* a well-circumscribed lytic lesion with an irregular lobulated cortex (± sequestrum)
- *High-grade lesion:* a lytic ill-defined lesion ▶ permeative bony destruction ▶ extraosseous mass

MRI T1WI: intermediate-to-low SI ▶ T2WI: heterogeneous high SI: T1WI + Gad: variable enhancement

Scintigraphy Increased uptake

PEARL

- It may be indistinguishable from a malignant fibrous histiocytoma

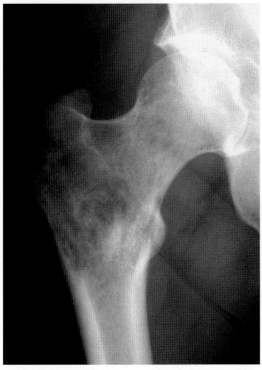

Osseous MFH. AP XR of the proximal femur showing a moth-eaten destructive lesion with no characteristic features.*

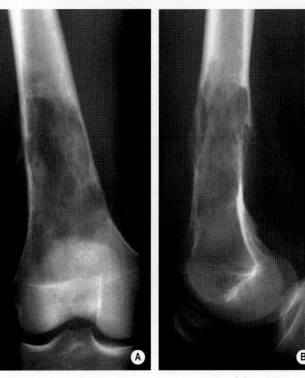

Malignant fibrous histiocytoma. Anteroposterior (A) and lateral (B) radiographs show an aggressive lytic lesion of the distal femoral diaphysis with absent mineralization and periosteal new bone formation. ©35

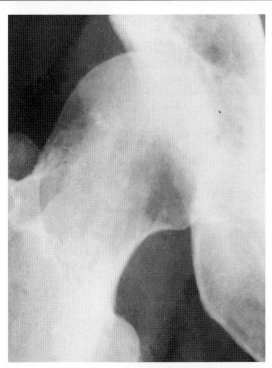

Fibrosarcoma arising in the medulla of the femoral head and neck. At presentation an ill-defined area of bone destruction in the medial aspect of the head and neck is seen, with preservation of the cortex and no new bone formation.[†]

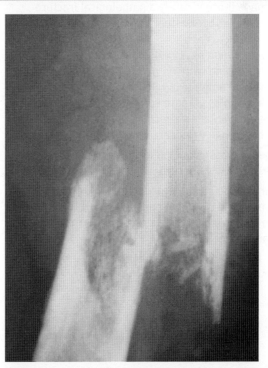

Fibrosarcoma presenting with a pathological fracture of the femur. Ill-defined bone destruction, particularly of the medulla, is associated with very minor periosteal new bone formation and no sclerosis.[†]

EWING'S SARCOMA

DEFINITION

- A highly malignant neoplasm derived from undifferentiated bone marrow mesenchymal cells or primitive neuroectodermal cells
- It arises from bone (usually medullary in origin) or extraskeletally

CLINICAL PRESENTATION

- Presentation is between 5 and 15 years, with 90% of patients presenting under the age of 30 years (M : F, 2 : 1)
- Local pain and swelling ▶ systemic symptoms (including pyrexia and an elevated ESR) are present if there is disseminated disease – this indicates a poor prognosis

RADIOLOGICAL FEATURES

Location It usually involves a single bone (it is multiple in 10% as Ewing's sarcoma is one of the few tumours that readily metastasizes to bone) ▶ it affects the diaphysis or metadiaphysis of a long bone (femur and humerus > pelvic bones > ribs) ▶ typically central/medullary in origin

XR Permeative lytic bone destruction with a wide zone of transition ▶ rapid extension through the cortex producing a large extraosseous subperiosteal mass ▶ cortical thickening ▶ occasionally a mixed or mainly sclerotic appearance (especially in the flat bones) mimicking an osteosarcoma ▶ there is rarely a pathological fracture

- *'Saucerization':* subperiosteal tumour eroding through the outer cortex
- *Multilaminar 'onion peel' periosteal reaction:* uncommon ▶ this is in keeping with the periodic activity of the lesion (although an incomplete laminar reaction with marginal Codman's triangles is more commonly seen)
- *'Hair-on-end' periosteal reaction:* this is also classical ▶ can also be seen in osteosarcoma

CT A large extraosseous (soft tissue) component is visualized ▶ aggressive periosteal reaction

MRI Accurately defines the medullary infiltration and soft tissue extension ▶ T1WI: intermediate-to-low SI compared with muscle ▶ T2WI: high SI compared with muscle ▶ T1WI + Gad: enhancement

FDG-PET More sensitive than bone scintigraphy ▶ can be used for assessing treatment response and for recurrence

PEARLS

- Together with an osteosarcoma, it represents 90% of paediatric primary malignant bone tumours
- There is early spread to the lungs and bones (30% at presentation)
- An extraosseous (soft tissue) Ewing's sarcoma is rare
- **Differential:** osteomyelitis ▶ stress fracture ▶ lytic osteosarcoma ▶ primary bone lymphoma ▶ Langerhans' cell histiocytosis
- **Treatment:** surgical resection (with wide margins) if there has been a good response to chemotherapy
- **Primitive neuroectodermal tumour (PNET):** this is a more differentiated form of Ewing's sarcoma (although it is more common in females) ▶ it includes soft tissue and bone neoplasms that were previously reported as a peripheral neuroepithelioma, adult neuroblastoma, or a small cell tumour of the chest wall (Askin's tumour) ▶ it cannot be differentiated from a Ewing's sarcoma on imaging
  - **Askin's tumour:** a rare PNET of the chest wall occurring in children and young adults ▶ it presents as a lytic extrapleural mass with rib involvement ▶ the soft tissue mass tends to be slightly hyperintense to muscle on T1WI

Staging classification for MSK tumours	
Stage	**Description**
IA	Low grade ▶ intracompartmental
IB	Low grade ▶ extracompartmental
IIA	High grade ▶ intracompartmental
IIB	High grade ▶ intracompartmental
IIIA	Low or high grade ▶ intracompartmental ▶ metastases
IIIB	Low or high grade ▶ extracompartmental ▶ metastases

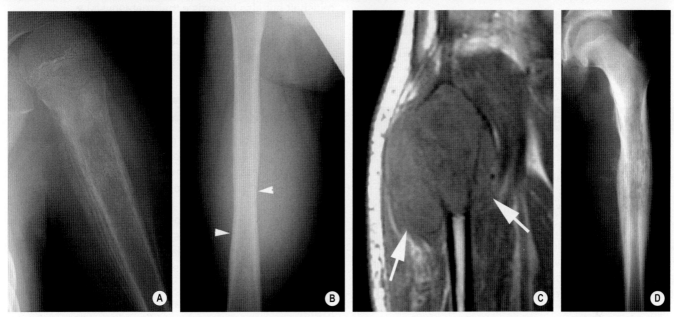

Ewing's sarcoma. (A) Typical appearance in the proximal humeral metadiaphysis with permeative marrow destruction, 'hair-on-end' and multilaminated periosteal reaction. (B) AP XR of the femur showing cortical 'saucerization' (arrowheads). (C) Coronal T1WI shows a large extraosseous mass (arrows).* (D) AP radiograph of an Ewing's sarcoma. Typical features include a central diaphyseal location, permeative bone destruction, a lamellar (onion skin) periosteal reaction with spiculation medially.**

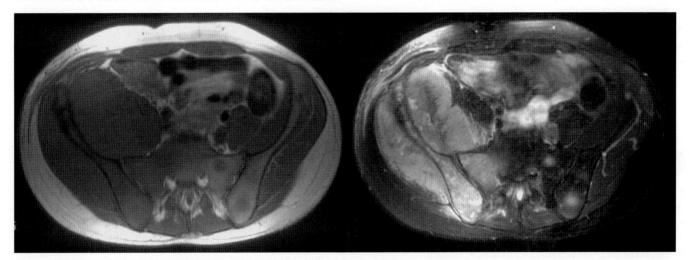

Axial T1- and T2-weighted fat-suppressed images at initial presentation showing a primary Ewing's sarcoma infiltrating the right ilium with a large intra- and extrapelvic soft-tissue mass. There is also evidence of disseminated disease with foci in the sacrum and left ilium.**

CHORDOMA

DEFINITION

- A slow-growing locally aggressive neoplasm originating from ectopic cellular remnants of the notochord
- It therefore arises from the midline axial skeleton

CLINICAL PRESENTATION

- It usually presents between 50 and 70 years of age: M = F (< 40 years), M:F, 2:1 (> 40 years)
- Symptoms are usually present for > 1 year before presentation ▶ pain and local pressure effects:
  - *Sacral:* bladder dysfunction and constipation
  - *Clival:* cranial nerve palsies

Location A predilection for the sacrococcygeal (50%) and clival (40%) regions >1 vertebral body involved in 50% of cases ▶ midline location is helpful in distinguishing from other sacral tumours (e.g. chondrosarcoma/metastases)

RADIOLOGICAL FEATURES

XR A large area of bone destruction with well-defined margins ▶ occasional amorphous calcification ▶ destruction of the dorsal aspect of the sella and clivus with spheno-occipital lesions

MRI Essential for local staging ▶ it is almost always associated with a large soft tissue mass

- T1WI: variable SI with areas of high SI (focal haemorrhage or a high protein content) ▶ T2WI: a lobulated, high SI mass with internal septations and well-defined margins with areas of low SI (haemosiderin) ▶ T1WI + Gad: heterogeneous or septal enhancement

PEARL

- It is the 2nd commonest primary spine malignancy, accounting for > 50% of sacral tumours
- Wide excision is the treatment of choice ▶ radiotherapy for inoperable cases
- Local recurrence (multifocal) in 40% ▶ distant metastases uncommon

ADAMANTINOMA

DEFINITION

- A locally aggressive bone tumour of epithelial origin

CLINICAL PRESENTATION

- The average age at presentation is 35 years (M:F, 5:4)
- Local pain and tenderness (several years)

Location 85% occur within the tibia (mostly in the midshaft but also towards either metaphysis) ▶ synchronous involvement of the tibia and fibula in 10% ▶ initially eccentric but eventually involves the whole depth of the shaft ▶ occasionally multifocal lesions within the same long bone

RADIOLOGICAL FEATURES

XR Typically multiple well-defined lucencies with interspersed sclerosis ▶ eccentric involvement of the tibial diaphysis is classical ▶ The majority are intracortical with geographic cortical destruction (lytic with a sclerotic lobulated margin) ▶ there can be internal ossification and septations ▶ there can be a multilocular appearance with satellite lesions ▶ extracortical extension is seen in 15% of cases

- *Rare findings:* anterior tibial bowing ▶ moth-eaten destruction ▶ ground-glass mineralization ▶ bony expansion

MRI Ideal for assessing marrow extension (60%), extraosseous extension and multifocal lesions ▶ no specific signal characteristics (a lobulated growth pattern is typical) ▶ T1WI + Gad: intense uniform enhancement

PEARL

- It readily recurs if it is incompletely removed ▶ lung metastases are seen in 10% of cases

MALIGNANT VASCULAR TUMOURS

Haemangioendothelioma

- A low-grade malignant endothelial tumour presenting with local pain and swelling ▶ multifocal in 25% (multifocal disease is a clue to the diagnosis)
- *Epithelioid haemangioendothelioma:* multifocal but limited to a single anatomic region in 40% ▶ a lytic lesion (with a small extraosseous mass in 40%)

XR Non-specific ▶ lytic or mixed lytic and sclerotic lesions
- *Rarely seen:* periosteal reaction ▶ cortical destruction and extraosseous extension

Angiosarcoma

- A high-grade vascular neoplasm (unifocal or multifocal) ▶ presents during the 3rd or 4th decades

XR Non-specific imaging features (an aggressive lytic destructive process) ▶ sclerotic lesions, periosteal reaction and pathological fractures are uncommon

Anaplastic sarcoma

- This is highly malignant (sometimes the tissue of origin cannot be identified)

XR A lytic and locally aggressive process with no specific features

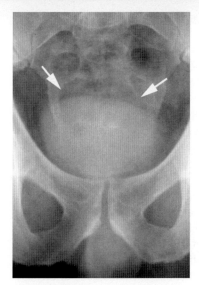

Sacral chordoma. AP XR shows a central, lytic destructive sacral lesion (arrows).*

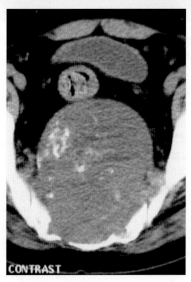

Sacral chordoma. CT shows a predominantly lytic mass with small foci of calcification.*

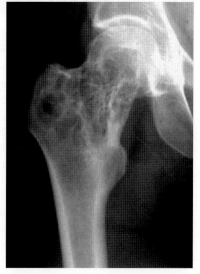

Angiosarcoma. AP XR of the proximal femur shows an aggressive, lytic destructive lesion with no specific features.*

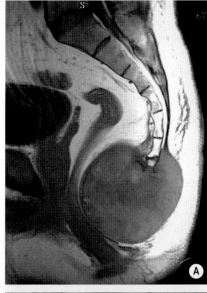

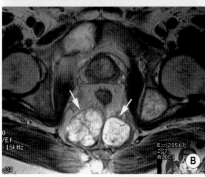

Sacrococcygeal chordoma. (A) Sagittal T1WI shows the intraosseous extent of the lesion and the relationship to the anterior pelvic viscera. (B) Axial T2WI shows the classical hyperintense, lobulated nature of the lesion (arrows).*

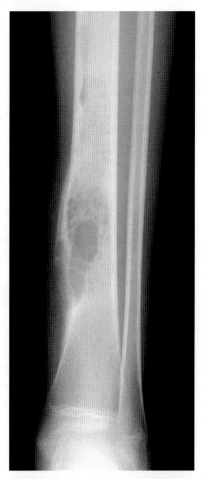

Adamantinoma. AP XR of the tibia showing a multiloculated, lytic lesion expanding the cortex.*

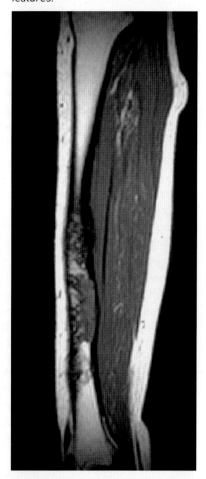

Adamantinoma. Sagittal T1WI showing a lobulated diaphyseal lesion with extension into the medullary cavity.*

BONE METASTASES

DEFINITION

- Distant metastases result from venous tumour emboli either from a primary tumour, regional nodes or other metastases ▶ they are related to the vascularity of the primary tumour and if there is access to a valveless venous plexus (e.g. Batson's vertebral plexus)
- They are common and often multiple (although 10% are solitary) ▶ they are usually a late occurrence as the lungs will trap most tumour emboli (unless there is transpulmonary passage of malignant cells or paradoxical embolism with passage of cells through a patent foramen ovale, or occult lung metastases)

Location   The commonest metastatic sites are bones containing red marrow – therefore the axial skeleton (vertebrae, pelvis, proximal femur, humerus, ribs) is more commonly involved than the appendicular skeleton

- *Thoracic vertebrae:* the commonest site for spinal metastases (pelvic malignancies favour the lumbosacral spine)
- *Peripheral metastases:* these are rare (50% arise from the bronchus)

RADIOLOGICAL FEATURES

- Metastases are commonly multiple and lytic ▶ osteoblastic change is a tissue response of the host bone rather than bone tumour production by a metastasis

XR   This can only visualize lesions > 2 cm ▶ larger lesions can cause cortical destruction ▶ any periosteal reaction is usually less pronounced than with a primary bone tumour (exceptions include prostate) ▶ soft tissue masses may develop with large bone metastases ▶ metastases can have a geographic, moth-eaten or permeative appearance

Scintigraphy   It is highly sensitive compared to XR but has a poor specificity (correlation with XR, CT or MRI is required) ▶ trauma can cause increased activity

- Increased activity reflects increased osteoblastic activity
- Lesions that infarct or stimulate no osteoblastic response (e.g. renal metastases) will be photopenic as any increased activity relies on a combination of local blood flow and osteoblastic activity
- *'Superscan':* this is caused by diffuse osteoblastic metastatic disease (e.g. breast or prostate) with associated reduced or absent renal activity
- 'Flare phenomenon': increased activity secondary to a normal healing response

MRI   This is more sensitive than XR, and more specific than scintigraphy ▶ most metastases are located within the medulla

- T1WI: low SI ▶ T2WI: high SI (a hyperintense halo around a lesion is highly specific)

FDG PET-CT   This is sensitive and specific for metastases

Typical features
- **Breast:** these are mostly lytic (10% are osteoblastic and 10% are mixed) ▶ it is the commonest cause of osteoblastic metastases in women ▶ it commonly involves the vertebrae, pelvis and ribs ▶ increasing sclerosis may indicate a treatment response
- **Prostate:** these are predominantly osteoblastic (lytic lesions are rare) ▶ there can be a florid 'sunburst' periosteal reaction which can mimic an osteosarcoma ▶ bone metastases rare if PSA <10 ng/mL
- **Lung:** this commonly affects the axial skeleton (however it is also the commonest cause of metastases to the hands and feet) ▶ the majority are lytic (usually a squamous cell or small cell carcinoma) ▶ focal or diffuse osteoblastic disease can be seen with bronchial carcinoid or adenocarcinoma
- **Renal:** these are usually lytic and expansile ▶ there is a marked predilection for the pelvis and lumbar spine ▶ they are hypervascular, often slow growing, and can be excised if solitary
- **Thyroid:** these are usually lytic and expansile (± miliary lung involvement)
- **Colon:** these are usually lytic (but can be sclerotic and demonstrate calcification) ▶ they occur in < 7% of patients
- **Bladder:** these are usually lytic ▶ there can be exuberant periosteal new bone ▶ they have an unusual predilection for the lower limbs
- **Cervix, pancreas, melanoma:** these are usually lytic
- **Uterus, carcinoid, stomach, medulloblastoma, neuroblastoma/Hodgkin's lymphoma:** these are osteoblastic

PEARLS

- A solitary lesion in a middle-aged or elderly patient is more likely to be an atypical metastasis than a typical primary malignant bone tumour
- A lesser trochanter avulsion fracture in an adult should be considered pathological until proven otherwise ▶ a transverse fracture in a long bone (especially without significant trauma) may be pathological
- *A solitary metastasis can mimic:* a primary malignant bone tumour, an aggressive benign tumour (e.g. giant cell tumour), infection, or Paget's disease
- **Paediatric skeletal metastases:** neuroblastoma ▶ leukaemia ▶ osteosarcoma ▶ Ewing's sarcoma ▶ medulloblastoma

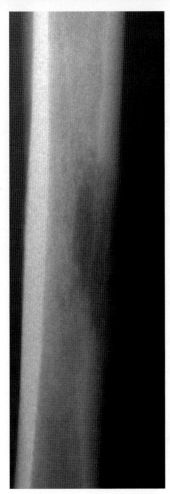

Detail of an AP radiograph of the tibia showing a cortically based metastasis from carcinoma of the bronchus.**

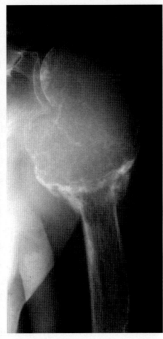

AP radiograph of the proximal humerus showing an expansile thyroid metastasis.**

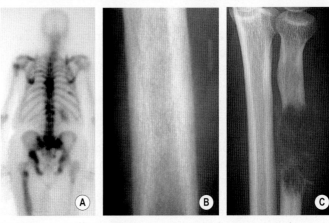

(A) Whole body ^{99m}Tc-MDP bone scintigram (posterior view) showing multiple regions of increased uptake due to prostatic carcinoma metastases. (B) Sunburst periosteal reaction. AP XR of the femoral diaphysis showing a spiculated periosteal reaction mimicking osteosarcoma in a patient with prostatic metastasis. (C) AP XR showing a mineralized squamous carcinoma metastasis to the radius.*

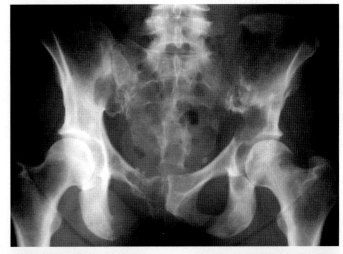

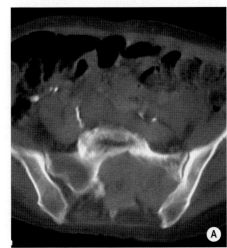 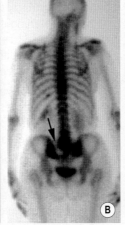

Cold metastasis due to hypernephroma metastasis to the sacrum. CT (A) shows a lytic destructive lesion of the left sacrum that also manifests as a 'cold' spot on the bone scintigram (arrow) (B).*

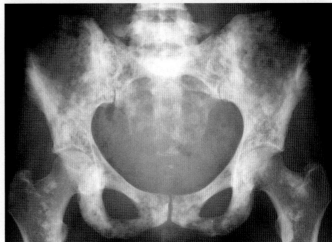

AP radiograph of the pelvis showing multiple sclerotic breast metastases.**

OSTEOPOROSIS

Definition

- A systemic skeletal disease characterized by a low bone mass and micro-architectural deterioration of the bone tissue with a consequent increase in bone fragility and an associated susceptibility to fracture
- It is the most common metabolic disorder affecting 50% of woman and 20% of men (> 50 years old) ▶ due to:
  - Reduced bone accumulation during development
  - Bone resorption outstrips new bone formation during later life (the ratio of osteoid matrix to hydroxyapatite mineral is normal)
- **WHO definition:** this is based on the bone mineral density (BMD) ▶ a T-score is the standard deviation of the BMD compared to a young healthy reference ▶ it is not appropriate for use in children (where you use > 2SD below the mean BMD matched for age, gender and ethnicity)
  - *Normal:* BMD > -1SD below the young adult mean (peak bone mass)
  - *Osteopenia:* BMD between -1 and -2.5SD below the young adult mean
  - *Osteoporosis:* BMD > -2.5SD below the young adult mean

Clinical presentation

- It can be asymptomatic ▶ there can be insufficiency fractures presenting with pain (e.g. vertebral crush fractures) ▶ the pain resolves spontaneously after 6–8 weeks unlike a more sinister pathology ▶ vertebral fractures may result in an increasing thoracic kyphosis
- Bone loss typically begins during the 4th decade (females) or 5th and 6th decades (males)

Location It is more prominent in areas rich in trabecular bone (e.g. the vertebrae, pelvis, ribs and sternum)

Radiological features

XR A reduced bone density (50% of bone density has to be lost to be visible) ▶ thin or absent trabeculae (with thickened remaining trabeculae due to increased stresses) ▶ thinned, irregular or a scalloped cortex (due to endosteal resorption) ▶ intracortical tunnelling and porosity (representing enlarged Haversian systems and Volkmann's canals)

- **Spine:** a vertical 'striated' appearance to the vertebral bodies due to preferential loss of the horizontal trabeculae (this is seen within most vertebrae, in comparison with a haemangioma that affects a single vertebra)
  - *Wedge, biconcave ('cod-fish') or crush deformities:* the vertebral anterior and central mid-portions withstand any compressive forces relatively poorly ▶ with a posterior fracture, consider metastases/myeloma
- **Sacrum:** insufficiency fracture lines are parallel to the SI joint on CT
  - *'Honda' sign:* a characteristic 'H' pattern of radionuclide uptake

MRI/scintigraphy This is sensitive at detecting femoral neck/pelvis insufficiency fractures before they are evident radiographically

Pearls

Insufficiency fractures These are low trauma fractures due to increased bone fragility
- *Common sites:* pubic rami ▶ sacrum ▶ vertebrae ▶ calcaneus ▶ distal forearm ▶ proximal femur ▶ vertebral bodies
- The axial skeleton is affected more frequently than the appendicular skeleton (and most commonly within the thoracic and thoracolumbar regions) ▶ fractures are uncommon above the level of T7 (consider metastases)

Postmenopausal osteoporosis (type I) This is due to an oestrogen lack ▶ it occurs 15–20 years after the menopause ▶ *there is a disproportionate loss of trabecular bone*

Senile osteoporosis (type II) This affects men and women (≥ 75 years) ▶ it is due to age-related impaired bone formation associated with secondary hyperparathyroidism (there is a reduced vitamin D production in the elderly) ▶ *there is a proportionate loss of trabecular and cortical bone*

Disuse and reflex sympathetic dystrophy (RSD/Sudeck's atrophy) Overactivity of the sympathetic nervous system causing pain, soft tissue swelling and hyperaemia with excessive bone resorption (particularly peri-articularly) ▶ it is precipitated by a variety of causes (e.g. following a fracture or related to tumour)

Transient osteoporosis of the hip A self-limiting condition affecting young and middle-aged patients (M>F) ▶ there is a sudden onset of pain with no associated trauma

XR Reduced proximal femoral bone density

MRI This is sensitive for detecting early marrow changes (T2WI: increased SI)

Idiopathic juvenile osteoporosis This is rare and affects prepubertal children with an acute variable course over a period of 2–4 years (it is reversible and spontaneously remits) ▶ it affects the vertebral bodies and the long bones (particularly the distal tibial metaphysis) ▶ it may be life threatening if thoracic involvement leads to a kyphoscoliosis (± respiratory failure)
- It needs to be differentiated from osteogenesis imperfecta (there are no blue sclerae)

Osteoporosis of young adults A mild condition leading to multiple fractures of the vertebrae, metatarsals, ribs and hips (M = F) ▶ it is possibly due to inadequate bone mass formation during development

Secondary osteoporosis See table of main causes

Treatment For painful osteoporotic vertebral fractures:
- *Vertebroplasty:* cement (methylmethacrylate) is injected under image guidance into a fractured vertebral body ▶ a minimum of 4 weeks has to have elapsed
- *Kyphoplasty:* a balloon is first used to decompress a fracture prior to cement injection

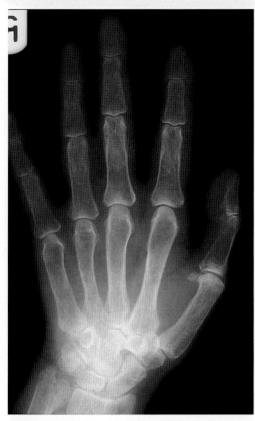

Osteoporosis. Reduced bone density, thinned cortex and reduced number of trabeculae, those which remain appearing more prominent.*

Main causes of osteoporosis*		
Primary		
	Juvenile	
	Idiopathic of young adults	
	Postmenopausal	
	Senile	
Secondary		
Endocrine	Glucocorticoid excess	
	Oestrogen/testosterone deficiency	
	Hyperthyroidism	
	Hyperparathyroidism	
	Growth hormone deficiency (childhood onset)	
Nutritional	Intestinal malabsorption	
	Chronic alcoholism	
	Chronic liver disease	
	Partial gastrectomy	
	Vitamin C deficiency (scurvy)	
Hereditary	Osteogenesis imperfecta	
	Homocystinuria	
	Marfan's syndrome	
	Ehlers–Danlos syndrome	
Haematological	Thalassaemia	
	Sickle-cell disease	
	Gaucher's disease	
Tertiary		
Other	Rheumatoid arthritis	
	Haemochromatosis	

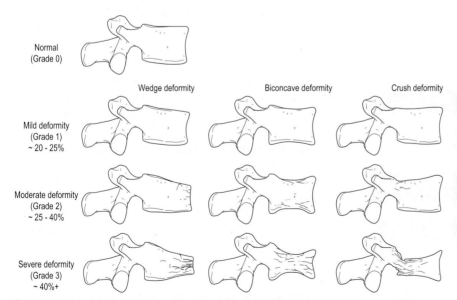

Osteoporosis – grading vertebral fractures. Vertebral fractures are strong predictors of future fractures (×5 for vertebral fracture and ×2 for hip fractures) so it is important that they are accurately and clearly reported by radiologists. The higher the grade of vertebral fracture, the higher the risk of future fracture.*

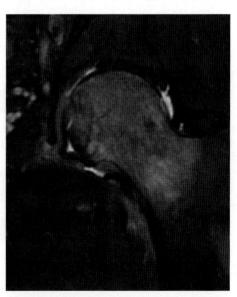

Transient osteoporosis of the hip. STIR image of the left hip in a 42-year-old man with transient osteoporosis. Note homogeneous bone marrow oedema pattern without focal linear signal abnormalities, which would suggest a fracture, or deformities as might occur in avascular necrosis of the femoral head with subchondral fracture.**

595

OSTEOMALACIA

DEFINITION

- Vitamin D deficiency resulting in defective mineralization of osteoid in the **mature** skeleton
- *Causes:* nutritional deficiency ▶ malabsorption states and biliary disease (vitamin D is fat soluble and absorbed in the small bowel) ▶ chronic liver disease (affecting the initial prohormone hydroxylation step) ▶ chronic renal disease (the active metabolite is not produced) ▶ drug therapy (e.g. long-term anticonvulsants)

RADIOLOGICAL FEATURES

Looser's zone (pseudofracture/Milkman's fracture)
Translucent areas within bone (unmineralized osteoid) are a pathognomonic feature ▶ typically bilateral and symmetrical

- *Location:* typically found at sites of stress: medial aspect of the femoral neck ▶ pubic rami ▶ lateral border of the scapula and ribs

XR A radiolucent line perpendicular to the cortex with a slightly sclerotic margin (it does not extend across the entire bone shaft)

- There is no callus formation unless it has been treated with vitamin D (osteoporotic insufficiency fractures often show florid callus formation) ▶ fractures occur medially on the concave side of a bone (incremental fractures in Paget's disease tend to occur on the convexity of a bone)
- Osteomalacic bone is soft: it can result in bowing of the long bones, protrusio acetabuli and a triradiate deformity of the pelvis

Scintigraphy Radionuclide bone scans are more sensitive than XR

PEARL

- Features of secondary hyperparathyroidism (the hypocalcaemia acts as a stimulus) can be seen

RICKETS

DEFINITION

- Vitamin D deficiency resulting in defective mineralization of osteoid in the **immature** skeleton ▶ abnormalities predominate at the growing ends of bones where endochondral ossification is occurring
- *Causes:* as for osteomalacia but also including inborn errors of vitamin D metabolism

Location The most obvious changes are at the metaphyses (the area of most rapid growth) ▶ commonly seen around the knee and wrist, the anterior ends of the middle ribs, the proximal femur and the distal tibia

RADIOLOGICAL FEATURES

XR Initially loss of the normal 'zone of provisional calcification' adjacent to the metaphysis

- *Later features:* a widened growth plate ▶ indistinct metaphyseal margins ('frayed' metaphyses) ▶ metaphyseal splaying and cupping (following weight bearing on uncalcified bone) ▶ indistinct and relatively osteopenic epiphyses (± Looser's zones) ▶ thin 'ghost-like' rim of mineralisation at the periphery of the metaphysis
- There may be features of secondary hyperparathyroidism (in response to the hypocalcaemia)
- *Harrison's sulcus:* rib in-drawing near the diaphragm
- *Craniotabes:* softening of the cranial vault
- *Rachitic rosary:* expanded long bone metaphyses can cause anterior rib enlargement
- **Bone deformities:** skull bossing ▶ delayed fontanelle closure ▶ bowing of the long bones (particularly the lower limbs) ▶ thoracic kyphosis with a 'pigeon chest' ▶ genu valgus and varum ▶ coxa vara and valga ▶ protrusio acetabuli ▶ a triradiate pelvis
- **Post treatment:** XR features of healing lag behind biochemical and clinical improvements (2 weeks)
  - *Harris growth arrest line:* with treatment mineralization of the zone of provisional calcification gives a dense white line adjacent to the metaphysis (as a marker of the age at which the rickets occurred) ▶ initially separated by translucent osteoid, which may be mistaken for a metaphyseal fracture (NAI)

PEARLS

Vitamin D resistant rickets This follows defective renal tubal reabsorption of phosphate (with increased renal excretion of calcium and phosphate) ▶ normal or elevated vitamin D levels ▶ radiographically similar to rickets but refractory to vitamin D therapy ▶ it may be seen with X-linked hypophosphataemia or Fanconi's syndrome

Vitamin D dependent rickets A group of autosomal recessive conditions

- *Type I:* a defect in the renal production of the active metabolite
- *Type II:* end-organ resistance to the active metabolite

Acquired hypophosphataemic rickets (tumour-induced oncogenic rickets) Seen in association with bone or soft tissue tumours that produce FGF23, a phosphate and vitamin D regulating hormone (e.g. a haemangiopericytoma, non-ossifying fibroma, giant cell tumour, fibrous dysplasia, or an osteoblastoma) ▶ there is a normal serum calcium

Metaphyseal chondrodysplasias Mild (Schmit type) or severe (Jansen type) ▶ this can mimic rickets but is differentiated by a normal serum biochemistry

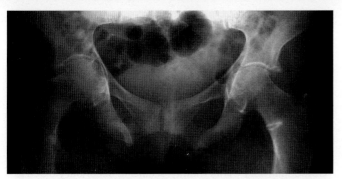

Osteomalacia. The pathognomonic XR feature is the Looser's zone – radiolucent, unmineralized linear areas perpendicular to the cortex and which may have a sclerotic margin (demonstrated in the medial aspect of the left femoral neck).*

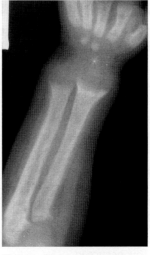

Rickets. There is 'fraying' of the visible metaphyseal margins.[†]

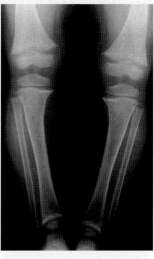

Rickets. There is splaying of all the visible metaphyses, with widened epiphyseal plates. In addition there is bowing of the femora and bones of the lower leg.[†]

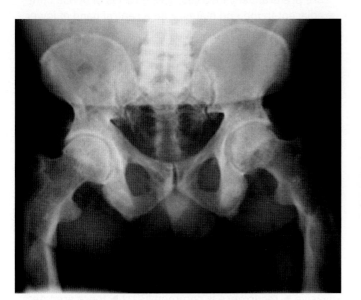

Patent sacroiliac joints, dense bones, and bowed femora in X-linked hypophosphatemic osteomalacia.©35

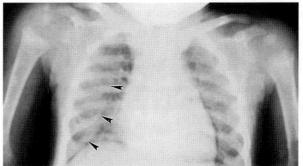

Rickety rosary. Widening of the anterior ribs is demonstrated (arrows). Metaphyseal changes are also seen in the proximal humeri.[†]

	Serum			Urine
	Calcium	Phosphorus	Alkaline phosphatase	Calcium
Osteoporosis	N	N	N	N
Hyperparathyroidism				
Primary	↑		N or ↑	N or ↑
Secondary	N or ↑	↑	↑	↓
Tertiary	↑	N or ↓	N or ↑	N or ↑
Hypoparathyroidism	↓	↑	N	↓
Pseudohypoparathyroidism	↓	↑	N	↓
Rickets/osteomalacia				
Vit D deficient	↓	↓	↑	
Vit D refractory	N	↓	↑	↓
Hypophosphatasia	N or ↑	N	↓	N or ↑

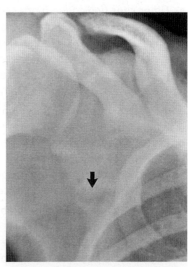

Looser's zone. There is lucency with surrounding sclerosis in the lateral border of the scapula.[†]

HYPERPARATHYROIDISM

DEFINITION

Primary hyperparathyroidism This is due to increased parathyroid hormone production (most parathyroid tumours are functionally active)

- *Causes:* a single parathyroid adenoma (80%)* ►
  hyperplasia (15–20%) ► carcinoma (1%)
    - * multiple adenomas are seen in 4% of cases

Secondary hyperparathyroidism This is induced by a fall in the serum calcium

- *Causes:* vitamin D deficiency ► intestinal malabsorption of calcium ► chronic renal failure (causing a lack of the active vitamin D metabolite)

Tertiary hyperparathyroidism This occurs in long-standing secondary hyperparathyroidism when an autonomous adenoma develops within the hyperplastic parathyroid glands

CLINICAL PRESENTATION

- It is often asymptomatic, but can present with: renal stones and nephrocalcinosis ► hypertension ► pseudogout (chondrocalcinosis) ► osteoporosis ► peptic ulcers ► acute pancreatitis ► depression ► proximal muscle weakness ► lethargy

RADIOLOGICAL FEATURES

- 95% have no radiological abnormalities (as a result of effective early therapy)
- **Subperiosteal erosions of cortical bone:**
  pathognomonic ► initially affects the radial aspects of the middle phalanges of the index and middle fingers – if it is not seen here then it is unlikely to be identified elsewhere ► tufts of the distal phalanges
- *Other sites (indicating more severe and long-standing disease):* distal phalanges (acro-osteolysis) ► proximal medial tibial cortex ► outer ends of the clavicles ► symphysis pubis ► ribs ► vertebral bodies (Schmorl's nodes) ► sacroiliac joints ► proximal humeral shaft
    - There can be loss of the lamina dura of the teeth

Intracortical bone resorption (cortical 'tunnelling') This is not specific and may also be seen in Paget's disease or acute osteoporosis ► cortical 'tunnelling': linear translucencies within the cortex

- A 'pepper pot' or 'salt and pepper' skull: a characteristic granular or mottled appearance of the skull

Chondrocalcinosis Deposition of calcium pyrophosphate dehydrate (CPPD) within articular cartilage and fibrocartilage (e.g. the TFCC of the wrist, knee menisci, and symphysis pubis) ► this can present with acute pain (pseudogout)

- It is a feature of *primary* but not secondary hyperparathyroidism

Brown tumours (osteitis fibrosa cystica) These are so called due to the presence of haemorrhage or altered blood seen at surgery, giving it a brown appearance

- Rare ► mainly seen with primary disease

XR Low-density, multiloculated and well-defined cysts ► occur within any skeletal site with associated bone expansion

Osteosclerosis This mainly occurs in secondary disease due to excessive accumulation of poorly mineralized osteoid (which is more dense than normal bone) ► it particularly affects the axial skeleton

- 'Rugger jersey' spine: the vertebral body end plates are preferentially involved, giving bands of dense bone adjacent to the end plates, with a central band of lower normal bone density

Osteoporosis This can occur with excessive bone resorption (postmenopausal and the elderly) ► there is preferential involvement of the cortical rather than the trabecular bone ► It is seen with primary disease

Metastatic calcification Soft tissue calcification (other than cartilage) does not occur in primary disease unless there is reduced glomerular filtration with the precipitation of calcium phosphate within the organs, blood vessels or soft tissues

PEARLS

- It can form part of a familial hyperplasia, multiple endocrine neoplasia (MEN) syndrome

Parathyroid carcinoma This is slow growing but locally invasive ► recurrence is common (30%) ► there are late metastases to the regional nodes, lungs, liver and bone (30%)

- Treatment: primary hyperparathyroidism – surgery ► secondary hyperparathyroidism – dietary change

CUSHING'S

Cushing's syndrome Increased free circulating glucocorticoid

- *Causes:* adrenal adenoma or carcinoma ► iatrogenic ► ectopic ACTH production (e.g. a bronchial carcinoma)

Cushing's disease Increased free circulating glucocorticoid from a basophil pituitary adenoma

Clinical presentation Truncal obesity ► hirsutism ► cutaneous striae

XR Osteoporosis (axial skeleton) ► low-trauma fractures ► exuberant callus formation ► avascular necrosis of the hip

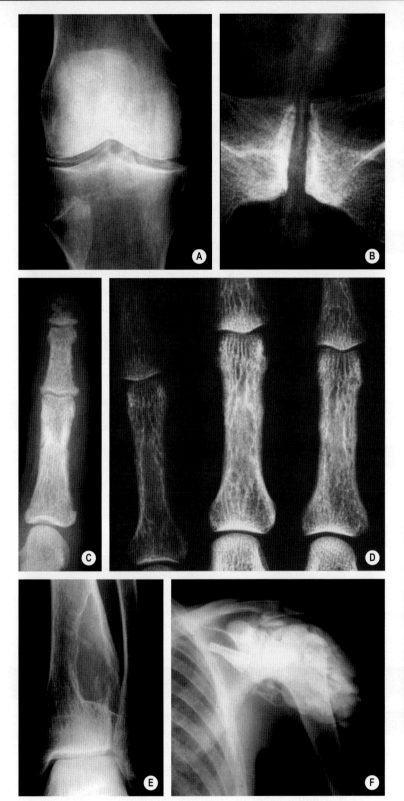

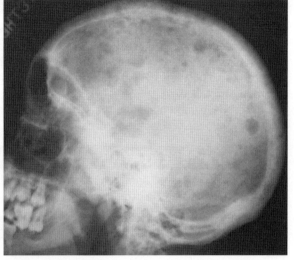

'Pepper pot' skull. Multiple characteristic lucencies throughout the skull.[†]

Primary hyperparathyroidism	Secondary hyperparathyroidism
Chondrocalcinosis	
Brown tumours	Metastatic calcification
Osteoporosis	Osteosclerosis

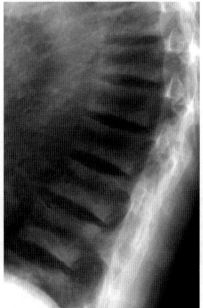

Hyperparathyroidism. Chondrocalcinosis in the knee menisci (A) and (B) the symphysis pubis. (C) Subperiosteal erosions along the radial side of the middle phalanx of the 2nd finger. Acro-osteolysis is also present. Metastatic calcification of the digital artery confirms this is secondary hyperparathyroidism. (D) cortical 'tunnelling' in the proximal phalanges. (E) Brown tumour within the distal tibia. (F) Precipitation of amorphous calcium phosphate in the soft tissues of the shoulder (hyperparathyroidism secondary to chronic renal disease).*

Secondary hyperparathyroidism. Lateral radiograph of the thoracic spine demonstrating increased sclerosis along the end-plates and increased lucency of the central part, giving a 'rugger jersey' spine appearance. Also note deformity of the vertebral bodies, with loss of height and increased diameter, in addition to wedge-shaped deformities at the upper thoracic spine related to decreased stability and weakness of the abnormal bone.**

HYPOPARATHYROIDISM

DEFINITION

- Hypoparathyroidism can result from reduced or absent parathyroid hormone (PTH) production, or from end organ resistance
- *Causes:* developmental abnormality ▶ post surgical ▶ autoimmune disorders ▶ end-organ resistance

CLINICAL PRESENTATION

- The resultant hypocalcaemia causes neuromuscular symptoms and signs (e.g. tetany and fits)

RADIOLOGICAL FEATURES

XR Generalized or localized osteosclerosis (particularly affecting the skull with a thickened vault) ▶ dense metaphyseal bands ▶ hypoplastic dentition ▶ metastatic calcification (e.g. within the basal ganglia and subcutaneous tissues around the hips and shoulders, interosseous membranes and tendinous insertions) ▶ enthesopathy with extraskeletal ossification in a paraspinal distribution (mimicking DISH) ▶ premature epiphyseal closure

PEARLS

- Ankylosing spondylitis can mimic hypoparathyroidism (but the latter has no erosive arthropathy and normal SI joints)

Pseudohypoparathyroidism (PHP) A group of autosomal dominant genetic disorders characterized by end-organ (bone and kidney) resistance to PTH ▶ normal parathyroid glands but an elevated PTH, with hypocalcaemia and hyperphosphataemia

- **Clinical features:** short stature ▶ reduced intellect ▶ rounded face ▶ tetany ▶ cataracts ▶ nail dystrophy

XR Premature epiphyseal fusion ▶ calvarial thickening ▶ bone exostoses ▶ bowing of the long bones ▶ basal ganglia calcification ▶ soft tissue calcification (plaque-like and within the subcutaneous tissues) ▶ shortened metacarpals – particularly the 4th and 5th resulting in a positive metacarpal sign

Pseudopseudohypoparathyroidism (PPHP) The features are the same as for PHP but there is no biochemical abnormality ▶ there remains an osseous response

THYROID DISEASE

DEFINITION

- High or low thyroid activity (thyrotoxicosis and myxoedema, respectively)

RADIOLOGICAL FEATURES

XR

- **Hyperthyroidism:** generalized osteoporosis
  - *Signs of thyroid acropachy:* painless diaphyseal periostitis predominantly involving the tubular bones of the hand (cf. painful HPOA)

- **Hypothyroidism:** congenital or childhood-onset (cretinism) results in delayed skeletal maturation and growth retardation ▶ fragmented ('stippled') epiphyses ▶ 'bullet-shaped' vertebrae ▶ wormian bones within the skull ▶ a small sella ▶ underdeveloped paranasal sinuses ▶ dense metaphyseal bands

PEARL

- **Thyroid acropachy:** the triad of pretibial myxoedema + thyroid eye disease (exophthalmos) + finger clubbing ▶ it usually occurs following therapy for hyperthyroidism

ACROMEGALY

DEFINITION

- This is due to an eosinophilic adenoma of the pituitary gland (leading to gigantism in children) ▶ it causes overgrowth of all tissues and organs with resultant premature osteoarthritis (hypertrophied cartilage is liable to fissuring and degeneration)

RADIOLOGICAL FEATURES

XR Generalized osteoporosis ▶ prominence of the muscle attachments (tuberosities) ▶ chondrocalcinosis ▶ widened joint spaces ▶ increased number of sesamoid bones

- **Skull:** enlarged mastoid air cells and sinuses ▶ frontal bossing (overgrowth of frontal sinuses) ▶ pituitary fossa enlargement ▶ prognathism (jaw protrusion)
- **Spine:** vertebral body enlargement ▶ posterior scalloping ▶ lordosis
- **Hands:** spade-like terminal tufts or arrowhead distal phalanges ▶ widened joints are best seen at the MCP joints
- **Feet:** increased heel pad thickness (> 25 mm) ▶ increased sesamoid bones

PEARL

- Cord compression can occur with spinal involvement

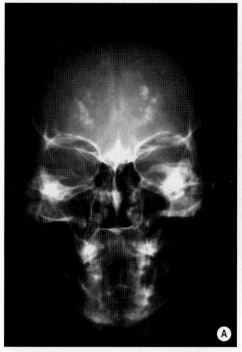
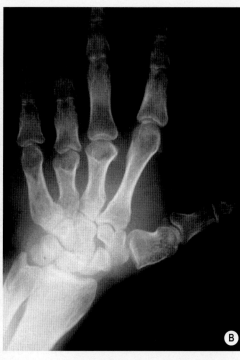

Hypoparathyroidism. (A) Soft tissue calcification may be present, seen here in the basal ganglia. (B) In pseudohypoparathyroidism there are shortened metacarpals, particularly the 4th and 5th.*

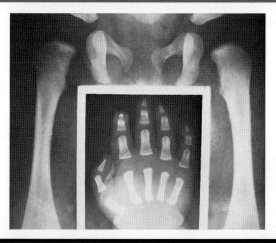

Cretinism. Marked skeletal retardation present in this 12-month-old child. Note the carpal and proximal femoral centres have not yet appeared.†

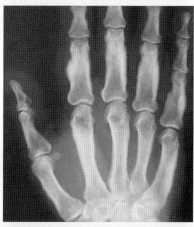

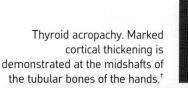

Thyroid acropachy. Marked cortical thickening is demonstrated at the midshafts of the tubular bones of the hands.†

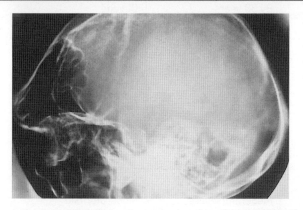

Acromegaly. The frontal sinuses are markedly enlarged with frontal bossing. A double floor is seen in the pituitary fossa with 'ballooning'.†

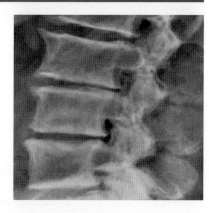

Acromegaly. The vertebral bodies show bony overgrowth. Mild posterior scalloping is also seen at several levels.†

OSTEOGENESIS IMPERFECTA (BRITTLE BONE SYNDROME)

Definition
- An inherited disorder of connective tissue resulting in osteoporosis ▶ it is due to genetic mutations affecting type I collagen

Clinical presentation
- It presents at birth, childhood or adulthood depending on its severity ▶ the fracture incidence declines following puberty
- It is characterized by bone deformity, fractures, osteopenia and blue sclera

Radiological features
- These vary according to the type of disease and its severity

XR Osteopenia ▶ fractures (with florid callus formation that can mimic an osteosarcoma) ▶ thin and under-tubulated (gracile) bones which are normal in length or shortened ▶ thickened or deformed bones (due to multiple fractures) ▶ intrasutural (wormian) bones that can be identified on a skull XR ▶ dentinogenesis imperfecta

Pearls
- **Type I (> 70%):** *autosomal dominant* ▶ the mildest and commonest form (which can present in adulthood)
  - Short stature ▶ joint laxity ▶ blue sclera ▶ dentinogenesis imperfecta ▶ presenile hearing loss ▶ vertebral fractures (4th decade)
  - There can be recurrent fractures with a normal or reduced bone density (and which may resemble NAI in infancy)
- **Type II (lethal perinatal) (10%):** *spontaneous dominant mutation* ▶ this is due to defective endochondral and membranous ossification

- Infants are small for dates ▶ blue sclerae ▶ shortened and deformed limbs due to multiple fractures (with a 'concertina' deformity of the lower limbs – there can also be 'beaded' ribs due to multiple fractures) ▶ severely under-mineralized cranial vault, distorted with moulding + Wormian bones ▶ platyspondyly
- Death occurs within 3 months (due to pulmonary insufficiency)
- **Type III (severe progressive) (15%):** *autosomal recessive/dominant*
  - Blue sclerae at birth turning white as an adult ▶ fractures are present from birth (affecting the long bones, clavicles, ribs and cranium) ▶ growth retardation ▶ increasing calvarial deformity (with facial distortion, malocclusion, prognathism, basilar invagination, progressive hearing loss) ▶ vertebral fractures (with progressive and severe kyphoscoliosis) ▶ expanded epiphyses with islands of calcified 'popcorn' cartilage ▶ pulmonary insufficiency (due to distortion of the thorax)
- **Type IV (moderately severe) (5%):** *autosomal dominant* ▶ it can be of variable severity
  - Blue sclerae at birth, which may turn white as an adult ▶ short stature ▶ basilar invagination ▶ dysplastic bones (with scoliosis and deformity particularly within the pelvis) ▶ joint laxity (particularly ankle or knee dislocation)
  - It can be confused with type I (but it is generally associated with more severe osteopenia and extensive bone deformities)

Osteogenesis imperfecta clinical (based on the Sillence classification) and radiological findings

	I	II	III	IV
Clinical findings				
Incidence	1:30 000	1:30 000	Rare	Unknown (rare)
Severity	Mild	Lethal	Severe	Mild/moderately severe
Death	Old age	Stillborn	By 30 years	Old age
Sclerae	Blue	Blue	Blue, then grey	White
Hearing impairment	Frequent	–	Rare	Rare
Teeth (dentinogenesis)	IA normal IB abnormal	– –	Abnormal –	IVA normal IVB normal
Stature	Short	–	Short	Normal/mildly short
Inheritance	Autosomal dominant	Autosomal dominant	Autosomal dominant/ autosomal recessive	Autosomal dominant
Radiological findings				
Fractures at birth	< 10%	Multiple	Frequent	Rare
Osseous fragility	Moderate/mild	Severe	Moderate/severe	Moderate/mild
Deformity	Mild	–	Severe	Variable

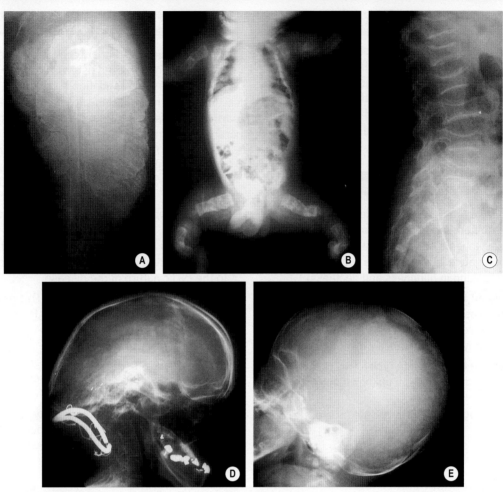

Osteogenesis imperfecta. (A) Exuberant callus formation around the fractured left femur. (B) Osteogenesis imperfecta type III in a neonate. This is the severe deforming type. Long bones are broad, angulated and short, and the ribs are beaded, secondary to multiple fractures. (C) Biconcave flattening of the vertebral bodies giving rise to the 'codfish' appearance. (D) Surgical stabilization for severe platybasia. Multiple wormian bones in the lambdoid suture. This skull vault shape is described as a 'Tam O'Shanter' appearance. Dentinogenesis imperfecta is also present. (E) Multiple wormian bones in neonate.*

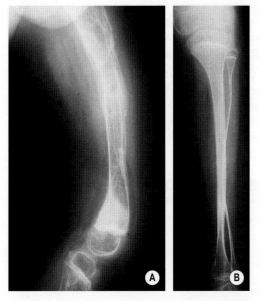

Osteogenesis imperfecta.
(A) Osteopenia with a fracture resulting in bowing and periostitis.
(B) The long bones are gracile and bowed with marked osteopenia.†

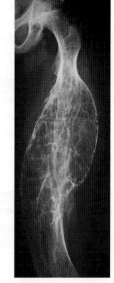

Osteogenesis imperfecta. The skeleton is immature. The femur is expanded and bowed at the site of previous fractures. The midshaft has a cystic, or soap bubble, appearance.†

OSTEOPETROSIS (MARBLE BONE DISEASE)

DEFINITION

- This is due to defective osteoclastic resorption of the primary spongiosa of bone (the osteoclasts are devoid of the ruffled borders through which they adhere to bone and through which they express their resorptive activity) ▶ in the presence of continued bone formation, there is generalized osteosclerosis and abnormalities of metaphyseal modelling

CLINICAL PRESENTATION

Autosomal recessive lethal type This demonstrates early manifestations ▶ obliteration of the marrow cavity leads to anaemia, thrombocytopenia and recurrent infections
- Hepatosplenomegaly ▶ hydrocephalus ▶ cranial nerve involvement (resulting in blindness and deafness)

Autosomal dominant benign type (Albers–Schönberg disease) It is often asymptomatic with late manifestations
- Pathological fractures ▶ anaemia ▶ facial palsy and deafness ▶ osteomyelitis (particularly mandibular)

Autosomal recessive intermediate type This is rare ▶ it presents during childhood with an unknown outcome on life expectancy
- Anaemia ▶ pathological fractures ▶ short stature ▶ hepatomegaly

RADIOLOGICAL FEATURES

Autosomal recessive lethal type Dense brittle bone (due to a generalized osteosclerosis) ▶ a lack of corticomedullary differentiation ▶ horizontal pathological fractures (with normal callus formation) ▶ skull sclerosis (particularly affecting the skull base) ▶ poorly developed paranasal and mastoid air cells
- *Erlenmeyer flask deformity:* abnormal bone modelling with undertubulation and expanded metaphyses (particularly affecting the distal femur and proximal humerus)
- *'Sandwich' appearance:* sclerosis of the vertebral end plates
- *'Bone within a bone' appearance:* alternating sclerotic and radiolucent bands at the ends of the diaphyses due to the cyclic nature of the disease

Autosomal dominant benign type This has similar radiological features to the recessive form (but they are less severe)
- *Type I:* fractures are unusual
- *Type II:* fractures are common, as are transverse metaphyseal bands and a raised serum acid phosphatase

Autosomal recessive intermediate type Diffuse osteosclerosis (skull base and facial bone involvement) ▶ abnormal bone modelling ▶ 'bone within a bone' appearance

HYPOPHOSPHATASIA

DEFINITION

- A normally autosomal recessive and rare genetic disorder
- There are reduced levels of serum alkaline phosphatase, with raised levels of blood and urine phosphoethanolamine (but normal serum calcium and phosphorus levels)

CLINICAL PRESENTATION

- There is a variable onset and severity (but it tends to be more severe if it presents during childhood)
- It can be fatal in the neonate because of inadequate thoracic or cranial ossification and support

RADIOLOGICAL FEATURES

Less severely affected children There are features of rickets but with larger lucent defects extending into the metaphysis and diaphysis ▶ generalized osteopenia with a coarse trabecular pattern (± fractures) ▶ bowing deformities and limb shortening

Severely affected neonates There is poor (if any) mineralization except for the skull base ▶ widened skull sutures ▶ wormian bones ▶ there can be later premature fusion (craniostenosis) with subsequent hydrocephalus

Adult onset Osteomalacia with Looser's zones ▶ a coarse trabecular pattern ▶ bowing deformities ▶ low-impact fractures with slow healing and little callus formation (particularly affecting the metatarsals) ▶ extraskeletal ossification of the ligaments and tendons ▶ chondrocalcinosis

PEARL

- There is no effective treatment

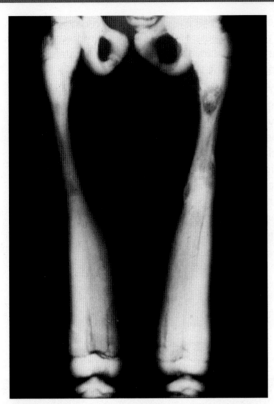

Osteopetrosis. Dense sclerotic brittle bones with abnormal modelling of the distal femora (Erlenmeyer flask deformity) due to the failure of normal osteoclastic periosteal bone resorption which remodels the bones as they grow in length by endochondral ossification.*

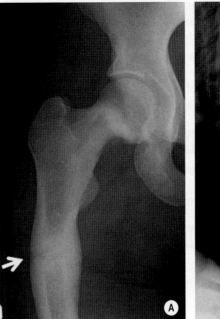 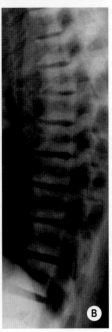

Osteopetrosis. Osteoclastic function is defective, resulting in dense sclerotic bones which are brittle and prone to fracture. There is evidence of abnormal modelling of the long bones due to the failure of normal osteoclastic periosteal bone resorption which remodels the distal shafts of bones as they grow in length by endochondral ossification. In (A) the AP radiograph of the hip and femur shows increased density of the proximal femur with a remote diaphysis fracture (arrow) and cortical thickening. The lateral thoracic spine radiograph in (B) demonstrates increased sclerosis along the end-plates with a 'sandwich' appearance.**

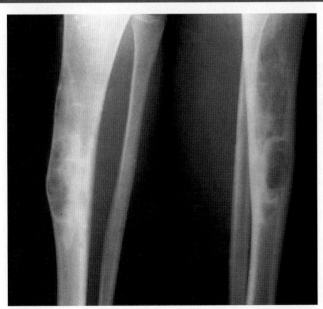

Hypophosphatasia. The appearances resemble a very severe form of rickets, with changes especially affecting the metaphyses but extending further into the diaphyses than is normal with rickets.†

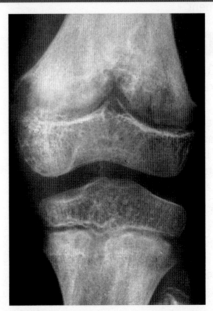

Hypophosphatasia. Affected patients may have rickets in childhood and osteomalacia in adulthood. The AP XR shows widened growth plates, particularly in the distal femur, and rather more patchy deficiency of calcification of the metaphysis than is characteristic of rickets due to vitamin D deficiency.*

HYPERPHOSPHATASIA

DEFINITION

- A rare genetic disorder resulting from mutations in osteoprotegerin ▶ there are markedly elevated serum alkaline phosphatase levels
- There is an increased rate of bone turnover with woven bone failing to mature into lamellar bone

CLINICAL PRESENTATION

- Fever ▶ bone pain ▶ progressive skull enlargement ▶ pathological fractures
- There is an onset from 2 years onwards

RADIOLOGICAL FEATURES

- It radiographically resembles Paget's disease of bone (it is sometimes called 'juvenile' Paget's disease)

– however Paget's disease is rare before 40 years of age and demonstrates monostotic or asymmetrically polyostotic skeletal involvement (there is whole skeletal involvement with hyperphosphatasia)

XR A decreased bone radiodensity with coarsening and disorganization of the trabecular pattern (due to increased bone turnover) ▶ widened diploic spaces with patchy skull sclerosis ▶ expanded long bone diaphyses with cortical thickening (affecting the concave aspect) ▶ long bone bowing resulting in a short stature ▶ coxa vara and protrusio acetabulae ▶ biconcave vertebrae with reduced height and radiodensity ▶ premature dentition loss (resorption of dentine with pulp replacement by osteoid)

Scintigraphy A 'superscan': generalized increased uptake (due to increased osteoblastic activity)

RENAL OSTEODYSTROPHY

DEFINITION

- Bone disease associated with chronic renal impairment
- Historically, radiological features were secondary to vitamin D deficiency and secondary hyperparathyroidism ▶ with improved management, features are now usually secondary to treatment

RADIOLOGICAL FEATURES

Untreated Vitamin D deficiency (rickets or osteomalacia) ▶ secondary hyperparathyroidism (erosions, osteosclerosis and brown cysts)

Treated Extensive vascular and soft tissue calcification is a complication of disease (phosphate retention) and treatment (phosphate binders) ▶ extreme soft tissue calcification may lead to ischaemic necrosis of the skin, subcutaneous tissues and muscle ('calciphylaxis')

Chronic renal failure, long-term haemodialysis and renal transplantation

- *Arthropathy:* this resembes a Charcot joint (without extensive debris) ▶ it is due to amyloid and crystal deposition, and is commonest within the shoulder and spine

- *Crystal deposition* (e.g. calcium hydroxyapatite, monosodium urate, calcium oxalate): this induces a synovitis and bursitis
- *Aluminium accumulation:* this produces similar changes to osteomalacia ▶ it commonly affects the ribs, vertebra, hips and pelvis
- *Effects secondary to steroid use:* avascular necrosis (commonly affecting the femoral head) ▶ osteomyelitis and septic arthritis

PEARLS

Renal tubular defects This involves either the proximal (responsible for absorption of glucose, inorganic phosphate and amino acids) or distal (responsible for urine concentration and acidification) tubule ▶ it results in a spectrum of biochemical disturbances that may result in the loss of phosphate, glucose, or amino acids alone or in combination with additional defects in urine acidification and concentration

- **Congenital:** Fanconi's syndrome ▶ cystinosis ▶ X-linked hypophosphataemia
- **Acquired:** Wilson's disease ▶ toxins ▶ interstitial nephritis ▶ oncogenic rickets

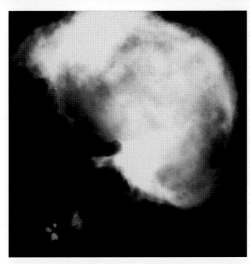

Hyperphosphatasia (juvenile Paget's disease). In the lateral skull XR there is sclerosis, thickening of the skull vault and evidence of bone softening with basilar invagination.*

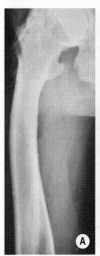
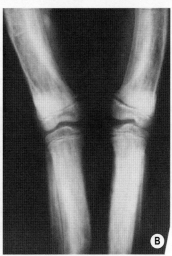

Familial hyperphosphataemia. (A) The femur is abnormal with some bowing, increased width, and prominent but irregular cortex, somewhat resembling Paget's disease. (B) The radiological appearances in this child are diagnostic. The bones are widened with loss of differentiation of cortex and medulla. A coarse trabecular pattern and bowing are also evident. Again, these features resemble those of Paget's disease.†

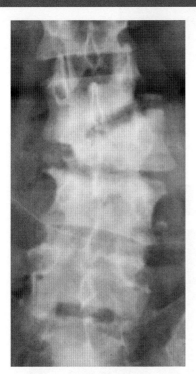

Chronic renal failure in a haemodialysis patient. An appearance resembling a Charcot spine.†

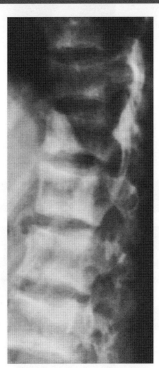

Renal osteodystrophy with a 'rugger jersey' spine due to end-plate sclerosis with alternating bands of lucency.†

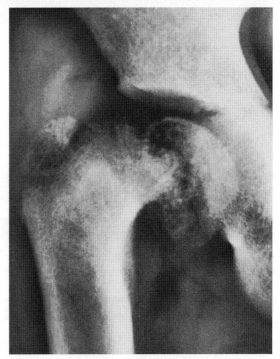

Uraemic osteodystrophy. The combination of rickets and secondary hyperparathyroidism is affecting this paediatric skeleton. The femoral metaphysis is irregular and the capital epiphysis shows considerable displacement (likened to a 'rotting fence post').†

HYPERVITAMINOSIS A

DEFINITION

- This occurs in patients receiving vitamin A or one of its synthetic derivatives (retinoic acids) for the treatment of skin disorders (e.g. refractory acne or psoriasis)

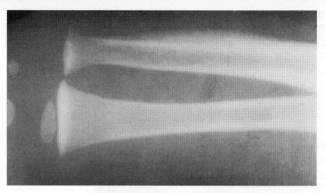

RADIOLOGICAL FEATURES

XR Large bony outgrowths from the spine (particularly affecting the cervical region) ▶ a mild enthesopathy involving the peripheral skeleton
- *Children:* cupping and splaying of the metaphyses ▶ diaphyseal periostitis (particularly affecting the metatarsals and ulna) ▶ widened cranial sutures

Hypervitaminosis A. There is increased cortical density and periosteal reaction, most marked in the ulna.

TOXIC POISONING

Lead poisoning

- This occurs in children following the ingestion of lead-containing paint or water (from lead-containing pipes) ▶ the lead is deposited within the growing metaphyses

XR Modelling deformities ▶ increased bone density ▶ dense metaphyseal bands ▶ widened sutures (secondary to raised intracranial pressure) ▶ radio-opacities seen on an AXR
- Lead encephalopathy is a serious complication

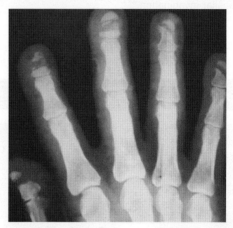

Vinyl chloride poisoning

- This is used during PVC manufacture and results in Raynaud's phenomenon and acro-osteolysis (± sacroiliitis and/or a liver haemangiosarcoma)

Vinyl chloride poisoning. Characteristic resorption of the central portions of the terminal phalanges (acro-osteolysis).

FLUOROSIS

DEFINITION

- This is due to long-term ingestion of excessive fluoride with an osteoclastic response to the ingested fluoride

RADIOLOGICAL FEATURES

XR Osteosclerosis (particularly affecting the axial skeleton) ▶ cortical thickening with encroachment on the medullary cavity ▶ enthesopathy with ligamentous ossification ▶ large spinal osteophytes
- Paraspinal ossification may cause a compression myelopathy

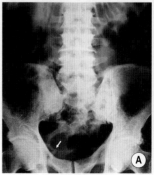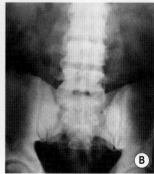

Fluorosis: axial skeletal abnormalities. (A) Osteosclerosis with a coarsened trabecular pattern, vertebral osteophytosis, and sacrotuberous ligament ossification (arrow) are the observed radiographic changes. (B) Osteosclerosis and vertebral osteophytosis are evident in a different patient with fluorosis. Note the bony eburnation about the sacroiliac joints.©35

SCURVY

DEFINITION

- A deficiency (usually dietary) of vitamin C (ascorbic acid) ▶ this leads to defective osteoid production by osteoblasts with reduced endochondral bone ossification
- Infants typically present between 6 and 9 months of age (when the maternal supplies have been exhausted)

RADIOLOGICAL FEATURES

XR The bones are generally osteopenic ▶ there is exuberant periosteal reaction (due to recurrent episodes of subperiosteal bleeding) ▶ haemarthroses can develop
- *Wimberger's sign:* a small epiphysis sharply marginated by a pencil-thin sclerotic rim (where the mineralization of osteoid continues)
- *Frankel's line:* a dense zone of provisional calcification at the growing metaphysis
- *Trummerfeld's zone:* a lucent zone (representing a lack of osteoid mineralization) beneath Frankel's line
- *Pelkan's spurs:* as Trummerfeld's zone weakens it is prone to fractures, which manifest themselves at the cortical margin as Pelkan's spurs

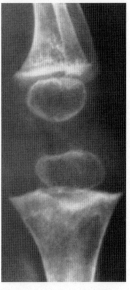
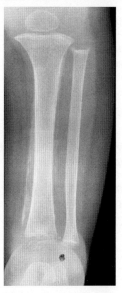

The epiphyseal margins are sclerotic (Wimberger's sign). There is a narrow epiphyseal plate, with increased density of the zone of provisional calcification (Frankel's line). The lucent zone beneath this is due to a lack of mineralized osteoid (Trummerfeld's zone).

Scurvy. Subperiosteal haemorrhage has elevated the periosteum. The healing stage shows marked periosteal new bone formation. Trummerfeld's zone is again visible, as is Pelkan's spur at the medial border of the proximal tibial metaphysis.

VITAMIN D INTOXICATION

DEFINITION

- Historically this followed vitamin D treatment (e.g. for sarcoidosis, TB and rheumatoid arthritis, and recently for cancer and psoriasis) ▶ it is now less common with the introduction of $1,25(OH)_2D$

CLINICAL PRESENTATION

- The resultant hypercalcaemia causes hypercalciuria, hypercalcaemia, impaired renal function and hypertension
- *Other symptoms and signs:* fatigue ▶ malaise ▶ weakness ▶ thirst ▶ polyuria ▶ anorexia ▶ nausea and vomiting

RADIOLOGICAL FEATURES

XR Metastatic calcification within tendons, ligaments, fascial planes, arteries and the periosteum (resulting in periostitis and bone sclerosis) ▶ nephrocalcinosis

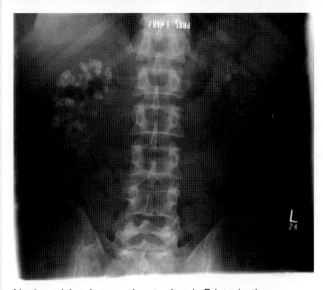

Nephrocalcinosis secondary to vitamin D intoxication.

5.8 JOINT DISEASE

CLINICAL AND RADIOLOGICAL FINDINGS IN JOINT DISEASE

Condition	Site of involvement	Discriminatory findings
Primary osteoarthritis (F>M ▶ > 45 years)	Hands	PIP and DIP joint involvement (Heberden's and Bouchard's nodes) ▶ no osteopenia
	Large joints (e.g. hip, knee)	Joint space narrowing ▶ subchondral sclerosis ▶ subchondral cysts ▶ marginal osteophytes
	Spine	Degenerative disc disease ▶ spondylosis deformans ▶ apophyseal joint involvement ▶ spinal stenosis ▶ foraminal stenosis
Erosive osteoarthritis (affects middle-aged females)	Hands	PIP and DIP joint involvement ▶ joint ankylosis ▶ 'gull-wing' deformities (central erosions and marginal osteophytes)
Rheumatoid arthritis (F>M ▶ Rh factor positive)	Hand and wrist	Symmetrical arthritis ▶ MCP and PIP joint involvement ▶ periarticular (early) and diffuse (late) osteopenia ▶ marginal erosions ▶ subluxation (swan neck and boutonnière deformities) ▶ periostitis is uncommon
	Large joints	Joint space narrowing ▶ marginal erosions ▶ synovial cysts ▶ protrusio acetabulae
	Spine	Atlantoaxial subluxation
Juvenile idiopathic arthritis (M = F ▶ affects children)	Hands	Joint ankylosis ▶ florid periosteal reaction ▶ osteopenia
	Large joints (e.g. knee)	Abnormalities of growth and maturation ▶ epiphyseal overgrowth and premature closure of the physis ▶ widened intercondylar notch
	Cervical spine	Apophyseal joint fusion ▶ atlantoaxial subluxation
Psoriatic arthritis (M>F ▶ nail changes ▶ HLA-B27 +ve)	Upper extremities (e.g. hands and feet)	'Sausage' digit ▶ DIP joint involvement ▶ terminal tuft erosion ▶ pencil-in-cup deformity ▶ joint ankylosis ▶ arthritis mutilans ▶ periosteal reaction ▶ no osteopenia
	SI joints	Asymmetric or unilateral sacroiliitis
	Spine	Coarse syndesmophytes
Reiter's syndrome (affects young male adults)	Lower extremities (e.g. foot)	Hallux involvement ▶ periosteal reaction ▶ calcaneal erosions ▶ osteopenia not prominent
	Spine	Coarse syndesmophytes
	SI joints	Asymmetric or unilateral sacroiliitis
Ankylosing spondylitis (M>F ▶ affects young adults ▶ HLA-B27 +ve in 95%)	SI joints	Bilateral symmetrical sacroiliitis ▶ ankylosis
	Spine	Anterior vertebral body squaring ▶ syndesmophytes ▶ paravertebral ossification ▶ bamboo spine
	Pelvis	'Whiskering' of the iliac crests and ischial tuberosities
Enteropathic arthropathies	SI joints	Symmetrical sacroiliitis
Gout (M>F)	Hands and feet (especially the great toe)	MTP joint of the great toe ▶ juxta-articular erosions ▶ punched-out lesions with an overhanging margin ▶ no periarticular osteopenia ▶ tophi

Condition	Site of involvement	Discriminatory findings
CPPD crystal deposition disease (M = F)	Any peripheral joint ▶ predilection for the knee	Degenerative changes ▶ chondrocalcinosis ▶ paucity of subchondral sclerosis
HA crystal deposition disease (M = F)	Predilection for the shoulder (supraspinatus tendon)	Periarticular calcification
Haemochromatosis (M>F)	Hands	2nd and 3rd MCP joint involvement ('squared' metacarpal heads) ▶ joint space narrowing ▶ 'hook-like' osteophytes ▶ numerous subchondral cysts
Alkaptonuria (ochronosis) (M = F)	Intervertebral discs ▶ SI joints ▶ large joints	Degenerative changes: disc calcification ▶ joint space narrowing ▶ periarticular sclerosis
Systemic lupus erythematosus (F>M ▶ affects young adults)	Hands	Reversible MCP joint subluxation
Scleroderma (F>M ▶ affects adults)	Hands	IP joint arthritis ▶ acro-osteolysis ▶ soft tissue calcifications
Mixed connective tissue disease (overlap syndrome)	Hands	PIP joint, MCP joint, mid-carpal involvement ▶ soft tissue swelling, calcifications or atrophy
Multicentric reticulohistiocytosis (F>M)	Hands and feet	DIP joint and carpal involvement ▶ soft tissue swelling ▶ articular erosions ▶ no osteopenia
Polymyositis / dermatomyositis	Proximal extremities Hands	Soft tissue calcification DIP joint erosions
Sarcoidosis	Distal and middle phalanges of the hands and feet	Punched-out cyst-like lesions ▶ 'lace-like' appearance
Haemophilic arthropathy (affecting males – but with female carriers)	Predilection for large joints (e.g. knee)	Epiphyseal overgrowth ▶ juxta-articular osteopenia ▶ erosion and cartilage destruction ▶ widened intercondylar and trochlear notches ▶ squared patella
Neuropathic arthropathy	Any joint	5 'D's': normal bone **D**ensity ▶ joint **D**istension ▶ bony **D**ebris ▶ joint **D**isorganization ▶ **D**islocation
Hypertrophic osteoarthropathy	Tubular bones (radius and ulna > tibia and fibula)	Diaphyseal and metaphyseal painful periostitis

OSTEOARTHRITIS

DEFINITION

- This is the most common joint disorder – it is a balance between degenerative joint destruction (stressed bone) and repair (non-stressed bone)
- **Primary OA:** there is no underlying cause ▶ it occurs in the context of normal biomechanical forces
  - *The joints most at risk:* thumb base ▶ DIP joints ▶ acromioclavicular joints ▶ knees ▶ hips ▶ 1st MTP joints ▶ spinal apophyseal joints
- **Secondary OA:** joints are damaged by previous disease
  - *Causes:* trauma ▶ systemic, metabolic or endocrine disorders (e.g. rheumatoid arthritis, ochronosis, haemochromatosis) ▶ crystal deposition disease ▶ neuropathic disorders ▶ congenital hip dislocation ▶ bone dysplasias

CLINICAL PRESENTATION

- Pain ▶ reduced movement ▶ joint crepitus (± effusion) ▶ early morning stiffness

RADIOLOGICAL FEATURES

Location It is typically asymmetrical and affects the hands, spine and large weight-bearing joints ▶ primary and secondary OA have similar radiological appearances

XR Localized joint space narrowing ▶ subchondral cysts and sclerosis ▶ marginal osteophytes ▶ loose bodies ▶ chondrocalcinosis

- Deformity and subluxation are uncommon ▶ osteoporosis and ankylosis are not features

Hand *The commonly affected joints:* 1st MCP joint, scaphotriquetral joint, IP joints ▶ distal and proximal IP joint prominences are commonly seen (Heberden's and Bouchard's nodes, respectively)

Knee Tibial spine spiking is an early sign ▶ the medial joint compartment shows the greatest narrowing (as it is subject to greater stressors) leading to a varus deformity ▶ it usually affects the *lateral* facet of patellofemoral joint ▶ there is articular and meniscal cartilage chondrocalcinosis

- *Chondromalacia patellae:* this is a related condition in younger patients with softening of the patellar cartilage (due to repetitive trauma)
- *Pellegrini–Stieda disease:* ossification of the medial collateral ligament is associated with degenerative change or may occur in isolation

Hip Loss of the superior weight-bearing joint space with marginal osteophytes, subchondral acetabular cysts (Egger's cyst) and sclerosis formation ▶ there is a tendency for superolateral femoral head subluxation (but there may be lateral restraining osteophytes) ▶ rarely medial migration can lead to protrusio acetabuli ▶ 'buttressing': osseous hypertrophy along the medial femoral neck

Foot/ankle The 1st MTP joint is the most commonly affected site (and is associated with hallux valgus)
- *'Talar beak':* the talonavicular joint is also commonly involved with formation of a dorsal bone spur

Spine See degenerative spinal disease Section 7 Chapter 6

PEARLS

Erosive OA This characteristically affects middle-aged women ▶ destructive changes outstrip productive changes and can mimic an erosive arthritis (such as psoriatic arthropathy)

XR Central erosions and marginal osteophytes (a 'gull wing' pattern) affecting the PIP + DIP joints (although large joint involvement has been described)
- *Differential:* psoriasis and rheumatoid arthritis – however these will have no 1st CMC joint involvement and will have marginal (as opposed to central) erosions with no true osteophyte formation

Plain radiographic findings in primary osteoarthritis and corresponding underlying pathophysiological causes*

Radiological finding	Pathological cause
Localized joint space narrowing	Articular cartilage fibrillation, ulceration and erosion lead to changes in collagen and protein polysaccharide structure of cartilage. This results in reduced turgor
Subchondral bony sclerosis	Increased osteoblastic activity resulting in new bone formation and increased cellularity of the subchondral bone
Osteophyte formation (most commonly marginal)	Cartilage and bone proliferation and revascularization of remaining cartilage
Bone cysts and bone collapse	Subchondral micro-fractures and passage of synovial fluid under pressure through the damaged cartilage to excavate a subchondral cyst
Gross deformity with subluxation	Ligamentous laxity resulting from mechanical force applied after the distortion of capsular structures
Loose bodies	Fragments of bone and cartilage become separated and, if not resorbed, become loose in the joint. They may reattach to the membrane, become vascularized and undergo endochondral ossification
Fibrocartilage or hyaline cartilage calcification	This is usually due to calcium pyrophosphate deposition disease (CPPD). The reparative response is usually quite florid

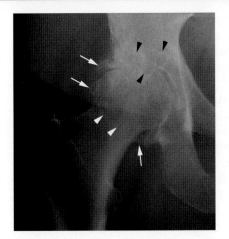

Severe osteoarthritis of the hip. There is joint space narrowing which has occurred asymmetrically within the joint, in this case affecting the superior joint (the most common pattern of hip involvement). Note also subchondral cyst formation (black arrowheads) and osteophytosis (arrows). The osteophytes form a rim around the femoral head/neck junction and are superimposed over the neck visible as a sclerotic line (white arrowheads), which should not be mistaken for a fracture.**

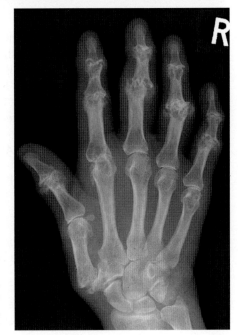

Erosive osteoarthritis. DP radiograph: in addition to the typical osteoarthritis changes seen in multiple joints, including the thumb base carpometacarpal joint, there is erosive change seen at many of the interphalangeal joints. The majority of these are central in location (subchondral) and give rise to the characteristic 'seagull wing' appearance of the distal articular surface (seen for example at the index, middle and ring distal interphalangeal joints).**

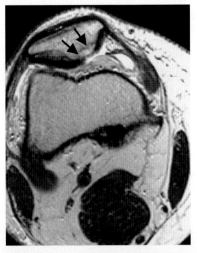

Chondromalacia patellae. T2WI MRI demonstrates denuded cartilage on the medial patella facet, with cystic change in the underlying bone (arrows).*

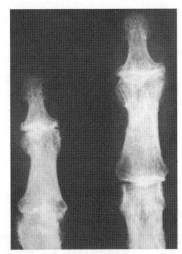

Osteoarthritis with joint narrowing and osteophyte formation (Heberden's nodes).†

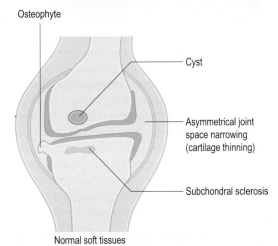

Osteophyte

Cyst

Asymmetrical joint space narrowing (cartilage thinning)

Subchondral sclerosis

Normal soft tissues

Schematic diagram showing typical joint changes associated with osteoarthritis.

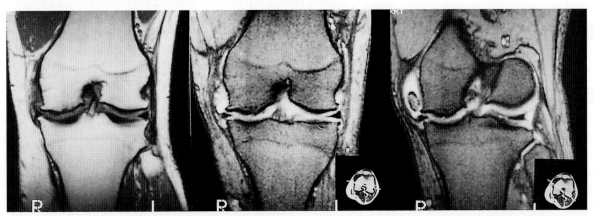

Osteoarthritis. MRI demonstrates degenerative changes of the knee with an effusion, loss of the medial meniscus, marginal osteophytosis and a large loose body lying medially within the joint.†

HAEMOPHILIC ARTHROPATHY

Definition

- There is recurrent bleeding into a joint due to a deficiency of blood clotting factors ▶ the repeated intra-articular bleeding leads to villous synovial hypertrophy with the accumulation of haemosiderin within macrophages ▶ with recurrent bleeds there is no longer complete recovery (restricted joint motion/ contractures/muscle atrophy)
  - *Classic haemophilia (haemophilia A):* X-linked recessive ▶ factor VIII deficiency
  - *Christmas disease (haemophilia B):* X-linked recessive ▶ factor IX deficiency

Clinical presentation

- Painful and swollen joints ▶ joint deformities
- It is only expressed in males (females can be carriers)

Radiological features

Location It particularly affects the knee, elbow, ankle and shoulder ▶ small peripheral joints are rarely involved

XR Hyperaemia causes epiphyseal overgrowth and accelerated maturation in the immature skeleton ▶ pannus similar to that in rheumatoid arthritis causes marginal erosions ▶ there is neither uniform nor symmetrical joint involvement
- **Acute:** joint effusion and oedema
- **Chronic:** juxta-articular osteoporosis resulting from haemorrhage and periarticular hyperaemia ▶ increased radio-opacity of the periarticular soft tissues·and synovium (due to haemosiderin deposition) ▶ articular erosion and cartilage destruction (due to a thickened synovium) ▶ secondary osteoarthritis (subchondral cysts are common)
  - *Knee:* a widened intercondylar notch ▶ a squared patella ▶ enlarged femoral condyles ▶ it demonstrates similar appearances to juvenile rheumatoid arthritis

- *Elbow:* an enlarged radial head, erosion of the trochlear notch and olecranon fossa
- Hip osteonecrosis ▶ protrusio acetabuli ▶ slipped epiphysis ▶ coxa valga
- **5 stages:**
  - *Stage I:* soft tissue swelling (± joint effusion) ▶ normal joint surfaces
  - *Stage II:* stage I + periarticular osteoporosis ▶ epiphyseal overgrowth
  - *Stage III:* erosions, sclerosis and subchondral cysts ▶ the joint space is preserved
  - *Stage IV:* stage III + focal or diffuse joint space narrowing
  - *Stage V:* a stiff contracted joint with significant degenerative change

MRI This can detect early synovial thickening and hypervascularity, and cartilaginous changes ▶ it can differentiate between acute and chronic soft tissue bleeding
- T1WI/T2WI: a thickened and irregular synovium with fibrosis and haemosiderin deposition
  - *Haemosiderin:* this generates low SI foci, with a blooming artefact on gradient-echo (GE) sequences

Pearls

- Septic arthritis is a rare complication of haemophilia

Intraosseous subperiosteal or soft tissue pseudotumours

These can develop following the encapsulation of episodes of repeated haemorrhage ▶ it occurs particularly within the femur and around the pelvis ▶ it presents as a painless expanding mass, with soft tissue and bone destruction ▶ can be calcified ▶ mural nodules are characteristic

MRI T1WI: a low SI thick fibrous capsule ▶ T2WI: central high SI (due to blood breakdown products)

NEUROPATHIC ARTHROPATHY (CHARCOT JOINT)

Definition

- A destructive and productive articular abnormality following a loss of pain sensation and/or proprioception

Clinical presentation

- Painless joint deformity and destruction on a background of neurological disease

Radiological features

Location The distribution helps determine the cause (see table)

Atrophic form This occurs early and is more acute ▶ resorption of the ends of affected bones results in sharp pointed ends ▶ there is an absence of osteoporosis, sclerosis, fragmentation or soft tissue debris ▶ it may lead to joint dislocation

Hypertrophic form This occurs later with a slow progression ▶ it begins with a joint effusion ▶ the joint spaces are initially widened but then narrowed ▶ there is marked bony sclerosis (and no osteoporosis) ▶ fragmentation of the articular surfaces results in bony debris, which may later fuse into a large dense and well-organized corticated bony mass (± fusion with the underlying bone or dissection into the muscle planes) ▶ there is periosteal new bone formation ▶ subluxation and dislocation preceeds total joint disorganization ▶ pathological fractures can occur
- **5 'D's':** normal bone **D**ensity ▶ joint **D**istension ▶ bony **D**ebris ▶ joint **D**isorganization ▶ **D**islocation

Pearl

- *Differential:* the pseudoneuropathic form of CPPD

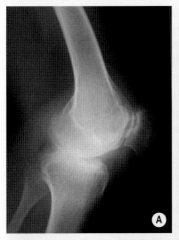 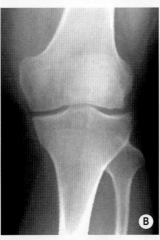 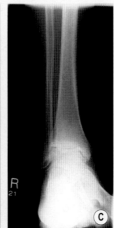

Classic radiographic findings in hemophilia. (A) Note squaring of inferior pole of the patella. (B) Enlarged femoral condyles. (C) Tibiotalar slant.©35

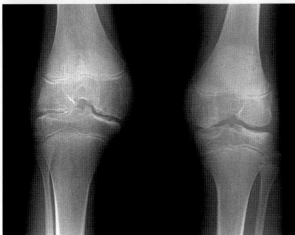

Bleeding into the joints in haemophilia. AP XR demonstrating widened intercondylar notches, narrow joint spaces and erosive change. The right knee is more severely affected.*

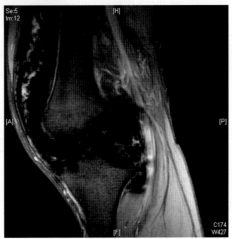

Gradient echo (GE) MR images of the knee in a patient with advanced haemophilia. There is low signal abnormality in the synovium, secondary to hemosiderin deposition. GE images are the most sensitive to susceptibility, and this can be seen in the marked 'blooming' artefact.©35

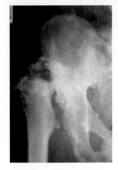 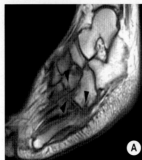 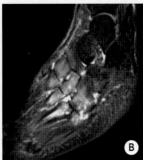

Syphilitic neuropathic arthropathy of the hip. There is destruction and fragmentation of the right femoral head leading to bony dislocation and joint disorganization.*

Acute neuropathic osteoarthropathy. (A) Sagittal, T1WI shows marginal erosions (arrowheads) at the Lisfranc joint and intertarsal joints. Note that the surrounding subcutaneous fat is preserved, a finding that would be unlikely in the setting of infection. (B) Sagittal, T2W, fat-suppressed MR image of the same patient shows bone marrow edema with extensive regional distribution around the Lisfranc and intertarsal joints that contain small effusions.©35

Conditions associated with neuropathic arthropathy*		
Condition	Prevalence of arthropathy	Joints most commonly affected
Congenital insensitivity to pain	100%	Ankle, tarsal, knee, hip
Syringomyelia	20–50%	Shoulder, elbow, wrist, cervical spine
Neurosyphilis	5–10%	Knee, hip
Diabetes mellitus	1%	Midfoot, forefoot
Alcohol related	Rare	Foot

JUVENILE IDIOPATHIC ARTHRITIS (JIA)

Definition

- This is otherwise known as juvenile rheumatoid arthritis or juvenile chronic arthritis
- It is an inflammatory disorder of the connective tissues characterized by joint swelling, pain and tenderness affecting ≥ 1 joints for at least 6 weeks in patients who are < 16 years of age

Clinical presentation

- **Acute systemic onset type (Still's disease):** constitutional symptoms ▶ hepatosplenomegaly ▶ there is little joint involvement
- **Oligoarthritis:** ≤ 4 joints involved during the 1st 6 months, usually progressing to:
- **Polyarthritis:** ≥ 5 joints involved (both presentations are equally common) ▶ there is often asymmetrical involvement of the peripheral joints
- **Systemic arthritis:** arthritis + a systemic illness ▶ there can also be a psoriatic arthritis and an enthesitis-related arthritis

Radiological features

Location Knee > wrist ▶ also involved: feet, shoulders, elbows and hips

Early Soft tissue swelling ▶ synovitis ▶ synovial hyperplasia and pannus formation ▶ a widened joint space (secondary to an effusion) ▶ periarticular osteopenia
- Initially there is cartilage preservation

Late Epiphyseal overgrowth and premature closure of the physis (due to a prolonged synovitis and hyperaemia) ▶ cartilage loss ▶ there is often extensive ankylosis (affecting the CMC and mid-carpal joints) ▶ joint space narrowing
- Bone erosions are uncommon

Peripheral joints Marked radial head enlargement may be seen ▶ a widened intercondylar notch of the knee ▶ overtubulated diaphyses ▶ enlarged and osteoporotic epiphyses with compression fractures ▶ florid periosteal new bone formation within the phalanges, metacarpals and metatarsals (cf. RA) ▶ enlarged, irregular and squared carpal bones (due to erosion and repair)
- Misalignment and subluxation are uncommon

Spine/sacroiliac joints The cervical spine is the most commonly affected region (it is rare within the thoracolumbar spine or sacroiliac joints) ▶ atlantoaxial subluxation is common ▶ compression fractures ▶ scoliosis (with advanced disease)
- There can be underdevelopment and block fusion of the vertebral bodies and intervertebral discs (due to disc and apophyseal joint ankylosis which can also mimic Klippel–Feil syndrome)

Pearls

- Rheumatoid factor is positive in 10% of cases
- *Complications:* leg length discrepancy due to growth plate disturbance ▶ contractures ▶ AVN (due to JIA or the resultant steroid therapy)
- In some children isolated hip involvement with bilateral protrusio acetabuli has been documented

DIFFUSE IDIOPATHIC SKELETAL HYPEROSTOSIS (DISH) (FORESTIER'S DISEASE)

Definition

- Marked hyperostosis at multiple sites ▶ involvement typically at enthesis sites
- A multifocal entity characterized by 'flowing' ligamentous spinal ossification involving ≧ 4 contiguous vertebrae with preservation of the underlying disc height (cf. degenerative disc disease)
- There is no apophyseal or sacroiliac joint fusion (cf. ankylosing spondylitis) ▶ there is hyperostosis of certain ligamentous attachments

Clinical presentation

- Asymptomatic ▶ back pain and stiffness ▶ tendinosis (commonly affecting the elbow and heel)

Radiological features

Spine T7 to T12 are commonly affected (it is typically right sided as the pulsating aorta inhibits ossification on the left) ▶ ossification of the anterior longitudinal ligament is seen at the affected level (up to 2 cm)
- New bone formation within the cervical spine can cause dysphagia
- Ossification of the posterior longitudinal ligament can cause spinal stenosis

Extraspinal features

- *Enthesopathy:* heel and elbow spurs and a whiskered pelvic appearance
- *Ossification:* pelvic tendons and ligaments ▶ superior $\frac{1}{3}$ of the sacroiliac joints ▶ symphysis pubis ▶ calcaneus ▶ tarsal bones ▶ patella ▶ olecranon ▶ humerus ▶ hands

Pearl

- DISH is a reaction to stress and not an arthritis as such

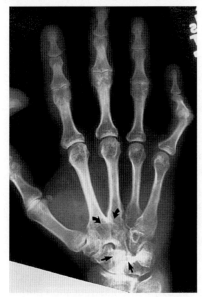

Wrist fusion in juvenile rheumatoid arthritis. Posteroanterior (PA) view of the wrist shows fusion at the second and third carpometacarpal joints (curved arrows). Some of the carpal bones (arrows) are also fused.©34

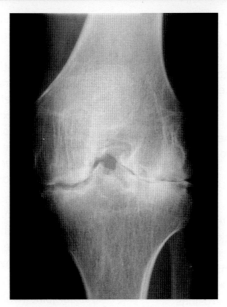

JIA of the knee. There is secondary degenerative change with loss of joint space, subchondral sclerosis associated with epiphyseal overgrowth, and widening of the intercondylar notch.*

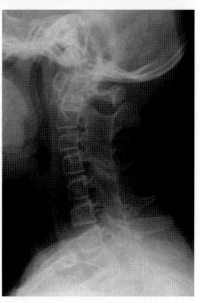

Lateral radiograph of the cervical spine. There is squaring of the vertebral bodies. Note the extensive ankylosis of the facet joints posteriorly and widening of the space anterior to the odontoid.

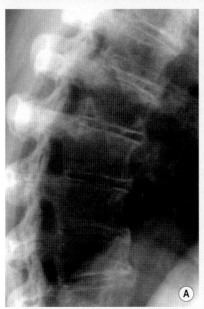

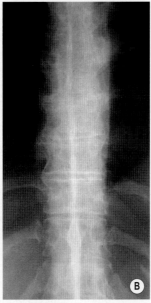

(A)

(B)

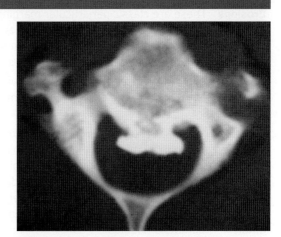

DISH. CT demonstrating ossification of the posterior longitudinal ligament.†

DISH. (A) Lateral and (B) AP XRs show bridging osteophytes at multiple levels, out of proportion to the degree of underlying degenerative change.*

RHEUMATOID ARTHRITIS

Definition

- An inflammatory polyarticular synovitis (with synovial hypertrophy) of unknown aetiology ▶ it is a multisystem disease, with a positive rheumatoid factor identified in the majority ▶ joint destruction with late disease

Clinical presentation

- Joint pain ▶ morning stiffness ▶ symmetrical joint swelling ▶ rheumatoid nodules ▶ tendon rupture (F > M)

Radiological features

Location A *symmetrical* polyarthritis of the small joints of the hands and feet > larger joints > axial skeleton (usually affecting the cervical spine)

- **Early:** juxta-articular osteopenia ▶ symmetrical soft tissue swelling ▶ joint space widening ▶ tenosynovitis
- **Later:** diffuse osteoporosis ▶ marginal erosions involving the bare area (the bone between the edge of the articular cartilage and the joint capsule attachment) ▶ joint space narrowing ▶ reduced soft tissue swelling ▶ subchondral cysts ▶ joint subluxation and dislocation ▶ joint ankylosis (this is uncommon but typically affects the carpus)
- **End stage:** pancompartmental loss of the joint spaces ▶ resorption of the carpal bones and 'arthritis mutilans'

Osteopenia *Early:* periarticular ▶ *late:* it becomes generalized due to steroid use or limitation of movement

Joint space changes Early widening (due to synovial hypertrophy, effusion or pannus interposition between the articular surfaces) is followed by narrowing (due to cartilage destruction by pannus) ▶ joint alignment abnormalities are caused by tendonitis, tendon rupture or synovitis weakening the capsule

Erosions These are classic periarticular marginal erosions involving the 'bare areas' of bone ▶ they less commonly involve the larger joints but are often more destructive in nature due to the greater stresses involved

Periostitis This is less commonly seen than with a seronegative arthropathy ▶ if present it is commoner within the feet

Soft tissue changes Fusiform swelling (due to capsular distension and oedema) over the IP and MCP joints ▶ swelling over the ulnar styloid (due to local involvement of the extensor carpi ulnaris tendon sheath) ▶ distension of the knee joint capsule (due to lateral displacement of the normally barely visible fat planes adjacent to the distal femur) ▶ rheumatoid nodules

Hand Proximal distribution (carpal/MCP/PIP joints) with sparing of the DIP joints (cf. OA and psoriatic arthritis) ▶ commonly affected sites: the 2nd and 3rd MCP joints (initially affecting the radial side – more distal erosions are less commonly seen) ▶ the ulnar and radial styloid processes ▶ the distal radioulnar joint and carpus

- Ulnar deviation (due to MCP subluxation)
- Volar subluxation and dislocation of the phalanges at the MCP joint
- Rotary subluxation of the scaphoid and drift of the entire carpus in an ulnar (± volar) direction
- *Boutonnière deformity:* proximal IP joint flexion and distal IP joint extension
- *Swan neck deformity:* proximal IP joint extension and distal IP joint flexion
- *'Telescope' fingers:* phalangeal dislocation with subsequent shortening

Foot Changes lag behind those in the hands ▶ disease initially involves the MTP joints (particularly the 4th and 5th) with erosions on the bare areas of the metatarsal heads ▶ lateral phalangeal subluxation with PIP joint dorsiflexion deformities ▶ bony ankylosis with chronic disease

Hips There is predominantly medial joint involvement (cf. superior joint involvement in OA) ▶ medial migration and acetabular resorption results in protrusio acetabuli

Shoulder Lateral clavicular resorption ▶ upward subluxation of the humeral head

Spine Disease usually affects the cervical spine (the thoracic and lumbar spine are rarely involved) ▶ cervical spine facet joint erosions may result in subluxation and nerve entrapment ▶ basilar invagination is a late feature

- *Atlantoaxial subluxation:* this is due to cruciate ligament damage (separation in flexion of > 2.5 mm in adults or 5 mm in children is abnormal)
- *Odontoid erosion:* this results from involvement of the synovial joint between the odontoid peg and cruciate ligament or involvement of the small bursa adjacent to the odontoid
- *Odontoid fracture:* this is due due to erosions or osteopenia

MRI This can detect early bone marrow oedema and early erosions (compared with XR)

Pearls

- **Complications:** secondary infection ▶ insufficiency fractures and avascular necrosis (due to steroid use) are commonly seen in the hip
- **Extra-articular manifestations:** pleural effusions ▶ interstitial fibrosis ▶ pulmonary nodules ▶ pericarditis ▶ myocarditis
- *Felty's syndrome:* RA + splenomegaly + neutropenia
- *Caplan's syndrome:* RA + pneumoconiosis

Jaccoud's arthritis This is not related to RA, but causes a severe non-destructive symmetrical polyarthropathy in the hands ▶ it follows rheumatic fever and is an uncommon disease

- *Early:* reversible ulnar deviation ▶ bone is not usually involved although erosions may occur in some cases
- *Late:* 'hook-like' projections and pseudocysts at the radio-palmer aspects of the metacarpal heads ▶ contractures

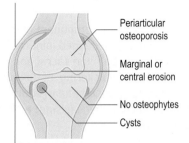

Symmetrical soft tissue swelling

Periarticular osteoporosis

Marginal or central erosion

No osteophytes

Cysts

Diffuse joint space narrowing (erosions of cartilage)

Diagram showing the typical radiographic changes in rheumatoid arthritis.

Plain radiographic findings in rheumatoid arthritis and corresponding pathophysiological causes*	
Radiological findings	**Pathological cause**
Periarticular osteoporosis	This reflects localized hyperaemia and is most pronounced during the acute stages of the disease
Soft tissue swelling	This represents synovial hypertrophy, joint effusion and periarticular soft tissue oedema, and is typically symmetrical
Erosions	These are marginal in location caused by the inflammatory and erosive effect of the inflamed synovium on the 'bare area' of the joint (that part of the joint adjacent to the synovium which is not covered by cartilage)
Joint space narrowing	This results from cartilage loss. Early uniform cartilage loss results from interruption of the flow of synovial fluid nutrients by the pannus. Later the hypertrophied synovium causes direct destruction with undermining of the cartilage and destruction of the subchondral bone. There may be joint widening in the early stages or ankylosis in the end stages of the disease
Subchondral cysts	These result from destruction of the subchondral plate by pannus, which allows joint fluid to be forced into the subchondral bone under pressure
Joint subluxation and dislocation	These are due to damage or destruction to tendons and ligaments as a result of the inflammatory pannus. In the early stages the deformity may be reversible and therefore underestimated on plain films
Generalized regional osteoporosis	This results from pain-induced disuse and may be exacerbated by the effects of therapy (e.g. steroids)

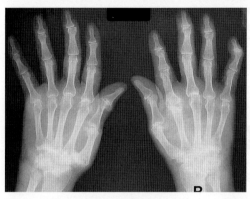

Rheumatoid arthritis. Bilateral symmetrical changes with soft tissue swelling (especially over the ulnar styloids). Erosions are seen at the carpus, MCP joints, distal radius and ulna with joint space narrowing and bone collapse. There is a swan neck deformity of the right 5th DIP joint.[†]

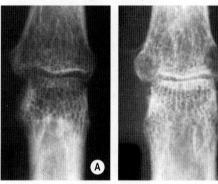

Rheumatoid arthritis. (A) Initial XR shows early trabecular loss around the finger PIPJ with joint space preservation. (B) Subsequently there is erosive change with joint space narrowing.[†]

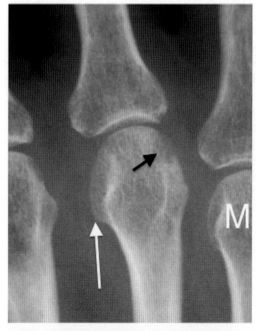

Rheumatoid arthritis with the earliest feature of erosive change seen along the radial border of this middle metacarpal head. There is localised osteopenia with a 'dot-dash' pattern of deossification (white arrow). Note also the symmetrical soft-tissue swelling and frank erosion of the ulna border (black arrow).**

619

ANKYLOSING SPONDYLITIS

DEFINITION

- This is a progressive chronic spondyloarthropathy with a proliferative chronic synovitis involving the diarthrodial joints
- The disease hallmark is a relatively rapid onset of joint ankylosis (sacroiliitis and enthesitis of the axial skeleton)

CLINICAL PRESENTATION

- There is an insidious onset of back pain and stiffness
- The peak age of onset is between 25 and 35 years (M:F, 10:1)

RADIOLOGICAL FEATURES

Location

- The lower ⅔ of the sacroiliac joints ▶ the spine (affecting the apophyseal joints, annulus fibrosus, and deep layers of the anterior longitudinal ligament)
- *Other sites:* hips ▶ shoulders ▶ knees ▶ ankles ▶ costovertebral joints ▶ manubriosternal joint ▶ symphysis pubis ▶ temporomandibular joints
- Involvement of the small joints of the hands and feet is unusual

Spine

- Involvement begins within the thoracolumbar region and progresses cranially (preceding any sacroiliitis), with eventual ankylosis of the apophyseal joints ▶ cervical involvement is rare
- **'Shiny or ivory corner':** the disease is characterized by early erosion and sclerosis adjacent to the vertebral end plates of the anterior vertebral body corners
- **Anterior vertebral body 'squaring':** mineralization of the anterior longitudinal ligament fills in the anterior vertebral body concavity
- **Romanus lesion:** sclerotic healing of any vertebral end-plate erosive change stands out in marked contrast to the remaining vertebral body
- **Andersson lesion:** destructive sclerotic inflammation of an intervertebral disc can resemble an infective discitis
- **Syndesmophytes:** these represent ossification of the outer lamellae of the annulus fibrosus and immediately adjacent anterior longitudinal ligament
  - Complete fusion of the vertebral bodies and sacroiliac joints produces the classic 'bamboo' spine
  - It is differentiated from an osteophyte by its vertical rather than horizontal origin
  - It is distinguished from DISH by the lack of a radiolucent line between the calcified ligament and the anterior margin of a vertebral body
- **Other features:** secondary degenerative changes between fused segments ▶ thoracic kyphosis ▶ demineralization of the entire spine

Sacroiliac joints

- There is bilateral and symmetrical involvement

XR Sacroiliitis involves the synovial component of the sacroiliac joint ▶ there are initially ill-defined joint margins within the ligamentous portion as both the sacral and iliac cortices become indistinct due to 'whiskering' of the bone ▶ the joint space then becomes widened and irregular with focal erosions (particularly affecting the iliac side) ▶ there is sclerosis and ultimately ankylosis

MRI Detects early subchondral bone marrow oedema

Peripheral joints (30%)

- It mainly affects the hips, shoulders and knees (the hands and feet are rarely involved)

XR Compared with rheumatoid arthritis, bony ankylosis predominates rather than erosions ▶ there is less demineralization and more reactive sclerosis

Enthesitis

- An enthesis is a region of a bone where a tendon, capsule or ligament attaches ▶ enthesitis is also seen in psoriatic arthritis, enteropathic spondylitis and Reiter's syndrome

XR Irregular new bone proliferation (a 'whiskering' effect) is seen at an enthesis – this is sometimes associated with a reactive sclerosis ▶ it is commonly found at the ischial tuberosity, iliac margins and calcaneum

PEARL

- Ankylosing spondylitis is strongly linked to the HLA-B27 histocompatability antigen

Complications

- Fracture of a rigid osteoporotic spine (relatively common) can lead to a pseudoarthrosis, which is an unstable injury ▶ there may be an associated spinal cord injury
- *Visceral complications:* aortic valve disease ▶ upper zone pulmonary fibrosis
- *Differential diagnosis:* enteropathic arthropathy
  - This affects up to 10% of patients with ulcerative colitis and Crohn's disease ▶ bowel disease usually precedes any arthropathy
- **Central type (predominant form):** there is a sacroiliitis and spondylitis identical to that seen with ankylosing spondylitis
  - The course is independent of any underlying bowel disease
- **Peripheral type:** periarticular osteopenia ▶ joint space narrowing affecting the hands, wrists and feet
  - Recurrent acute mild synovitis coincides with exacerbations of bowel disease ▶ it tends to resolve following colectomy

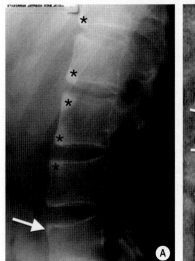

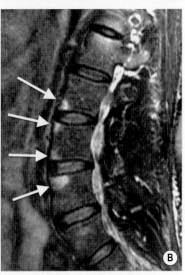

(A) Ankylosing spondylitis (AS) with sclerosis of the vertebral corners (Romanus lesions). The radiograph shows advanced lesions (*) and an early lesion (arrow). (B) STIR sagittal MR image of a different AS patient with oedema of the vertebral corners (arrows) termed MR Romanus lesions.**

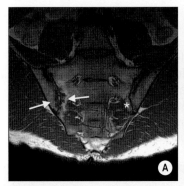

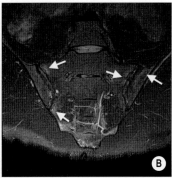

T1-weighted (A) and T2 fat-supressed (B) coronal MR images of the sacroiliac joints (SIJ) in ankylosing spondylitis. The T1-weighted image readily demonstrates erosion (arrows) in the right SIJ with joint space loss on the left (*), all indicative of damage. Note how poor the T2-weighted image is at demonstrating erosion; however, it shows subchondral oedema (arrows) more reflective of disease activity.**

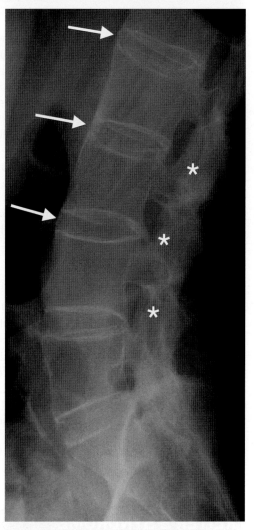

Ankylosing spondylitis with bamboo spine. Bridging vertical syndesmophytes are seen around the intervertebral discs (arrows). Note no facet joint spaces are visualised, indicating fusion of the posterior joints between L3 and S1 (*).**

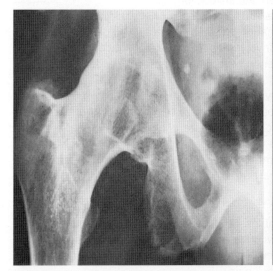

Ankylosing spondylitis. Bone ankylosis across the joint cartilage.†

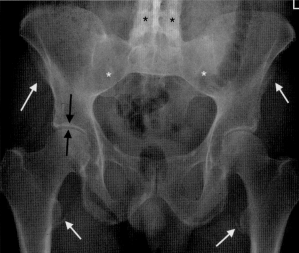

Patient with ankylosing spondylitis with spinal fusion (black*) and SIJ fusion (white*). There is hip arthropathy with diffuse loss of joint space (black arrows) and flattened configuration of the femoral heads. Widespread entheseal new bone formation is noted around the pelvis (white arrows).**

621

PSORIATIC ARTHROPATHY

Definition

- This is a seronegative spondyloarthropathy
- Skin changes typically precede the arthropathy (7%)
  - **Asymmetrical oligoarthritis** (70%): this affects ≥1 random joints ▶ often associated with dactylitis
  - **Symmetrical polyarthritis:** this is indistinguishable from rheumatoid arthritis (15%)
  - **Oligoarthritis:** distributed symmetrically and involving any synovial joint
  - **Inflammatory arthritis of the spine:** a pattern of spinal and large joint disease similar to ankylosing spondylitis
  - **Arthritis mutilans:** a severe destructive arthropathy mainly involving the small joints of the hands and feet with digit shortening and telescoping

Radiological features

Location Hands ▶ feet ▶ spine ▶ SI joints

- **Hands and feet:** a bilateral, *asymmetrical* destructive arthropathy predominantly affecting the DIP joints ▶ periarticular erosions ▶ any soft tissue swelling precedes bone changes ▶ periarticular osteopenia is not a feature (cf. RA) ▶ widened joint spaces ▶ fluffy reactive new bone formation or periosteal reaction along the diaphysis (cf. RA) ▶ terminal tuft resorptions (acro-osteolysis) ▶ subluxation or cartilage loss (affecting a minority) ▶ spontaneous bony ankylosis of the IP joints (late feature) ▶ tenosynovitis ▶ pancarpal involvement with carpal erosion, destruction and fusion
  - *'Pencil-in-cup' appearance:* tapering of the phalanx head
  - *'Sausage' digit:* swelling of the entire finger
- **Calcaneus:** similar features to Reiter's disease (fluffy sclerosis + erosions at the Achilles tendon insertion)
- **Larger joints:** asymmetrical and monoarticular involvement ▶ soft tissue swelling and effusions ▶ marginal erosions ▶ uniform joint space narrowing (no osteopenia) ▶ new bone formation + periosteal new bone formation at the entheses
- **Spine (25%):** Coarse *asymmetrical* non-marginal syndesmophytes ▶ multiple levels (with skip areas) ▶ occasional 'squared' vertebral bodies ▶ atlantoaxial subluxation
- **Syndesmophytes:** these originate from the mid-vertebral body (and are not always attached to a vertebral body) ▶ more superficially situated than with ankylosing spondylitis ▶ vertically orientated (cf. horizontal osteophytes)
- **Sacroiliac joints (25%):** A *bilateral and asymmetrical* sacroiliitis ▶ involvement of the iliac side of a joint first

Pearls

- Sacroiliac involvement is indistinguishable from Reiter's disease ▶ sacroiliac involvement is more asymmetrical than that seen with ankylosing spondylitis
- *Differential:* rheumatoid arthritis ▶ psoriatic arthritis is more likely if there is preserved bone density, periosteal reaction, asymmetrical involvement, a sausage digit, spontaneous bony ankylosis and enthesitis

REITER'S SYNDROME

Definition

- A seronegative spondyloarthropathy tending to affect young men
- *Reiter's triad:* conjunctivitis + urethritis + arthritis
  - Additional features include balanitis and a specific dermatitis (keratoderma blennorrhagicum affecting the palms of the hands and soles of feet)
- It is associated with infectious agents, particularly sexually transmitted diseases (e.g. *Chlamydia*) ▶ it can also follow dysentery-like symptoms (e.g. *Salmonella, Shigella, Yersinia, Campylobacter*)

Radiological features

Location Similar appearances to psoriatic arthritis but affecting the lower extremities as opposed to the upper extremities with psoriatic disease

- MTP > calcaneus > ankle > knee
- **Peripheral skeleton:** prominent bone proliferation ▶ periosteal reactions are common ▶ periarticular osteopenia is only seen in the acute inflammatory phase (osteoporosis is not a prominent feature) ▶ random asymmetrical joint involvement (although the 1st MTP joint is the most commonly involved) ▶ uniform joint space narrowing and marginal erosions followed by joint destruction and dislocation
- **Calcaneus (50%):** erosions or fluffy periosteal new bone formation and spurs ▶ increased density and size ▶ typical involvement of the site of attachment of the Achilles tendon and plantar surface (plantar aponeurosis insertion)
- **Spine:** asymmetric coarse non-marginal syndesmophytes with a discontinuous distribution
- **Sacroiliac joints:** a *bilateral and asymmetrical* sacroiliitis (the iliac side is affected first) ▶ involvement is less commonly seen than with psoriasis ▶ complete fusion is rare

Pearl

- There is an association with the HLA-B27 antigen ▶ patients with the antigen have more acute disease, a higher prevalence of sacroiliitis, and more frequent and chronic back pain

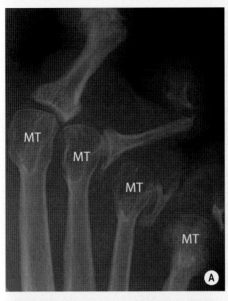

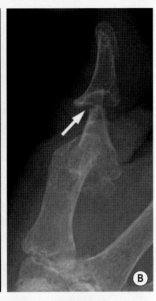

Psoriatic arthritis. (A) There is arthritis mutilans present with subluxation and erosion of the metacarpophalangeal joints and marked bone loss with a peg-like appearance to the phalanges. MT, metatarsal heads. (B) There is a severe deforming arthritis of the thumb and the 'pencil in cup' pattern of erosive change is appreciated at the interphalangeal joint (arrow).**

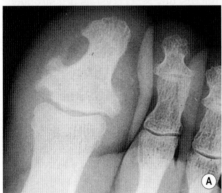

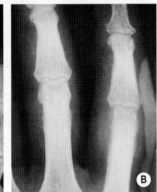

(A) Psoriasis. The erosions at the bases of the distal phalanges are on the articular, rather than periarticular, surface, producing a 'gulls wing' appearance. (B) A 'sausage digit'. There is soft tissue swelling and periostitis is demonstrated.†

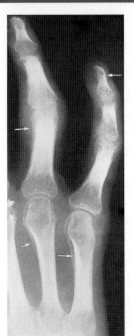

Acute Reiter's syndrome with marked osteoporosis and periosteal reaction (arrows).†

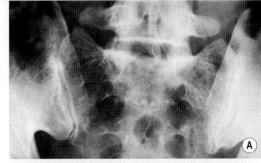

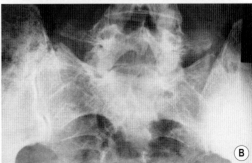

Reiter's syndrome. XRs (A, B) taken over a 12-year period demonstrate the progression of a unilateral left sacroiliitis.†

GOUT (PODAGRA)

DEFINITION

- An inborn error of purine metabolism which causes hyperuricaemia and the deposition of monosodium urate (MSU) crystals within the joints and soft tissues – this results in recurrent episodes of acute arthritis
- **Primary gout:** an autosomal dominant condition ▶ it usually occurs during the 3rd decade of life (with a low penetrance in women)
- **Secondary hyperuricaemia:** this is due to an excessive breakdown of nuclear proteins (e.g. with blood dyscrasias, leukaemia or myeloma), or decreased renal excretion of uric acid (e.g. with chronic renal disease or diuretic use)

CLINICAL PRESENTATION

- *4 stages:*
  - Asymptomatic hyperuricaemia
  - Acute gouty painful arthritis
  - Intercritical (between attacks) gout
  - Chronic tophaceous gout
- *Intercritical periods:* these are initially symptom free and can last many months ▶ with recurring attacks there is shortening of the intercritical period with incomplete recovery

RADIOLOGICAL FEATURES

Location The 1st attack is usually monoarticular (classically affecting the 1st MTP joint of the foot) ▶ it also affects the hand, ankle, wrist, elbow, knee, sacroiliac joints and spine

- **Early:** an intense inflammatory response and joint effusion (which is not radiologically observed)
- **Late:** radiological findings only occur in chronic tophaceous gout: there are typical erosions and eccentric soft tissue swelling
- Periarticular osteopenia is not a common feature
- **Peripheral joints**
- It predominantly affects the small joints of the lower extremities
- The joint space may be uniformly narrowed with associated chondrocalcinosis ▶ there can be adjacent eccentric soft tissue swelling which may be calcified (tophi) ▶ bony ankylosis may occur
  - Periarticular, marginal and subchondral erosions: these are remote from the articular surface (cf. RA) ▶ they appear as cyst-like or 'punched-out' lesions with a sharp overhanging margin and a thin sclerotic rim (with little surrounding sclerosis)

- *Hand:* there is asymmetric and random joint involvement ▶ the CMC compartment is the most commonly involved region within the wrist ▶ during treatment, telescoping of the digits can lead to a severe deformity (due to the rapid resorption of osseous tophi without replacement by bone matrix)
- *Foot:* the hallmark location is the MTP joint of the great toe ▶ hallux valgus is common ▶ osteoporosis is seen with late-stage disease
- *Shoulders/elbows/hips:* involvement is uncommon
- *Spine (rarely involved):* intervertebral disc narrowing ▶ erosion of the odontoid peg ▶ atlantoaxial subluxation
  - Sacroiliac joint involvement is more common with sclerosis, marginal irregularity, erosions and cyst-like changes (with sclerotic margins)

PEARLS

- Under polarizing microscopy MSU crystals are strongly *negatively* birefringent
- **Tophi:** these are soft tissue lumps containing monosodium urate crystals ▶ they appear approximately 10 years into the disease process ▶ a chronic inflammatory reaction can erode cartilage and subchondral bone leading to a deforming arthritis

Related conditions

Lesch–Nyhan syndrome This is an X-linked recessive condition due to a metabolic enzyme deficiency ▶ it presents in male children with hyperuricaemia and mental retardation

Saturnine gout This is due to a decreased renal urate clearance following a lead nephropathy ▶ its features are similar to primary gout

Other types of depositional arthropathy

Multicentric reticulohistiocytosis (lipoid dermatoarthritis)
This is of unknown aetiology and due to the deposition of giant multinucleated vacuolated histiocytes within the soft tissues ▶ cutaneous xanthomas are associated with an erosive arthritis leading to severe deformity

Location DIP and carpal joints of the hands and feet MCP joints (bilateral and symmetrical)
- *Also affected:* shoulder, elbow, wrist, hip and cervical spine (with atlantoaxial subluxation)

XR Sharply demarcated marginal erosions ▶ articular and subchondral bone destruction with little osteoporosis ▶ an unremitting progression to an arthritis mutilans is common

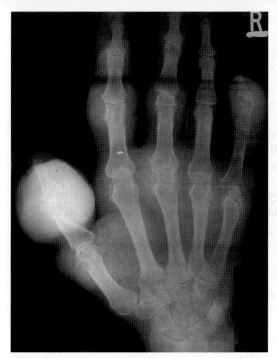

Chronic tophaceous gout. Asymmetric large eccentric soft tissue lumps (tophi). Underlying gouty erosions are seen at several sites, particularly the DIP joint of the right little finger and the CMC joint of the thumb.*

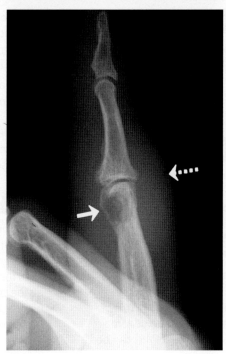

A large periarticular erosion is noted at the volar aspect of the proximal phalanx (solid arrow). The adjacent joint space is preserved, there is no osteopenia, and a tophus is evident on the extensor surface (dashed arrow).©58

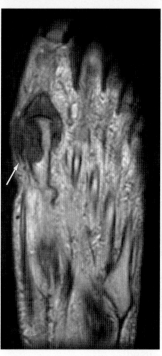

MRI examination of the forefoot in a patient with gout involving the first metatarsophalangeal joint. Long-axis, T1-weighted MR image shows a low signal tophus and/or synovitis present intra-articularly and eroding the medial aspect of the first metatarsal and proximal phalanx (arrow).©35

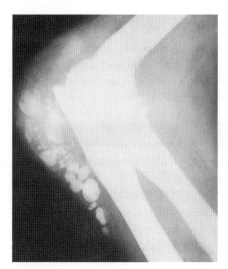

Gout: large calcified tophi within the olecranon bursa.†

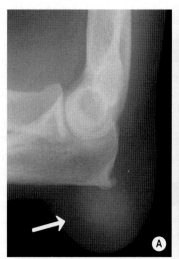
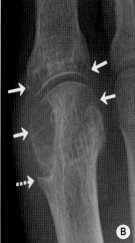

(A) Gouty olecranon bursitis in a 55-year-old man. A rounded soft tissue mass (arrow) containing 'cloud-like' calcifications surrounds the olecranon. The elbow joint is normal. Olecranon bursitis is a common finding in gout. (B) Classic radiographic findings of gout in a 69-year-old man. Note the asymmetric, well-marginated erosions in the head of the first metatarsal and lesser erosions in the opposing phalanx (solid arrows). The medial erosions are characteristically larger than the lateral erosions. There is a 'hook' sign on the inferior margin of the large medial erosion of the head of the metatarsal (dashed arrow). The joint space is preserved, and there is no osteopenia.©35

CALCIUM PYROPHOSPHATE DEPOSITION DISEASE (PSEUDOGOUT)

DEFINITION

- This results from the deposition of calcium pyrophosphate dihydrate (CPPD) crystals in joints, bursae, tendon sheaths and the annulus of the intervertebral discs (cf. nucleus pulposus deposition with ochronosis)

CLINICAL PRESENTATION

- Asymptomatic ▶ if symptomatic, it is known as pseudogout (with an acute intermittent synovitis or a chronic pyrophosphate arthropathy)

RADIOLOGICAL FEATURES

Location It commonly involves the knee (particularly the patellofemoral articulation) ▶ it can also affect the radiocarpal, metacarpophalangeal and elbow joints
- **Acute attack:** a joint effusion and soft tissue oedema which is not well appreciated on XR (US or MRI can be used)
- **Chronic disease (XR):** uniform cartilage thinning ▶ multiple subchondral cysts and osteophytes with a bilateral and symmetrical distribution ▶ giant cysts ▶ structural collapse ▶ subchondral plate fragmentation ▶ periarticular calcific deposits which can have an erosive pressure effect on the adjacent bone (tophaceous pseudogout)

Chondrocalcinosis This is frequently present, and refers to the deposition of a calcium salt within the hyaline or fibrocartilage ▶ this is commonly CPPD (but hydroxyapatite and other calcium salts are radiologically indistinguishable)

XR Streaking of the affected soft tissues with calcium ▶ it is commonly seen within the knee menisci and TFCC of the wrist
- *Also seen in:* gout ▶ hyperparathyroidism ▶ haemachromatosis ▶ Wilson's disease ▶ degenerative joint disease

PEARLS

- Pseudogout has many similar features to osteoarthritis (and can be misdiagnosed as such)
  - *Suggestive features of a pyrophosphate arthropathy:* an unusual distribution (e.g. affecting the patellofemoral, radiocarpal, or elbow joints) ▶ prominent subchondral cysts ▶ a lack of subchondral sclerosis ▶ a relative paucity of osteophytes ▶ erosions are not a feature of pyrophosphate arthropathy
- Under polarizing microscopy MSU crystals are weakly *positively* birefringent

'Crowned dens' syndrome Tophaceous pseudogout at the atlantoaxial joint with progressive cervical cord compression

BASIC CALCIUM PHOSPHATE (BCP) DEPOSITION DISEASE

DEFINITION

- This is also called calcium hydroxyapatite deposition disease (HADD)
- It commonly involves calcium hydroxyapatite crystals (but also octacalcium phosphate and tricalcium phosphate crystals) ▶ it is thought to be due to repetitive trauma with associated dystrophic calcification

CLINICAL PRESENTATION

- **Periarticular deposition:** occurs in small and large joints ▶ common within the supraspinatus tendon (calcific tendinitis) and is associated with a sudden onset of severe local pain due to release of crystals into the surrounding tissues ▶ in small joints deposition is usually pericapsular or peritendinous
- **Intra-articular deposition:** this results in acute pain and swelling with no chondrocalcinosis (unless there is additional CPPD) ▶ it ranges from a monoarticular

periarthritis to joint destruction ▶ Milwaukee shoulder (cranial migration of the humeral head/rapid humeral head bone loss/ remodelling of the acromial undersurface) is linked with HA deposition

RADIOLOGICAL FEATURES

- There is predominantly periarticular deposition (cf. intra-articular deposition with CPDD)

XR Amorphous calcification (up to several cm) seen around and within the joints, tendons and bursae (which may change in size over time) ▶ larger periarticular deposits are associated with metabolic disease (e.g. hyperparathyroidism)
- Synovial and capsular calcification is seen with articular disease
- Joint space narrowing is followed by subchondral sclerosis and destructive changes (subchondral cysts and osteophytes are absent unless secondary OA is also present)

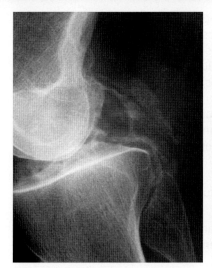

In cases in which deposition is heaviest, entheseal and capsular calcification may be seen outside the confines of the joint.©35

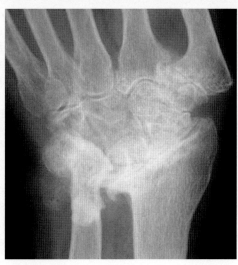

Marked osteophyte formation in the wrist. This huge osteophyte is a marker of hypertrophic osteoarthritis and is part of the spectrum of CPPD.©35

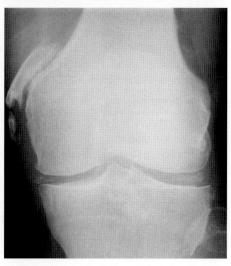

Chondrocalcinosis of the menisci. Ossification adjacent to the medial femoral condyle indicates old medial collateral ligament injury (Pellegrini–Stieda lesion).*

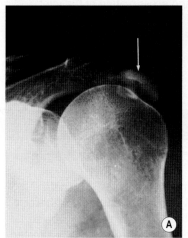
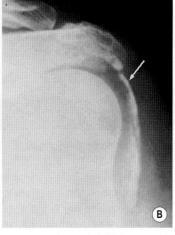

(A) Calcification within the supraspinatus tendon (arrow). (B) Same patient. Following sudden cessation of pain there has been extrusion of calcareous material (arrow) from the tendon.†

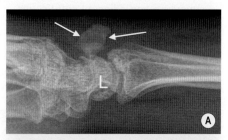
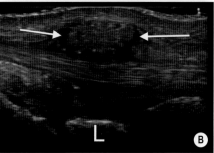

Hydroxyapatite deposition in the wrist. The lateral wrist radiograph (A) demonstrates a large amorphous calcific deposit (arrows) with no internal architecture typical of an HA deposit. The ultrasound of the same patient (B) shows the deposit has a somewhat heterogeneous echotexture containing bright foci without acoustic shadowing (arrows). L, Lunate.**

HAEMOCHROMATOSIS

Definition

- A chronic disease of iron overload – excess iron is deposited within the parenchymal tissues
- It is acquired or inherited (secondary to a deficiency of hepatic xanthine oxidase)

Clinical presentation

- Liver cirrhosis ▶ 'bronze diabetes' (skin pigmentation + cirrhosis + diabetes)
- It presents between the ages of 40 and 60 years (M:F, 10:1)

Radiological features

Location It is a distinct arthropathy involving the hands

XR A symmetrical arthropathy involving the 2nd and 3rd MCP joints ('squared metacarpal heads) ▶ joint space narrowing ▶ well-defined 1–3 mm subarticular cysts and erosions ▶ 'hook-like' osteophytes from the medial aspects of the metacarpal heads ▶ sclerosis and irregularity of the articular surface (± subluxation, flattening and widening of the metacarpal heads) ▶ diffuse osteoporosis ▶ chondrocalcinosis

- Can resemble OA, but the pattern of joint disease, particularly in the hands, is different (relative sparing of the IP joints, and involvement of the MCP joints)

Pearls

Wilson's disease Accumulation of copper within the basal ganglia, liver and joints

XR Premature osteoarthritis ▶ chondrocalcinosis ▶ osteochondritis dissecans

AMYLOIDOISIS

Definition

- A systemic disease with deposition of insoluble fibrillar protein within extracellular tissues
- It may be primary or secondary (e.g. associated with multiple myeloma, long-term haemodialysis and connective tissue disorders)

Clinical presentation

- Renal failure ▶ organomegaly ▶ respiratory and gastrointestinal tract involvement ▶ pericardial and myocardial disease
- Bone or joint involvement (in approximately 10% of cases) can occur with deposition of amyloid within bone, synovium and adjacent soft tissues

Radiological features

Location It commonly affects the large peripheral joints
- Wrists, elbow, shoulder > knees, hips
- Bilateral and symmetrical involvement

XR Sharply marginated erosions and subchondral intraosseous cysts ▶ osteoporosis ▶ joint space narrowing is not an expected feature
- Spondyloarthropathy manifests as disc space narrowing and end-plate irregularity
- Soft tissue deposition results in large bulky nodules, particularly around the wrists, elbows and shoulders
- *'Shoulder pad' sign:* bulky nodules superimposed on atrophic shoulder musculature

Pearl

- Both rheumatoid arthritis and amyloid arthopathy may coexist (although amyloidosis will frequently have well-defined erosions and preservation of the joint space)

OCHRONOSIS (ALKAPTONURIA)

Definition

- A rare autosomal recessive hereditary disorder of tyrosine metabolism leading to homogentisic acid accumulation within the tissues (particularly connective tissues)
- This leads to black or brown cartilage pigmentation (ochronosis) ▶ the affected cartilage becomes brittle, predisposing to early degenerative change

Clinical presentation

- Severe early degenerative change
- It is commonly seen during the 5th decade (M:F, 2:1)

Radiological features

Location Spinal involvement (spondylosis) is more common than a peripheral arthropathy (lumbar > thoracic > cervical spine) ▶ the apophyseal joints are not involved
- The shoulders, hips and knees are occasionally affected – other peripheral joints are rarely involved

XR/CT Intervertebral disc space narrowing (with dense calcification from any associated CPPD disease) ▶ diffuse osteoporosis, kyphosis and scoliosis ▶ there may be marked joint space narrowing without marked osteophyte formation or sclerosis
- Advanced disease may resemble an ankylosing spondylitis

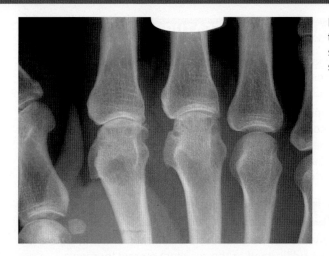

Haemochromatosis. Joint space narrowing is seen affecting specifically the MCP joints of the 2nd and 3rd digits with well-defined 1–3 mm subarticular cysts and erosions, hook-like osteophytes and articular surface irregularity.*

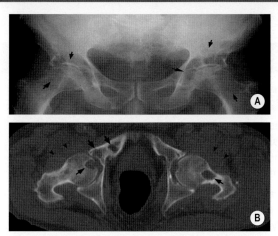

(A) Anteroposterior view of the pelvis demonstrates multiple lytic lesions on both sides of the joint space affecting the hips bilaterally (arrows). (B) Noncontrast CT image of the hips demonstrates multiple punched-out lesions with a thin sclerotic rim on both sides of the joint (arrows). Soft tissue density is present within the joint space representing synovial deposition (arrowheads) and within the punched-out lesions.©35

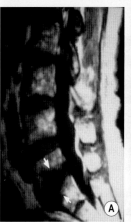

T1WI (A) and T2WI (FS) (B) MR images of the lumbar spine in a long-term dialysis patient demonstrate a lesion centered at the L5/S1 disc space that is predominantly low in signal intensity on both sequences. This appearance is typical of amyloid deposition and helps to differentiate amyloidosis from infectious spondylodiscitis.©35

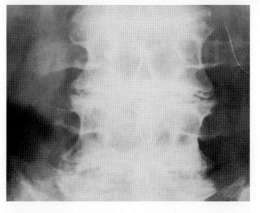

Ochronosis. The intervertebral discs are narrowed and calcified.†

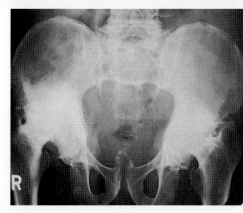

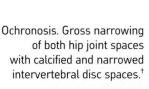

Ochronosis. Gross narrowing of both hip joint spaces with calcified and narrowed intervertebral disc spaces.†

SYSTEMIC LUPUS ERYTHEMATOSUS

DEFINITION

- A systemic autoimmune disease characterized by the production of antibodies directed against the cell nucleus (± its components)
- Deforming non-erosive arthropathy (no erosions) ▶ deformities secondary to ligamentous laxity

CLINICAL PRESENTATION

- It has an undulating course with exacerbations and remissions ▶ joint effusions are uncommon ▶ it tends to affect young adults (F>M)
- 'Butterfly' skin rash over the cheeks ▶ pleurisy and pericarditis

RADIOLOGICAL FEATURES

Location A symmetrical arthritis of the hands, wrists and knees ▶ hands/wrists > feet

XR The findings may be normal ▶ severe soft tissue atrophy (with concave thenar and hypothenar borders) ▶ osteoporosis (periarticular or diffuse)

- Severe disease causes reversible joint subluxation or dislocation in the absence of erosions (the hallmark sign is reversible ulnar devation at the MCP joints)

PEARL

- **Avascular necrosis:** this is common and may due to the vasculitis itself or the resultant steroid therapy

SCLERODERMA (PROGRESSIVE SYSTEMIC SCLEROSIS)

DEFINITION

- An autoimmune systemic connective tissue disease with excessive deposition of collagen within the soft tissues, resulting in fibrosis of the skin, small vessels and internal organs ▶ soft tissue calcification (calcinosis)

CLINICAL PRESENTATION

- It is often accompanied by Raynaud's phenomenon and skin changes

RADIOLOGICAL FEATURES

Location It is commonly seen in the hands

XR Progressive soft tissue atrophy ▶ acro-osteolysis (due to terminal phalangeal resorption from the pressure exerted by the tightened skin) ▶ soft tissue calcinosis (periarticular or at the fingertips) ▶ occasionally there is ligamentous or intra-articular calcification ▶ contractures ▶ generalized osteopenia

- *Calcinosis circumscripta:* discrete dense plaques of calcification

PEARLS

- **Changes of an erosive arthropathy suggest progressive systemic sclerosis:** erosions with a 'pencil-in-cup' deformity involving the DIP and PIP joints, distal ulna and radius

CREST syndrome This is a combination of calcinosis, Raynaud's phenomenon, oesophageal dysmotility, sclerodactyly, telangiectasia and Thibierge–Weissenbach syndrome (calcinosis and digital ischaemia)

Mixed connective tissue disease This is a combination of scleroderma, polymyositis, rheumatoid arthritis and SLE

- Arthritis with variable features is reported in 75% of cases
- *Hands:* osteoporosis (periarticular and diffuse) ▶ soft tissue swelling ▶ marginal erosions ▶ flexion deformities ▶ subluxation and marked ulnar deviation of the phalanges ▶ terminal phalangeal resorption
  - Soft tissue atrophy and calcification may mimic scleroderma
- Large joint involvement is rare

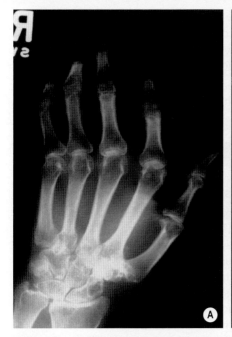

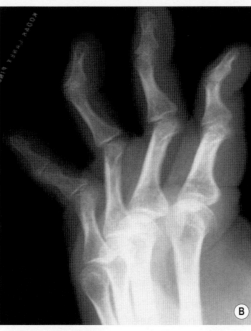

Reducible 'swan neck' deformities in the finger of the right hand in a patient with systemic lupus erythematosus. (A) Posteroanterior view of the right hand shows periarticular osteopenia, but the finger deformities are not obvious. (B) Oblique view of the right hand shows the typical 'swan neck' deformities in fingers 2 through 5.©34

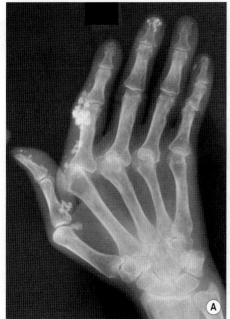

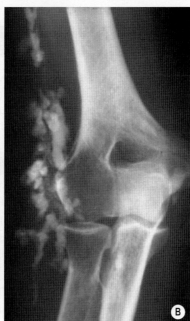

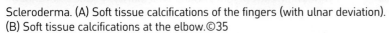

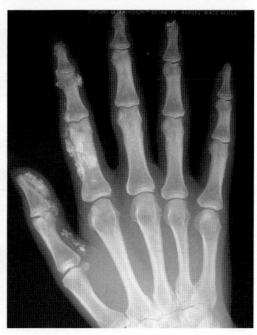

Scleroderma. (A) Soft tissue calcifications of the fingers (with ulnar deviation). (B) Soft tissue calcifications at the elbow.©35

Scleroderma. There is soft tissue atrophy, particularly over the terminal tufts, with extensive soft tissue calcinosis, both along the shafts of several phalanges and also related to the terminal tuft of the 4th and 5th digits.*

HYPERTROPHIC OSTEOARTHROPATHY (HPOA)

DEFINITION

- This is a triad of periosteal new bone formation, painful finger clubbing and synovitis
- It is associated with intrathoracic tumours (e.g. bronchogenic carcinoma, pleural mesothelioma, benign pleural fibroma), infections (e.g. bronchiectasis), cyanotic heart disease and inflammatory bowel disease

CLINICAL PRESENTATION

- Stiff, swollen and painful fingers ▶ finger clubbing ▶ periostitis and arthralgia
- The onset may be acute and hyperhydrosis may occur if it is associated with a bronchogenic carcinoma

RADIOLOGICAL FEATURES

Location Distal $\frac{1}{3}$ of the radius and ulna > tibia and fibula > humerus and femur > metacarpals and metatarsals > proximal and middle phalanges

XR Periosteal new bone formation along the tubular bones (affecting the diaphyses and metaphyses with sparing of the epiphyses) ▶ long-standing periostitis results in cortical thickening

Scintigraphy Increased uptake is seen symmetrically along the shafts of the affected bones (paralleling the cortices)

PEARLS

Pachydermoperiostosis

An autosomal dominant condition which is a primary or idiopathic form of HPOA (accounting for < 5% of cases) ▶ it occurs predominantly in black men

- *Clinical presentation:* finger clubbing ▶ generalized pachydermia (with characteristic deep facial and scalp furrows) ▶ excessive sweating
- It can resemble acromegaly (with associated enlargement of the extremities) but there is no associated elevated growth hormone levels
- Marrow failure can occur due to endosteal cortical thickening

PIGMENTED VILLONODULAR SYNOVITIS (PVNS)

DEFINITION

- An uncommon benign disorder resulting from proliferation of the entire synovium of the joints, bursae and tendons ▶ there can be diffuse and focal forms

CLINICAL PRESENTATION

- It usually affects young adults with intermittent pain and joint swelling

RADIOLOGICAL FEATURES

Location It usually affects a single joint (most commonly the knee)

XR Periarticular bone erosions with sclerotic margins (in approximately 50%) affecting both sides of a joint ▶ in the hip erosions can lead to narrowing of the femoral neck ('apple-core' configuration)

- Articular surface and joint space are preserved until late
- Disuse osteoporosis and osteophyte formation are not features

CT High attenuation (due to haemosiderin) within the mass

- Synovial calcification is very rare (cf. a malignant synovioma)

MRI 'Black synovium': repeated haemarthrosis leads to haemosiderin deposition, which is hypointense on all MRI sequences (particularly gradient-echo sequences where areas of haemosiderin deposition are seen to 'bloom')

PEARLS

Giant cell tumour of tendon sheath

- This describes PVNS affecting the synovium of a tendon sheath ▶ soft tissue calcification and osteophytes are not features ▶ usually painless but can affect function ▶ common in the fingers (flexor tendon sheath)

XR Bony erosion ± periosteal reaction

US This will identify a solid mass in association with the tendon sheath (hypoechoic ± vascularity) ▶ does not move with the tendon

MRI Low SI mass (haemosiderin) related to the tendon

Lipoma arborescens

- A rare benign synovial metaplastic condition

MRI There are delicate branching fronds of fat identified within synovial hypertrophy (T1WI: high SI)

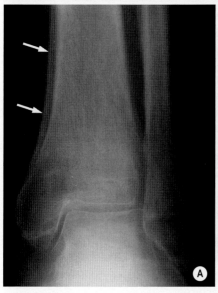
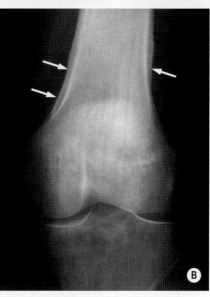

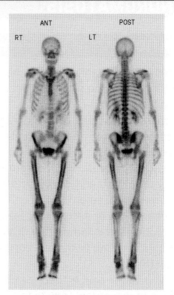

Hypertrophic pulmonary osteoarthropathy (HPOA) in a patient with a bronchogenic neoplasm. (A) AP radiograph of the distal tibia and fibula showing a lamellar pattern of new bone formation along the medial tibial cortex (arrows). (B) AP radiograph of the distal femur: involvement was severe and relatively unusually there was also femoral involvement.**

A 63-year-old woman presented with secondary hypertrophic osteoarthropathy from lung cancer. Whole-body bone scintigram demonstrates increased radionuclide uptake with the 'parallel tract' sign in the femora. Linear cortical uptake is also present in both tibiae.©35

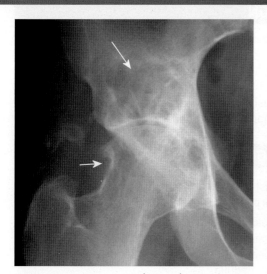
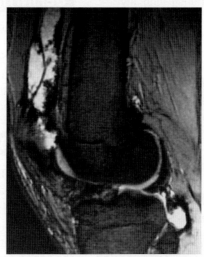
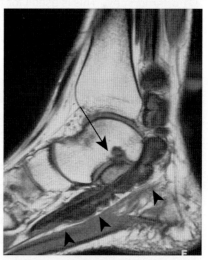

PVNS. Erosions are seen (arrows) on both sides of the joint. Along the femoral neck, erosion is maximal at the site of capsular insertion.*

PVNS. Sagittal GE image. There is a joint effusion and multiple areas of signal void from haemosiderin deposition and synovial thickening.†

PVNS. Sagittal T1WI. This concerns the flexor hallucis longus tendon sheath (arrowheads) with involvement of the sinus tarsi (arrow) and subtalar joints.†

SYNOVIAL (OSTEO-) CHONDROMATOSIS

DEFINITION

- This describes metaplastic cartilage formation that can occur throughout the synovium (including joints, bursae and tendon sheaths)
  - *Chondromatosis:* the cartilage fragments that form become detached and float freely within the joint or bursal cavity
  - *Osteochondromatosis:* the fragments are nourished by synovial fluid and grow ▶ the cartilage eventually becomes calcified or ossified
- It can be primary or secondary (due to trauma, degenerative and inflammatory disease)
- It presents in young or middle-aged adults, and rarely in children (M>F)
- There is minimal pain ▶ there can be swelling or limitation of movement (due to the loose bodies)

RADIOLOGICAL FEATURES

Location Typically monoarticular (affecting the knee, hip, elbow and shoulder)

XR Multiple intra-articular small calcified oval or rounded loose bodies (which may not be detected in the early stages) ▶ these are usually similarly sized loose bodies

CT arthrography This is useful for demonstrating any loose bodies

Scintigraphy This may demonstrate increased uptake indicative of active ossification

PEARLS

- **Differential:** osteoarthritis (but these loose bodies are of differing sizes and are associated with joint space narrowing)
- Chondrosarcoma is a very rare complication

POLYMYOSITIS/DERMATOMYOSITIS

DEFINITION

- **Polymyositis:** an inflammatory condition of unknown aetiology affecting striated muscle
- **Dermatomyositis:** polymyositis accompanied by a typical (pathognomonic) rash ▶ calcification within skin and skeletal muscle (along muscle or fascial planes)
- *Diagnosis:* this requires the presence of the rash and any 3 of the following 4 criteria:
  - A symmetrical proximal muscle weakness
  - Elevated muscle enzymes
  - Diagnostic histopathology findings
  - Characteristic features on electromyogram (EMG)

CLINICAL PRESENTATION

- **Acute phase:** soft tissue oedema and atrophy ▶ bone erosions are not a feature
- **Healing phase:** non-specific subcutaneous or sheet-like calcification along the fascial and muscle planes (particularly affecting the proximal large muscles)
- **Chronic phase:** flexion contractures
- There is a bimodal age distribution, with the condition seen in children and the elderly (F>M)

RADIOLOGICAL FEATURES

MRI T2WI/STIR: high SI within the affected muscles and subcutaneous fat (perimuscular oedema)

PEARLS

- Steroid administration or limb disuse can lead to osteopenia and fractures
- It is associated with various malignancies (e.g. bronchus, breast, stomach and ovary), as well as interstitial lung disease
- There is a normal calcium and phosphate metabolism

SARCOIDOSIS

DEFINITION

- A generalized systemic disease of unknown aetiology characterized by granulomatous changes in the skin, lungs, lymph nodes and viscera ▶ bone involvement in 10% of patients at some time
- The diagnosis is usually made on CXR (with lymphadenopathy ± pulmonary fibrosis)

RADIOLOGICAL FEATURES

Location Distal and middle phalanges of the hands and feet > metacarpals and metatarsals

Diffuse sarcoidosis Tubular bone is widened with a reticular or honeycomb appearance to the spongiosa (a 'lace-like' appearance) ▶ there is loss of definition between the cortex and medulla

Circumscribed sarcoidosis Punched-out cyst-like lesions (up to 5 mm in diameter)

Mutilating sarcoidosis This is rare ▶ punched-out areas coalesce to form larger areas of destruction

Other features Sclerosis ▶ periosteal reaction ▶ soft tissue nodules (which are much more common than bone involvement) ▶ resorption of the distal phalanges ▶ sclerosis (which may be disseminated) ▶ periarticular calcification (due to the associated hypercalcaemia)

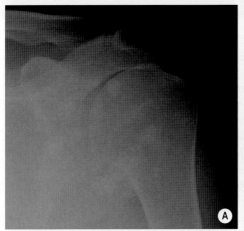

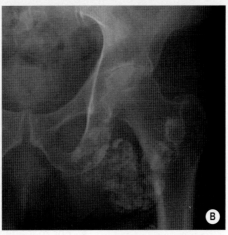

Synovial osteochrondomatosis. Multiple calcified intra-articular bodies are seen in (A) AP XR of left shoulder and (B) AP XR of left hip.

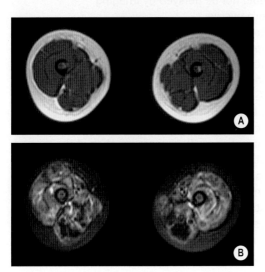

Juvenile dermatomyositis. (A) T1WI of the thighs. (B) STIR image of the thighs. There is bilateral active myositis with no significant loss of muscle bulk.*

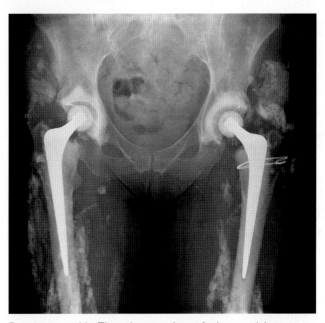

Dermatomyositis. There is extensive soft-tissue calcium deposition. Note how this is associated with the muscle groups and can be seen tracking along these groups and in the associated fascial planes.**

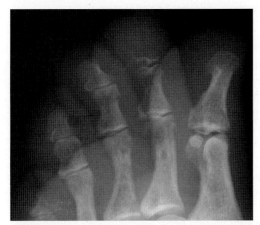

Sarcoidosis of bone. There is widening of the proximal phalanx of the 2nd digit with a reticular or honeycomb appearance to the spongiosa of the proximal phalanges of the 2nd and 3rd digits, associated with areas of destruction particularly affecting the distal phalanx and the distal portions of the proximal and middle phalanges of the 2nd digit. These are associated with soft tissue swelling.*

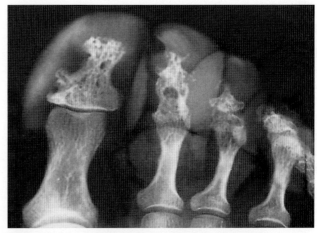

Sarcoid of the foot showing typical cyst-like lesions and absorption of the tufts of the distal phalanges.†

635

5.9 BONE AND SOFT TISSUE INFECTION

ACUTE OSTEOMYELITIS

Definition

- Acute infection of the bone diagnosed within 2 weeks of symptoms (subacute if diagnosed > 2 weeks) ▶ causes:
  - *Staphylococcus aureus*: commonest organism in any age group (80%)
  - Gram-negative organisms (*Pseudomonas/ Enterobacter*): remaining 20%
  - *Acute infections prosthetic implants: S. aureus*
- Spontaneous MSK infections in adults are less common than in children and are usually die to trauma, previous surgery or underlying immunodeficiency ▶ in adults haematogenous infection is mostly responsible for vertebral osteomyelitis (cf. common in childhood osteomyelitis)

Clinical presentation

- Local pain ▶ soft tissue redness and swelling (± discharging abscess) ▶ reduced function and mobility ▶ pyrexia and systemic ill health
- The presence of any infected dead bone or debris makes treatment difficult

Radiological features

- *NB: The appearance of acute (and chronic) osteomyelitis can simulate almost the entire spectrum of bone tumour appearances*

Early

XR / CT   This is often normal (soft tissue gas is an ominous sign)

Skeletal scintigraphy   This is sensitive but non specific ▶ there is early increased uptake ▶ it can be problematic in children as the growth plates are often adjacent to any involved areas

US   A subperiosteal fluid collection

MRI   May be positive as early as 3–5 days ▶ STIR/T2WI (fat-suppressed): high SI within bone marrow (oedema) ▶ it initially extends beyond the limits of the true bone infection ▶ T1WI + Gad: enhancement

Intermediate (after several days)

XR   New periosteal reaction with a thin, thick or laminated ('onion peel') appearance (it can also have a 'fluffy' margin) ▶ a Codman's triangle may also be present ▶ lytic lesions with a narrow zone of transition usually in the metaphyseal region

US   Increasing soft tissue oedema and subperiosteal fluid ▶ thickened synovium ▶ thickened bursae with increased Doppler flow and fluid

- *Pyomyositis:* abnormal echogenicity in the early stages, abscess formation in the later stages

MRI   T1WI: 'penumbra' sign (representing granulation tissue) ▶ T2WI/STIR: a double line observed at the lesion margin

- *Differentiating between acute osteomyelitis and acute medullary bone infarction:*
  - *Osteomyelitis:* thick, irregular peripheral enhancement around a non-enhancing centre
  - *Infarction:* thin, linear rim enhancement or a long segment of serpiginous central medullary enhancement

Pearls

- For management purposes the diagnosis is a clinical one – it should not be delayed by imaging
- Causative organisms:
  - **Haematogenous**: Staphylococcus aureus (the most important) ▶ Haemophilus influenzae (in immunocompromised patients) ▶ Streptococcus pneumoniae ▶ beta-haemolytic streptococci ▶ aerobic Gram-negative rods
  - **Foreign body or implant**: coagulase-negative staphylococci (skin commensals of low virulence)
    - Most infections reflect contamination at the time of operation
  - **Open fracture**: aerobic Gram negative rods (e.g. Pseudomonas) and anaerobic Gram-positive rods (eg. Clostridium spp.)
    - Early sepsis reflects direct implantation with environmental organisms

General patterns

- *Bacterial infection:* this is rapid and destructive
- *Fungal infection:* this occurs in immunocompromised patients ▶ there is a slow, chronic, infiltrative pattern that may mimic malignancy ▶ it is hard to eradicate
- *TB*: an aggressive, indolent or reparative pattern
- **Location:**

Differential diagnosis

- **Tumour**: this tends to demonstrate a more homogenous appearance than infection ▶ infection is more likely to produce soft tissue fluid filled cavities ▶ diagnosis is often only resolved with biopsy
- **Langerhan's histiocytosis**: with disseminated disease multiple lesions of the same age are less likely to be infective
- **Aggressive degenerative disease**: Milwaukee shoulder (rapidly progressive osteoarthritis) may mimic a septic arthritis
- **Irradiation**: subsequent bone necrosis with osteopaenia traversing a joint can mimic infection
- **SAPHO syndrome**

Haematogenous osteomyelitis of tubular bones†

Features	Infant	Child	Adult
Localization	Metaphyseal with epiphyseal extension	Metaphyseal	Epiphyseal
Involucrum	Common	Common	Not common
Sequestration	Common	Common	Not common
Joint involvement	Common	Not common	Common
Soft tissue abscess	Common	Common	Not common
Pathological fracture	Not common	Not common	Common*
Fistulas	Not common	Variable	Common

*Neglected areas

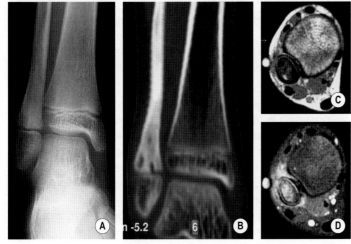

Acute osteomyelitis. (A) Plain radiograph of a child showing ill-defined lucency adjacent to the growth plate of the distal fibula with surrounding sclerosis. (B) Coronal CT reconstruction demonstrating the lucent areas adjacent to the growth plate with prominent surrounding sclerosis. Axial T1WI (C) and T1WI (FS), gadolinium-enhanced (D) MR images. The abnormal infected marrow is of low signal intensity on the T1-weighted pulse sequence. After administration of the gadolinium chelate, osteomyelitis is demonstrated by the high signal-enhancing area adjacent to the growth plate in the distal fibula associated with periosteal new bone formation.©35

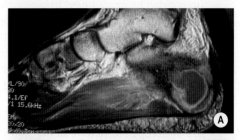

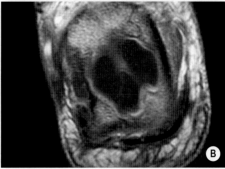

Penumbra sign. Sagittal (A) and coronal (B) MR images of the calcaneus show a circumscribed area of bone destruction with a halo or penumbra of granulation tissue and oedema.*

Imaging findings in osteomyelitis

	Plain radiograph	CT	MRI	NM
Acute	Minimal findings. Soft-tissue swelling may be seen	Not useful	Bone marrow oedema can occur as early as 24–48 h, seen as low T1, and high T2 signal	May show increased uptake, but takes a few days
Subacute	Lucent or sclerotic lesion, periosteal reaction, soft-tissue swelling	Cortical and marrow abnormalities, including abscess, periosteal reaction, soft-tissue oedema and abscess	Bone marrow changes, cortical abnormalities seen as thickening, bone abscess, periosteal reaction, increased T2 signal in soft tissues, abscess formation. Post-gadolinium T1W sequences outline abscess cavities clearly	Three-phase bone scintigram, ¹¹¹indium WBC scan and combined studies are useful, especially to assess multifocal involvement. PET-CT generally not used in this context, but may be useful in exceptional circumstances
Chronic	Bone sclerosis, cortical thickening, sequestrum and cloaca, bone destruction, resorption and deformities	Much better than plain radiographs to demonstrate cloaca and sequestrum, periosteal new bone formation and abscess	Better soft-tissue and bone marrow resolution to demonstrate medullary and cortical changes, sequestra and cloaca well demonstrated, useful to outline soft-tissue abscess and sinus tracts	Generally useful if there is a problem with diagnosis. Combined WBC and bone marrow scintigram is useful. May highlight multiple sites of involvement

CHRONIC OSTEOMYELITIS

Definition

- Bone (marrow) infection > 6 weeks in duration

Clinical presentation

- Asymptomatic or intermittent flare ups:
  - Pain ▶ swelling ▶ general debility ▶ weight loss ▶ a discharging sinus ▶ anaemia
  - There is rarely renal dysfunction secondary to amyloid deposition

Radiological features

- If an abscess cavity forms within bone pus can interfere with the local blood supply and lead to necrotic bone that is surrounded by granulation tissue:
  - **Sequestrum**: a mechanically separate avascular bone fragment ▶ it appears dense (due to surrounding hyperaemia) ▶ it is a foci for recurrence
  - **Involucrum**: a shell of thickened sclerotic living bone surrounding dead bone ▶ it is formed beneath vital periosteum that is elevated by pus
  - **Cloaca:** a defect within the involucrum that can allow pus to escape (sometime to the skin via a sinus)

US Increasing soft tissue oedema and subperiosteal fluid ▶ thickened synovium ▶ thickened bursae with increased Doppler flow and fluid

- *Tenosynovitis:* thickening of the tendon sheath with fluid surrounding the tendon itself ▶ non-compressible thickening of the tendon sheath with increased Doppler flow

XR/CT Local osteopaenia is present with a superimposed mixed pattern:

- *Aggressive or rapidly changing features:* lysis ▶ cortical breach ▶ fracture
- *Slower, more indolent and reparative reactions:* sclerosis ▶ heterotopic new bone ▶ periosteal reaction of increasing maturity

CT Periosteal reaction ▶ subtle bone erosion ▶ cortical destruction ▶ abscess formation ▶ soft tissue swelling ▶ trabecular thickening and medullary abnormalities

99mTc-MDP This has a high sensitivity but a low specificity ▶ it allows differentiation from cellulitis (which will have increased uptake during the 'blood pool' image but no bone uptake on delayed imaging)

111In-labelled white cell studies and 99mTc-sulphur colloids >90% accuracy in diagnosing prosthetic infection

MRI T2WI / STIR: high SI ▶ necrotic areas: loss of SI with no enhancement

- *Periostitis:* thin linear pattern of oedema with enhancement
- *Chronic periostitis and periosteal reaction:* thickening of low SI of cortical bone (T1WI and T2WI)
- *Sequestrum:* cortical bone: low SI (higher if derived from cancellous bone) ▶ any exudate which may surround the sequestrum shows low T1WI and high T2WI SI ± enhancement

- *Involucrum:* SI of normal living bone (commonly thickened and sclerotic and may show oedema)
- *Cloaca:* high SI defect within cortical bone

Pearls

Brodie's abscess A walled off intraosseous abscess ▶ it is seen in paediatric acute on chronic or chronic osteomyelitis ▶ it is usually located within a metaphysis (± epiphyseal extension)

XR An oval lytic lesion with a well-defined reactive sclerotic border

MRI Central fluid (T1WI: low SI, T2WI: high SI) surrounded by a sclerotic rim (T1WI + T2WI: low SI)

- *Differential:* an osteoid osteoma

Sickle cell disease A homozygous disease associated with dactylitis and bone infarction ▶ there is a higher incidence of Salmonella osteomyelitis (sickling in the gut vasculature leads to impaired gut defence and organism entry)

Infected prosthesis It usually mimics chronic aseptic loosening ▶ there is peri-implant osteopaenia with periosteal reaction and progressive bone destruction

- *Early* (within 3 months): due to contamination during surgery of the early postoperative period (*S. aureus*)
- *Subacute* (3–24 months): virulent coagulase-negative staphylococci or S. epidermis
- *Chronic* (>24 months): haematogenous spread from other sources

USS Diagnoses fluid collections and the prosthesis

MRI Limitations due to associated prosthesis artefacts ▶ IV contrast can demonstrate bone marrow oedema and fluid collections

Gallium imaging Increased uptake, but this can have a significant false positive rate

Combined labelled leucocyte and 99mTc-sulphur colloid Is the current gold standard:

- Sulphur colloid is taken up in normal marrow ▶ labelled leucocytes accumulate at sites of infection as well as normal marrow ▶ hence prosthetic infection if activity in the labelled leucocyte images without activity on sulphur colloid imaging
- Squamous metaplasia or even carcinoma can developing within a chronic sinus ▶ chronic infection may result in sarcomatous transformation (very rarely)
- **Specific infections:**
  - **Leprosy**: this is common in the hands, feet and face ▶ thickened nerves can be seen with US
    - *Osteitis leprosa:* granulomas causing focal cortical and medullary destruction
    - *'Licked candy stick' appearance:* neuropathic long term effects leading to a Charcot joint or neuropathic resorption

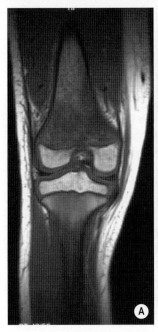
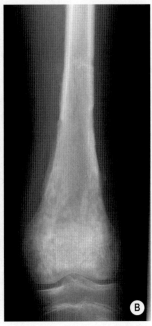

Osteomyelitis of the distal femur. The early MRI (T1WI) study (A) shows sparing of the epiphyses. The XR taken some months later (B) shows chronic osteomyelitis with sclerosis from the metaphyses and epiphysis. There are cortical defects and periosteal new bone.*

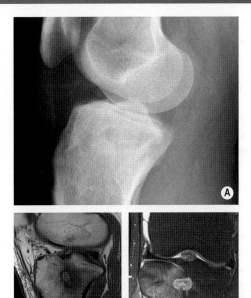

Brodie's abscess of the tibia. (A) Lateral plain radiograph of the right tibia shows a well-defined lucent lesion with surrounding sclerosis, features of Brodie's intramedullary bone abscess. (B) Sagittal T1-weighted and (C) coronal PD-weighted with fat suppression show the well-defined Brodie's abscess with surrounding bone oedema.**

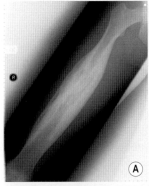
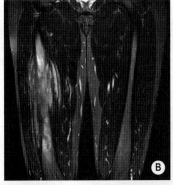
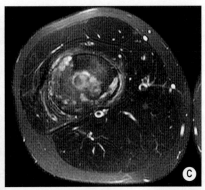

Chronic osteomyelitis of the femur. (A) Plain XR. (B) Coronal FS STIR. (C) Axial T2WI with fat suppression. This degree of periosteal new bone takes months if not years to develop.*

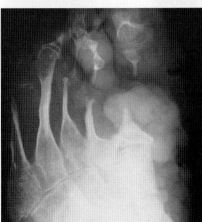

Leprosy. 'Licked candy stick' appearance with associated thickened soft tissues.†

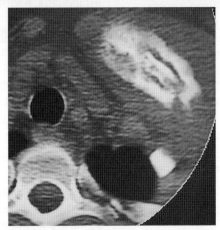

Osteomyelitis of the clavicle (CT) with an involucrum and sequestrum.†

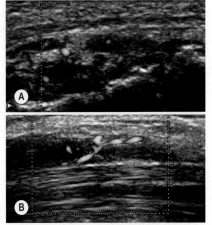

Ultrasound extremities. (A) Increased colour Doppler flow over the dorsum of the foot. (B) Tenosynovitis of extensor tendons with synovial thickening and fluid around the extensor tendons of the hand. There is also increased colour Doppler flow suggesting active inflammation.

PAEDIATRIC MSK INFECTIONS

Definition Paediatric bone infections more commonly occur in healthy bones without pre-existing trauma; usual mode of infection is haematogenous

- Acute haematogenous osteomyelitis (AHO) is the most common form of bone infection in children
  - *50% occur < 5 years of age ▶ 2M > F*
- *Organisms: S. aureus* (commonest) ▶ *Haemophilus influenza* type b ▶ *S. pneumonia* ▶ *S. pyogenes*

Clinical presentation A systemic illness is more common in younger patients

- *Acute osteomyelitis:* pain ▶ reluctance to use the affected limb ▶ pain, redness and swelling may not be present initially
- *Chronic osteomyelitis:* a more insidious course ▶ more difficult to diagnose ▶ minimal loss of function ▶ systemic signs usually absent ▶ local tenderness

Radiological features

Location Infection usually starts in the metaphysis due to its rich blood supply ▶ the subsequent pattern of infection differs depending on the patients age:

- **Blood supply to a long bone:** 1) Nutrient artery: the major source supplying the marrow and inner cortex ▶ 2) Periosteal vessels: these supply the outer cortex ▶ 3) Metaphyseal and epiphyseal vessels
- **Infants up to 12 months**: vessels penetrate the growth plate in both directions allowing infection to easily pass to the epiphysis and joint space (pyogenic arthritis is a common sequelae of osteomyelitis in infants) ▶ the loose periosteum also allows pus to extend along the shaft to the epiphyseal plate (resulting in septic arthritis if the metaphysis is intracapsular)
- **Older children**: metaphyseal vessels terminate in slow flowing sinusoids (promoting blood borne infections) but few vessels cross the epiphyseal plate (resulting in less frequent epiphyseal and joint infections)
- **Adults:** after growth plate fusion the metaphyseal and epiphyseal vessels are reconnected allowing a septic arthritis ▶ periosteum now well bound down and articular infections via a metaphyseal route less likely
- Infections commonest in long bones ▶ most cases limited to a single site ▶ lower limbs usually involved in acute osteomyelitis ▶ <10% involve ≥ 2 bones (multifocal involvement does not exclude acute osteomyelitis)

XR
- *Acute:* excludes other pathologies (e.g. fracture) ▶ joint space initially expanded with fluid (USS is more reliable)
- *Subacute:* periosteal reaction ▶ new bone formation ▶ occasional lucent lesions (Brodie's abscess) in the metaphyseal region
- *Chronic:* bone sclerosis, destruction and periosteal new bone formation

USS Sensitive for demonstrating increased joint fluid in acute septic arthritis ▶ can guide aspiration ▶ fluid may be echoic with debris ▶ subperiosteal abscess can be seen as hypoechoic fluid along the bone surface

CT Less useful in the paediatric population (radiation dose)

MRI
- *Acute:* bone marrow oedema (T1WI: low SI, T2WI/STIR: high SI)
- *Abscesses:* well defined fluid collections ± rim enhancement ▶ they can extend through the cortex into surrounding soft tissues with the formation of sinuses
- *Septic arthritis:* joint effusion ▶ abnormal bone marrow signal either side of the joint ▶ synovial thickening ± enhancement
- *Physeal involvement:* T1WI: low SI, T2WI: high SI along the growth plate with widening of the growth plate ± enhancement
- *Chronic:* 'rim' sign: low SI area of fibrosis surrounding an area of active infection ▶ thickening and remodeling of the cortex ± periosteal reaction

NM 99m-Tc-MDP skeletal scintigraphy: increased activity in the dynamic perfusion, early blood pool and delayed images (uptake is non specific and can be seen with tumours)

Pearls

Chronic recurrent multifocal osteomyelitis (CRMO)

Definition Uncommon non-bacterial inflammatory osteomyelitis occurring in children ▶ unknown aetiology but may be related to autoimmune disorders

Clinical presentation Vague symptoms, presenting as a monoarthritis or poly arthritis ▶ recurrent bouts of inflammatory arthritis and features of osteomyelitis with spontaneous remission

Location Metaphyseal lesions (75%) ▶ more common in lower limbs ▶ may be symmetrical

XR Osteolytic lesions with surrounding sclerosis

MRI Periostitis ▶ bone marrow oedema ▶ transphysitis

SAPHO syndrome

Definition A form of CRMO occurring in children and young adults

Clinical presentation **S**ynovitis/**A**cne/**P**ustulosis/**H**yperostosis/**O**steitis (SAPHO) ▶ skin manifestations (acne and palmoplantar pustolosis) and osteoarticular involvement common ▶ bilateral symmetric pain and boen and joint swelling

Location Metaphyses of the tubular bones (flat bones and the axial skeleton may also be affected)

Sclerosing osteomyelitis of Garré

Definition Chronic osteomyelitis, usually occurring in children and commonly affecting the mandible (a form of CRMO affecting the mandible)

Clinical presentation Pain ▶ hard mandibular swelling

XR Lytic lesions of the mandible associated with sclerosis ▶ with disease progression a non-suppurative ossifying periostitis with subperiosteal new bone formation and sclerosis

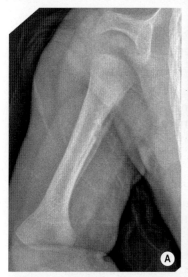
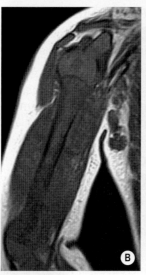
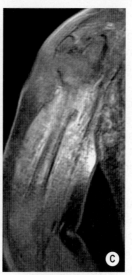

Osteomyelitis of the humerus in a child. (A) Plain radiograph of a child with humeral osteomyelitis showing abnormal texture of medullary bone, with cortical destruction and periosteal reaction. (B) Coronal T1 and (C) fat-suppressed PD-weighted images show low T1 signal in bone marrow, which is hyperintense on the fat-suppressed PD image. Periosteal reaction, cortical destruction and adjacent soft-tissue oedema (seen as low T1 and high T2 signal abnormality) is also evident.**

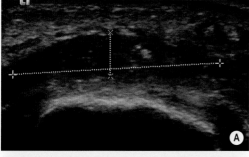
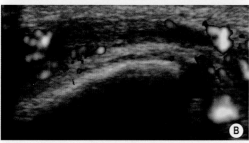

Septic arthritis in a child. (A) Ultrasound of the right knee in a limping 3-year-old child demonstrates the presence of echogenic fluid in the prepatellar bursa. (B) There is increased colour Doppler flow in the surrounding soft tissues and wall of the bursa. The finding of an infected bursa should arouse the possibility of adjacent septic arthritis.**

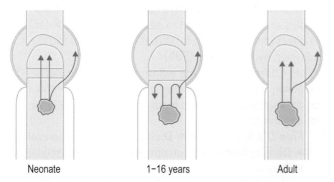

| Neonate | 1–16 years | Adult |

Osteomyelitis. The three ages of infection and how change involves the joint.

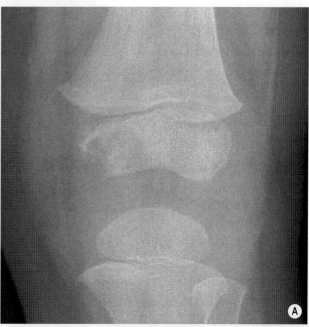
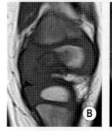
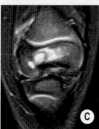
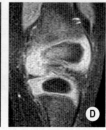

Osteomyelitis in an 18-month-old child. (A) AP radiograph shows irregularity, erosion and rarefaction of the femoral epiphysis. (B) Coronal T1W image showing low T1 signal at the site of epiphyseal destruction, loss of normal fat signal and destruction of medial aspect of left femoral epiphysis. (C) Coronal STIR image demonstrates high signal in the affected epiphysis. (D) Coronal T1 fat-saturated enhanced image demonstrates abnormal enhancement in the affected medial epiphysis due to active infection.**

SOFT TISSUE INFECTION

Abscess

Definition A focal collection of pus ▶ this can be from an extrinsic source (e.g. a puncture wound) or an intrinsic source (e.g. haematogenous spread, an adjacent fistula or an infected joint)

US A predominantly cystic lesion (which is often complex and multiloculated) ▶ there are varying degrees of internal echogenicity depending upon the internal contents ▶ there is posterior acoustic enhancement ▶ the surrounding tissues may be hypervascular ▶ a foreign body may be identified

CT Non-enhancing areas of low attenuation (haemorrhage or proteinaceous fluid may increase the attenuation)

MRI T1WI: low or intermediate SI ▶ T2WI: high SI (oedematous change within the surrounding tissues appears as feathery ill-defined high SI) ▶ T1WI + Gad: peripheral enhancement

Pyomyositis

Definition A muscular infection (usually in an immunocompromised patient)

US A generalized alteration in muscle echogenicity

MRI T2WI: heterogeneous increased SI throughout the muscle ▶ there is formation of fluid pockets with disease progression (with similar imaging characteristics to an abscess)

Cellulitis

Definition A superficial subcutaneous infection

US Thickened skin and subcutaneous tissues ▶ low reflective septa (fluid tracking between subcutaneous fat lobules)

MRI T2WI: thickened septa yield increased SI ▶ there is increased SI within the skin and underlying fascia

NECROTIZING FASCIITIS

Definition A progressive rapidly spreading deep fascial inflammatory infection ▶ there is secondary necrosis of the subcutaneous tissues

- It is often life threatening and commonly follows surgical procedures or a relatively minor trauma
- Group A haemolytic streptococci and *S. aureus* are commonly the initiating factors ▶ other organisms can also be present (e.g. *Clostridium, Pseudomonas*)

Clinical presentation Initially there is pain and localized swelling, with rapidly spreading erythema and necrosis ▶ the patient is systemically unwell

Radiological features

CT/MRI Asymmetric fascial thickening ▶ large areas of soft tissue and muscle destruction and necrosis (± gas within the tissues) ▶ no enhancement

Pearls

- **Treatment:** aggressive surgical debridement and a broad-spectrum antibiotic is required
- **Fournier gangrene:** a necrotizing fasciitis localized to the scrotum and perineum

DIABETIC ARTHROPATHY

Definition Diabetic-induced vasculaitis and microangiopathy, together with p[eripheral neuropathy leads to chronic ulceration with secondary infection (due to loss of protective sensation, autonomic changes and abnormal biomechanics due to motor neuropathy)

Clinical presentation Swollen erythematous foot
- *Charcot neuroarthropathy:* warm, swollen foot with intact skin
- *Osteomyelitis:* a cutaneous ulcer that can be probed down to underlying bone

Radiological features Changes of osteomyelitis are superimposed on a destructive neuropathic arthropathy, with florid osteophytes and sclerosis

XR A triad of osteolysis/periosteal reaction/bone destruction ▶ progression to cortical destruction, increased bone sclerosis, bone resorption and auto-amputation

MRI Investigation of choice for pedal osteomyelitis ▶ demonstrates bone marrow oedema/periosteal reaction/

cellulitis/joint effusion ▶ can demonstrate ulcers and sinus tracts

Pearls

- *Neuropathic changes:* joint deformity ▶ subluxation or dislocation ▶ cortical fragmentation ▶ intra-articular bodies are more common in neuropathic joints ▶ tends to affect intertarsal and tarsometatarsal joints (60%) followed by MTP joints (30%)
- *Acute Charcot Joint:* acute inflammation (particularly involving the midfoot) following minor trauma ▶ this can be an aggressive process leading to major structural re-organisation
  - **Five D's: D**estruction ▶ **D**islocation ▶ **D**isorganization ▶ **D**ensity (florid heterotropic new bone and sclerosis) ▶ **D**ebris
- Bone destruction tends to be faster with infection than with a Charcot joint

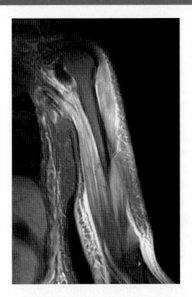

Muscle infection is rare but dramatic on MRI. Pyomyositis is seen as edema and swelling within a muscle group. Later necrosis and abscess formation may change the imaging appearances.©35

Pyomyositis of the thigh with perhaps less dramatic muscle involvement than was seen in the case of necrotizing fasciitis. The distinction between these conditions is dependent on clinical presentation and speed of progression.©35

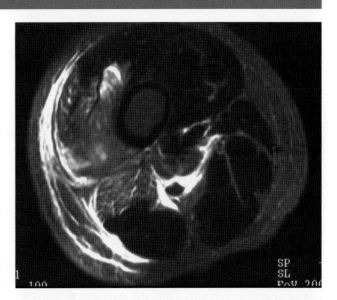

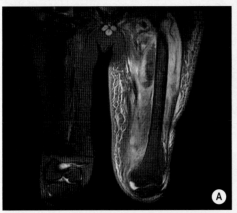

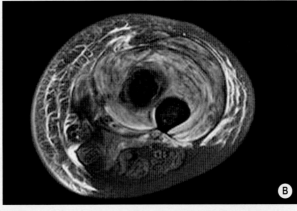

Extensive muscle and soft tissue necrosis in a case of severe necrotizing fasciitis. (A) Coronal STIR (FS) image shows the extent of tissue damage. (B) Axial STIR (FS) image.©35

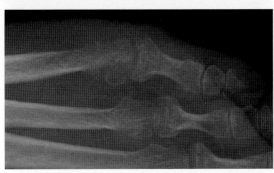

Diabetic foot osteomyelitis. Cortical bone destruction is evident along the lateral edges of the fifth metatarsal head and base of the adjacent proximal phalanx, with overlying soft-tissue abnormality due to cutaneous ulceration.**

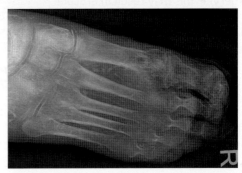

Diabetic foot complication. Oblique radiograph of the foot shows extensive vascular calcification. There is gas in the soft tissues of the great toe; this more commonly occurs due to air forced in through an open ulcer than a gas-forming organism infection. The loss of soft tissue around the great toe indicates ischaemic mummification of the toe.**

TUBERCULOUS INFECTION

Definition

- This follows haematogenous spread (and is usually from the lung with active chest disease in < 50% of cases)

Clinical presentation

- There is a myriad of clinical presentations and appearances ▶ large 'cold' abscesses can occur with the patient feeling surprisingly well and unaware of any ill health
- The diagnosis is usually made after some delay, with radiographic changes often seen at presentation (radiographic changes occur 2–3 weeks following presentation with pyogenic infections)

Radiological features

Bone Infection is typically slow growing and indolent ▶ it is initially located within the metaphysis (diaphyseal lesions are rare) and soon crosses into the epiphysis ▶ there is little surrounding sclerosis ▶ sequestration and periostitis are not prominent features

- *Phemister triad:* joint space narrowing + marginal erosions + osteoporosis

Vertebral bodies Most lesions occur in or below the mid-thoracic spine ▶ two or more vertebrae may be involved ▶ it tends to affect the anterior vertebral body, where a local kyphus or gibbus can occur (the subperiosteal type of infection begins anteriorly, spreading under the anterior longitudinal ligament) ▶ ultimately this results in vertebral body ankylosis (and occasionally a vertebra plana)

- There can be an anterior concavity to the vertebral bodies (this is due to transmitted aortic pulsations through an anterior paraspinal abscess)
- The discs are destroyed late (early destruction is seen with simple infections)
- Sclerosis and reactive bone formation are not prominent features (there is, however, marked collapse)
- Lumbar abscesses may cause psoas bulging
- Prominent tracking can easily be seen if subsequently calcified (which is characteristic of TB)

Tuberculous dactylitis (spina ventosa) The affected phalanx is characteristically widened by medullary expansion (cf. a syphilitic dactylitis with widened new cortical bone)

Joints It usually affects the major joints (hip and knee) ▶ early radiographic signs are non-specific (capsular thickening, synovial effusion, surrounding osteoporosis) ▶ chronic hyperaemia can cause early epiphyseal fusion

- Late signs include surface bone erosions and loss of the joint space

CT Demonstrates any bone destruction

MRI T2WI: subchondral bone marrow oedema ± enhancement ▶ T1WI + Gad: smooth synovial thickening (cf. irregular thickening in pyogenic arthritis) ▶ thin walled abscess cavities with little inflammation 'cold abscess' – cf. pyogenic abscess

SEPTIC ARTHRITIS

Definition

- Joint infection due to haematogenous spread, direct spread from adjacent osteomyelitis, or from direct intervention (e.g. surgery) ▶ this may result in articular damage
- It can have a bacterial, viral or fungal aetiology (the latter 2 generate more chronic changes)

Clinical presentation

- Patients usually present with sudden onset of monoarticular arthritis, systemic symptoms and a joint effusion ▶ pain ▶ effusion ▶ reduced movement ▶ it is very rarely asymptomatic

Radiological features

Location The hip is the commonest site in children

- **Early:** synovial thickening ▶ joint effusion (US is the best method of detecting joint fluid)
- **Intermediate:** joint effusion and osteopenia ▶ adjacent bone marrow oedema ▶ early cartilage thinning on all imaging
- **Late:** marginal destruction and bone erosion ▶ joint narrowing ▶ eventually ankylosis may occur

MRI This is the most sensitive at showing the true extent of soft tissue and bone involvement ▶ T2WI/STIR: bone marrow oedema appears as high SI ▶ synovial thickening ▶ effusion

US Joint effusion ▶ synovial thickening ▶ increased vascularity ▶ this is non-specific – aspiration is the only reliable means of determining the nature of an effusion

Pearls

- The articular cartilage (with its poor blood supply) is particularly susceptible to damage from the inflammatory response to infection
- Septic arthritis is especially common in children
  - The growing epiphysis is at risk of secondary growth arrest ▶ in chronic infection hyperaemia may lead to epiphyseal overgrowth
- Bacterial septic arthritis may present with a normal white cell count and CRP
- Septic arthritis is a surgical emergency usually requiring arthrotomy and lavage ▶ delayed diagnosis can lead to cartilage and bone destruction

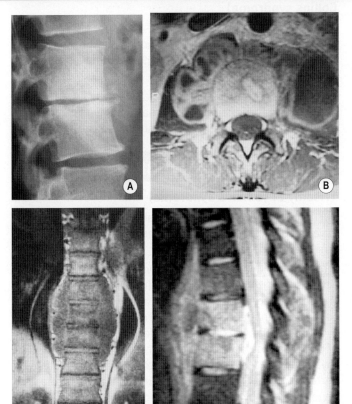

Tuberculous discitis. (A) The plain XR changes are similar to a normal discitis with end-plate irregularity and reactive sclerosis. (B) Axial T1WI shows the end-plate defect well as well as psoas abscesses with central necrosis. (C) Coronal image in a different patient demonstrates intervertebral disc destruction at the point of maximal paraspinal widening and associated vertebral body signal change. (D) With fat suppression there is increased SI in adjacent vertebral bodies together with anterior and posterior masses (the latter compressing the spinal cord).[†]

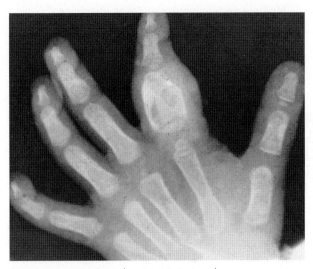

Spina ventosa of the 2nd proximal phalanx.[†]

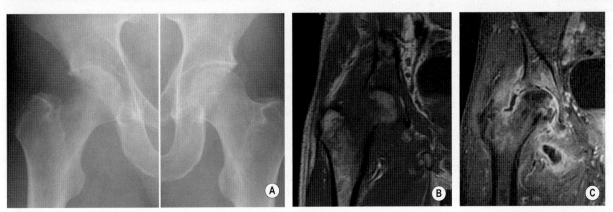

Septic arthritis. Late presentation, three weeks after onset of symptoms in an intravenous drug user. (A) Plain radiograph demonstrates loss of joint space, marked reduction in bone density of the femoral head and partial destruction of the subchondral bone plate in the lateral part of the femoral head. (B) Coronal T1W and (C) enhanced fat-suppressed T1W images show a joint effusion with surrounding enhancement, enhancing bone marrow oedema and an abscess in the adjacent medial soft tissues. Despite immediate surgical arthrotomy and joint washout, the prognosis for this articulation is poor.**

5.10 CONGENITAL SKELETAL ANOMALIES

OSTEOCHONDRODYSPLASIAS

- These are classified into 33 groups (1–33) ▶ abnormalities are intrinsic to bone and cartilage and will continue to evolve throughout life
  - *Dysplasias:* abnormalities of bone ± cartilage growth
  - *Osteodystrophies:* abnormalities of bone ± cartilage texture
- **Conditions referenced elsewhere**
  - Group 25 *(dysplasia with increased bone density)*
    - Osteogenesis imperfecta (Section 5 Chapter 7, Osteogenesis imperfecta)
  - Group 31 *(disorganized development of cartilagenous and fibrous skeletal components)*
    - Multiple cartilaginous exostoses (diaphyseal aclasis) (Section 5 Chapter 5, Osteochondroma)
    - Enchondromatoses (± haemangiomas) (Section 5 Chapter 5, Benign bone tumours: (En)chondroma)
    - Fibrous dysplasia (Section 5 Chapter 5, Fibrous dysplasia)

DYSOTOSES (LOCALIZED DISORDERS WITH PREDOMINANT CRANIAL AND FACIAL INVOLVEMENT)

- These are classified into 3 groups (A–C)
- They are due to altered blastogenesis occurring during the 1st 6 weeks of life ▶ previously normal bones will remain so (unlike an osteochondrodysplasia) ▶ more than 1 bone may be involved

Osteo-onychodysostosis (nail-patella syndrome, Fong syndrome)

Clinical presentation *Autosomal dominant* ▶ multiple skeletal abnormalities (dysplastic knees and elbows) ▶ dysplastic fingernails ▶ clinodactyly (curving of the 5th finger towards the 4th finger) ▶ renal disease

Radiological features Posterior iliac horns ▶ absent or hypoplastic patellae ▶ hypoplastic lateral femoral condyles ▶ genu valgum ▶ hypoplastic capitellum ▶ radial head dislocation ▶ short 5th metacarpals

Apert's syndrome

Clinical presentation *Sporadic (autosomal dominant in some families)* ▶ abnormalities are present from birth ▶ malformations of the skull, face, hands and feet ▶ proptosis ▶ high arched or cleft palate ▶ bifid uvula

Radiological features Progressive carpal and tarsal fusions ▶ progressive ankylosis of the phalangeal joints ▶ dislocated radial heads ▶ progressive fusion within the cervical spine (commonly C5/C6) ▶ progressive fusion of the large joints ▶ hypoplasia of the glenoid fossae

- *Craniosynostosis:* premature fusion of the skull sutures and facial bones
- *'Mitten' or 'sock' deformities:* these are due to syndactyly (fused digits) of the hands and feet

Mandibulofacial dysostosis (Treacher Collins syndrome)

Clinical presentation *Autosomal dominant* ▶ ear deformities ▶ deafness ▶ downslanting eyes ▶ lateral coloboma of the lower eyelid ▶ hypoplastic malar bone ▶ cleft palate

Radiological features Symmetrical stenosis or atresia of the external auditory meati ▶ maxillary hypoplasia ▶ mandibular hypoplasia ▶ hypoplastic paranasal sinuses

CHROMOSOMAL DISORDERS

Trisomy 21 (Down's syndrome)

Clinical presentation Craniofacial abnormalities (e.g. brachycephaly, microcephaly, hypertelorism and relatively small facial bones)

Radiological features The iliac wings are flared with relatively horizontal acetabulae ▶ frequently there are 11 pairs of gracile ribs ▶ there are often two ossification centres within the manubrium sterni (normally only one) ▶ atlantoaxial subluxation and instability with hypoplasia of the odontoid process (which is frequently a cause of myelopathy) ▶ generalized joint laxity ▶ relatively tall vertebral bodies ▶ short hands with clinodactyly of the little finger due to a hypoplastic middle phalanx

- *Associations:* congenital heart lesions (e.g. endocardial cushion defects and intra- and extracardiac shunts) ▶ duodenal atresia and stenosis ▶ Hirschsprung's disease ▶ anorectal anomalies

45XO (Turner's syndrome)

Clinical presentation Short stature ▶ cubitus valgus ▶ webbed neck ▶ widely spaced nipples ▶ lymphoedema

- Patients have a classical form of ovarian dysgenesis (with streak ovaries and a small uterus) ▶ a 25% incidence of associated ovarian tumours such as a dysgerminoma (occurring up to the age of 20 years)

Radiological features A short 4th metacarpal ▶ flattening of the medial tibial condyle with a transitory exostosis ▶ beaked vertebral bodies ▶ osteoporosis ▶ scoliosis ▶ coarctation of the aorta ▶ increased occurrence of urinary tract anomalies (e.g. a horseshoe kidney) ▶ delayed skeletal maturation

- *Madelung deformity:* a reduced angle between the distal radial and ulnar metaphyses

NEUROCUTANEOUS SYNDROMES

Neurofibromatosis

Clinical presentation *Autosomal dominant* ▶ multiple neurofibromas and schwannomas ▶ axillary freckling, café au lait spots and molluscum fibrosum

- Up to 85% of patients with neurofibromatosis manifest a musculoskeletal abnormality

Radiological features See table

Radiographic musculoskeletal features of neurofibromatosis	
Soft tissues	• Focal gigantism (soft tissue overgrowth or plexiform neurofibroma) • Neurofibrosarcomas
Skull	• Macrocrania • Aplasia/hypoplasia of the sphenoid wings ('bare' orbit) • Hypoplasia of the posterosuperior orbital wall (pulsatile exophthalmos) • Mesodermal dysplasia (calvarial defects) • Neuromas ± fibromas (with enlarged cranial foramina)
Spine	• Angular kyphoscoliosis • Posterior scalloping of the vertebral bodies (dural ectasia) • Dumb-bell neurofibromas/lateral meningoceles
Ribs	• 'Ribbon' ribs (mesodermal dysplasia) • Rib notching
Tubular bones	• Pseudoarthroses of the tibia, fibula, or clavicle • Anteromedial tibial bowing • Fibrous cortical defects (multiple and large) • Intraosseous cysts

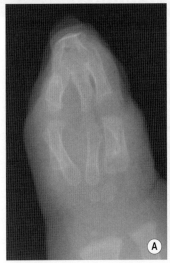
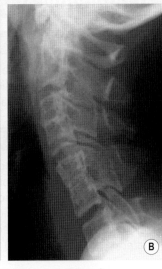

(A) Apert's syndrome. Radiograph of the hand. 'Mitten' polysyndactyly of soft tissues and bones. (B) Apert's syndrome. Lateral radiograph of the cervical spine. Progressive fusion of the cervical spine is a recognized feature of this condition.©35

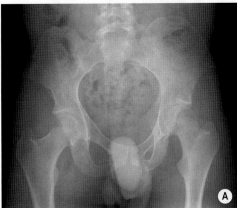
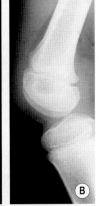

Nail-patella syndrome. (A) Radiograph of the pelvis showing hypoplastic pelvic wings (more pronounced on the right side) and a small iliac horn on the right ilium. (B) Lateral knee radiograph. Note absence of the patella bone.©35

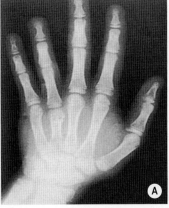
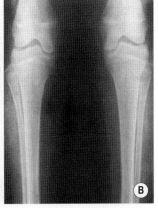

Turner's syndrome. (A) Typical shortening of fourth metacarpals. (B) The medial tibial plateau is depressed and the adjacent femoral condyle enlarged.[†]

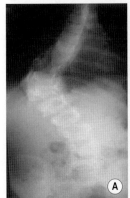
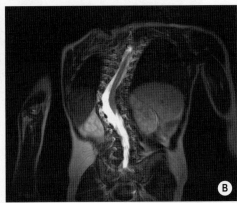
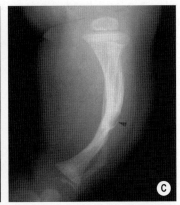

Type 1 neurofibromatosis with a short angular thoracolumbar curve as seen on an anteroposterior radiograph (A) and coronal T2-weighted MR image (B). There is scalloping of the posterior vertebral body wall and enlargement of the exit foramen. The MR image demonstrates dural ectasia with a widened spinal canal. (C) A cystic lesion (arrow) in the tibia at the prefracture stage. The distal fibula is dysplastic and bowed.©35,©34

ACHONDROPLASIA (GROUP 1)

DEFINITION

- This results from defective endochondral bone formation
- *Limb shortening:* rhizomelic (proximal) ▶ mesomelic (medial) ▶ acromelic (distal)

CLINICAL PRESENTATION

- *Autosomal dominant* ▶ short limbs and trunk ▶ narrowed thorax with respiratory distress in infancy ▶ bowed legs ▶ lumbar lordosis ▶ prominent forehead with a depressed nasal bridge ▶ hydrocephalus, brainstem and spinal cord compression (dilatation of lateral cerebral ventricles)

RADIOLOGICAL FEATURES

- A decreasing interpedicular distance within the lumbar spine (travelling caudally) ▶ short vertebral pedicles ▶ posterior vertebral body scalloping ▶ flat acetabular roofs ▶ short ribs and short wide tubular bones ▶ a large skull vault and a small foramen magnum ▶ relative overgrowth of fibula
  - *'Bullet-shaped' vertebral bodies:* with an antero-inferior anterior beak
  - *'Tombstone' appearance:* squared small iliac wings with a small sciatic notch
  - *'Champagne glass' pelvis:* the pelvic inlet resembles a champagne glass
  - *'Chevron' deformity:* V-shaped growth plate notches
  - *'Trident hand':* the fingers are all the same length and diverge into 2 pairs

PEARLS

Achondrogenesis This is a fatal autosomal recessive dwarfism where the abnormalities are similar to those seen in achondroplasia (but are much more severe)
- *Abnormalities include:* severe short limb dwarfism ▶ unossified vertebral bodies ▶ a large head with normal or reduced ossification
- *Type I:* severe
- *Type II:* less severe ▶ it is caused by type II collagen abnormalities leading to abnormal bone and cartilage formation

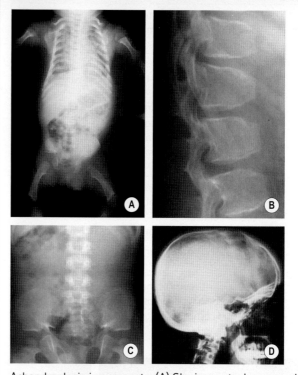

Achondroplasia in a neonate. (A) Sloping metaphyses, oval transradiant proximal femora and a narrow thorax with short ribs. (B) Mild kyphosis, posterior scalloping of the vertebral bodies, 'bullet-shaped' vertebral bodies and short pedicles with associated spinal stenosis. (C) Small square iliac wings, horizontal acetabular roofs, short sacrosciatic notches, progressive caudal narrowing of the lumbar interpedicular distances and low-set sacrum. (D) Short skull base with prominent frontal bone and narrow cervical canal.*

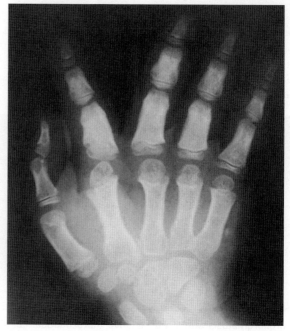

Trident hand in achondroplasia.[†]

HYPOCHONDROPLASIA (GROUP 1)

DEFINITION

- This is also known as 'achondroplasia tarda' with milder features than those seen with achondroplasia

CLINICAL PRESENTATION

- *Autosomal dominant* ▶ variable short stature and a prominent forehead

RADIOLOGICAL FEATURES

- No normal widening is demonstrated in the interpedicular distance within the lumbar spine (travelling caudally) ▶ short and relatively broad long bones ▶ elongation of the distal fibula and ulnar styloid process ▶ variable brachydactyly

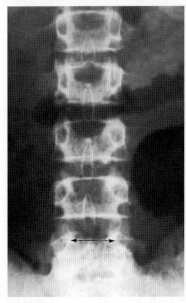
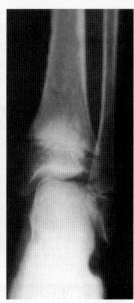

Hypochondroplasia. A narrowed interpedicular distance at L5.[†]

Overgrowth of the distal fibula in hypochondroplasia.[†]

THANATOPHORIC DYSPLASIA (GROUP 1)

CLINICAL PRESENTATION

- *Sporadic, autosomal dominant mutation* ▶ this is the most common lethal neonatal skeletal dysplasia ▶ short markedly curved limbs ▶ respiratory distress due to a (small thoracic cage)

RADIOLOGICAL FEATURES

- Short ribs with wide costochondral junctions ▶ severe platyspondyly ▶ horizontal acetabular roofs with medial spikes ▶ small sacroiliac notches ▶ marked shortness and bowing of the long bones ▶ irregular metaphyses ▶ short broad tubular bones in the hands and feet ▶ small scapulae
  - *'Telephone handle' appearance of the long bones:* this is due to metaphyseal flaring
  - *'Cloverleaf skull':* this is due to lateral temporal bulging
- Type 1: normal skull
- Type 2: 'clover leaf' skull

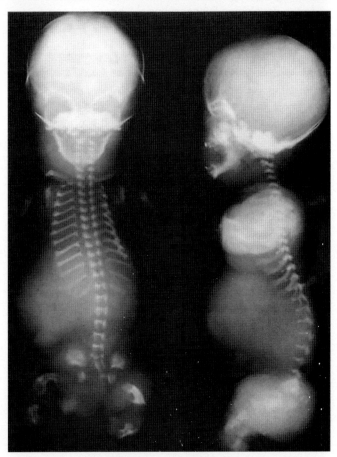

Thanatophoric dwarfism. A cloverleaf skull is present. The scapulae are hypoplastic and the clavicles high. Platyspondyly is shown, resulting in H-shaped vertebral bodies. The bones are short and bowed.[†]

ASPHYXIATING THORACIC DYSPLASIA (JEUNE'S) (GROUP 9)

CLINICAL PRESENTATION

- *Autosomal recessive* (often lethal) ▶ respiratory problems with a long narrow thorax ▶ short hands and feet ▶ nephronophthisis in later-life survivors

RADIOLOGICAL FEATURES

- Small thorax with short ribs (horizontally orientated) ▶ widened costochondral junctions ▶ high clavicles ▶ short iliac bones ▶ horizontal acetabula with medial and lateral 'spurs' ('trident' appearance) ▶ 'wineglass' pelvis ▶ premature appearance of the proximal femoral ossification centres ▶ cone-shaped phalangeal epiphyses ▶ may have polydactyly (10%)

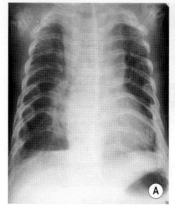
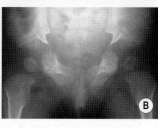

Asphyxiating thoracic dystrophy. (A) Narrow thorax and short ribs. (B) Horizontal acetabular roofs and pronounced medial spurs, less pronounced laterally ('trident' appearance).*

METATROPIC DYSPLASIA (GROUP 8)

DEFINITION

- The development of dwarfism changes over time – the trunk gradually shortens relative to the limbs (due to the developing kyphoscoliosis) – hence the name 'metatropic'

CLINICAL PRESENTATION

- *Variable inheritance (autosomal dominant or recessive)* ▶ short limbs ▶ relatively narrow chest ▶ small appendage in the coccygeal region (tail) ▶ progressive kyphoscoliosis

RADIOLOGICAL FEATURES

- Short tubular bones with marked metaphyseal widening ('dumb-bell') ▶ platyspondyly ▶ relatively large intervertebral discs ▶ flat acetabular roofs ▶ short iliac bones ▶ short ribs with anterior widening ▶ hypoplastic odontoid process

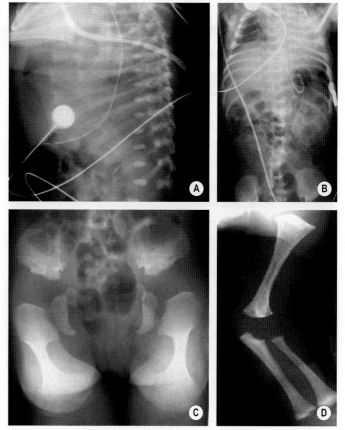

Radiographs in a newborn with metatropic dysplasia. (A) Spine: dense vertebral bodies and short ribs with anterior splaying. (B) Thorax: long trunk and small chest. (C) Pelvis: short iliac wings, narrow sciatic notches, irregular acetabular roofs and halberd (hunting ax)-shaped with trumpet-shaped metaphyses. (D) Upper extremities: flared proximal humeral and distal radial and ulnar metaphyses ▶ shortened long bones. ©24

METAPHYSEAL CHONDRODYSPLASIA (GROUP 13)

DEFINITION

- Severe short-limbed dwarfism
- *Schmid type:* more common ▶ mild ▶ predominantly involves the lower limbs
- *Jansen type:* less common ▶ more severe ▶ symmetrical involvement of all tubular bones

CLINICAL PRESENTATION

- *Autosomal dominant* ▶ short limbs, short stature, presenting in early childhood ▶ genu varum (bow legs) ▶ waddling gait

RADIOLOGICAL FEATURES

- Metaphyseal flaring ▶ irregular widened growth plates (most marked at the hips) ▶ increased density and unevenness of the metaphyses (particularly the upper femora and around the knees) ▶ large femoral capital epiphyses ▶ coxa vara ▶ femoral bowing ▶ anterior cupping of the ribs ▶ normal spine

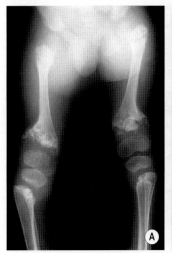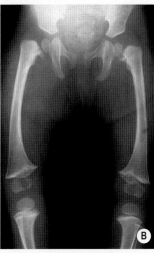

Metaphyseal chondrodysplasia (A) Jansen type. Femora are short with marked expansion, irregular ossification and some sclerosis of the metaphyses. Epiphyses are large and rounded. (B) Schmid type. There is bilateral coxa vara, the metaphyses are splayed and irregular and there is lateral bowing of the femora.*

ELLIS–VAN CREVELD (CHONDROECTODERMAL DYSPLASIA) (GROUP 9)

CLINICAL PRESENTATION

- *Autosomal recessive* ▶ short stature ▶ short limbs (more marked distally) ▶ polydactyly ▶ hypoplasia of the nails and teeth ▶ ectodermal dysplasia with sparse hair ▶ congenital cardiac defects (e.g. ASD) ▶ fusion of upper lip and gum

RADIOLOGICAL FEATURES

- Short ribs in infancy ▶ short iliac wings ▶ 'trident' appearance – the pelvis becomes more normal in childhood ▶ premature ossification of the femoral capital epiphyses ▶ laterally sloping proximal tibial metaphysis ▶ exostosis of the medial upper tibial shaft ▶ carpal fusions ▶ cone-shaped epiphyses (middle phalanges) ▶ polydactyly of the hands and feet

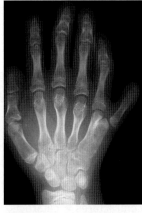

Postaxial polydactyly in a patient with chondroectodermal dysplasia (Ellis-van Creveld syndrome). The plain radiographs show an extra digit on the ulnar side of the right hand. Note also bony fusion of the fifth metacarpal digit and the metacarpal of the extra digit (bony syndactyly).©35

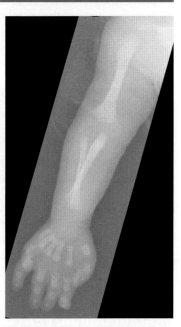

Ellis–van Creveld syndrome. Postaxial polydactyly, short middle and terminal phalanges, cupped metaphyses (the epiphyses will be cone-shaped when they ossify) and sloping of the proximal humeral metaphysis.**

SPONDYLOEPIPHYSEAL DYSPLASIA CONGENITA (GROUP 2)

CLINICAL PRESENTATION

- *Autosomal dominant* ▶ short stature ▶ cleft palate ▶ myopia ▶ maxillary hypoplasia ▶ thoracic kyphosis and lumbar lordosis ▶ barrel-shaped chest

RADIOLOGICAL FEATURES

- Ovoid, pear-shaped, irregular-sized vertebral bodies in infancy ▶ irregular platyspondyly in later life ▶ L5 smaller than L1 in infancy ▶ odontoid hypoplasia and cervical spine instability ▶ short long bones ▶ absent ossification of the epiphyses of the knees, talus and calcaneus at birth ▶ pubic and ischial hypoplasia ▶ severe coxa vara developing in early childhood ▶ horizontal acetabulum

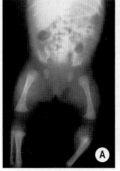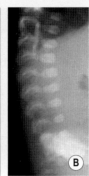

Spondyloepiphyseal dysplasia congenita in a neonate. (A) Absent ossification of the pubic rami, short femoral necks and absent ossification of the epiphyses at the knees. (B) 'Pear-shaped' vertebral bodies with posterior constriction.*

SPONDYLOEPIPHYSEAL DYSPLASIA TARDA (GROUP 8)

CLINICAL PRESENTATION

- *Several types with different modes of inheritance are recognized* ▶ usually presents in adolescence with short stature due to a short trunk ▶ joint limitation

RADIOLOGICAL FEATURES

- Characteristic mound of bone in the central and posterior parts of the vertebral end plates (X-linked dominant type) ▶ narrow intervertebral discs ▶ mild-to-moderate generalized epiphyseal dysplasia ▶ early osteoarthritis ▶ platyspondyly

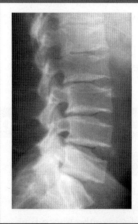

X-linked spondyloepiphyseal dysplasia tarda. Characteristic dense mounds of bone on the posterior $\frac{2}{3}$ of the vertebral end plates are seen.*

CHONDRODYSPLASIA PUNCTATA (CDP) (GROUP 12)

- Also known as congenital stippled epiphyses

CLINICAL PRESENTATION

- Flat nasal bridge ▶ high-arched palate ▶ cutaneous lesions (e.g. ichthyosis) ▶ asymmetrical or symmetrical shortening of the limbs ▶ joint contractures ▶ cataracts
  - Rhizomelic type *(autosomal recessive):* lethal type
  - Non-rhizomelic type (Conradi-Hünermann syndrome)
    - *Autosomal dominant:* common and mild
    - *X-linked dominant:* lethal in males

RADIOLOGICAL FEATURES

- Shortened long bones (symmetrical or asymmetrical) ▶ short digits in some types ▶ vertebral bodies show coronal clefting ▶ stippled cartilaginous calcification (particularly around the joints and in the laryngeal and tracheal cartilage) – this eventually disappears in later life
- *Punctate calcification may also be seen in:* Pacman dysplasia ▶ Zellweger syndrome ▶ fetal alcohol and warfarin embryopathies ▶ some chromosomal abnormalities and mucolipidoses

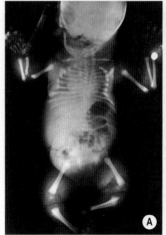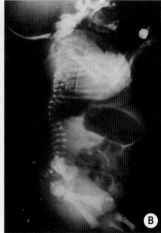

(A,B) Chondrodystrophia calcificans congenita. There is irregularity of vertebral bodies and of the neural arches and spinous processes in association with soft-tissue stippled calcification. These changes are also seen at the joints. The long bones are markedly shortened. The humeral metaphyses are irregular.[†]

PSEUDOACHONDROPLASIA (GROUP 10)

CLINICAL PRESENTATION

- *Autosomal dominant* ▶ short limbs with a normal head and face ▶ accentuated lumbar lordosis ▶ genu valgum (knock knees) or varum (bow legs) ▶ joint hypomobility

RADIOLOGICAL FEATURES

- Platyspondyly with a tongue-like anteroinferior protrusion of the vertebral bodies ▶ biconvex configuration of the upper and lower vertebral end plates ▶ atlantoaxial dislocation ▶ small femoral capital epiphyses ▶ short iliac bones ▶ wide Y-shaped cartilage ▶ irregular acetabulum ▶ small pubis and ischium ▶ pointed proximal metacarpals ▶ shortening of the tubular bones with expanded, markedly irregular metaphyses ▶ small irregular epiphyses ▶ wide costovertebral joints ▶ relatively long distal fibula

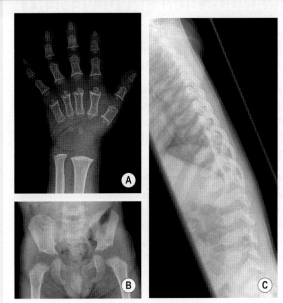

Pseudoachondroplasia in a 3 year old. (A) Short tubular bones of the hand, small epiphyses with delayed bone age, pointed bases of the metacarpals with pseudoepiphyses, irregular metaphyses, flared metaphyses of distal radius and ulna. (B) Irregularity of acetabula and proximal femoral metaphyses, delayed ossification of femoral heads with short femoral necks, wide triradiate cartilages. (C) Mild platyspondyly with anterior protrusions of the vertebral bodies.**

MULTIPLE EPIPHYSEAL DYSPLASIA (FAIRBANK'S DISEASE) (GROUP 10)

DEFINITION

- Delayed ossification and irregularity of the epiphyses of the tubular bones, carpus and tarsus

CLINICAL PRESENTATION

- *Autosomal dominant* ▶ joint stiffness and a limp ▶ early osteoarthritis ▶ mild shortening of the limbs

RADIOLOGICAL FEATURES

- Short tubular bones of the hands and feet ▶ double-layered patella ▶ only mild irregularity of the vertebral end plates ▶ mild wedging of the vertebral bodies ▶ mild acetabular hypoplasia ▶ symmetrical flattening and fragmentation of the femoral capital epiphyses (mimicking bilateral Legg–Calvé–Perthes disease) ▶ tibiotalar slant ▶ hypoplastic femoral and tibial condyles ▶ shallow intercondylar notch ▶ early joint degenerative changes

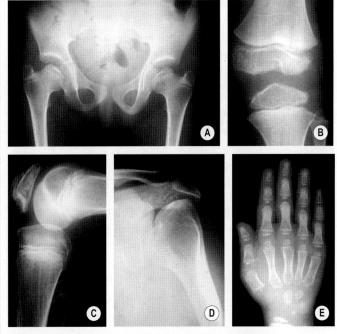

Multiple epiphyseal dysplasia. (A) Small flattened capital femoral epiphyses with short femoral necks and coxa vara. (B) Small flattened irregularly ossified knee epiphyses. (C) Layered ossification of the patella. (D) The left shoulder shows a 'hatchet' deformity of the proximal humerus. (E) Delayed bone maturation with small carpal centres and flattened small and fragmented epiphyses.*

653

CLEIDOCRANIAL DYSPLASIA (GROUP 32 – DYSPLASIAS WITH PREDOMINANT MEMBRANOUS BONE INVOLVEMENT)

DEFINITION

- Delayed ossification of the midline structures

CLINICAL PRESENTATION

- *Autosomal dominant* ▶ large head and fontanelles (with delayed closure) ▶ excessive mobility of the shoulders ▶ a narrow chest

RADIOLOGICAL FEATURES

- Frontal bossing ▶ wide skull sutures with multiple wormian bones ▶ persistently open anterior fontanelle ▶ prominent jaw with multiple supernumerary teeth ▶ variable hypoplasia or pseudoarthrosis of the clavicles (particularly the lateral end) ▶ small scapulae ▶ narrow thorax with incompletely ossified sternum ▶ the vertebral bodies retain an infantile biconvex shape ▶ absent or delayed ossification of the pubic bones ▶ hypoplastic iliac wings, short middle phalanges with cone-shaped epiphyses and tapering of the terminal phalanges ▶ undermodelling of the shafts of the long bones ▶ pseudoarthrosis of the long bones (rare)

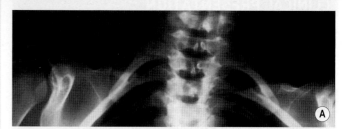
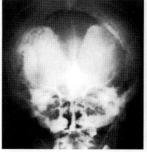
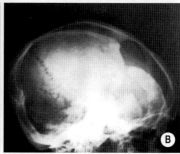

Cleidocranial dysplasia. (A) Absent ossification of the lateral portions of the clavicles, the glenoid fossae are hypoplastic and there is dysraphism in the lower cervical spine. (B) Wide fontanelles and sagittal suture with multiple wormian bones in the lambdoid suture.*

CAMPOMELIC DYSPLASIA (GROUP 21 – BENT BONE DYSPLASIAS)

CLINICAL PRESENTATION

- *Autosomal dominant* (sex reversal has been reported)
- *Neonatal:* respiratory distress ▶ cleft palate ▶ prenatal bowing of the lower limbs ▶ pretibial dimpling
- *Survivors:* short stature ▶ learning difficulties ▶ recurrent respiratory infections

RADIOLOGICAL FEATURES

- *Neonatal:* 11 pairs of ribs ▶ hypoplastic scapulae ▶ femoral angulation at the junction of the proximal ⅓ and distal ⅔ ▶ tibial angulation at the junction of the proximal ⅔ and distal ⅓
- *Survivors:* short fibulae ▶ progressive kyphoscoliosis ▶ dislocated hips ▶ deficient ossification of the ischium and pubis ▶ hypoplastic patellae

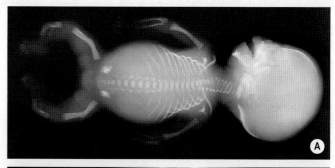
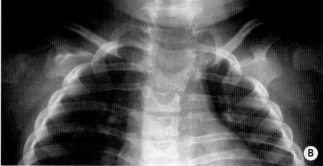

(A) Radiograph in a fetus of 21 weeks' gestation with campomelic dysplasia. Findings include a large skull with a small face ▶ hypoplastic/absent scapular bodies ▶ 11 ribs ▶ poorly ossified thoracic pedicles ▶ tall, narrow iliac wings ▶ and short extremities with proportionately long, bent femurs. (B) Three-year-old girl with campomelic dysplasia demonstrating hypoplastic scapulae.©24

MUCOPOLYSACCHARIDOSES (GROUP 27 – DYSOSTOSIS MULTIPLEX)

DEFINITION

- Abnormality of mucopolysaccharide and glycoprotein metabolism resulting in mucopolysaccharide accumulation in the bone marrow, liver and brain
  ▶ differentiation between types is dependent upon laboratory analysis (e.g. urine, leucocytes)
- *Commonest types:* Hurler and Morquio syndromes

CLINICAL PRESENTATION

- *Autosomal recessive except MPS type II (Hunter), which is X-linked recessive* ▶ presents in early childhood (variable manifestations) ▶ short stature is associated with a distinctive coarse facial appearance with mental retardation, corneal opacities, joint contractures, hepatosplenomegaly and cardiovascular problems

RADIOLOGICAL FEATURES

- *All have features of dysostosis multiplex (DM):* short stature ▶ macrocephaly ▶ a thickened vault with 'ground-glass' opacity ▶ 'J'-shaped sella ▶ ovoid, hook-shaped vertebral bodies with a thoracolumbar gibbus ▶ wide ribs, short wide clavicles and poorly modelled scapulae ▶ lack of normal modelling of the long bones (with thin cortices and a coarse trabecular pattern) ▶ short wide phalanges with a characteristic proximal pointing of the metacarpals ▶ flared iliac wings with constricted bases to the iliac bones ('goblet shaped' or 'wineglass' pelvis) ▶ coxa valga ▶ small, irregular femoral capital epiphyses
- DM is also seen with other storage diseases, such as Gaucher's disease

Hurler syndrome (MPS type 1) DM beginning during the first few years ▶ also known as 'gargoylism' due to the associated everted lips and protruding tongue
- Anterior *lower* vertebral body 'beak'

Morquio syndrome (MPS type IV) The only form *not* to cause mental retardation ▶ DM + joint laxity ▶ short stature ▶ corneal opacities ▶ an absent odontoid peg (with associated cervical instability leading to spinal cord compression) ▶ platyspondyly (flattened vertebral bodies) with posterior scalloping of the vertebral bodies ▶ delayed appearance of fragmented stippled epiphyses ▶ proximal pointing of the 2nd to 5th metacarpals ▶ progressive disappearance of the femoral heads ▶ irregular ossification of long bone metaphyses
- Anterior *central* vertebral body 'beak'

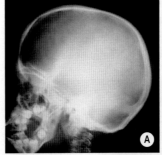
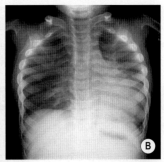
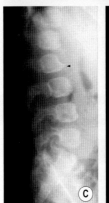
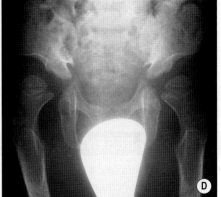
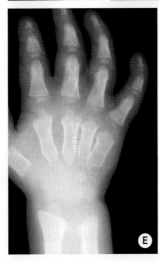
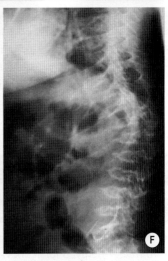

Mucopolysaccharidosis. (A) Elongated (J-shaped) sella. The vault shows an overall ground-glass opacity. (B) The ribs are broad, and the clavicles short and broad. Varus deformity of the upper humeri is seen. (C) Inferior hook (arrowhead) on the body of L2 with a mild kyphosis. (D) The iliac wings are flared laterally and the acetabular roofs are shallow. Bilateral hip subluxation with long femoral necks and coxa valga. (E) Flexion deformities of the fingers. The short bones are undermodelled, and there is proximal pointing of the 2nd to 5th metacarpals and a V-shaped deformity of the metaphyses at the wrist. (F) MPS IV (Morquio–Brailsford syndrome). The lateral view of the spine shows osteopenia and platyspondyly with anterior beaking. There is a thoracolumbar kyphosis.[†]

PYKNODYSOSTOSIS (GROUP 23)

CLINICAL PRESENTATION

- *Autosomal recessive* ▸ short limbs ▸ propensity to fracture ▸ respiratory problems ▸ irregular dentition

RADIOLOGICAL FEATURES

- Wormian bones ▸ delayed closure of the fontanelles ▸ generalized increase in density of the skeleton (particularly the calvarium, skull base and orbital rims) ▸ hypoplastic facial bones and a straight mandible ▸ prognathism ▸ deficient ossification of the distal phalanges ▸ reabsorption of the lateral end of the clavicle ▸ pathological fractures

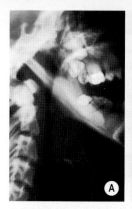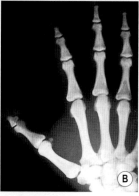

Pyknodysostosis. (A) The mandibular angle is obtuse (straight). (B) Generalized osteosclerosis. The terminal phalanges show varying degrees of hypoplasia and tapering.*

OSTEOPOIKILOSIS (GROUP 23)

CLINICAL PRESENTATION

- Often asymptomatic ▸ may present with cutaneous or subcutaneous nodules ▸ M = F

RADIOLOGICAL FEATURES

- Multiple sclerotic foci (islands), especially around the pelvis and metaphyses of long bones ▸ these are situated parallel to the long axis of the affected bone

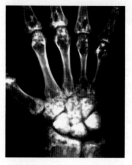

Osteopoikilosis. Multiple discrete islands of sclerosis, especially affecting the carpus, metaphyses and epiphyses.*

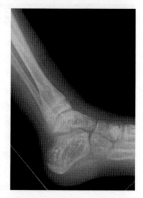

Osteopoikilosis. Multiple sclerotic bone islands.**

OSTEOPETROSIS (GROUP 23)

CLINICAL PRESENTATION

- *More severe types are autosomal recessive, although a milder delayed form shows autosomal dominant inheritance* ▸ hepatosplenomegaly ▸ bone fragility ± fractures ▸ cranial nerve palsies ▸ blindness ▸ osteomyelitis ▸ anaemia

RADIOLOGICAL FEATURES

- Generalized increase in skeletal density ▸ abnormal modelling of the metaphyses, which are widened with alternating bands of radiolucency and sclerosis, a 'bone within a bone' appearance ▸ rickets and basal ganglia calcification in a recessive form with carbonic anhydrase deficiency

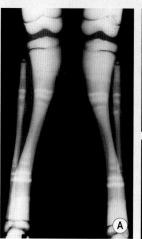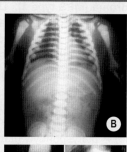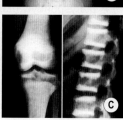

Osteopetrosis. (A) Increased bone density with deformity and abnormal modelling, as well as alternating bands of radiolucency and sclerosis. (B) Increased bone density with relative radiolucent bands at the metaphyses of the humeri and also in the iliac wings. (C). Bands of increased bone density especially seen at the vertebral end plates.*

MELORHEOSTOSIS (LÈRI'S DISEASE) (GROUP 23)

CLINICAL PRESENTATION

- *Non-genetic* ▶ sclerodermatous lesions over the bony lesions ▶ asymmetry of the affected limbs ▶ vascular anomalies ▶ abnormal pigmentation ▶ muscle contractures and wasting

RADIOLOGICAL FEATURES

- Dense irregular bone running down the cortex of a long bone (± overgrowth and bowing) ▶ 'dripping candle wax' appearance ▶ likened to 'molten wax running down the side of a candle' ▶ the distribution corresponds to a sclerotome ▶ there is usually a segmental and unilateral distribution ▶ it particularly involves the long bones (less commonly other bones)

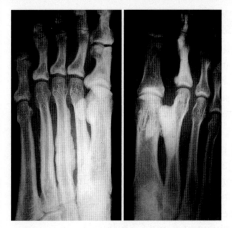

Melorheostosis (two patients). There is dense irregular cortical bone: this is sometimes described as the 'flowing candle wax' appearance. One patient demonstrates a 'ray' distribution (asymmetrical changes).*

DIAPHYSEAL DYSPLASIA (CAMURATI-ENGELMANN DISEASE) (GROUP 24)

DEFINITION

- Abnormal intramembranous bone formation resulting in diaphyseal thickening ▶ also affects the skull (affecting the passage of nerve and blood vessels)

CLINICAL PRESENTATION

- *Autosomal dominant* ▶ muscle weakness ▶ pain in the extremities ▶ gait abnormalities ▶ exophthalmos

RADIOLOGICAL FEATURES

- Sclerotic skull base ▶ progressive endosteal and periosteal diaphyseal sclerosis ▶ narrowing of the medullary cavity of tubular bones ▶ bone scintigraphy: increased activity

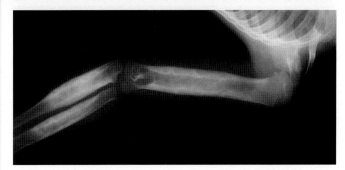

Diaphyseal dysplasia. Anteroposterior radiograph of left arm. Cortical thickening and sclerosis of diaphyses are seen. The metaphyses and epiphyses are relatively spared.©35

CAFFEY'S DISEASE (INFANTILE CORTICAL HYPEROSTOSIS) (GROUP 22)

DEFINITION

- A self-limiting proliferative bone disease of infancy

CLINICAL PRESENTATION

- *Autosomal dominant is suggested in some families (also a lethal recessive form)* ▶ usually appears in the first 5 months of life ▶ hyperirritability ▶ soft tissue swelling

RADIOLOGICAL FEATURES

- It commonly affects the mandible, clavicles and ulna ▶ it may be asymmetrical ▶ massive periosteal new bone and cortical thickening ▶ when tubular bones are affected, the abnormality is limited to the diaphyses ▶ proximal pointing of the 2nd to 5th metacarpals

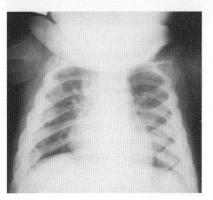

Caffey's disease. Gross periostitis affects the ribs, and the mandible is also thickened.†

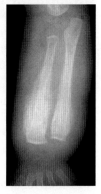

Infantile cortical hyperostosis. Anteroposterior radiographs of forearm.©35

657

SPRENGEL'S DEFORMITY (CONGENITAL ELEVATION OF THE SCAPULA)

DEFINITION

- This is due to failure of the normal descent of the scapula from its initial mid-cervical to its final mid-thoracic position ▶ it occurs in isolation or with cervical spine fusion in the Klippel–Feil deformity
- It can be unilateral (left > right) or bilateral ▶ M = F

XR The scapula is elevated and rotated with the inferior edge of the glenoid pointing towards the spine ▶ the affected scapula is larger than the normal scapula

- *Omovertebral bone:* a bony or fibrous connection between the superomedial angle of the scapula and the spinous process, lamina or transverse process of a vertebral body between C4 and C7 ▶ (50%)

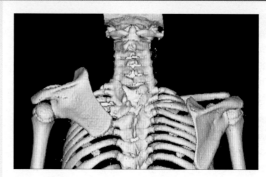

Sprengel's deformity. 3D CT of thorax on bone windows. Elevated right scapula (Sprengel's deformity). Note also the spinal dysraphism (C5–T3) and failure of segmentation (T4/T5).*

MADELUNG'S DEFORMITY

DEFINITION

- This results from premature fusion of the medial half of the distal radial epiphysis ▶ it demonstrates an autosomal dominant inheritance or occurs as an isolated disorder
  - **Reverse Madelung's deformity:** bowing of the forearm bones in association with a shortened and abnormal ulna
- *Causes:* trauma ▶ hereditary multiple exostoses ▶ diaphyseal aclasis

XR The radii are short and bowed ▶ the distal ulna is dorsally prominent ▶ there is a reduction of the carpal angle and wedging of the carpal bones between the distal radius and ulna

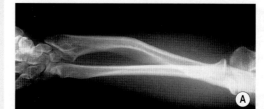
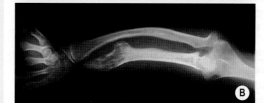

(A) Madelung's deformity. The distal radial metaphysis is sloping and there is dislocation of the distal end of the ulna. The radius is bowed laterally. (B) Reverse Madelung's deformity.*

FEMORAL DYSPLASIA (IDIOPATHIC COXA VARA)

DEFINITION

- This ranges from a mild idiopathic coxa vara to severe forms of proximal focal femoral deficiency in which only the distal femoral condyles develop

Idiopathic coxa vara Reduction of the femoral neck/shaft angle ▶ a separate fragment of bone from the inferior portion of the femoral neck (Fairbank's triangle) is characteristic ▶ if the neck/shaft angle is <100°, then without surgical intervention a varus deformity will progress

Proximal focal femoral deficiency (PFFD) Varying degrees of agenesis of the proximal femur can occur ▶ there is an association between the severity of the femoral dysplasia and the severity of the acetabular dysplasia ▶ it is bilateral in only 10% of cases

- The lower leg may also be short, and the fibula may be absent or hypoplastic

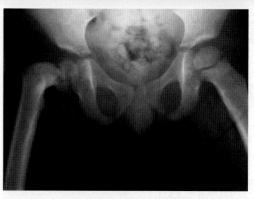

Femoral dysplasia. Right coxa vara deformity.*

DEVELOPMENTAL DYSPLASIA OF THE HIP

DEFINITION

- This can occur as an isolated disorder or in association with other conditions (e.g. a sternomastoid tumour, torticollis, talipes calcaneovalgus, arthrogryposis multiplex or trisomy 21)

RISK FACTORS

- Female sex ▶ breech presentation ▶ firstborn children ▶ oligohydramnios ▶ a positive family history

RADIOLOGICAL FEATURES

Static and dynamic US examination this is performed on all newborn infants with a positive Ortolani (± a Barlow) test, breech presentation or a positive family history
- It is performed at about 6 weeks ▶ measurements include the Graf angles (normal: β <77° ▶ α >60°)

FOLLOW-UP

- XR should be performed if ossification of the proximal femoral epiphysis renders a US examination difficult

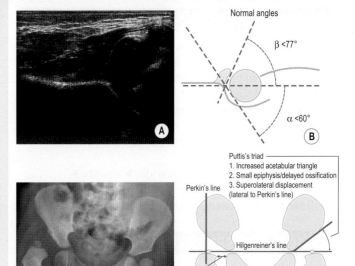

Developmental dysplasia of the hip (DDH). (A) Ultrasound of a dislocated hip. (B) Normal Graf angles. (C) Dysplastic right acetabulum with dislocated femoral head.** (D) Measurements in DDH. Hilgenreiner's line: horizontal line through the superior aspect of the triradiate cartilages. Perkin's line: drawn perpendicular to Hilgenreiner's line. The upper femoral epiphysis should normally be seen below Hilgenreiner's line and medial to Perkin's line.*

TIBIA VARA

DEFINITION

- Bowing of the legs (which can be bilateral or unilateral) ▶ the bowing may occur at the level of the knee joint or proximal tibia
- *Causes:* physiological bowing (bilateral and self-resolving) ▶ Blount's disease ▶ rickets ▶ trauma ▶ infection ▶ neurofibromatosis ▶ Ollier's disease ▶ Maffucci's syndrome ▶ fibrous dysplasia ▶ focal fibrocartilaginous dysplasia

Blount's disease A tibial growth disorder (due to the effects of weight on the growth plate) ▶ it affects the medial aspect of the proximal tibial epiphyses (with tibial bowing below the level of the knee) ▶ it is a progressive condition (unlike 'bow-legs' which will straighten with age) ▶ initial beaking of the medial proximal tibial metaphysis progresses to irregularity fragmentation and premature fusion of the medial aspect of the proximal tibial growth plate
- It is unilateral in 40% ▶ there can be infantile and adolescent presentations

Focal fibrocartilaginous dysplasia Affects the proximal tibia causing bowing, but is benign and usually self-limiting
- A linear radiolucency extending inferolaterally from the proximal tibial metadiaphysis

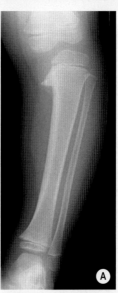
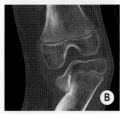
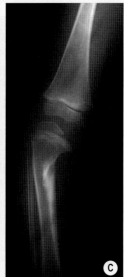

Blount's disease. (A) Plain XR and (B) coronal CT. (C) Focal fibrocartilaginous dysplasia. Note the pathognomonic appearance of the radiolucent band.*

659

SLIPPED CAPITAL FEMORAL EPIPHYSIS (SCFE)

DEFINITION

- Anterolateral and rotational forces of the hip muscles on the femoral shaft result in anterosuperior translation of the proximal femoral metaphysis relative to the epiphysis (it occurs through the non-rachitic physis) ▶ it is the commonest hip disorder of adolescence
- Unilateral > bilateral (left > right) ▶ bilateral slips occur in 25% of Caucasian and up to 50% of Afro-American children
- **Risk factors:** Afro-American origin ▶ obesity ▶ endocrine disorders (hypothyroidism, growth hormone deficiency, hypogonadism and panhypopituitarism)

CLINICAL PRESENTATION

- It is more common in boys than girls ▶ it usually occurs during puberty (when there is a relative growth spurt and therefore increased forces on a relatively immature skeleton)
- Two classifications can be used:
  - *Duration of symptoms:* acute (symptoms <3 weeks) ▶ chronic (symptoms >3 weeks) ▶ acute on chronic
  - *Patient mobility:* stable (patient able to walk ± crutches) ▶ unstable (patient unable to walk ± crutches)

RADIOLOGICAL FEATURES

`AP XR` Disuse osteopenia ▶ a widened growth plate with indistinct borders ▶ malalignment of the epiphysis and proximal femoral metaphysis objectively, which is assessed with Klein's line:

- *Klein's line:* a line drawn along the outer border of the femoral neck ▶ when extended upwards this line should intersect approximately $\frac{1}{6}$ of the femoral epiphysis ▶ in SCFE Klein's line may not intersect the proximal femoral epiphysis

`Frog lateral view` This allows an assessment of the severity of the slip using a 'slip angle': SCFE can be classified as mild (<30°), moderate (31–50°), or severe (≥51°)

`US`

- *Stable SCFE:* no joint effusion or evidence of remodelling at the physeal–epiphyseal junction (e.g. periosteal reaction) is demonstrated
- *Unstable SCFE:* a joint effusion is present with no signs of remodelling

PEARL

- **Complications:** chondrolysis (narrowing of the joint space) ▶ AVN ▶ osteoarthritis

SCOLIOSIS

DEFINITION

- Lateral curvature of the spine (>10°)
- **Idiopathic:** there is a strong hereditary component and it is subdivided into:
  - Infantile (onset <3 years of age)
  - Juvenile (3–10 years of age)
  - Adolescent (from 10 years to skeletal maturity)
- **Congenital**
  - *Vertebral anomalies:* hemivertebrae and butterfly vertebrae (failure of formation) ▶ block vertebrae (failure of segmentation)
  - *Syndromes:* Alagille ▶ Jarcho–Levin ▶ VACTERL ▶ Goldenhar ▶ Klippel–Feil
  - *Connective tissue disorders:* Marfan's ▶ Ehlers–Danlos ▶ homocystinuria
  - *Neurological conditions:* cerebral palsy ▶ tethered cord ▶ syringomyelia ▶ meningocele ▶ myelomeningocele ▶ neurofibromatosis
- **Other causes:** any cause of a leg length discrepancy ▶ post radiotherapy ▶ painful scoliosis (e.g. an osteoid osteoma, spinal tumour or infection)

RADIOLOGICAL FEATURES

`CT/MRI` This excludes any underlying vertebral and spinal cord anomalies

- MRI is advised whenever there is a left thoracic curve, pain, abnormal neurological examination, or other unexpected findings (to exclude causes such as tumour, syringomyelia, or spondylolisthesis)

PEARLS

- *The prognosis (risk of curve progression) depends upon:* the patient's gender (it is worse in girls) ▶ the severity of the curve ▶ the child's growth potential
  - The magnitude of the curve is determined by measuring the Cobb angle
  - An estimation of the growth potential can be made by an assessment of the Tanner stage (clinical) and the Risser grade
    - *Risser grade:* this is based on the degree of maturation of the iliac crest apophysis, giving an estimation of how much growth remains ▶ it correlates directly with the risk of curve progression

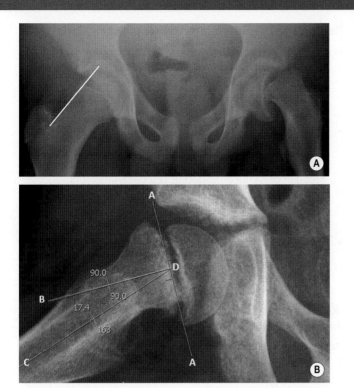

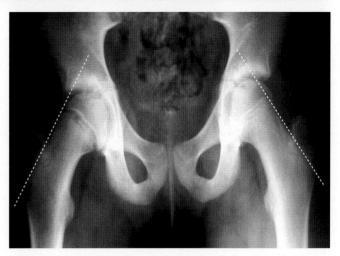

Slipped capital femoral epiphysis. Klein's line.*

Slipped capital femoral epiphysis. (A) Left slipped capital femoral epiphysis. Klein's line is shown on the right. This line should normally intersect approximately the lateral sixth of the capital femoral epiphysis in the AP projection. (B) The slip angle – between (1) a line [BD] perpendicular to the plane of the growth plate [AA] and (2) a line [CD] parallel to the longitudinal axis of the femoral shaft in the frog lateral projection – is 17.4°.**

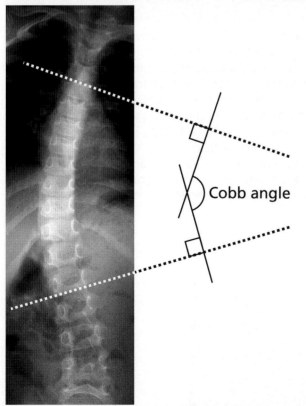

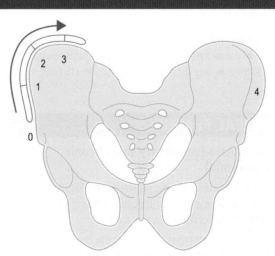

Line diagram of the Risser grades (0 = iliac crest yet to ossify ▶ 4 = full closure of apophysis).

Scoliosis. AP XR of the spine showing measurement of the Cobb angle.*

SICKLE CELL ANAEMIA

DEFINITION

- Normal haemoglobin (HbA) is composed of 2 α and 2 β globin chains
- An autosomal recessive genetic mutation (involving the short arm of chromosome 11) leads to the formation of abnormal β globin chains and the production of sickle cell haemoglobin (HbS) ▶ this affects 1% of the black population (and is rarely seen in Caucasians)

Sickle cell disease (homozygous HbSS)

- With low oxygen tensions, dehydration, acidosis or infection the deoxygenated HbS becomes insoluble with an associated reduced red cell flexibility and a characteristic 'sickle' shape ▶ as well as occluding small vessels, these cells are more fragile with an associated short circulating life (and are subsequently removed by the RES)
- The anaemia is not as marked as seen with thalassaemia major

Sickle cell trait (heterozygous HbAS)

- This generates a milder anaemia, and any vaso-occlusive crises are rare

CLINICAL PRESENTATION

- **Acute sickle crisis:** bone pain ▶ an acute abdomen ▶ hand–foot syndrome (usually affecting patients <4 years old) ▶ acute chest syndrome (due to pulmonary infarction)
- **Other presentations:** cholelithiasis (due to pigment gallstones) ▶ cardiomegaly (secondary to high-output failure) ▶ stroke ▶ leg ulcers ▶ priapism ▶ chronic anaemia

RADIOLOGICAL FEATURES

Marrow hyperplasia (secondary to a chronic haemolytic anaemia)

- Osteopenia ▶ widened diploic space of the skull (the 'hair-on-end' appearance is infrequent) ▶ significant bone modelling abnormalities are rare

  MRI Replacement of normal fatty marrow by intermediate SI T1WI tissue which can extend to the epiphyses

Bone infarcts (due to microvascular occlusions)

- This predominantly affects the medullary diaphyseal and metaphyseal bone (especially the femoral and humeral heads) ▶ the repairing bone is brittle and prone to collapse ▶ it can mimic Legg–Calvé–Perthes disease in children
- Asymmetrical tubular bone shortening is a common sequelae to childhood sickling crises ▶ in adults infarction occurs more in the metaphyses and epiphyses
- *'Hand–foot' syndrome* (sickle cell dactylitis): this describes infarctions of the small tubular bones of the hand and feet ▶ there is massive and painful soft tissue swelling, together with a florid periosteal reaction
- *Vertebral bodies:* 'cod-fish' or 'H-shaped' vertebrae (venous thromboembolism within the central vertebral end plate causes collapse) ▶ it is almost pathognomonic for SCD (but is also seen with Gaucher's disease)

  XR A laminar periosteal reaction ▶ patchy medullary destruction ▶ healing leads to reactive sclerosis

  MRI T2WI/STIR: high SI oedematous medullary cavities ▶ fibrosis and medullary sclerosis generates low SI

Other manifestations

- Papillary necrosis (± chronic renal failure) ▶ an atrophic calcified spleen (due to autoinfarction) ▶ dental complications (caries and mandibular osteomyelitis) ▶ chronic arthritis ▶ growth failure (secondary to involvement of the growth plate)

PEARL

- **Superadded infection:** osteomyelitis is commonly due to salmonella or staphylococcal infection ▶ it usually involves the diaphysis of the humerus, femur and tibia ▶ it can be difficult to distinguish from an infarct (although infarcts are much more common)
- **MRI** Poorly defined bone marrow oedema, periostitis and soft tissue oedema ▶ T1WI + Gad: geographic marrow enhancement
- Long bone marrow infarction can mimic osteomyelitis
- Sickle cell disease is the commonest cause of femoral head necrosis in children

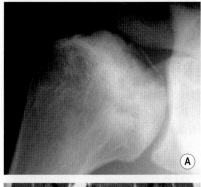

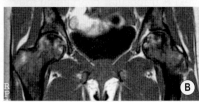

Sickle cell disease. (A) Infarction of the humeral head has led to the separation of an osteochondral fragment of the subarticular bone with adjacent reactive medullary sclerosis. (B) Coronal T1WI of the proximal femora showing patchy hypointensity within the marrow due to marrow hyperplasia and bilateral femoral head osteonecrosis.*

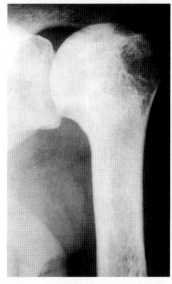

Sickle cell disease. Endosteal bone deposition has resulted in diffuse sclerosis beneath the articular surface (the 'snow cap' sign) due to medullary infarction.[†]

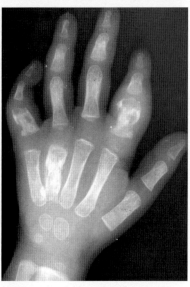

Sickle cell disease. Infarction in several of the metacarpals and proximal phalanges has resulted in bone destruction and swelling of the soft tissues.*

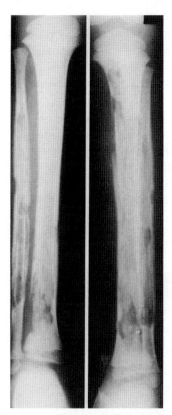

Sickle cell disease with salmonella osteomyelitis. Extreme destructive changes in the long bones have been caused by infection superimposed upon infarction. Numerous sequestra are present.[†]

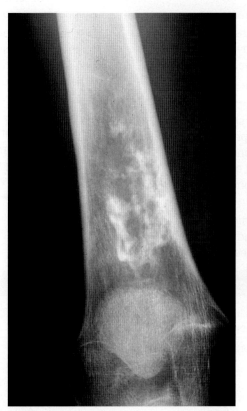

Anteroposterior radiograph of the distal femur demonstrates peripheral sclerosis related to a chronic or healed medullary bone infarct.©35

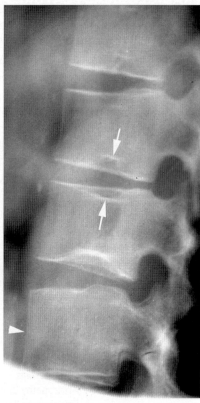

Sickle cell disease. The classical 'stepped depression' ('H-shape') of the vertebral end plates is seen (arrows). Note increased height of the adjacent 'tower' vertebra (arrowhead).*

THALASSAEMIA

DEFINITION

- An inherited defect of HbA synthesis (autosomal dominant) with diminished manufacture of either the α or β chains (leading to α-thalassaemia and β-thalassaemia, respectively) ▶ none of the substitute haemoglobins is as an effective oxygen carrier as HbA and are short-lived (resulting in an erythroid hyperplasia)
  - *Homozygous:* thalassaemia major
  - *Heterozygous:* thalassaemia minor and intermedia

CLINICAL PRESENTATION

Thalassaemia major (β-thalassaemia)

- This is the most severe form, and presents with severe anaemia in infants and young children (with death often in childhood) ▶ characteristically there are rodent facies and hepatosplenomegaly (+ extramedullary erythropoiesis)
- Thalassaemia minor and the other variants show widespread osteopenia only
- Patients are usually of Mediterranean origin

RADIOLOGICAL FEATURES

- The skeletal changes seen in thalassaemia arise from the chronic anaemia and marrow hyperplasia ▶ most commonly seen after the age of 1 year

XR features (untreated thalassaemia major)

Skull Widened diploic spaces (except the occiput) with thinning of the outer table of the skull vault ▶ the trabecular markings are oriented perpendicular to the inner and outer tables (the 'hair-on-end' appearance)
- *'Rodent facies':* frontal bossing and overgrowth of the facial bones with reduced pneumatization of the paranasal sinuses

Spine Marked osteoporosis and cortical thinning results in fractures of the vertebral bodies and platyspondyly ▶ biconcave vertebral bodies are also seen ▶ scoliosis

Extramedullary erythropoiesis Paraspinal (commonly thoracic) cord compression can result if a paraspinal mass extends into the extradural space
- **MRI:** T1WI: diffuse and reduced marrow SI

Ribs Rib expansion ▶ osteoporosis
- *'Rib within a rib' appearance:* subperiosteal extension of haematopoietic tissue at the mid and anterior ribs

Medullary bone Initial trabecular thinning, followed by trabecular coarsening due to new bone formation (most marked in the metacarpals and phalanges, which become cylindrical or even biconvex) ▶ trabecular coarsening may also be seen in the pelvis and vertebrae

Long bones Medullary hyperplasia results in bony expansion and cortical thinning ▶ premature growth plate fusion (particularly of the proximal humerus and distal femur) ▶ Erlenmeyer flask appearances of the long bones (due to marrow expansion with cortical thinning)

PEARLS

Hypertransfusion Repeated transfusion therapy may produce iron overload ▶ this can lead to cartilage abnormalities (symmetrical joint space loss/cystic change/subchondral collapse/osteophytosis) ▶ chondrocalcinosis ▶ osteoporosis secondary to bone iron deposition

DFX therapy Iron chelation therapy can cause dysplastic changes in the spine and long bones + growth retardation – changes typically occur at the metaphysis/physis/epiphysis of the proximal humerus, distal femur, proximal tibia and distal radius and ulna

MRI Irregularity of the metaphyseal–physeal junction with dense sclerotic metaphyseal bands (extending in a 'flame-shaped' manner towards the diaphysis ▶ later features: splaying of the metaphysis and growth plate widening ▶ severe dysplasia at the proximal femur and around the knee ▶ spine: platyspondyly/kyphosis/biconvex vertebral bodies

Skeletal manifestations of anaemias		
	Thalassaemia	**Sickle cell disease**
Skull	*Severe* 'hair-on-end' appearance	*Mild infrequent* 'hair-on-end' appearance
Vertebral bodies	Biconcave vertebral bodies ▶ less common than in sickle cell disease	'H-shaped' vertebrae almost pathognomonic
Other bones	Osteoporosis Arthropathy (haemochromatosis, gout) Erlenmeyer flask deformity	Osteonecrosis Osteomyelitis Growth arrest (decreased blood flow)
Spleen	Large (splenomegaly)	Small (infarction)
Heart	Cardiomegaly	Cardiomegaly
Other	Extramedullary haematopoiesis	Pulmonary crises

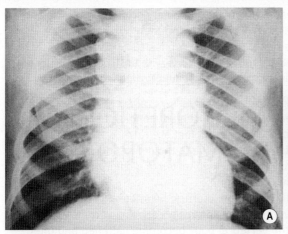
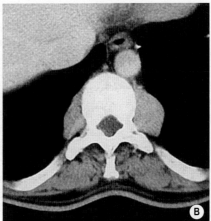

Thalassaemia. (A) Lobulated soft tissue masses due to extramedullary haematopoiesis are present adjacent to the thoracic spine. (B) In another patient, paravertebral extramedullary haematopoietic tissue is shown in the lower sections of a CT examination of the thorax.[†]

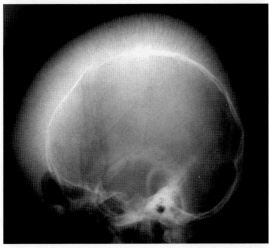

Thalassaemia. Lateral SXR (skull X-ray) showing gross expansion of the diploë and loss of definition of the outer table with sparing of the occipital bone. A gross 'hair-on-end' appearance is shown.*

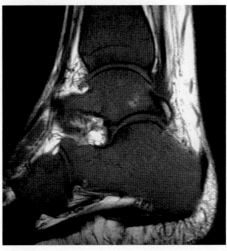

Thalassaemia. Sagittal T1WI of the ankle showing diffuse reduction of marrow signal intensity due to reconversion.*

Thalassaemia. (A) Considerable bone expansion, cortical thinning and simplification of the trabecular pattern. (B) Considerable marrow expansion has produced a flask shape of the distal femur. The coarsened trabecular pattern and cortical thinning are obvious.[†]

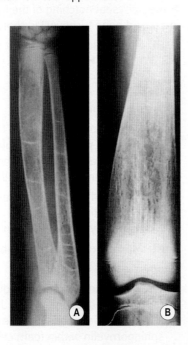
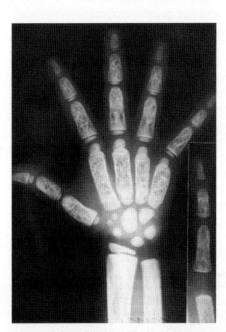

Thalassaemia (boy aged 7). Gross marrow hyperplasia has expanded and thinned overlying cortical bone. Medullary trabeculae have been destroyed and the residual ones are coarsened. Inset – early changes of the same type in a finger of a child aged 4.[†]

5.11 MYELOPROLIFERATIVE DISORDERS

LANGERHANS CELL HISTIOCYTOSIS

Definition

- A non-neoplastic proliferation of Langerhans cells

Letterer–Siwe disease (acute disseminated histiocytosis)

Rare and usually fatal ▶ it affects children <2 years of age ▶ splenomegaly, hepatomegaly and lymphadenopathy with anaemia predominate (patients usually die before any bone lesions are identified) ▶ patients present with fever and a failure to thrive

Hand–Schüller–Christian disease (chronic multifocal histiocytosis)

A disorder of childhood ▶ a classical triad of calvarial lesions + exophthalmos (due to bony orbit histiocytosis) + diabetes insipidus

Eosinophilic granuloma (lesions mainly confined to bone)

The commonest type ▶ benign and self-limiting ▶ 80% present before 10 years of age (2M:1F) ▶ multiple lesions in 10% at presentation ▶ pain and local tenderness (± a moderately elevated ESR) ▶ pathological fractures are rare

Radiological features

Letterer–Siwe disease

XR Destructive medullary lesions within the flat bones and long bone metaphyses

Hand–Schüller–Christian disease

XR Skeletal lesions similar to, but more numerous than, eosinophilic granuloma ▶ long bone metaphyseal and diaphyseal lesions are initially lytic but later heal with periosteal reaction and medullary sclerosis ▶ pelvic and vertebral body lesions are common

- Large geographic areas of destruction within the calvaria
- *'Floating' teeth:* jaw lesions with destruction mainly of the alveolar margins leading to 'floating' teeth (40%)

Eosinophilic granuloma

XR Geographic destruction of bone is characteristic ▶ lesions of the hands and feet are rare

- **Skull:** a bevelled edge to the defect, indicating destruction of the two tables to a differing degree ('hole within a hole' sign)
- **Paediatric spine:** thoracic > lumbar > cervical involvement ▶ it classically causes a vertebra plana, with the vertebral body becoming flattened and often wafer-thin
- **Flat or long bones:** typically diaphyseal involvement with an ill-defined medullary lesion ▶ endosteal erosion and a linear periosteal reaction is common
- **Unusual features:** epiphyseal lesions ▶ transphyseal lesions ▶ extracranial 'button' sequestra ▶ posterior vertebral arch lesions

Scintigraphy 'Hot' or 'cold' spots

MRI A non-specific focal lesion with extensive marrow and soft tissue oedema (± fluid–fluid levels or dural extension of spinal lesions) ▶ T1WI: low SI ▶ T2WI/STIR: high SI ▶ extraosseous involvement in 30%

GAUCHER'S DISEASE

Definition

- The most common lipid storage disorder due to an autosomal recessive genetic enzyme (glucocerebrosidase) deficiency ▶ this leads to accumulation of the lipid glucocerebroside within the lysosomes of monocytes and macrophages of many organs (Gaucher cells)
  - *Type 1:* non-neuronopathic (common)
  - *Type 2:* neuronopathic (acute)
  - *Type 3:* neuronopathic (subacute)
- **Infantile form:** hepatosplenomegaly, lymphadenopathy, neurological complications, anaemia and haemorrhage ▶ death usually occurs at <2 years of age (mainly due to CNS involvement) ▶ it mainly affects non-Jews
- **Adult form:** hepatosplenomegaly, abdominal pain, ascites, dull bone pain or acute painful crises due to bone infarction (± fever, leucocytosis and a raised ESR) ▶ many patients are Ashkenazi Jews

Radiological features

XR Lipid accumulation within the marrow space results in osteopenia (± pathological fractures), lytic lesions, a 'soap bubble' appearance and endosteal scalloping ▶ an Erlenmeyer flask deformity (due to loss of normal modelling) ▶ osteosclerosis (due to a healing bone infarct) ▶ metaphyseal notching of the humerus (secondary to increased bone turnover) is characteristic

MRI This evaluates the extent of any marrow infiltration ▶ T1WI: low SI ▶ T2WI: high SI

Pearls

Bone infarction (AVN)

- This is due to an interrupted blood supply or a fat embolism ▶ particularly involves subarticular bone of the femoral and humeral heads, the metaphyseal regions of the long bones and vertebral bodies

XR 'H-shaped' vertebral bodies (following collapse) ▶ periosteal reaction

- **Scintigraphy:** focal photopenic areas

MRI Marrow oedema ▶ possible cord compression

Niemann–Pick disease

- A rare autosomal recessive disorder of phospholipid metabolism affecting mainly Jewish infants ▶ it resembles Gaucher's disease but there is deposition of sphingomyelin within foam cells

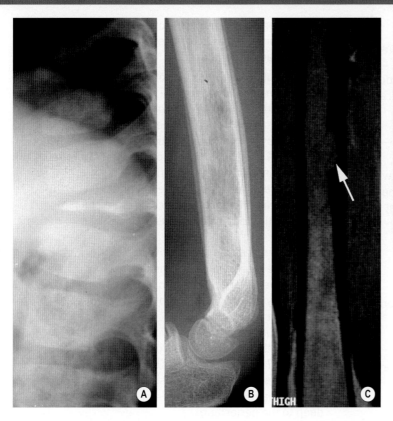

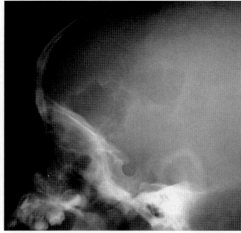

Langerhans cell histiocytosis. Geographic lytic lesions of the skull vault in Hand–Schüller–Christian disease.*

Langerhans cell histiocytosis. (A) Vertebra plana of T11 is demonstrated. (B) Distal humeral metadiaphyseal lesion showing permeative destruction and periosteal reaction. (C) Coronal T1WI of the femur showing a focal lesion causing endosteal scalloping (arrow).*

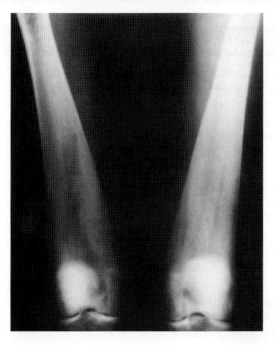

Gaucher's disease. Abnormal modelling of the distal femora has resulted in a typical Erlenmeyer flask deformity. An osteolytic lesion with a coarse trabecular pattern is present in the right femur.†

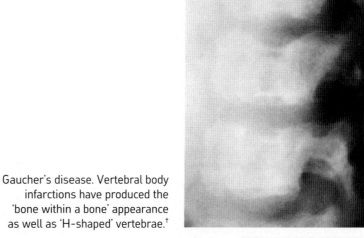

Gaucher's disease. Vertebral body infarctions have produced the 'bone within a bone' appearance as well as 'H-shaped' vertebrae.†

LEUKAEMIA

Definition

- Cancer of the blood-forming cells of the bone marrow (usually affecting leucocytes)
  - *Acute lymphocytic leukaemia (ALL):* this affects adults and children although it is more common in children (75% of paediatric acute leukaemias)
  - *Acute myeloblastic leukaemia (AML):* the most common adult acute leukaemia (20%)
  - *Chronic lymphocytic leukaemia (CLL):* an adult disorder (predominantly affecting the elderly) ▶ twice as common as CML ▶ characterized by enlargement of the spleen and lymph nodes and rarely skeletal involvement (except as a terminal event)
  - *Chronic myeloid leukaemia (CML):* this is more common in adults

Clinical presentation

- Bone pain at presentation is five times more common in children than adults
- **Acute leukaemia:** the commonest malignancy of childhood ▶ it presents with non-specific malaise, anorexia and weight loss ▶ bone lesions are common, as is limb pain and pathological fractures
- **Chronic leukaemias:** these predominate in adults ▶ bone lesions are uncommon and focal (simulating metastases)
- It can sometimes terminate in an acute blastic form

Radiological features

- Adult skeletal lesions affect sites of residual red marrow: the axial skeleton and the proximal ends of the femora

and humeri ▶ they are less commonly seen than in children and have to be differentiated from metastases or a primary bone tumour

XR (children) Overproduction of leukaemic cells: trabecular and endosteal cortical destruction and eventually extraosseous extension ▶ diffuse osteopenia (due to marrow infiltration with leukaemic cells, steroids or chemotherapy) ▶ mixed osteolytic or osteoblastic lesions (affecting 18% of children) ▶ osteosclerosis (rarely seen) ▶ osteonecrosis following treatment

- *Metaphyseal lucent bands:* these primarily affect the sites of maximum growth (such as the distal femur, proximal tibia and distal radius) ▶ typically 2–15 mm in width
- *Diffuse permeative bone destruction:* this occurs with more extensive involvement ▶ osteolytic bony destructive lesions have a 'moth-eaten' appearance commonly affecting the long bone metaphyses ▶ cortex eroded on its endosteal surface
- *Non-specific cortical destruction:* this affects the medial aspect of the proximal humerus, tibia and femur
- *Periosteal reaction (up to 50%):* this occurs in isolation or with destructive cortical lesions ▶ it is due to haemorrhage and proliferation of leukaemic deposits deep to the periosteum
- *Chloroma:* a paediatric focal expanding geographical tumour (seen in AML) ▶ it is due to a collection of leukaemic cells and is usually located within the skull, spine, ribs or sternum

MRI Diffuse marrow infiltration ▶ T1WI: low SI (normal to nodular, then diffuse low SI)

MASTOCYTOSIS (MAST CELL RETICULOSIS/URTICARIA PIGMENTOSA)

Definition

- A clonal disorder of mast cell proliferation within different body tissues that can result in a variety of clinical syndromes, including:
  - *Urticaria pigmentosa (80–90%):* self-limiting and typically affects children ▶ bone changes in 10%
  - *Systemic mastocytosis (<10%):* this typically affects adults ▶ bone changes in 70%
  - *Mast cell leukaemia*

Clinical presentation

- Clinical symptoms resemble lymphoma or leukaemia and can be fatal
- Hepatosplenomegaly (the lymph nodes, skin and bone marrow can also be affected) ▶ bone marrow involvement in 90%

Radiological features

XR Changes are always seen within the spine (± vertebral compression fractures) as well as in the skull, ribs and pelvis

- Diffuse generalized osteosclerosis (due to trabecular and cortical thickening) ▶ there can be a superimposed fine reticular or nodular sclerosis ▶ multifocal sclerotic lesions can mimic osteoblastic metastases
- Small osteolytic or osteoblastic lesions which may disappear spontaneously ▶ small (4–5 mm) lytic lesions may be surrounded by a rim of sclerosis (commonly seen in the spine/ribs/skull/pelvis/tubular bones)
- Diffuse osteopaenia is a common pattern (commonly affecting the axial skeleton)

MRI T1WI: homogeneous or heterogeneous low SI within the bone marrow

Pearls

- **Other features:** jejunal fold thickening ▶ peptic ulcers ▶ hepatosplenomegaly ▶ pulmonary fibrosis and nodules
- *Differential:* myelofibrosis ▶ fluorosis ▶ carcinomatosis ▶ lymphoma

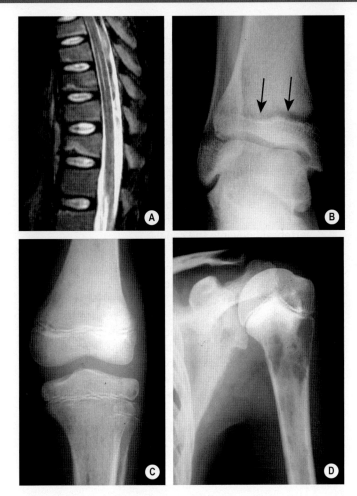

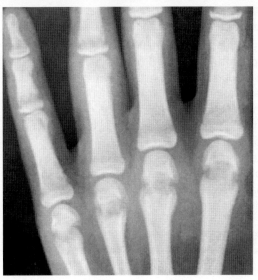

Acute leukaemia. Extensive metaphyseal radiolucencies are present with adjacent periosteal new bone formation.†

Acute leukaemia. (A) Sagittal fat-suppressed T2WI MRI of the thoracic spine showing multilevel wedge compression fractures due to osteopenia as the presenting feature of AML. (B) Metaphyseal lucent bands (arrows) in the distal tibia in a patient with acute lymphocytic leukaemia (ALL). (C) Permeative pattern of bone destruction in the distal femoral and proximal tibial metaphyses. (D) Multiple lytic areas of bone destruction in the proximal humeral metaphysis and scapula.*

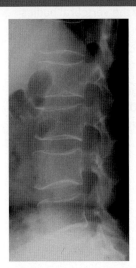

Mastocytosis. Lateral radiograph of the lumbar spine showing diffuse osteopenia and multilevel mild compression fractures.**

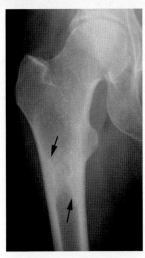

Mastocytosis. AP radiograph of the right hip showing endosteal sclerosis in the proximal femur (arrows).**

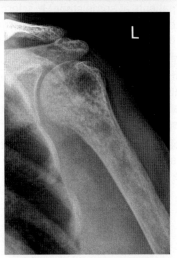

Mastocytosis. AP radiograph of the left shoulder showing nodular sclerosis in the ribs and proximal humerus.**

MULTIPLE MYELOMA (MM)

DEFINITION

- This is due to monoclonal proliferation of the antibody-producing plasma B cells with an associated increased production of a single immunoglobulin
- It is the most common primary malignant neoplasm of bone and is the predominant plasma cell dyscrasia (representing 10% of all haematological malignancies) ▶ it is incurable
- Protein electrophoresis: there will be a wide M-band because of the abnormal paraprotein ▶ Bence Jones proteinuria is present in over 50% (due to light chain immunoglobulin production)

CLINICAL PRESENTATION

- The median age at presentation is 65 years (M:F 2:1) ▶ it can present with fever, pain, backache and weakness ▶ there is an elevated ESR
- *Risk factors for acute renal failure:* hypercalcaemia ▶ dehydration ▶ infection ▶ amyloidosis
- Chronic renal failure is a major cause of death

RADIOLOGICAL FEATURES

Location There is widespread involvement of the skeleton in 80% of cases (especially the axial skeleton and proximal ends of the long bones)

XR There are two common appearances:
- *The classically well-defined small 'punched-out' lesions throughout the skeleton* (most characteristically affecting the skull)
- *Diffuse osteopenia* (usually involving the spine and which may result in multiple compression fractures in 50% of patients at some stage) ▶ sclerotic or mixed lesions are rare in untreated patients (marginal sclerosis may be observed following radiotherapy)

CT Purely marrow lesions appear as focal areas of soft tissue density – diffuse osteopaenia of MM may be indistinguishable from osteoporosis ▶ progressive disease results in endosteal scalloping, cortical destruction and soft tissue masses

Scintigraphy This may underestimate the disease extent (many lesions show normal uptake or photopenia as they are non-osteoblastic)

^{18}FDG-PET This is more sensitive than a skeletal survey in demonstrating the disease extent

MRI Variable appearances ▶ there is normal marrow at presentation in 50–75% of cases with untreated early disease (and 20% of advanced cases)
- It can distinguish between benign vertebral body collapse (in ⅔ of patients this is due to diffuse osteopenia) and a pathological collapse (due to tumour infiltration):
  - *Benign:* band-like marrow oedema (acute stage) ▶ normal marrow SI (chronic stage) ▶ normal SI within the pedicles ▶ homogeneous contrast enhancement, retropulsion of the posteriosuperior corner of the vertebral body into the canal
  - *Pathological:* T1WI: diffuse low SI throughout the vertebral body ▶ neural arch involvement ▶ soft tissue extension ▶ posterior bulging of the vertebral body cortex
- *Focal disease:* T1WI: localized areas of reduced SI ▶ T2WI/STIR: corresponding increased SI
- *Diffuse disease (poorer outcome):* T1WI: generalized reduced marrow SI (the intervertebral discs appear hyperintense relative to the vertebral bodies) ▶ T2WI/STIR: high SI marrow ▶ T1WI + Gad: diffuse enhancement
- *'Variegated' (early) disease:* T1WI: multiple tiny foci of reduced SI on a background of normal marrow ▶ T2WI/STIR: corresponding high SI

PEARLS

- Unlike metastatic disease, myeloma can involve the intervertebral discs and mandible and produce a large soft tissue mass
  - *Myeloma:* this will also destroy the vertebral bodies before the pedicles
  - *Metastatic disease:* this will destroy the pedicles first

Poems syndrome

- A purely sclerotic myeloma may occur and may be associated with **P**olyneuropathy, **O**rganomegaly, **E**ndocrinopathy, **M**onoclonal gammopathy and **S**kin changes

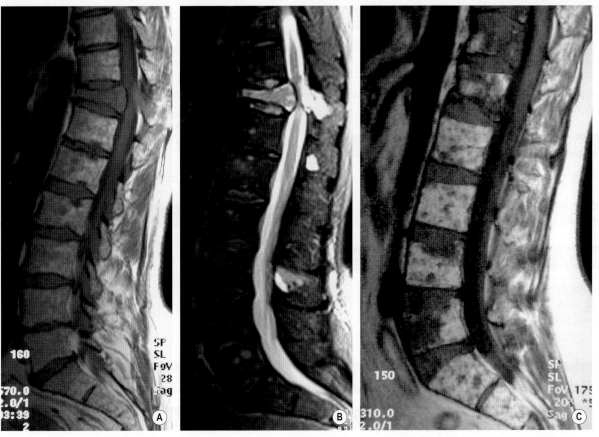

Multiple myeloma. (A) Sagittal T1WI and (B) fat-suppressed T2WI showing pathological collapse of T11 with cord compression and multiple smaller areas of focal marrow involvement. (C) Sagittal T1WI showing the variegated pattern of marrow involvement.*

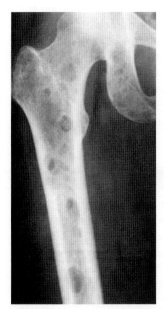

Myeloma. Typical localized lesions which are sharply defined rounded defects with endosteal erosion of the cortex.†

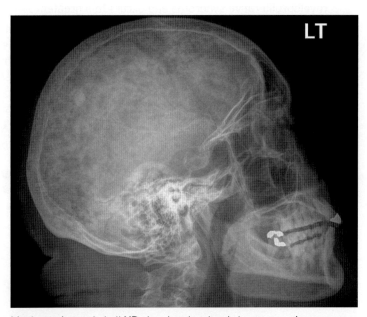

Myeloma. Lateral skull XR showing the classic 'pepper-pot' appearance of the skull.*

PLASMACYTOMA (SOLITARY MYELOMA)

DEFINITION

- A solitary destructive bony lesion due to the pathological proliferation of B lymphocytes ▶ it accounts for approximately 2% of all plasma cell dyscrasias
- It can remain localized for many years, but 30% progress rapidly to a generalized myelomatosis

CLINICAL PRESENTATION

- It is asymptomatic or can present with pain (e.g. backache)
- It has an earlier and wider age range at presentation than with multiple myeloma

RADIOLOGICAL FEATURES

Location Usually sites where there is persistent red marrow (e.g. the axial skeleton, pelvis, proximal femur, proximal humerus and ribs) ▶ peripheral lesions are rare

XR An expansile lytic destructive lesion arising within the medulla (± a soft tissue mass) ▶ sclerosis is rare ▶ it often has a well-defined margin (as it is slow growing) ▶ there is cortical thinning ▶ there can be a 'soap bubble' appearance (due to apparent trabeculation) ▶ it may resemble an ABC or expanding osteolytic metastasis in the long and flat bones

- *Vertebral bodies:* involvement is common ▶ it can lead to early collapse ▶ there is rarely extension across the disc space

MRI/¹⁸FDG-PET This can detect occult lesions

PEARL

- Protein electrophoresis is often normal (as there is a relatively small tumour mass)

PRIMARY MYELOFIBROSIS (MYELOID METAPLASIA/MYELOSCLEROSIS)

DEFINITION

- A slowly progressive marrow disorder of unknown aetiology ▶ secondary causes of myelofibrosis should be excluded
  - Secondary myelofibrosis is the end stage of the myeloproliferative syndrome and occurs to a greater or lesser degree in leukaemia, lymphoma, Gaucher's disease, toxic exposure, carcinomatosis and even infection

CLINICAL PRESENTATION

- It presents between the ages of 20 and 80 years, with a median age of 60 years (M = F) ▶ death typically occurs <2–3 years after diagnosis
- It presents with an insidious onset with weakness, dyspnoea and weight loss ▶ antecedent polycythaemia is common, but obliteration of the marrow by fibrosis or bony sclerosis soon leads to a moderate normochromic normocytic anaemia ▶ there is a leucocytosis with immature white cell forms
  - Hepatosplenomegaly ▶ extramedullary haematopoiesis also occurs within the lymph nodes, lungs, choroids plexus and kidneys

RADIOLOGICAL FEATURES

XR Bone sclerosis is the major finding and is due to trabecular and endosteal new bone formation resulting in a reduced marrow diameter (30–70%) – this is typically diffuse but can occasionally be patchy in nature ▶ in established disease lucent areas are due to fibrous tissue reaction ▶ it predominantly affects the red marrow containing bones (e.g. the axial skeleton and metaphyses of the femur, humerus and tibia) ▶ periosteal reaction is seen in ⅓ of cases and affects the medial aspects of the distal femur and proximal tibia ▶ a mixed sclerotic and lytic pattern can be seen in the skull

MRI T1WI/T2WI: the high SI fatty marrow is replaced by low SI material

PEARLS

- *Other features:* arthropathy due to haemarthrosis and secondary gout (5–20%) ▶ polyarthralgia and polyarthritis due to infiltration of the synovium by bone marrow elements ▶ leukaemic conversion manifests as development of an extraosseous soft tissue mass
- Increased bone density is also seen with: osteopetrosis ▶ fluorosis ▶ mastocytosis ▶ carcinomatosis ▶ adult sickle cell disease
  - A combination of bone sclerosis, anaemia and splenomegaly suggests myelofibrosis

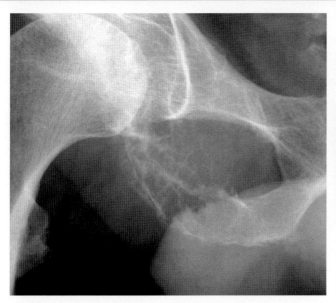

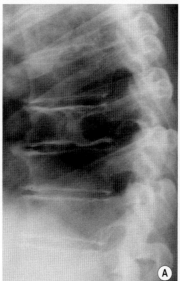

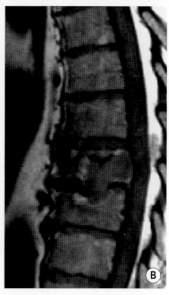

Plasmacytoma. AP XR shows a slightly expanded lytic lesion with apparent trabeculation in the inferior pubic ramus.*

Plasmacytoma of the spine. (A) Lateral XR shows a lytic destructive lesion exhibiting minor collapse. (B) Sagittal T1WI MRI demonstrates extension across the disc space.*

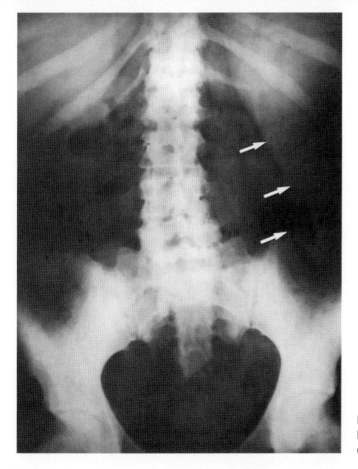

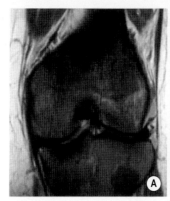

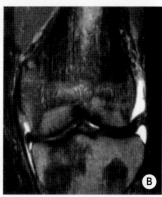

Myelosclerosis. Coronal intermediate (A) and T2W (B) images of the knee showing replacement of the normal high SI fatty marrow by fibrosis. This, and abnormal bone deposition around the trabeculae, results in the diffuse low SI from the medullary cavity.†

Myelosclerosis. All the bones are dense with a lack of distinction between cortical and medullary bone. The spleen is grossly enlarged (arrows).†

WOMEN'S IMAGING

6.1 BREAST

NORMAL ANATOMY

- The breast lies on the chest wall and on the deep pectoral fascia ▶ the superficial pectoral fascia envelops the breast ▶ suspensory ligaments (Cooper's ligaments) connect the two layers

2 components

- **Nipple–areolar complex:**
  - Collecting ducts open onto the tip of the nipple
  - Sebaceous glands within the nipple–areolar complex are called Montgomery's glands ▶ ducts open onto the skin surface (and are seen as small raised nodular structures called Morgagni's tubercles)
- **Glandular tissue:**
  - This is divided into 15–25 lobes, each consisting of a branching duct system leading from the collecting ducts to the terminal duct lobular units (TDLUs)
  - Each duct drains a lobe made up of 20–40 lobules
  - Young women usually have dense glandular breast tissue ▶ this is usually replaced by fatty tissues in older women with loss of the lobular units
  - Lymphatic drainage is usually to the axillary and internal mammary nodes

METHODS OF IMAGING

Imaging in mammography

- *High spatial resolution is required to detect microcalcification:* a short exposure time limits any movement artefact ▶ it requires a very small focal spot (0.1–0.3 mm) ▶ grids are used to reduce scatter and increase contrast ▶ digital mammography is now used
- *There is a narrow range of inherent breast densities* (as it is predominantly fatty tissue): low molybdenum energy peaks (17.5 and 19.6 keV) provide high contrast (filtering reduces extraneous radiation)
- *Breast compression:* this reduces geometric and movement unsharpness ▶ it improves contrast (it reduces scatter) ▶ it reduces radiation dose (less tissue needs to be penetrated) ▶ it achieves uniform image density ▶ it separates superimposed breast tissues ▶ it highlights rigid tumours (glandular tissue is compressible)

Mammography (digital/analogue) (MMG)

- **Indications:**
  - Evaluation of breast symptoms and signs, including masses, skin thickening, deformity, nipple retraction, nipple discharge and nipple eczema
  - Breast cancer screening
  - Follow-up of breast cancer patients
  - Guidance for biopsy or localization of lesions not visible on ultrasound
- **Mediolateral oblique (MLO) view (standard):**
  - The XR beam is directed from superomedial to inferolateral (usually at 30–60°) ▶ compression is applied obliquely across the chest wall and perpendicular to the long-axis pectoralis major
  - The only view demonstrating the entire breast tissue on a single image
  - *Well positioned if:* the inframammary angle is demonstrated ▶ the nipple is in profile ▶ the nipple is positioned at the level of the lower border of the pectoralis major, with the muscle across the posterior border of the film at 25–30° to the vertical
- **Craniocaudal (CC) view (standard):**
  - The XR beam travels from superior to inferior ▶ the breast is pulled forward and away from the chest wall with compression applied from above
  - *Well positioned if:* the nipple is in profile ▶ it demonstrates virtually all of the medial tissue and the majority of the lateral tissue (with exclusion of the axillary tail of the breast) ▶ the depth of breast tissue should be <1 cm of the distance from the nipple to the pectoralis major on the MLO projection
- **Paddle views (supplementary):**
  - Localized compression applied with a compression paddle
  - It distinguishes a real lesion from superimposition of normal tissues ▶ it defines the margins of a mass
- **True lateral view (supplementary):**
  - The mammography unit is turned through 90° and a mediolateral or lateromedial XR beam used
  - It distinguishes superimposition of normal structures from real lesions ▶ it increases the accuracy of wire localizations of non-palpable lesions
- **Magnification views (supplementary):**
  - Performed in the craniocaudal and lateral projections
  - These interrogate areas of microcalcification and can demonstrate 'teacups' with benign calcification
- **Eklund technique (supplementary):**
  - For use with subpectoral breast implants (displacement of the implant posteriorly)

Ultrasound (US)

- Use a high-frequency transducer (e.g. 7.5–15 MHz) for greater resolution at a cost of reduced penetration
- Image breast tissue in two planes (perpendicular to each other)
- **Indications:**
  - Characterization of palpable mass lesions
  - Assessment of abnormalities detected on a mammogram
  - The primary technique for the assessment of breast problems in younger patients
  - Guidance for biopsy and wire localizations

Elastography Assesses tissue 'stiffness' (tumours tend to be stiff) ▶ strain elastography: operator manually compresses the breast ▶ shear wave elastography: pulses are produced by the transducer

MRI Adjunctive diagnostic tool – see Section 6 Chapter 1, Contrast enhanced MRI in breast cancer

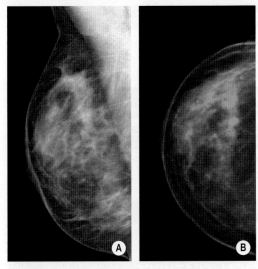

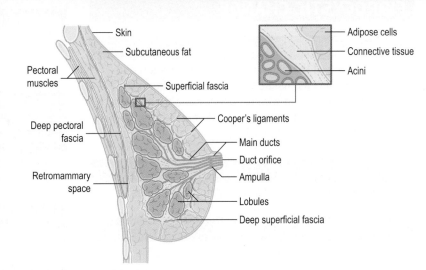

A standard set of mammograms consists of the mediolateral oblique (MLO) view (A) and the craniocaudal (CC) view (B). This normal breast contains a moderate amount of dense glandular tissue.*

Gross anatomy of the breast.

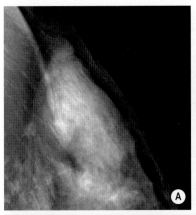

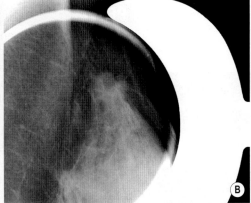

Additional mammographic views. (A) An area of concern was identified in the lateral aspect of the left breast on initial mammography. (B) A 'paddle view' was performed and two suspicious spiculated mass lesions were demonstrated much more clearly.*

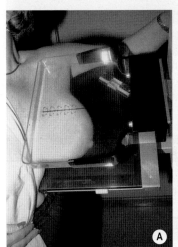

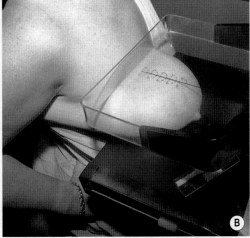

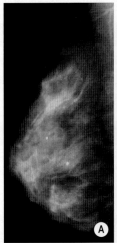

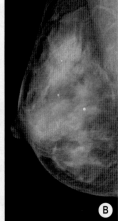

Breast positioning. Positioning for the (A) mediolateral oblique and (B) craniocaudal views.*

Screening mammogram of a 57-year-old, with dense breast parenchyma and scattered benign microcalcifications. This MLO view has been performed on (A) a conventional screen/film system and (B) a digital mammography system.*

FIBROCYSTIC CHANGE

DEFINITION

- Exaggeration of the normal cyclical proliferation and involution of breast tissue with the development of fibrosis ▶ regression with pregnancy and menopause ▶ increased risk for developing certain types of cancer (e.g. ductal carcinoma in situ (DCIS))

CLINICAL PRESENTATION

- Breast fullness, tenderness and palpable nodules

RADIOLOGICAL FEATURES

US Ill-defined focal lesions

MRI T1WI: diffuse low SI ▶ T2WI: diffuse high SI (2nd half of cycle): T1WI + Gad: patchy enhancement

- **Adenosis:** hyperplasia and hypertrophy of the glandular elements
- **Sclerosing adenosis:** adenosis + reactive fibrosis ▶ diffusely scattered calcifications
- **Lobular hyperplasia:** adenosis + cystic lobule dilatation ▶ a 'teacup' configuration of calcium within the cystic spaces

CYSTS

DEFINITION

- The most common cause of a discrete breast mass

CLINICAL PRESENTATION

- Often multiple and bilateral masses ▶ common between 20 and 50 years old (peak between 40 and 50 years old)

RADIOLOGICAL FEATURES

MMG Well-defined round or ovoid masses ± a halo

US Well-defined round or oval anechoic lesions + posterior acoustic enhancement

PEARL

US-guided aspiration can be performed if symptomatic ▶ perform cytology only if there are suspicious imaging features or if the aspirate is bloodstained

FAT NECROSIS (OIL CYST)

DEFINITION

- This occurs following local trauma (due to fat saponification by tissue lipase after local cell destruction), appearing as single or multiple lesions

RADIOLOGICAL FEATURES

MMG An ill-defined spiculated mass ▶ coarse mural curvilinear calcification

PAPILLOMA

DEFINITION

- A benign neoplasm arising within a duct (either centrally or peripherally within the breast)

CLINICAL PRESENTATION

- Watery nipple discharge (which may be bloodstained)

RADIOLOGICAL FEATURES

MMG A well-defined mass, commonly in a retroareolar location ± microcalcification

US A filling defect within a dilated duct or cyst

PEARL

- Impossible to differentiate papillomas from papillary carcinoma on imaging alone
- Papillomas may be associated with an increased risk of malignancy, particularly if they are multiple or occur in a more peripheral location within the breast (papillomatosis)
  - It requires surgical excision (or piecemeal percutaneous excision using a vacuum-assisted biopsy device if there is no cellular atypia following percutaneous biopsy)

HAMARTOMA

DEFINITION

- Benign breast masses composed of normal breast components (lobular structures, stroma and adipose tissue) ▶ they can occur at any age and are often palpable

RADIOLOGICAL FEATURES

MMG Large (3–5 cm) well-circumscribed masses containing a mixture of dense and lucent areas

PEARL

- These may be indistinguishable on imaging from other benign masses (e.g. a fibroadenoma) ▶ on histology it may be reported as normal breast tissue

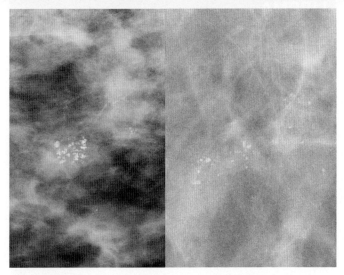

Sclerosing adenosis. Clusters of fine granular pleomorphic calcifications.†

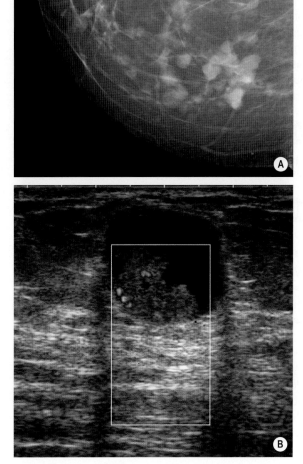

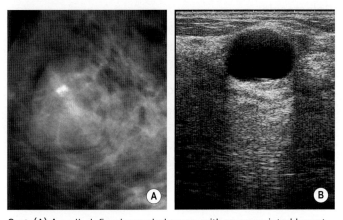

Cyst. (A) A well-defined rounded mass, with an associated lucent halo. (B) US. The absence of internal echoes and posterior enhancement is diagnostic of a cyst.*

(A) Multiple small papillomas. Papillomas are frequently well defined on mammography, although part of the mass may have an irregular or ill-defined contour. (B) US: the presence of a filling defect within a cystic structure suggests the diagnosis. Colour Doppler can be useful to distinguish debris within a cyst from a soft tissue mass.*

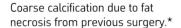

Coarse calcification due to fat necrosis from previous surgery.*

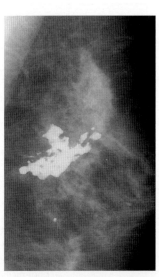

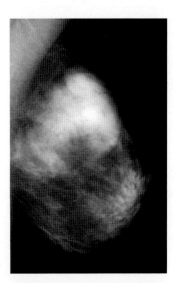

Hamartomas are frequently encountered on screening mammograms as large, lobulated masses with areas of varying density reflecting the presence of elements which are of fat and soft tissue density.*

FIBROADENOMA

DEFINITION

- A benign tumour arising from the TDLU (fibrous stroma + epithelial ductal structures) ▶ it often enlarges during pregnancy and regresses after the menopause ▶ it is the most common cause of a benign solid mass in the breast
- Requires biopsy for diagnosis unless <25 years old (to exclude malignancy)

CLINICAL PRESENTATION

- Smooth, well-demarcated, mobile lumps ▶ peak incidence – 3rd decade ▶ multiple in 10–20%

RADIOLOGICAL FEATURES

MMG Well-defined, rounded or oval masses ▶ coarse calcifications may develop (particularly in older women)

US Well-circumscribed, gently lobulated, smooth oval lesion ▶ isoechoic or mildly hypoechoic relative to fat ± a thin echogenic pseudocapsule ▶ a surrounding halo (Mach effect) ▶ displaced normal vessels around the edge of the lesion

- *Juvenile fibroadenoma:* a more cellular variant occurring at a younger age
- *Phyllodes tumour:* a fibroepithelial tumour similar to a giant fibroadenoma, affecting an older age group ▶ <25% are locally aggressive requiring clear surgical margins ▶ large fibroadenomas or those rapidly increasing in size are excised to avoid missing a phyllodes tumour

LIPOMA

DEFINITION

- Benign tumours composed of fat, and seen in older patients

CLINICAL PRESENTATION

- Soft, lobulated masses

RADIOLOGICAL FEATURES

MMG A radiolucent mass

US A well-defined lesion, and hyperechoic compared to adjacent fat

OTHER BENIGN MASS LESIONS

Galactocele

- Milk-containing cysts resulting from inspissated milk obstructing a duct ▶ they occur shortly after or during lactation (within the retroareolar area)

Radial scar (sclerosing duct hyperplasia)

- A benign idiopathic scarring process which is rarely palpable ▶ it requires excision for diagnosis as it is difficult to distinguish from lobular carcinoma

    MMG An irregular spiculated non-calcified lesion without a central mass

Typical US characteristics of solid breast lesions[†]		
	Benign	**Malignant**
Shape	Oval/ellipsoid	Variable
Alignment	Wider than deep ▶ aligned parallel to tissue planes	Deeper than wide
Margins	Smooth/thin echogenic pseudocapsule with 2–3 gentle lobulations	Irregular or spiculated ▶ echogenic 'halo'
Echotexture	Variable-to-intense hyperechogenicity	Low-level Marked hypoechogenicity
Homogeneity of internal echoes	Uniform	Non-uniform
Lateral shadowing	Present	Absent
Posterior effect	Minimum attenuation/posterior enhancement	Attenuation with obscured posterior margins
Other signs		Calcification Microlobulation Intraductal extension Infiltration across tissue planes and increased echogenicity of surrounding fat

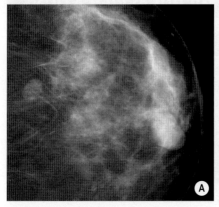
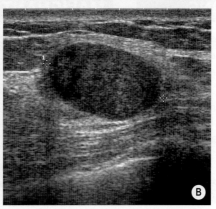

Fibroadenoma. (A) Two well-defined masses on mammography. (B) US showed a well-defined oval mass.*

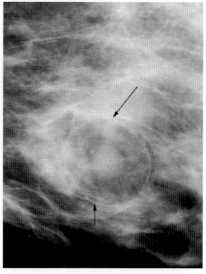

Galactocele. A circumscribed mixed-density lesion with a capsule (arrows).†

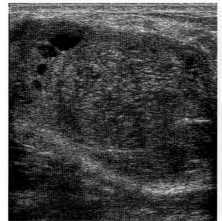
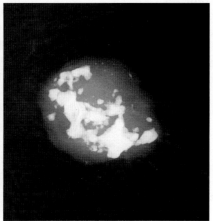

Phyllodes tumour. The presence of several cystic spaces within this large, well-defined mass suggested the possibility of a phyllodes tumour.*

Fibroadenomas may develop coarse 'popcorn'-type calcifications.*

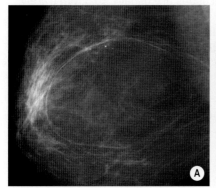
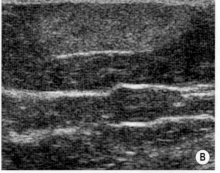

Lipoma. (A) On mammography, a lipoma may be seen as a well-defined mass of fat density, contained within a thin capsule. (B) US: a well-defined hyperechoic lesion characteristic of a lipoma.*

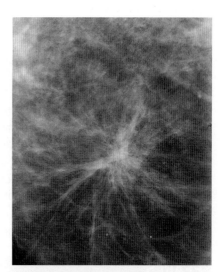

Architectural distortion (stellate lesion) due to a benign complex sclerosing lesion/radial scar.†

BENIGN MICROCALCIFICATIONS

DEFINITION

- Small breast calcifications seen on MMG of benign aetiology
- *Causes:* normal stroma ▶ fibrocystic change ▶ duct ectasia ▶ fat necrosis ▶ fibroadenomatoid hyperplasia ▶ fibroadenomas ▶ papillomas ▶ vascular calcification ▶ skin calcification ▶ atrophic breast lobules

RADIOLOGICAL FEATURES

Vascular calcification A 'tramline' appearance (calcification of both walls)

Duct ectasia *'broken-needle' appearance:* bilateral coarse dense rod and branching calcifications with well-defined margins (representing calcification of debris within dilated ducts) ▶ this is seen within the anterior $\frac{1}{3}$ of the breast

- *'Lead-pipe' appearance:* if debris is extruded from the ducts into the adjacent parenchyma, then an inflammatory-type reaction can occur with fat necrosis: calcifications then take on this characteristic appearance

Fibrocystic change Sedimented milk of calcium within microcysts

- *CC view:* round 'smudge' shadow
- *Lateral magnification view:* a characteristic 'teacup' sign due to a calcium-fluid level (layering of calcific fluid within microcysts)

Fat necrosis This occurs following trauma or surgery ▶ eggshell calcification is seen within the wall of an oil cyst, or coarse dystrophic calcification is associated with areas of scarring

Fibroadenoma Calcification with a coarse 'popcorn' appearance (occurring especially after the menopause) ▶ occasionally any calcification is small and punctuate

Fibroadenomatoid hyperplasia Histologically there are features of both a fibroadenoma and fibrocystic change ▶ any microcalcification has a non-specific appearance

Skin calcification These are round, well-defined and have a lucent centre ▶ they are very often bilateral and symmetrical ▶ talcum powder, deodorants and tattoos can mimic microcalcification

Calcified suture material Dense, curvilinear calcification

PEARLS

- Indeterminate microcalcifications require biopsy to exclude DCIS (e.g. with fibroadenomatoid hyperplasia, fibrocystic change, or atypical fibroadenomas)
- Talcum powder, deodorants on skin and tattoo pigments can mimic microcalcifications

MALIGNANT MICROCALCIFICATIONS

DEFINITION

- Many breast cancers arise from areas of ductal carcinoma in situ (DCIS) and are associated with microcalcification on MMG – particularly true for high-grade invasive ductal carcinomas associated with high-grade DCIS

RADIOLOGICAL FEATURES

- Microcalcifications are more likely to be malignant if they are clustered, vary in size and shape (pleomorphic) or are found in a ductal or linear distribution

High histological grade DCIS 'Casting' or comedo microcalcifications: microcalcifications are classically linear, fragmented, rod shaped and branching

- These represent calcified necrotic debris within ducts (hence their linear and branching structure)
- The greater the number of microcalcification flecks associated with an area of DCIS, the greater the risk of invasive disease

Low histological grade DCIS Microcalcifications are much less frequent as there is usually no intraductal necrosis

- *'Cribriform' pattern:* when present they are clustered in appearance, but otherwise non-specific appearance

PEARLS

- The greater the number of flecks of microcalcification associated with an area of DCIS, the greater the risk of invasive disease:
  - <5 calcifications per cm^3 have a low probability for malignancy
  - Malignant calcifications are usually <0.5 mm (rarely >1 mm)
- The sensitivity of ultrasound for detecting DCIS is significantly lower than MMG (hence US is not a good screening tool)

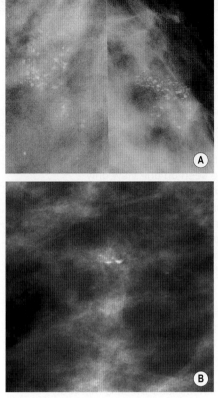

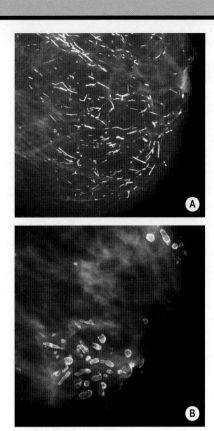

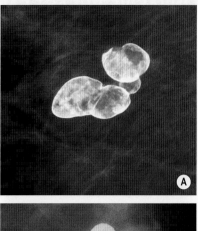

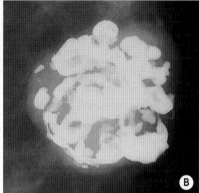

Fibrocystic change. (A) On the CC view the calcifications appear as round 'smudge' shadows. (B) On the lateral view 'teacups' representing the layering out of calcific material in the dependent portion of microcysts is seen.*,†

Duct ectasia. (A) Broken-needle appearance, typical of duct ectasia. (B) Sometimes thicker, more localized calcifications can be seen, giving a 'lead-pipe' appearance.*

(A) 'Eggshell' calcifications of fat necrosis. (B) Coarse 'popcorn' calcification in an involuting or degenerating fibroadenoma.*

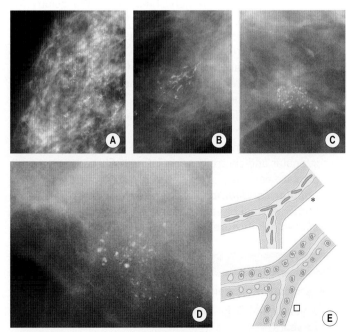

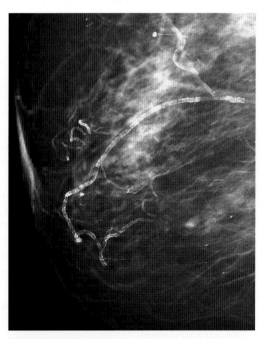

Ductal carcinoma in situ. (A-C) high-grade comedo type with an irregular linear branching microcalcification. (D) Intermediate/ low-grade DCIS with irregular polymorphic microcalcification. (E) Microcalcification in ductal carcinoma in situ. Comedo type (*), cribriform type (□).†

Vascular calcifications.*

683

INVASIVE BREAST CARCINOMA

DEFINITION

- A malignant tumour originating in the epithelial cells that line the terminal ductal lobular unit (TDLU) ▶ aetiology:
  - *Genetic defects:* mutations in the *P53* tumour suppressor gene (chromosome 17) ▶ *BRAC1* (chromosome 17) ▶ *BRAC2* (chromosome 13)
  - *Environmental risk factors:* age ▶ early menarche ▶ late 1st pregnancy ▶ late menopause ▶ nulliparity (tumour is sensitive to unopposed cyclical oestrogen) ▶ radiation exposure before 30 years
- **Classification**
  - Tumours with specific features: invasive carcinoma of special type ▶ remainder: no special type (NST or ductal NST)

Invasive   Malignant cells have extended across the basement membrane of the TDLU into the surrounding normal breast tissue

Non-invasive   Malignant cells are contained by basement membrane

- *Invasive ductal carcinoma (NOS):* this probably arises from DCIS with a strong fibrotic component (and therefore palpable) ▶ it is multifocal in 15% and bilateral in 5% ▶ it has a worse prognosis than other ductal tumours
- *Medullary carcinoma:* it demonstrates low-grade infiltrative properties and is well circumscribed ▶ it is soft to palpation (little desmoplastic response) ▶ it has a good prognosis
- *Mucinous/colloid carcinoma:* there is abundant extracellular mucin and colloid formation ▶ there is a good prognosis
- *Papillary carcinoma:* this occurs around the menopause with a central breast location ▶ it forms papillary structures with associated nipple (blood-tinged) discharge ▶ there is a good prognosis
- *Tubular carcinoma:* there is conspicuous tubule formation ▶ it is the most benign and slow-growing tumour type
- *Invasive lobular carcinoma:* a multicentric tumour with a poor prognosis due to a late diagnosis (it is difficult to detect clinically and mammographically)
- *Inflammatory breast carcinoma:* this is due to tumour emboli within dermal lymphatics and is seen in older patients ▶ it is aggressive with a poor prognosis
  - *Signs:* nipple retraction ▶ skin oedema ('peau d'orange') ▶ erythema ▶ induration of breast tissue
  - *Paget's disease:* tumour involving the nipple
- *DCIS:* a premalignant condition
- *LCIS:* this is not premalignant (affecting younger women) ▶ it is a risk factor for subsequent invasive breast carcinoma

RADIOLOGICAL FEATURES

Mammography (MMG)
- This tends to overestimate tumour size

- *High-grade tumour:* an ill-defined mass (if rapidly growing it may appear relatively well defined) ▶ microcalcifications are associated with high-grade DCIS
- *Lower-grade tumour:* a spiculated mass (due to the associated desmoplastic reaction in the adjacent stroma)
- *Lobular carcinoma:* this may be difficult to detect as it diffusely infiltrates fatty tissue ▶ it is often seen as an ill-defined mass or an area of asymmetrically dense breast tissue (microcalcifications are less common) ▶ it is more likely to be seen on one view only
- *Tubular and cribriform cancers:* architectural distortion (with abnormal trabecular markings) or a small spiculated mass
- *Papillary, mucinous and medullary neoplasms:* these may appear as new or enlarging multilobulated masses and may be well defined (simulating a benign lesion)

US
- This tends to underestimate tumour size
- It is useful in preoperative local staging ▶ it is a better predictor of tumour size than MMG ▶ it may detect intraductal tumour extension and satellite foci not seen with MMG
- *Findings:* an ill-defined mass which is markedly hypoechoic compared to surrounding fat ▶ if poorly differentiated, a high-grade tumour is more likely to be well defined with no acoustic shadowing – hence the importance of biopsy even if appears benign
  - A mass which is taller than it is wide (anterior to posterior dimension > transverse diameter)
  - ± an ill-defined echogenic halo around the lesion (particularly the lateral margins)
  - ± distortion of the adjacent breast tissue (analogous to MMG spiculation)
  - ± posterior acoustic shadowing (due to a reduction in through transmission of sound through the dense tumour tissue)
  - ± microcalcifications (arising in areas of high-grade DCIS)
- *Doppler:* this may show abnormal vessels that are irregular and centrally penetrating ▶ fibroadenomas will displace vessels
- *Lobular carcinoma:* this can be difficult to demonstrate on US: normal or vague abnormalities such as subtle altered echotexture

PEARLS

Breast cancer screening in the UK
- 3-yearly MMGs for women between the ages of 47 and 73 years
- Women over 70 are encouraged to attend by self-referral
- A 2-view MMG is used (MLO and CC)
- The majority of MMGs are double read by experienced radiologists or radiographers

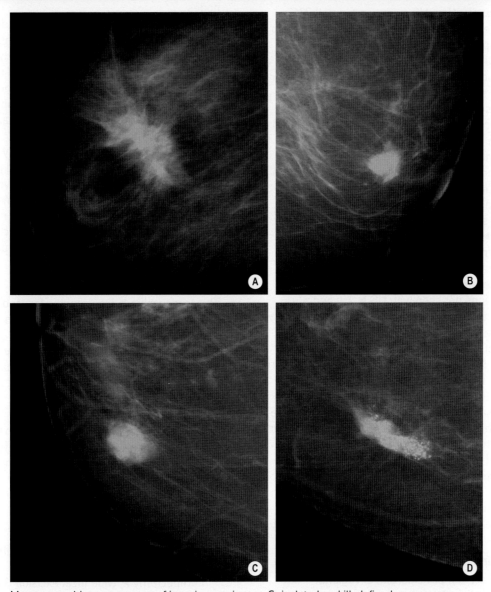

Mammographic appearances of invasive carcinoma. Spiculated and ill-defined masses are typical features of malignancy. (A) Spiculated and (B) ill-defined masses. (C) Sometimes high-grade tumours that exhibit rapid growth may appear more well-defined. (D) Calcifications typical of high-grade DCIS may be found in association with invasive carcinomas.*

Invasive breast carcinoma		
Ductal carcinoma (arising from the terminal ducts)	Non-invasive	Ductal carcinoma in situ (DCIS)
	Invasive	Invasive ductal carcinoma (NOS*) (70%)
		Medullary carcinoma (2%)
		Mucinous (colloid) carcinoma (2%)
		Papillary carcinoma (4%)
		Tubular carcinoma (10%)
Lobular carcinoma (arising from the terminal lobules)	Non-invasive	Lobular carcinoma in situ (LCIS)
	Invasive	Invasive lobular carcinoma (5–10%)
Other		Inflammatory carcinoma (5%)
*Not otherwise specified: invasive ductal carcinomas with no specific histological features.		

Interventional breast radiology

- *Fine-needle aspiration:* US guidance: a small 23G needle is passed repeatedly through an abnormality to sheer off clumps of cells
- *Core biopsy:* US guidance: a 14G needle (on a spring-loaded device) is used ▶ it demonstrates better sensitivity and specificity than FNAC
- *Vacuum-assisted mammotomy (VAM):* US, MRI or XR stereotactic guidance: an 11 to 8G vacuum-assisted needle system is used ▶ multiple cores are obtained without removing the needle from the breast ▶ after needle placement, suction is applied pulling tissue into a sampling chamber – a rotating cutting inner cannula automatically advances
  - Indications: small mass lesions ▶ architectural distortions ▶ failed core biopsy ▶ microcalcifications ▶ papillary/mucocele-like lesions ▶ diffuse non-specific abnormalities
- *XR-guided stereotactic biopsy:* this is used for impalpable lesions not seen with US ▶ x, y and z coordinates of the lesion are calculated from the relative positions of the target lesion compared to a fixed reference point
- *Preoperative localization of impalpable lesions:* wire (with retaining hook) localization on the day of surgery ▶ it employs similar techniques as for image-guided biopsy ▶ permits less normal surrounding tissue to be removed ▶ other techniques include skin marking over the lesion, or injection of carbon dye or radioisotope labelled colloid
- *Specimen radiography:* this ensures that representative material containing any microcalcifications has been sampled ▶ it is also used for post-surgical samples (ensuring adequate surgical margins)

Axillary LN staging

- Axillary nodes are the principal site of regional metastatic deposits with a direct correlation with primary tumour size ▶ 40% of patients have axillary involvement at diagnosis
- *Abnormal nodes (US):* hypoechoic ▶ round rather than ovoid ▶ >1 cm
- *Axillary node levels* (usually sequentially involved):
  - *Level 1:* inferolateral to the inferior border of pectoralis minor
  - *Level 2:* beneath pectoralis minor
  - *Level 3:* superior to the superior border of pectoralis minor (with a poor prognosis)
- Internal mammary nodes are often seen with inner or central tumours ▶ supraclavicular node involvement represents late disease with a poor prognosis
- Lymph node involvement is determined traditionally at the time of surgery by lymph node sampling procedures, sentinel node biopsy, or clearance of the axillary lymph nodes
  - *Sentinel node:* the 1st lymph node to demonstrate metastatic disease (absence of disease has a negative predictive value of 98%) ▶ the sentinel node is identified by injection in or around the tumour with blue dye (the sentinel node is then identified visually perioperatively) or with technetium sulphur colloid (which can be identified with an intraoperative gamma probe)
  - *Alternative approach:* US can identify abnormal nodes preoperatively ▶ nodes are biopsied percutaneously (under US guidance) ▶ a preoperative diagnosis of lymph node involvement can be made in just over 40% of patients who are lymph node positive – this allows a more radical axillary clearance to be targeted to those patients with a preoperative diagnosis of axillary disease

Metastatic disease

- This is incurable ▶ treatment is focused on symptom relief ▶ it is unusual to detect distant metastases at the time of diagnosis
  - *Chest:* lung metastases can have a variable appearance (well or ill defined ▶ small or large) ▶ mediastinal adenopathy ▶ pleural effusions ▶ lymphangitic spread
  - *Bone:* lytic and sclerotic deposits
  - *Liver:* this is generally less common than bone or lung metastases ▶ they are usually low attenuation lesions (CT) ▶ they can be diffuse and infiltrating and therefore difficult to detect
  - *Brain:* this is not uncommon ▶ it can also involve the meninges and spinal cord

Treatment options

- Surgical options to provide disease control in the breast and axilla:
  - Lumpectomy ▶ wide local excision (1 cm clearance margin) ▶ quadrantectomy (2–3 cm clearance by resecting a breast quadrant) ▶ mastectomy ▶ axillary clearance (± postoperative radiotherapy)
- Chemotherapy and hormone therapy (e.g. the anti-oestrogen tamoxifen) is used for distant disease

Differential diagnosis

- *Surgical scar:* a spiculated mass or architectural distortion
- *Infection and inflammation:* abscess formation in a lactating woman ▶ granulomatous mastitis
- *Radial scar:* this is also called a complex sclerosing lesion ▶ it is associated with epithelial atypia, DCIS and invasive carcinoma
  - A spiculated lesion ± microcalcification

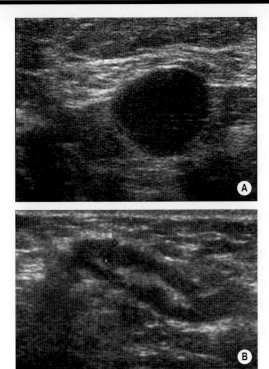

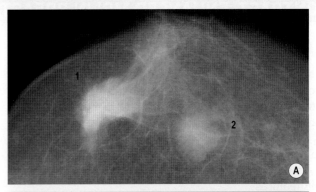

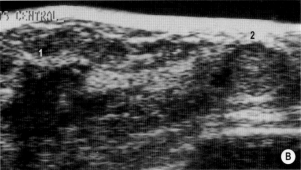

(A) Nodes are likely to contain tumour if their longitudinal-to-transverse diameter is <2 (the node appears round rather than oval). Nodes are more likely to contain tumour if the cortex is thickened to >2.5–3 mm. (B) The node has a normal shape, but part of the cortex had a thickness of 3 mm. Both these axillary lymph nodes were found to contain tumour.*

Mucinous carcinoma and invasive ductal carcinoma. (A) MMG shows a poorly defined spiculate mass: (1) due to invasive ductal carcinoma and a circumscribed soft tissue mass ▶ (2) due to a mucinous carcinoma. (B) US shows a typical low reflectivity mass: (1) due to invasive ductal carcinoma, and a circumscribed mass with posterior acoustic enhancement due to mucinous carcinoma (2).†

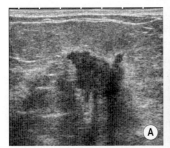

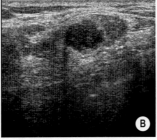

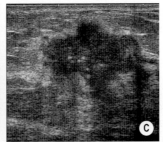

US appearances of invasive carcinoma. (A) This irregular hypoechoic mass with acoustic shadowing and an echogenic halo is typical of a carcinoma. (B) Occasionally high-grade tumours may appear well defined, mimicking benign lesions. This shows the importance of performing a core biopsy even on apparently benign-appearing mass lesions. (C) Small echogenic foci of microcalcification associated with malignant lesions may be identified.*

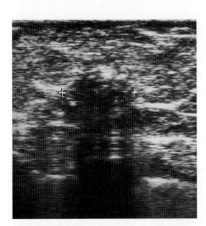

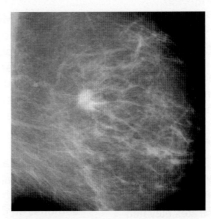

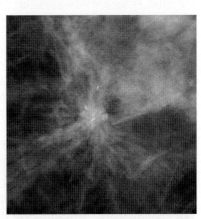

US showing an echo-poor mass with irregular margins and posterior acoustic enhancement due to a carcinoma.†

Spiculate mass due to an invasive carcinoma.†

A spiculate mass with microcalcification due to a complex sclerosing lesion/radial scar.†

CONTRAST-ENHANCED MRI IN BREAST CANCER

INDICATIONS

- For local staging of primary breast cancer ▶ the most accurate technique for sizing a tumour ▶ it can demonstrate unsuspected multifocal disease in the same breast or additional tumour foci in the contralateral breast
- A high sensitivity for detecting invasive breast cancer (up to 100%) but a lower specificity: some benign lesions and even normal breast tissue can demonstrate worrying MR features
- *MRI is usually reserved for the following indications:*
  - Patients where estimating tumour size is proving difficult by conventional methods
  - Patients with mammographically dense breasts
  - With significant discrepancy between size at MMG, US and clinical examination
  - Patients who have a carcinoma with lobular features: these are more likely to be multifocal ▶ they are also more difficult to detect and their size is more difficult to measure by conventional methods because of their infiltrating growth pattern
  - Identifying an occult primary tumour if there is malignant axillary adenopathy (but a normal MMG/US)
  - Differentiating surgical scarring from tumour recurrence
  - Assessing the response to neoadjuvant chemotherapy for locally advanced primary breast cancers
  - Screening younger women with a high familial risk of breast cancer (MMG is difficult in dense breasts – however MMG remains more sensitive for DCIS)

TECHNIQUE

- The technique uses a ≥1.5T magnet with a dedicated breast coil and compression devices ▶ the patient is imaged prone with the breasts hanging down into the coil
- Fat suppression is required to increase the conspicuity of enhancement

Dynamic IV gadolinium imaging The morphology of a lesion is more important than the enhancement characteristics

  - Images are acquired dynamically every minute over a period of 6–7 min after injection
  - Optimum contrast between malignancy and normal breast tissue is achieved within the first 2 min
  - At later times normal breast tissue may start to show non-specific enhancement
  - Malignant tumours show rapid uptake of contrast agent followed by a 'washout' phase

DWI Cancers generally have lower ADC values, but there is overlap between benign and malignant lesions

MR spectroscopy Breast cancer demonstrates elevated choline levels (choline peak)

LESION CHARACTERIZATION

Lesion morphology

Benign lesions Well defined with smooth margins

Malignant lesions Poorly defined ▶ they may show spiculation or parenchymal deformity
- Characteristic ring enhancement ▶ invasive cancer can be effectively excluded if no enhancement is seen

Assessment of enhancement kinetics

Benign lesions (type I enhancement) Steady increase in SI throughout the time course of the examination

Indeterminate lesions (type II enhancement) Rapid uptake of contrast agent during the initial phase ▶ this is followed by a slower subsequent rise in uptake

Malignant lesions (type III enhancement) Rapid uptake of contrast agent during the initial phase ▶ this is followed by a washout or plateau in the intermediate and late periods after injection

Pearls

- Dedicated biopsy coils and MRI-compatible needles are now becoming commercially available

MRI pitfalls

- There can be overlap in the enhancement characteristics of benign and malignant lesions:
  - Sinister patterns of contrast enhancement have been observed in benign conditions, including fibroadenomas, fat necrosis and fibrocystic change
  - Normal breast tissue may enhance (which is more likely in the middle of the menstrual cycle – optimum time to image is during the second week of the menstrual cycle)
  - Recent surgery or radiotherapy can interfere with image interpretation ▶ enhancement patterns return to normal approximately 3–6 months after radiotherapy

Unenhanced MRI for imaging breast implants

- MRI is the technique of choice for assessing the integrity of breast implants
- **Intracapsular rupture:** silicon has escaped from the plastic shell of the implant, but is contained within the fibrous implant capsule
  - *'Wavy line', 'linguini', 'keyhole'* and *'salad oil' signs:* these can sometimes be mistaken for normal implant folds
- **Extracapsular rupture:** silicon is demonstrated outside the fibrous capsule ▶ free silicon, silicon granulomas or silicon within the axillary lymph nodes can be demonstrated
  BI RADS reporting: characterizes lesions into: (1) a focus (a lesion <5 mm, not worth investigating further) ▶ (2) a mass (>5 mm) ▶ non-mass enhancement

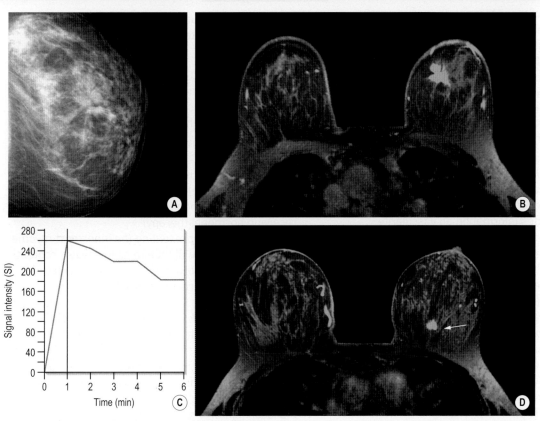

MRI for local tumour staging. Mammography showed a spiculated lesion lying centrally within the breast, best appreciated on the CC view (A). MRI confirmed the presence of a malignant spiculated lesion (B) with a typically malignant enhancement curve (rapid uptake of contrast agent followed by a washout phase) (C). An additional tumour focus was identified away from the primary tumour site (D). Biopsy indicated a carcinoma with lobular features.*

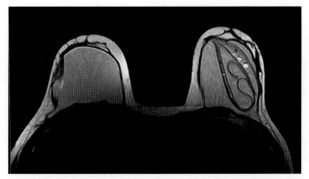

Intracapsular implant rupture. On these T2WI, the plastic shell of the left breast implant can be seen floating within the silicon, producing a 'wavy line' or 'linguini' sign. Note the presence of a couple of bright dots of water-like material, the 'salad oil' sign.*

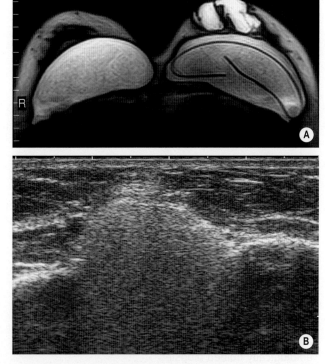

Extracapsular implant rupture. (A) A collection of free silicon is seen anterior to this ruptured left breast implant. (B) US may be useful in the diagnosis of extracapsular rupture, with free silicon or silicon granulomas having a typical 'snowstorm' appearance.*

6.2 GYNAECOLOGY

Ultrasound (US)

Indications Evaluation of a pelvic mass, uterine enlargement, endometrial abnormalities, ovarian masses or acute pelvic pain ▶ it allows transabdominal and transvaginal guidance of fluid or tissue sampling ▶ it allows transvaginal-guided drain placement and guidance for placement of brachytherapy for cervical and endometrial malignancy ▶ it allows intraoperative assessment for the completion of evacuation of products of conception

- *Transabdominal US (TAS):* a full bladder is required ▶ a 3.5–5 MHz transducer is used
- *Transvaginal US (TVS):* an empty bladder is required ▶ a 5–8 MHz transducer is used ▶ it allows closer apposition to the pelvic organs
- *Doppler US:* this provides information on vascularity

Normal US anatomy

- **Premenopausal**
  - **Uterus:** 5–9 cm in length
  - **Endometrium:** *proliferative phase:* ≤8 mm ▶ *midcycle:* a trilaminar appearance measuring up to 12–16 mm ▶ *secretory phase:* hyperechoic due to the increasing glandular complexity ▶ ≤16 mm
  - **Ovaries:** these are anterior to the iliac vessels ▶ they typically measure 30 mm in any two dimensions but may measure ≥50 mm in one plane ▶ the ovarian volume is usually <10 cm³
- **Postmenopausal**
  - **Endometrium:** <5 mm (unless on hormonal therapy, when it can measure ≤8 mm)

Computed tomography (CT)

Indications The distant staging of gynaecological malignancies ▶ the detection of persistent and recurrent pelvic tumour ▶ for biopsy guidance

Normal CT anatomy

- **Uterus:** a triangular or ovoid soft tissue structure located behind the urinary bladder ▶ the myometrium enhances with contrast (helping to delineate the endometrium, which is of lower attenuation)
- **Cervix:** a rounded structure inferior to the uterine corpus
- **Vagina:** a flat rectangular structure at the level of the fornix
- **Broad and round ligaments:** these are seen coursing laterally and anteriorly (respectively)
- **Ovaries:** these are posterolateral to the uterine corpus ▶ they are of soft tissue density with small cystic regions ▶ they are atrophic in postmenopausal women

Magnetic resonance imaging (MRI)

Indications For the evaluation of Müllerian duct anomalies ▶ for the local staging of uterine and cervical cancer ▶ as a problem-solving tool in the evaluation of adnexal masses ▶ allowing differentiation between radiation fibrosis and recurrent tumour ▶ permitting radiologically guided biopsies

Normal MRI anatomy

T1WI The pelvic musculature and viscera are of homogeneous low-to-intermediate SI

T1 + Gad

- The endometrium and outer myometrium enhances more than the junctional zone
- The inner cervical mucosa and outer smooth muscle enhances more than the fibrocervical stroma

T2WI The zonal anatomy is demonstrated as follows:

- **Uterus:**
  - *Endometrium:* this is of high SI ▶ ≤8 mm (proliferative phase) ▶ ≤16 mm (secretory phase) ▶ <5 mm (postmenopausal women that are not receiving hormonal therapy)
  - *Junctional zone (representing the innermost myometrium):* this is of low SI (due to its low water content)
  - *Peripheral myometrium:* this is of intermediate SI (and higher than striated muscle)
- **Cervix:**
  - *Endocervical glands and mucus:* central high SI
  - *Stroma:* low SI (as it is composed of elastic fibrous tissue)
  - *Periphery of cervix:* intermediate SI similar to myometrium (as it is composed of smooth muscle)
- **Vagina:**
  - *Mucosa:* high SI
  - *Vaginal wall:* intermediate SI
- **Ovaries:** The follicles demonstrate higher SI than the surrounding stroma

Other imaging techniques

FDG-PET and FDG-PET/CT This uses a glucose analogue, 2-[¹⁸F]-fluoro-2-deoxy-D-glucose (FDG) ▶ it is not widely available but can be used in cervical and ovarian cancer

Hysterosalpingography (HSG) Radiopaque contrast medium is instilled into the uterus and Fallopian tubes ▶ it is used for the evaluation of infertility

- *Cervical canal:* 3–4 cm long and ⅓ the length of the uterus (it shortens after childbirth) ▶ it is often spindle shaped and there may be glandular filling
- *Cavity of uterine body:* this is triangular in shape ▶ the average length and intercornual diameter is approximately 35 mm
- *Fallopian tubes:* these are 5–6 cm long ▶ the isthmus is of uniform diameter and opens laterally into a wide ampulla

Sonohysterography A 5F catheter is placed through the cervix ▶ distension of the uterine cavity is obtained with sterile saline under direct US visualization

- This is more accurate than endovaginal US alone ▶ focal pathology can be differentiated from diffuse endometrial conditions with increased accuracy ▶ it can differentiate between intracavitary, endometrial and subendometrial pathology ▶ it can evaluate tubal patency

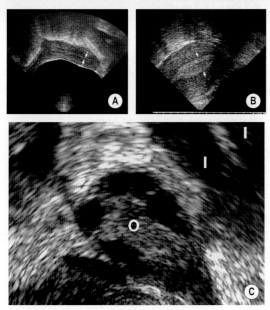

(A) Transvaginal US shows normal endometrium (arrows) in proliferative phase and (B) in follicular phase (arrows). (C) Sagittal transvaginal US shows a normal ovary (O) with follicles. Note the location of the ovary anterior and medial to the internal iliac vessels (I) within the ovarian fossa.*

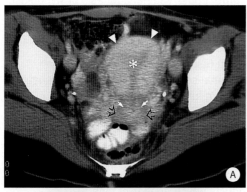

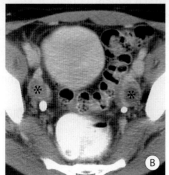

CT. (A) Normal uterus with a low attenuation endometrial canal (*) flanked by enhancing myometrium (arrowheads). Enhancing endocervical mucosa (short solid white arrows) surrounds the endocervical canal. The fibrous cervical stroma (open black arrows) enhances less than the uterine corpus myometrium. (B) Bilateral physiological ovarian cysts (*) in their expected location (anterior to the internal iliac vessels and posterior to the external iliac vessels).*

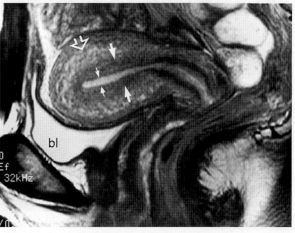

Zonal anatomy of the uterus. Sagittal T2WI. The central, high SI stripe represents the endometrium (small arrows) ▶ the band of low SI subjacent to the endometrial stripe represents the inner myometrium or junctional zone (arrows). The outer layer of the myometrium is of intermediate SI (open arrow). bl = bladder.*

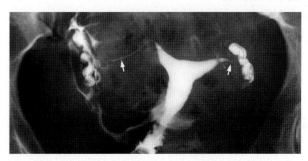

Normal hysterosalpingogram. Cervix and uterine body are delineated by contrast media. Both Fallopian tubes are shown (arrows), with early peritoneal spill.*

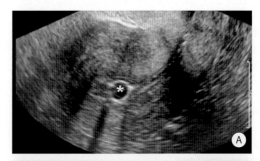

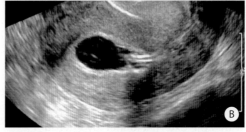

Sonohysterography. Sagittal transvaginal US (A) demonstrates the inflated balloon of the sonohysterographic catheter (*) within the endometrial canal. Following the instillation of 40 ml of sterile saline (B), fluid distends the endometrial canal.*

CONGENITAL ANOMALIES OF THE FEMALE GENITAL TRACT

Definition

- **Embryology:** the uterus, upper ⅔ of the vagina and Fallopian tubes are derived from the paired Müllerian ducts ▶ at approximately 10 weeks following conception the ducts migrate caudally and undergo fusion and subsequent canalization ▶ congenital anomalies arise when this process is interrupted:
  - *Non-development:* uterine agenesis
  - *Varying degrees of non-fusion:* a didelphys or bicornuate uterus
  - *Non-resorption of the Müllerian ducts:* septate uterus

Clinical presentation
Asymptomatic ▶ menstrual disorders ▶ infertility ▶ obstetric complications
- Congenital anomalies are present in 1–15% of women, with associated renal anomalies in up to 50% of cases

Radiological features (MRI)

Uterine anomalies

Class I: Müllerian (uterine) agenesis or hypoplasia
- *Due to non-development or rudimentary development of the Müllerian ducts*
  - *Uterine hypoplasia:* a small uterus with an atrophic endometrium ▶ T2WI: the myometrium is of lower SI than normal ▶ ovaries are normal
  - *Uterine agenesis:* MRKH Syndrome

Class II: unicornuate uterus
- *Due to non-development or rudimentary development of one Müllerian duct ▶ the remaining Müllerian duct is fully developed ▶ increased obstetric complications/ renal abnormalities*
- T2WI: a 'banana-like configuration' of the normal duct: there is a curved, elongated uterus with tapering of the fundal segment off the midline ▶ the normal uterine zonal anatomy is maintained ▶ the rudimentary horn demonstrates lower SI

Class III: uterus didelphys
- *Due to non-fusion of the two Müllerian ducts*
- T2WI: there are two widely separate normally sized uterine horns with two cervices ▶ the endometrial and myometrial widths are preserved ▶ vaginal septum (75%)
- T1WI: haemorrhage may be seen if there is a transverse septa causing obstruction

Class IV: bicornuate uterus
- *Due to partial fusion of the Müllerian ducts (with incomplete fusion of the cephalad extent of the uterovaginal horns with resorption of the uterovaginal septum) ▶ obstetric complications relate to the degree of horn fusion*
- The uterine horns are separated by an intervening cleft (>1 cm) within the external fundal myometrium ▶ a normal zonal anatomy is seen within each horn + a dividing septum composed of central myometrium
  - *Bicornuate unicollis:* the central myometrium extends to the internal os
  - *Bicornuate bicollis:* the central myometrium extends to the external os ▶ there is some fusion between the two horns (cf. complete separation with didelphys)

Class V: septate uterus
- *Due to incomplete resorption of the final fibrous septum between the two uterine horns*
- *The septum may be partial, or it may be complete and extend to the external cervical os*
- T2WI (parallel to uterine long axis): a convex, flat or concave (<1 cm) external uterine contour (+ fibrous septa)

Class VI: arcuate uterus
- *Single uterine cavity with a convex / flat uterine fundus*
- Uterine cavity demonstrates a small fundal cleft ▶ often considered a normal variant ▶ no effect on pregnancy

Class VII: in utero diethylstilbestrol (DES) exposure
- *Uterine hypoplasia with a 'T-shaped' uterus*

Vaginal anomalies

Congenital absence of Müllerian ducts (vaginal aplasia, MRKH syndrome)
- Due to failure of the vaginal plate to form, or a failure of cavitation
- **MRKH syndrome:** upper vaginal agenesis or hypoplasia (with normal ovaries and Fallopian tubes) accompanied by variable anomalies of uterus (class 1), urinary tract and skeletal system

Disorder of vertical fusion
- A transverse vaginal septum prevents loss of menstrual blood and results in haematocolpos
- T2WI: a dilated vagina with intraluminal fluid of intermediate or high SI (± fluid and debris levels) ▶ the lower ⅓ of the vagina is replaced by low SI fibrous tissue with loss of the normal zonal anatomy
- T1WI (+ fat suppression): this confirms the presence of any blood products which appear of high SI

Disorder of lateral fusion
- This often presents with an incidental asymptomatic vaginal septum

Vaginal cysts
- *Gartner duct cysts:* anterolateral upper vagina above pubic symphysis
- *Bartholin gland cysts:* posterolateral lateral vaginal introitus below pubic symphysis
- *Nabothian cysts:* cervical cysts

Pearls

- Compared to a bicornuate uterus, a septate uterus is associated with a higher rate of reproductive complications
  - A collagenous septum cannot support a pregnancy as well as a myometrial septum
- A transverse vaginal septum in adolescence with cyclical abdominal pain + a pelvic mass

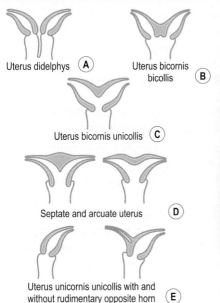

Uterus didelphys (A)

Uterus bicornis bicollis (B)

Uterus bicornis unicollis (C)

Septate and arcuate uterus (D)

Uterus unicornis unicollis with and without rudimentary opposite horn (E)

Congenital abnormalities of the uterus.

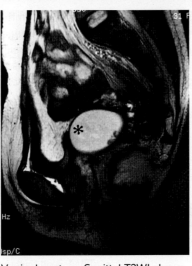

Vaginal septum. Sagittal T2WI shows the presence of haematometra (*) caused by a transverse vaginal septum.*

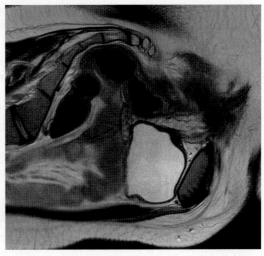

Uterus bicornuate. Coronal T2WI demonstrating two endometrial canals (*).*

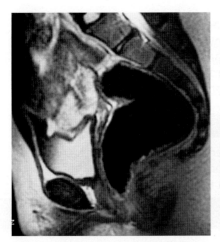

Absence of the uterus. Sagittal T2WI shows no uterine tissue.*

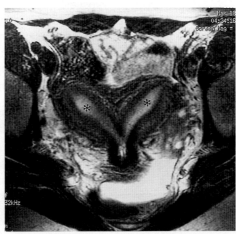

Uterine and vaginal agenesis. Sagittal T2-weighted MRI of the pelvis showing absent uterus and vagina.**

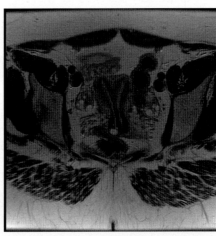

Uterus didelphys. T2-weighted axial oblique MRI elegantly demonstrates two separate normal-sized uterine horns and cervices.**

LEIOMYOMA (FIBROID)

DEFINITION

- A benign tumour arising from uterine smooth muscle cells (± varying amounts of fibrous tissue) ▶ it is oestrogen dependent, and therefore regresses after the menopause
- It is the most common uterine tumour (seen in up to 40% of premenopausal women) ▶ they are usually multiple
  - *Intramural:* the most common type
  - *Submucosal:* this is the most likely to be symptomatic
  - *Subserosal:* this may be pedunculated (± torsion)

CLINICAL PRESENTATION

- Menorrhagia (if there is a submucosal location) ▶ dysmenorrhoea ▶ subfertility (due to narrowed Fallopian tube or interference with implantation) ▶ urinary frequency
  - *Red degeneration:* this follows acute impairment of the blood supply (often during pregnancy), and presents with acute abdominal pain and tenderness
  - *Hyaline degeneration:* there is gradual impairment of the blood supply, and it is asymptomatic
  - *Obstetric complications:* malposition ▶ a retained placenta ▶ interference with vaginal delivery ▶ premature uterine contractions
- Fibroids are more prevalent amongst black women

RADIOLOGICAL FEATURES

US An enlarged uterus (± an irregular and lobular outline) ▶ a well-marginated, hypoechoic, rounded mass within the uterine body ▶ distortion of the endometrial complex if there is a submucosal component

- Depending on the proportion of smooth muscle, fibrosis and degeneration, appearances can range from hypoechoic to echogenic, and homogeneous to heterogeneous ▶ there can be acoustic shadowing or shadowing echogenic foci due to the presence of calcification
- Submucosal leiomyomas may mimic endometrial lesions on US – US HSG may aid in the diagnosis

CT A fibroid has a soft tissue density similar to that of normal myometrium ▶ necrosis or degeneration may result in low attenuation (± calcification or uterine contour deformity)

MRI This allows the precise determination of the size, location and number of leiomyomas ▶ it can differentiate a pedunculated subserosal leiomyoma from an adnexal mass
- T1WI: well-circumscribed, rounded lesions with intermediate SI
- T1WI (FS): this can demonstrate haemorrhagic degeneration (with high SI)
- T1WI + Gad: the enhancement is less than that of the adjacent myometrium ▶ any degenerated areas may not enhance
- T2WI: there is lower SI relative to the myometrium or endometrium ▶ signal voids represent calcification or vessels
- Cystic degeneration: well-defined non-enhancing areas of fluid density ▶ myxoid degeneration: very high signal on T2WI (non-enhancing) ▶ red degeneration: massive haemorrhagic infarction + necrosis (peripheral low T2WI rim + high T1WI signal)

PEARL

- *Treatment:* hysterectomy, myomectomy or uterine arterial embolization (UAE) ▶ MR-guided ultrasound ablation is a recent innovation

ENDOMETRIAL POLYPS

DEFINITION

- A benign polypoid tumour consisting of a stromal core with the mucosal surface projecting above the level of the adjacent endometrium
- Although it can occur at any age, it is commonest in older (>50 years) females

RADIOLOGICAL FEATURES

TVS This will often not reveal any endometrial polyps

US HSG The homogeneous polyp is isoechoic to (and continuous with) the endometrium ▶ there is a preserved

endomyometrial interface ▶ there can be central cystic areas and feeding vessels (best seen with colour Doppler)

MRI This is rarely employed due to the high cost ▶ T1WI: the polyp is isointense to the endometrium (± hypointense foci) ▶ T2WI: the polyp is hypo- to isointense to the endometrium (± cystic changes) ▶ if pedunculated there can be a central hypointense core (± a stalk) ▶ T1WI + Gad: there is homogeneous or heterogeneous enhancement

Hysteroscopy The diagnostic technique of choice

PEARL

- *Differential:* submucosal leiomyoma ▶ malignant neoplasm

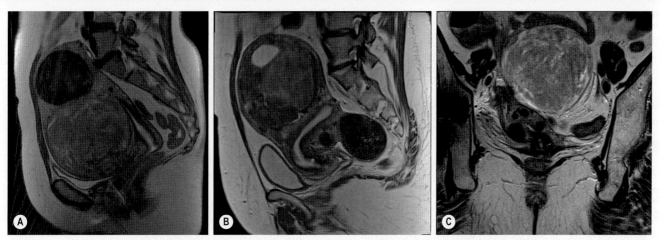

Variable appearance of fibroids on MRI. (A) Sagittal T2-weighted MRI showing an intermediate signal anterior myometrial fibroid. Patchy high signal areas indicate degeneration. A second fibroid at the fundus is of characteristic low signal. (B) There is cystic degeneration in the anterior fibroid, and a low signal intensity posterior fibroid that has displaced the rectum. Note retroverted uterus. (C) A large pedunculated fibroid is of mixed signal, indicating degeneration. Note multiple small low signal fibroids in the myometrium.**

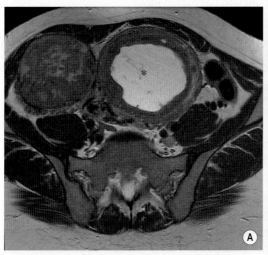

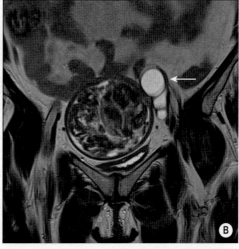

Myxoid and red degeneration of fibroids on MRI. (A) Axial T2-weighted image. There is myxoid degeneration of a large fibroid with central very high signal. (*) A second fibroid on the right is of mixed signal. (B) Red degeneration with massive haemorrhagic infarction and necrosis of the entire leiomyoma, with a peripheral rim of low signal on this coronal T2-weighted image. Note also left hydrosalpinx (arrow).**

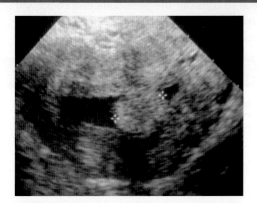

Saline hysterography. Endometrial polyp outlined by saline.[†]

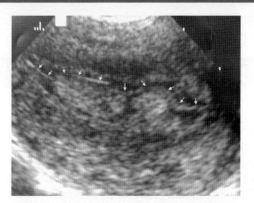

TVUS. Multiple endometrial polyps. Note the midline echoes due to the endometrial interface (arrows) displaced by the polyps. This is a useful feature in differentiating polyps from endometrial hyperplasia.[†]

ADENOMYOSIS

Definition

- The presence of endometrial tissue within the myometrium, with secondary smooth muscle hypertrophy and hyperplasia
- It can be diffuse or focal, and is seen in 15–27% of hysterectomy specimens (there is an increased incidence in multiparous women)

Clinical presentation

- Dysmenorrhoea and dysfunctional uterine bleeding

Radiological features

TVS

- An enlarged globular uterus, often with antero-posterior asymmetry ▶ myometrial heterogeneity (due to the endometrial implants and intervening smooth muscle hypertrophy) ▶ endometrial implants can present as diffuse echogenic nodules, subendometrial echogenic linear striations, or 2–6 mm subendometrial cysts (representing haemorrhage within an implant)

- *'Endometrial pseudowidening'*: this is due to poor definition of the endomyometrial junction
- *'Rain shower' appearance:* multiple fine areas of attenuation throughout the lesion

Doppler US There is a speckled pattern of increased vascularity within a heterogeneous area

MRI

- **T2WI**: areas of low myometrial SI, presenting as focal or diffuse thickening of the junctional zone (JZ)
  - *JZ >12 mm:* this will diagnose disease with a high accuracy
  - *JZ <8 mm:* this excludes disease with a high accuracy
  - *JZ 8–12 mm (intermediate cases):* this requires ancillary criteria for diagnosis:
    - High SI linear striations (finger-like projections) extending out from the endometrium and into the myometrium
    - T1WI: high SI foci representing endometrial rests (± punctate haemorrhages)

ENDOMETRIAL HYPERPLASIA

Definition

- This describes the proliferation of the endometrial glands (due to unopposed oestrogen stimulation)
  - *Causes:* polycystic ovaries ▶ anovulation ▶ obesity ▶ exogenous hormones ▶ functioning oestrogen-secreting ovarian tumours
- Subdivisions:
  - *Cystic hyperplasia:* this is simple and predominantly seen in premenopausal females
  - *Adenomatous hyperplasia:* this is complex and predominantly seen in postmenopausal females
  - *Atypical hyperplasia:* hyperplasia is a precursor to endometrial carcinoma

Clinical presentation

- Abnormal uterine bleeding ▶ infertility ▶ postmenopausal bleeding

Radiological features

TVS Endometrial thickening ≥5 mm in postmenopausal women

- Premenopausal women: ≥8 mm (proliferative phase) ▶ ≥16 mm (secretory phase)

US HSG Focal or more commonly diffuse endometrial thickening without a localized mass or abnormality

MRI T2WI: diffuse thickening of the endometrial stripe ▶ the stripe is isointense or slightly hypointense relative to the normal endometrium (this is a non-specific sign which is also seen with endometrial carcinoma) ▶ can see heterogeneous T2WI signal, with lattice-like enhancement traversing the endometrial canal

Pearl One needs to consider the possibility of a coexisting endometrial or ovarian carcinoma, or progression to an endometrial carcinoma

UTERINE INFECTIONS

Definition

- Uterine infections usually occur in the puerperium, postoperatively, or after a septic abortion (endometritis)
- Pyometra (pus within endometrial cavity) is seen in patients with a cervical stenosis due to a cervical carcinoma, following radiotherapy, or as a complication of endometritis

Radiological feature

US/CT/MRI A thick-walled, and distended uterus

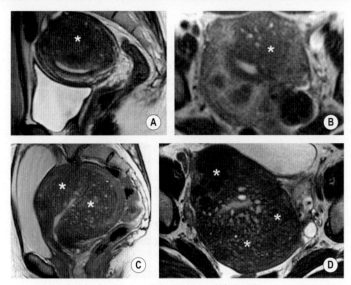

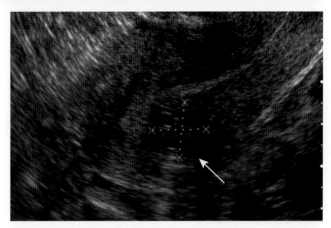

US of focal adenomyosis. Sagittal transvaginal US showing focal adenomyosis as a poorly defined echogenic nodule (arrow).**

Focal adenomyosis. Sagittal (A) and axial (B) T2WI demonstrate focal junctional zone widening and multiple punctate high SI foci with the areas of thickening (* A and B). Diffuse adenomyosis. Sagittal (C) and axial (D) T2WI in a different patient demonstrate widening of the entire junctional zone (* C and D) which contains multiple foci of high SI that represent endometrial rests.*

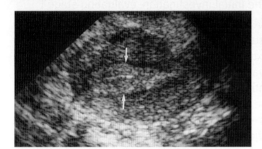

Endometrial echo complex. The distance between the outer lines of the echogenic endometrial echo (arrows) is measured on a sagittal endovaginal US. In postmenopausal women, this distance should not exceed 5 mm.†

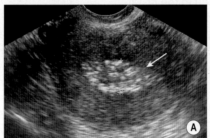

Endometrial hyperplasia. US in a patient with postmenopausal bleeding who is taking tamoxifen following breast cancer surgery. The endometrium (A) is thickened and hyperechoic, measuring more than 10 mm. (B) Sagittal T2-weighted MRI shows non-specific heterogeneous endometrial thickening. Endometrial biopsy is indicated to exclude endometrial cancer. In this case the histological diagnosis was endometrial hyperplasia.**

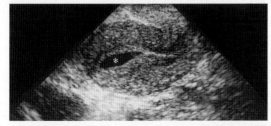

TVUS of endometritis. Sagittal image of the uterus demonstrates a thickened endometrial echo and focal distension of the endometrial cavity by fluid (asterisk).ʃ

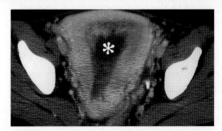

Helical CT shows a distended fluid-filled endometrial canal (*) in a postpartum patient with endometritis and pyometra. Without the presence of gas, it may be impossible to differentiate a pyometra from a hydrometra.*

ENDOMETRIAL CARCINOMA

Definition

- A malignant adenocarcinoma arising from the endometrium ▶ 90% are well differentiated (grade I)
  - It is the most common malignancy of the female reproductive tract
- The main risk factors are a chronic exposure to unopposed oestrogen: tamoxifen ▶ nulliparity ▶ obesity ▶ polycystic ovarian syndrome

Clinical features Postmenopausal bleeding – therefore most women present with early-stage disease

- The peak age of presentation is 55–65 years

Radiological features

TVUS There is non-specific thickening of the endometrium (≥5 mm in postmenopausal women) ▶ can be indistinguishable from hyperplasia/polyps ▶ there can be a disrupted endometrial or myometrial junction or an irregular endometrial surface

- *Evaluation of any myometrial invasion:* assess the presence and continuity of the hypoechoic halo that surrounds the outer layer of the endometrium (i.e. intact, focally disrupted, or totally disrupted) ▶ the extent of any myometrial invasion is estimated by measuring the distance from the central uterine lumen to the distal junction between the tumour and normal myometrium
- **Sonohysterography:** an intracavitary polyp or asymmetric thickening of the endometrial lining

CECT Tumour is seen as a hypodense mass relative to the normally enhancing myometrium

MRI T1WI: tumour is isointense with normal endometrium

- T2WI: this may demonstrate high SI – it is typically heterogeneous and may even be of low SI
- T1 + Gad (dynamic imaging): there is early and avid enhancement of the normal myometrium ▶ endometrial cancer enhances at a slower rate than the adjacent normal myometrium ▶ during the later phases of enhancement the tumour appears hypointense relative to the myometrium
  - **Stage 1A** (*tumour extends <50% into the myometrium*): there is disruption of the junctional zone (JZ) and of the subendometrial enhancement (SEE) by tumour ▶ there is an irregular tumour–myometrium interface
    - If tumour is limited to the endometrium, a normal or widened (focally or diffuse) endometrium is seen
    - An intact JZ and a band of early SEE excludes deep myometrial invasion
  - **Stage IB** (*tumour extends ≥50% into the myometrium*): low SI tumour is seen within the outer myometrium during the later phases of enhancement

- **Stage II**
  - *Endocervical glandular involvement:* invasion of the endocervix appears as widening of the internal os and endocervical canal with preservation of the normally low SI fibrocervical stroma
  - *Cervical stromal invasion:* there is disruption of the fibrocervical stroma by high SI tumour (T2WI) ▶ there is disruption of the normal enhancement of the cervical mucosa by low SI tumour (early dynamic contrast-enhanced MRI)
- **Stage IIIA** (*serosal ± adnexal involvement*): uterine serosal disruption ▶ irregular uterine contour ▶ sigmoid serosal deposits ▶ ovarian deposits
- **Stage IIIB** (*vaginal ± parametrial involvement*): tumour extends into the upper vagina (with loss of the low SI vaginal wall)
- **Stage IIIC** (*pelvic ± para-aortic metastases*): pelvic or para-aortic adenopathy is demonstrated (>1 cm)
- **Stage IV** (*bladder or bowel invasion, distant metastases*): tumour extends beyond the true pelvis or invades the bladder or rectum

Imaging approach This is used to facilitate treatment planning

TVS This is the initial investigation, evaluating stage I disease

MRI This is superior to US and CT in the evaluation of both tumour extension into the cervix and depth of any myometrial invasion

- The differentiation between revised stage IA and revised stage IB disease has prognostic as well as morbidity implications – stage IA patients undergo lymph node sampling whereas stage IB patients undergo radical lymph node surgical resection
- Gross cervical invasion requires preoperative radiation therapy or a different treatment plan (i.e. a radical hysterectomy instead of a total abdominal hysterectomy)

CT This can confirm any parametrial and side-wall extension in stage III tumours ▶ it can detect pelvic lymphadenopathy and distant metastases ▶ it is used for screening for lymphatic or peritoneal metastases in patients with a poorly differentiated carcinoma or sarcoma ▶ it can confirm stage III or stage IV disease

FDG-PET This has a role in the post-treatment surveillance of endometrial cancer patients

Pearls Staging is based upon the recently revised FIGO classification (see Section 9)

Patterns of tumour spread

- *Upper uterine body:* common iliac and para-aortic nodes
- *Lower uterine body and cervix:* parametrial, paracervical and obturator nodes ▶ then via the iliac to the retroperitoneal nodes

Diagnosis Endometrial biopsy or dilatation and curettage

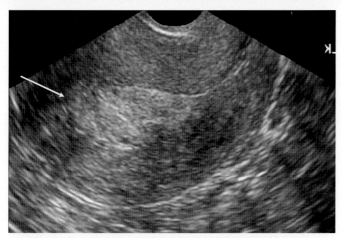

Endometrial carcinoma, transvaginal US. The endometrium is thickened and irregular in this postmenopausal patient. Near the fundus, the endometrial–myometrial junction is indistinct, indicating myometrial invasion (arrow).*

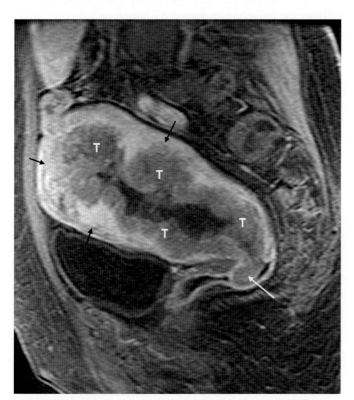

Endometrial carcinoma, MRI. Sagittal gadolinium-enhanced T1WI fat-suppressed image shows an endometrial cancer (T) with deep myometrial invasion. Note the thin rim of normal myometrium (black arrows). The disease extends to the upper third of the vagina (white arrow).*

Stage IIIa endometrial carcinoma. Sagittal T2-weighted MRI demonstrates a heterogeneous intermediate signal intensity endometrial tumour (T) distending the endometrial cavity. A serosal deposit (S) is seen on the sigmoid colon, superior to the bladder.**

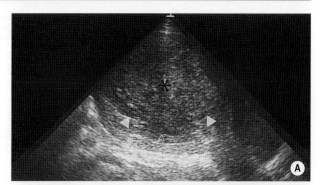

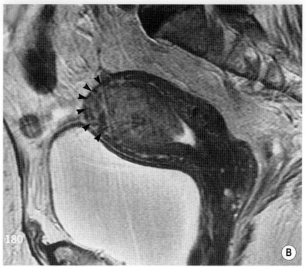

TVUS and MRI of deep myometrial invasion of endometrial carcinoma. (A) Sagittal US image shows a large endometrial mass (*). Deep myometrial invasion is suggested by focal interruption (open triangles) of the inner myometrium (closed triangles). (B) Sagittal T2W MRI shows tumour is relatively hyperintense compared with myometrium. There is marked thinning of the fundal myometrium (arrowheads) at the site of deep myometrial invasion.ʃ

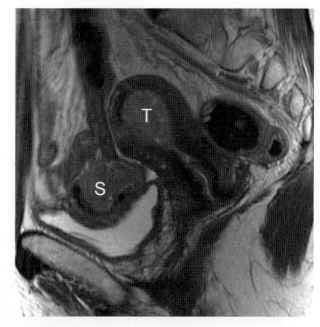

CARCINOMA OF THE CERVIX

DEFINITION

- This is usually a primary malignant squamous cell carcinoma of the cervix (accounting for up to 95% of cases) ► it is the $\frac{1}{3}$ most common gynaecological malignancy
  - An adenocarcinoma can arise from the glandular elements
- *Risk factors:* early sexual activity (especially with multiple partners) ► cigarette smoking ► immunosuppression ► infection with human papilloma viruses 16 and 18

CLINICAL PRESENTATION

- Abnormal uterine bleeding (especially after intercourse) ► vaginal discharge
- A cervical smear screening programme is in place

RADIOLOGICAL FEATURES

US This has a limited role
- **TAS:** This can detect hydronephrosis (with advanced disease)
- **Transrectal/TVS:** this can assess local disease but there is limited detection of parametrial disease and pelvic side-wall involvement ► the cervix appears as an enlarged, irregular, hypoechoic mass (± a hydro- or haematometra if the endocervical canal is obstructed)

CECT This is of greater value with higher stages of disease ► it is used for distant staging
- An enlarged cervix with low attenuation areas within the tumour (representing necrosis and ulceration) ► an ill-defined interface between the cervix and parametrium (it may be difficult to distinguish tumour from normal cervix and parametrium) ► an obstructed endocervical canal can lead to uterine enlargement with a fluid-filled endometrial cavity

MRI This is the method of choice for loco-regional staging ► it can accurately determine the tumour location (exophytic or endocervical), the tumour size, the depth of stromal invasion and any extension into the lower uterine segment ► it is better than CT for demonstrating parametrial invasion
- **T1WI:** the tumour is usually isointense to the normal cervix (and may not be visible) ► this is used to assess the nodal status (>1 cm is considered abnormal)
  - *Imaging with ultra small iron oxide contrast agents:* normal nodes have a uniform reduction in SI – involved nodes demonstrate relatively high SI
- **T2WI:** tumour demonstrates relatively high SI (cf. the low SI cervical stroma)
  - **Stage IA** *(microinvasive tumour):* this is not seen on MRI
  - **Stage IB** *(macroscopic tumour):* IB1: <4 cm, IB2: >4 cm ► T2WI: a high SI cervical mass ► a surrounding low SI fibrocervical stromal ring is a good indicator of a confined tumour

- **Stage IIA** *(vaginal involvement – not the lower $\frac{1}{3}$):* IIA1: <4 cm, IIA2: >4 cm ► T2WI: segmental disruption of the upper $\frac{2}{3}$ of the low SI vaginal wall by high SI tumour (without parametrial invasion)
- **Stage IIB** *(parametrial invasion):* T2WI: parametrial invasion is indicated by a lack of preservation of the low SI cervical stroma, together with parametrial fat stranding/soft tissue extension/encasement of peri-uterine vessels
- **Stage IIIA** *(involvement of the lower $\frac{1}{3}$ of vagina)*
- **Stage IIIB** *(pelvic wall invasion):* tumour extends to the pelvic musculature (within 1 cm), iliac vessels or causing hydronephrosis
- **Stage IVA** *(bladder or rectal invasion):* tumour invades the adjacent organs or extends outside the true pelvis
- **Stage IVB** *(distant spread):* including para-aortic or inguinal node metastases

FDG-PET This can assess nodal disease and tumour recurrence ► it has a higher sensitivity and specificity than MRI for the detection of metastatic lymph nodes

PEARLS

- The recently revised FIGO clinical staging system is used (see Section 9)
- Because of the relatively high likelihood of parametrial invasion (± lymph node metastases), cross-sectional imaging is recommended for evaluating clinical stage IB disease or greater (or when the primary lesion is larger than 2 cm)
- Accurate tumour staging is important not only for prognosis but also for determining the appropriate therapy
  - Imaging must distinguish early disease from advanced disease:
    - Early disease (stages I and IIA) is treated with surgery
    - Advanced disease is treated with radiation alone or in combination with chemotherapy
- **Pattern of spread:**
  - *Direct invasion:* there is direct invasion of the uterus, vagina, bladder, pouch of Douglas and rectum ► tumour can spread along the uterine ligaments to the pelvic side wall (± ureteric involvement)
  - *Nodal spread:* parametrial and paracervical nodes ► external, internal and common iliac nodes ► there is late retroperitoneal nodal involvement
  - *Haematogenous spread:* this is unusual but can be to the lungs, bone and liver
- **Tumour recurrence (MRI):**
  - T2WI (<6 months): a high SI soft tissue mass can be recurrent tumour or radiation fibrosis
  - T2WI (>6 months): radiation fibrosis demonstrates progressively lower SI
  - Dynamic contrast enhancement: there is more rapid contrast uptake within tumour than with radiation fibrosis

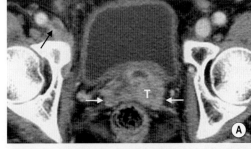
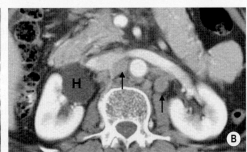
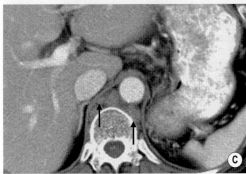
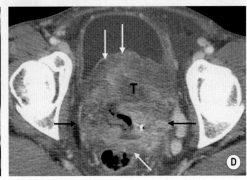

Cervical cancer, CT. Axial CT images (A–C) show a cervical cancer (T, A) which is contiguous with the adjacent parametrial fat, indicating parametrial invasion (white arrows, A). Note the presence of a filling defect within the right external femoral vein suggesting a DVT (black arrow, A). There is bilateral para-aortic (black arrows, B) and retrocrural lymphadenopathy (black arrows, C). Also, note the presence of right hydronephrosis (H, B). Axial CT image (D) of extensive cervical cancer (T, D) in a different patient. The tumour extends to both parametria (black arrows, D) and invades the posterior aspect of the bladder (white arrows, D) and anterior rectal wall (bottom white arrow, D).*

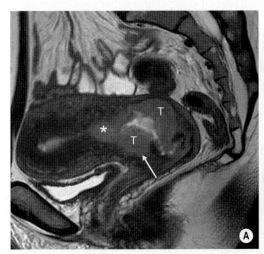
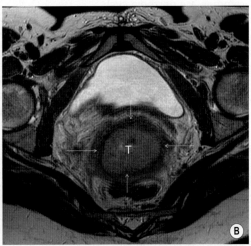

Cervical cancer, MRI. Sagittal (A) and axial oblique (B) T2-weighted images show a large cervical cancer (T) involving the anterior fornix of the vagina (arrow, A). The fibrocervical stroma (arrows, B) is intact, which excludes parametrial invasion. The tumour extends into the lower endometrial canal (asterisk, A).**

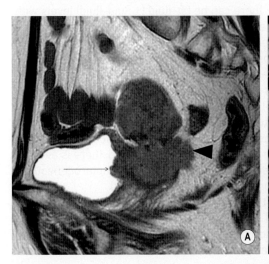
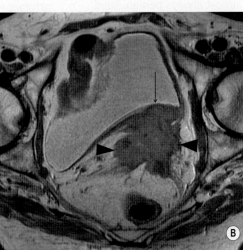

Cervical cancer, MRI. Sagittal (A) and axial (B) T2-weighted images show a large cervical cancer (T) invading the posterior aspect of the bladder (arrows, A and B). Bilateral parametrial invasion and posterior tumour extension is seen (arrowheads, A and B).**

BENIGN OVARIAN TUMOURS

Definition Benign ovarian neoplasms of various histological types – they account for 90% of all ovarian tumours

Histological types

- **Benign epithelial tumours:** these arise from the surface epithelium
  - *Serous cystadenoma:* the most common benign epithelial tumour ▶ 60% are benign
  - *Mucinous cystadenoma:* the epithelium consists of mucin-secreting cells ▶ it is the 2nd most common epithelial tumour ▶ 80% are benign
  - *Endometrioid cystadenoma:* these are often malignant ▶ it can mimic endometriosis
  - *Brenner tumour:* this is rare (1–2%), and arises from Wolffian metaplasia of the surface epithelium ▶ the vast majority are benign
- **Germ cell tumour:** this is the most common ovarian tumour in women <30 years old (accounting for 70% of cases) ▶ it accounts for 20% of *all* ovarian neoplasms ▶ only 2–3% of germ cell tumours are malignant
  - *Dermoid cysts (mature benign cystic teratoma):* the vast majority of ovarian teratomas are dermoid cysts ▶ it forms 40% of all ovarian tumours and arises from cells that differentiate into embryonic tissues ▶ the median age at presentation is 30 years
    - Malignant immature teratomas are rare aggressive tumours
  - *Other malignant GCTs (see ovarian carcinoma):* dysgerminoma ▶ yolk sac tumours ▶ choriocarcinoma
- **Sex cord-stromal tumours:** tumours developing from the ovarian stroma and sex cords ▶ they can develop in a testicular direction (Sertoli or Leydig cells), in an ovarian direction (granulose-theca cells), or in a stromal direction (fibromatous cells) ▶ they can synthesize oestrogen, progesterone, testosterone and steroids ('functioning' tumours) ▶ they can present throughout the reproductive years and beyond the menopause
  - *Theca cell tumour:* this is almost always benign, solid and unilateral ▶ it usually affects postmenopausal women ▶ it produces oestrogen (leading to precocious puberty, postmenopausal bleeding, endometrial hyperplasia and endometrial cancer)
  - *Sertoli–Leydig cell tumours:* this is a rare, low-grade malignancy tumour ▶ unilateral and large tumours, that are usually solid but can be partly cystic ▶ it usually affects premenopausal women ▶ it produces androgens (leading to virilization)
  - *Fibroma and thecoma:* derived from stromal cells ▶ it presents during the 4th to 5th decades ▶ unilateral solid encapsulated masses ▶ it is associated with the basal cell naevus syndrome
    - *Fibroma:* composed of fibroblasts ▶ can be mistaken for malignant tumours due to their solid nature
    - *Thecoma:* composed of spindle cells with lipid droplets (may secrete oestrogen) ▶ often unilateral + solid ▶ can produce oestrogen in sufficient amounts to produce systemic effects
    - *Fibrothecoma:* a combination of both cell types
    - *Meigs' syndrome:* fibroma + ascites + pleural effusion
    - *Gorlin's syndrome:* fibroma + BCC + jaw keratocysts + dural calcification

Radiological features Most benign ovarian tumours are non-specific in appearance, however some have more characteristic features:

TVS

- **Dermoid cyst:** variable appearances:
  - A cystic mass with echogenic nodules projecting into the lumen
  - A predominantly echogenic mass with posterior sound attenuation owing to the presence of sebaceous material and hair
  - A cystic mass with fine internal echogenic lines also representing hair
  - A fluid–fluid level (representing sebaceous material floating on fluid)
- **Serous cystadenoma:** a smooth thin-walled unilocular cyst (measuring up to 50 cm) ▶ papilliferous processes on the inner (and occasionally outer) surface
- **Mucinous cystadenoma:** a multilocular cyst with thin septations ▶ can grow to a large size
- **Brenner tumour:** this is usually a small (<5 cm) hypoechoic solid mass ▶ there is posterior acoustic shadowing due to extensive calcification ▶ seldom bilateral ▶ rarely cystic
- **Fibroma/thecoma/fibrothecoma:** a solid hypoechoic mass (US) ▶ a hyperattenuating mass (CT)

MRI

- **Dermoid cyst:** the fat component parallels the SI of fat on all pulse sequences (with loss of SI with fat saturation sequences) ▶ there will be a fat–water chemical shift artefact ▶ there can be fat–fluid (± fluid–fluid) levels with layering debris ▶ low SI regions represent calcification (e.g. formed teeth)
  - *Rokitansky nodules or dermoid plugs:* soft tissue protuberances attached to the cyst wall
- **Mucinous cystadenoma:** T2WI: a multilocular cyst with variable SI (a 'stained glass' appearance)
- **Brenner tumour:** T1WI: a solid mass of low SI ▶ T2WI: a solid mass of very low SI (with a cystic component if borderline or malignant) ▶ T1WI + Gad: there is avid homogeneous enhancement (which is heterogeneous if the tumour is borderline or malignant)
- **Fibroma/thecoma/fibrothecoma:** T1WI: low SI ▶ T2WI: low SI ▶ T1WI + Gad: there is little enhancement ▶ there can be calcification, cystic areas or fat (with a thecoma) demonstrated

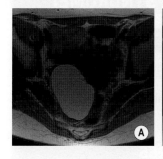
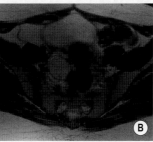
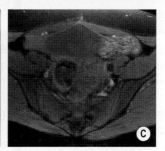

MRI of a dermoid cyst. (A) T1-, (B) T2- and (C) T1-weighted fat saturation axial images which demonstrate the typical findings of a dermoid cyst on MRI. There is a right adnexal mass with areas of high and intermediate signal on the T1-weighted image, intermediate signal on the T2-weighted image and suppression of the high signal from fat on the T1-weighted fat saturation sequence.**

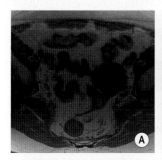
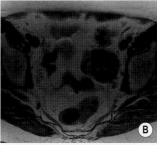
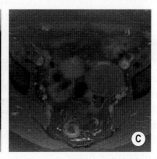

MRI of an ovarian fibroma. (A) T1-, (B) T2- and (C) T1-weighted post-contrast fat saturation axial images showing the typical findings of a fibroma on MRI, with low signal on T1- and T2-weighted images and little enhancement.**

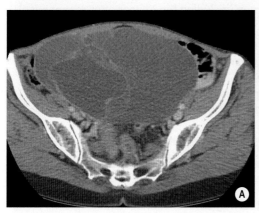
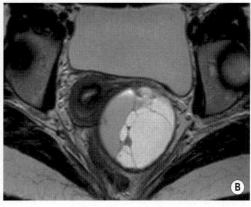

Mucinous cystadenoma. (A) CT of mucinous cystadenoma of the pelvis. Note subtle changes in attenuation between the cyst locules. (B) T2-weighted axial MRI of the pelvis elegantly demonstrates variable signal of the locules due to differing amounts of proteinaceous and mucinous material within.**

	T1W	T2W	FST1W	CET1W
Simple cyst				
Haemorrhagic cyst				
Endometrioma				
Dermoid				
Fibroma/ Brenner				
Cystic epithelial neoplasm				
Solid malignant neoplasm				

Diagram of enhancement patterns of adnexal lesions.** (Image kindly supplied by Dr John Spencer, Consultant Radiologist, Leeds, UK.)

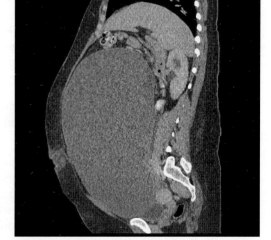

CT of a serous cystadenoma. A 25-year-old woman complained of abdominal distension. There is a huge unilocular cyst arising from the pelvis with no discernible papillary projections or mural nodules. Axial image.**

ENDOMETRIOSIS

DEFINITION

- The presence of endometrial epithelium and stroma outside of the endometrium and myometrium (possibly due to retrograde menstruation through the Fallopian tubes)
  - *Endometrioma:* ectopic endometrium is influenced by circulating hormones and undergoes repeat haemorrhage with the development of a blood-filled cyst
  - *Common locations:* ovaries (80%) ▶ uterosacral ligaments ▶ Fallopian tubes ▶ rectovaginal septum ▶ pouch of Douglas ▶ bladder wall ▶ umbilicus

CLINICAL PRESENTATION

- It can be asymptomatic, but symptoms can include dysmenorrhoea, dyspareunia, abdominal pain, dysfunctional uterine bleeding, infertility and bowel obstruction ▶ it can also present with an endometrioma, adhesions, or endometrial implants
  - It accounts for up to 65% of cases of chronic pelvic pain ▶ it usually affects women of reproductive age

RADIOLOGICAL FEATURES

US (endometrioma) A cystic mass with diffuse uniform low-level echoes – after repeated episodes of bleeding it may develop irregular walls and echogenic mural nodules ▶ fluid–fluid levels or fluid–debris levels represent blood products ▶ with thin or thick septations it may be difficult to differentiate this from a malignant ovarian mass

MRI

- **Endometrioma** ('chocolate cyst'): T1WI: high SI ▶ T2WI: low or heterogeneously high SI (the high SI is caused by the high iron content) ▶ there is increased conspicuity with fat suppression ▶ T2WI 'shading sign' representing old blood products may help differentiate from haemorrhagic corpus luteum cysts
- **Endometrial implants:** these may be detected (but MRI is inferior to laparoscopy, which is the gold standard for diagnosis and evaluation of disease extent) ▶ irregular/indistinct masses ± cystic/haemorrhagic areas ▶ minimal enhancement ▶ thickened/nodular pelvic ligaments ▶ adhesions ▶ 'kissing' ovaries ▶ hydro/haemato salpinx

PEARLS

Atypical sites

- *Lung:* catamenial pneumothorax ▶ cyclic haemoptysis
- *GI tract:* it commonly affects the inferior sigmoid margin and anterior rectosigmoid ▶ it appears as a extramucosal mass with a crenulated or spiculated mucosal margin ▶ it can present with catamenial diarrhoea

POLYCYSTIC OVARIAN DISEASE (STEIN–LEVENTHAL SYNDROME)

DEFINITION

- Two of the following three required for diagnosis:
  (1) oligo- ± anovulation
  (2) hyperandrogenism (clinical or biochemical)
  (3) polycystic ovaries

RADIOLOGICAL FEATURES

US Enlarged ovaries (>10 ml in volume) with an echogenic central stroma and >12 peripherally placed cysts (measuring <9 mm in diameter) ▶ need to reference cycle stage

FOLLICULAR CYST

Definition

- A physiological cyst that follows a failure of fluid resorption within an incompletely developed follicle ▶ it is a common asymptomatic finding and occurs in premenopausal women (including the 1st year after menopause)
  - It usually spontaneously regresses (after <2 months)

US A 3–8 cm simple cyst ▶ the wall becomes thicker and more vascular towards ovulation ▶ it may undergo haemorrhage

- A follow-up US is recommended in 6 weeks (immediately post menstruation)

LUTEIN CYSTS

Definition

- **Corpus luteum cyst:** a functional, non-neoplastic physiological enlargement of the ovary following ovulation ▶ may demonstrate internal haemorrhage (giving a complex appearance on US) ▶ if it persists it may cause local pain, tenderness and either amenorrhoea or delayed menstruation ▶ it can mimic an ectopic pregnancy
  - It usually spontaneously regresses (after <2 months)

US It appears as a thick-walled unilocular cyst with a vascular wall (± haemorrhagic content)

MRI High T1WI signal

Definition

- **Theca lutein cyst:** these are medium-sized physiological cysts, which are usually bilateral and filled with straw-coloured fluid ▶ result from excessive BHCG stimulation or hypersensitivity
  - *Associations:* polycystic ovarian disease ▶ hydatidiform mole ▶ choriocarcinoma ▶ chorionic gonadotrophin or clomifene therapy

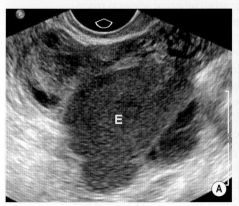
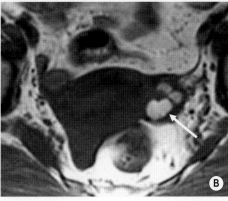
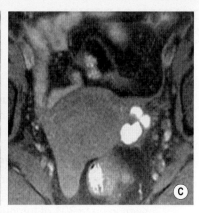

Endometrioma. Transvaginal sagittal US (A) demonstrates a complex left ovarian cystic mass (E) consistent with an endometrioma. Although similar to a haemorrhagic cyst, the irregular contour, internal echo homogeneity and persistence over time favours an endometrioma. Axial T1W (B) and T1W fat-suppressed (C) images show multiple high SI lesions within the left ovary (arrow, B), suggesting either endometriosis or haemorrhagic cysts. The fat suppression increases the conspicuity of haemorrhagic lesions and helps differentiate them from dermoids.*

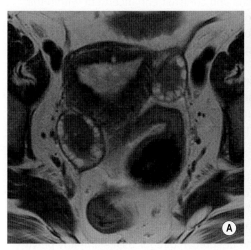
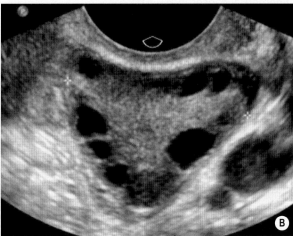

Polycystic ovaries. (A) Axial T2-weighted MRI demonstrating the classic appearances of polycystic ovaries with 12 or more follicles of 2–9 mm in diameter, and increased ovarian volume.** (B) Transverse TVUS of the left ovary depicting multiple subcentimetre peripherally placed follicles in enlarged ovaries with echogenic central stroma.*

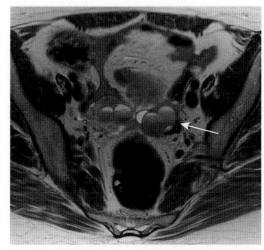
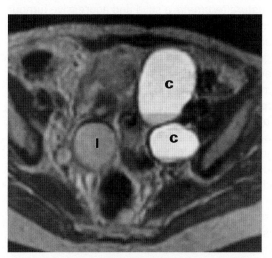

Endometriosis 'kissing ovaries'. Axial T2-weighted sequence of the pelvis which shows the ovaries tethered by adhesions in the mid-line ('kissing ovaries'). There are bilateral endometriotic cysts with classic layering of haemorrhagic debris (arrow).**

Multiloculated thin-walled haemorrhagic benign ovarian cysts (c) showing fluid–fluid levels on a transverse T2WI. There is a coincidental uterine leimyoma (l).†

OVARIAN CARCINOMA

Definition

- A primary malignant tumour of the ovary (usually affecting postmenopausal women)
- **Histological types:**
  - **Malignant surface epithelial tumours:** tumours of surface epithelial origin ▶ accounting for up to 70% of all primary ovarian tumours and 90% of all malignant ovarian cancers:
    - *Serous cystadenocarcinoma* (50%): predominantly cystic and can be unilocular or multilocular
      - *Psammoma bodies:* microscopic calcification seen in up to 30% of tumours
    - *Mucinous cystadenocarcinoma* (20%): typically multilocular with numerous thin-walled cysts ▶ less likely to be malignant or bilateral than a serous tumour
    - *Endometrioid tumour* (20%): usually invasive ▶ it is associated with endometrial cancer in 20–30%
    - *Clear cell tumour* (10%): tends to remain confined to the ovary with a good prognosis ▶ usually unilocular with a few mural nodules
    - *Undifferentiated tumour* (1%): very poor outcome ▶ usually advanced at presentation
  - **Germ cell tumours (GCT):** 70% of tumours presenting during the first 2 decades ▶ the vast majority are benign
    - *Dysgerminoma:* the most common malignant GCT (although only 2% of all primary ovarian tumours) ▶ it is comparable to a testicular seminoma or a pineal gland germinoma ▶ it is bilateral in 15% of cases ▶ solid ± cystic areas ▶ presents during the 2nd and 3rd decades
    - *Endodermal sinus (yolk sac) tumour:* the 2nd most common malignant GCT ▶ usually unilateral and rapidly growing ▶ solid ± cystic areas ▶ presents during the 2nd and 3rd decades
    - *Immature teratoma:* a solid and aggressive tumour demonstrating widespread dissemination
    - *Embryonal carcinoma/choriocarcinoma:* rare aggressive tumours ▶ usually metastasized to the liver, lungs and bone at presentation ▶ presents at a young age (<20 years)
  - **Sex cord-stromal tumours:**
    - *Granulosa cell tumour:* usually confined to the ovary at presentation ▶ grows very slowly with a good prognosis (but recurs frequently) ▶ usually unilateral and solid ▶ associated with endometrial cancer ▶ usually presents following the menopause ▶ oestrogen secretion can lead to postmenopausal bleeding or precocious puberty
  - **Metastases:** commonly from the breast, endometrium and GI tract
    - *Krukenberg tumours:* bilateral ovarian mucin-producing metastases from the stomach

Radiological features

US (TAS and TVS) This is the primary technique for the detection and characterization of adnexal masses

- **Features suspicious for malignant adnexal mass:**
  - Wall irregularity ▶ thick septations (>3 mm) ▶ papillary projections ▶ solid components ▶ size >9 cm ▶ ascites ▶ peritoneal deposits
    - *Approximate abnormal ovarian volumes:* >18 cm^3 (premenopausal) ▶ >8 cm^3 (postmenopausal)
  - *Neovascularity on Doppler US:* a RI <0.4 (due to new vessels having little smooth muscle within their walls)

CT *Indications:* preoperative staging ▶ assessment of any related complications (bowel or renal obstruction) ▶ determining the extent of cytoreductive surgery required to optimize a subsequent chemotherapeutic response

- **Adnexal masses:** these are frequently bilateral
  - A multilocular cyst with thick internal septations and solid mural or septal components ▶ a partially cystic and solid mass ▶ a lobulated papillary heterogeneous solid mass (± an irregular outer border, coarse calcifications and contrast enhancement within the cyst wall or soft tissue components)
  - Calcification suggests a serous tumour ▶ high density within a multilocular tumour suggests a mucinous tumour
- **Peritoneal implants:** usually indicates peritoneal disease ▶ there can be difficulty detecting lesions <1 cm
  - Nodular or plaque-like enhancing soft tissue masses
  - *Location:* pouch of Douglas ▶ paracolic gutters ▶ surface of the small and large bowel (± obstruction) ▶ greater omentum ('tumour cake') ▶ liver surface (perihepatic implants) ▶ subphrenic space
- **Pseudomyxoma peritonei:** rupture or metastasis of a mucinous tumour leads to the filling of the peritoneal cavity with mucinous material akin to the cyst contents

MRI This is the best technique for assessing any pelvic side-wall invasion ▶ it requires contrast-enhanced protocols and Buscopan (hyoscine) to limit bowel motion

- **Primary criteria for malignant adnexal mass:**
  - Size >4 cm
  - A cystic lesion with a solid component
  - An irregular wall thickness >3 mm
  - Septa >3 mm (± vegetations or nodularity)
  - A solid mass with necrosis
- **Ancillary criteria:**
  - Involvement of the pelvic organs or side wall
  - Peritoneal, mesenteric, or omental disease
  - Ascites
  - Adenopathy
- The presence of at least one of the primary criteria coupled with a single criterion from the ancillary group correctly characterizes 95% of malignant lesions
- Ovarian metastasis tend to be more solid in appearance than a primary ovarian neoplasm ▶ peritoneal/serosal implants are best seen on delayed images (5 min) – longer delays should be avoided as ascites can enhance

FDG-PET/PET/CT This can evaluate patients for recurrent ovarian cancer, particularly those with negative CT or MRI findings and rising tumour markers

- It can detect implants that are difficult to assess by conventional imaging studies

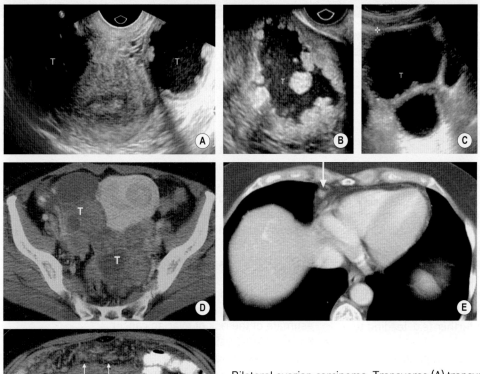

Bilateral ovarian carcinoma. Transverse (A) transvaginal ultrasound image of the pelvis shows bilateral cystic adnexal masses (T). Sagittal images of right (B) and left (C) ovaries demonstrate cystic mass (T) with mural nodularity (B) and multiple septations (C). MDCT of a different patient shows bilateral complex solid and cystic adnexal masses (T, D), highly suggestive of ovarian carcinoma, and demonstrates the presence of omental tumour implants (white arrows, F). Note also the presence of left para-aortic, interaortocaval (black arrows, F) and superior diaphragmatic (arrow, E) lymphadenopathy.*

Borderline serous cystadenocarcinoma. (A) Axial T1-weighted MRI showing enhancement of the solid components (arrowheads). (B) Sagittal T2-weighted MRI showing bilateral multiseptated adnexal masses (arrows) with mural nodules and papillary projections (arrowheads).

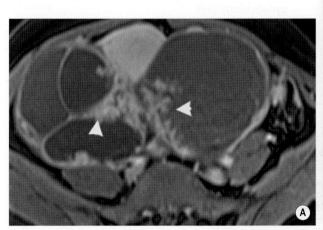

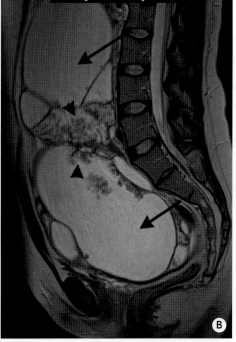

OVARIAN CARCINOMA

PEARLS

- 10% of ovarian tumours are due to hereditary syndromes: *BRAC1* and *BRAC2* mutations (with an associated risk of breast cancer) ▶ Lynch syndrome II (with a risk of colon cancer)
- **Protective factors:** anovulation ▶ multiparity ▶ a history of breastfeeding
- **Staging:** the TNM and FIGO staging systems are used ▶ imaging cannot replace surgical staging (see Section 9)
- **Patterns of tumour spread:**
  - *Local extension:* uterus ▶ rectum ▶ colon ▶ bladder ▶ pelvic side wall
  - *Transcoelomic spread:* vascularized peritoneal deposits can shed malignant cells which are carried predominantly towards the undersurface of the right hemidiaphragm (due to the inherent peritoneal fluid flow dynamics) ▶ here the lymphatics can absorb the deposits and disseminate them further (e.g. leading to a pleural effusion)
  - *Lymphatic drainage:* via the ovarian lymphatics that travel with the ovarian vessels ▶ their blockage leads to ascites
  - *Haematogenous spread:* this is late and is to the liver, lungs and bone
  - Bilateral ovarian involvement is seen in 50% of cases (25% of these represent spread from an initial tumour ▶ 25% are multicentric tumours)
- **Tumour markers:** CA-125 lacks sensitivity or specificity to be used alone ▶ germ cell tumours may produce AFP and hCG ▶ tumour markers may have a screening role in the future
- **Imaging approach:**
  - *US:* the primary technique for detection and characterization
  - *MRI:* this is a problem-solving tool ▶ it can assess for any side-wall involvement
  - *CT:* this is used for preoperative staging and follow up
  - *FDG-PET/CT:* this is used for assessing recurrent disease, and for the assessment of peritoneal deposits
- **Non-resectable disease is indicated if:**
  - There is pelvic side-wall invasion (suspect if the primary tumour lies <3 mm within the pelvic side wall or when the iliac vessels are surrounded or distorted by tumour)
  - There is invasion of the urinary bladder or urinary obstruction
  - There are tumour deposits >1 cm within the gastrosplenic ligament, lesser sac, ligamentum teres, porta hepatis, subphrenic space and small bowel mesentery
  - There are retroperitoneal nodes above the renal hilar
  - There are distant metastases (e.g. liver/lung/spleen)

- **Treatment:**
  - **Early ovarian cancer:** a comprehensive staging laparotomy + a transabdominal hysterectomy and bilateral salpingo-oophorectomy (± an omentectomy, retroperitoneal lymph node sampling, peritoneal and diaphragmatic biopsies and cytology of the peritoneal washings)
  - **Advanced but operable disease (stage I/II):** primary cytoreductive surgery followed by adjuvant chemotherapy
  - **Non-resectable disease (stage III/IV):** neoadjuvant (preoperative) chemotherapy prior to debulking ▶ radiotherapy has a decreasing role

THE RISK OF MALIGNANCY INDEX (RMI)

- RMI is used as tool to triage women with adnexal masses for referral to a cancer centre ▶ it allows an estimate of the risk of ovarian cancer
- It is calculated using US findings (U), menopausal status (M) and CA-125 value
  - $RMI = U \times M \times CA\text{-}125$
- ***US findings are scored with 1 point for each of the following:***
  - Multilocular cyst ▶ evidence of solid areas ▶ evidence of metastases ▶ presence of ascites ▶ bilateral lesions
    - U = 0 (US score of 0)
    - U = 1 (US score of 1)
    - U = 3 (US score of 2–5)
- ***Menopausal status:***
  - M = 1 (premenopausal)
  - M = 2 (postmenopausal)
- ***Guidelines for referral:***
  - RMI <25: surgery at a local gynaecology unit
  - RMI 25–1000: specialist USS
    - No suspicious US features: surgery at a local gynaecology unit
    - Suspicious US features: MRI scan
      - No suspicious MRI features: surgery at a local gynaecology unit
      - Suspicious MRI features: surgery at a cancer centre
  - RMI >1000: CT for staging ▶ surgery at a cancer centre

Risk	RMI*	Women (%)	Cancer risk
Low	<25	40	<3%
Moderate	25–1000	30	Up to 20%
High	>1000	30	>80%

*This value can be centre-dependent.

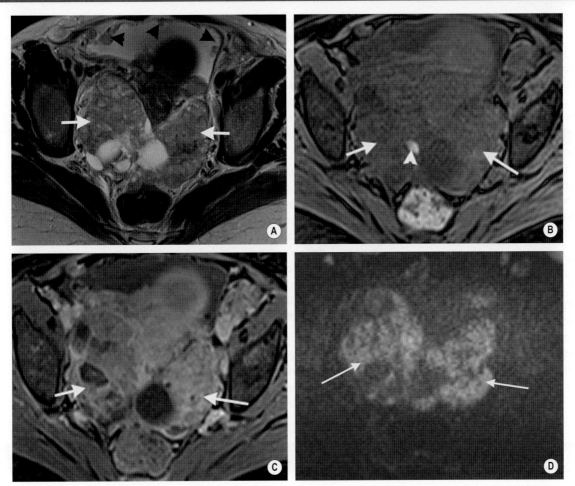

Bilateral serous cystadenocarcinoma. (A) Axial T2-weighted MRI showing bilateral solid/cystic adnexal masses (arrows) and peritoneal implants (arrowheads) with ascites. (B) Axial T1W MRI with fat saturation shows adnexal masses of intermediate-to-low signal intensity (arrows) with focus of hemorrhage within them (arrowhead). (C) Axial T1-weighted MRI with fat saturation following gadolinium shows enhancement of solid components (arrows) ▶ (D) diffusion-weighted image (B = 1000) shows masses to be of high signal intensity.

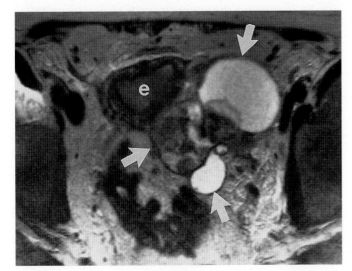

Axial T2WI. Complex large left adnexal mass with a solid and cystic component (arrows) compressing and displacing the uterus. There is also distension of the endometrial cavity due to a coexisting endometrial tumour (e). Endometrioid carcinoma is associated with endometrial carcinoma.[†]

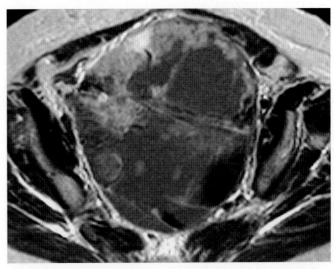

Axial T2WI. Mucinous cystadenocarcinoma of the ovary producing a large mass, with mixed contents, filling the pelvis. The area of signal void in the tumour is due to either blood products or mucin.[†]

PELVIC INFLAMMATORY DISEASE

Definition An acute clinical syndrome associated with the ascending spread of micro-organisms (e.g. *Chlamydia trachomatis* and *Neisseria gonorrhoeae*) from the vagina or cervix to the endometrium, Fallopian tubes (± any contiguous structures) ▶ the associated adhesions can lead to the formation of a pyosalpinx, hydrosalpinx or tubo-ovarian abscess

Clinical presentation It can be asymptomatic or present with subacute lower abdominal pain, fever, a purulent vaginal discharge, bilateral adnexal tenderness with cervical excitation and an elevated ESR ▶ delayed recognition and treatment may lead to infertility ▶ associated with IUCD use

US

- **Uterus:** this can be slightly enlarged, and more hypoechoic than normal ▶ ill defined uterine margins ('indefinite uterus') ▶ thickened endometrium (>14 mm) with variable echogenicity ▶ poorly defined endometrial/myometrial interface ▶ hypoechoic myometrium ▶ there can be prominent adnexa ▶ pelvic free fluid
- **Pyosalpinx/hydrosalpinx:** thickened adnexal tubular structure progressing to an elongated convoluted configuration ± internal echoes (debris)

  - *Hydrosalpinx (4 distinct features):* tubular shape/folded configuration/well defined echogenic wall/short linear echoes protruding into the lumen
- **Tubo-ovarian abscesses:** unilocular or multilocular adnexal mass with a thickened echogenic wall (± sepatations and hypoechoic areas) ▶ a septic abortion, intrauterine manipulation or pelvic operation may also provoke a pyogenic adnexal abscess

CT

- **Early PID:** subtle findings: mild pelvic oedema/bulky uterus/abnormal endometrial enhancement
- **Salpingitis:** thickened fallopian tubes/enlarged and abnormally enhancing ovaries
- **Pyosalpinx:** wall thickening and enhancement of the fallopian tubes distended with complex fluid
- **Pelvic abscess:** a soft tissue mass with central areas of low attenuation and thick irregular walls ▶ it may be difficult to differentiate from a necrotic tumour or an endometrioma

MRI

- **Abscess:** thick-walled, fluid-filled adnexal mass (± wall enhancement)
- **Abscess/pyosalpinx contents:** T1WI: high SI ▶ T2WI: low SI

GESTATIONAL TROPHOBLASTIC DISEASE

DEFINITION

- This includes the tumour spectrum of a hydatidiform mole, an invasive mole (choriocarcinoma destruens) and a choriocarcinoma
  - It arises from fetal tissue within the maternal host and is composed of both syncytiotrophoblastic and cytotrophoblastic cells
- The tumour produces human chorionic gonadotrophin (hCG) and is highly curable by chemotherapy

RADIOLOGICAL FEATURES

- Imaging is used for staging metastatic disease and evaluating persistent disease ▶ it is unable to differentiate between a complete mole, an invasive mole or a choriocarcinoma

US Large-for-gestational-age uterus with an echogenic soft tissue mass distending the endometrial canal ▶ the mass is punctuated by multiple small cystic spaces

(corresponding to hydropic villi in cases of a complete hydatidiform mole)

CT An enlarged uterus demonstrating heterogeneous contrast enhancement ▶ irregular hypodense regions may be seen within the myometrium ▶ bilateral ovarian enlargement by multilocular theca lutein cysts

- Locoregional spread is characterized by an enhancing soft tissue density within the parametria (± obliteration of the pelvic fat or muscle planes)

MRI

- T1WI: an iso- or hyperintense mass (cf. the adjacent myometrium)
- T2WI: a heterogeneous, predominantly high SI mass that obliterates the normal uterine zonal anatomy ▶ enlarged vessels within the broad ligament and the uterus are depicted as signal voids on both T1WI and T2WI
- T1WI + Gad: there is avid enhancement

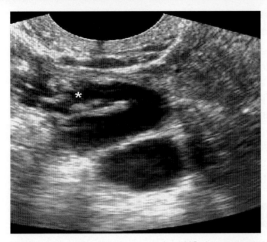

Hydrosalpinx. Sagittal transvaginal US demonstrates a cystic lesion of tubular appearance within the pelvis. Small internally projecting nodules are compatible with the fimbriae and give the cyst (*) a 'cogwheel' appearance, typical of hydrosalpinx.*

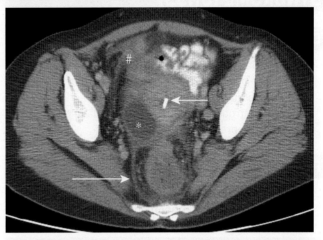

CT of pelvic inflammatory disease. This CT shows some of the typical features of PID on CT. The presence of an IUCD (small arrow), inflammatory changes (#), thickening of the uterosacral ligaments (large arrow) and right adnexal cystic mass (*) are all suggestive of PID.**

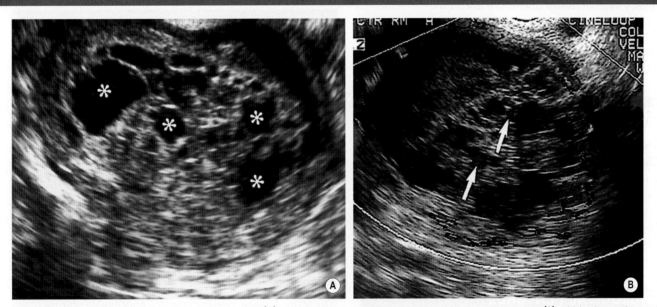

Gestational trophoblastic disease. Transverse TVS (A) shows an echogenic mass with multiple cystic spaces (*) within the endometrial cavity in a woman with a hydatidiform mole. Sagittal TVS with colour flow (arrows, B) shows flow to the mole.*

OVARIAN HYPERSTIMULATION SYNDROME (OHSS)

DEFINITION

- Ovarian enlargement (>5 cm) with multiple follicular and theca lutein cysts and an oedematous stroma ▶ there is also associated ascites and pleural effusions
  - *Causes:* iatrogenic hCG therapy ▶ hydatitiform mole ▶ multiple pregnancies

PEARL

- There is a risk of death from intra-abdominal haemorrhage or a thromboembolic event

VULVAR AND VAGINAL MALIGNANCIES

DEFINITION

Vulvar carcinoma

- This demonstrates metastatic spread to the superficial inguinal nodes, and then subsequently to the deep inguinal and external iliac groups
- CT and MRI are usually performed for distant and locoregional staging

Vaginal malignancies

- Primary vaginal malignancies are uncommon
- Metastatic tumours to the vagina are more frequent – these originate usually from carcinoma of the endometrium and cervix (followed by melanoma and carcinoma of the colon and kidney)

PERITONEAL INCLUSION CYSTS

DEFINITION

- Cystic non-neoplastic reactive mesothelial proliferation that is seen in premenopausal women
  - Pelvic adhesions from previous surgery, pelvic inflammatory disease (PID), or endometriosis results in impaired clearing of the peritoneal fluid that is normally produced by the ovaries

RADIOLOGICAL FEATURES

US/MRI Simple or complex cystic structure(s) that are contiguous with the ovary (and which may mimic a hydrosalpinx or pyosalpinx) ▶ adhesions extending to the ovarian surface (giving a 'spider web' appearance with an entrapped ovary)

CERVICAL INCOMPETENCE

DEFINITION

- A shortened and widened endocervical canal
- It is responsible for approximately 15% of all 2nd and 3rd trimester abortions
  - *Primary:* congenital (associated with diethylstilbestrol exposure) ▶ secondary to reduced collagen within the cervix
  - *Secondary:* multiple gestations ▶ gynaecological or obstetric trauma ▶ increased prostaglandin production

RADIOLOGICAL FEATURES

US (gravid patient)

- A cervical length <3 cm ▶ a cervical canal width >2 cm during the 2nd trimester
- Bulging of the membranes into the cervical canal leads to an unfavourable prognosis
- No criteria have been established for a non-gravid patient

MRI This can diagnose incompetence in the non-gravid patient – one of more of the following is required:
- A shortened endocervical canal (<3 cm)
- A widened internal cervical os (>4 mm)
- Asymmetric widening of the endocervical canal
- Thinning or absence of the low SI cervical stroma

UTERINE SARCOMAS

DEFINITION

- These are rare, accounting for 3–5% of all uterine malignancies ▶ they are often highly malignant and commonly metastasize to the lungs and liver
- **Leiomyosarcoma:** a primary malignant uterine smooth muscle tumour
- **Endometrial sarcoma:** a malignant endometrial mesenchymal tumour
- **Malignant mixed Müllerian tumour (carcinosarcoma):** a malignant uterine tumour composed of tissues that can differentiate into both carcinoma and sarcoma

RADIOLOGICAL FEATURES

US/MRI A large, heterogeneous, aggressive uterine mass

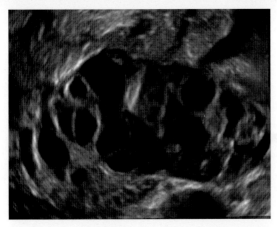

Ovarian hyperstimulation. The ovary is massively enlarged and contains several follicular cysts and stromal oedema.*

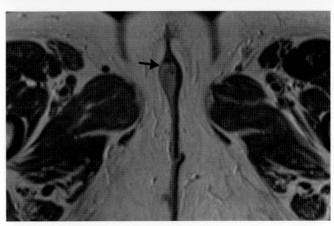

Axial T2W MRI showing intermediate signal tumour in the right labia (arrow) in a patient with vulval carcinoma.

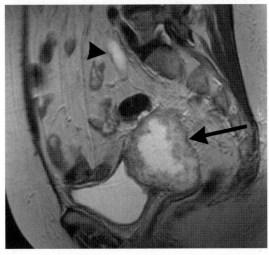

Sagittal T2W MRI in a patient with a large solid/cystic mass (arrow) to the vaginal vault following previous total abdominal hysterectomy (TAH) and bilateral salpingo-oophorectomy (BSO) for endometrial carcinoma. Biopsy confirmed metastatic deposit. There is a hydroureter (arrowhead) secondary to the mass.

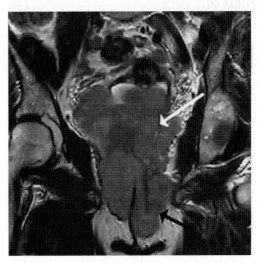

A patient with vaginal lymphoma. Coronal T2WI shows a mass of homogeneous intermediate signal intensity extending down into the perineum (black arrow) and superiorly into the pelvis (white arrow).

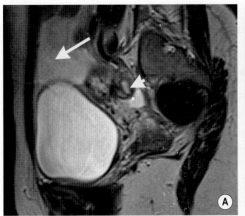

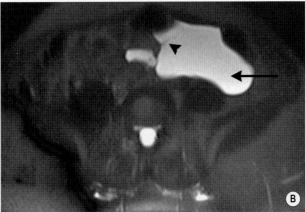

Peritoneal inclusion cyst in a patient with adhesions following pelvic surgery. (A) Sagittal T2W MRI and (B) axial fat-saturated T2W MRI shows a large cyst arising from the pelvis to lie superior to the bladder (arrows). The left ovary is seen within this (white arrowhead). A single septation is seen (black arrowhead).

NEURORADIOLOGY

7.1 INTRACRANIAL TUMOURS

COMPUTED TOMOGRAPHY

NECT

- **Intra-axial tumours:** usually of low attenuation on NECT ▶ high attenuation areas within a tumour indicate tumour calcification or recent intratumoural haemorrhage
- **Extra-axial tumours:** associated with bone erosion or hyperostosis

CECT
Improved visualization of an enhancing mass lesion (e.g. a meningioma or metastases)

CT perfusion
This can assess tumour relative cerebral blood volume (rCBV) and permeability changes ▶ it provides a limited area of coverage (compared with MRI) ▶ unlike MRI it can provide a direct relationship between the CT attenuation value and tissue contrast material concentration

MAGNETIC RESONANCE IMAGING

Usual tumour appearance

- T1WI: low SI ▶ T2WI/FLAIR: high SI
- FLAIR: this provides particularly good contrast between normal brain tissue and glial tumours ▶ signal loss is seen within any cystic tumour components
- *Highly cellular tumours* (e.g. lymphoma): a corresponding decreased water content (relatively low SI on T2WI)

Extra-axial enhancement

- Vascular extra-axial tumours (e.g. meningioma)

Intra-axial enhancement

- Following disruption of the blood–brain barrier (generally high-grade tumours) ▶ it may also be seen with certain low-grade tumours (e.g. pilocytic astrocytomas)

T2*/susceptibility images

- Haemorrhage/calcification becomes more conspicuous

Intratumoural haemorrhage or calcification

- T2WI: low SI ▶ this is more conspicuous on T2*WI (stronger magnetic susceptibility effects)

High SI (T1WI)

- If there is haemorrhage, proteinaceous fluid, melanin (e.g. metastatic melanomas) or fat

Dynamic susceptibility-weighted contrast-enhanced (DSC) MR perfusion imaging

- This can assess tumour blood vessel density (an indirect measure of tumour neovascularity malignancy)
  - rCBV measurements correlate closely with markers of tumour vascularity and angiogenesis
    - indirect measure of tumour neovascularity

- Higher rCBV values with high-grade tumours
- rCBV maps can aid stereotactic tumour biopsies
- In radiation necrosis the residual enhancing lesion has a low rCBV (higher with tumour recurrence due to new vessel formation)
- DSC imaging differs from contrast enhancement, which is an indicator of vascular endothelial (blood–brain barrier) integrity

Dynamic contrast-enhanced (DCE) imaging   T1WI + Gad
▶ DCE imaging can generate time–signal intensity curves, and analysed with mathematical models (e.g. K^{TRANS})

Permeability imaging – the 'transfer coefficient' (K^{TRANS})

- This quantifies tumour microvascular permeability and correlates with tumour grade
- Measured using T1W steady-state or first-pass T2*W gradient-echo imaging

Arterial spin labelling

- Labelled endogenous hydrogen measures cerebral blood flow (rCBF)

MR diffusion imaging

- Useful in identifying acute infarcts or abscesses (which can mimic brain tumours)
- ADC measurements correlate inversely with the histological glioma cell count
  - ADC measurements of any enhancing components in radiation necrosis are significantly higher than with recurrent tumour (mirroring the higher cellular density with a recurrent neoplasm)
- Diffusion tensor imaging (DTI) provides additional information about the direction of water diffusion ▶ the normally high anisotropy within white matter tracts can be lost if infiltrated by tumour

MR spectroscopy (MRS)

- MRS is a sensitive but not specific technique
- The common pattern seen with brain tumours:
  - *Decreased:*
    - N-acetylaspartate (NAA): a neuron-specific marker
    - Creatine (Cr)
  - *Increased:*
    - Lipids (L)
    - Lactate (Lac): a marker of tumour tissue hypoxia
    - Choline (Cho): a reflection of cell membrane turnover (increased with neoplastic activity)

fMRI

- BOLD imaging detects changes in regional cerebral blood flow during various forms of brain activity
- This is used for preoperative localization of important cortical regions that may have been displaced by tumour

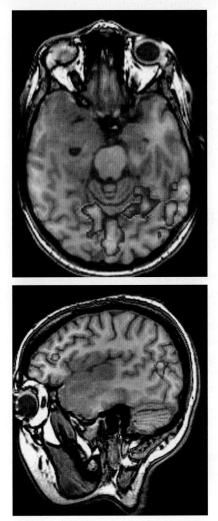

fMRI in a patient with a right peri-insular and temporal lobe tumour. Images acquired during a picture-naming task show activation in the visual cortex and in the left Broca's area, which lies outside the tumour.*

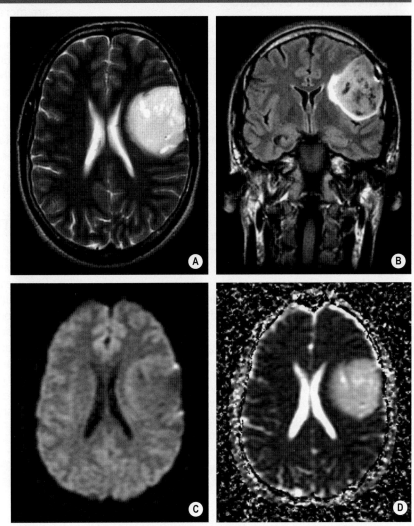

WHO grade II astrocytoma. Axial T2W (A), FLAIR (B) images showing a left frontal hyperintense mass lesion with well-defined borders and small cystic areas. On the trace-weighted DW image (C) the tumour is not very conspicuous as T2 effects and diffusion effects cancel each other out. On the ADC map (D) the glioma is easily identified as an area of increased diffusivity compared to normal brain parenchyma.*

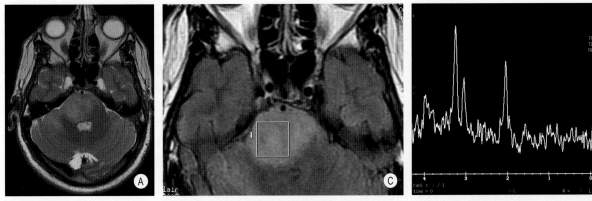

Proton magnetic resonance spectroscopy. (A) Single voxel magnetic resonance spectroscopy. Diffusely infiltrative brainstem glioma which is hyperintense on T2WI. A magnified FLAIR image (C) demonstrates placement of the spectroscopy voxel within the tumour. The spectrum (D) demonstrates that the choline peak (3.22 ppm) is elevated and much higher than the creatine peak (3.03 ppm) and the N-acetylaspartate peak (2.01 ppm). (CHO = choline, PCr/Cr = creatine, NAA = N-acetylaspartate).**

INTRA-AXIAL TUMOURS

Definition Tumours arising from the brain parenchyma
- *Glioma:* a broad category including tumours arising from either astrocytes (astrocytoma), oligodendrocytes (oligodendroglioma) or ependymal cells (ependymoma)

EXTRA-AXIAL TUMOURS

Definition Tumours arising from the tissues covering the brain (e.g. the dura or arachnoid) ▶ these occur much more frequently in adults than children (accounting for the majority of the primary infratentorial adult tumours)
- Tissues of origin:
  - *Meningioma:* meningothelial arachnoidal cells
  - *Haemangiopericytoma:* mesenchymal pericytes
  - *Schwannomas and neurofibromas:* cranial nerves
  - *Epidermoid and dermoid cysts:* developmental cysts or tumour-like lesions
  - *Choroid plexus papillomas:* choroid plexus cells
- Intracranial tumours are classified according to the WHO classification

Patient age and tumour site are useful indicators to the likely tumour type

- *Children:* primary tumours usually occur infratentorially and within the posterior fossa between the ages of 2 and 10 years (e.g. pilocytic astrocytoma, pontine glioma, ependymoma and medulloblastoma) ▶ below

2 and above 10 years of age supratentorial tumours are more common (paediatric supratentorial tumours will preferentially affect the midline structures) ▶ intracranial metastases are rare
  - *Astrocytoma:* this is the most common primary childhood brain tumour (the majority are pilocytic astrocytomas and characteristically occur within the cerebellum, hypothalamus and optic nerves)
- *Adults:* 70% of intracranial tumours are primary (30% are metastases) ▶ the vast majority of tumours are supratentorial – the posterior fossa is rarely affected by a primary tumour (a metastasis is more likely at this location)

RADIATION NECROSIS

- Late complication of radiotherapy or gamma knife surgery
- Can present as an enhancing mass lesion (difficult to distinguish from recurrent tumour)
- Radiation necrosis:
  - Enhancing area has low FDG uptake/low rCBV
  - Dynamic contrast enhancement: lower max enhancement slope than recurrence
  - ADC measurements: enhancing components have higher values than recurrence (lower relative cellular density)

Features distinguishing an extra- from an intra-axial tumour		
	Extra-axial tumour	**Intra-axial tumour**
'Buckling' and medial displacement of the grey–white matter interface	Yes	No
CSF cleft separating the base of the mass from adjacent brain	Yes	No
Broad base along a dural or calvarial surface	Yes	No
Associated bone changes	<ul><li>*Meningioma:* hyperostotic bone reaction</li><li>*Dermoid cyst/ schwannoma:* bone thinning (with enlargement of the middle cranial fossa or internal auditory meatus)</li></ul>	Rare
Grey–white matter junction	Preserved	Destroyed

Intraventricular lesions*	
Tumour	**Typical site**
Colloid cyst	Foramen of Monro/third ventricle
Meningioma	Trigone of lateral ventricle
Choroid	Fourth ventricle
Ependymoma	Lateral ventricle (more common in children) and fourth ventricle
Neurocytoma	Lateral ventricles (involving septum pellucidum)
Metastases	Lateral ventricles, ependyma and choroid plexus

Primary cerebral tumours and age groups†	
Tumour	**Age group**
Brainstem glioma, optic nerve glioma	0–5
Medulloblastoma, cerebellar astrocytoma, papilloma choroid plexus, pinealoma, craniopharyngioma	5–15
Ependymoma	15–30
Glioma, meningioma, acoustic neuroma, pituitary tumour, hemangioblastoma	30–65
Meningioma, acoustic tumour, glioblastoma	65+

The 2007 WHO classification of tumours of the central nervous system (abridged)

TUMOURS OF NEUROEPITHELIAL TISSUE

Astrocytic tumours
Anaplastic astrocytoma
Diffuse astrocytoma
Glioblastoma
Gliomatosis cerebri
Pilocytic astrocytoma
Pleomorphic xanthoastrocytoma
Subependymal giant cell astrocytoma

Oligodendroglial tumours
Oligodendroglioma
Anaplastic oligodendroglioma

Oligoastrocytic tumours
Oligoastrocytoma
Anaplastic oligoastrocytoma

Ependymal tumours
Ependymoma
Subependymoma
Anaplastic ependymoma
Myxopapillary ependymoma

Choroid plexus tumours
Choroid plexus papilloma
Choroid plexus carcinoma

Other neuroepithelial tumours
Astroblastoma
Chordoid glioma of the third ventricle
Angiocentric glioma

Neuronal and mixed neuronal-glial tumours
Ganglioglioma and gangliocytoma
Desmoplastic infantile ganglioglioma
Dysembryoplastic neuroepithelial tumour
Central neurocytoma and extraventricular neurocytic tumours

Tumours of the pineal region
Pineoblastoma
Pineocytoma

Embryonal tumours
Medulloblastoma
CNS primitive neuroectodermal tumour
Atypical teratoid/rhabdoid tumour

TUMOURS OF CRANIAL AND PARASPINAL NERVES
Schwannoma (neurilemoma, neurinoma)
Neurofibroma
Perineurioma
Malignant peripheral nerve sheath tumour (MPNST)

TUMOURS OF THE MENINGES
Tumours of meningothelial cells
Meningioma

Mesenchymal tumours

Primary melanocytic lesions

Other neoplasms related to the meninges
Haemangioblastoma

LYMPHOMAS AND HAEMATOPOIETIC NEOPLASMS
Malignant lymphomas
Plasmacytoma
Granulocytic sarcoma

GERM CELL TUMOURS
Germinoma
Embryonal carcinoma
Yolk sac tumour
Choriocarcinoma
Teratoma
Mixed germ cell tumour

TUMOURS OF THE SELLAR REGION
Craniopharyngioma
Granular cell tumour
Pituicytoma
Spindle cell oncocytoma of the adenohypophysis

METASTATIC TUMOURS

Differentiating between an infarct and tumour ©12

	Tumour	Infarct
Grey matter changes	This is usually centred on the cerebral white matter and spares the overlying grey matter	This often simultaneously involves the cerebral cortex and juxtacortical white matter
Shape	Spherical or ovoid	Wedge or box shaped (with its base towards the brain surface)
Distribution	Not confined to a vascular territory	Confined to a vascular territory
Contrast enhancement	Gyriform enhancement is rare	Gyriform enhancement can be present

ASTROCYTOMA

DEFINITION

- A benign or malignant tumour arising from an astrocyte
- *Astrocyte:* a structural or supporting cell type within the brain
- This is the largest group of primary brain neoplasms (75% of all glial tumours)
- **Location:** supratentorial (50%) ▸ cerebellum (35%) ▸ brainstem (15%)

WHO classification (the majority will eventually progress to a more malignant type over time):

- *Grade I (benign pilocytic astrocytoma):* non-invasive ▸ occur mainly in young patients ▸ this is potentially resectable with a low proliferative potential (up to 40% of all paediatric intracranial tumours)
  - It characteristically occurs within the cerebellum in children ▸ it can also occur within the hypothalamus and optic nerves (optic nerve involvement is a feature of NF-1)
- *Grade II (diffuse astrocytoma):* an infiltrating (rather than destroying) low-grade tumour ▸ it results in a relatively mild neurological deficit and a generally good prognosis ▸ typically found in the cerebral hemisphere of young adults
- *Grade III (anaplastic astrocytoma):* although there is increased mitotic activity and anaplasia there is no necrosis
- *Grade IV (glioblastoma multiforme):* this is the commonest primary adult intracranial neoplasm ▸ 90% arise de novo ▸ 10% from lower grade astrocytoma transformation ▸ it is very malignant (with the worst prognosis) ▸ tumour necrosis is a hallmark
  - It occurs de novo or from a pre-existing lower-grade astrocytoma

RADIOLOGICAL FEATURES

Pilocytic astrocytoma

- **Cerebellar pilocytic astrocytoma:** this occurs equally within the vermis and cerebellar hemispheres and commonly presents with the effects of hydrocephalus ▸ can be mistaken for haemangioblastoma in adults

CT A well-circumscribed and encapsulated large mass ▸ predominantly cystic (70%) or solid (30%) ▸ an associated strongly enhancing mural nodule when cystic ▸ calcification is rare ▸ no adjacent oedema

- *Differential:* a medulloblastoma is a hyperdense solid lesion (NECT)

MRI Cystic component: T1WI: low SI ▸ T2WI: high SI ▸ T1WI + Gad: avid homogeneous enhancement of any solid component

- **Optic pathway pilocytic astrocytoma:** occurs anywhere along the optic tract (usually at the chiasm) ▸ hypothalamic or chiasmatic tumours may be more aggressive

CT An enlarged optic nerve (variable enhancement) ▸ often large and lobulated when at the chiasm and can extend into the hypothalamus ▸ haemorrhage and necrosis is uncommon

- No calcification (unlike an optic nerve sheath meningioma or craniopharyngioma)

MRI An expanded chiasm and hypothalamus ▸ T1WI: low SI ▸ T2WI: high SI

Diffuse astrocytoma This is less well defined than a pilocytic astrocytoma and with variable mass effect

CT An iso- or hypodense mass ▸ poor enhancement (there is an intact blood–brain barrier) ▸ calcification in 20%

MRI T1WI: low-to-intermediate SI ▸ T2WI/FLAIR: high SI ▸ T1WI + Gad: enhancement suggests progression to a higher histological grade

Anaplastic astrocytoma

CT More extensive infiltration of peritumoural tissues than with a grade II tumour (+ vasogenic oedema) ▸ ⅓ may be non-enhancing

Glioblastoma multiforme (GBM) Contrast enhancement and vasogenic oedema are much more extensive than with an anaplastic astrocytoma ▸ although tumours may appear well-defined they are always infiltrative (commonly extending along the white matter tracts)

MRI Solid ± central necrosis ± oedema ▸ T1WI/T2WI: heterogeneous SI appearances due to necrosis and haemorrhage ▸ T1WI + Gad: an irregularly thick enhancing peripheral 'ring' (active mitosis) ▸ a multicentric tumour with seeding via the CSF space (5%) ▸ a lower ADC than with a low-grade glioma

- *'Butterfly lesion':* tumour commonly crosses the midline via the corpus callosum (as can a CNS lymphoma)
- *Pseudoprogression:* due to an inflammatory reaction following chemoradiation (increased enhancement and oedema) ▸ spontaneous improvement
- *Pseudoresponse:* decreased enhancement and oedema without improved survival

PEARLS

Gliomatosis cerebri Diffuse infiltration of large areas of brain or spinal cord tissue by glial tumour cells with preservation of the underlying architecture (no definitive mass) ▸ it typically involves the hemispheric white matter ▸ it presents between the 2nd and 4th decades (M = F)

MRI A diffuse ill-defined 'mass-like' lesion with ventricular effacement ▸ T1WI: a homogeneous intermediate-to-low SI infiltrating mass ▸ T2WI/FLAIR: a homogeneous high SI infiltrating mass ▸ T1WI + Gad: no or minimal enhancement

- *Differential:* lymphomatosis cerebri ▸ viral encephalitis ▸ acute disseminated encephalomyelitis (ADEM) ▸ vasculitis

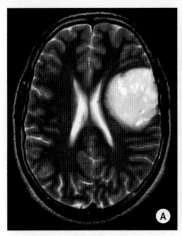
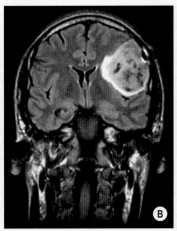
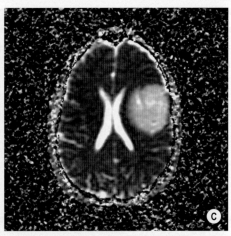

Low-grade glioma (WHO grade II astrocytoma). Axial T2W (A), FLAIR (B) images showing a left frontal hyperintense mass lesion with well-defined borders and small cystic areas. On the ADC map (C) the glioma is easily identified as an area of increased diffusivity compared to normal brain parenchyma.**

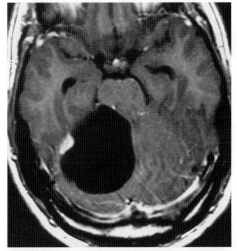

Cerebellar pilocytic astrocytoma. Axial T1W postgadolinium MRI. There is a cystic lesion in the cerebellum with a small, enhancing mural nodule but otherwise non-enhancing cyst wall. The fourth ventricle is compressed, causing hydrocephalus (note enlargement of the temporal horns). The differential diagnosis of this lesion is a cerebellar haemangioblastoma.**

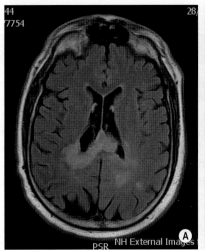
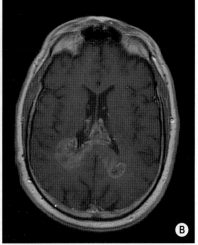

Glioblastoma. A 55-year-old patient with a 'butterfly' glioblastoma. The tumour appears hyperintense on FLAIR images (A) and infiltrates and thickens the splenium of the corpus callosum and surrounds the trigones of both lateral ventricles. On the post-contrast T1WI (B) the glioblastoma shows widespread inhomogeneous enhancement of the tumour.**

	Pilocytic astrocytoma	Diffuse astrocytoma	Anaplastic astrocytoma	Glioblastoma multiforme
Malignant potential	Benign	Low grade	High grade	Very malignant
Age (approximate)	Children	3rd or 4th decade	5th decade	6th decade
Location	Optic chiasm or hypothalamus > cerebellum > brainstem*	Hemispheres (cortex + white matter)	Hemispheres (cortex + white matter)	Hemispheres (cortex + white matter)
Enhancement	Mild	Mild	Moderate (ring)	Intense
Vasogenic oedema	Minimal	Minimal	Moderate	Significant
Calcification	Common	Up to 20%	Occasional	Rare

*It is typically cystic with a mural nodule and located within the posterior fossa – it tends to be solid or lobulated when seen elsewhere.

OLIGODENDROGLIOMA

DEFINITION

- A relatively benign slow-growing neoplasm arising from the oligodendrocyte
  - *Oligodendrocyte:* a cell that insulates the central nervous system axons and which is equivalent to a Schwann cell within the peripheral nervous system
- It is classified as a WHO grade II (well-differentiated, low-grade) or WHO grade III (anaplastic high-grade) tumour ▶ it is chemosensitive
- It occurs predominantly in adults (during the 4th decade) and accounts for 5–10% of all intracranial neoplasms

RADIOLOGICAL FEATURES

Location It is a diffusely infiltrating neoplasm found almost exclusively within the cerebral hemispheres and typically involving the subcortical white matter and cortex (85% are seen within the frontal lobes)

- It is well circumscribed, unencapsulated and less infiltrative than a diffuse astrocytoma ▶ it may erode the calvarium

CT A hypodense lesion which may involve the cortex (with associated cortical thickening) ▶ cysts or haemorrhage can be seen in 20% but necrosis and oedema is rare

- 50% of tumours will demonstrate variable (and often heterogeneous) contrast enhancement – this is not a reliable indicator of tumour grade (unlike for an astrocytoma)
- Intratumoral haemorrhage
- Calcification is present in up to 90% of cases – this is central, peripheral or gyriform in nature

MRI T1WI: heterogeneous low-to-intermediate SI ▶ T2WI/FLAIR: heterogeneous high SI ▶ T1WI + Gad: variable and often heterogeneous

EPENDYMOMA

DEFINITION

- A low-grade tumour arising from the ependyma ▶ usually intraventricular – extraventricular rests of ependymal cells may give rise to hemisphere tumours
  - *Ependyma:* this forms the epithelial lining of the ventricular system, cerebral hemispheres, brainstem and cerebellum, central canal of the spinal cord and tip of the filum terminale
- It accounts for 5% of all intracranial tumours (a higher incidence is seen in the paediatric population)

Location 65% are infratentorial (most commonly arising from the *floor* of the 4th ventricle) ▶ 25% are supratentorial (arising from white matter ependymal cells) ▶ 10% arise within the spinal cord

  - *Supratentorial tumours:* these are commonly extraventricular (involving the periventricular white matter) ▶ they predominantly affect young adults
  - *Infratentorial tumours:* these are commonly intraventricular (affecting the 4th ventricle) ▶ there are two age peaks at 5 and 35 years of age
  - Uncommonly disseminates by leptomeningeal spread

RADIOLOGICAL FEATURES

CT An isodense-to-hyperdense, well-demarcated, lobulated mass lesion which takes on the shape of the 4th ventricle (originating from the roof or floor) and frequently extends through the foramina of Magendie and Luschka to seed via the subarachnoid space (a 'plastic' ependymoma) ▶ calcification is seen in >50% of cases and cystic elements can also be demonstrated ▶ there can be an associated obstructive hydrocephalus

- *Cerebral hemisphere ependymoma:* this tends to arise adjacent to the ventricular system (characteristically adjacent to the trigone of the lateral ventricle) and can resemble an astrocytoma ▶ it is more frequently calcified or cystic than an infratentorial tumour

MRI There are mixed signal intensities ▶ T1WI: normal-to-low SI ▶ T2WI: predominantly high SI ▶ T1WI + Gad: mild-to-moderate enhancement (which is often heterogeneous)

PEARLS

Treatment

- Surgical resection (although the tendency of posterior fossa tumours to infiltrate around the cranial nerves makes total resection difficult with associated high recurrence rates)

Subependymoma

- A variant containing both ependymal and astrocyte cells ▶ it occurs mainly in elderly males and presents as an intraventricular mass in the lateral or 4th ventricle ▶ it is relatively benign and does not disseminate

Differentiating features of a medulloblastoma

- An important differential of a posterior fossa ependymoma
- It calcifies less frequently ▶ it arises from the *roof* of the 4th ventricle ▶ it demonstrates a rounded shape compared with an ependymoma (that moulds to the ventricular margins)

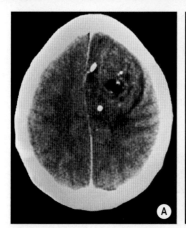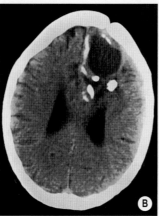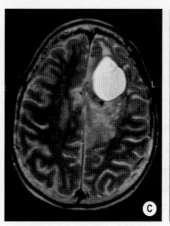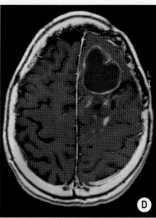

Oligodendroglioma. CECT (A) shows a large left frontal tumour that involves the cortex. It is predominantly solid with irregular enhancement, but there are also cysts and coarse calcification. Follow-up after 2 years with CT (B), T2WI (C) and T1WI + Gad (D) shows more extensive cyst formation and calcification (C). Note the left frontal craniotomy.*

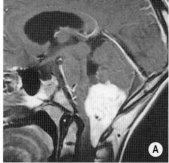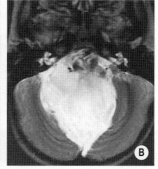

A large avidly enhancing ependymoma is shown on the sagittal T1WI + Gad (A) occupying the lower part of the 4th ventricle, compressing the medulla and extending through the foramen of Magendie into the upper cervical canal. The axial T2WI (B) shows that the mass is high SI and also extends out through the lateral recesses into the cerebellopontine angles, particularly on the right.†

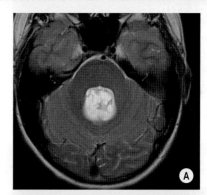
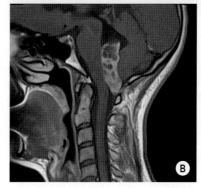

Ependymoma of the fourth ventricle. (A) The axial T2WI demonstrates a relatively well-circumscribed hyperintense partially solid and cystic mass expanding the fourth ventricle. (B) Sagittal post-contrast T1WI shows a heterogeneously enhancing mass expanding the inferior part of the fourth ventricle and extending through the foramen of Magendie. There is dilatation of the ventricular system in keeping with obstructive hydrocephalus.**

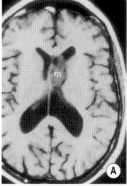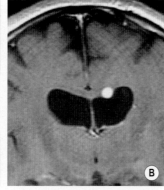

Supratentorial subependymoma. (A) A mass (m) is attached to the septum pellucidum and enlarges the left frontal horn. (B) A different enhancing lesion, on the outer surface of the ventricle.+

723

CEREBELLAR HAEMANGIOBLASTOMA

DEFINITION

- A benign tumour of endothelial origin that is composed of thin-walled blood vessels ▶ it is predominantly found within the posterior fossa (supratentorial lesions are rare) and is the commonest primary intra-axial and infratentorial adult tumour
- 10% of adult infratentorial masses are haemangioblastomas

CLINICAL PRESENTATION

- It usually presents in young adults (M>F)
- Common symptoms include headache, ataxia, nausea, vomiting and vertigo
- 20% are associated with von Hippel–Lindau (VHL) disease – these generally present at an earlier age
- Multiple haemangioblastomas are only seen with von Hippel–Lindau disease ▶ it is an unusual paediatric tumour unless in the context of von Hippel–Lindau disease

RADIOLOGICAL FEATURES

CT/MRI It usually appears as a cystic mass with an intensely enhancing mural nodule (± haemorrhage) ▶ there is little surrounding oedema ▶ cyst wall enhancement indicates tumour extension (as for a pilocytic astrocytoma)

- It may only consist of strongly enhancing solid components
- Multiple signal voids may be seen with MRI (as the lesion is highly vascular)

Angiography A vascular nodule within an avascular mass ▶ there may be draining veins present

Differentiating between a haemangioblastoma and a juvenile pilocytic astrocytoma		
	Haemangioblastoma	**Juvenile pilocytic astrocytoma**
Age	30–40 years	5–15 years
Pial attachment	Yes	No
A tiny nodule with a huge cystic component	More likely	Less likely
Arteriogram	Hypervascular nodule	Hypovascular nodule
Multiplicity and association with VHL disease	More likely	Less likely

BRAINSTEM GLIOMA

DEFINITION

- This accounts for up to 30% of all paediatric infratentorial tumours (they may occur in adults) ▶ 80% of tumours are high grade, but symptoms occur late as the tumour infiltrates rather than destroys adjacent tissues (hydrocephalus is a late feature)
  - Pons > midbrain > medulla

Diffuse type

- This is the most common pontine lesion and has a poor prognosis

CT/MRI It is an expansile and poorly defined pontine lesion (± haemorrhage) ▶ there is poor enhancement ▶ it can encase the basilar artery

Focal type

- This is more common than diffuse disease within the midbrain and medulla

CT/MRI This has similar imaging features to a pilocytic astrocytoma seen elsewhere

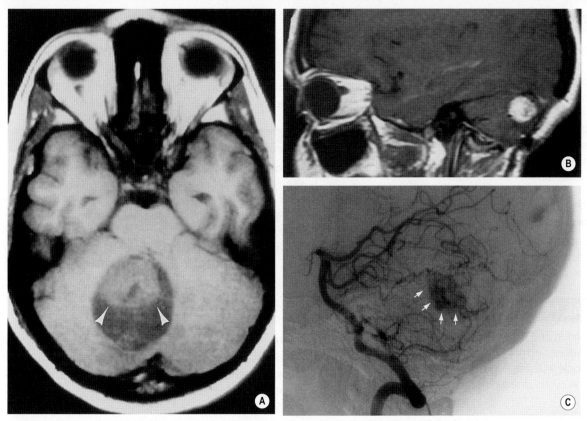

Haemangioblastoma of the cerebellum. (A) T1WI demonstrating a haemangioblastoma with both a cyst and mural nodule (arrowheads). (B) T1WI + Gad demonstrates an enhancing solid haemangioblastoma with small flow voids along its circumference. (C) A vertebral artery angiogram demonstrates a tumour stain (arrows) with the vascular supply from the posterior inferior cerebellar artery and branches of the superior cerebellar artery.[+]

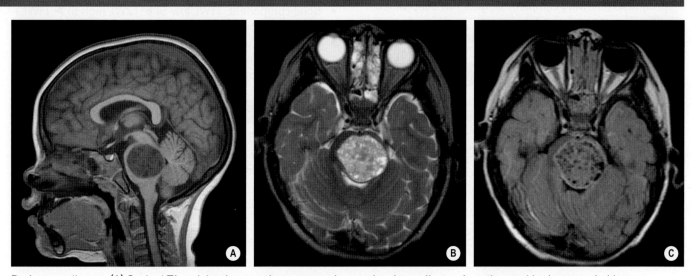

Brainstem gliomas. (A) Sagittal T1-weighted magnetic resonance image showing well-marginated central brainstem primitive neuroectodermal tumours. (B) Axial T2-weighted image showing heterogeneous signal of tumour. (C) Axial fluid-attenuated inversion recovery (FLAIR) image showing multiple small central cysts. ©24

MEDULLOBLASTOMA

DEFINITION

- This is an aggressive tumour, accounting for 30-40% of all posterior fossa tumours ▶ it is also known as the PNET of the posterior fossa
- It classically arises from the *roof* of the 4th ventricle and is therefore usually a midline cerebellar mass (a lateral cerebellar location is more common in older children and adults) ▶ subsequent hydrocephalus is common ▶ occasionally intracranial or intraspinal leptomeningeal disease at presentation

CLINICAL PRESENTATION

- There is a peak age of presentation at 7 years (M>F) ▶ a 2nd peak is seen in young adults who present with a 'desmoplastic' and less aggressive form

RADIOLOGICAL FEATURES

NECT A well-defined and hyperdense (due to its high cellular density) midline vermian mass abutting the roof of the 4th ventricle ▶ there is perilesional oedema (± hydrocephalus) ▶ cystic change, haemorrhage and calcification are frequently seen ▶ brainstem usually displaced anteriorly rather than directly invaded

MRI T2WI: intermediate-to-low SI ▶ T1WI + Gad: variable patchy enhancement ▶ DWI: restricted diffusion

MRS There is a reduced N-acetylaspartate (NAA) peak with an increased choline-to-creatine ratio

PEARLS

- Intracranial and intraspinal subarachnoid dissemination is seen in $\frac{1}{3}$ of patients at presentation ▶ this can appear as:
  - Irregular, and nodular leptomeningeal enhancement
  - A communicating hydrocephalus
  - Nodularity and clumping of the nerve roots
  - Pial 'drop' metastases along the spinal cord surface

Associations

- Li–Fraumeni, Gorlin's, basal cell naevus, Turcot and Cowden syndromes

Treatment

- Surgical resection + adjuvant radiotherapy (only for those patients who are >3 years old due to the susceptibility of the infant brain)

CEREBELLAR LOW-GRADE ASTROCYTOMA

DEFINITION

- A benign tumour that is associated with an excellent prognosis following complete surgical removal (with a >90% 5-year survival rate)
- Usually a pilocytic tumour (WHO grade 1)

RADIOLOGICAL FEATURES

- The typical cerebellar astrocytoma seen in the paediatric age group is cystic (up to 80%), with tumours more likely to be solid with increasing age
- Well-circumscribed, cerebellar vermian or hemispheric tumour

MRI

- A mural enhancing nodule may be present, mimicking the appearances of a haemangioblastoma
- Solid component: T1WI: low SI ▶ T2WI: high SI ▶ T1WI + Gad: avid enhancement
- They may occasionally present with diffuse nodular enhancement of the leptomeninges (indicating intracranial or intraspinal pial dissemination)

PEARL

- Although 60% of pilocytic astrocytomas occur within the posterior fossa, they can also occur within the optic pathways and hypothalamus

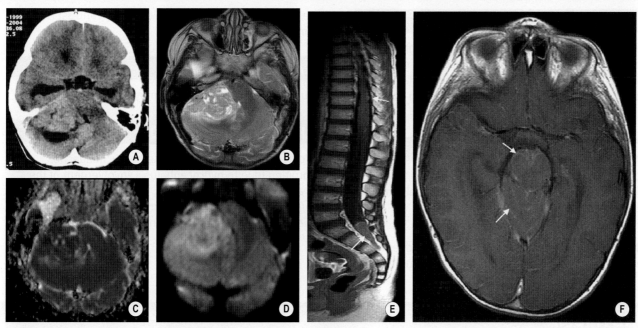

Medulloblastoma. (A) CT and (B–D) axial T2, ADC, and diffusion MRI show a mixed solid and cystic mass within the right cerebellopontine angle encroaching on the pons and fourth ventricle and causing hydrocephalus. The solid component is hyperdense on CT, hypointense on the T2WI and demonstrates restricted diffusion in keeping with a cellular tumour. It does demonstrate some less typical features, such as lateral site (more usually seen in older patients and associated with the desmoplastic variant) and cystic components. (E) There is nodular enhancement over the conus medullaris and a mass within the thecal sac. (F) In addition to pial enhancement over the midbrain and cerebellar folia (arrows), this is indicative of metastatic disease.*

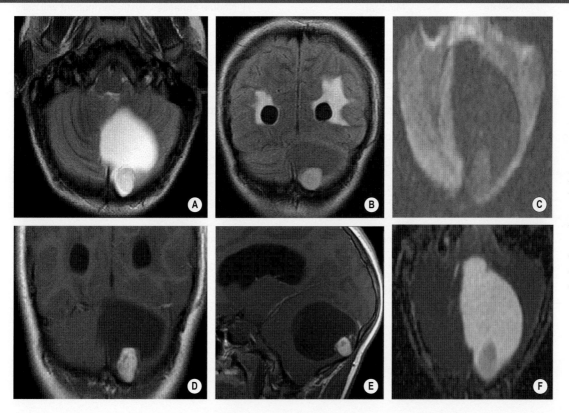

Cerebellar pilocytic astrocytoma. Axial T2W, coronal FLAIR, coronal and sagittal T1W-enhanced MRI (A,B,D,E) show a left cerebellar hemispheric tumour with a large cystic component and solid homogeneously enhancing component which is bright on T2WI. The solid component is not restricted on the diffusion-weighted image (C) and ADC map (F) and there is free diffusion in the cystic component.*

ATYPICAL TERATOID/RHABDOID TUMOURS

DEFINITION

- An unusual malignant tumour with a poor prognosis ▶ it is often large at the time of presentation and occurs in slightly younger children than with a medulloblastoma (typically <2 years of age) ▶ it may also be supratentorial (40% of cases)

RADIOLOGICAL FEATURES

- Imaging features are indistinguishable from a medulloblastoma or primitive neuroectodermal tumour (PNET)

NECT A hyperdense lesion

CT/MRI There is a heterogeneous appearance due to haemorrhage, necrosis, calcification or cyst formation ▶ there is patchy enhancement following IV contrast medium administration

PEARL

- Subarachnoid dissemination may occur

CLINICAL PRESENTATION

- 'Posterior fossa' syndrome – lethargy, headache, vomiting (due to hydrocephalus ± involvement of the brainstem emetic centre)
- *Infants:* macrocephaly and 'sunsetting' eyes
- *Older children and adults:* truncal and gait ataxia

EPENDYMOMA

- See Section 7, Gliomas

Distinguishing among a posterior fossa medulloblastoma, ependymoma and astrocytoma			
Feature	Medulloblastoma	Ependymoma	Astrocytoma
NECT	Hyperdense	Isodense	Hypodense
Enhancement	Moderate	Minimal	Nodule enhances, cystic component will not
Calcification	Uncommon	Common	Uncommon
Site of origin	Vermis	4th ventricle ependyma	Hemisphere
T2WI	Intermediate SI	Intermediate SI	High SI
Site	Midline	Midline	Eccentric
Subarachnoid seeding	Common	Uncommon	Rare
Age (years)	5–12	2–10	10–20
Foraminal spread	No	Yes (Luschka and Magendie)	No
Haemorrhage	Rare	10%	Rare
NAA (MRS)	Low	Intermediate	Intermediate
Lactate (MRS)	Absent	Often present	Often present
Choline (MRS)	High	Less elevated	High

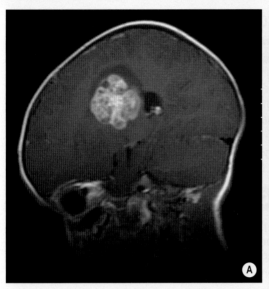

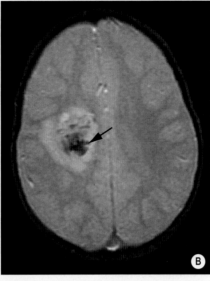

Atypical teratoid/rhabdoid tumor. (A) Sagittal T1-weighted image after gadolinium administration shows heterogeneously enhancing solid and cystic right frontal mass with surrounding edema. (B) Axial gradient-echo image shows haemosiderin (arrow) from punctate tumoural hemorrhage. ©24

Paediatric infratentorial tumours	Adult infratentorial tumours
Juvenile pilocytic low-grade cerebellar astrocytoma: the most common paediatric infratentorial primary tumour **Medulloblastoma:** accounting for >⅓ of paediatric posterior fossa neoplasms **Brainstem glioma:** this accounts for 20% of all paediatric posterior fossa masses **Ependymoma:** this accounts for 10% of all paediatric posterior fossa tumours **Other posterior fossa tumours:** • extra-axial tumours (e.g. dermoid and epidermoid cysts, schwannoma, neurofibroma and meningioma) • skull base lesions (e.g. Langerhans' cell histiocytosis, Ewing's sarcoma and glomus tumours)	**Metastases:** the most common adult infratentorial neoplasm **Haemangioblastoma:** the most common primary adult infratentorial tumour **Astrocytic tumour:** these are usually supratentorial but can occur within the posterior fossa **Medulloblastoma:** although typically a paediatric tumour, 20% can occur in adults **Ependymal tumour:** e.g. a subependymoma **Neuronal and mixed neuronal/glial tumours**

Paediatric supratentorial intra-axial tumours	Adult supratentorial intra-axial tumours*
Pleomorphic xanthoastrocytoma Hemispheric astrocytoma Embryonal tumours: • *a supratentorial primitive neuroectodermal tumour (PNET)* Giant cell subependymal astrocytoma (tuberous sclerosis) Neuronal and mixed neuronal/glial tumours: • *ganglioglioma ▶ gangliocytoma ▶ desmoplastic infantile ganglioglioma ▶ dysembryoplastic neuroepithelial tumour (DNET)* Germ cell tumours	Metastases Astrocytomas: • *ranging from a circumscribed astrocytoma through to a glioblastoma multiforme* Oligodendroglioma Lymphoma Giant cell subependymal astrocytoma (tuberous sclerosis) Neuronal and mixed neuronal/glial tumours: • *e.g. a central neurocytoma* Gliomatosis cerebri
*Multiple adult supratentorial masses are usually metastases – a single mass is equally likely to be a metastasis or an astrocytoma (as metastases are usually multiple and an astrocytoma is the most common single primary tumour)	

SUPRATENTORIAL TUMOURS

PLEOMORPHIC XANTHOASTROCYTOMA

DEFINITION

- An uncommon astrocytoma of children and young adults that does not demonstrate any infiltrative features
- It arises from the subpial astrocytes and is therefore located near the cerebral hemispheric surface

CLINICAL PRESENTATION

- As it is commonly seen within the temporal lobe, it often presents with epilepsy

RADIOLOGICAL FEATURES

- It may be radiologically indistinguishable from a ganglioglioma or other glioneuronal tumour subtypes

CT/MRI Frequently cystic with a mural nodule (± scalloping of the adjacent skull vault due to its slow growth) ▶ usually little associated oedema ▶ haemorrhage or calcification is uncommon ▶ it may enhance strongly

EMBRYONAL TUMOURS

DEFINITION

- This is a high-grade (WHO grade IV) tumour of neuroectodermal origin – also known as a primitive neuroectodermal tumour (PNET)
- It includes supratentorial PNETs (cerebral neuroblastoma) and infratentorial PNETs of the posterior fossa (medulloblastoma).

RADIOLOGICAL FEATURES

Supratentorial PNET

- This has a poor prognosis with a high rate of recurrence and subarachnoid seeding ▶ 80% of patients present at <10 years old (the younger the age at presentation the worse the prognosis)
  - *Sites:* cerebral hemisphere > suprasellar or periventricular regions

NECT A large (3–10 cm) hyperdense mass with a heterogeneous appearance (cysts, calcification and haemorrhage)

CECT Heterogeneous enhancement

Other tumour types

- Medulloepithelioma and ependymoblastoma – both of these are WHO grade IV tumours occurring in infants
  - Usually supratentorial tumours ▶ can contain cysts, haemorrhage, necrosis and calcification

GANGLIOGLIOMA/GANGLIOCYTOMA

DEFINITION

- A slow-growing low-grade tumour usually located within the temporal lobe (F>M) ▶ it can cause epilepsy in young adults
- *Ganglioglioma:* a mixture of neural and glial elements ▶ there is a potential for malignant change
- *Gangliocytoma:* neuronal elements only ▶ there is no potential for malignant change

RADIOLOGICAL FEATURES

CT/MR A peripherally located mixed solid or cystic lesion that commonly calcifies ▶ associated bone remodelling and mild associated oedema ▶ variable and peripheral enhancement

DESMOPLASTIC INFANTILE GANGLIOGLIOMA (DIG)

DEFINITION

- A variant of a ganglioglioma that usually occurs within the 1st 2 years of life ▶ associated with a good prognosis

RADIOLOGICAL FEATURES

CT/MRI A predilection for the frontal and parietal lobes ▶ the tumour has a meningeal base

- Cyst formation is the rule ▶ peripheral rim or nodular enhancement is present (± a calcified rim)

DYSEMBRYOPLASTIC NEUROEPITHELIAL TUMOUR (DNET)

DEFINITION

- A highly polymorphic WHO grade I tumour arising during embryogenesis
- Preferentially located within the supratentorial cortex (and commonly the temporal lobe)

CLINICAL PRESENTATION

- It frequently manifests through intractable complex partial seizures in children or young adults

RADIOLOGICAL FEATURES

CT/MRI A focal intracortical mass superimposed upon a background of cortical dysplasia ▶ it can demonstrate a 'bubbly' appearance due to multiple small intratumoural cysts ▶ calcification (25%) ▶ no associated oedema or mass effect

NECT A hypodense mass ▶ scalloping of the overlying bone in 50% of cases (due to extremely slow tumour growth)

T1WI low SI ▶ T2WI: high SI ▶ T1WI + Gad: enhancement is uncommon (if present it is faint or patchy)

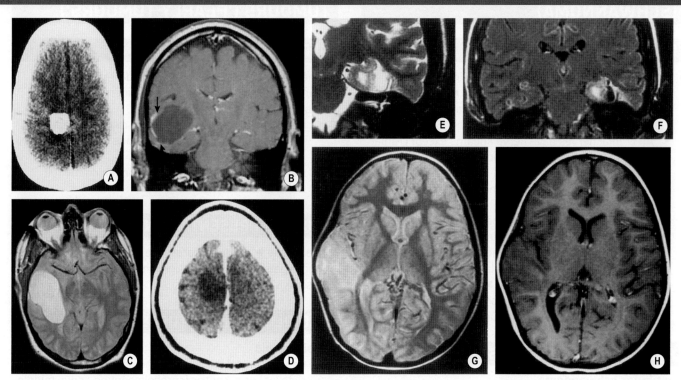

Ganglioglioma. (A) NECT shows a well-defined calcified mass in the right hemisphere. (B) T1WI + Gad shows a cystic mass with a small rim of enhancement (arrows). (C) PDWI. The lesion is well defined without white matter oedema. (D) NECT demonstrating a low-density lesion. (E) T2WI showing a cystic/solid left temporal lobe mass. (F) FLAIR confirms hippocampal infiltration. (G) T2WI demonstrating temporal bone remodelling. (H) No enhancement characterized this mass.[+]

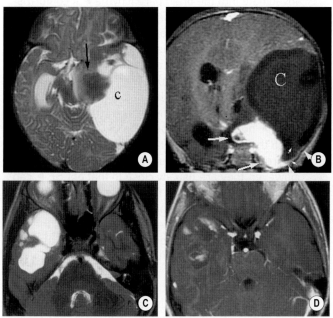

DIG. (A) This large cystic mass (c) in the frontotemporal region has a solid component (arrows) more medially seen as intermediate signal on the T2WI. (B) Typical of a DIG, there is a peripheral solidly enhancing component to the mass which has a dural attachment (arrows) and a huge cyst C. (C) T2WI showing a multifocal abnormality with involvement of cortex subcortical regions (small arrows) and white matter. (D) The enhancement is faint and peripheral.[+]

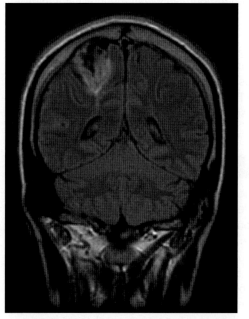

Coronal FLAIR of a dysembryoplastic neuroepithelial tumour (DNET) showing a right parietal, pyramidal-shaped, predominantly cortically based, tumour. It has peripheral cystic areas and a linear area of hyperintensity extends towards the right lateral ventricle.*

CRANIAL NERVE SHEATH TUMOURS (SCHWANNOMA)

DEFINITION

- A benign slow-growing neoplasm arising from the Schwann cells of the nerve sheath ▶ it arises eccentrically from the sheath and compresses the nerve rather than invading it
  - All cranial nerves have nerve sheaths except cranial nerves I (olfactory) and II (optic) – these are white matter tracts of the cerebrum
  - It accounts for 6–8% of all primary intracranial tumours
- Schwannomas usually involve the sensory nerves – pure motor cranial nerves are rarely involved
  - *Acoustic neuroma*: a schwannoma usually involving the superior vestibular division of the vestibulocochlear (VIII) nerve ▶ the trigeminal, glossopharyngeal and lower cranial nerves are affected with decreasing frequency

RADIOLOGICAL FEATURES

Vestibular schwannoma

- **MRI**: this is much more sensitive than CT ▶ high resolution T2W imaging of the posterior fossa can demonstrate focal thickening of the 7th and 8th nerves ▶ tumour forms an acute angle with the petrous bone ▶ if large enough tumour can widen the internal auditory meatus:
  - *'Ice cream cone' appearance*: IAM extension represents the cone with the main tumour mass representing the ice cream scoop
  - T1WI: an iso- or hypointense mass ▶ T2WI: high SI mass ▶ T1WI+Gad: there is marked enhancement (which is solid in $\frac{2}{3}$, and ring-like or heterogeneous in $\frac{1}{3}$)

PEARLS

- Schwannomas account for >80% of cerebellopontine lesions (bilateral vestibular schwannomas are pathognomonic for NF2) ▶ the differential includes:
  - *Meningioma* (10% of CP angle tumours): this usually forms an *obtuse* angle with the petrous bone ▶ it may also extend into the internal auditory meatus
    - NB: acoustic schwannomas may also demonstrate the 'dural tail' sign
  - *Epidermoid* (5% of CP angle tumours): there is no enhancement ▶ they tend to 'creep' around the brainstem with a very different morphological appearance to either a meningioma or schwannoma
- **Neurofibroma**: a benign tumour derived from Schwann cells and fibroblasts ▶ it usually involves cutaneous or spinal nerves (and is associated with NF1)

EPIDERMOID AND DERMOID TUMOURS ('PEARLY TUMOURS')

DEFINITION

- These result from inclusion of ectodermal elements during neural tube closure ▶ an epidermoid is much more common than a dermoid
  - *Epidermoid*: tumours with a thin capsule of epidermis – the desquamated epithelial debris gives rise to their 'pearly' sheen
  - *Dermoid*: tumours with a wall containing the full width of the dermis

CLINICAL PRESENTATION

- Headache ▶ seizure ▶ pressure effects (e.g. cranial nerve palsies, cerebellar signs, hypopituitarism, diabetes insipidus, visual symptoms)

RADIOLOGICAL FEATURES

- **Epidermoid**
  - Can be central (chiasmatic and quadrigeminal plate cisterns) or eccentric (cerebellopontine angle, middle cranial fossa, Sylvian fissure)
  - This grows slowly from birth and can expand its occupying cistern and distort the adjacent neural structures (e.g. the pons and medulla) ▶ can invaginate into the brain parenchyma ▶ it conforms to the shape of the adjacent subarachnoid space ▶ it can infiltrate widely around vessels and nerves (an arachnoid cyst will displace rather than engulf adjacent structures) ▶ it grows slowly (accumulating desquamated epithelium)
  - **CT**: well-circumscribed, lobulated, non-enhancing, homogeneously hypodense lesion (similar density to CSF) ▶ no surrounding oedema
  - **MRI**: the signal characteristics usually depend upon the relative proportions of keratin and cholesterol – however, they are usually close to that of CSF ▶ can be difficult to distinguish from other cystic lesions (e.g. arachnoid cyst, which tends to have better defined margins and causes bone thinning) ▶ DWI is the most helpful sequence for diagnosing epidermoid tumours (appearing bright on DWI, cf. dark with arachnoid cysts)
- **Dermoid**
  - The wall may contain hair, sebaceous glands and an outer layer of connective tissue ▶ there may be an associated occipital bone defect
  - Often asymptomatic ▶ can rupture and release contents into the subarachnoid space with fatty globules within the basal cisterns or ventricles (aseptic meningitis)
  - **MRI**: heterogenous signal characteristics
  - **Differential**: arachnoid cyst

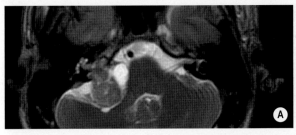
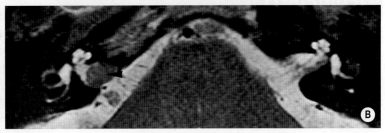

(A) Cystic vestibular schwannoma. T2WI reveals a large right cerebellopontine angle tumour with a medial cystic component. The mass extends into and expands the internal auditory meatus and distorts the right middle cerebellar peduncle. (B) Vestibular schwannoma. Axial T2WI. There is a small soft tissue mass (arrowhead) in the right internal auditory meatus.*

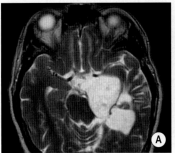
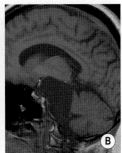

Epidermoid tumour. Axial T2WI (A) and sagittal T1WI + Gad (B) shows a large non-enhancing lesion of similar signal intensity to CSF, which occupies the chiasmatic and ambient cisterns, and distorts the medial aspect of the left temporal lobe.*

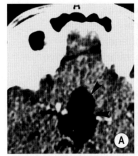
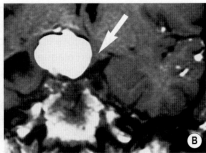

Suprasellar dermoid tumours. In this CT (A) there is a midline, fat density tumour (arrowheads) in the suprasellar region. (B) Coronal T1W I of a different patient with a ruptured dermoid tumour. There is a lobulated high SI mass in the chiasmatic cistern compressing and displacing the optic chiasm to the left (arrow). Fat globules are seen as high SI foci in the left sylvian fissure.*

	Epidermoid	Dermoid	Arachnoid
Composition	A thin capsule of epidermis containing epithelial debris and cholesterol	It contains all skin elements (including hair and fat)	An intra-arachnoid sac filled with CSF ▶ it does not connect with the ventricular system
Location	Eccentric (commonly the cerebellopontine angle, middle cranial fossa or sylvian fissure)*	Midline (commonly the posterior fossa within the 4th ventricle or the spinal canal)	Middle cranial fossa (50%) ▶ cerebellopontine angle (10%) ▶ suprasellar region (10%)
Presentation	Adults	Children	Children (75%)**
CT	Low attenuation (fat content) or similar attenuation to CSF	Low attenuation (fat content)	Identical attenuation to CSF ▶ hyperattenuating if there is haemorrhage (rare)
MR	Similar signal characteristics as CSF$^\alpha$	The fat content leads to high signal intensity (T1WI)	Identical signal characteristics to CSF$^\alpha$
Enhancement	Occasionally peripheral	None	None
Calcification	Unusual	More commonly seen (arc-like type, similar to that seen in aneurysms)	None
Rupture	Rare	It may rupture, releasing fat globules that can float within the CSF space (a chemical meningitis)	No

* Can also be within the midline (e.g. chiasmatic and quadrigeminal plate cisterns)
$^\alpha$ DWI allows differentiation of an epidermoid from an arachnoid cyst: restricted diffusion within an epidermoid generates high SI (free diffusion within an arachnoid cyst leads to low SI)
** Often asymptomatic

MENINGIOMA

Definition

- A tumour originating from arachnoid cell rests (which are related to the dura mater arachnoid granulations)
  - *WHO grade I:* the majority (90%) and representing a typical 'benign' tumour
  - *WHO grade II:* demonstrating atypical features (e.g. increased mitotic activity and necrosis)
  - *WHO grade III:* an anaplastic (malignant) tumour
- The commonest non-glial intracranial neoplasm (20% of all primary intracranial tumours) ▶ a peak prevalence during the 5ᵗʰ and 6ᵗʰ decades (F>M)
- *90% are supratentorial* and arise from the:
  - Parasagittal region (falx) > cerebral convexities (adjacent to the suture lines) > sphenoid ridge (commonly the 'en plaque' type) > olfactory groove > tentorium > optic nerve sheath (commonly seen in adult females)
- *Infratentorial meningiomas:* these are most frequently located on the posterior surface of the petrous bones or clivus and can mimic an acoustic neuroma
  - Bone sclerosis is in favour of a meningioma, whereas enlargement of the internal auditory meatus is in favour of an acoustic neuroma

Radiological features

- There are two common types: a spherical well-circumscribed mass or a flat, infiltrating ('en plaque') lesion

Angiography Occasionally performed for preoperative blood supply assessment (± preoperative embolization)
- *Cardinal findings:* a meningeal blood vessel supply ▶ a 'spokewheel' appearance ▶ a dense, homogeneous and persistent blush

CT A hyperdense extra-axial mass (60%) ± calcification (20%) ▶ intense and uniform enhancement ▶ bone hyperostosis indicates the site of meningeal attachment (and is particularly common when the skull base or anterior cranial fossa is involved)

MR 'capping cysts' of similar SI to CSF ▶ T1WI and T2WI: the mass is frequently isointense to the cerebral cortex and therefore requires IV contrast medium for evaluation ▶ T1WI + Gad: vivid and homogeneous enhancement (except for the uncommon cystic or very densely calcified tumours) ▶ MRS: alanine peak (characteristic) but seen in <50% of cases ▶ PWI: elevated rCBV (cf. lower rCBV in dural metastases)
- *Vasogenic oedema:* this is frequently seen – the extent does not correlate with tumour size
- *'Dural tail sign':* a linear, contrast-enhancing 'dural tail' extending from the tumour along the dura mater
  - This can also be seen with a schwannoma or a metastasis

PET High uptake of ⁶⁸Ga-DOTATOC

Pearls

- Multiple meningiomas and cranial nerve tumours are found in neurofibromatosis type 2 ▶ meningiomas are uncommonly seen in children and their presence suggests NF-2
- Meningiomas abutting the superior sagittal or transverse sinuses can compress or invade these venous structures

CHORDOMA

Definition

- This originates from malignant transformation of notochordal cells – the most frequent location is at the clivus, followed by the basiocciput and petrous apex ▶ it can also be seen within the sacrum
- A slow-growing, locally invasive lesion which destroys adjacent bone ▶ uncommonly metastasize ▶ it presents with pain (± lower cranial nerve palsies) and is rarely seen in children
- Partial encasement or displacement of intracranial vessels is common but arterial narrowing or stenoses are rare

Radiological features

CT A midline lobulated mass with associated bone destruction and calcification

MR Mixed and heterogeneous SI (low SI tumour will replace the normal high SI of the adjacent bone marrow) ▶ T1WI: intermediate to low SI ▶ T2WI: very high SI ▶ it may have a 'soap-bubble' appearance (septae of low SI) ▶ there is often variable but marked enhancement of the solid components
- T1WI (fat suppressed): this is particularly good for distinguishing pathological enhancement from the high SI of adjacent clival fat

GLOMUS JUGULARE TUMOUR (CHEMODECTOMA)

Definition

- This arises from paraganglion cells (chemo- and baroreceptor precursors) ▶ it is most commonly seen at the jugular bulb

Clinical presentation

- Pulsatile tinnitus ▶ deafness ▶ vertigo ▶ lower cranial nerve palsies ▶ It frequently obstructs and causes thrombosis of the internal jugular vein

Radiological features

CT Associated moth-eaten bone destruction ▶ enlargement of the pars vasorum of the jugular foramen

MRI T1WI: isointense to brain ▶ T2WI: high SI and areas of flow void corresponding to dilated vessels (a 'salt and pepper' appearance) ▶ T1WI + Gad: intense enhancement

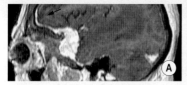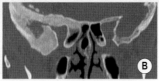

Sphenoid wing meningioma. (A) Sagittal T1WI + Gad. The dural tail arising from the enhancing sphenoid meningioma can clearly be seen (arrow). (B) Coronal NECT. In addition, there is marked associated hyperostosis of the sphenoid bone.

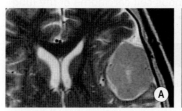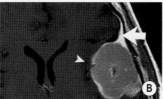

Meningioma. Axial T2W (A), gadolinium-enhanced T1W (B). A grey-matter isointense mass deeply indents the left cerebral convexity (A). Its broad dural base, the surrounding displaced cerebral sulci and the small pial vessel between the tumour and the brain surface (arrowhead) are all features of an extra-axial lesion. The tumour enhances and there is a 'dural tail' (arrow) (B).*

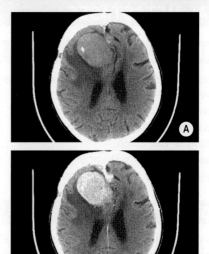

Falcine meningioma. (A) NECT demonstrating a hyperdense spherical midline mass, with associated oedema and tumoural calcification. (B) Following contrast medium administration, there is intense enhancement.

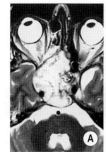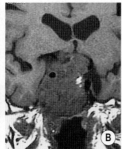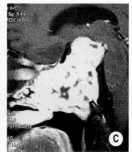

Clivus chordoma. Axial T2WI (A), coronal T1WI (B) and sagittal T1WI + Gad (C). A large heterogeneous SI mass, with irregular enhancement, has destroyed the clivus and extends superiorly compressing the midbrain and hypothalamus. It invades the right cavernous sinus, encasing the internal carotid artery, and extends into the nasopharyngeal soft tissues, posterior ethmoid air cells, optic canals and pontine cistern.*

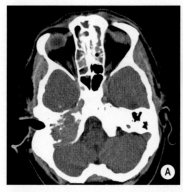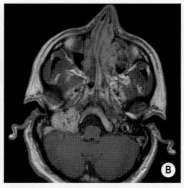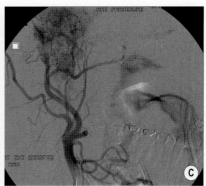

Glomus jugulare tumour. An axial CT (A) demonstrates expansion of the right jugular foramen and bone destruction in the adjacent petrous bone by a mass that is markedly enhancing on axial T1WI + Gad (B). The mass contains flow voids, corresponding to the dilated tumour vessels seen on the right external carotid artery angiogram (C). (Courtesy of Dr M. Adams.)*

CEREBRAL METASTASES

DEFINITION

- **Primary *adult* neoplasms commonly metastasizing to the brain:**
  - lung ▶ breast ▶ malignant melanoma
- **Primary *paediatric* neoplasms commonly metastasizing to the brain:**
  - neuroblastoma ▶ Wilms' tumour ▶ rhabdomyosarcoma ▶ osteosarcoma

RADIOLOGICAL FEATURES

- Metastases generally appear as multiple well-defined rounded lesions with significant surrounding vasogenic oedema (which is often disproportionate to the tumour size)
  - *Vasogenic oedema:* low SI on trace-weighted DWI ▶ T2WI and FLAIR: high SI

NECT Metastases are usually of a similar or lower attenuation to normal brain tissue (melanoma metastases can be hyperdense) ▶ calcification is very rare (and should suggest another diagnosis)

- *Calcified metastases:* mucin-producing neoplasms (e.g. GI tract or breast) ▶ osteosarcoma

CECT There is strong enhancement with IV contrast medium: this can be uniform or ring-like (if the metastasis has outgrown its blood supply with subsequent central necrosis)

MR T1WI: low SI ▶ T2WI: high SI
- *Haemorrhage (10% of cases):* T1WI: high SI ▶ T2WI: low or high SI (depending upon the blood age)
- *Haemorrhagic metastases:* melanoma ▶ renal ▶ choriocarcinoma ▶ thyroid ▶ lung ▶ breast
  - Non-haemorrhagic melanoma metastases can appear similar due to the paramagnetic properties of melanin
- *Cystic metastases:* squamous cell carcinoma of the lung ▶ adenocarcinoma of the lung

PEARLS

- 80% of metastases are supratentorial ▶ they are multiple in 66% of cases
- There is a tendency to seed peripherally within the cerebral substance (at the grey/white matter junction) ▶ there can also be spread to the meninges
- DWI is helpful to differentiate a cerebral abscess from a cystic metastasis:
  - *Cerebral abscess:* this contains more viscous fluid and pus than a necrotic tumour ▶ it will therefore show a more marked restriction of water diffusion, appearing high SI on trace-weighted DWI and low SI on ADC maps
  - *Cystic metastasis:* this will be of low SI on the trace-weighted DWI and high SI on the ADC map

MENINGEAL METASTASES

DEFINITION

- Metastatic disease may involve the pachymeninges (dura mater) or leptomeninges (arachnoid and pia mater)

Carcinomatosis of the dura mater

- This is commonly seen with breast carcinoma
- It manifests as focal curvilinear or diffuse contrast enhancement closely applied to the skull inner table (it does not follow the gyral convolutions)
- Focal segmental lesions may be difficult to distinguish from an en plaque meningioma

Leptomeningeal carcinomatosis

- This is commonly seen with leukaemia, lymphoma, breast and lung cancer
- It manifests as linear or finely nodular contrast enhancement of the brain surface which extends into the sulci
- It may be indistinguishable from infective meningitis or neurosarcoidosis

PEARL

- Contrast-enhanced MRI is much more sensitive than CECT

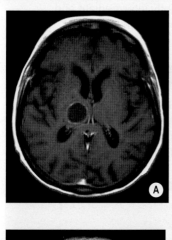
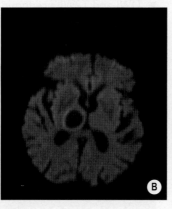
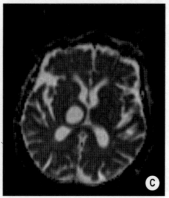

Cystic metastasis from breast cancer. Axial T1WI + Gad (A) demonstrates a peripherally enhancing, centrally necrotic lesion in the right thalamus. The lesion appears dark on the trace-weighted DWI (B) and bright on the ADC map (C), which is consistent with a relatively unrestricted diffusion in the centre of the mass.*

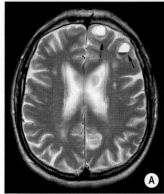
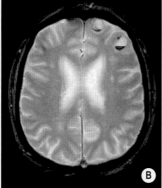
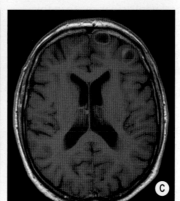

Haemorrhagic brain metastasis. (A) T2WI demonstrating a clear fluid level secondary to haemorrhage (arrows), which is more evident on the gradient-echo sequence (B). (C) These metastases also show thin rim enhancement following gaddinium.

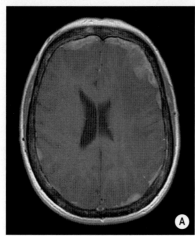
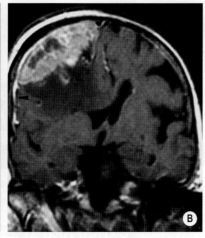

(A) Axial T1WI + Gad demonstrating heterogeneously enhancing dural metastases. (B) Dural metastasis from breast carcinoma. Coronal T1WI + Gad. There is a heterogeneously enhancing mass that arises from the dura over the right cerebral convexity with dural tail (arrowhead). It displaces the underlying brain and causes considerable low SI oedema within it.*

NEUROEPITHELIAL TISSUE ORIGIN – CENTRAL NEUROCYTOMA

DEFINITION

- A relatively benign slow-growing intraventricular tumour of purely neuronal origin ▶ it typically arises from the septum pellucidum and therefore occupies the frontal horns or bodies of the lateral ventricles (sometimes it extends through the foramen of Monro) ▶ rarely arise outside the ventricular system

CLINICAL PRESENTATION

- It occurs predominantly during the 2nd and 3rd decades of life (it is the commonest lateral ventricular mass in this age group) ▶ an obstructive hydrocephalus is common

RADIOLOGICAL FEATURES

CT A relatively dense lobulated mass which frequently demonstrates calcification and the presence of small cysts

MRI A heterogeneously enhancing mixed SI mass containing septated cysts, susceptibility artefact from calcification and grey matter isointense nodules

NEUROEPITHELIAL TISSUE ORIGIN – CHOROID PLEXUS PAPILLOMA

DEFINITION

- A benign tumour of the choroid plexus ▶ it can demonstrate drop metastases to the spine

CLINICAL PRESENTATION

- It is relatively more common in childhood (accounting for 3% of primary paediatric brain tumours and is also the commonest brain tumour in children <1 year old) ▶ it presents with hydrocephalus due to CSF overproduction and obstruction

RADIOLOGICAL FEATURES

CT An iso- to hyperdense mass ('frond-like') with punctate calcification and homogeneous enhancement
- *Children:* a 'cauliflower-like' mass within the trigone of the lateral ventricle
- *Adults:* it is predominantly located within the 4th ventricle or cerebellopontine angle

MRI A well-defined, lobulated, intraventricular mass ▶ T1WI and T2WI: predominantly intermediate and heterogeneous SI ▶ T1WI + Gad: intense contrast enhancement (flow voids are often seen)

PEARL

- **Choroid plexus carcinoma:** a rare but highly malignant tumour ▶ it is radiographically indistinguishable from a papilloma (but will invade the adjacent brain parenchyma to a greater degree)

NEUROEPITHELIAL TISSUE ORIGIN – EPENDYMOMA

- See Section 7, Gliomas

NON-NEUROEPITHELIAL TISSUE ORIGIN – COLLOID CYSTS

DEFINITION

- This occurs exclusively at the foramen of Monro (between the 3rd and lateral ventricles) – it therefore tends to cause hydrocephalus by intermittently or continuously obstructing CSF outflow from the lateral ventricles

RADIOLOGICAL FEATURES

NECT A characteristically hyperdense benign, smooth and spherical lesion

MRI Its appearance will vary depending upon the cyst contents (e.g. calcium, cholesterol, or haemosiderin) ▶ it can generate similar SI to CSF but is usually of high SI on both T1WI and T2WI

NON-NEUROEPITHELIAL TISSUE ORIGIN – MENINGIOMA

DEFINITION

- This is the commonest cause of a mass within the trigone of the lateral ventricle (after the 1st decade)

RADIOLOGICAL FEATURES

CT/MRI The appearances are similar to an extraventricular meningioma

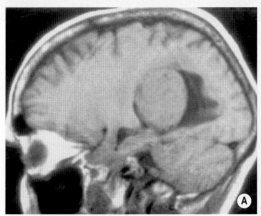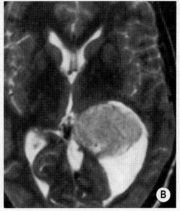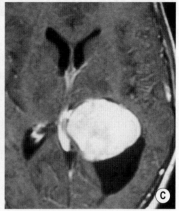

Intraventricular meningioma. (A) Sagittal T1WI shows a well-defined large mass in a dilated left lateral ventricular trigone. (B) The mass is isointense to grey matter and centred on the choroid. (C) T1WI + Gad demonstrating marked enhancement.[+]

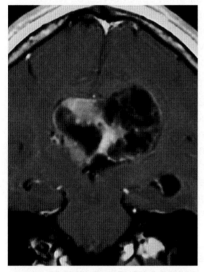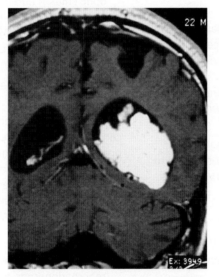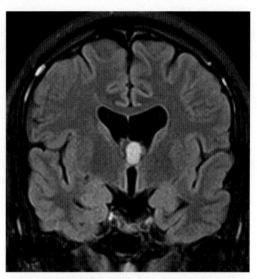

Central neurocytoma. Coronal T1WI + Gad. A partly cystic, multiseptated, enhancing mass, which is related to the septum pellucidum, fills the bodies of both lateral ventricles and causes hydrocephalus with dilatation of the left temporal horn.*

Choroid plexus papilloma. Coronal T1WI + Gad. There is a lobulated, strongly enhancing tumour in the trigone of the left lateral ventricle. Both lateral ventricles are dilated due to associated hydrocephalus.*

Colloid cyst. FLAIR image shows a well-circumscribed mass at the foramen on Monro, which is homogeneously hyperintense due to proteinaceous cyst content.**

Intraventricular masses by site			
	Lateral	**3rd**	**4th**
Choroid plexus papilloma	Common (paediatric)		Common (adult)
Ependymoma			Common
Medulloblastoma			Common
Meningioma	Common (glomus and atrium)		Along choroid plexus
Craniopharyngioma		Common (suprasellar growth)	

PITUITARY ADENOMAS

Definition

- A benign slow-growing tumour derived from cells of ectodermal endothelial origin and originating from the anterior hypophysis ▶ as they are not encapsulated, they will displace adjacent tissues
- It is the most common tumour found within the sellar region
  - *Microadenoma:* this has a diameter <1 cm (and is often endocrinologically active)
  - *Macroadenoma:* this has a diameter >1 cm (and is often non-functional)

Clinical presentation

Asymptomatic Hypopituitarism is rare and a non-functioning microadenoma is often an incidental finding on MRI

Endocrine activity This is seen with microadenomas and functioning macroadenomas ▶ they can produce prolactin (prolactinoma), ACTH (Cushing's disease) or growth hormone (gigantism or acromegaly)

- *Prolactinoma:* this is the commonest functioning microadenoma and tends to arise laterally within the anterior pituitary lobe

Mass effect This is seen with non-functioning macroadenomas, and can lead to visual symptoms (due to compression of the optic chiasm) or cranial nerve palsies

Radiological features

MRI The investigation of choice ▶ a fat-saturated T1W sequence obtained after the administration of IV contrast medium eliminates any confounding high SI from the fat within the clivus and clinoid processes

- *Normal pituitary gland appearance:* T1WI and T2WI: the anterior gland demonstrates homogeneous SI (which is isointense to white matter) ▶ T1WI: the posterior gland demonstrates high SI (due to the stored neurosecretory material)

Microadenoma

- This may depress the floor of the sella turcica or expand one side of the gland (causing a subtle upwardly convex bulge of the gland or contralateral displacement of the infundibulum)

MRI T2WI: there may be high SI ▶ T1WI + Gad: microadenomas usually enhance later and to a lesser degree than normal pituitary tissue (therefore appearing as focal areas of low SI) ▶ dynamic pituitary MRI will exploit the time differences in enhancement between the adenoma and normal gland

Macroadenoma

- This will balloon the pituitary fossa ▶ any suprasellar component may lead to elevation (± compression) of the optic chiasm and intracranial optic nerves, as well as upward displacement of the 3rd ventricle (± obstruction of the foramen of Monro) ▶ inferior extension into the sphenoid sinus or clivus can occur ▶ large tumours may compress the brain parenchyma

NECT A hyperdense mass

MRI T1WI: low SI ▶ T2WI: high SI ▶ T1WI + Gad: there is uniform or heterogeneous enhancement ▶ cystic change can be present ▶ cavernous sinus extension is a poor prognostic sign ▶ enhancement/thickening of the dura ('dural tail') can be seen with large macroadenomas and implies an aggressive lesion

- *Haemorrhagic change:* this will appear as high SI (on both T1WI and T2WI)

Pearls

- Most microadenomas are treated medically – macroadenomas are treated surgically ▶ inferior petrosal/cavernous sinus venous sampling can localize an adenoma if MRI is inconclusive

Pituitary apoplexy Acute haemorrhage can lead to rapid expansion of the pituitary gland resulting in acute compression of the optic chiasm ▶ this is commonly seen with a macroadenoma

RATHKE'S CLEFT CYSTS

Definition

- This arises from an embryologic remnant of Rathke's pouch (which itself is a precursor of the anterior lobe and pars intermedia of the pituitary gland) ▶ it usually lies within the pituitary gland and can be found adjacent to the infundibulum (above the sella)

Clinical presentation

- It is usually an asymptomatic lesion (symptomatic lesions are much less common than with a craniopharyngioma)

Radiological features

MRI T1WI: a high SI cyst (but which may exhibit similar signal characteristics to CSF) ▶ T2WI: variable SI ▶ T1WI + Gad: no enhancement is usually seen (cyst wall enhancement is possible) ▶ thin and uniform walls (in contradistinction to a craniopharyngioma)

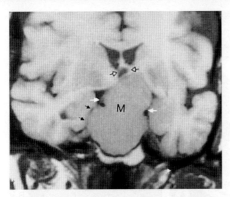

Pituitary macroadenoma. Coronal T1WI demonstrating a large macroadenoma (M) extending from the sella superiorly to distort the 3rd ventricle (open arrows). The right cavernous sinus is bowed (black arrows). When the tumour grows through the diaphragma sellae, it can be constricted by the dural margins (white arrows) just above the carotid flow voids.[+]

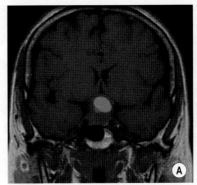
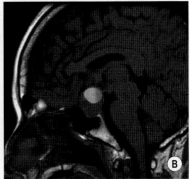

Pituitary apoplexy due to haemorrhage into a pituitary macroadenoma. Coronal (A) and sagittal (B) T1W images demonstrate a hyperintense area at the superior aspect of the tumour that contains a fluid level and is consistent with a recent intratumoural haemorrhage. The optic chiasm is stretched across the apex of the mass.[**]

Primary tumours in the sellar and parasellar region*	
Tumour	**Typical features**
Pituitary macroadenoma	Enlarged sella turcica, strong enhancement, sometimes haemorrhage
Meningioma	Broad dural base, enhancement along planum sphenoidale Hyperostosis, 'blistering' of sphenoid sinus
Schwannoma	T1-hypo- and T2-hyperintense, strong (e.g. of 5th nerve) enhancement
Chordoma	Bone destruction on CT, heterogeneous signal and enhancement on MRI
Chondrosarcoma	Bone destruction and calcification on CT, T2 hyperintense on MRI
Crangiopharyngioma	Calcification, cysts, nodular enhancement
Rathke's cleft cyst	T1-hyperintense on MRI, smooth peripheral enhancement
Dermoid	Hypodense on CT and T1 hyperintense on MRI
Epidermoid	Isodense to CSF on CT and isointense to CSF on T1 and T2 weighting, brighter than CSF on FLAIR and DWI
Tuber cinerum	Grey matter isointense on T1 weighting and T2 hamartoma hyperintense
Optic glioma	Thickening of chiasm, spread along optic pathways
Germ cell tumours	Located in midline, intense enhancement ▶ can be synchronous with pineal germinomas

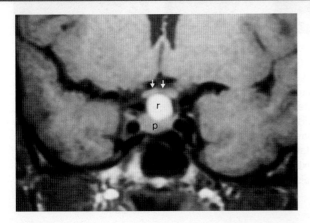

Rathke's cleft cyst. Coronal T1WI of a Rathke's cyst (r), which is in the suprasellar cistern and of high SI. The pituitary (p) and optic chiasm (arrows) are identified.[+]

CRANIOPHARYNGIOMA

Definition A benign suprasellar tumour arising from squamous epithelial remnants of Rathke's pouch (from which the anterior pituitary develops)

- It is the most common paediatric tumour of the suprasellar cistern

Clinical presentation Visual failure (due to optic chiasm compression) ▶ headache (secondary to raised intra-cerebral pressure following obstruction of the foramen of Monro) ▶ endocrine disturbances (due to pituitary compression) ▶ large tumours may cause hydrocephalus

- Although it occurs most frequently during childhood, a further peak is seen during the 6th decade

Radiological features The tumour tends not to expand the pituitary fossa unless it is very large (which is a differentiating feature from a pituitary macroadenoma)

Location It is commonly located within the hypothalamic region ▶ it less commonly involves both the suprasellar and intrasellar regions (with a smaller intrasellar component) ▶ a purely intrasellar region is rare

CT A cystic and calcified suprasellar tumour (calcification is often present in childhood tumours but less commonly seen in adult tumours)

MRI Although usually cystic, there can also be a solid or mixed cystic/solid appearance ▶ solid components show intense contrast enhancement

- *Cystic components:* T1WI: slightly hyperintense to CSF (due to the protein content) ▶ T2WI: high SI ▶ MR spectroscopy: high lipid peak

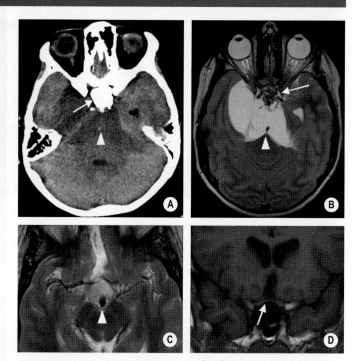

Craniopharyngiomas in two children. (A,B) The first child has a large suprasellar, prepontine and middle cranial fossa tumour which is causing considerable mass effect on the brainstem and is encasing the basilar artery (arrowheads). There are calcified components (arrows). The cystic components are of higher density on CT in keeping with proteinacous contents. The second child has a smaller suprasellar lesion, which is also calcified (arrowhead) (C). The optic chiasm (arrow) is clearly separate from the lesion and is draped over the top (D).*

PARASELLAR MENINGIOMA

Definition This arises from the dura mater of the cavernous sinus, tuberculum, dorsum or diaphragma sellae

Clinical presentation Cranial nerve palsies or visual symptoms

Radiological features

CT/MRI A strongly enhancing mass expanding the cavernous sinus ▶ it frequently encases and narrows the cavernous internal carotid arteries

Pearl A suprasellar meningioma often shows forward extension along the dura mater of the anterior cranial fossa, with dilatation ('blistering') of the sphenoid sinus ▶ intracranial extension of optic nerve sheath meningiomas characteristically involves the planum sphenoidale

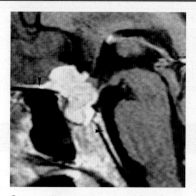

Suprasellar meningioma. Sagittal T1WI + Gad. A lobulated, enhancing suprasellar mass arises from the region of the tuberculum sellae and extends down into the pituitary fossa displacing the pituitary stalk posteriorly. Enhancing dural 'tails' (arrowheads) can be seen extending over the planum sphenoidale and clivus.*

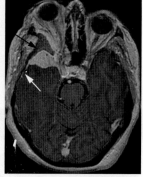

Axial MR image demonstrating a menigioma overlying the right sphenoid and extending into the suprasellar region. A dural tail (white arrow) is demonstrated as is hyperostosis of the underlying sphenoid bone (black arrow). There is also associated proptosis on this side.*

OPTIC NERVE GLIOMA

DEFINITION

- An astrocytic tumour (pilocytic astrocytoma) occurring in childhood and involving the optic nerves, optic chiasm and optic tracts ▶ chiasmal tumours often extend into the hypothalamus and may be of a higher histological grade
- It is associated with NF-1 (although chiasmatic tumours are more frequently seen in patients without NF-1)

CLINICAL PRESENTATION

- There is usually a very indolent course (although chiasmatic tumours tend to be more aggressive)

RADIOLOGICAL FEATURES

MRI T1WI: an iso- to hypointense SI mass ▶ T2WI: a hyperintense mass ▶ T1WI + Gad: variable enhancement ▶ there may be diffuse fusiform expansion of the nerve from subarachnoid dissemination of tumour around the optic nerve

PEARL

- A craniopharyngioma will tend to present later, is usually calcified, and is adherent to the chiasm rather than arising from it and causing expansion

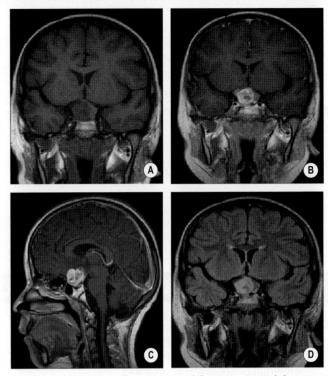

Hypothalamic–optic pathway glioma. (A) coronal T1W, (B) coronal, and (C) sagittal T1W + Gad images and (D) coronal FLAIR show an optic chiasm glioma. The chiasm is not identified separately from the tumour.*

INFUNDIBULAR TUMOURS

Germinomas and Langerhans' cell histiocytosis

- Both of these conditions can cause expansion and enhancement of the pituitary infundibulum

MRI The onset of diabetes insipidus correlates with an absence of high T1WI SI within the posterior pituitary

Hypothalamic hamartoma

- This is a congenital lesion of non-neoplastic heterotropic grey and white matter ▶ it presents with precocious puberty and gelastic seizures
- It presents as a sessile or pedunculated lesion arising from the floor of the 3ʳᵈ ventricle, with extension into the suprasellar or interpeduncular cisterns

CT An isodense, well-circumscribed, non-enhancing mass

MRI T1WI/T2WI: intermediate SI ▶ T1WI + Gad: there is no enhancement

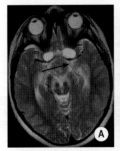
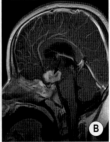

Langerhans' cell histiocytosis. (A) Axial T2WI. (B) Sagittal T1WI + Gad. There is a suprasellar T2 low SI and enhancing mass (arrows) with associated oedema extending superiorly along white matter tracts.*

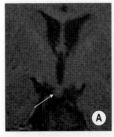
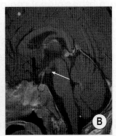

Hypothalamic hamartoma. (A) Coronal T1WI and (B) sagittal T1WI + Gad shows a non-enhancing lesion arising from the floor of the third ventricle posterior to the pituitary infundibulum and projecting inferiorly into the suprasellar cistern (arrows).*

743

CLINICAL PRESENTATION

- Pineal region tumours account for 10% of all paediatric brain tumours, and 1% of all adult tumours
- They present with obstructive hydrocephalus (due to aqueduct compression), problems with eye movements or accommodation (due to compression of the tectal plate), or precocious puberty

Parinaud's syndrome Paralysis of upward gaze

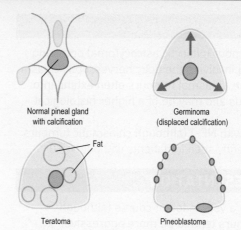

Schematic diagram showing different patterns of calcification in pineal tumours.

TUMOURS OF GERM CELL ORIGIN (60%)

Germinoma This is the most common pineal tumour (and is equivalent to a testicular seminoma or an ovarian dysgerminoma) ▶ it can demonstrate diffuse subependymal or subarachnoid spread

- It is usually seen in young males (90% of cases)
- It may be multifocal (the hypothalamic region is the 2nd commonest site with diabetes insipidus and the more common location when seen in females) ▶ can show diffuse subependymal and subarachnoid spread

NECT An iso- or hyperdense rounded mass ▶ the tumour itself is rarely calcified, but will engulf any normal pineal calcification

MRI T1WI and T2WI: the tumour is isointense to grey matter (due to the dense cell packing) ▶ T1WI + Gad: there is marked and homogeneous contrast enhancement ▶ DWI: restricted diffusion (dense cellularity)

Teratoma As for a germinoma, this is much more frequently seen in males

CT/MRI The tumour appears more lobulated and inhomogeneous than a germinoma (reflecting its fat content and calcification) ▶ it often demonstrates irregular tumour margins ▶ there is poor enhancement

Choriocarcinoma This tumour is often haemorrhagic and is associated with a poor prognosis (M>F)

- It will be human chorionic gonadotrophin and human placental lactogen positive on immunochemistry

Yolk sac tumours and embryonal carcinoma Yolk sac tumours are often cystic ▶ embryonal tumours are usually solid

TUMOURS OF PINEAL CELL ORIGIN (40%)

Pineocytoma This is a benign tumour of young adults (with a good prognosis)

CT/MRI A well-defined mass (± calcification ± enhancement) ▶ it lacks specific imaging features, allowing a differentiation from other pineal region neoplasms

Pineoblastoma This is a highly malignant tumour (behaving like a cerebellar medulloblastoma with frequent CSF seeding) ▶ it most frequently presents during the 1st two decades of life

- *Trilateral retinoblastoma*: bilateral retinoblastomas + a pineoblastoma

CT An 'exploded calcification' along the margins of the mass (due to displaced pre-existing central pineal

calcification) ▶ there is rarely haemorrhage ▶ hyperdense mass

MRI T2WI: low SI ▶ DWI: high SI ▶ T1WI + Gad: there is marked contrast enhancement

PEARLS

- Common and benign pineal cysts must be differentiated from pineal tumours:
  - Cysts are smooth and well defined ▶ they can exhibit rim enhancement
  - T1W/PD/FLAIR images: cysts may be of higher SI to CSF (protein content)
  - Cysts do not cause hydrocephalus or a midbrain syndrome

Pineal region masses					
	Pineoblastoma	**Pineocytoma**	**Germinoma**	**Choriocarcinoma**	**Teratoma**
Sex	M = F	M = F	M ≫ F	M > F	M = F
NECT	Hyperdense	Hyperdense	Hyperdense	Variable (haemorrhage)	Variable (fat, calcification)
Calcification	Exploded calcification	A higher intrinsic rate of calcification than a pineoblastoma	Engulfs pineal calcification	Rare	Frequent (± teeth formation)
Enhancement	Moderate	Moderate	Marked	Moderate	Minimal
Heterogeneity	Homogeneous	Homogeneous	Homogeneous	Heterogeneous	Heterogeneous
Haemorrhage	Yes	No	Yes	Yes (+++)	Possible

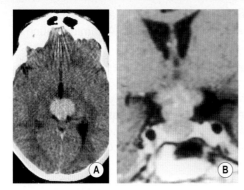

Germinoma. (A) A hyperdense pineal region mass is seen on this enhanced CT. (B) Coronal T1WI. An enhancing suprasellar germinoma is seen infiltrating the optic chiasm.[+]

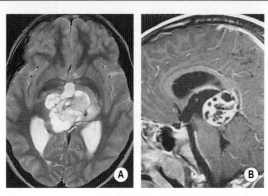

Pineal region teratoma. T2WI demonstrating a large heterogeneous SI mass in the pineal region (A). The mass comprises both solid and cystic components, there is heterogeneous enhancement on the sagittal T1WI + Gad (B) and the mass results in obstructive hydrocephalus.[†]

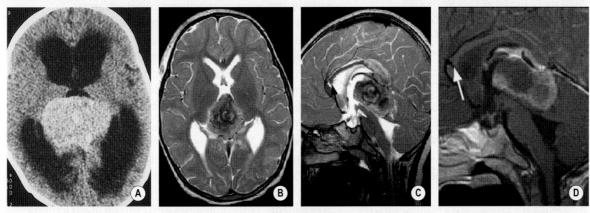

Pineoblastoma. (A) CECT, (B) axial T2WI, (C) sagittal T2WI and (D) T1WI + Gad show a pineal region tumour effacing the tectal plate. The hydrocephalus is treated by a frontal extraventricular drain (track through the genu of the corpus callosum marked by the arrow). The tumour is low SI on the T2WI with rings of lower signal consistent with calcification and haemorrhagic products, and peripheral rim enhancement.[†]

7.2 CEREBROVASCULAR DISEASE AND NON-TRAUMATIC HAEMORRHAGE

CEREBRAL ISCHAEMIA

Definition

Stroke A sudden persistent neurological deficit of vascular origin

Causes *Large vessel thromboembolic stroke (40%)*
- Most commonly due to thrombus at the site of atherosclerotic plaque or embolization more distally ▶ sites: carotid bifurcation > intracranial internal carotid artery (ICA) > proximal MCA (> anterior cerebral artery (ACA)) ▶ vertebral artery origins > distal vertebral artery (VA) > basilar artery
- *Vasculopathy* (dissection / FMD / vasculitis)
- *Haematological* (rotein C deficiency / pregnancy / OCP)
- *Cardioembolic stroke (15–30%)*
  - Intracardiac thrombu or tumour / valvular disease / cardiac
- *Small vessel / lacunar stroke (15–30%)*
- Deep white matter infarcts are typically small vessel in nature ▶ MCA territory infarcts can arise from emboli from the heart or carotid artery, or from in situ MCA thrombosis ▶ small peripheral infarcts in a vascular territory are usually embolic

Transient ischaemic attack (TIA) By definition this describes neurology resolving within 24 hours (including amaurosis fugax)

Penumbra This describes a peripheral rim of underperfused salvageable ischaemic tissue (surrounding already infarcted tissue) ▶ it is liable to infarct without prompt intervention
- Large core infarcts (70 ml) have a poor outcome regardless of penumbra characteristics
- *'Matched' defects* (core infarct with a small penumbra) have reduced reperfusion benefit ▶ *'mis-matched' defects* (large areas of salvageable tissue – penumbra >20% of core) are likely to benefit ▶ patient selection using penumbral imaging may extend therapeutic window >4.5 hrs

Watershed ischaemia (border zone infarction) This occurs at the boundaries of major vessel territories, possibly due to global hypoperfusion (e.g. between collaterals of the MCA / ACA and MCA / PCA) ▶ uncommon in the posterior fossa

CLINICAL OUTCOME

Proximal occlusions These cause infarcts of an entire arterial territory (unless a sufficient collateral circulation exists, in which case there may be deep infarcts with sparing of the overlying cortex)

Emboli / occlusions of terminal branch These cause cortical peripheral wedge-shaped infarcts

Perforator vessel occlusion These cause lacunar infarcts
- Most carotid territory infarcts involve the middle cerebral artery
- The anterior cerebral artery (ACA) collateral flow is

generally excellent and emboli are relatively rare ▶ the commonest cause of an ACA infarct is vasospasm following a subarachnoid haemorrhage
- Brainstem infarcts: these are commonly due to occlusion of a short perforating vessel
  - *'Top of the basilar' syndrome:* a combination of an infratentorial, thalamic and occipital infarct suggesting a distal basilar arterial occlusion
- Multiple infarcts within different arterial territories suggest a cardiac rather than a carotid embolic source (or a haemodynamic hypotensive stroke if the distribution conforms to the arterial border 'watershed' zones)

IMAGING STRATEGIES IN ACUTE STROKE

- Diagnostic imaging plays an important role as an ischaemic or haemorrhagic stroke cannot be distinguished clinically (and also around 30% of stroke-like episodes have a nonvascular cause)

Benefits of urgent neuroimaging This allows exclusion of a haemorrhagic stroke, allowing rapid tPA administration ▶ can exclude an underlying mass or AVM

Objectives of penumbral imaging Determine size of core infarct ± penumbra salvageable tissue
- Assessment of suitability for thrombolytic therapy in cases presenting at 3–6 hrs, or in cases with an unclear time of onset (tissue infarcted <3 hrs normal: subtly abnormal on FLAIR, tissue infarcted >4.5 hrs: hyperintense on FLAIR)
- Assessing clinically severe strokes to determine whether the deficit can be accounted for by a large area of reversible ischaemia
- If considering mechanical thrombectomy as a rescue therapy if IV treatment failed

CT This is usually the first-line investigation and is more widely available outside routine working hours
- *MRI:* this is better at showing the extent of the ischaemic change
- *DWI:* this is more sensitive for early infarcts, demonstrating a new infarct on a background of chronic ischaemic damage, or for diagnosing a TIA

MRA/CTA These allow a full assessment of the arterial tree from the aortic arch to the circle of Willis ▶ identifies embolic sources ▶ excludes dissection ▶ assesses potential for intra arterial thrombolysis / endovascular mechanical embolectomy (acute stroke therapy)

Doppler US Will not clearly show arterial segments that are anatomically inaccessible or heavily calcified
- *Surgical candidates:* a symptomatic (70–99%) stenosis of the internal carotid artery

Treatment IV thrombolysis (tPA) can be given (criteria: haemorrhage excluded / <4.5 h of onset / infarct <$\frac{1}{3}$ MCA territory / <80 years old) ▶ intra-arterial thrombolysis or endovascular mechanical embolectomy

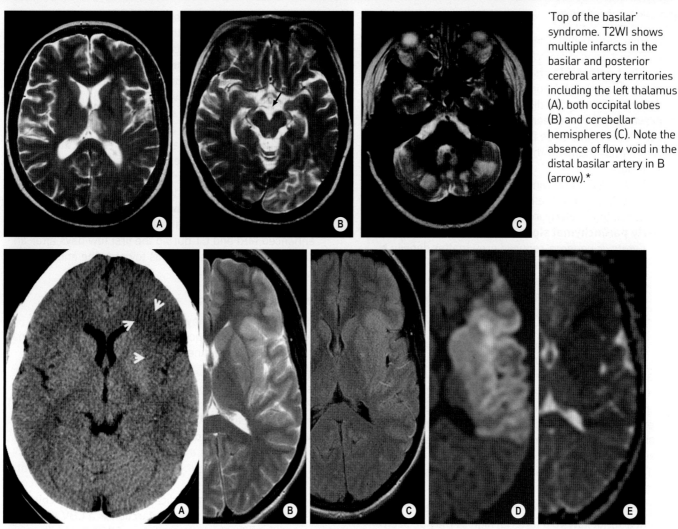

'Top of the basilar' syndrome. T2WI shows multiple infarcts in the basilar and posterior cerebral artery territories including the left thalamus (A), both occipital lobes (B) and cerebellar hemispheres (C). Note the absence of flow void in the distal basilar artery in B (arrow).*

An acute left MCA territory infarct presenting 7 h after onset is visible on CT (A) as low attenuation in the left frontal operculum and left insula. At this stage, not only is the infarct shown as T2 hyperintensity and gyral swelling but also more extensive involvement of the left MCA territory is identified on T2-weighted and FLAIR imaging (B, C). However, the full extent of involvement—including the basal ganglia—is only clearly demonstrated on DWI (D) as hyperintensity and on the corresponding ADC map (E) as hypointensity.**

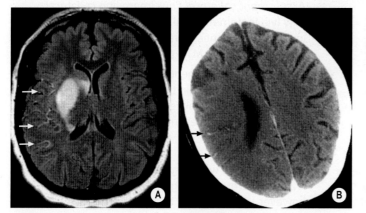

Vascular signs in acute infarcts. (A) FLAIR axial image of an acute right striatocapsular infarct. Note asymmetrical high signal returned from patent right MCA cortical branches due to compromised flow (arrows). (B) CECT shows early infarct changes of mild low density and local swelling in posterior part of right MCA territory. There is asymmetrical enhancement of MCA cortical branches because of sluggish flow (arrows).*

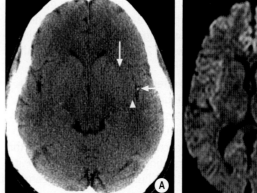

Sylvian 'dot' sign. (A) CT shows dense MCA branch due to occlusive acute thrombus (short arrow). There is very subtle loss of grey–white differentiation between the insular cortex and lateral border of putamen posteriorly (arrowhead), whereas more anteriorly it is preserved (long arrow). (B) DWI confirms a small acute cortical infarct adjacent to the thrombosed vessel.*

CEREBRAL ISCHAEMIA

Radiological features

CT Poor sensitivity for infarcts – consider using the ASPECTS scoring system

- **Earliest detectable change**: *the 'dense artery' sign*: this is due to fresh thrombus occluding a vessel (as thrombus can rapidly disperse this sign is not always present) ▶ if this is seen within the proximal MCA it correlates with a large infarct ▶ better prognosis if within MCA branch within sylvian fissue (sylvian fissure 'dot' sign)
  - MCA calcification can also mimic this sign but it is often bilateral ▶ the basilar artery may also appear dense (particularly in the 'top of basilar' syndrome)
- **Early parenchymal signs**:
  - *Cytotoxic oedema*: reduced grey matter density ▶ brain swelling (sulcal effacement)
  - *Early MCA infarcts*: a reduction in the clarity of the lentiform nucleus and cortex (particularly the insula) ▶ >50% involvement of MCA territory has a high mortality rate
    - *'Insular ribbon' sign*: this is demonstrated if the insular cortex is involved
- **Late signs**: encephalomalacia and atrophy with enlargement of the adjacent sulci and ventricles
- A region of swelling without an area of associated low density (resulting from a compensatory increase in CBV) can be a sign of compromised perfusion that may be reversible
- CT is much more sensitive than MRI for detecting acute haemorrhage

MRI **Early changes**: thrombus can cause loss of the normal arterial flow void (arterial high SI may be seen with FLAIR imaging due to altered flow – this is a useful qualitative sign of reduced perfusion when the parenchyma still appears normal)

- **Early parenchymal signs**: there is structural breakdown and disruption of the blood-brain barrier with fluid leaking into the extracellular space ▶ this manifests as cortical swelling and T1/T2 prolongation (this is more obvious with T2WI and especially FLAIR imaging)
  - T2 hyperintensity is often absent or very subtle in infarcts only a few hours old
- **Subacute stage**: contrast enhancement is commonly seen on MRI (as well as CT) due to disruption of the blood–brain barrier ▶ occurs in almost all cases by the end of the 1st week, persisting for several months ▶ it can have a variable pattern but gyriform enhancement is characteristic of a cortical infarct
  - This is seen with MRI in almost all cases by the end of the 1st week and persists for several months
- **Late signs**: these are as for CT (MRI signal intensities and CT attenuation values approach that of CSF) ▶

Wallerian degeneration is sometimes visible as faint T2 hyperintensity within the isilateral corticospinal tract together with asymmetrical brainstem atrophy

- **Haemorrhagic transformation**: this follows secondary bleeding into areas of reperfused ischaemic tissue ▶ it occurs during the first 2 weeks in up to 80% of infarcts seen on MRI ▶ it is often seen within the basal ganglia and cortex (with possibly a gyriform pattern) ▶ the severity of the haemorrhage correlates with the size of the infarct and the degree of contrast enhancement in the early stages
  - T1WI: high SI ▶ T2WI: low SI
- **Intravascular enhancement (due to sluggish flow)**: this may be seen within affected vessels on contrast enhanced MRI and CT during the first few days after an infarct (becoming less obvious towards the end of the 1st week)

Advanced techniques

Proton MR spectroscopy (MRS) *Infarcted regions*: increased lactate ▶ reduced N-acetylaspartate (a neuronal marker) and total creatine

Perfusion CT (CTP) / perfusion-weighted MRI (PW-MRI) This utilizes dynamic bolus tracking techniques

- PW-MRI produces maps of time-to-peak contrast (TTP), mean transit time (MTT), cerebral blood volume (CBV) and cerebral blood flow (CBF) – (CBF = CBV/MTT)
  - *TTP*: this provides a qualitative overview of brain perfusion ▶ a delay >4 s seems to indicate tissue at risk
  - *A reduced CBV*: this indicates an inadequate collateral supply and a high risk of infarction ▶ a CBV defect seems to be the best predictor of the initial infarct size (and final size if it successfully reperfused)
  - *MTT and CBF*: this indicates the tissue at risk (i.e. the final infarct volume unless reperfusion occurs)
  - *Assessment collateral flow*: improving collateral flow (via leptomeningeal vessels) is associated with improved outcomes ▶ in these areas CBF / CBV likely to be preserved ▶ MTT prolonged

DWI This has a pre-eminent role in acute stroke imaging (with a high sensitivity within the first few hours when T2WI is usually normal) ▶ DWI hyperintense / ADC hypointense areas almost always represent areas of irreversible ischaemia

- **Pitfalls**:
  - *Chronic lesions with very long T2 relaxation times*: 'T2 shine through' may generate high SI on DWI – however in comparison to an acute infarct it will also generate high SI on an ADC map
  - *Acute haemorrhage*: this can generate high SI resembling an infarct – however there is often a low SI margin produced by susceptibility effects

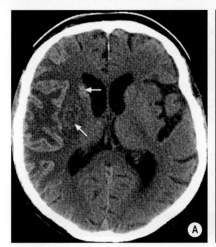
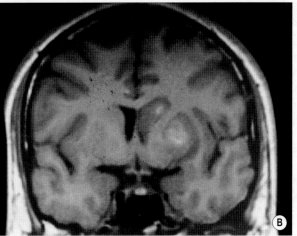

Haemorrhagic transformation. (A) NECT 2 weeks after a large right MCA territory infarct shows a gyriform pattern of haemorrhagic transformation in the right cerebral cortex. There is also haemorrhage in the basal ganglia (arrows). (B) Coronal T1WI shows swelling and signal alteration of the caudate and lentiform nuclei. Sparing of the cortex is due to adequate leptomeningeal collateral circulation. The central T1–high SI area within the infarct indicates haemorrhagic transformation.*

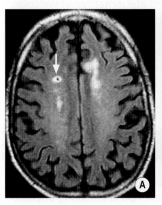
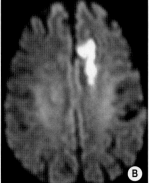
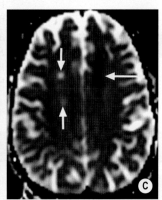

New and old infarcts on DWI. (A) FLAIR shows high signal ischaemic change of indeterminate age in both frontal lobes. There is a small mature lacunar infarct on the right with a low SI central cavity (arrow). (B) DWI shows an acute high SI lesion on the left. (C) The ADC map confirms the left-sided lesion is acute (dark indicates low ADC ▶ long arrow). The infarcts on the right are bright, indicating increased ADC and therefore older lesions (short arrows).*

Ischaemic stroke

	T1WI	T2WI	DWI	ADC
Hyperacute (0–6 h)	Isointense	Isointense	Bright	Dark
Acute (6 h to 4 days)	Hypointense (+ oedema mass effect)	Hyperintense (+ oedema mass effect)	Bright	Dark
Subacute (4–14 days)	Hypointense	Hyperintense	Dark (It may be bright secondary to T2 shine through)	Pseudonormalization
Chronic	A smaller area of low intensity + encephalomalacia	Hyperintense	Hypointense Dark (It may be bright secondary to T2 shine through)	Bright

Ischaemic stroke

	Vasogenic oedema	Cytotoxic oedema
Cause	Tumour ▶ abscess ▶ haemorrhage ▶ trauma	Ischaemia (e.g. stroke)
Mechanism	Disruption of the blood–brain barrier ▶ increased capillary endothelial permeability leads to fluid extravasation	Failure of membrane ATP-dependent sodium pumps ▶ accumulation of intracellular sodium and water
Imaging	Characteristic finger-like pattern with cortical sparing	Involvement of both cortex and white matter

SMALL VESSEL ISCHAEMIC DISEASE

DEFINITION

- A normal variant seen in older people predominantly affecting the periventricular and deep cerebral white matter, basal ganglia and ventral pons ▶ it is due to arteriolar occlusion of the long penetrating arteries with the outcome dependent upon vessel size:
  - *Large vessel:* a lacunar infarct (with an associated cavity)
  - *Small vessels:* ischaemic demyelination and gliosis

CLINICAL PRESENTATION

- It is usually clinically silent unless it arises within an eloquent area
- Severe ischaemic damage is associated with cognitive impairment

RADIOLOGICAL FEATURES

- *Acute lacunar infarct:* rounded with a hazy outline ▶ may fluctuate in size (enlarging)

- *Mature lacunar infarct:* sharply delineated ▶ shrink in size (<1.5 cm) ▶ cavity like

CT Periventricular white matter hypodensities (leukoaraiosis)

MRI T2WI: high SI within the white matter (FLAIR sequences are particularly sensitive) ▶ white matter changes are non-specific and can be encountered in vasculitis

DWI This will confirm the site of an acute subcortical infarct even if there is widespread pre-existing ischaemic change

PEARLS

- Microbleeds (foci of old haemorrhage) can occur with hypertensive small vessel and are a marker of vascular fragility ▶ small foci of susceptibility artefact on T2*GRE and SWI
- *Risk factors:* age ▶ hypertension ▶ elevated haemoglobin levels ▶ diabetes ▶ smoking ▶ hyperlipidaemia

MOYAMOYA

DEFINITION

- An idiopathic arteriopathy whereby dilated collateral vessels (particularly the lenticulostriate and thalamoperforator arteries) develop secondary to a progressive stenosis of the terminal internal carotid artery and its proximal intracranial segments (particularly the anterior circulation) ▶ primarily involves the supraclinoid ICAs, often progressing to the proximal anterior and middle cerebral arteries (occasionally the posterior circulation)
- Moyamoya is Japanese for 'puff of smoke' (describing the angiographic appearance of the collateral vessels)

ASSOCIATIONS

- As well as being idiopathic it is associated with:
- Sickle cell disease ▶ secondary to NF-1 ▶ cranial irradiation ▶ Down's syndrome ▶ HIV ▶ tuberculous meningitis

- In post-infective angiitis associated with varicella zoster the terminal ICA and proximal MCA are usually affected and there is infarction of the basal ganglia

MRA/CTA/MRI Abnormal dilated and irregular collateral vessels (± infarcts, usually in the border zones)

PEARL

- It accounts for up to 30% of the cerebral vasculopathy in paediatric stroke

Treatment

- External to internal carotid bypass

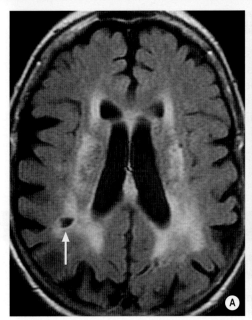
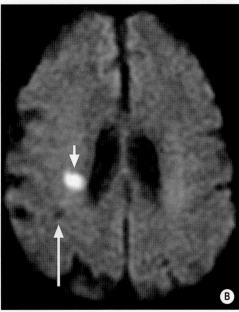

Small vessel disease. (A). Axial FLAIR of a patient shows diffuse high signal indicating small vessel ischaemic change in deep and periventricular cerebral white matter. There is a mature lacunar infarct in the right parietal lobe (arrow). (B). Axial DWI shows an acute infarct as high signal (short arrow) and the mature lacuna as low signal (long arrow). Only DWI can differentiate the acute infarct from the surrounding signal abnormality.*

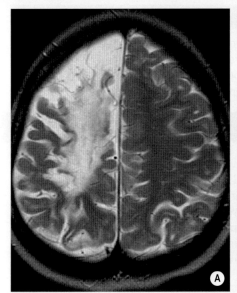
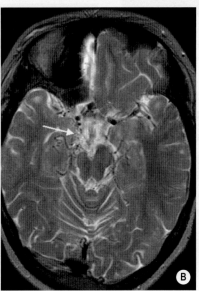
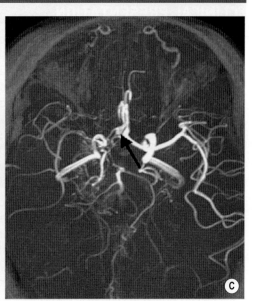

Sickle cell disease and Moyamoya syndrome. (A) Child with extensive frontal, deep and posterior watershed infarction. (B) Extensive perimesencephalic 'Moyamoya' collaterals (arrow) and attenuated right middle cerebral artery (MCA) flow voids. (C) Compressed maximum intensity projection image shows narrowed terminal internal carotid artery (ICA), reduced filling of right MCA and A1 segment of the anterior cerebral artery. There is an aneurysm at the A1/anterior communicating artery (ACOM) junction (arrow).*

GLOBAL CEREBRAL HYPOPERFUSION AND ANOXIA

DEFINITION

- An inadequate oxygen supply due to severe hypotension or impaired blood oxygenation
- Global hypoperfusion can result in watershed infarcts: these are wedge-shaped lesions within the frontal or parietal lobes at the junctions of the ACA/MCA and MCA/PCA arterial territories, respectively
- Anoxia due to defective blood oxygenation (e.g. carbon monoxide poisoning) tends to cause infarcts within especially sensitive regions (e.g. the basal ganglia)

RADIOLOGICAL FEATURES

MRI DWI is especially sensitive (CT and MRI can miss early disease as the changes are frequently symmetrical)
- FLAIR: diffuse high S1 (diffuse swelling)
- DWI: diffuse grey matter restricted diffusion ▶ obvious grey–white differentiation

VEIN OF GALEN ANEURYSMAL MALFORMATIONS

DEFINITION

- A unique congenital malformation of the intracranial circulation characterized by an enlarged midline venous structure (a persistent embryological remnant) with multiple arteriovenous communications leading to aneurysmal dilatation (presumably secondary to a high arteriovenous flow) ▶ it accounts for 30% of vascular malformations in children and is a rare cause of paediatric stroke

CLINICAL PRESENTATION

- Neonates may present with severe cardiac failure
- In infants the degree of shunting is much smaller ▶ they present with hydrocephalus and cerebral atrophy
- Older children can present with headaches, seizures, intracerebral or subarachnoid haemorrhage

RADIOLOGICAL FEATURES

CT Parenchymal calcification associated with the chronic venous hypertension

MRI This demonstrates a dilated venous sac (± thrombus), the location of fistulous connections, the arteries involved and the venous drainage ▶ it also determines the extent of any parenchymal damage (infarction or atrophy)

Angiography This is the gold standard ▶ it ideally should be performed at the time of endovascular treatment

FOLLOW-UP

- Look for evidence of significant arteriovenous shunting, progressive cerebral damage or atrophy ▶ jugular venous occlusion can occur (as a chronic effect of the venous hypertension)

CEREBRAL VENOUS THROMBOSIS (CVT)

DEFINITION

- An infarct due to venous occlusion (commonly thrombotic) ▶ it will not conform to an arterial territory, and the resultant infarcts are often haemorrhagic and multifocal ▶ the superior sagittal sinus is the most commonly involved, leading to bilateral parasagittal infarcts (isolated occlusions of the transverse sinus or deep cerebral veins can also occur)
  - *Causes:* trauma ▶ infection (particularly a subdural empyema) ▶ hypercoagulability disorders (including oral contraceptive use) ▶ smoking ▶ vasculitis

RADIOLOGICAL FEATURES

NECT An expanded and hyperdense venous sinus

CECT *'Empty delta' sign:* there is more intense enhancement of the venous sinus walls than the sinus contents (the 'empty delta' represents the venous filling defect)

MRI A lack of flow void in an affected sinus
- *Caution:* normal slow-flowing blood may appear bright (simulating a thrombus) ▶ acute thrombus can generate low SI (mimicking a flow void)
  - Therefore a phase-contrast MR venogram (MRV) is usually required
- Thrombosed vessel (T1WI + T2WI): hyperintense

PEARL

Appearance of parenchymal lesions depends on venous hypertension ± infarction ± secondary haemorrhage (disproportionate swelling + oedema is typical) ▶ distribution:
- *Internal cerebral vein/straight sinus:* bilateral thalami ± basal ganglia
- *Vein of Labbé/lateral venous sinus:* posterolateral temporal lobe/inferior parietal lobe
- *Superior sagittal sinus:* bilateral (asymmetric) cortical + subcortical lesions

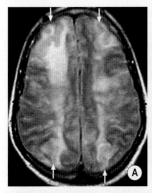
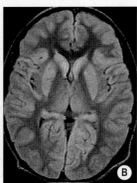
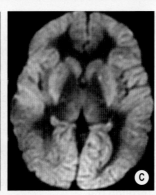

Global hypoperfusion. (A) Acute watershed infarcts and diffuse brain swelling on FLAIR axial image after a cardiac arrest (arrows). (B) FLAIR axial image in a different patient with a generalized hypoxic ischaemic brain insult after self-hanging shows diffuse high SI. (C) DWI shows diffuse grey matter restricted diffusion markedly different from white matter SI, alerting the observer that the scan is abnormal despite its symmetry. Obvious grey–white differentiation is not a normal feature of DWI.*

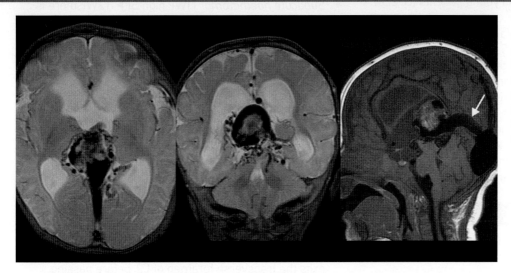

Vein of Galen malformation (partly occluded by embolization glue) showing residual flow through the promesencephalic vein, containing a combination of glue and thrombus, via the falcine sinus (arrow) towards the venous confluence. Arterial supply is via a number of choroidal vessels.*

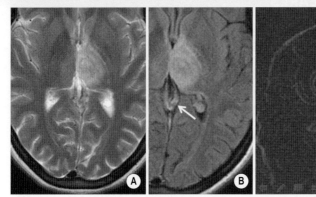

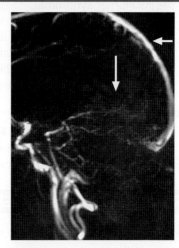

Deep venous thrombosis. This young female patient presented with headache and right-sided hemiparesis whilst playing in a prolonged hockey competition in summer, followed by reduced consciousness. The initial MRI examination (A) demonstrates signal abnormality and swelling consistent with venous hypertension, oedema and ischaemia in the left thalamus. There is abnormal signal within and expansion of the left internal cerebral vein and straight sinus on FLAIR (B, white arrow) in keeping with thrombus. The MR venogram does not show any flow in the deep venous system (C).**

Acute deep venous system thrombosis. A phase contrast MR venogram shows a normal superior sagittal sinus (short arrow) but no flow in the deep venous system (position indicated by long arrow).

CAROTID AND VERTEBRAL ARTERY DISSECTION

DEFINITION

- Arterial dissection occurs when the intima and media of the arterial wall is disrupted, resulting in an intramural haematoma (direct haemorrhage into the media can also occur from disruption of the vasa vasorum)
  - A dissection may be subintimal (causing luminal narrowing or occlusion) or subadventitial (with pseudoaneurysm formation)
  - A dissection of an intracranial vessel is rare and has a worse prognosis than an extracranial dissection ▶ an intracranial dissection may rupture through the adventitia and lead to a subarachnoid haemorrhage
- It is a major cause of stroke in young adults and children, accounting for 20% of strokes in young patients (cf. 2.5% of strokes in older patients)
- It usually affects the *extra*cranial great vessels ▶ a carotid arterial dissection is 3–5 times more common than a vertebral arterial dissection (internal carotid artery dissection is the most common)
- *Risk factors:* hereditary connective tissue diseases (e.g. Marfan's syndrome, Ehlers–Danlos syndrome, fibromuscular dysplasia, osteogenesis imperfecta type I, autosomal dominant polycystic kidney disease, Menkes' disease) ▶ migraine ▶ hypertension ▶ smoking ▶ oral contraceptives ▶ trauma or manipulation to the neck

CLINICAL FEATURES

- Dissection may follow blunt trauma to the neck or abrupt head turning or hyperextension

Carotid arterial dissection

- Ipsilateral headache ▶ neck pain ▶ ipsilateral visual symptoms (e.g. a transient monocular visual loss or a painful Horner syndrome)
- Cerebral ischaemia resulting in a transient ischaemic attack or stroke (this is usually due to thromboemboli and the majority recover with little sequelae)
- Occasionally they can be asymptomatic as the bilateral cerebral circulation can maintain brain perfusion

Vertebral arterial dissection

- A unilateral occipital headache ▶ posterior neck pain ▶ brainstem, cerebellar or occipital infarcts
- The majority have a good outcome

RADIOLOGICAL FEATURES

US An echogenic dissection flap with a double lumen

CECT This may demonstrate a dissection flap ▶ there may be an enhancing narrowed eccentric lumen associated with an increased overall diameter (due to the haematoma causing mural thickening)
- *'Fried egg' appearance:* seen on CT (expanded vessel with crescentic hyperdensity) and MRI (a true lumen with variable patency ranging from normal flow void to abnormal signal due to occlusion or slow flow) with a surrounding crescent of intramural haemorrhage in the false lumen

MRI An expanded artery with high SI eccentric intramural haematoma surrounding a narrow, often eccentric, signal void (indicating the true lumen) ▶ the signal characteristics of intramural haemorrhage follow those of parenchymal haemorrhage (but haemosiderin deposition is rare)
- *Acute haematoma:* T1/T2: intermediate-to-low SI
- *Subacute haematoma:* T1WI: high SI ▶ T2WI: there is later development of high SI
- *Chronic haematoma:* T1WI/T2WI: low SI

Digital subtraction angiography (DSA) / CT angiography (CTA) / MR angiography (MRA)

- A *'rat's tail' appearance:* a tapered stenosis or occlusion of the true lumen
- An intraluminal flap or pseudoaneurysmal dilatation
- There may be differential opacification and contrast washout in the true and false lumens (if they are both patent)
- A dissection within the internal carotid arteries often starts at or just above the carotid bifurcation and sometimes extends intracranially
- A dissection within a vertebral artery is most commonly found at the C1–2 level as the vertebral artery exits the transverse foramen of C2, before passing posterolaterally over the lateral masses of C1 to enter the foramen magnum

PEARLS

- Internal carotid arterial dissections often involve the vessel just below the skull base
- Death may occur in up to 10% of patients during the acute episode (due to extensive intracranial arterial dissection, brainstem infarction or subarachnoid haemorrhage)

Fibromuscular dysplasia (FMD)

Occurs predominantly in middle-aged women ▶ cervical ICA (75%) ▶ vertebral artery (12%) ▶ bilateral (60%) ▶ angiography: 'string of beads' (luminal narrowing and dilatation) typically affecting mid ICA usually 2 cm distal to the bulb ▶ FMD occasionally seen intracranially

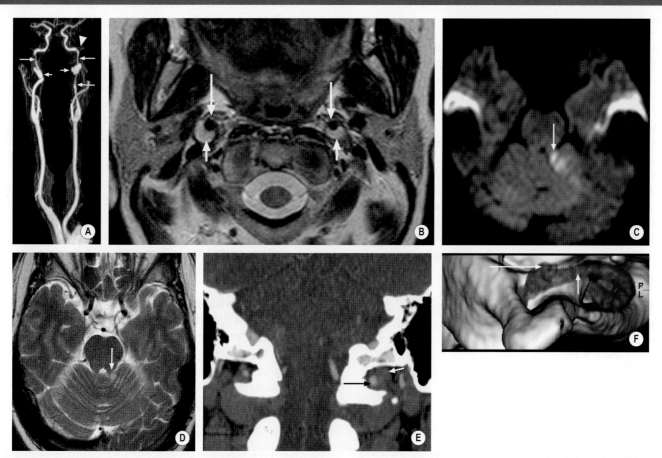

Cervical arterial dissection on MRA and CTA. (A) CEMRA. There are bilateral ICA dissections with irregular narrowing (long arrows), extending into the proximal petrous canal on the left (arrowhead). There are also pseudoaneurysms on both sides (short arrows). (B) Axial T2WI through the neck at C2 level in a different patient. On both sides there is high signal mural thrombus (short arrows) with eccentric flow void indicating the position of the true lumen (long arrows). (C) DWI in a different patient shows a small left superior cerebellar infarct (arrow), which would be easily overlooked on D, the corresponding T2WI (arrow). (E) Coronal reformat from CTA shows expanded left vertebral artery at C1 with mural thrombus (short arrow) and eccentric enhancing lumen (long arrow), analogous to the MRI appearance in B. (F) Volume rendering from the same examination shows the left vertebral artery (short arrow) as it passes around the left lateral mass of C1, viewed from the left and slightly in front. A small pseudoaneurysm is shown (long arrow).*

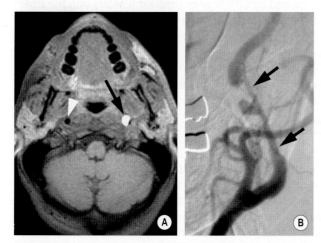

Spontaneous carotid dissection. (A) T1WI showing the true lumen of the left ICA lumen compressed by a false lumen that demonstrates high SI (arrow) consistent with thrombus or slow flow. The right ICA (arrowhead) is normal. (B) DSA in the same patient showing the compressed true lumen of the left ICA (arrows). The false lumen does not fill.¶¶

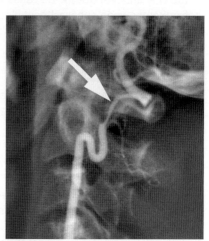

Lateral angiogram of a patient with neck pain following a boxing match. There is segmental narrowing of the vertebral artery (arrow) characteristic of dissection.¶¶

INTRACEREBRAL HAEMORRHAGE

Definition

- **Causes:** vascular malformations ▶ 'recreational' drugs (e.g. cocaine) ▶ coagulopathies or anticoagulation ▶ vasculitis ▶ venous infarcts ▶ haemorrhagic transformation of an arterial infarct ▶ primary or secondary neoplasms ▶ aneurysms (these are usually associated with a SAH)
    - Occasionally a ruptured aneurysm can cause an apparently isolated intracerebral clot
- *Older patients:* haemorrhage is frequently due to rupture of a small perforating vessel (secondary to hypertension or amyloid angiopathy) – this occurs preferentially within the basal ganglia, thalamus or pons
- *Amyloid:* peripheral or lobar haemorrhage suggests an amyloid angiopathy (particularly if multifocal)

Radiological features

CT Acute intracerebral clot is usually of homogeneous hyperdensity (it is rarely isodense in very anaemic patients) ▶ hyperacute unclotted blood will appear less dense (± a blood–fluid level) ▶ extensive haemorrhage may form an intraventricular haematoma or a blood–fluid level within the occipital horns

- An untreated haematoma will become less dense over several days (from the periphery inwards and therefore appearing smaller) – small haemorrhages can mimic an infarct by day 8–9
    - Blood products become hypodense after several weeks, leaving a focal cavity or area of atrophy
- Vasogenic oedema may develop within the surrounding white matter and contrast medium will usually produce a halo of enhancement
- *Features favouring a neoplastic haemorrhage:* a complex structure ▶ extensive surrounding oedema ▶ enhancing areas not immediately adjacent to the clot

MRI

- **Acute haemorrhage:** CT has a much higher sensitivity than spin-echo MRI (although T2-weighted gradient-echo sequences have equivalent or better sensitivity than CT)
- **Chronic haemorrhage:** gradient-echo imaging is much more sensitive to magnetic field inhomogeneities induced by paramagnetic blood products

CTA/MRA These are easier and quicker to perform than DSA in very sick patients ▶ it is not yet established whether small arteriovenous fistulas or malformations (AVMs) can be reliably excluded using these techniques

SUBARACHNOID HAEMORRHAGE

Definition

- Blood located within the subarachnoid space – this can be following trauma or due to a spontaneous cause
- *Spontaneous causes:* a ruptured arterial aneurysm (80%) ▶ an AVM (10%) ▶ no cause identified (10%) – most frequently when subarachnoid blood is confined to the perimesencephalic basal cisterns 'non-aneurysmal perimesencephalic SAH'

Clinical presentation

- A sudden and very severe (occipital) headache ▶ photophobia ▶ unresponsiveness ▶ focal neurology (30%)

Radiological features

CT This is positive in 98% of cases within 12 h of onset (and positive in <75% by the 3rd day)

- Increased density of the CSF spaces – blood is usually seen within the basal cisterns (as most aneurysms are near the circle of Willis)
- The entire intracranial subarachnoid space may be opacified (intraventricular blood is common)
- Lumbar puncture is required if there is a negative CT and a strong clinical suspicion persists (within 6 hrs)

MRI This may be used following a normal CT

- *Spin-echo sequences:* these are unreliable

- *FLAIR sequences:* these are reasonably sensitive in the acute and subacute periods ▶ they are less sensitive at low CSF red blood cell concentrations following a normal CT ▶ the CSF will generate high signal due to its increased protein content (artefactual high signal can be caused by CSF flow or contrast leakage into the CSF space following an infarct) ▶ FLAIR images may remain positive for at least 45 days (when blood has long since become invisible on CT)
- *Gradient-echo sequences:* areas of haemorrhage demonstrate low SI (due to the susceptibility effects of paramagnetic iron)

Pearls

Complications

- **Communicating hydrocephalus:** this is due to ventricular obstruction ▶ mild dilatation of the ventricles (particularly the temporal horns) is very common at presentation
- **Vasospasm:** this usually occurs 4–11 days post haemorrhage ▶ it is a significant cause of morbidity (due to the associated ischaemia)
- **Chronic repeated SAH:** this may develop a superficial siderosis with leptomeningeal haemosiderin staining (particularly around the midbrain and posterior fossa) ▶ it often presents with lower cranial nerve symptoms, ataxia or a gradual cognitive decline

Imaging characteristics of maturing haematoma on MRI					
	Hyperacute (<12 h)	**Acute (hours to days)**	**Early subacute (few days)**	**Late subacute (up to 1 month)**	**Chronic (1 month +)**
Underlying pathology	Extravasation	Deoxygenation	Clot retraction + deoxy-Hb is oxidized to met-Hb	Cell lysis	Clot digestion (macrophages)
Erythrocyte status	Intact	Intact – hypoxic	Intact – severely hypoxic	Lysis	Absent
Haemoglobin status	Intracellular oxy-Hb	Intracellular deoxy-Hb	Intracellular met-Hb	Extracellular met-Hb	Haemosiderin/ ferritin
T1WI	$\leftrightarrow$ or $\downarrow$	$\leftrightarrow$ or $\downarrow$	$\uparrow\uparrow$	$\uparrow\uparrow$	$\leftrightarrow$ or $\downarrow$
T2WI	$\uparrow$	$\downarrow$	$\downarrow\downarrow$	$\uparrow\uparrow$	$\downarrow\downarrow$

deoxy-Hb, deoxyhaemoglobin ▶ met-Hb, methaemoglobin ▶ oxy-Hb, oxyhaemoglobin.©31

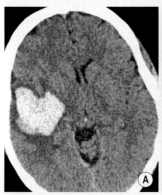
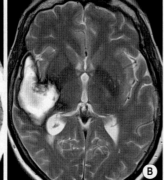

Evolution of intraparenchymal haemorrhage. (A) Acute primary haematoma on CT. Note the homogeneous appearance with only a small peripheral rim of hypodensity. (B) MRI at 1 month. The haematoma remains prominent but the surrounding oedema has resolved. There is a peripheral haemosiderin rim.**

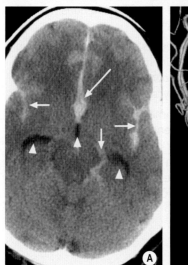
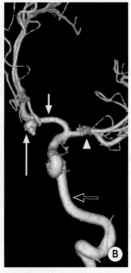

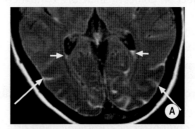
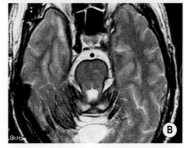

Anterior communicating artery aneurysm rupture. (A) CT shows diffuse subarachnoid haemorrhage (short arrows) and a small haematoma in the septum pellucidum indicating the likely source is an aneurysm of the anterior communicating artery (long arrow). The temporal horns of the lateral ventricles and anterior recesses of the 3rd ventricle are enlarged (arrowheads) due to secondary communicating hydrocephalus. (B) A 3D angiogram shows a lobulated aneurysm in the predicted location (long arrow). The left proximal anterior cerebral artery (short arrow), middle cerebral artery (arrowhead) and internal carotid artery (open arrow) are clearly shown.*

(A) Subarachnoid haemorrhage on FLAIR. Blood is shown as high SI in occipital sulci (long arrows) and layered in the occipital horns of both lateral ventricles (short arrows). (B) Superficial siderosis. Axial T2WI shows the pons, mesial temporal lobes and cerebellar folia are outlined by a low SI haemosiderin rim indicating repeated SAH.*

757

CEREBRAL ARTERY ANEURYSMS

Definition

Aneurysm types

- **Saccular ('berry aneurysm'):** this is the most common type (80% of cases) ▶ it is usually a degenerative round or lobulated lesion arising from an arterial bifurcation ▶ it is often an incidental finding usually in the circle of Willis
- *An increased incidence is seen with:* adult polycystic disease ▶ aortic coarctation ▶ Marfan's and Ehlers–Danlos syndromes
- **Fusiform:** this can be regarded as an extreme form of focal ectasia due to arteriosclerotic disease ▶ it is usually found within the vertebrobasilar system
- **Dissecting:** following a dissection the resultant intramural haematoma may organize and the resultant wall weakness may lead to an aneurysm ▶ it can be spontaneous or follow trauma or a vasculopathy
- **Giant:** by definition these are >25 mm in diameter (accounting for 5% of aneurysms) ▶ they often contain layers of organized thrombus
- **Mycotic:** these are caused by septic emboli (e.g. a bacterial endocarditis or IV drug abuse) ▶ they tend to occur peripherally (typically on MCA branches) ▶ they commonly present with haemorrhage with an associated peripheral intraparenchymal clot (in a septic patient this is highly suggestive of a mycotic aneurysm) ▶ there can be intense enhancement adjacent to the involved vessel

Clinical presentation

- *Severe headache:* due to a subarachnoid haemorrhage
- *Mass effect on adjacent structures:* most commonly a posterior communicating artery aneurysm causing a 3rd nerve palsy
- Up to 20% of aneurysms are multiple

Radiological features

Carotid circulation (90%) ▶ vertebral or basilar arteries (10%)

- *Anterior and posterior communicating arteries:* approximately 33% each
- *Middle cerebral arteries:* 20%
- *Basilar termination:* 5%

Anterior circulation aneurysms

- *Anterior communicating artery:* a clot within the septum pellucidum is virtually diagnostic
- *Aneurysms of the distal anterior cerebral artery:* these are related to the pericallosal branches and are less common
- *Middle cerebral artery:* this can cause bleeding into the sylvian fissure (with occasionally a temporal lobe clot)
- *Posterior communicating artery:* this is a frequent cause of SAH but can also present with an isolated 3rd nerve palsy (due to pulsatile pressure on the nerve)

Posterior circulation aneurysms

- These are commonly located at the basilar artery bifurcation ▶ rupture leads to blood within the interpeduncular fossa, brainstem or thalamus (with a poor prognosis)
- The 2nd commonest site is the posterior inferior cerebellar arterial origin – this is associated with haemorrhage into the ventricular system (via the 4th ventricle) and also downwards into the spinal subarachnoid space

DSA Traditionally a 'four vessel' angiogram is performed with bilateral common or internal carotid injections and injection of one or both vertebral arteries ▶ a limited angiogram can be performed if the bleeding territory has been indicated with cross-sectional imaging

- Ruptured aneurysms often have an irregular shape (and may show a 'nipple' indicating the rupture site) ▶ generally the largest aneurysm is frequently responsible
- DSA should be performed as soon as possible following a SAH: the aneurysm rebleed rate is greatest during the first 48 h and vasospasm can adversely affect the angiogram quality

CT A rounded enhancing lesion ▶ any haematoma or SAH is usually adjacent to the bleeding aneurysm ▶ giant aneurysms have an enhancing lumen and a wall of variable thickness (which often contains laminated calcified thrombus)

CTA This outperforms DSA for aneurysms that are <5 mm (as well as being easier and quicker to perform it also avoids an arterial puncture and the associated risks of ischaemic stroke from catheter angiography)

- It is preferable to MRA with an acute SAH: the vessel lumen is properly opacified with CTA and does not suffer from flow-related artefacts

MRI A patent aneurysm appears as an area of flow void ▶ increased SI within an aneurysm may represent mural thrombus or turbulent/slow flow ▶ surrounding white matter oedema suggests a mycotic aneurysm

MRA Preferred method for imaging in the non-acute setting ▶ this has a modest sensitivity for aneurysms >5 mm (and a poor sensitivity <3 mm) ▶ a recent SAH may cause image degradation on a TOF MRA (due to T1 shortening from haemorrhage) ▶ giant aneurysms are rarely fully visualized on 3D TOF MRA (because of slow or turbulent fundal flow)

Pearl

Aneurysm complications

- Rupture (+ bleeding) ▶ vasospasm (typically occurring 5 days after rupture) ▶ mass effect (if large) ▶ rebleeding (50% will rebleed within 6 months)

Treatment

- Surgical clipping or endovascular coiling (debate exists regarding the risk–benefit of treating an anterior circulation aneurysm <7 mm in a patient without a prior SAH)

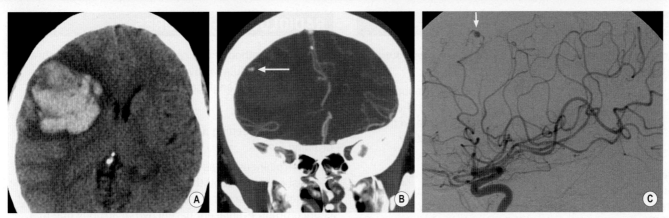

Mycotic aneurysm. (A) CT of a patient with infective endocarditis shows an acute right frontal intraparenchymal haemorrhage. (B) Coronal MIP from a CTA shows pooling of contrast at the periphery of the haematoma, suggesting an aneurysm (arrow). (C) Lateral right ICA arteriogram confirms a peripheral mycotic aneurysm (arrow).*

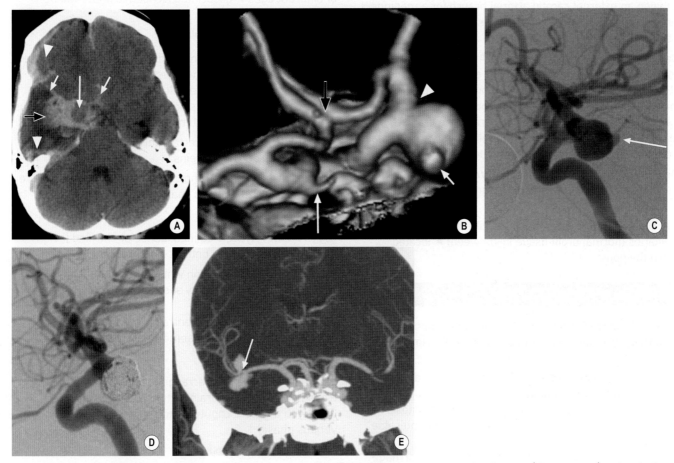

Aneurysms on CTA. (A) CT shows acute subarachnoid blood in interhemispheric and right sylvian fissures (short arrows) and a clot in the right side of the chiasmatic cistern extending into the temporal lobe (black arrow). Within this is a rounded area of lower density, suggesting an aneurysm (long arrow). There is also an acute right subdural haematoma (arrowheads). (B) CTA viewed from above, behind and the left shows a large right distal ICA aneurysm arising at the level of the posterior communicating artery (not visible as anatomically hypoplastic). The neck is clearly shown (arrowhead) and there is a small lobule (short arrow) on the fundus possibly indicating the site of rupture. Note the left posterior communicating (long arrow) and anterior communicating arteries (black arrow). The decision to treat by endovascular coiling was based on this examination. (C, D) Lateral right ICA arteriograms from coiling procedure, immediately before and after occlusion of the aneurysm. Note confirmation of aneurysm anatomy as shown on CTA, including terminal lobule (arrow). (E) Coronal MIP from CTA in a different patient with a complex right middle cerebral artery aneurysm. Note the anatomical detail of separate lobules and artery arising from the neck of the superior aneurysm (arrow).*

ARTERIOVENOUS MALFORMATIONS

DEFINITION

An abnormal collection of arteries and veins without a normal intervening capillary bed

- *Arteriovenous shunting present:* cerebral (or subpial) arteriovenous malformation (AVM) ▶ dural fistula
- *Arteriovenous shunting absent:* developmental venous anomaly (DVA) ▶ cavernous angioma ▶ capillary telangiectasia

Cerebral (subpial) AVM Probably a congenital anomaly consisting of a direct arteriovenous shunt without a normal intervening capillary bed ▶ some are essentially fistulous ▶ 80% are parenchymal and 10% are dural in location ▶ supplied by branches of the internal carotid artery or vertebrobasilar system

Dural arteriovenous fistulae An acquired direct shunt between an external carotid arterial branch (or a meningeal cerebral arterial branch) and a dural sinus ▶ it may be the result of a prior venous thrombosis

Cavernous angioma (cavernoma) A mulberry-like lesion consisting of multiple vascular spaces (with little intervening normal brain) and haemorrhage of different ages ▶ 80% are supratentorial and multiple (they are occasionally intraventricular or can arise on a cranial nerve) ▶ previous bleed/infratentorial location are the main prognostic factors for recurrent haemorrhage

Developmental venous anomaly (DVA) This is not a malformation and represents a benign variation in venous drainage

Capillary telangiectasia Benign nests of dilated capillaries (normal brain tissue in-between) ▶ located within the pons

CLINICAL PRESENTATION

Cerebral (subpial) AVM Cerebral haemorrhage (commonest) ▶ epilepsy ▶ headache ▶ focal neurological deficit

Dural arteriovenous fistulae The presentation depends upon the location and venous drainage pattern
- *Lesions shunting into the cavernous sinus:* proptosis
- *Shunting into the transverse or sigmoid sinus:* pulsatile tinnitus
- *Reflux into the cortical veins:* intracranial haemorrhage

Cavernous angioma Epilepsy ▶ often an incidental finding

DVA Asymptomatic ▶ commonly seen near a frontal horn

Capillary telangiectasia Asymptomatic

RADIOLOGICAL FEATURES

DSA The method of choice for investigating a cerebral AVM or dural fistula (a cavernous angioma and a telangiectasia are angiographically occult)

Cerebral AVM

DSA Dilated feeding arteries ▶ early opacification of the draining veins

CT Serpiginous areas of high density (with marked contrast enhancement) that may be calcified ▶ surrounding low attenuation areas of ischaemic damage ▶ mass effect is uncommon ▶ adjacent parenchymal atrophy due to a 'vascular steal' phenomenon

MRI Serpiginous areas of mixed SI ▶ areas of flow void and high SI (thrombosis) ▶ areas of haemorrhage of different ages ▶ associated ischaemic areas will be hyperintense (T2WI)

Dural arteriovenous fistulae

DSA Required for a definitive diagnosis ▶ there may be associated aneurysms or venous varices or stenoses
- Increased haemorrhage risk in the presence of an intranidal aneurysm, a single draining vein, deep venous drainage or a venous stenosis

CT/MRI It may go undetected unless there are enlarged dural sinuses or cortical veins

CTA/MRA These may show any abnormal vessels more clearly ▶ it currently lacks spatial resolution

Cavernous angioma

CT A relatively well-defined, dense or calcified lesion demonstrating patchy contrast enhancement

MRI A multilobular lesion which may be multiple ▶ gradient-echo susceptibility sequences are the most sensitive
- *'Popcorn' appearance:* central mixed signal intensity surrounded by a dark haemosiderin rim

DVA

DSA/CT/MRI Radially arranged and dilated transmedullary veins draining into a large transcortical vein (with a typical 'caput medusa' appearance during the venous phase)

Capillary telangiectasia

MRI Occasionally visible as areas of very subtle T2WI high SI ▶ they demonstrate ill-defined enhancement with no associated haemorrhage

PEARLS

- *Cerebral AVM treatment options:* surgery/radiosurgery/ endovascular embolization

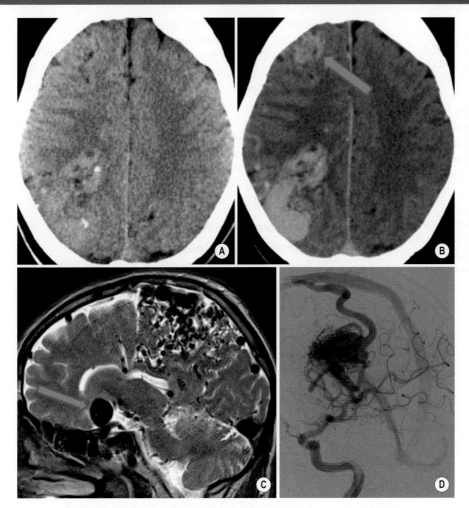

CT in a young female patient who presented with a seizure. (A) Unenhanced study shows lobulated hyperdensity with focal areas of calcification. (B) Following contrast administration there is avid enhancement in two distinct areas of the right frontal and parietal lobes. The appearances are typical of an AVM. Multiple AVMs suggest hereditary haemorrhagic telangiectasia (HHT). In this case there was no parenchymal haemorrhage. (C) MRI in a different patient shows a diffuse parietal AVM with large superficial draining veins. Note the large flow aneurysm related to the terminal ICA (arrow). (D) DSA shows an AVM with a compact nidus. It is supplied by branches of the middle cerebral artery and drains via both the superficial and deep venous systems.**

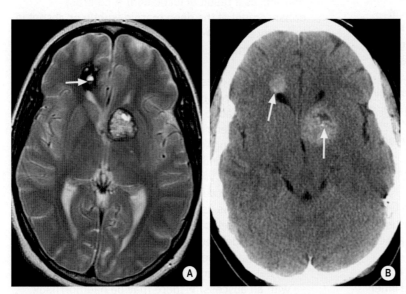

Cavernous haemangioma. (A) T2WI showing typical mixed SI lesions. High SI is due to methaemoglobin and the low SI rim of haemosiderin indicates an old haemorrhage. The 'popcorn' appearance of the larger lesion is typical of a 'cavernoma'. Note the blood–fluid level in the smaller lesion (arrow). (B) NECT of the same patient shows the lesions to be predominantly high density with tiny foci of calcification (arrows).

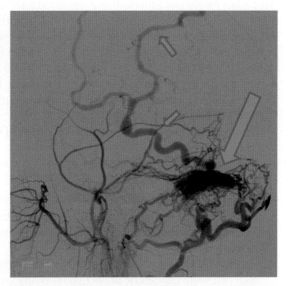

DSA injection of the external carotid circulation shows a fistulous connection between ECA branches (occipital and meningeal) with an isolated transverse sinus (long arrow). There is retrograde venous drainage via a hypotrophied vein of Labbé and the vein of Trolard (short arrows) into the superior sagittal sinus.**

BRAIN ABSCESS

Definition

- A focal encapsulated pus-containing cavity ▶ in immunocompetent patients it is usually due to a streptococcal bacterial infection (multiple in 10–50%)
  - It usually arises by haematogenous dissemination ▶ it can also occur following penetrating trauma or due to direct spread from a contiguous infection
  - *Fungal cerebral abscesses:* these typically affect immunocompromised patients ▶ they are similar to a pyogenic abscess but are more likely to demonstrate areas of haemorrhage
- The abscess site depends on the cause:
  - *Frontal sinusitis:* adjacent frontal lobe abscess
  - *Mastoiditis:* temporal lobe or cerebellar abscess
  - *Blood-borne infection:* a predilection for the middle cerebral arterial territory (particularly the frontoparietal region)

Clinical presentation

- Fever ▶ headache ▶ a focal neurological deficit

Radiological features

- Abscesses are frequently subcortical or periventricular
- 4 stages: early and late cerebritis, early and late capsule formation
- A rim-enhancing mass is a non-specific finding and may be mimicked by a metastasis, a glioblastoma, a resolving haematoma, or a subacute infarct
  - A thick irregular rind of enhancement is more suggestive of tumour

CT There is central low attenuation pus or necrotic debris but rarely gas (unless there has been a surgical intervention or a gas-forming organism is present) ▶ following IV contrast medium administration the ring of enhancement corresponds to the abscess capsule (and is surrounded by low attenuation vasogenic oedema)

- The enhancing rim typically has a smooth inner margin with thinning of its medial aspect (as the white matter is perfused less than the grey matter)
- The abscess centre never enhances on delayed images (cf. cerebritis)
- The degree of enhancement is diminished in immunocompromised patients

MRI A similar pattern of rim enhancement as with CT

- *Abscess centre:* high DWI/low ADC (pus) ▶ restricted diffusion techniques are unable to distinguish an abscess from a tumour
- *Susceptibility-weighted imaging:* very low SI rim ▶ 'dual rim' sign: concentric outer hypointensity and inner hyperintensity
- *Dynamic contrast-enhanced perfusion MRI:* abscesses have a lower relative cerebral blood volume within their enhancing rim than a glioma

- *Resolution post treatment:* this is indicated by resolution of any rim enhancement or disappearance of the low SI rim (T2WI) ▶ a low SI on DWI correlates with a good clinical response (increasing SI implies pus reaccumulation)

Pearls

- A rim-enhancing mass is a nonspecific finding and may be mimicked by a metastasis, a glioblastoma, a resolving haematoma or a subacute infarct
  - A thick irregular rind of enhancement is more suggestive of tumour

Other intracranial infections

- *Intracranial epidural abscess:*
  - A collection of pus between the skull inner table and skull endosteum ▶ usually direct spread from contiguous infection (e.g. sinusitis) ▶ slow growing
  - CT / MRI: lentiform collection of fluid constrained by the dura at the sutures ▶ can cross the midline (cf. subdural empyemas which do not) ▶ the dura at the deep margin shows thick and irregular enhancement ▶ internal pus can show restricted diffusion
- *Subdural empyema:*
  - A collection of pus in the potential space between the inner layer of the dura mater and the arachnoid mater ▶ most common predisposing causes: sinusitis/otogenic infection
  - CT/ MRI: crescentic fluid collection overlying the cerebral convexity or in the interhemispheric fissure along the falx cerebri (irregular and scalloped margins as a result of loculation) ▶ contrast enhancement at the deep margin (subtle or absent in the early stages) ▶ adjacent brain can show oedema ± enhancement
- *Ventriculitis:*
  - Uncommon ▶ causes: trauma/intraventricular abscess rupture/shunt infection/haematogenous infection spread to the ependymal or choroid plexus
  - CT/MRI: intraventricular debris (slightly hyperattenuating with restricted diffusion) ▶ periventricular and subependymal high SI ▶ enhancement of ventricular margins
  - **Cerebritis:** a focal infection without a capsule or pus formation ▶ it is usually pyogenic in origin and can resolve or develop into a frank abscess
    - **CT:** an ill defined area of low attenuation with thick ring enhancement that may progress centrally on delayed images (cf. no central enhancement with an abscess) ▶ there may be haemorrhagic transformation

	Abscess centre*	Abscess rim	Surrounding vasogenic oedema
T1WI	SI between CSF and white matter	Slightly higher SI than white matter	Low SI
T2WI	SI similar or slightly higher than CSF	Relatively low SI	High SI

*DWI: high SI (due to restricted diffusion within the viscous pus) ▶ ADC map: low SI

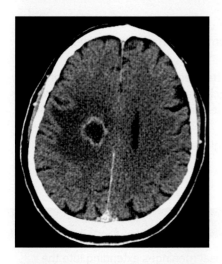

Cerebral abscess. CT: low attenuation central abscess cavity surrounded by an enhancing rim and white matter vasogenic oedema. The medial aspect of the enhancing rim is subtly thinned.*

Subdural empyema. Coronal T1WI + Gad shows the empyema is loculated and also extends along the right tentorial leaflet.*

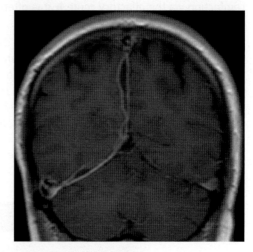

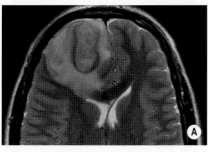
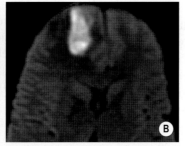

Streptococcal abscess due to penetrating trauma. (A) Axial T2WI. Note low signal of the abscess capsule and extensive high signal perilesional oedema. (B) DWI shows high signal in the abscess centre, indicating restricted diffusion.*

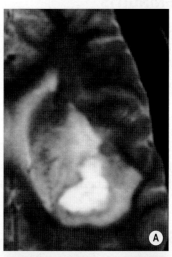

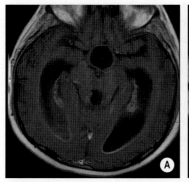
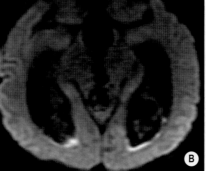

Ventriculitis. (A) Subependymal enhancement, most marked posteriorly, extends along the margins of the dilated ventricles. (B) DWI shows restricted diffusion as high SI.*

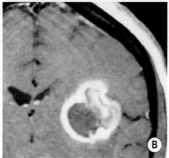

Fungal abscess. (A) Axial T2WI. Central high SI abscess cavity with surrounding vasogenic oedema. (B) Coronal T1WI + Gad. Large multiloculated abscess cavity with enhancement of the capsule and abscess wall. Note relative thinness of the medial wall compared with the thicker, more irregular, lateral component.*

ENCEPHALITIS

Herpes encephalitis

Definition Diffuse inflammation of the brain parenchyma caused by the herpes simplex virus

Adult

Definition This is due to the reactivation of latent herpes simplex (type 1) within the trigeminal ganglion or by reinfection via the olfactory route ▶ it is often fatal without treatment

CT Abnormalities usually visible within 3 days ▶ this is followed by low attenuation within the anteromedial temporal lobe (± involvement of the insula or the orbital surface of the frontal lobe) ▶ haemorrhage is not usually prominent and is a late feature ▶ there can be patchy or gyriform enhancement ▶ initially unilateral, progressing to bilateral

- *Perfusion CT:* this is increased during the acute phase

MRI T2WI/FLAIR: there is high SI within the antero-medial temporal lobe within 2 days of onset ▶ the abnormal SI is mainly cortical (with secondary subjacent white matter involvement) ▶ it is more sensitive than CT for detecting haemorrhagic foci (particularly with T2* or SWI)

- **DWI:** cortical high SI

Neonate

Definition Intrapartum infection with the herpes simplex virus (type 2)

CT Patchy white matter oedema ▶ cortical areas of increased density (which are not limited to the temporal lobes) ▶ there can be lesion progression to a multicystic encephalomalacia

MRI T2WI: low SI regions

MENINGITIS

PYOGENIC MENINGITIS

Definition Bacterial infectious inflammatory infiltration of the leptomeninges ▶ common causes in adults are *S. pneumoniae* and *N. meningitidis*

CT This is usually normal in uncomplicated pyogenic meningitis ▶ CT is useful for detecting any complications (e.g. hydrocephalus, a subdural empyema, an abscess or a cerebral infarction)

MRI FLAIR: high SI (this is non-specific and can also be seen with SAH and leptomeningeal metastases) ▶ FLAIR + Gad: meningeal enhancement (this may be more sensitive than T1WI + Gad)

TUBERCULOSIS

Definition CNS involvement is seen in 5% of cases (predominantly affecting patients <20 years old) ▶ tuberculous meningitis is the most frequent manifestation (involving the basal leptomeninges)

- A tuberculoma can also develop (usually at the corticomedullary junction) ▶ a tuberculous abscess is a rare finding

Tuberculous meningitis

CT There is obliteration of the basal cisterns by isodense or slightly hyperdense exudates ▶ there is avid enhancement of the basal meninges extending into the ambient, sylvian, pontine and chiasmatic cisterns

- This meningeal exudate obstructs CSF resorption and causes a communicating hydrocephalus ▶ meningeal calcification is rarely seen with healing
- An arteritis of the penetrating arteries at the base of brain can lead to infarctions of the basal ganglia and internal capsule

MRI This is more sensitive than CT for the above signs

- *Differential:* fungal meningitis ▶ neurosarcoid ▶ carcinomatous meningitis

Tuberculoma (parenchymal granuloma)

CT A small rounded lesion which is isodense or hypodense to brain ▶ there is variable surrounding oedema ▶ there is homogeneous enhancement (with solid lesions) or rim enhancement (with central caseation or liquefaction) ▶ lesions rarely calcify with healing ▶ brainstem involvement is uncommon

- The 'target sign' of central high attenuation with rim enhancement is not pathognomonic for a tuberculoma

MRI T1WI: low SI ▶ T2WI: high SI (but low SI with caseation) ▶ T1WI + Gad: solid lesions demonstrate homogeneous enhancement ▶ ring enhancement is seen with caseation

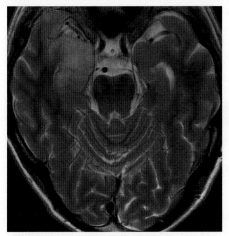

Herpes simplex encephalitis. Axial T2WI shows swelling and high SI in the anteromedial right temporal lobe with normal appearance on the left.*

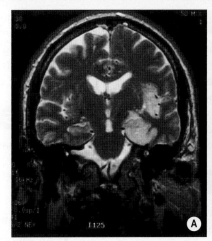 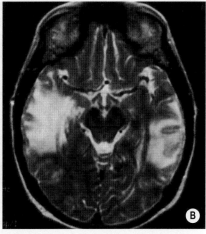

(A) Herpes encephalitis. Coronal T2WI shows swelling of the left temporal lobe with sparing of the basal ganglia. (B) T2WI demonstrating bilateral disease.*

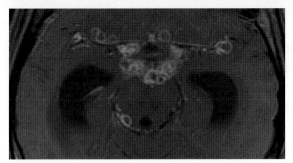

Tuberculous meningitis. T1WI + Gad shows basilar meningeal enhancement, and multiple ring-enhancing tuberculomas in the suprasellar and ambient cisterns and the medial sylvian fissures. Marked dilatation of the temporal horns indicates hydrocephalus.*

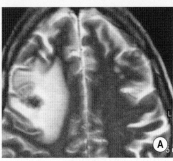

Axial T2WI image (A) showing a low SI caseating tuberculous granuloma in the right frontal lobe in association with vasogenic oedema. The lesion is situated at the grey–white matter junction and on the T1WI + Gad image (B) it has a multiloculated ring-enhancing appearance.†

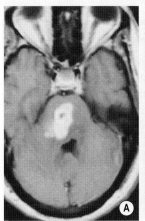 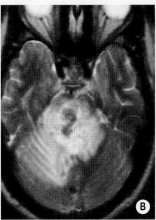 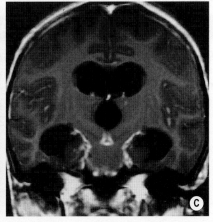

An irregular enhancing tuberculoma is shown within the pons on the postcontrast axial T1-weighted MR image. (A) The lesion is of relatively low signal on the T2 axial image (B) and there is extensive vasogenic oedema and some modest mass effect with distortion of the 4th ventricle. On the coronal T1 postcontrast image (C) there is nodular meningeal thickening and enhancement around the brainstem and cerebellum.†

765

ACUTE DISSEMINATED ENCEPHALOMYELITIS (ADEM)

DEFINITION

- Usually a monophasic demyelinating disorder occurring after vaccination or a viral illness ▶ predominantly affects brain white matter and spinal cord
- A fulminant course results in encephalopathy and focal neurological deficits ▶ usually 7–14 days between febrile illness and neurology ▶ it usually resolves without long-term sequelae ▶ children > adults, M=F

RADIOLOGICAL FEATURES

MRI Multiple large, patchy and poorly marginated lesions ▶ usually asymmetrical involvement of subcortical and central white matter and cortical grey–white junction of cerebral hemispheres, cerebellum, brainstem and spinal cord ▶ symmetrical involvement thalami grey matter and basal ganglia ▶ spinal cord lesions tend to be large ± enhancement

- T2WI: high SI ▶ T1WI + Gad: variable enhancement
- *Differential*: a viral encephalitis will be more cortically based ▶ a vasculitis will demonstrate restricted diffusion

PEARLS

- ADEM has similar imaging appearances to MS – however, ADEM is less likely to be periventricular (MS also rarely affects the thalami and is polyphasic in nature)

Acute haemorrhagic leukoencephalopathy

- An aggressive ADEM variant (which is often fatal within 1 week) ▶ it has similar appearances to ADEM but there is more oedema, mass effect and small haemorrhages are present

PARASITIC INFECTION – NEUROCYSTICERCOSIS

Cysticerci

- Caused by the encysted larvae of the tapeworm *Taenia solium* ▶ they are commonly located at the corticomedullary junction
- **Vesicular stage:** a live parasite incites little perilesional oedema ▶ there is minimal enhancement
  - The cyst is of similar SI to CSF ▶ the scolex is of similar SI to white matter
- **Colloidal vesicular stage:** the larva dies inciting an immune response ▶ lesions now show ring enhancement with surrounding oedema ▶ increasing proteinaceous cyst contents increase T1WI signal
- **Granular nodular stage:** as the larva dies, the cyst collapses with a marked host response, thick enhancing cyst walls and progression of oedema

- **Nodular calcified stage:** non-active form ▶ small calcified lesions (2–10 mm) ▶ mild oedema/enhancement

Intraventricular cysticercosis

- 3rd/4th ventricles > lateral ventricles ▶ intraventricular cysts can cause obstruction and hydrocephalus

Subarachnoid cysticercosis

- Basal cisterns/sylvian fissures/cerebellopontine angle

Racemose form

- Multilobular cysts located within the subarachnoid space (typically within the cerebellopontine angles, suprasellar region, basal cisterns and sylvian fissures)
- Can enhance and coexist with a leptomeningitis
- 'Bunch of grapes': clustered cysts separated by septae

PARASITIC INFECTION – HYDATID CYSTS

DEFINITION

- **Cystic echinococcosis**: large, isolated, unilocular, well-defined thin walled cysts ± daughter cysts
- **Alveolar echinococcosis**: numerous irregular small cysts ▶ heterogeneous nodular, cauliflower enhancement

RADIOLOGICAL FEATURES

CT/MRI A well-defined spherical lesion with the attenuation and signal characteristics of CSF ▶ enhancement and perilesional oedema only occurs if the cyst is superinfected ▶ calcification occurs late (cyst death)

- T2WI: there is a low SI cyst wall

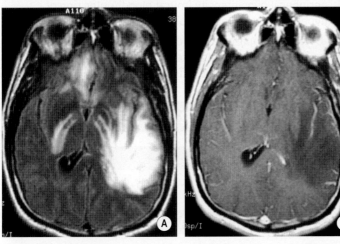
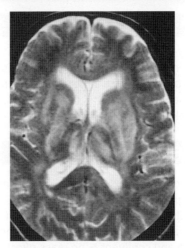

ADEM. (A) FLAIR image demonstrating high SI within the right frontal, internal capsule and left temporal regions. (B) T1WI + Gad: There is significant mass effect but no enhancement.[+]

Multiple T2 high SI lesions in the basal ganglia, thalami, internal capsules and periventricular white matter are present in this patient with ADEM.[†]

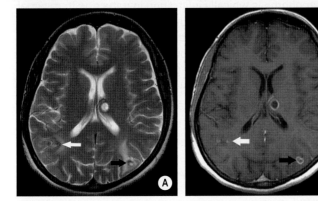
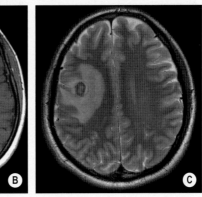
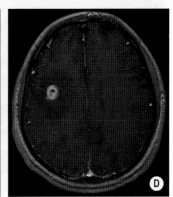

Neurocysticercosis. T2 image (A) and contrast-enhanced T1 image (B) showing the vesicular stage (lesion in the left lateral ventricle), colloidal vesicular stage (black arrows) and calcified nodular stage (white arrows) of cysticercosis. T2 image (C) and enhanced T1 image (D) demonstrating the granular nodular stage with a partially collapsed cyst associated with marked immune reaction from the host evidenced by a thick enhancing wall and marked surrounding oedema.[**]

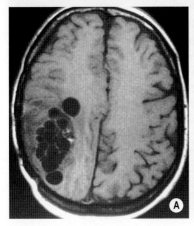
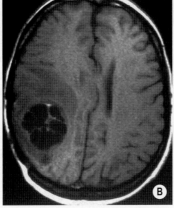
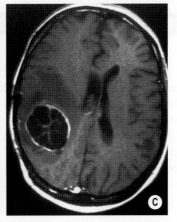

Echinococcus (hydatid). Non-enhanced T1 (A, B) show multiple well-defined cysts corresponding to a hydatid cyst with multiple daughter cysts. There is also some associated oedema which appears hypointense. The contrast-enhanced T1 (C) demonstrates a thin outer rim of enhancement, which together with the oedema indicates that this is an active hydatid cyst.[**]

HIV ENCEPHALOPATHY

DEFINITION

- HIV encephalopathy (HIV-associated dementia) can lead to myelin loss, macrophage infiltration and gliosis ▶ affected patients present with a subcortical dementia (10–20% of AIDS cases)
- Increased stroke risk (ischaemic > haemorrhagic)

RADIOLOGICAL FEATURES

CT/MRI Cerebral atrophy (the extent of the volume loss correlates with the cognitive impairment)
- *White matter:* low attenuation lesions located within the centrum semiovale and periventricular regions ▶ they may become diffuse and confluent ▶ no mass effect ▶ no enhancement
- T2WI: high SI lesions

MRI High SI lesions (T2W1) ▶ lesions can be ill defined, diffuse and symmetrical, or patchy and scattered – involvement of the deep grey matter is also seen

MR spectroscopy Decreased N-acetylaspartate levels (neuronal loss) ▶ increased choline levels (increased membrane turnover)

PET/SPECT Hypermetabolism within the basal ganglia and thalami ▶ cortical hypermetabolism in advanced cases

CEREBRAL TOXOPLASMOSIS

DEFINITION

- This is caused by reactivation of a latent infection with *Toxoplasma gondii* ▶ characterized by a mutifocal haemorrhagic necrotizing encephalitis with organizing abscesses ▶ it can appear similar to a primary CNS lymphoma ▶ diagnosis is usually made by the response to empirical treatment
- It is the commonest (and most treatable) cause of a cerebral mass lesion in an AIDS patient

RADIOLOGICAL FEATURES

CT/MRI Multiple lesions (1–4 cm) located at the corticomedullary junction or within the basal ganglia (single lesions within the brainstem or cerebellum are uncommon)
- Ring or nodular enhancement with associated oedema and mass effect (diminished enhancement in severely immunocompromised patients) ▶ enhancement can be absent if the patient is severely immunocompromised
- Treated lesions may calcify

T2WI *'Target' sign:* central hyperintensity (fluid)/peripheral hypointensity (mural blood)/outer ring of hyperintense perilesional oedema

DWI In comparison with a pyogenic abscess, cerebral toxoplasmosis demonstrates low SI to white matter (indicating no restricted diffusion)

PRIMARY CEREBRAL LYMPHOMA

DEFINITION

- Usually a high-grade B-cell non-Hodgkin's lymphoma

RADIOLOGICAL FEATURES

- The tumour is usually multifocal and located deep within the paramedian cerebral hemispheres (typically within the periventricular cerebral white matter, corpus callosum and basal ganglia) ▶ the thalami and hypothalamus can also be affected
- Lesions usually abut the ependyma or leptomeninges
- Lymphoma is typically infiltrating in nature, with minimal mass effect and peritumoural oedema ▶ it can cross anatomic boundaries and also midline structures (infiltration across the corpus callosum can mimic the appearances of a butterfly glioma)

NECT A well-defined round or oval high attenuation lesion (due to its dense cellularity) ▶ calcification is only seen post treatment

MRI Little mass effect or oedema for its size ▶ haemorrhage is unusual
- T2WI: a lower SI than grey matter (due to its dense cellularity)
- T1WI + Gad: smooth or nodular ring enhancement surrounding a zone of central necrosis (solid enhancement is seen in immunocompetent patients)
- DWI: this is of limited value in distinguishing lymphoma from toxoplasmosis

PEARLS

- Metastases from a systemic lymphoma typically involve the meninges (parenchymal disease without leptomeningeal involvement is rare)
- Features favouring a diagnosis of lymphoma over toxoplasmosis: a periventricular location ▶ a *single* enhancing mass ▶ a large lesion ▶ callosal involvement ▶ a lesion with a central low T2W SI ▶ subependymal spread
- Lymphoma may respond dramatically to radiotherapy (± corticosteroids) but it is usually associated with a poor prognosis

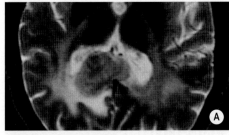
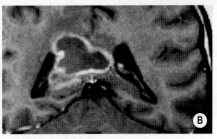

Primary cerebral lymphoma involvement of the corpus callosum. Axial T2WI (A) and coronal T1WI + Gad (B). Lymphomatous masses may involve the corpus callosum, as in this patient who had multifocal primary cerebral lymphoma. Rim enhancement of the mass is seen.*

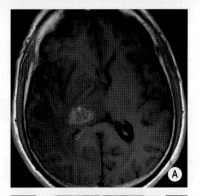

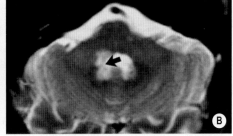
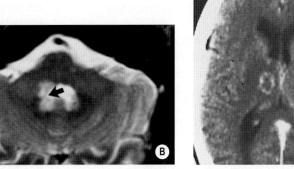

Multifocal primary cerebral lymphoma. Transverse T2WI. Multiple masses, most of which show mixed SI on T2WI, are present. Like multiple toxoplasmosis, they involve the basal ganglia. However, subependymal tumour spread is clearly seen around the lateral and the 4th ventricles (arrows), which favours the diagnosis of lymphoma.*

Enhancement in toxoplasmosis. (A) T1WI + Gad. Toxoplasma abscess in the right thalamus shows extensive surrounding vasogenic oedema and irregular peripheral enhancement. (B) CT demonstrating multiple ring-enhancing abscesses.*,†

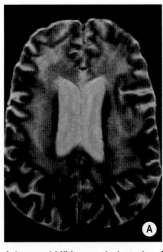
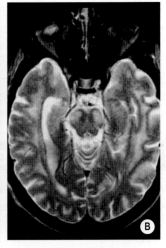

Advanced HIV encephalopathy. Axial T2WI. There is diffuse confluent and symmetrical abnormal high signal returned from the white matter of the cerebral hemispheres (A), which is also extending into the brainstem to involve the cerebral peduncles (B). In this patient there is also generalized atrophy. Features that help to differentiate HIV from PML are the symmetry of the changes and the lack of signal abnormalities on T1WI.*

Differentiating between lymphoma and toxoplasmosis in HIV patients		
	Lymphoma	**Toxoplasmosis**
Hyperdense on NECT	Yes	No
T2WI	Isointense (50%)	Hyperintense
Periventricular	50%	3%
Subependymal	40%	0%
Basal ganglia involvement	Uncommon	Common
Haemorrhage	Rare	More common (especially after treatment)
²⁰¹Thallium SPECT	Positive	Negative
MR perfusion	Increased	Decreased
MRS	Increased choline ► low NAA	Increased lactate
Steroid treatment	Sensitive	Not sensitive
*Unreliable in distinguishing lesions <2 cm		

CRYPTOCOCCOSIS

DEFINITION

- This is the 2nd commonest opportunistic CNS infection

CLINICAL PRESENTATION

- Headache ▶ fever ▶ an altered mental state

RADIOLOGICAL FEATURES

MRI The earliest imaging manifestation is dilatation of the perivascular spaces (this is usually seen within the basal ganglia but can also be seen within the brainstem and cerebral white matter)

- *'Gelatinous pseudocysts'*: these spaces are distended by mucoid material, organisms and inflammatory material which appears as multiple foci of high SI on T2WI ▶ with disease progression cryptococcomas can develop at these sites
- *Cryptococcoma*: these are 3 mm to several cm in size ▶ they lack surrounding oedema and there is no restricted diffusion
  - T1WI: low-to-intermediate SI ▶ T2WI: high SI
  - T1WI + Gad: lesions rarely enhance as the patient is usually severely immunocompromised

PEARL

Immune reconstitution inflammatory syndrome (IRIS): a paradoxical clinical deterioration attributable to immune recovery following antiretroviral therapy

- **CT/MRI**: transient increase in parenchymal signal (FLAIR/T2) ▶ hypoattenuation on CT + contrast enhancement

PROGRESSIVE MULTIFOCAL LEUKOENCEPHALOPATHY (PML)

DEFINITION

- A central demyelinating disease resulting from reactivation of a latent oligodendrocyte infection with a JC polyomavirus (seen in 4–5% of AIDS cases) ▶ it commonly affects the parieto-occipital regions and pathologically there is demyelination and astrocytosis

CLINICAL PRESENTATION

- Limb weakness with an insidious onset ▶ visual field defects ▶ speech abnormalities ▶ ataxia and dementia

RADIOLOGICAL FEATURES

MRI Multifocal, bilateral (but asymmetric) white matter lesions ▶ there is rarely mild mass effect and peripheral enhancement ▶ apparent basal ganglia involvement can

result from lesions affecting the white matter tracts that course through this region

- T1WI: low SI ▶ T2WI: high SI
- *'Scalloped' appearance*: this is due to extension to the subcortical U-fibres
- DWI: characteristic peripheral hyperintense rim

OTHER CNS INFECTIONS

Tuberculosis

- This is usually seen amongst IV drug abusers with similar radiological manifestations to those seen in immunocompetent patients (although tuberculomas and abscesses are more frequent with HIV infection)

Candidiasis

- CNS involvement is rare ▶ haematogenous dissemination results in meningitis (± cerebral abscesses) ▶ these demonstrate non-specific imaging appearances

Herpes viruses

- This can cause an encephalitis, necrotizing ventriculitis or myelitis
  - *Encephalitis:* imaging may be normal, but may also demonstrate non-specific white matter or focal enhancing lesions
  - *Ventriculitis:* ependymal enhancement
  - *Myelitis:* non-specific swelling and signal changes within the spinal cord

Neurosyphilis

- Meningovascular disease causes a small vessel endarteritis (with associated basal ganglia infarction) ▶ this appears as segmental 'beading' on angiography

MRI The rare cerebral gummas (typically arising from the meninges) appear as mass lesions with variable signal characteristics and enhancement

SPINAL CORD DISORDERS

AIDS-associated vacuolar myelopathy

- There is an insidious presentation progressing to a severe paraparesis (commonly affecting the thoracic cord)

MRI This is usually normal or demonstrates nonspecific changes (e.g. diffuse symmetrical cord signal abnormalities)

Primary HIV myelitis

- This is rare and presents acutely with a paraparesis and a sensory level

MRI Multifocal asymmetrical cord signal change

Other diseases affecting the spinal cord in AIDS

- Herpes virus infection ▶ toxoplasmosis ▶ tuberculosis

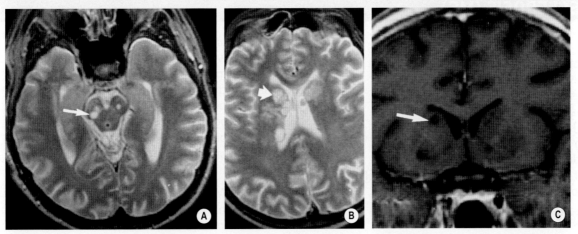

Cryptococcomas. Axial T2WI (A, B) and coronal T1WI (C). Expanded Virchow–Robin spaces (arrow) of high SI on T2 and low SI on T1 are seen in the brainstem and the basal ganglia, so that the ganglia look like 'Swiss cheese'.*

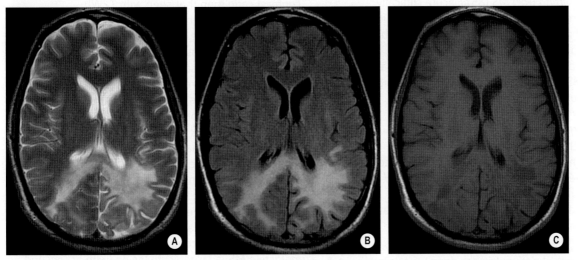

Progressive multifocal leukoencephalopathy. Axial T2WI (A), FLAIR (B) and T1WI (C). Asymmetrical signal abnormalities in the parieto-occipital white matter of both hemispheres extend to the subcortical U-fibres. There is no mass effect associated with the lesions.*

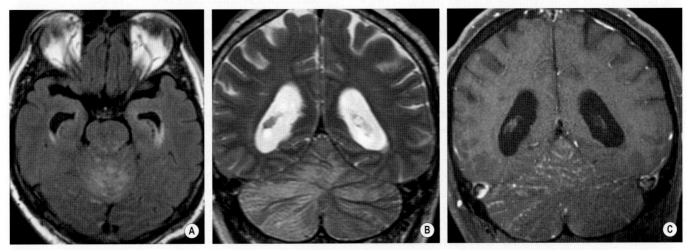

Crypotcoccus neoformans meningitis and cerebellitis in a renal transplant recipient. (A) Axial FLAIR images show high signal intensity of the subarachnoid spaces in the region of the cerebellar vermis. (B) High signal in the cerebellum on both sides was demonstrated on the coronal T2 MR image. (C) Strong leptomeningeal enhancement is nicely shown on axial and coronal post-contrast T1 images.**

MULTIPLE SCLEROSIS (MS)

Definition

- A chronic, persistent inflammatory–demyelinating disease of the CNS, characterized by areas of inflammation, demyelination, axonal loss and gliosis
  - Acute plaques (representing perivascular inflammation) progress to chronic plaques (representing demyelination)
- MS is a *clinical* diagnosis requiring evidence of dissemination of lesions in space and time ► the role of imaging is supportive only

Clinical presentation

- **Clinical course**: acute worsening episodes (relapses), gradual progressive deterioration of neurological function, or a combination of both
  - *Relapsing-remitting (RR) MS (85%):* acute clinically isolated syndrome (mono- or multifocal CNS lesion) ► episodes of acute worsening followed by variably complete recovery
  - *Secondary progressive (SP) MS:* after several years, >50% of RR MS cases develop progressive disability with or without relapses or remissions
  - *Primary progressive (PP) MS (10%):* progressive disease with occasional plateaus and relapses
- Predilection for the optic nerves (optic neuritis), brainstem (internuclear ophthalmoparesis), spinal cord (acute transverse myelitis), cerebellum (gait ataxia)/periventricular white matter
- 2F:M ► peak incidence between 25–35 yrs ► men have a later onset with a generally poorer prognosis

Radiological features

MS lesions are commonly located within the subependymal periventricular deep white matter (cf. ischaemic lesions affecting the subcortical white matter) ► they are typically round to ovoid lesions with their long axis perpendicular to the ventricle wall (few mm to >1 cm) ► become confluent as disease progresses

- *Other common sites:* callososeptal interface along the inferior surface of the corpus callosum/cortico-juxtacortical regions/infratentorial regions ► focal involvement of the anterior temporal lobe periventricular white matter is typical for MS
  - Juxtacortical lesions involving the 'U' fibres characteristic in early disease (best seen with FLAIR imaging)
  - Posterior fossa lesions preferentially involve the floor of the 4th ventricle, middle cerebellar peduncles and the brainstem ► most brainstem lesions are contiguous with cisternal or ventricular CSF
- *Spinal cord involvement is common:* single or multiple lesions ► lesions are generally <2 vertebral segments long and aligned along the cord axis (characteristic 'cigar' shape) ► typically occupy the lateral and posterior white matter columns, extending to the central grey matter, and rarely occupying >½ the cord area ► there is a predilection for the cervical cord ► acute lesions can cause mass effect ± enhancement
  - *RR MS:* multifocal lesions
  - *Secondary progressive MS:* diffuse and more extensive lesions ± cord atrophy
  - *PP MS:* cord > brain abnormalities

MRI

- T2WI/FLAIR/PDWI: high SI
  - PDWI/T2WI: this is better for infra-tentorial lesions which tend to occur within the brainstem and middle cerebellar peduncles
  - FLAIR: this is very sensitive for supra-tentorial lesion detection (as it provides an increased lesion-to-CSF contrast ratio than that seen with T2WI)
  - 'Dawson's fingers': these represent inflammation along the axis of the periventricular collecting veins ► characteristic lesions which are perpendicular to the ventricular axis on sagittal FLAIR imaging
- T1WI: 'T1 black holes': representing oedema in acute lesions, which resolves as acute inflammation settles ► chronic black holes more common in severe/progressive disease rather than RR disease ► more common in the supratentorial white matter
- T1WI + Gad: mainly seen during the acute and relapsing stages ► solid or incomplete ring enhancement (with the open border facing the grey matter) of acute lesions which generally resolves within weeks (inactive plaques do not enhance) ► enhancement more common during relapses in RR and secondary progressive MS
- *Tumefactive MS:* a large acute lesion (with associated oedema and mass effect) that may mimic the appearances of a glioma ► its enhancement pattern often forms an incomplete ring
- *Optic neuritis:* high SI within the optic nerve (± swelling) ► intense enhancement in acute disease

Pearls

- Patient disability correlates poorly with the T2WI lesion load – there is an improved correlation with the number of low SI lesions seen on T1WI ('black holes')
  - A better correlation is seen with the brain and spinal cord atrophy that develops later during the disease
- *Differential diagnosis:* ADEM ► a vasculitis (e.g. lupus, anti-phospholipid syndrome, Behçet's disease) ► sarcoidosis ► small vessel ischaemia
- **Tumefactive or pseudotumoral MS:** single or multiple focal lesions that can be difficult to differentiate from a brain tumour ► features distinguishing from a tumour: incomplete ring enhancement (open border facing grey matter)/minimal mass effect

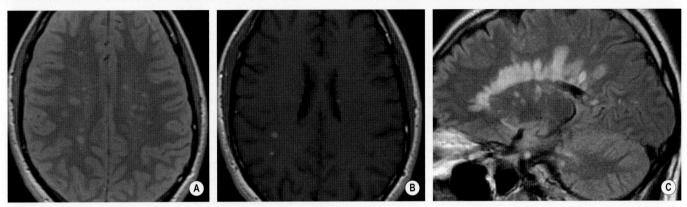

Multiple sclerosis. (A) Axial PD and (B) T1WI + Gad show multiple lesions in the periventricular white matter, two of which are in the acute phase and enhance. (C) Sagittal T2 image in a different patient showing typical 'Dawson's fingers'.*

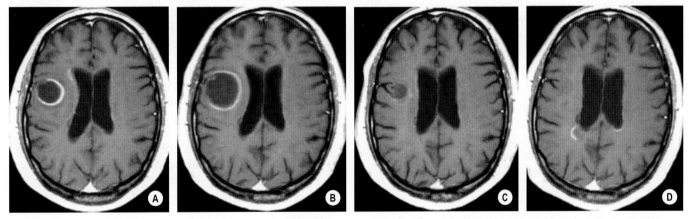

Tumefactive form of relapsing-remitting MS. Contrast-enhanced T1-weighted (A–D) serial MR images of the brain acquired over 12 months in a patient with the relapsing-remitting form of MS. Note the initial increase, and later decrease in size of the right frontal lobe pseudotumoural lesion, which is almost imperceptible on the 12-month imaging. The lesion shows an open ring-enhancing pattern of contrast uptake, with the open margin facing the grey matter. This pseudotumoural lesion was asymptomatic.**

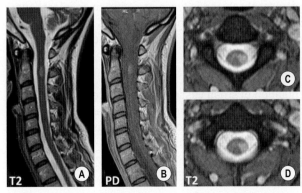

(A–D) Relapsing-remitting MS with plaques in the cervical spinal cord. Sagittal T2 and proton-density and transverse T2 MR images. Observe the small focal lesion that does not exceed two vertebral segments in length and does not affect more than half the cross-sectional area of the cord.**

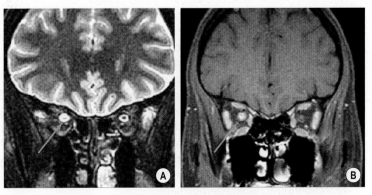

Right optic neuritis. Coronal fat-suppressed T2-weighted fast spin-echo (A) and fat-suppressed contrast-enhanced T1-weighted MR images. There is hyperintensity of the right optic nerve, with diffuse enhancement (arrows) (B).**

OTHER DISEASES

Neurosarcoidosis

- **Definition:** symptomatic CNS involvement is seen in 5% of patients ► no known cure – treatment is supportive ► cranial neuropathy, particularly facial nerve palsy, often multifocal with other neuropathies, is the most common clinical presentation ► commonly presents as meningeal disease but can lead to the appearance of small enhancing granulomas:
  - *Meningeal disease:* plaque-like dural thickening and masses that can mimic a meningioma ► enhancement of the basal and suprasellar meninges ► subependymal granulomatous infiltration that can rarely cause hydrocephalus
  - *Small enhancing granulomas:* these are usually located within the superficial brain parenchyma bordering the basal cisterns (non-enhancing lesions within the periventricular white matter can mimic MS)
  - *Other MRI findings:* T2WI: high SI non-enhancing lesions in the periventricular white matter and brainstem that can mimic MS lesions ► optic nerve enhancement ► intramedullary spinal cord lesions

Behçet's disease

- Multisystemic vascular inflammatory disease affecting larger vessels ► classical triad of oral and genital ulcerations and uveitis ► isolated optic neuritis, aseptic meningitis and intracranial haemorrhage secondary to ruptured aneurysms are rare
- CNS involvement most often occurs as a chronic meningoencephalitis, with typical reversible inflammatory parenchymal lesions located within the brainstem, with occasional extension to the diencephalon or basal ganglia

Systemic lupus erythematosus

- Autoimmune disorder
- Neuropsychiatric systemic lupus erythematosus (NPSLE) is associated with an increased morbidity and mortality, with multifocal micro-infarcts, cortical atrophy, gross infarcts, haemorrhage, ischaemic demyelination and patchy MS-like areas of demyelination
- Can present with psychosis, stroke or epilepsy
- Lupus patients are also at risk for a wide range of CNS events related to immunosuppression (e.g. infection)
- CNS vasculitis ± cerebritis = a severe form of NPSLE
- **MRI:** non-specific small punctate focal lesions in the white matter ► more severe findings: cortical atrophy/ventricular dilatation/cerebral oedema/cerebral infarction/intracranial haemorrhage

TOXIC BRAIN DISORDERS

Ethanol intoxication

- Characteristic distribution of volume loss: initially infratentorial predominance with atrophy of the vermis and cerebellum ► frontal and temporal atrophy subsequently evident, followed by diffuse brain atrophy
  - **Wernicke's encephalopathy:** caused by a deficiency of thiamine (vitamin B₁) ► FLAIR/T2WI: bilateral and symmetrical high SI within the mamillary bodies and thalami ► T1WI: mamillary body haemorrhage is a bad prognostic sign ► T1WI + Gad: marked mamillary body enhancement

Hepatic encephalopathy

- Most cases associated with cirrhosis and portal hypertension or portal-systemic shunts
- T1WI: high SI in the globus pallidum ► T2WI: bilateral symmetric high SI abnormalities involving cortical grey matter – involvement of subcortical white matter and basal ganglia, thalami and midbrain also seen

Osmotic myelinolysis

- **Definition:** precipitous correction of severe hyponatraemia leading to acute demyelination in the pons ► it can also affect extrapontine structures such as the cerebellum, subinsular regions, basal ganglia and thalami
- **MRI:** this is often initially normal
  - T2WI: the later stages can demonstrate swelling and high SI within the basal pons
  - DWI: this is more sensitive in the acute stage with restricted diffusion seen as early as 24 hours

Cocaine

- Most CNS complications are ischaemic and haemorrhagic strokes
- Ischaemic strokes caused by cocaine-induced vasoconstriction and vasculitis/thrombosis
- Bleeding can be localized in the subarachnoid space or be intracerebral, and is twice as common as infarctions ► 50% of patients have underlying AVMs or aneurysms
- Cerebral atrophy (frontal > temporal lobe) associated with chronic use

Ecstasy

- Stimulation of small vessel 5-HT 2A receptors can lead to prolonged vasoconstriction and areas of brain necrosis ► the occipital cortex and globus pallidus are the most vulnerable areas

Opioids (heroin/morphine)

- Acute and chronic effects: neurovascular disorders/leucoencephalopathy (more common with inhalation)/atrophy ► also complications secondary to the addition of additives (e.g. cutting of heroin)
- Ischaemic strokes are the most frequent complication (similar mechanisms to cocaine), often affecting the globus pallidus ► white matter changes from microvascular pathology in chronic abuse

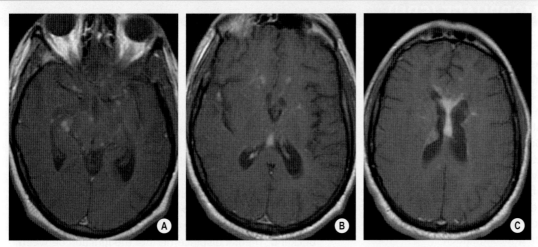

Axial post-contrast-enhanced T1-weighted images of the brain in a 40-year-old woman with neurosarcoidosis demonstrate multiple contrast-enhancing lesions on the leptomenginal surfaces (A), and subependymal lesions (B, C) with slight enlargement of the lateral ventricles (C).**

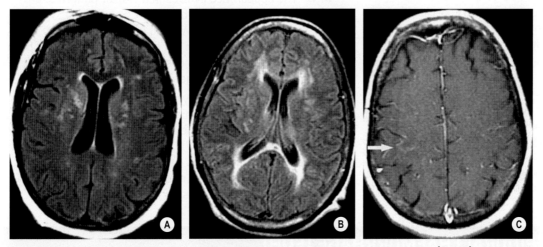

Brain MRI in a 45-year-old woman with SLE. Axial fluid-attenuated inversion recovery (FLAIR) demonstrates small foci of increased signal in the periventricular and deep white matter (A) and more confluent areas of increased signal in the periventricular white matter (B). Axial post-contrast-enhanced image demonstrates diffuse faint pathological contrast enhancement (arrow) in a systemic lupus erythematosus female patient with vasculitis (C).**

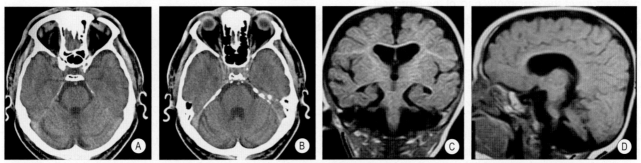

(A, B) CT demonstrates atrophic changes selectively involving the cerebellum in a chronic alcoholic subject. In the initial stages, volume reduction is caused by water loss and brain tissue shrinkage, and is therefore reversible. (C, D) T1-weighted MRI images show global cerebellar hypotrophy in a baby born from an alcoholic. Alcohol inhibits development of Bergmann's fibres and consequently impairs processes of neuroblastic migration and normal cerebellar development.**

SUBDURAL HAEMORRHAGE (SDH)

Definition Traumatic bleeding between the dura mater and arachnoid mater ▶ it usually arises from rupture of the veins crossing the subdural space (vault fractures are an uncommon cause) ▶ often associated with brain damage

- These may be extensive – although the haemorrhage is of low pressure, the blood is unrestricted and can spread over the entire brain surface
  - *Acute:* this can be caused by rupture of a posterior communicating artery aneurysm or a dural arteriovenous fistula bleeding into the subdural space
  - *Chronic:* these are frequently bilateral and occur in elderly patients, alcoholics with underlying brain atrophy, or patients on anticoagulation
  - *Common sites:* over the cerebral convexities ▶ under the temporal and occipital lobes ▶ along the falx cerebri

Clinical presentation It may follow a minor head injury or develop spontaneously

- Increasing confusion or a reduction in conscious level
  - Large bleeds requiring operative evacuation are associated with a reduced conscious level

Radiological features

CT (acute bleed) There can be a characteristic 'comma' shape on axial images (the subdural haematoma extends along the falx cerebri and spreads onto the tentorium)

- Acute lesions are usually hyperdense but become progressively less dense over time – as a rule of thumb it remains denser than brain for 1 week and is less dense after 3 weeks (ending up as CSF density within a few weeks or months)

- An 'isodense subdural' haematoma (occurring at approximately 2 weeks) can be easily missed
- Acute bleeding can be isodense in very anaemic patients

CT (chronic bleed) Chronic subdural collections are usually biconvex and approach CSF density ▶ fluid–fluid levels may be seen (denser blood elements within the dependent regions are due to acute or chronic haemorrhage)

- *Indirect signs:* midline shift (with compression of the ipsilateral ventricle) ▶ contralateral ventricular enlargement ▶ effacement of the cerebral sulci ▶ 'buckling': medial displacement of the junction between the white and grey matter
- Some of these signs can be absent if there are bilateral collections – the frontal horns may then lie close together (with a 'rabbit's ears' configuration)

MRI The appearance evolves in a similar pattern to an intraparenchymal haemorrhage

- There can be low SI (T1WI) and high SI (T2WI) with chronic bleeds (which do not become isointense to CSF due to their high protein content) ▶ repeated bleeding produces variable changes in signal intensity

Pearls The high morbidity (particularly within the elderly) is due to the associated brain swelling, contusion or laceration ▶ dilatation of the contralateral ventricle is a bad prognostic sign

- **Pseudomembrane:** this can form around a chronic subdural haematoma ▶ it may show marked contrast enhancement or haemosiderin staining

EXTRADURAL (EPIDURAL) HAEMORRHAGE (EDH)

Definition

- Traumatic bleeding between the cranial vault and dura mater
- This is often associated with a skull fracture, which is often a fracture of the squamous part of the temporal bone (with an associated injury to the middle meningeal artery)

Radiological features

CT A lenticular biconvex hyperdense area immediately beneath the skull vault which is convex towards both the brain and skull vault

- As the dura mater tends to adhere to the skull, the haematoma will not cross any cranial sutures but may cross a dural reflection (e.g. the falx) ▶ the underlying brain is displaced but often appears intrinsically normal

- The temporoparietal convexity is the commonest site (the haematoma often lies beneath a fractured squamous temporal bone)
- Internal areas of low density may indicate continuing bleeding

Pearl

- **Skull fractures:** compared with vascular markings, skull fractures are straighter, more angulated, more radiolucent and do not have corticated margins
  - *Compound fracture:* a fracture passing through a sinus or air cell is a compound fracture
  - *Depressed fracture:* usually comminuted and compound ▶ risk of post-traumatic epilepsy
  - *Leptomeningeal cyst:* the dura mater underlying a linear fracture is torn – exposure of the remodelling bone to CSF pulsations results in progressive fracture line widening

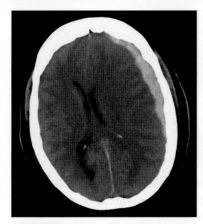

CT. Acute SDH overlying the left cerebral convexity with quite severe mass effect.*

Differentiation between an extradural and subdural haematoma		
	Extradural haematoma	**Subdural haematoma**
Location	Between the skull and dura mater	Between the dura and arachnoid mater
Cause	Trauma (fracture)	Tear of cortical bridging veins
Acute shape	Lenticular biconvex	Crescentic concave
Chronic shape	Crescentic	Elliptical
Crosses suture lines	No	Yes
Crosses a dural reflection	Yes	No

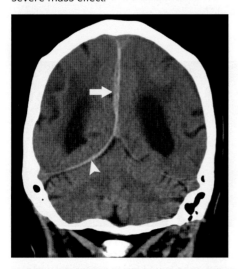

CT: Coronal reformatted image demonstrates a subtle parafalcine subdural haematoma (arrow) with layering over the tentorium cerebelli (arrowhead). Reformatted coronal images are useful for identifying the latter, which may be difficult to identify on axial images.**

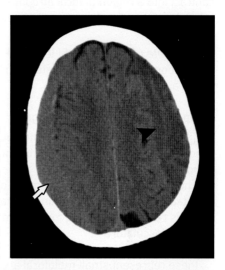

Bilateral subacute haematomas. CT: The subdural haematoma overlying the right cerebral convexity is isodense to brain parenchyma (arrow), and results in mass effect with effacement of the adjacent cortical sulci. The subdural collection overlying the left convexity (arrowhead) is of lower attenuation than brain parenchyma but denser than CSF, and is therefore older than that on the right side.**

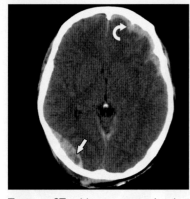

Trauma. CT: a biconvex extradural haematoma overlies the right parieto-occiptal region. Note the central low attenuation (arrow) within the haematoma, indicative of active haemorrhage. A crescent of fresh subdural blood is also seen overlying the left frontal and temporal lobes (curved arrow).**

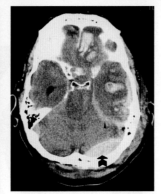

Trauma. CT: A biconvex density of blood over the left cerebellar hemisphere indicates an extradural haematoma (thick arrow). A crescent of fresh subdural blood spreads over the left temporal lobe and tracks along the tentorium in a comma-shaped fashion (arrowhead); this feature differentiates it from an extradural. Typical sites of haemorrhagic contusions are also seen; gyrus recti and temporal lobe.**

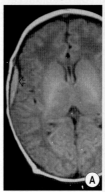
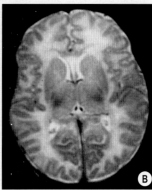

Acute extradural haematoma. MRI in a neonate with traumatic delivery. (A) Axial T1-weighted image (750/16). Slightly hyperintense epidural collection (arrow) in the right temporal region. (B) Axial T2-weighted image (3000/120), epidural collection is hypointense and is invisible except for deformation of the underlying cortex. This is the MR signature of deoxyhaemoglobin.**

PRIMARY CEREBRAL INJURY

Superficial primary cerebral damage

Definition This includes cerebral contusions and cortical lacerations which are usually quite extensive

- The injury mechanism is brain rotation with respect to the skull – it typically involves the inferior frontal lobes and the anterior temporal lobes as the sphenoid ridges and the anterior cranial fossae have irregular margins adjacent to the brain surface
- *'Contrecoup' contusion:* cerebral damage lying diametrically opposite the site of impact (as defined by the skull fracture and scalp haematoma)

CT This is often normal ▶ there can be superficial low-density areas with a mild-to-moderate mass effect – these tend to increase in the initial period and subsequently contract into a region of focal atrophy (± cavitation) ▶ small hyperdense haemorrhages can be present within the early stages

MRI *Acute phase:* mixed SI lesions ▶ *chronic phase:* contraction to regions of persistent (and mainly cortical) cerebral damage

Deep primary cerebral damage

Definition These are less common but have a worse prognosis ▶ they occur more commonly in high-speed accidents

- The injury mechanism is the result of differential rates of rotational acceleration within the brain substance itself – this results in shearing forces damaging the axons and microvasculature
- One may have to rely on so-called 'marker' lesions – these represent small multifocal areas of microvascular damage (with haemorrhage or infarction) and are a reliable guide to the presence of DAI but not its extent
- *Characteristic sites:* the high parasagittal cerebral white matter ▶ the corona radiata ▶ the posterior corpus callosum ▶ the subcortical white matter

CT The lesions are not usually visible ▶ there may be hypodense foci (oedema) or hyperdense foci (petechial haemorrhages)

MRI This is more sensitive (even if a lesion is not haemorrhagic)

- T2WI: multifocal areas of high SI
- T2* imaging: this is more sensitive still (even long after the event) ▶ it will demonstrate small dark patches of haemosiderin with characteristically normal surrounding brain

Diffuse axonal injury (DAI)

Definition This describes larger haemorrhages located within the basal ganglia and elsewhere ▶ they result from a more severe vascular component of the shearing injury and are associated with loss of consciousness at the time of injury

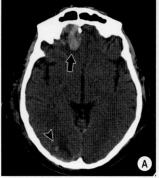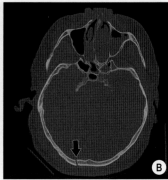

Contrecoup injury. (A) Haemorrhagic 'contrecoup' contusion is demonstrated within the anterior right frontal lobe (arrow). A 'coup' contusion of the occipital lobe resulting from the direct impact is also seen (arrowhead), adjacent to a fracture of the right occipital bone (B, arrow).**

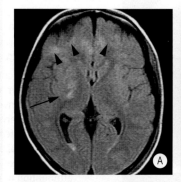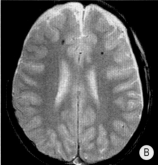

Diffuse axonal injury. (A) FLAIR high SI foci in the posterior limb of internal capsule (arrow) and subcortical white matter (arrowheads). (B) Gradient-echo low SI foci in subcortical white matter indicative of haemorrhages were not evident on other sequences. Note IVH in occipital horns of lateral ventricles.++

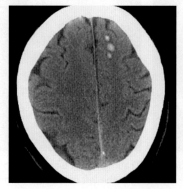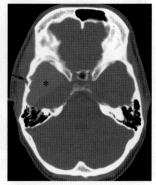

NECT. Shear haemorrhages of diffuse axonal injury in left superior frontal gyrus following blunt head trauma.++

Right middle cranial fossa extra-axial haemorrhage (*) secondary to a fracture through the temporal bone (arrow).

SECONDARY CEREBRAL INJURY

Hyperaemic brain swelling (brain oedema)

Definition Diffuse cerebral swelling occurring 2–3 days after a major head injury ▶ it is caused by an increased cerebral blood volume as a result of abnormal cerebrovascular autoregulation and is a potent cause of raised intracranial pressure

CT/MRI It can be difficult to detect on imaging alone ▶ there may be effacement of the sulci and cisterns with loss of the grey/white matter interface

Cerebral herniation

Definition Herniation of brain from one compartment to another

- *Causes:* intracranial haemorrhage ▶ brain tumours ▶ cerebral oedema following a stroke or anoxic injury

Subfalcine herniation Displacement and impingement of the cingulate gyrus underneath the falx ▶ compression of the ipsilateral lateral ventricle and obstruction of the foramen of Monro with dilatation of the contralateral ventricle ▶ associated with anterior cerebral arterial infarcts

Transtentorial (uncal) herniation Herniation of the medial temporal lobe through the incisura

- **Descending:** the uncus is initially displaced medially and occupies the ipsilateral suprasellar cistern ('uncal' herniation) ▶ eventually the whole medial temporal lobe is displaced through the incisura

  CT/MRI Enlarged ipsilateral and effaced contralateral ambient cisterns ▶ compression of the ipsilateral cerebral peduncle ▶ compression of the contralateral peduncle against the tentorium with ipsilateral motor weakness (a false localizing sign)

  - *Kernohan's notch:* brainstem compression against the contralateral tentorium
  - *Duret haemorrhage:* due to anterior midbrain compression against the contralateral tentorium
  - *Bilateral mass effect:* this can cause bilateral descending herniation with compression of the posterior cerebral artery and oculomotor nerve

- **Ascending:** less common and due to a mass effect within the posterior fossa causing superior displacement of the cerebellum and brainstem through the incisura ▶ associated hydrocephalus due to an obstructed cerebral aqueduct

Tonsillar herniation Downward displacement of the cerebellar tonsils through the foramen magnum and into the spinal canal (>5 mm below the foramen is abnormal) ▶ there can be a 'peg-like' configuration to the tonsils ▶ an obstructive hydrocephalus can result from compression of the 4th ventricle

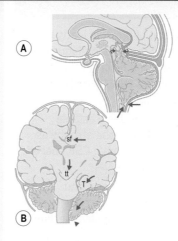

Herniations of the brain. (A) Cerebellar herniation with curved arrows demonstrating upward herniation of the superior cerebellum and superior vermis, with the straight arrows demonstrating tonsillar and inferior vermian herniation. (B) Temporal lobe herniation (T), central transtentorial herniation (tt), tonsillar herniation (arrowhead) and subfalcine herniation (sf). Lines of force are demonstrated by arrows.

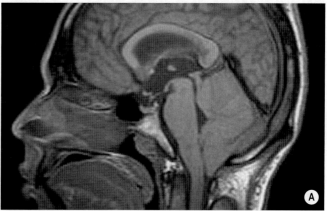

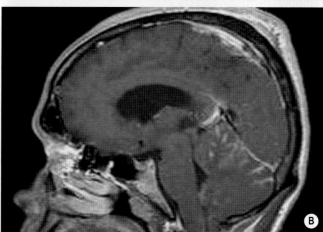

Tonsillar herniation (A) Sagittal T1WI shows pegged appearance of cerebellar tonsils through foramen magnum simulating a Chiari I malformation. (B) T1WI + Gad shows cerebellar leptomeningeal enhancement due to cryptococcal menginoencephalitis in this patient with AIDS.++

DEMENTIAS – ALZHEIMER'S DISEASE (AD)

Definition Abnormal aggregation of amyloid leads to impaired nerve function, formation of amyloid plaques and neurofibrillary tangles ▶ a generalized disorder which may affect the medial part of the temporal lobe (especially the hippocampus) during the early stages

CT/MRI This is usually normal (excludes treatable causes) ▶ occasionally medial temporal lobe atrophy as indicated by widening of the perihippocampal CSF spaces

Regional cerebral blood flow (rCBF) SPECT Characteristic symmetrical posterior temporal and parietal perfusion defects with established disease ▶ rCBF reduction correlates with the degree of cognitive decline

FDG PET Reduced glucose uptake that is not explained by atrophy alone

DEMENTIAS – FRONTOTEMPORAL DEMENTIA (E.G. PICK'S DISEASE)

Definition A dementia characterized by the presence of Pick bodies within neurons, accounting for <10% of the primary degenerative dementias ▶ behavioural, motor or speech disorders tend to dominate the early clinical stages rather than memory loss ▶ 3 types: (1) behavioural variant, (2) progressive non-fluent aphasia, (3) semantic dementia

CT/MRI Abnormal in >50% of clinically confirmed cases ▶ markedly asymmetric atrophy seen within the anterior and medial temporal lobes (diminishing posteriorly) ▶ asymmetric frontal lobe atrophy may be present

rCBF SPECT Predominantly frontal and anterior temporal perfusion defects

DEMENTIAS – LEWY BODY DEMENTIA

Definition A dementia characterized by the presence of Lewy bodies (composed of α-synuclein and ubiquitin proteins) within neurons ▶ the 2nd most common degenerative dementia after AD (20% of all dementias)

CT/MRI/rCBF SPECT Unable to distinguish from AD

HMPOA SPECT Reduced frontal perfusion compared with AD

FDG PET Reduced cerebellar and visual cortex uptake compared with AD

DEMENTIAS – VASCULAR DEMENTIA

Definition Dementia following chronic impaired blood supply to the brain ▶ heterogeneous entity, and can be due to small or large vessel involvement

CT/MRI Although evidence for ischaemic change is mandatory for a diagnosis, ischaemic changes are very commonly seen in elderly non-demented patients

Functional imaging Patchy cortical and basal ganglia perfusion defects ▶ this does not always reliably distinguish from a frontotemporal dementia

Pearl Small vessel vascular dementia: extensive white matter lesions/multiple lacunes/bilateral thalamic lesions ▶ white matter lesions tend to spare U-fibres (cf. MS)
- **MRI:** FLAIR most sensitive (thalamic lesions best seen on T2WI) ▶ hyperintense white matter lesions vs. hypointense lacunes ▶ increased DWI with acute lesions

DEMENTIAS – PRION DISEASES

Definition A prion is an infectious agent composed primarily of protein ▶ prions cause neurodegenerative disease by accumulating extracellularly within the CNS and forming amyloid plaques – these plaques disrupt the normal tissue function with the formation of vacuoles within the neurons ('holes') ▶ the diseases so caused include Creutzfeldt–Jakob disease (CJD ▶ sporadic, iatrogenic, familial) and new variant CJD (nvCJD)
- Presents initially with behavioural disturbances, then rapidly progressive dementia (+/− myoclonus)

CT Normal in the early stages but a rapidly progressive atrophy develops

MRI Symmetrical increased SI demonstrated within the putamen and caudate nuclei (10% of sporadic CJD cases) and posterior thalamus (>50% of nvCJD cases)

CHRONIC EPILEPSY

Definition There are usually repeated seizures over a number of years ▶ there may be no detectable underlying structural lesion (cryptogenic epilepsy) or a variety of non-progressive lesions:
- *Scars:* infarcts ▶ post-traumatic
- *Vascular lesions:* cavernomas ▶ arteriovenous malformations
- *Malformations of cortical development:* focal cortical dysplasia ▶ cortical hamartomas (tuberous sclerosis) ▶ neuronal heterotopias ▶ schizencephaly
- *Neoplasms:* grade 1 tumours (particularly within the temporal lobe)
- *Hippocampal sclerosis:* this is the commonest cause and is associated with temporal lobe epilepsy
- Infections: bacterial/viral/fungal/mycobacterial/parasitic

MRI The recommended investigation of choice for detecting a structural lesion
- **Hippocampal sclerosis:** the hippocampus shows volume loss (best detected on thin-section volumetric acquisitions in the coronal plane) ▶ dilatation of the adjacent temporal horn ▶ T2WI: high SI

Functional imaging Abnormalities of cortical metabolism (FDG-PET) may be larger than on a structural MRI

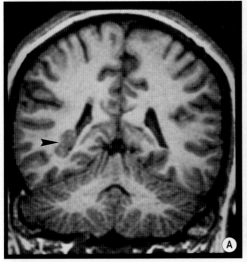

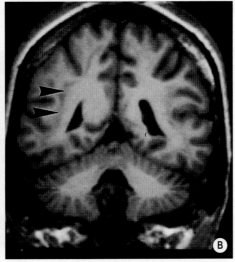

Neuronal heterotopia as a cause of chronic epilepsy. Coronal T1WI from a volumetric acquisition ► slice thickness is 1.5 mm. (A) Subependymal (nodular) heterotopia (arrowhead), (B) laminar heterotopia (arrowheads).*

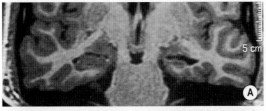

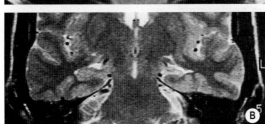

Diagnosis of hippocampal sclerosis. (A) T1WI and (B) T2WI through the temporal lobes. In (A) the left hippocampus is smaller than the right and (B) is of higher SI.*

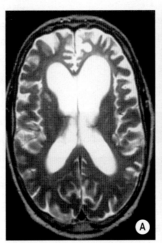

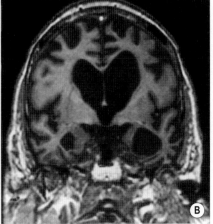

Pick's disease. (A) Axial T2-weighted image (T2WI) is remarkable for the dilated subarachnoid space over the frontal lobes, signifying atrophy. The frontal horns of the lateral ventricle enlarge to fill the void. The atrophy is striking in its frontal predominance. This is typical of Pick's disease. (B) The coronal T1WI again shows the striking frontal and anterior temporal atrophy. The patient was in his late 50s.[+]

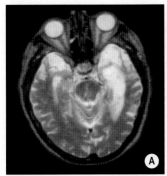

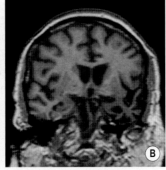

Pick's disease. (A) Axial T2WI and (B) coronal T1WI (from a volumetric acquisition) showing severe rather generalized mainly anterior temporal lobe atrophy, most marked on the left side.*

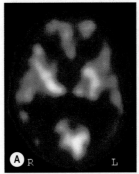

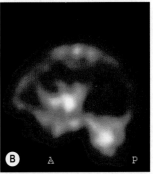

(A) Axial (L) and (B) sagittal (R) 99mTc-HMPAO SPECT in Alzheimer's disease showing typical perfusion defects in the posterior temporal and parietal regions.*

FIBROUS DYSPLASIA

Sclerotic form

- This is more common than the cystic form (especially in polyostotic fibrous dysplasia) and is the commonest cause of 'leontiasis ossea'
  - *Differential:* meningioma (although with a meningioma, sclerosis is often more marked than expansion, and extension from the sphenoid bones into the facial skeleton is much less common)

SXR/CT

- An expanded and dense skull base (± the facial skeleton) which can sometimes demonstrate the classical featureless 'ground-glass' pattern ▶ lower-density masses within the sclerotic bone represent cysts or fibrotic masses and are a good indication of the true diagnosis

Cystic form

- This usually produces a small skull vault lesion with outer table expansion and a 'blistered' appearance
  - *Differential:* epidermoid – this has a finer, better-defined border and a more homogeneously radiolucent centre

PAGET'S DISEASE

DEFINITION

- A chronic disease of osteoblasts and osteoclasts resulting in progressive bone remodelling deformities ▶ it consists of an active lytic phase and an inactive sclerotic phase

CLINICAL PRESENTATION

- This is rare before middle age (M>F) ▶ the skull is involved in ⅔ of cases that present clinically

RADIOLOGICAL FEATURES

XR/CT A mixture of sclerosis and lysis is most commonly seen ▶ the middle and outer tables are the most affected and thickened with course trabeculation ▶ early manifestations include a spotty 'cotton-wool pledget' increase in bone density or a generalized thickening of the skull vault

- A thickened skull vault (which may appear irregular due to patchy sclerosis)
- *Osteoporosis circumscripta:* a portion of the skull vault is demineralized (from the base upwards) with a very sharp border between normal and abnormal bone

MRI This can demonstrate basilar invagination (sagittal images)

PEARLS

Complications

- *Basilar invagination:* this is due to bone softening and may lead to a 'Tam O'Shanter' deformity
- *Basal foraminal narrowing:* this can cause cranial nerve lesions (especially deafness)
- *Malignancy:* osteo- or fibrosarcomas are seen in 1% of patients and manifest as irregular bone destruction

TUMOURS OF THE SKULL VAULT

Haemangioma

XR/CT A well-circumscribed lucent area with a characteristic stippled appearance and no associated bone expansion (although it may present as a lump on the head or local tenderness) ▶ it is a non-progressive tumour that does not require treatment

External carotid arteriography This sometimes demonstrates a vascular blush

Intraosseous epidermoid

XR/CT A well-corticated vault lesion ▶ it may expand the inner and outer tables away from each other

Osteoma

- A benign condensation of cortical bone which can project external to the skull (exostosis) or towards the cranial cavity (enostosis)

XR/CT An osteoma is typically denser, more circumscribed, and without an abnormal bone texture when compared with a meningioma or fibrous dysplasia

Myelomatosis

XR/CT 'pepper pot' skull: widespread well-defined small lytic deposits

Tumours

- These are usually metastatic or due to local invasion (e.g. a nasopharyngeal or basal cell carcinoma)

XR/CT Metastases demonstrate irregular lysis (± sclerosis) and are often multiple ▶ focal osteolytic skull defects are a common manifestation of paediatric Langerhans' cell histiocytosis

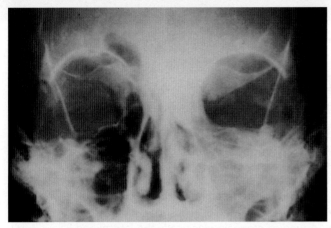

Fibrous dysplasia of the skull base. Dense 'ground-glass' appearance, with loss of the normal bone texture, extending from the nasion to the clivus into the sphenoid wings on both sides, and into the left maxilla.*

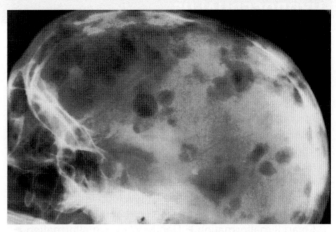

Multiple lytic deposits in the skull vault in a patient with carcinoma of the breast.†

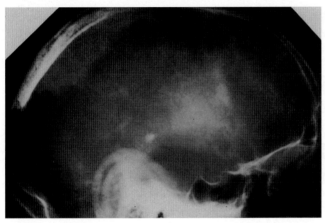

Osteoporosis circumscripta (Paget's disease). Extensive loss of bone density affects the lower part of the cranial vault ▶ the margin between abnormal and normal bone is characteristically sharp, as seen in the upper posterior parietal region.*

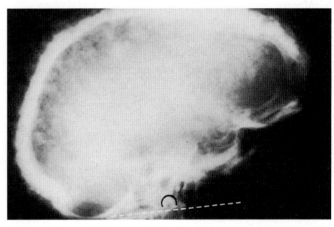

Advanced Paget's disease, with basilar invagination. Skull lateral projection: gross thickening and alteration of bone texture affects the entire skull. Basilar invagination is manifest as extension of the odontoid peg (outlined in black) above Chamberlain's line (dotted line).*

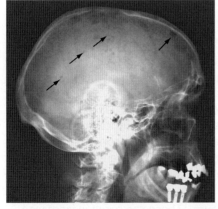

Radiograph of the skull yields the typical multiple punched-out osteolytic lesions in a patient with multiple myeloma (arrows).©35

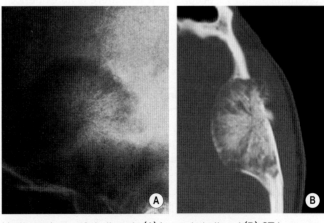

Haemangioma of skull vault. (A) Lateral skull and (B) CT bone windows. The well-defined lucency in the parietal bone has a typical 'spoke wheel' appearance due to prominent vascular impressions.*

HYDROCEPHALUS

Definition

- Hydrocephalus literally means 'water on the brain' – a non-specific term referring to any condition in which the ventricles are enlarged (including cerebral atrophy)

Non-communicating (obstructive) hydrocephalus This represents an intraventricular obstructive hydrocephalus

- The narrowest parts of the ventricular system are the most susceptible (e.g. the foramen of Munro, cerebral aqueduct and 4th ventricle outflow foramina)
- *Congenital:* aqueduct stenosis (developmental or acquired secondary to infection or haemorrhage) ▶ Chiari II malformation ▶ Dandy–Walker malformation ▶ congenital midline tumours
- *Masses affecting the foramen of Munro:* suprasellar tumours ▶ arachnoid cysts ▶ colloid cysts ▶ giant cell astrocytomas
- *Masses affecting the cerebral aqueduct:* tectal plate gliomas ▶ posterior fossa tumours ▶ brainstem astrocytomas ▶ pineal region tumours
- *Diffuse obstruction:* following intraventricular haemorrhage or meningitis ▶ disseminated intraventricular tumour ▶ reparative fibrosis

Communicating hydrocephalus This represents an extraventricular obstructive hydrocephalus

- The barrier to absorption is distal to the foramina of Magendie and Lushchka and usually at the tentorial hiatus within the basal cisterns or over the cerebral convexity
- *Causes:* trauma ▶ subarachnoid haemorrhage ▶ meningitis ▶ carcinomatosis ▶ spinal tumours
- *Raised intracranial venous pressures:* craniosynostosis (leading to stenosis of the jugular outflow foramina) ▶ venous thrombosis ▶ a vein of Galen aneurysmal malformation ▶ dural arteriovenous shunts

Normal pressure hydrocephalus A form of communicating hydrocephalus where there is no evidence of increased intracranial pressure

- It is characterized by dementia, urinary incontinence and gait disturbances

Clinical presentation

Children <2 years old (open fontanelles) An enlarging and disproportionate head circumference ▶ frontal bossing, calvarial thinning ▶ a tense, bulging anterior fontanelle ▶ sutural diastasis ▶ enlarged scalp veins ▶ sunsetting eyes ▶ lateral rectus palsies ▶ leg spasticity (stretched cortiospinal tracts)

- *Commonest causes:* post-haemorrhagic and infective hydrocephalus ▶ congenital causes

Older children or adults (closed fontanelles) Early morning headache ▶ nausea ▶ vomiting ▶ papilloedema ▶ leg spasticity ▶ cranial nerve palsies ▶ altered conscious level

- *Commonest causes:* posterior fossa neoplasms and aqueduct stenosis

Radiological features

Non-communicating or obstructive hydrocephalus

CT/MRI Dilatation of the temporal horns disproportionate to any lateral ventricular dilatation ▶ enlargement of the anterior and posterior recesses of the 3rd ventricle (with inferior convexity of its floor) ▶ transependymal (periventricular interstitial) oedema

- Effacement of the sulci, fissures and basal cisterns
- *Aqueduct stenosis:* classically the lateral and 3rd ventricles are dilated with a normal 4th ventricle
- *Unreliable features of chronic hydrocephalus:* erosion of the dorsum sellae ▶ a 'copper beaten' skull

Communicating hydrocephalus

CT/MRI Generalized symmetrical ventricular dilatation with variable interstitial cerebral oedema ▶ prominent basal cisterns or fissures

- The cerebral sulci are not enlarged

Normal pressure hydrocephalus

CT/MRI Dilated ventricles ▶ prominent cerebral aqueduct flow voids

Pearls

Treatment External ventricular drainage ▶ ventriculoperitoneal or ventriculoatrial shunt ▶ a 3rd ventriculostomy

Shunt complications

- **Shunt malfunction:** due to discontinuity within the shunt tubing or obstruction with choroid plexus or glial tissue

  CT/MRI Recurrence of hydrocephalus ▶ fluid tracking along the length of the shunt tubing ▶ calcification seen at either end of the shunt (secondary to inflammation and fibrosis)

- **Shunt infection** (1–5%): this can cause a ventriculitis which may progress to a devastating cerebritis

  CT/MRI Enlarged ventricles with a hyperdense ependyma ▶ ependymal enhancement and debris within the ventricular system

- **'Slit ventricle' syndrome:** shunted patients may develop symptoms without any ventricular dilatation
  - *Causes:* overdrainage of CSF ▶ poorly compliant ventricles allowing a raised intraventricular pressure without associated dilatation ▶ intermittent shunt malfunction

Choroid plexus tumours These can result in increased CSF production (with a communicating hydrocephalus) ▶ they may also obstruct the lateral ventricle due to mass effect or haemorrhage (with a non-communicating hydrocephalus)

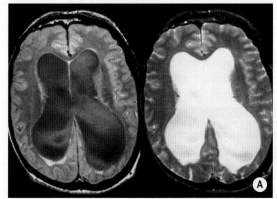

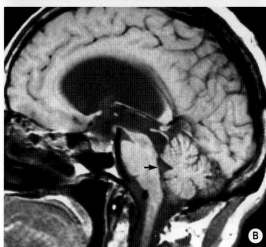

Hydrocephalus secondary to aqueduct stenosis: MRI. (A) Axial PD and T2WI. Marked enlargement of the lateral ventricles, with a thin 'halo' of interstitial oedema. (B) Sagittal T1WI demonstrating massive enlargement of lateral ventricles, outpouching of the suprasellar recesses of the 3rd ventricle impinging upon the sella and 'ventricularization' of the proximal aqueduct just above the level of obstruction and above the 4th ventricle. Note the normal size of the 4th ventricle (arrow).*

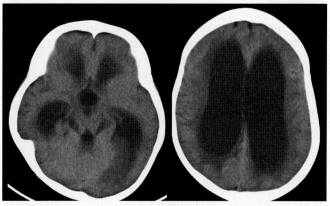

Child with mucopolysaccharidosis type I and hydrocephalus. The temporal horns and anterior recesses of the 3rd ventricle are dilated. There is transependymal oedema and the cerebral sulci are effaced.*

Differentiation between hydrocephalus and atrophy		
	Hydrocephalus	**Atrophy**
Temporal horns	Enlarged	Normal (except in Alzheimer's disease)
3rd ventricle	Convex ▶ distended anterior recess	Concave ▶ normal anterior recess
4th ventricle	Normal or enlarged	Normal
Transependymal CSF migration	Presents acutely	Absent
Sulci	Flattened	Enlarged out of proportion to age

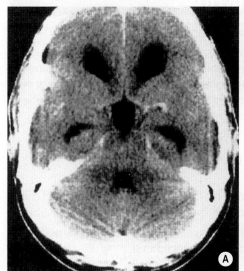

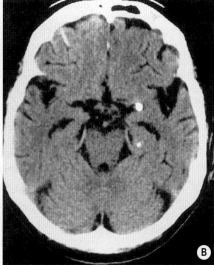

Hydrocephalus versus atrophy. (A) Hydrocephalus. There is dilatation of the frontal horns of the lateral ventricles, the temporal horns of the lateral ventricles and the 3rd ventricle. There is a normal 4th ventricle. No sulcal dilatation exists. (B) Atrophy. There is sulcal prominence and mildly enlarged temporal horns. In comparison with (A), the temporal horns, although enlarged, are not enlarged to the same degree. Furthermore, there is obvious sulcal prominence which is not demonstrated with a communicating hydrocephalus.+

CEREBELLAR HYPOPLASIA

Definition

- The cerebellum may be small due to a congenital lack of formation or from subsequent atrophy
  - *Causes:* infection (especially congenital cytomegalovirus) ▶ inborn errors of metabolism (e.g. glycolysation disorder)
  - *Other rarer causes:* carbohydrate-deficient glycoprotein syndrome ▶ infantile neuroaxonal dystrophy ▶ pontocerebellar hypoplasia ▶ spinocerebellar atrophies ▶ Friedreich's ataxia

Clinical presentation

- Variable hypotonia or ataxia

Radiological features

MRI Symmetrical atrophy of the cerebellar folia with widened cerebellar fissures ▶ variable cerebellar SI ▶ vermis more frequently affected

DANDY–WALKER COMPLEX

Definition

- This encompasses a spectrum of cystic posterior fossa malformations from the complete Dandy–Walker malformation to a mega cisterna magna
  - Membranous obstruction to the foramina of Magendie / Luschka causes cystic dilatation of the 4th ventricle
  - All have an apparently focal extra-axial CSF collection which is continuous with the 4th ventricle (with a variable degree of cerebellar hypoplasia)
- It is associated with hydrocephalus and other midline abnormalities (e.g. agenesis or a lipoma of the corpus callosum)

Clinical presentation

- Developmental delay ▶ seizures ▶ hydrocephalus

Radiological features

Dandy–Walker malformation

- There is cystic dilatation of the 4th ventricle (which almost fills an entire enlarged posterior fossa) ▶ the cerebellar vermis is hypoplastic as well as rotated or aplastic ▶ the tentorium and venous confluence of the torcula are elevated

Dandy–Walker variant

- This describes cases where the above lesions are less marked and the posterior fossa is not enlarged

Mega cisterna magna

- This forms the mildest end of the spectrum and is of dubious clinical significance

- It consists of an infracerebellar CSF collection and occasionally an enlarged posterior fossa ▶ the cerebellum and 4th ventricle are normal

Pearl

Differential: a posterior fossa arachnoid cyst (this will not communicate with the 4th ventricle)

JOUBERT'S SYNDROME

Definition

- Total aplasia of the cerebellar vermis reflecting the failure of formation of the decussation of the superior cerebellar peduncles, a lack of the pyramidal decussations and other anomalies of the midbrain crossing tracts and their nuclei
- Occasionally a genetic locus has been identified
- Many syndromes with additional features (e.g. renal cysts, ocular abnormalities, liver fibrosis, hypothalamic hamartomas and polymicrogyria) have been classified with this anomaly

Clinical presentation

- Tachypnoea ▶ abnormal eye movements ▶ ataxia
- Patients may occasionally be clinically normal

Radiological features

MRI A cleft is present within the vermis ▶ the midbrain is small ▶ the superior peduncles appear enlarged

- *'Molar tooth' appearance:* seen on axial images arising from the lack of the superior cerebellar decussation
- *'Batwing' appearance:* this is due to an enlarged 4th ventricle with cerebellar hypoplasia, midline vermian cleft and a dysplastic small vermis

OTHER CEREBELLAR MALFORMATIONS

Rhombencephalosynapsis

- A very rare cerebellar malformation where the cerebellar hemispheres are fused across the midline and there is hypoplasia or aplasia of the vermis ▶ it is associated with other midline supratentorial anomalies (e.g. absence of the septum pellucidum and corpus callosum, as well as holoprosencephaly)

Lhermitte–Duclos or dysplastic cerebellar gangliocytoma

- A developmental mass lesion with enlargement of the cerebellar cortex ▶ this usually affects one hemisphere

MRI A non-enhancing mass with diffusely enlarged cerebellar folia (± pial enhancement)

	Dandy–Walker malformation	Dandy–Walker variant	Mega cisterna magna
Posterior fossa	Enlarged	Normal	Normal or enlarged
Vermis	Absent or very hypoplastic	Hypoplastic	Normal
Hypoplastic cerebellar hemisphere	Yes	Rare	No
Hydrocephalus	75%	25%	Unusual
Supratentorial abnormalities	Common	Uncommon	Rare
Falx cerebelli	Absent	Present (32%)	Present (63%)
4th ventricle	Opens into cyst	Cyst dilatation	Normal
Prognosis	Poor	Good	Good

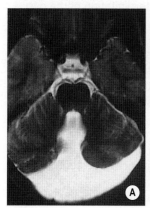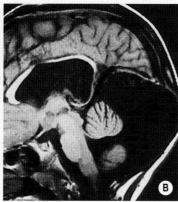

Axial T2WI (A) and sagittal T1WI (B) in a patient with the Dandy–Walker syndrome showing an enlarged posterior fossa with a high tentorium, and a large fluid-filled 4th ventricle–cisterna magna complex in association with vermian hypoplasia.†

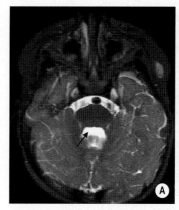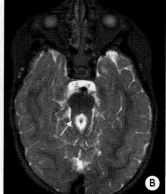

Child with Joubert's syndrome. (A) Typical batwing appearance to the 4th ventricle (arrow) and (B) prominent superior cerebellar peduncles with failure of the normal midline decussation (arrow). This gives the typical 'molar tooth' appearance. The midbrain is hypoplastic in this condition.*

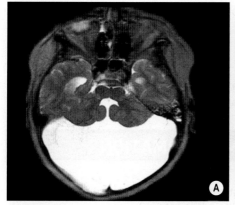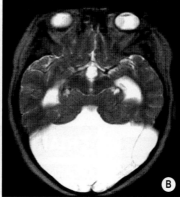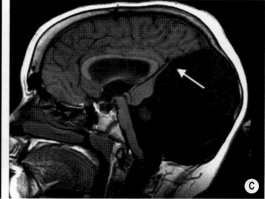

Dandy–Walker malformation. (A, B) The 4th ventricle opens into a large posterior fossa cyst. There is associated hydrocephalus. (C) The cerebellum is hypoplastic and a thin rim of cerebellar tissue is seen forming the wall of the posterior fossa cyst (arrow). The vein of Galen, straight sinus and venous confluence are elevated above the level of the lambdoid suture.*

DEFINITION

- **Chiari malformation:** A group of abnormalities characterized by dislocation of the hindbrain into the spinal canal

CHIARI I MALFORMATION (CEREBELLAR ECTOPIA)

Definition

- A form of hindbrain deformation rather than a true malformation characterized by tonsillar descent through a normal-sized foramen magnum ▶ it may be an acquired condition due to raised intracranial pressures, lowered intraspinal pressures or diminished posterior fossa volumes (e.g. basilar invagination)
- It is often an isolated hindbrain abnormality of little consequence
- It is not related to the Chiari II or III malformations

Clinical presentation

- There are usually no symptoms during childhood unless there is an associated syringomyelia or hydrocephalus
- Clinical symptoms are more likely when there is >5 mm of descent below the foramen magnum (children between 5 and 15 years can have normal tonsillar descent of up to 6 mm)
- Symptoms may include a cough-induced headache, cranial nerve palsies and a disassociated peripheral anaesthesia

Radiological features

MRI It is usually associated with 'peg-like' cerebellar tonsils ▶ an elongated medulla oblongata can be seen with a kink sometimes forming on its posterior surface

Associations

- Syringohydromyelia (50%) ▶ basilar invagination (30%) ▶ hydrocephalus (25%) ▶ Klippel–Feil anomaly (10%)
- It is not associated with a myelomeningocele

CHIARI II MALFORMATION

Definition

- A congenital malformation of the hindbrain (with a dysplastic cerebellum) that is almost always associated with a neural tube defect (usually a lumbosacral myelomeningocele)
- The inferior vermis is everted (rather than inverted) so that the nodulus becomes its most inferior aspect and the 4th ventricle is reduced to a coronal cleft (the cerebellar herniation consists mainly of the cerebellar vermis) ▶ the medulla is invariably elongated and kinked

Clinical presentation

- Affected children usually present with hydrocephalus following repair of a myelomeningocele after birth
- *Other symptoms:* upper airway problems ▶ feeding problems ▶ dysphagia

Radiological features

CT/MRI Inferior displacement of the cerebellum, pons, medulla oblongata and cervical cord ▶ medullary kinking ▶ a small slit-like 4th ventricle (which is inferiorly displaced and elongated) and a small posterior fossa ▶ scalloping of the clivus ▶ flattening of the ventral pons and a low attachment of the tentorium ▶ the falx is partially absent or fenestrated with consequent interdigitation of the gyri across the midline ▶ the foramen magnum is enlarged and 'shield-shaped'

- *'Tectal beaking':* this follows fusion of the midbrain colliculi into a single beak pointing posteriorly
- *'Towering cerebellum':* the tentorial incisura is enlarged and the cerebellum herniates superiorly into the supratentorial space
- *'Batwing' configuration of the frontal horns* (coronal view): this is due to impressions from prominent caudate nuclei
- *'Hourglass ventricle':* a small biconcave 3rd ventricle due to a large massa intermedia
- *'Cervicomedullary kink':* herniation of the medulla posterior to the spinal cord
- *'Banana' sign:* the cerebellum is wrapped around the posterior brainstem (seen during obstetric US)

Associations

- Lacunar membranous skull dysraphism ('luckenschadel') ▶ disorders of neuronal migration ▶ malformation of the corpus callosum ▶ a dorsal midline cyst ▶ absence of the septum pellucidum ▶ colpocephaly (occipital horn enlargement)

Complications

- Hydrocephalus ▶ an isolated 4th ventricle ▶ hydro-syringomyelia ▶ compression of the craniocervical junction

CHIARI III MALFORMATION

Definition

- This is the most severe abnormality (and unrelated to the Chiari II or III malformations)
- It consists of a high cervical or low occipital meningoencephalocele (in addition to an intracranial Chiari II malformation)

CHIARI IV MALFORMATION

Definition

- Extremely rare severe cerebellar hypoplasia

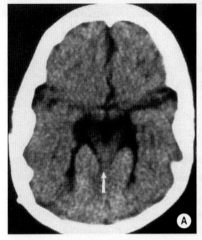
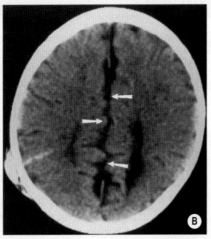

Chiari II malformation. (A) Imaging through the level of the midbrain reveals tectal beaking (arrow) with the cerebellum wrapping around the posterolateral aspect of the midbrain. The cerebellum is towering between the leaves of the tentorium. (B) Imaging through the supraventricular region shows interdigitation of the gyri (arrows) with hypoplasia of the falx.[+]

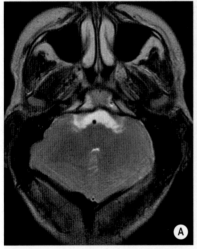
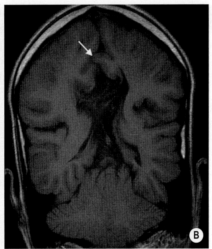

Chiari II malformation. (A) The posterior fossa is enlarged and 'shield shaped'. The 4th ventricle is small and slit-like. (B) The cerebellum towers superiorly through the tentorium and there is interdigitation of a cerebral gyrus through the fenestrated falx (arrow).*

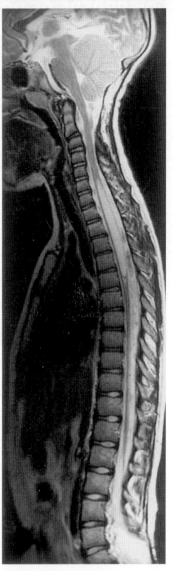

Chiari II malformation with tectal beaking, a cord syrinx and a treated myelomeningocele.[+]

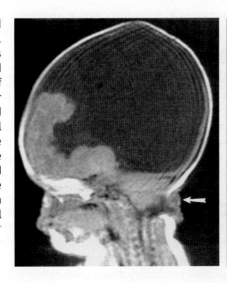

Chiari III malformation. T1WI shows downward herniation of the cerebellar tonsils associated with an occipital encephalocele (arrow). There is associated agenesis of the corpus callosum and maximal hydrocephalus.[+]

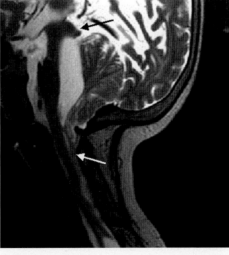

Chiari II malformation. The 4th ventricle, which should normally be small and slit-like in this condition, is enlarged, indicating hydrocephalus. There is cascading tonsillar tissue herniating through the foramen magnum (white arrow). Beaking of the tectal plate is also seen (black arrow), as well as a cervical spinal cord syringomyelic cavity.*

DISORDERS OF DORSAL INDUCTION

DEFINITION

- These are malformations considered to be consequences of abnormalities of dorsal induction (also including Chiari II malformations)

Anencephaly

- The most common fetal cerebral malformation which is incompatible with life ▶ there is no cerebral cortex present (unlike gross hydrocephalus)

Cephalocele

- An extracranial protrusion of intracranial structures through a congenital defect of the skull and dura mater ▶ unlike a spinal myelomeningocele there is usually no skin defect ▶ they tend to occur in the occipital and frontal regions and may be pulsatile ▶ mainly midline
- *Meningocele:* containing leptomeninges and CSF only
- *Encephalocele:* containing leptomeninges, CSF and neural tissue
- *Encephalocystocele:* containing leptomeninges, CSF, neural tissue and part of the ventricle

RADIOLOGICAL FEATURES

MRI This can establish: the presence of any neural tissue ▶ other intracranial malformations or hydrocephalus ▶ whether there is any ischaemia within the herniated neural tissue

DISORDERS OF VENTRAL INDUCTION

DEFINITION

- These are malformations following the formation of the neural tube

Holoprosencephaly

- A midline malformation of ventral induction of the anterior brain, skull and face (resulting from the failure of the embryonic prosencephalon to undergo segmentation and cleavage into two separate cerebral hemispheres) ▶ it is associated with chromosomal abnormalities, facial clefting and various teratogenic factors (including maternal diabetes)

MALFORMATIONS OF COMMISSURAL AND RELATED STRUCTURES

Definition

Agenesis of the septum pellucidum

- This may be associated with septo-optic dysplasia, agenesis of the corpus callosum, holoprosencephaly, Chiari II malformation, schizencephaly and other migration disorders

Septo-optic dysplasia (de Morsier's syndrome)

- A triad of: (1) hypopituitarism, (2) hypoplasia of the optic nerves, (3) absence of the septum pellucidum (the frontal horns have a typical 'box-like' configuration)

Agenesis or dysgenesis of the corpus callosum

- Fibres that normally travel across the corpus callosum now run in longitudinal bundles along the medial walls of the lateral ventricles (the bundles of Probst)

Associations Chiari II malformation ▶ Dandy–Walker malformation ▶ interhemispheric lipoma ▶ abnormalities of neuronal migration and organization ▶ dysraphic anomalies ▶ encephaloceles ▶ septo-optic dysplasia ▶ ocular anomalies ▶ midline facial anomalies

Radiological features

MRI Parallel widely spaced lateral ventricles with the 3rd ventricle elevated and seen between them (the interhemispheric cyst frequently seen is thought to originate from the 3rd ventricle but has lost continuity with this structure) ▶ vertically oriented sulci extend right down to the ventricle with no horizontally running cingulate sulcus ▶ small frontal horns ('bull's horn' appearance) with colpocephaly (large occipital horns)

Pearl The anterior part (the posterior genu and anterior body) of the corpus callosum is formed before the posterior part (the posterior body and splenium) ▶ thus a small or absent genu or body, with an intact splenium and rostrum, indicates secondary destruction rather than abnormal development

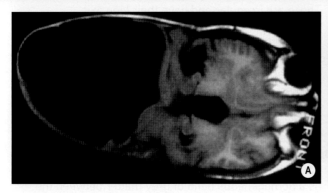 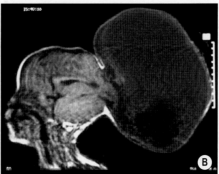

Parieto-occipital cephalocele with herniation of the brain and meninges through a calvarial defect. Most of the herniated component is in the form of a cerebrospinal fluid-containing meningocele.*

Holoprosencephaly			
	Alobar form *Severe form (often fatal)*	**Semilobar form** *Intermediate form*	**Lobar form** *Mild form*
Cleavage into two hemispheres	None (a 'cup'-shaped brain)	Partial posterior cleaving	Complete
Facial abnormalities (e.g. cyclopia[1] and hypotelorism[2])	Severe	Intermediate	None
Lateral ventricles	U-shaped monoventricle with a dorsal cyst	Partial anterior fusion (with partial occipital and temporal horns)	Normal (the frontal horns may be 'squared')
Falx and corpus callosum	Absent	Absent anteriorly	Normal (they may be incomplete or dysplastic)
Thalami	Fused	Partial separation	Normal
Septum pellucidum	Absent	Absent	Absent
[1]a single eye [2]the eyes are too close together			

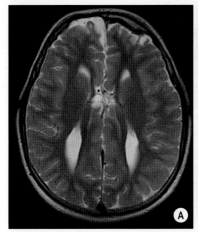 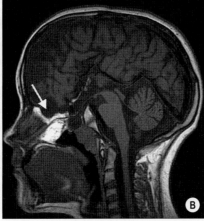 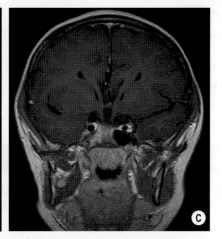

Callosal agenesis. (A) Axial T2WI shows separated ventricles with a parallel orientation. The superior part of the 3rd ventricle is just seen. (B) Sagittal T1WI through the midline confirms callosal agenesis. There is no cingulate sulcus and the vertically oriented cerebral sulci extend right down to the 3rd ventricle. This finding is associated with other midline anomalies such as a fronto-ethmoidal cephalocele (arrow). (C) The optic chiasm is absent.*

SCHIZENCEPHALY

Definition A cleft lined by grey matter and leptomeninges (cf. a transmantle infarction in which the defect is lined by white matter) ▶ it involves the complete cerebral mantle and connects the calvarium and the outer surface of the brain with the lateral ventricles

Location It is typically central (involving the pre- and postcentral gyri) ▶ it is also found within the parasagittal, frontal or occipital sites (with mild clinical manifestations)

Clinical presentation There are variable features depending on the site and size involved: severe seizures ▶ spasticity ▶ severe mental and psychomotor developmental delay (with bilateral clefts)

CT/MRI The adjacent thickened cortex demonstrates polymicrogyria ▶ it is associated with subependymal heterotopias (within the contralateral hemisphere) and subependymal or parenchymal calcification

- *'Open lip'*: a wide open defect
- *'Closed lip'*: if the cleft is closed but lined with grey matter entirely into the ventricle

LISSENCEPHALY–AGYRIA–PACHYGYRIA

Lissencephaly (a 'smooth' brain) (type 1)

- Very few or no gyri are present
- Opercularization (development of the sylvian fissures) is abnormal with shallow sylvian fissures ▶ it is associated with agenesis or hypoplasia of the corpus callosum and septum pellucidum

Cobblestone lissencephaly (type 2)

- This follows neuronal overmigration with thick meninges adherent to the smooth cortical surface ▶ heterotopias are prominent and there is often a delay in myelination ▶ it may be seen in congenital muscular dystrophies ▶ posterior fossa usually abnormal

Agyria (complete lissencephaly)

- Total absence of the gyri and sulci ▶ posterior fossa spared
- There are wide and vertically orientated sylvian fissures

Pachygyria (incomplete lissencephaly)

- The gyri are relatively few and unusually broad and flat
- There is an AP gradation of gyral development

GREY MATTER HETEROTOPIAS

Definition Grey matter found in an abnormal position anywhere from subependymal layer to cortical surface

MRI This is isointense with cortical grey matter demonstrated on all imaging sequences ▶ T1WI + Gad: there is no enhancement

Subependymal heterotopia

- This is smooth and ovoid with its long axis typically parallel to the ventricular wall

Subependymal hamartomas seen in tuberous sclerosis

- These are irregular and have their long axis perpendicular to the ventricular wall ▶ they are also more heterogeneous and may enhance

Focal subcortical heterotopia

- The overlying cortex is thin with shallow sulci and it is associated with variable motor and intellectual impairment ▶ it may coexist with schizencephaly, microcephaly, polymicrogyria, dysgenesis of the corpus callosum, or absence of the septum pellucidum

Band heterotopia or 'double cortex'

- This is located parallel to the ventricular wall and is seen as a homogeneous band of grey matter between the lateral ventricle and the cerebral cortex (separated from both by a layer of white matter) ▶ the overlying cortex is usually of normal thickness but has shallow sulci ▶ partial heterotopias predominantly affect frontal lobes
- It is commonly seen in girls with variable developmental delay or seizures

POLYMICROGYRIA

Definition A disorder of neuronal organization occurring after neuronal migration ▶ the extent varies from small, isolated, unilateral areas to larger areas of bilateral disease

MRI Appearances vary between broad and thickened gyri (mimicking pachygyria), overconvoluted and fused cortex of normal thickness ▶ overconvoluted multiple gyri

TRANSMANTLE CORTICAL DYSPLASIA

Definition Abnormal cells extend all the way from the wall of the ventricle to the cortex

MRI There is blurring of the junction between the cortex and the white matter ▶ there may calcification or abnormal venous drainage

- T2WI: high SI (compared to the white matter) extending from the lateral ventricular wall to the blurred cortex

HEMIMEGALENCEPHALY

Definition Hamartomatous overgrowth of all or part of one hemisphere – this is due to a structural malformation resulting from defective neuronal proliferation, migration and organization

- It can occur in isolation or be associated with proteus, epidermal naevus and Klippel–Trénaunay–Weber syndromes ▶ other associations include neurofibromatosis type 1 (NF-1) and tuberous sclerosis

MRI The affected hemisphere demonstrates pachygyria, polymicrogyria and heterotopias (as well as dysmyelination and gliosis) ▶ the affected hemisphere is usually (but not always) enlarged with diffuse cortical thickening, white matter signal abnormality and possibly calcification

- The ipsilateral ventricle is enlarged with characteristic straightening and pointing of the frontal horns

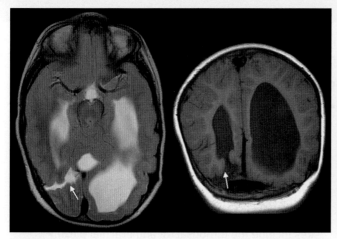

Schizencephaly with a grey matter-lined cleft (arrows) extending from the leptomeningeal surface through the brain parenchyma to the ventricular margin.*

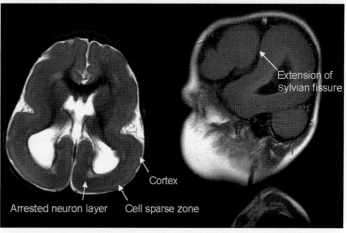

Lissencephaly. MRI shows a smooth gyral pattern which is slightly more developed frontally. The cerebral cortex is generally thin and there is a band of arrested neurons deep to the 'cell sparse zone'. The sylvian fissures are vertically oriented and extend into a vertical cleft.*

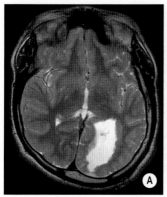
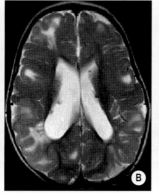

Subependymal grey matter heterotopia (A) and subependymal hamartomas of tuberous sclerosis (B). (A) Multiple subependymal continuous 'nodules' running along the ventricular margin with SI isointense to grey matter. (B) Scattered nodules which project into the ventricles and with variable SI. Some are markedly hypointense in keeping with calcification. Note also the multiple regions of cortical and subcortical white matter abnormality with slight mass effect in keeping with cortical tubers.*

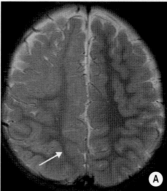
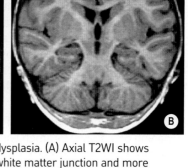

Right frontoparietal lobe cortical dysplasia. (A) Axial T2WI shows blurring of the right frontal grey–white matter junction and more extensive associated white matter signal high SI involving most of the hemisphere, including the parietal lobe at this level (arrow). (B) Coronal T1WI (part of the volumetric dataset) also shows grey–white matter junction signal abnormality (arrow) and more subtle white matter change.*

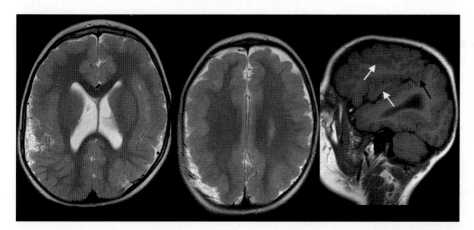

Extensive bilateral cerebral hemisphere polymicrogyria. Virtually no normal cortex is seen with an overconvoluted gyral pattern and a 'lumpy bumpy' grey–white matter interface noted (including regions marked by white arrows). The sylvian fissure is abnormally oriented with a parietal cleft that extends posteriorly (black arrow).*

NEUROFIBROMATOSIS TYPE 1 (NF-1)

Definition

- The neurocutaneous syndromes (or phakomatoses) are congenital malformations particularly affecting structures of neuroectodermal origin (i.e. the CNS, skin and eyes)
- Neurofibromatosis type 1 (autosomal dominant) is the commonest neurocutaneous syndrome and results from a mutation on chromosome 17 (50% are new mutations)

Optic pathway gliomas (OPGs)

- These are usually WHO grade I pilocytic astrocytomas and the commonest brain abnormality in NF-1 (affecting up to 15% of patients) ▶ they are more likely to affect the optic nerves rather than the chiasm or post-chiasmatic pathways (cf. non-NF-1 OPGs) and are associated with a better prognosis ▶ there is a risk of precocious puberty and visual deterioration with chiasm and hypothalamic involvement ▶ spontaneous tumour involution is recognized
- There is a small (1–3%) risk of associated grade I pilocytic astrocytomas (especially within the cerebellum and brainstem) ▶ brainstem tumours are more common within the medulla and midbrain (e.g. a tectal plate glioma) rather than the pons, and are usually less aggressive than a non-NF-1 brainstem astrocytoma ▶ a tectal plate tumour may cause aqueduct stenosis and hence hydrocephalus ▶ they may also regress spontaneously

CT/MRI Fusiform expansion of the optic nerve and widening of the optic foramen with characteristic sphenoid wing dysplasia and plexiform neurofibromata (± intraorbital extension of a plexiform neurofibroma) ▶ dilated optic nerve sheaths (due to dural ectasia) ▶ variable extension into the chiasm, the lateral geniculate bodies or optic radiations

- Tumour infiltration of the optic nerve causes variable enhancement of the expanded nerve within the optic nerve sheath
- Subarachnoid tumour leads to a rim of enhancing tumour around a minimally enhancing nerve

Non-neoplastic hamartomatous changes of NF-1

- These are also known as 'unidentified bright objects' (UBOs) and are seen in 60–80% of NF-1 cases ▶ the greatest number and volume occurs between 4 and 10 years of age (rarely >20 years)
  - *Typical sites:* the pons ▶ cerebellar white matter ▶ internal capsules ▶ basal ganglia ▶ thalami ▶ hippocampi
- Astrocytomas may develop within similar areas (but will demonstrate mass effect and enhancement)

MRI T1WI: lesions within the basal ganglia often demonstrate slightly high SI (elsewhere they demonstrate

intermediate SI) ▶ T2WI: multiple high SI lesions with minimal mass effect ▶ T1WI + Gad: no enhancement

Plexiform neurofibromas

- Multinodular lesions are formed when tumour involves either multiple trunks or multiple fascicles of a large nerve ▶ they are typically seen within the orbit and growing along the ophthalmic division of the trigeminal nerve (in association with progressive sphenoid wing dysplasia) ▶ they can extend along nerve pathways and into the pterygomaxillary fissure, orbital apex, superior orbital fissure and cavernous sinus (other characteristic sites include the lumbosacral and brachial plexi) ▶ malignant transformation is seen in 2–12% of cases

CT Hypodense lesions that do not enhance

MRI A more heterogeneous and diffuse appearance than a neurofibroma ▶ T1WI: low SI ▶ T2WI: high SI ▶ T1WI + Gad: variable enhancement

Neurofibromas

- These are more homogeneous and well-defined lesions which cause diffuse expansion of a nerve ▶ malignant transformation is less common (and is suggested by local pain, rapid growth, a large size and internal heterogeneity)

MRI T2WI: central low SI (target appearance) ▶ nodules seen along the spinal nerves of the cauda equina (extending out through, and enlarging, the neural exit foramina)

Non-CNS tumours

- Phaeochromocytoma ▶ carcinoid ▶ rhabdomyosarcoma ▶ childhood chronic myeloid leukaemia

Associated findings

- Lambdoid sutural dysplasia ▶ thinning of the long bone cortices ▶ kyphoscoliosis with a high thoracic acute curve ▶ dural ectasia with vertebral scalloping ▶ lateral CSF containing meningoceles
- *'Empty' or 'bare' orbit (XR):* the sphenoid wing dysplasia and associated bone defect allows herniation of the temporal lobe through the orbit, giving the appearance of an empty orbit
- Scoliosis may be seen in association with an intrinsic spinal cord tumour or a peripheral nerve neurofibroma

Neurofibromatosis type 2

- This is due to an abnormality on chromosome 2 and nearly all patients have bilateral vestibular schwannomas
- *Other tumours include:* meningiomas ▶ other cranial and peripheral nerve schwannomas and ependymomas (including spinal tumours)

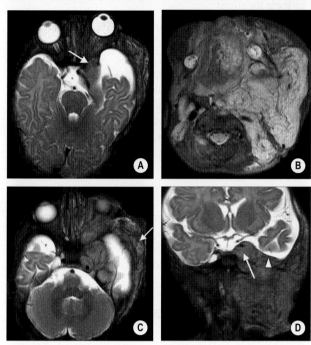

Infant with neurofibromatosis type 1. The diagnosis was made from these images. (A) There is sphenoid wing dysplasia causing expansion of the middle cranial fossa (arrow) and absence of the lateral orbital wall, which causes the 'bare orbit' sign (arrow) on AP XR. (B) There is an associated extensive plexiform neurofibroma involving the deep and superficial fascial spaces of the neck, tongue and orbit. (C,D) This is almost indistinguishable on imaging from multiple cranial nerve fibromas involving the left cavernous sinus (arrows) and middle cranial fossa. Note the neurofibroma has extended through the foramen ovale and is elevating the dura, seen as a black line (arrowhead).*

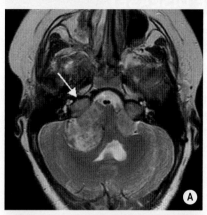

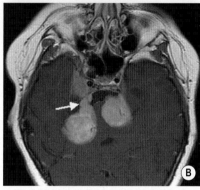

Neurofibromatosis type 2. (A) Bilateral cerebellopontine angle acoustic neuromas extend into the internal auditory meati and cause expansion (arrow). (B) Trigeminal schwannomas extending into the cavernous sinus on the right. The arrow indicates the cisternal component of the right trigeminal nerve.*

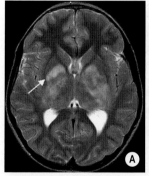
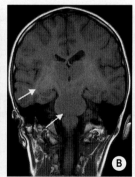
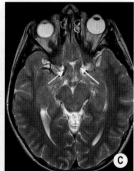

Child with neurofibromatosis type 1 (NF-1). (A,B) Characteristic hamartomatous lesions (unidentified bright objects) within the lentiform nuclei, brainstem and midbrain (arrows). They are high SI on T2WI, with minimal mass effect. Basal ganglia lesions may demonstrate some T1 shortening, as in this case, or are low SI on T1WI. (C) There are also bilateral optic nerve gliomas extending into the optic chiasm (arrows).*

Diagnostic criteria for neurofibromatosis type 1*	
Major criteria	**Minor criteria**
Café au lait spots Freckling in the inguinal or axillary areas One plexiform neurofibroma or two neurofibromas of any type* Visual pathway glioma* Two or more Lisch nodules of iris Distinctive osseous lesion, e.g. sphenoid dysplasia or thinning of cortex* First-degree relative with neurofibromatosis type 1 (NF-1)	Small stature Macrocephaly Scoliosis* Pectus excavates* 'Hamartomatous lesions' of NF-1* Neuropsychological abnormalities
*Radiologically detectable features	

TUBEROUS SCLEROSIS (BOURNEVILLE DISEASE)

DEFINITION

- A multisystem autosomal dominant neurocutaneous syndrome characterized by hamartomas, cortical tubers and benign neoplastic lesions (giant cell astrocytomas) ▶ 60–70% of cases are sporadic
- Genetic defects lead to abnormal migration of dysgenetic giant cells (capable of astrocytic or neuronal differentiation)
- *The most frequently affected organs:* skin ▶ brain ▶ retina ▶ lungs ▶ heart ▶ skeleton ▶ kidneys

CLINICAL PRESENTATION

- A clinical triad of intellectual impairment + epilepsy + adenoma sebaceum
- Infantile spasms or myoclonic seizures are the presenting symptom in 80%

RADIOLOGICAL FEATURES

Radiological criteria

- *Primary criteria:* calcified subependymal nodules and tubers ▶ *Secondary criteria:* non-calcified subependymal nodules and tubers ▶ cardiac rhabdomyoma ▶ renal angiomyolipoma

CNS lesions

Periventricular subependymal hamartomas or nodules These are seen in 98% of patients ▶ 90% are calcified and can be seen with CT or T2* MRI (calcification within a nodule increases with age but is rare if the patient is <1 year old)

MRI (infants <3 months old) T1WI: high SI ▶ T2WI: low SI

MRI (older children and adults) A reverse pattern of signal intensities ▶ T1WI + Gad: enhancement

Cortical and subcortical peripheral tubers These are most often seen within the frontal lobes ▶ they may demonstrate central umbilication

CT Low-density masses ▶ calcification with age

MRI A tuber has the same signal characteristics as a subependymal nodule

White matter hamartomatous lesions 50% are calcified ▶ often seen within the frontal lobes

MRI Variable appearances: curvilinear or straight thin bands radiating from the ventricles ▶ wedge-shaped lesions with apices near the ventricles ▶ tumefactive foci of abnormal signal intensity

Subependymal giant cell astrocytomas Located within the caudothalamic groove adjacent to the foramen of Monro (arising from a subependymal nodule) ▶ progressive

growth on serial imaging ▶ associated with hydrocephalus (due to their location)

MRI T1WI + Gad: homogeneous enhancement

Ocular manifestations

- Retinal hamartomas seen near the optic disc (15%) which are often bilateral and multiple (± micro-ophthalmia and leucocoria) ▶ subretinal effusions may be detected
- They appear as nodular masses originating from the retina, and when calcified may be difficult to distinguish from a retinoblastoma (unless there are also calcified subependymal nodules)

Other findings

- *Renal disease:* angiomyolipoma ▶ renal cell carcinoma
- *Pulmonary disease:* lymphangioleiomyomatosis ▶ bronchopneumonia
- *Cardiovascular disease:* rhabdomyosarcoma ▶ aneurysms

STURGE–WEBER SYNDROME

DEFINITION

- Congenital capillary venous angiomas of the face (a port wine naevus) + ipsilateral leptomeningeal cerebral angiomas with a primarily parieto-occipital distribution (occasionally bilateral)
- The abnormal venous drainage associated with a leptomeningeal angioma can cause chronic ischaemia (leading to cortical atrophy and calcification)

CLINICAL PRESENTATION

- Focal seizures (appearing during the 1st year) ▶ developmental delay with progressive hemiparesis, hemianopsia and intellectual impairment

RADIOLOGICAL FEATURES

SXR Tramline cortical calcifications, present by 2 years of age

CT/MRI The pial angioma is seen as diffuse pial enhancement of variable thickness ▶ enlargement of the ipsilateral choroid plexus ▶ dilatation of the transparenchymal veins that communicate between the superficial and deep cerebral venous systems ▶ progressive ipsilateral hemispheric atrophy

- Ipsilateral white matter: T1WI: low SI ▶ T2WI: high SI
- In 'burnt out' cases the pial angioma may no longer be detected after contrast enhancement, leaving only a chronically shrunken and calcified hemisphere

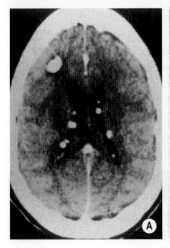
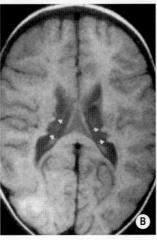
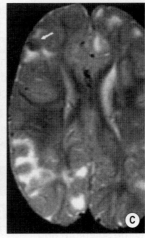

Tuberous sclerosis. (A) CT demonstrating periventricular calcified subependymal nodules. A cortical calcified tuber is also seen in the right frontal region. (B) T1WI demonstrating the subependymal nodules (arrows) lining the lateral ventricles (isointense to white matter). (C) T2WI demonstrating foci of abnormal SI throughout the subcortical white matter and in the cortex corresponding to cortical tubers. A right frontal tuber (arrow) is probably calcified (low SI).[+]

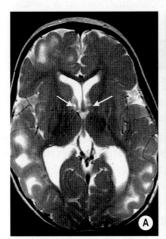
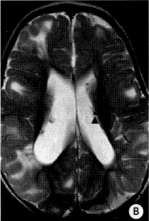
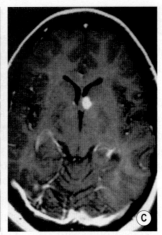

Intracranial manifestations of tuberous sclerosis. (A) Multiple tubers involving the cortex and subcortical white matter. Bilateral lesions are seen at the foramina of Monro, in keeping with giant cell astrocytomas (arrows). (B) Subependymal nodules project into the ventricles, some of which are markedly low SI, in keeping with calcification (arrowhead). (C) T1WI + Gad in a different patient shows an enhancing subependymal giant cell astrocytoma.[*]

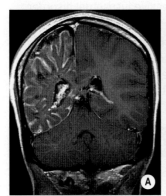
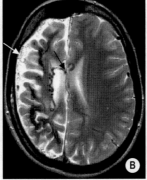
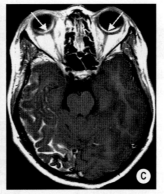

Sturge–Weber syndrome. (A) Coronal T1WI + Gad shows an enhancing pial angioma overlying the right cerebral hemisphere, which is atrophic. The right choroid plexus is enlarged. Foci of low SI within the gyri and adjacent white matter are due to calcification. (B) Axial T2WI shows in addition prominent superficial cortical veins and ependymal veins (arrows). (C) Axial T1WI + Gad shows bilateral choroidal angiomas (arrows) in addition to the pial angioma.[*]

X-LINKED ADRENOLEUKODYSTROPHY

Definition An X-linked disorder due to a defect in a peroxisomal membrane protein leading to defective incorporation of fatty acids into myelin

Clinical presentation Onset is between 5 and 10 years of age with learning and behavioural problems, a deteriorating gait and impaired visuospatial perception (± adrenal insufficiency)

- **Treatment:** Bone marrow transplantation replaces the defective gene ▶ Lorenzo's oil may delay disease progression

MRI T2WI: high SI changes are seen within the posterocentral white matter (particularly the splenium and peritrigonal white matter) progressing to the corticospinal tracts and visual/auditory pathways ▶ T1WI + Gad: enhancement of the leading edge of demyelination ▶ DWI: increased diffusion within the abnormal areas

ALEXANDER'S DISEASE

Definition A heterozygous (dominant) mutation of glial fibrillary acidic protein with neonatal, juvenile and adult forms

MRI T2WI: extensive abnormalities beginning within the frontal and periventricular white matter ▶ large cystic cavities are seen within the frontal and temporal regions (the basal ganglia may also be involved) ▶ T1WI + Gad: enhancement along the ventricular ependyma

CANAVAN DISEASE

Definition An autosomal recessive leukodystrophy with spongy white matter degeneration

Clinical presentation Hypotonia or spasticity ▶ seizures ▶ delayed development

MRI Symmetric white matter changes: T1WI: low SI ▶ T2WI: high SI

WILSON'S DISEASE

Definition An autosomal recessive disorder resulting from defective extracellular copper transport with resultant multiorgan copper deposition

Clinical presentation The onset is generally after the age of 12 years ▶ it is associated with liver cirrhosis and Kayser–Fleischer rings

MRI T1WI: low SI (basal ganglia) ▶ T2WI: high SI (basal ganglia ▶ midbrain and pons ▶ thalami and claustra ▶ white matter tracts)

MENKE'S DISEASE

Definition An X-linked disorder affecting transcellular copper metabolism with a systemic failure of copper-requiring enzymes (particularly those of the cytochrome c oxidase system)

Clinical presentation Connective tissue defects with 'kinky hair', inguinal herniae, hyperflexible joints and bladder diverticulae ▶ children can develop a severe cerebral vasculopathy where the vessels are prone to dissection

MRI Progressive cerebral atrophy which may allow subdural collections of CSF or subdural haematoma formation ▶ the basal ganglia may demonstrate T1 shortening

LEIGH'S DISEASE

Definition An inherited mitochondrial disorder (due to respiratory chain defects as well as enzyme disorders) with progressive neurodegeneration

MRI T2WI: bilateral and typically symmetrical high SI within the brainstem, deep cerebellar grey matter, subthalamic nuclei and basal ganglia

- The midbrain changes have been described as a 'panda face'

MELAS SYNDROME

Definition This is an inherited mitochondrial disorder: **M**itochondrial myopathy ▶ **E**ncephalopathy ▶ **L**actic **A**cidosis ▶ **S**troke-like episodes

Clinical presentation It typically occurs between 4 and 15 years of age ▶ acute metabolic decompensation may be provoked by an increased metabolic demand (e.g. during a febrile illness)

MRI Cerebral infarcts within non-vascular territories and symmetrical basal ganglia calcification

- **MERRF syndrome: M**yoclonic **E**pilepsy with **R**agged **R**ed **F**ibres

KRABBE' DISEASE

Definition An autosomal recessive lysosomal disorder (due to a galactocerebroside β-galactosidase deficiency)

MRI White matter changes (more severe posteriorly and centrally) ▶ basal ganglia and thalamic involvement (including low SI on T2WI) ▶ cerebellar white matter abnormalities (sparing the dentate nuclei) ▶ involvement of the brainstem pyramidal tracts

ZELLWEGER'S SYNDROME

Definition An autosomal recessive peroxisomal disorder

Clinical presentation The onset is shortly after birth ▶ it is associated with glaucoma, hepatomegaly, renal cortical cysts and stippled chondral calcification of the patella

MRI Hypomyelination ▶ subependymal periventricular cysts ▶ perisylvian polymicrogyria ▶ grey matter heterotopias

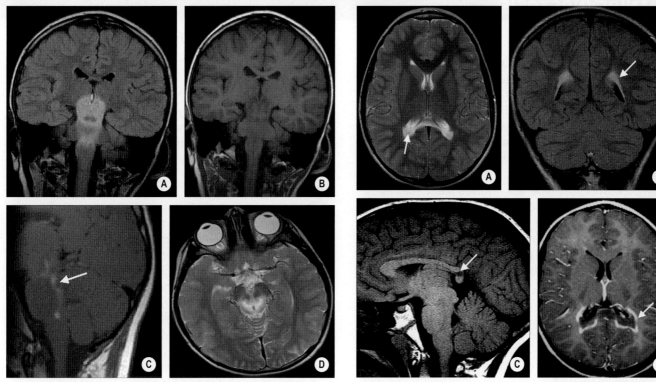

Leigh's disease. There is bilateral symmetrical high SI on the coronal FLAIR (A) and axial T2WI (D) matched by low SI on the coronal T1WI (B) affecting the midbrain, pons and medulla. Contrast enhancement (C) indicates breakdown of the blood–brain barrier in keeping with active disease (arrow).*

Adrenoleukodystrophy. There is peritrigonal and splenial signal abnormality (increased SI on T2WI and low signal on T1WI) (A, B, C, arrows) and marginal enhancement at the leading edges where there is active inflammation, typical of adrenoleukodystrophy (D, arrow).*

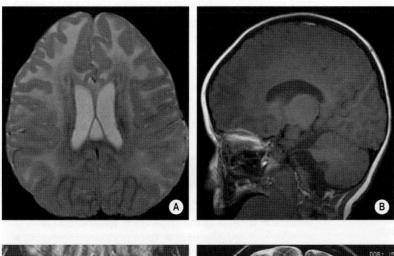

Child with Alexander's disease and macrocephaly. (A) Axial T2WI shows extensive bilateral symmetrical deep and subcortical white matter high SI with a frontal predominance and mild swelling. (B) Sagittal T1WI shows corresponding low signal in the affected areas without evidence of cavitation but in keeping with oedema.*

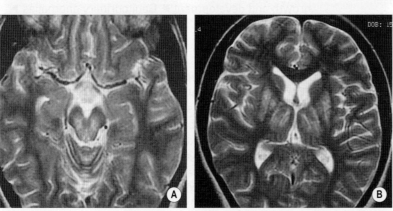

Wilson's disease. Axial T2WI demonstrating basal ganglia, thalamic and midbrain lesions.†

CRANIOSYNOSTOSIS

Definition

- A growth disorder with premature closure of one or more calvarial or skull base sutures ▶ the affected suture may be absent, indistinct, show bridging sclerosis, or a heaped-up or beaked appearance ▶ an affected suture may appear normal if the synostosis is fibrotic and not bony in nature
- *Primary simple non-syndromic type:* this usually involves one suture
- *Complex syndromic type:* this involves many sutures
- *Secondary craniosynostosis:* this is due to disrupted growth caused by drugs, metabolic bone disease, or an underlying small brain (microcephaly)
- Skull growth decreases perpendicular to the suture and increases parallel to it (therefore a normal skull shape makes craniosynostosis unlikely)

Clinical features

- An abnormal skull shape ▶ visual failure ▶ hydrocephalus

Radiological features

- *Sagittal synostosis:* an elongated head shape (scaphocephaly) ▶ the most common type
- *Bicoronal synostosis:* foreshortening in the AP direction (brachycephaly) ▶ it is associated with lateral elevation of the sphenoid wings (giving the characteristic 'harlequin' deformity), upward slanting of the petrous apices and hypertelorism
- *Unicoronal synostosis:* an oblique or slanting anterior skull (plagiocephaly) or an asymmetrical skull deformity ▶ it may be associated with compensatory growth on the unaffected side resulting in frontoparietal bossing
- *Metopic synostosis:* a triangular head (trigonoephaly – 'keel deformity') ▶ an AP view may show parallel and vertically oriented medial orbital walls

- *True unilateral lambdoid synostosis:* posterior plagiocephaly (the rarest form of a monosutural synostosis)

Pearl

- A posterior plagiocephaly must be distinguished from a positional or deformational plagiocephaly in which the suture is normal – the latter is due to a newborn lying on one side in preference to the other

Apert's syndrome

- This will demonstrate features of a brachycephaly due to a bicoronal synostosis ▶ there is a wide open midline calvarial defect from the root of the nose to the posterior fontanelle in what would normally be the sagittal and metopic sutures and anterior fontanelle ▶ the sutures never form properly with bone islands forming within the defect (coalescing to bony fusion at 36 months)
- *Additional features:* hypertelorism with shallow anterior cranial fossae ▶ a depressed cribriform plate ▶ maxillary hypoplasia causing midface retrusion with exorbitism (the globe may sublux onto the cheek) ▶ syndactyly, phalangeal fusion and a short radially deviated thumb producing the 'mitten' or more severe 'hoof' hand ▶ CNS abnormalities include callosal and septum pellucidum agenesis

Crouzon's syndrome

- This is a more complex syndromic synostosis involving the coronal, sagittal, metopic and squamosal sutures with early rather than late fontanelle closure ▶ there is no midline calvarial defect but there is maxillary hypoplasia, hypertelorism, exorbitism and dental malocclusion ▶ the limbs are usually clinically normal

CHOANAL ATRESIA/STENOSIS

Definition

- A congenital malformation of the anterior skull base characterized by failure of canalization of the posterior choanae ▶ it may be bony or fibrous

Clinical features

- *Unilateral atresia:* this presents in childhood with a chronic nasal discharge
- *Bilateral atresia:* this presents in newborns with respiratory distress (particularly during feeding) and is a surgical emergency ▶ bilateral forms are more likely to be syndromic (50%) and common associations are Crouzon's, Treacher Collins, CHARGE and Pierre Robin syndromes

- *CHARGE syndrome:* **C**olobomas of the eye ▶ **H**eart defects ▶ **A**tresia of the choanae ▶ **R**etardation of growth and development ▶ **G**enitourinary anomalies ▶ **E**ar anomalies

Radiological features

CT The nasal cavity appears funnel-shaped with a fluid level proximal to the obstruction ▶ the posterior vomer is thickened and the nasal septum is deviated to the side of the stenosis ▶ a bony, fibrous or membranous bridging bar across the posterior choana can be seen ▶ also congenital nasal pyriform aperture stenosis (focal stenosis of the nasal aperture anteriorly caused by medial displacement of the nasal process of the maxilla often associated with a single central maxillary incisor)

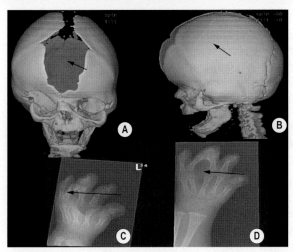

Apert's syndrome. (A,B) 3D CT surface-shaded display shows the wide open defect of the sagittal suture and brachycephaly with bicoronal synostosis typical of Apert's syndrome. The coronal sutures appear fused and are ridged. (C,D) Plain radiographs of the hands show the 'mitten hand' appearance with syndactyly and shortened metacarpals.*

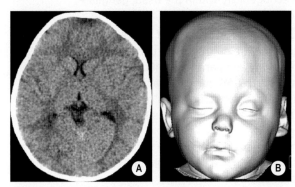

Unicoronal synostosis. (A) Axial CT and (B) 3D surface-shaded reformat show the asymmetrical head shape of left frontal plagiocephaly due to unicoronal craniosynostosis, with bossing seen on the right side.*

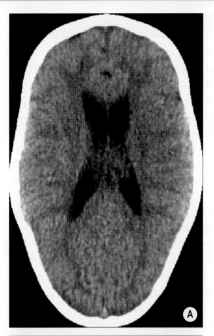

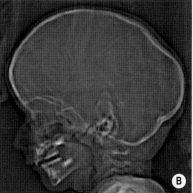

Sagittal synostosis. (A) Brain CT and (B) lateral scout view showing the typical 'boat-shaped' skull or scaphocephaly of sagittal synostosis.*

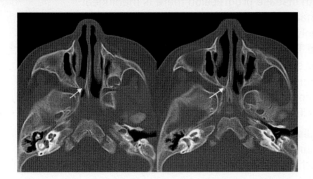

Choanal atresia. Axial skull base CT in a child with chronic nasal discharge shows right-sided choanal atresia. There is bony narrowing of the funnel-shaped posterior right choana down to a bony bridging bar (arrows) and pooling of secretions proximally.*

CONGENITAL INTRACRANIAL INFECTIONS

DEFINITION

- Intracranial infections acquired in utero or during passage through the birth canal ▶ TORCH infections (**TO**xoplasmosis ▶ **R**ubella ▶ **C**MV ▶ **H**erpes)
  - *Bacterial infections:* following spread from the cervix to the amniotic fluid
  - *Toxoplasmosis/rubella/cytomegalovirus (CMV)/ syphilis/HIV:* occurring via a transplacental route
  - *Herpes simplex virus (HSV):* following direct exposure to maternal type II herpetic genital lesions during delivery
- The pattern of brain injury depends upon the gestational age and stage of brain development at the time of infection (rather than the causative organism)
  - *<16–18 weeks:* neurons are forming within the germinal matrix and migrating to form the cerebral cortex
    - Infection results in spontaneous abortion, lissencephaly, or a small cerebellum
  - *18–24 weeks:* cortical neurons are organizing but no inflammatory response is possible
    - Infection results in localized areas of dysplastic cortex and porencephaly (a smooth-walled cavity, which is isointense to CSF on all sequences, is in continuity with the ventricular system, and without gliosis)
  - *24 weeks:* an inflammatory response is possible
    - Infection results in asymmetrical cerebral damage with gliosis, cystic change and calcification

CMV This is the commonest Western cause of serious viral infection in fetuses and neonates (affecting up to 1% of all births)

Toxoplasmosis A protozoan infection caused by ingestion by the mother of *Toxoplasma gondii* oocytes that are present within undercooked meat (it accounts for 1% of all still births)

HSV There is multifocal grey and white matter involvement

Rubella This is seen mostly in immigrant populations (following a mass vaccination programme)

HIV This follows vertical transmission

CLINICAL PRESENTATION

CMV Hepatosplenomegaly ▶ petechiae ▶ thrombocytopenia ▶ microcephaly ▶ chorioretinitis ▶ sensorineural deafness at birth (there is an increased risk of developing deafness and other neurological deficits up to 2 years after exposure)

Toxoplasmosis This is asymptomatic at birth ▶ seizures, hydrocephalus and chorioretinitis may appear at a later stage

Rubella *Infection during the first 8 weeks:* cataracts, glaucoma and cardiac malformations ▶ *infection during the 3rd trimester:* this may be asymptomatic

HIV This presents between the ages of 2 months and 8 years with hepatosplenomegaly and a failure to thrive
- *Progressive HIV encephalopathy:* dementia ▶ spasticity ▶ increasing head size
- *Static HIV encephalopathy:* cognitive and motor developmental delay predominate

RADIOLOGICAL FEATURES

CMV

- *Injury during the early 2nd trimester:* lissencephaly with a thin cortex ▶ a hypoplastic cerebellum ▶ ventriculomegaly and periventricular calcification
- *Injury during the late 2nd trimester:* polymicrogyria ▶ ventricular dilatation and cerebellar hypoplasia
- *Injury after the 2nd trimester:* parenchymal damage ▶ ventriculomegaly ▶ calcification and haemorrhage without an underlying structural brain malformation ▶ temporal pole cysts
- **Transfontanelle cranial US:** branching curvilinear hyperechogenicity within the basal ganglia ▶ 'lenticulostriate vasculopathy'

Toxoplasmosis The severity of any brain involvement correlates with the degree of earlier maternal infection ▶ microcephaly and parenchymal calcification is similar to that seen with CMV infection (although cerebellar hypoplasia and polymicrogyria is not seen)
- There can be a granulomatous meningitis or diffuse encephalitis
- Ventriculomegaly may be due to an active ependymitis (causing obstructive hydrocephalus) rather than diffuse cerebral damage

HSV This causes a rapidly disseminating encephalitis that is unlike the adult pattern (where disease starts within the medial temporal lobes)
- Within the paediatric population it appears as widespread asymmetrical regions of hypodensity or T2 high SI that is seen mainly within the white matter
- With disease progression there is meningeal enhancement as well as increasing swelling and cortical involvement (appearing as cortical hyperdensity on CT and T1W/T2W shortening)
- Any subsequent loss of brain parenchyma occurs early (often as early as the 2nd week) ▶ it eventually results in profound cerebral atrophy, cystic encephalomalacia and calcification

Rubella Imaging features are similar to the other congenital infections, although basal ganglia and parenchymal calcification predominates

HIV This usually presents with global atrophy and bilateral basal ganglia calcification ▶ diffuse symmetrical periventricular and deep white matter abnormalities are seen in 50% of patients with HIV encephalopathy and is usually associated with mild atrophy ▶ there may be corticospinal tract degeneration

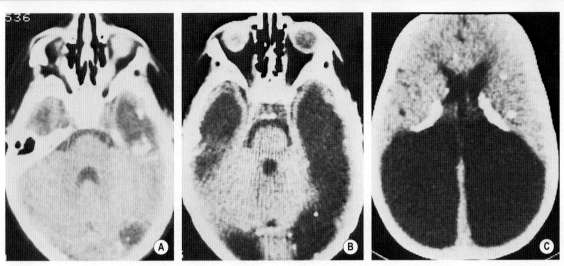

(A–C) Congenital toxoplasmosis. Grossly dilated ventricles and calcified granulomas in atrophic cortex and basal ganglia.[†]

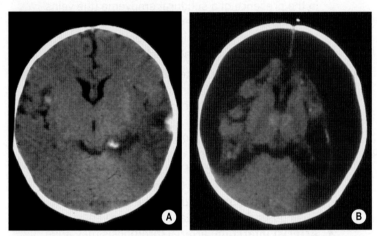

Herpes simplex type II encephalitis. (A) CT demonstrating the acute phase (including haemorrhages). (B) The chronic phase with atrophy and calcifications.[§]

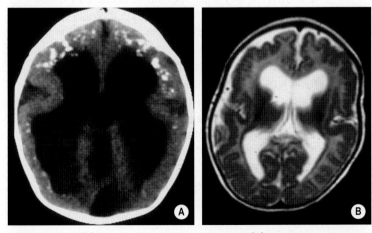

CMV infection. (A) CT demonstrating calcification. (B) T2WI demonstrating diffuse polymicrogyria.[§]

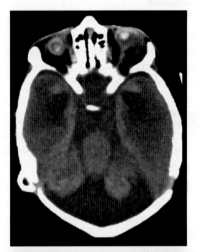

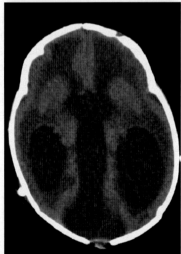

CT of a neonate with congenital TORCH infection. Both the optic globes are small and calcified (phthisis bulbi). There is a Dandy–Walker malformation and hydrocephalus with transependymal oedema.[†]

PAEDIATRIC MENINGITIS

Definition An infective or inflammatory process affecting the dura mater (pachymeningitis), pia and arachnoid maters (leptomeningitis) and CSF

Viral meningitis This is usually self-limiting

Pyogenic meningitis

- B streptococci
  - *Older children: Haemophilus influenzae ▶ E. coli ▶ Neisseria meningitides*
  - *Young adults: N. meningitidis ▶ Streptococcus pneumoniae*
- Organisms reach the meninges by five main routes: (1) direct spread from an adjacent infection (especially otitis media and sinusitis) ▶ (2) haematogenous spread ▶ (3) rupture of a superficial cortical abscess ▶ (4) passage through the choroid plexus ▶ (5) following a direct penetrating trauma

Clinical presentation

- *Neonate (1ˢᵗ few days of life):* overwhelming generalized sepsis ▶ often associated with a complicated labour
- *Neonate (after the 1ˢᵗ week):* a milder systemic sepsis but more meningitic features
- *Children/adults:* headache ▶ neck stiffness ▶ photophobia

Radiological features The diagnosis is made by the presence of clinical symptoms and a lumbar puncture ▶ neuroimaging is indicated if the diagnosis is unclear or to detect complications

Uncomplicated meningitis Imaging is usually normal

- T1WI + Gad: meningeal enhancement ▶ dense enhancing basal exudates are seen within the cisternal spaces in chronic and granulomatous meningitides

Complicated meningitis

- **Hydrocephalus:** ependymitis can cause an obstructive hydrocephalus due to debris and haemorrhage within the ventricular system ▶ purulent exudates can impair CSF absorption within the subarachnoid space resulting in a communicating hydrocephalus
- **Sterile subdural effusion:** this occurs especially in neonates with *S. pneumoniae* or *H. influenzae* ▶ it does not need surgical treatment
  - **CT/MRI** A subdural collection of CSF attenuation and signal characteristics ▶ there is rarely leptomeningeal enhancement
- **Subdural empyema:** a proteinaceous subdural collection requiring urgent surgical treatment
  - **CT** A hyperdense collection
  - **MRI** T1WI: intermediate SI ▶ T2WI: high SI ▶ T1WI + Gad: pachymeningeal and leptomeningeal enhancement
- **Ventriculitis:** this is usually spread via the choroid plexus with debris layering posteriorly within the ventricular system and hyperdense ependyma ▶ it is associated with subsequent hydrocephalus

- **Thrombosis of the deep venous sinuses and cortical veins:** this is common in the presence of a subdural empyema, infection or generalized sepsis ▶ the sagittal and transverse sinuses are the most commonly involved
  - **NECT** A hyperdense expanded sinus or hyperdense cortical vein
  - **CECT** The 'empty delta' sign (representing a filling defect within the sinus)
  - **MR venography**
    - *Acute phase:* T1WI: intermediate SI ▶ T2WI: low SI (cf a flow void that will not expand the sinus)
    - *Subacute phase:* T1WI: high SI
- A cavernous sinus thrombosis is more commonly seen with a paranasal sinus, dental or orbital infection ▶ it tends to present with ophthalmoplegia (due to involvement of cranial nerves II, IV and VI)
- **Venous infarction:** venous thrombosis is common in the presence of a subdural empyema (the veins thrombose as they traverse the infected subdural space) ▶ extension of infection into the brain parenchyma can result in a cerebritis or abscess formation
  - **MRI** Infarctions are often bilateral, conforming to the territory of the venous drainage (and are frequently haemorrhagic) ▶ DWI: there is a mixture of restricted and free diffusion
    - *Parasagittal infarction:* if the superior sagittal sinus is involved
    - *Thalamic infarction:* if the internal cerebral veins or straight sinus/vein of Galen are involved
    - *Temporal lobe infarction:* if the transverse or sigmoid sinus, or the vein of Labbé are involved
- **Arterial infarction:** arterial thrombosis may arise from the resulting arterial wall inflammation and necrosis, or from a similar process affecting the arteries that traverse any basal meningitic exudates ▶ small perforating branches from the circle of Willis can lead to small infarcts within the deep grey nuclei (the basal ganglia and thalami)
  - **CT** Wedge-shaped cortical and white matter hypodensities conforming to a major arterial territory
  - **MRI** T1WI: low SI ▶ T2WI: high SI
- **Labyrinthitis ossificans:** this is the most common cause of acquired deafness in childhood, and results from the direct spread of infection from the meninges into the inner ear
  - **CT** Increased density within the membranous labyrinth (due to fibrosis and ossification secondary to inflammation)
  - **MRI**
    - *Acute stage:* T1WI + Gad: faint enhancement of the membranous labyrinth
    - *Fibrous stage:* T2WI: signal drop-off

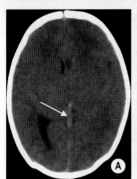 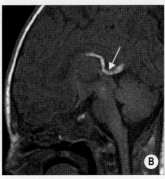 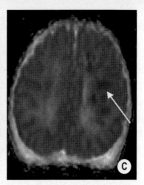

Venous sinus thrombosis in a child with recent history of vomiting. (A) CT shows hyperdense thrombus within the vein of Galen just reaching the internal cerebral veins (arrow). There is diffuse cerebral swelling with more hypodense change and swelling affecting the left hemisphere and thalami. (B) Sagittal T1WI confirms the diagnosis with T1 shortening in keeping with methaemoglobin in the internal cerebral veins and vein of Galen (arrow). (C) The ADC map shows patchy restricted diffusion (low signal) (arrow) within the deep white matter in keeping with infarction.*

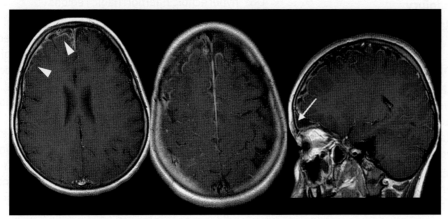

Bilateral subdural empyemas. There is leptomeningeal and pachymeningeal enhancement (arrowheads) most marked over the right cerebral convexity and extending back to the vertex (on the sagittal view). There is enhancing debris within the subdural space and the signal is slightly increased compared to cerebrospinal fluid. The source of infection was from the frontal sinus (arrow).*

Intracranial complications of meningitis in infants*	
Pathology	**Imaging**
Cerebritis	Diffuse hypodensity (CT) ▶ hyperintensity (T2-weighted MRI) involving the cortex and white matter ▶ gyral swelling ▶ ill-defined enhancement
Abscess formation	Peripheral rim enhancement surrounding a central necrotic cavity ▶ adjacent oedema
Effusion	Cerebrospinal fluid density/signal subdural collection ▶ no pathological enhancement
Empyema	Higher density (CT) ▶ restricted diffusion (MRI) subdural collection with pachymeningeal/dural enhancement
Deep venous thrombosis	Hyperdense expanded venous sinus (CT) ▶ lack of T2 flow void ▶ expanded sinus (MRI) ▶ variable haemorrhagic venous infarction
Cavernous sinus thrombosis	Expanded cavernous sinus ▶ filling defects on CTV ▶ signal drop off MRV
Arterial thrombosis	Large arterial territory infarct ▶ basal ganglia/thalamic small perforating arterial territory infarcts
Ventriculitis	Debris within the ventricular system ▶ hyperdense ependyma (precontrast) ▶ ependymal contrast enhancement ▶ ventricular isolation
Hydrocephalus	Obstructive intraventricular (foramen of Monro, cerebral aqueduct) ▶ obstructive extraventricular (communicating)
Deafness	CT/MRI evidence of labyrinthitis ossificans

HYPOXIC–ISCHAEMIC INJURY IN THE DEVELOPING BRAIN

PRETERM PATTERNS OF HYPOXIC–ISCHAEMIC INJURY

Definition Hypoxic–ischaemic injury tends to be seen in brains of about 20–35 weeks gestational age at the time of the precipitating insult ▶ it is a complication of prematurity (<1500 g birth weight) with a multifactorial aetiology:

- *Partial hypoxic–ischaemic injury:* this follows episode(s) of hypoxia or hypoperfusion to the developing brain
- *Profound hypoxic–ischaemic injury:* this follows a briefer episode of anoxia or circulatory arrest

Clinical presentation Neonatal encephalopathy ▶ spastic diplegia or quadriplegia ▶ visual impairment ▶ seizures

- Mental retardation is usually absent or mild (except in very severe cases)

Radiological features

Profound hypoxic–ischaemic injury

This affects the thalami with relative sparing of the other deep grey matter structures

Partial hypoxic–ischaemic injury

Periventricular leucomalacia (PVL) This describes ischaemic infarction of the periventricular deep white matter – this is the most sensitive part of the immature brain to hypoxia (and represents a 'watershed' region between the central and peripheral vascular supplies)

Focal (fPVL) Necrosis of all cell elements surrounding the lateral ventricles; a watershed infarct in the periventricular white matter giving rise to micro- and macrocysts

USS (early) Hyperechogenic periventricular white matter

USS (late) Development of coalescent macro- or microcysts (8–25 days) with transient small, often confluent, periventricular cysts ▶ there is associated atrophy of the damaged tissues (especially the white matter) with permanent secondary ventricular dilatation developing 4–8 weeks after injury

USS (end stage) Decreased periventricular white matter adjacent to the trigones ▶ ventricular dilatation with irregular ventricular markings (which is worse within the parieto-occipital regions with sparing of the front and temporal regions)

MRI (impending fPVL) Areas of restricted diffusion ▶ increased diffusion within cystic areas

MRI (established fPVL) Ventriculomegaly ▶ irregular lateral ventricles ▶ thinning of the periventricular white matter ▶ signal abnormalities of the white matter in the peritrigonal regions

- After 1 month, abnormal SI (low T1WI and high T2WI) in the posterior limb of the internal capsule predicts a poor motor outcome

Diffuse (dPVL) Injury of the premyelinating oligodendrocytes associated with astrocytosis and microgliosis ▶ injury results in decreased mature oligodendrocytes responsible for myelination (and changes in brain connectivity)

USS Initially usually normal

MRI Ventriculomegaly with regular outlines of the lateral ventricles

Germinal matrix or periventricular haemorrhage Secondary haemorrhage can occur following reperfusion of the damaged areas (the fragile vessels of the germinal matrix can easily rupture) ▶ this is probably less significant in terms of any subsequent handicap

US hyperechoic haemorrhagic regions

Intraventricular haemorrhage The proximity of the germinal matrix to the lateral ventricle (separated only by ependyma) may frequently result in rupture of any haemorrhage into the ventricles ▶ excessive blood can lead to ventricular dilatation (due to periventricular white matter congestions, venous infarction and secondary haemorrhage)

- Lesions are often unilateral and anterior and commonly occur in neonates that are <30 weeks' gestational age ▶ resolution of any parenchymal haemorrhage results in either paraventricular cavities which may communicate with the ventricle or focal ventricular dilatation

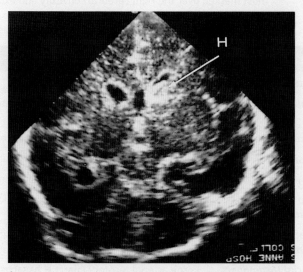

A coronal section in a premature infant showing a typical reflective haemorrhage (H) from the germinal matrix. A mass effect from the haemorrhage is distorting and elevating the lateral ventricle on this side.*

TERM PATTERNS OF HYPOXIC-ISCHAEMIC INJURY

Definition A hypoxic-ischaemic injury pattern seen in brains of about 36–42 weeks' gestational age at the time of the insult

Clinical presentation Sequelae include microcephaly with severe mental retardation and spastic quadriplegia (which may be asymmetric)

Radiological features

Profound hypoxic-ischaemic injury

Bilateral and symmetric changes affecting the most metabolically active regions ► posterolateral putamina ► ventrolateral thalami and adjacent capsular white matter ► hippocampi ► peri-Rolandic (motor and sensory) cortices ► visual cortex ► cerebellar vermis

Partial hypoxic-ischaemic injury

Bilateral (but not uncommonly asymmetric) injuries seen in a parasagittal distribution and typically involving a combination of the cortex and subcortical white matter (usually occurring across the frontoparietal regions) ► more prolonged insults are thought to result in cystic encephalomalacia

- A characteristic site is the posterior part of the Sylvian fissure with the greatest injury occurring at the base of the gyri (within depths of the sulci) and resulting in focal atrophy within these areas

Pearls Predominant involvement of the cerebral hemispheres with relative sparing of the posterior fossa structures is a pattern that favours a hypoxic-ischaemic injury over other causes of a global brain injury at term (such as perinatal or neonatal infection)

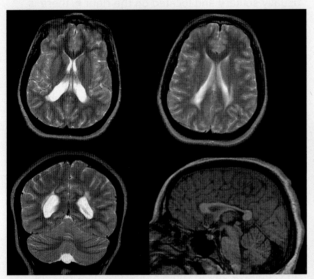

End-stage changes of periventricular leucomalacia. There is posterior periventricular increased signal on T2WI and enlargement of the ventricles posteriorly with irregular, scalloped margins, indicating white matter loss. The corpus callosum seen on the sagittal T1WI is markedly thinned, particularly affecting the posterior body.*

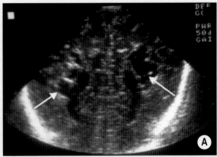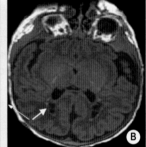

Early sign of periventricular leucomalacia. (A) US shows periventricular echolucencies (arrows), one of the earliest signs of periventricular leucomalacia. (B) On T1WI, these are seen posteriorly in the peritrigonal area and are lined by small focal regions of T1 shortening in keeping with haemorrhage (arrows).*

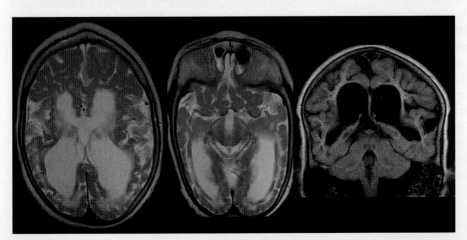

Hypoxic–ischaemia at term, imaged in childhood. The gyri are thinner at their bases than at their apices. This is known as ulegyria and dates the hypoxic–ischaemic event to term. Note the relative preservation of the cerebellum and brainstem.*

7.6 THE SPINE

SPINAL DYSRAPHISM

Definition This is also known as a neural tube defect (NTD), and are a group of congenital spine abnormalities that may cause progressive neurological damage (affecting 1:1000 live births)

- The common feature is an anomaly of the midline structures of the back
- It results from incomplete midline closure of the bony and neural spinal tissues following defective primary neural tube closure and persistence of the neural placode ▶ it is also associated with anomalous development of the caudal cell mass
- Neural placode: a flat segment of un-neurulated nervous tissue
- It can occur in closed (spina bifida occulta) and open (spina bifida aperta) forms
  - **Spina bifida occulta:** this is due to a failure of fusion of the posterior spinal bony elements ▶ the defect is covered by skin
    - *Without a tethered cord:* this is commonest at L5 or S1 ▶ it occurs in approximately 20% of the general population with no neurological problems (± back pain)
    - *With a tethered cord:* neurologic defects are uncommon ▶ a cutaneous lesion such as a dimple, sinus, hairy naevus or haemangioma may be a marker of an underlying defect and is seen in 50% of cases
      - *Associations:* meningocele ▶ lipomyelomeningodysplasia ▶ diastematomyelia ▶ neurenteric cyst ▶ dermoid and epidermoid cysts ▶ dorsal dermal sinus ▶ caudal agenesis ▶ myelocystocele ▶ spinal or filum terminale lipoma
  - **Spina bifida aperta**: the nervous tissue is exposed and neurologic defects are common
    - Most are myelomeningoceles and are virtually always associated with a Chiari II malformation ▶ they are usually found within the lumbosacral region
    - Usually the neural placode protrudes beyond the skin level with an expanded CSF containing sac lined by meninges ▶ occasionally it is a myelocele where the placode is flush with the surface and no meningocele component is present
    - Nerve roots (from the everted ventral placode) cross the widely dilated meningocele subarachnoid spaces to enter the neural exit foraminae ▶ the posterior elements of the vertebral column and the other mesenchymal derivatives (e.g. paravertebral muscles) remain everted
    - It is surgically repaired soon after birth, as untreated and exposed neural tissue is prone to ulceration and infection

MENINGOCELES

Definition Herniation of the spinal meninges through the intervertebral foramina or a vertebral body defect ▶ varying degrees of dural ectasia usually accompany spinal dysraphisms

- Generalized or focal dural ectasia may also be seen in: neurofibromatosis ▶ Ehlers–Danlos and Marfan's syndromes ▶ erosive arthropathies (e.g. ankylosing spondylitis)
- **Types of meningocele**
  - **Anterior thoracic meningocele with ventral herniation of the spinal cord**: this is most easily recognized with a midsagittal MRI of the thoracic spine where the spinal cord is displaced anteriorly and is in contact with a vertebral body near an intervertebral disc (commonly T6)
  - **Lateral thoracic meningocele:** this commonly presents as a paravertebral mass (CXR) ▶ it is usually solitary and located on the right ▶ there is an angular kyphoscoliosis towards the side of the meningocele with pressure erosion of the relevant intervertebral foraminal margins
    - Neurofibromatosis is present in up to 85% of cases
  - **Posterior meningocele:** herniation of the CSF sac (which is lined by dura and arachnoid) through a spinal defect results in a clinically apparent mass covered by skin ▶ it occurs mainly within the lumbosacral region
  - **Anterior sacral meningocele:** these are typically presacral and appear as a unilocular, complex lobular or multilocular cystic mass (the mass contains CSF which communicates with the intraspinal subarachnoid space) ▶ there is usually a large eccentric anterior lower sacral defect (with a pathognomonic scimitar appearance on XR) and an expanded sacral canal ▶ there can be varying degrees of sacral or coccygeal agenesis
    - It presents in older children and adults with low-back pain and bladder or bowel disturbance
  - **Terminal myelocystocele**: the central canal is dilated by a large hydromyelic cavity herniating into a posterior meningocele (through a posterior spinal bony defect) ▶ it is rare, and associated with syndromes such as VACTERL
  - **Myelomeningocele:** herniation of the spinal meninges and spinal neural tissue through a vertebral canal defect
  - **Myelocele:** the neural placode is flush with the skin surface but there is no skin covering

Pearl Hemimyelomeningoceles and hemimyeloceles may occur with diastematomyelia

Meningocele. (A) A huge CSF collection spills out through a defect in the spinal canal. (B) T2WI through the lumbosacral region shows no solid material within the fluid herniating through the dysraphic spine.[+]

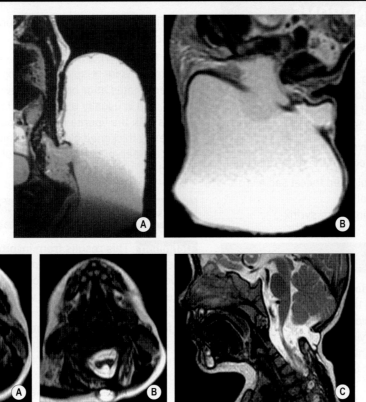

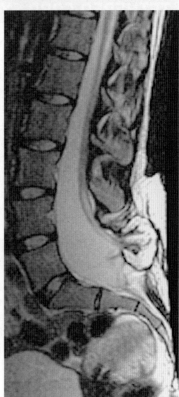

Cervical spinal cord diastematomyelia type II with associated craniocervical meningocele. (A) The meningocele is seen herniating through a bony defect in the vertebral posterior elements. (B) Axial T2WI shows that the cord has split into two hemicords. The apparent signal abnormality is in fact normal cerebrospinal fluid interspersed between the two hemicords. These reunite inferiorly. (C) Sagittal T2WI appears to show signal abnormality and thinning of the spinal cord, and is the clue to the diastematomyelia seen on the axial images.*

Myelomeningocele. Note the neural placode, enlarged spinal canal and spinal dysraphism. There is also a distal syrinx.[+]

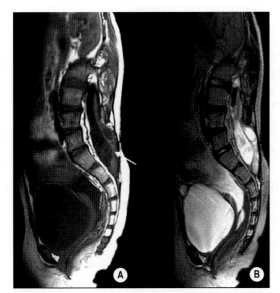

Repaired myelomeningocele in a child with Chiari II malformation. Sagittal T1WI (A) and T2WI (B) showing that the neural placode terminates inferiorly in the meningeal sac (arrow). The lumbosacral posterior vertebral elements have not formed.*

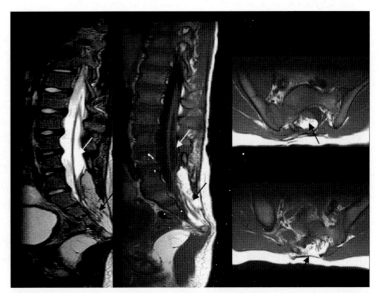

Closed spinal dysraphism. The spinal cord is too low and the neural placode terminates at the lumbosacral junction in a lipomyelocele (black arrows). There is an associated spinal cord syringomyelic cavity (white arrows). The posterior elements are deficient and everted.*

TETHERED CORD SYNDROME

Definition A low-lying conus medullaris tethered by a short thick filum terminale ▶ it is commonly a component of other spinal malformations (e.g. a spinal lipoma)

- The spinal cord reaches the adult position by term – the majority lie between T11/12 and L1/2 (it is abnormal if it is seen at or below the level of L3)

Clinical presentation Progressive neurological deterioration due to traction damage on the tethered cord

MRI A low-lying conus ▶ an enlarged thecal sac ▶ a thickened (>1.5 mm) filum terminale

- It may be associated with a spinal cord syrinx

SPINAL LIPOMA

- **Intramedullary/intradural lipomas:** a mass of adipose tissue located mainly between the posterior spinal cord columns (a tongue-like extension along the central canal can often be seen) ▶ the overlying dura mater is usually intact and the lipoma entirely intradural – however, there may be a dural defect to which the cord and lipoma become adherent
  - Its usual location is near the thoracocervical or craniovertebral junctions
  - CT and MR will demonstrate the fatty nature of the tumour
- **Filum terminale lipoma:** an asymptomatic fatty thickening of the filum terminale as a result of a disturbance of caudal regression ▶ it is considered a normal variant in the absence of a clinical tethered cord syndrome (and is seen in up to 5% of the normal population)

LIPOMYELOMENINGODYSPLASIAS

Definition These represent a spectrum of abnormalities ranging from an abnormally low conus medullaris (with minimal or even absent lipoma) to massive lipomatous formations involving all elements of the spinal and adjacent subcutaneous tissues

- *Lipomyelocele:* a lumbosacral neural lipomatous lesion continuous with the subcutaneous fat via a dysraphic spinal defect (tethering the spinal cord)
- *Lipomyelomeningocele:* a lipomyelocele + a meningocele

Clinical presentation These frequently present in adult life (sometimes with only back pain or minimal neurological signs)

XR There is non-fusion of ≥1 neural arches (± variable spinal canal expansion)

MRI T1WI/T2WI: a high SI lipoma continuous with the subcutaneous fat (± spinal canal extension) ▶ the spinal cord terminates at or below the level of L3 (in 80% of cases), and is usually tethered to the dorsal dura where it fuses with the lipoma ▶ nerve roots issuing from an apparently thickened filum terminale indicate it contains significant nervous tissue and should not be surgically divided

NEURENTERIC CYST

Definition This results from incomplete separation of the notochord from the endoderm, or from herniation of the endoderm into the dorsal ectoderm ▶ the cyst attachment to the notochord can prevent vertebral body fusion (leading to spinal anomalies)

- It forms part of the **'split notochord' syndrome**: this is a persistent connection between the endoderm and ectoderm resulting in splitting or deviation of the notochord:
  - *Dorsal enteric fistula:* the most severe form, representing a fistula connecting the intestinal cavity with the midline dorsal skin surface (therefore travelling through soft tissues and spine)
  - *Dorsal enteric (dermal) sinus:* this is a remnant of the posterior portion of the fistula with a blind ending tube opening onto the skin surface
  - *Dorsal enteric cyst (neurenteric cyst):* this is a trapped remnant of the middle portion of the fistula and is found within the intraspinal or paraspinal compartments
  - *Dorsal enteric diverticulum:* this is a remnant of the anterior portion of the fistula with a tubular diverticulum originating from the dorsal bowel mesentery
- **Intraspinal neurenteric cysts:** intradural (usually unilocular) cysts are lined by gastrointestinal or bronchial epithelium and are usually anterior to the spinal cord ▶ they occur within the cervical or lower thoracic regions and can compress the spinal cord (usually the anterior aspect)

XR A focal expansion of the spinal canal (butterfly or hemivertebrae are associated with thoracic lesions)

MRI T1WI / T2WI: the cyst contents are usually of high SI (relative to CSF)

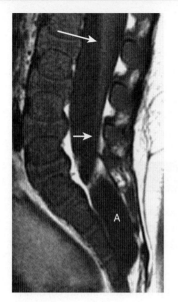

Tethered cord (long arrow), thick filum and lipoma (short arrows) and sacral extradural arachnoid cyst (A) on sagittal T1WI.[§]

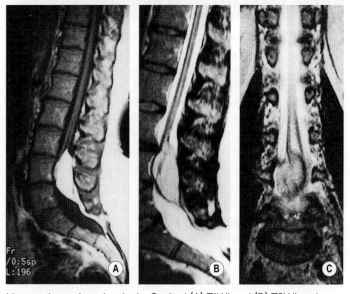

Lipomyelomeningodysplasia. Sagittal (A) T1WI and (B) T2WI and coronal (C) T2WI showing the lipoma, low position of the spinal cord and a cavity in the distal spinal cord.[*]

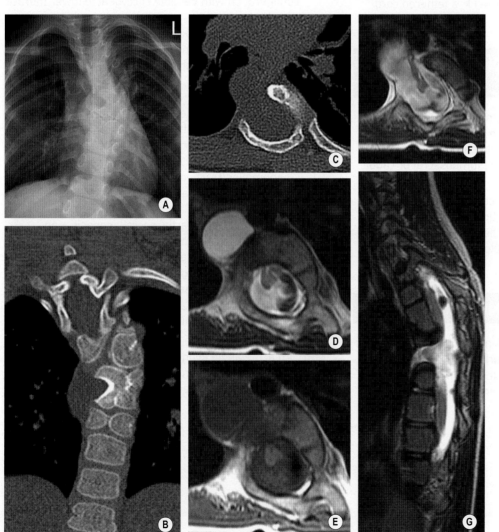

Neuroenteric cyst. (A) Chest radiograph and (B) coronal multiplanar reformat of CT thorax in same patient. There is a complex segmentation anomaly within the mid-thoracic region associated with kyphoscoliosis, consisting of congenital fusion and butterfly vertebrae. There is an associated right paraspinal mass. (C) Axial CT through the lesion shows that it is in direct continuation with the spinal canal through a large ventral bony defect. (D) Axial T2 and (E) axial T1 at the level of the lesion demonstrating that the lesion is cystic. (F) Axial T2 through the bony defect demonstrates the direct continuity of the cyst with the spinal canal. The appearances are in keeping with a neuroenteric cyst. The thoracic cord is also seen to extend through the bony defect. The neural tissue is seen to lie to the left of the neuroenteric cyst. (G) Sagittal T2 in the right paramidline demonstrating the direct communication with the spinal canal.[**]

DIASTEMATOMYELIA

Definition This forms part of the 'split notochord' syndrome: the spinal cord is split into two (usually unequal) hemicords ▶ each hemicord has a central canal and an anterior spinal artery but only gives off the ipsilateral spinal roots from one anterior and one posterior grey matter horn ▶ the hemicords nearly always re-unite caudally

- They are usually found within the thoracic cord, extending over several vertebral segments

XR A focal expansion of the spinal canal with narrowed intervertebral disc spaces ▶ there are varying degrees of laminar dysplasia and fusion

CT myelography/MRI The hemicords are enclosed within a common dural tube in 50% of cases but in the remainder each is enclosed within its own dural tube ▶ they are usually located within the cervical region ▶ a bony or cartilaginous midline extradural spur may arise from the malformed lamina which often lies between each hemicord

- Vertebral segmentation abnormalities are usually present (e.g. a hemivertebrae or bifid/fused vertebrae)
- Syringohydromyelia (50% of cases) ▶ a tethered cord (75% of cases)

SPINAL DERMOID/EPIDERMOID CYST

Definition A benign tumour arising from cells that can produce skin and its appendages ▶ it can be congenital or acquired (e.g. following a lumbar puncture)

- It is commonly located within the lumbosacral or cauda equina regions

CT/MRI A rounded intradural (occasionally intramedullary) lesion demonstrating fat (± calcification) ▶ in 20% a dorsal dermal sinus can be traced to a skin dimple on the lower back (this is a possible source of intradural sepsis)

DORSAL DERMAL SINUS

Definition An epithelial-lined skin opening with a variable fistulous extension to the dural surface ▶ it typically affects the lumbosacral region ▶ it is often associated with cutaneous stigmata (e.g. a hairy naevus or capillary haemangioma)

MRI A thin linear strip of tissue hypointense to the adjacent fat

- *Dermal openings at the sacrococcygeal level:* these are directed inferiorly below the thecal sac (sacrococcygeal pits) ▶ they do not require further imaging
- *Dermal openings above the intergluteal cleft:* these pass superiorly and may form a fistulous connection with the dural sac ▶ these warrant further investigation

CAUDAL AGENESIS

Definition This follows the abnormal development of the caudal cell mass as a result of apoptosis of notochordal cells which have not formed at the correct craniocaudal position

- **Caudal agenesis:** absence of the vertebral column at the affected level (as well as a truncated spinal cord, an imperforate anus and genital anomalies)
  - *Type I:* there is a high (often T12) abrupt spinal cord termination ▶ there is a characteristic wedge-shaped configuration with variable coccygeal to lower thoracic vertebral aplasia
  - *Type II:* the true notochord is not affected and only the caudal cell mass is involved ▶ the vertebral aplasia is less extensive (with up to S4 present as the last vertebra)
  - Associations:
    - *OEIS:* **o**mphalocele/**e**xstrophy/**i**mperforate anus/**s**pinal defects
    - *VACTERL:* **v**ertebral anomalies/**a**nal atresia/**c**ardiovascular anomalies/**t**racheoesophageal fistula/**o**esophageal atresia/**r**enal or **r**adial abnormalities/**l**imb anomalies
    - *Currarino triad:* Partial sacral agenesis + an anorectal malformation + a presacral mass (either a teratoma or anterior meningocele)
- **Segmental spinal dysgenesis:** a rare segmental abnormality affecting the spinal cord, segmental nerve roots and vertebrae
  - *Associations:* congenital paraparesis ▶ lower limb deformities

MRI An acute angle kyphus ▶ the spine and spinal cord may appear severed (the most severe cases) or focally hypoplastic (less severe cases)

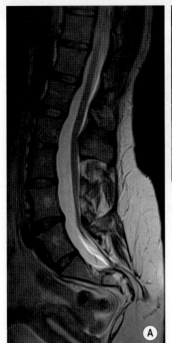

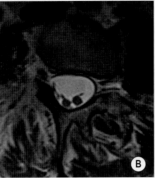

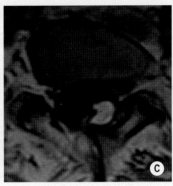

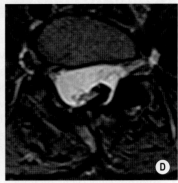

Diastematomyelia. (A) Sagittal T1 of the lumbar spine demonstrating an ill-defined low-lying conus at the L4–L5 level. The nerve roots are tethered caudally and herniate through a bony defect in the posterior elements. There is agenesis of the lower sacrum and of the coccyx. (B) Axial T2 through the lower thoracic spine clearly demonstrates the split cord. (C) Axial T1 through the lower dural sac demonstrates an intradural extramedullary left-sided high signal-intensity lesion. This suppresses on (D) fat-suppressed axial T2 at the same level. The appearances are in keeping with a lipoma.**

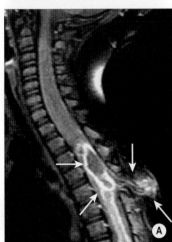

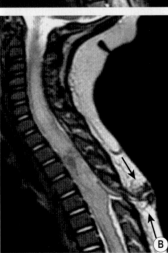

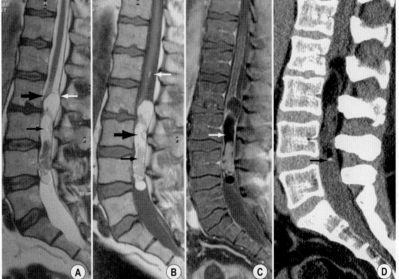

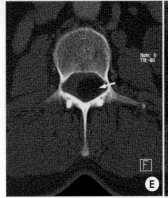

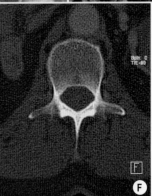

Intradural extramedullary dermoid in a 52-year-old man with backache, leg paresthesia, and anal incontinence. A, Sagittal T2W MR image depicts a large cystic intradural mass (thin black arrow) in the region of the conus medullaris and cauda equina. Note displacement of the dura mater (thin white arrow) posteriorly and the conus medullaris (thick black arrow) anteriorly. B, Sagittal T1W MR image shows an isointense solid component (thin black arrow) and a hyperintense fatty component (thick black arrow). A small fatty droplet is also visible in the subarachnoidal space (thin white arrow). C, Sagittal T1W MR image with fat suppression and administration of gadolinium affi rms the presence of fat (arrow) that is suppressed with this sequence. D, The sagittal CT image shows an additional small calcifi cation (arrow). E, The axial CT with bone window depicts a spinal canal widening in the region of the hypodense fatty component (at the level of L2) (arrow). In F, the spinal canal above it (at the level of L1) looks normal. This is a sign of a slowgrowing pathologic process with remodeling of the subjacent bony structures.■

Thoracic dermal sinus (posterior black and white arrows in (A) and (B)) and a cyst with an enhancing abscess (anterior white arrows in (B)) with cord oedema on the sagittal T1WI + Gad (A) and T2WI (B).§

813

SYRINGOMYELIA

Definition A longitudinal CSF filled cavity that is lined mainly by glial tissue ▶ it usually involves many segments (or the whole cord) ▶ it follows either cord damage (and subsequent cavitation) or CSF that has been abnormally driven into the cord (via the perivascular spaces) ▶ as a result of hydrodynamic forces the lesion is capable of propagating into normal cord tissue

- *Syringomyelia:* the cystic cavity is not continuous with the central cord canal
- *Hydromyelia:* cystic dilatation of the central cord canal
- *Syringohydromyelia:* features common to both of the above

Location It is commonly located within the cervical cord (only 10% extend cranial to C2)

Associations Cerebellar ectopia (70–90%) with the cerebellar tonsils usually lying at the level of C1 or C2

XR An expanded spinal canal (30–40%) ▶ scoliosis

MRI An enlarged spinal cord (affecting 80% of cases) which varies with changes in posture or respiration ▶ a well circumscribed CSF cavity often demonstrating prominent transverse ridges within its wall (giving a beaded or loculated appearance) ▶ pulsatile cysts can show flow-related signal changes

- There is a moderate correlation between the cavity location and the clinical features (but not between the clinical severity and the syrinx size relative to the remaining cord substance)
- T1WI/T2WI: a similar uniform SI to CSF (with slightly more variable SI on T2WI)

INTRASPINAL ARACHNOID CYST

Definition A loculated CSF fluid collection:
- *Extradural:* these arise from defects within the dura mater (congenital or inflammatory)
- *Intradural:* these arise from arachnoidal duplications or spinal arachnoiditis
- *Tarlov cyst:* a perineural arachnoid cyst occurring commonly within the sacrum (especially on the 2nd sacral root) ▶ can be large ▶ it is of doubtful clinical significance

Clinical presentation Pain or neurological disability if the spinal cord or cauda equina is compressed ▶ aspiration of cysts compressing the cord can improve symptoms

XR Spinal canal expansion (with extradural cysts)

MRI A well-defined cystic structure that often demonstrates higher SI than CSF (due to its reduced mobility) ▶ they can be multiple and are rarely associated with myelomalacia or syringomyelia ▶ extradural lesions can be overdiagnosed within the thoracic region (the thoracic spine is commonly wide and partly loculated)

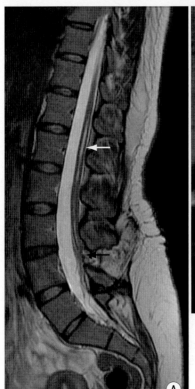

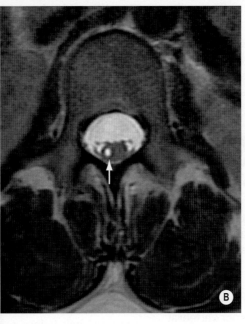

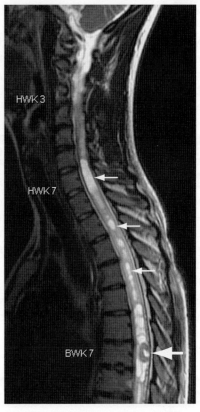

Syringohydromyelia, tethered cord, in a 21-year-old woman. Sagittal (A) and axial (B) T2W MR images show eccentric syringohydromyelia (white arrow) associated with tethered cord (black arrow).■

Syringohydromyelia associated with hemangioblastoma. T2W MR image shows the large sacculated syrinx extending in the thoracocervical spinal cord (thin white arrows), as well as thoracolumbar (not shown). Observe the nodule of the hemangioblastoma (thick white arrow).■

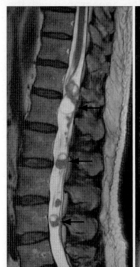

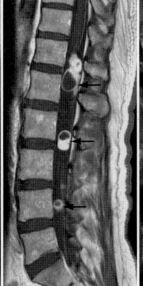

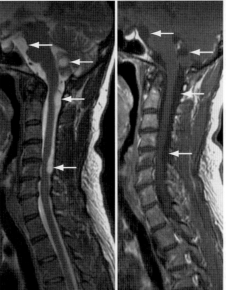

Cystic tumors usually show contrast enhancement (black arrows), whereas arachnoidal cysts (meningeal cyst type III) do not (white arrows).■

Multiple cystic tumor (presumed schwannoma)

Meningeal cyst, type III

815

ACHONDROPLASIA

Definition An autosomal dominant dwarfism affecting the spine and extremities

XR A decreasing lumbar spine interpedicular distance in the caudal direction ▶ bullet-shaped vertebral bodies ▶ short pedicles ▶ posterior vertebral body scalloping ▶ lumbar hyperlordosis ▶ a 'champagne glass' pelvis ▶ squared pelvic iliac wings

THE MUCOPOLYSACCHARIDOSES

Definition Inherited lysosomal storage disorders

Morquio–Brailsford type Instability and subluxation at the atlantoaxial joint and thoracolumbar junction (due to ligamentous laxity) ▶ upper spinal cord compression (due to ligamentous thickening) ▶ dens hypoplasia ▶ posterior vertebral body scalloping
• *Central* vertebral beaking

Hurler's type Especially marked thickening of dural and extradural tissues ▶ dens hypoplasia ▶ posterior vertebral body scalloping
• *Inferior* vertebral beaking

SPONDYLOEPIPHYSEAL DYSPLASIA

Definition
• Flattened or enlarged vertebrae in an AP dimension (especially with a thoracic kyphosis) ▶ there may be a severe scoliosis
• Neurological complications are uncommon

NEUROFIBROMATOSIS

Definition Neurofibromatosis type I is usually associated with a skeletal dysplasia:
• Severe scoliosis (50%) ▶ dysplastic vertebrae (10%) – often consisting of ≥1 absent or hypoplastic pedicles ▶ dural ectasia (10%) ▶ C1/2 or C2/3 subluxation or spinal compression (16%)

VERTEBRAL FUSION ANOMALIES

Definition
• Narrowed intervertebral discs which are partly bridged by regions where the disc material never formed early in development
• The fused segments usually show varying degrees of hypoplasia ▶ marked dysplasias (e.g. hemivertebrae) can occur if multiple segments are involved

Klippel–Feil syndrome The cervical region is predominantly involved

Spondylothoracic and spondylocostal dysplasia The thoracic spine is predominantly involved

TRANSITIONAL VERTEBRAE

Transitional lumbosacral vertebrae Complete or partial fusion of L5 with the sacrum ▶ there are enlarged L5 transverse processes with a narrowed L5–S1 disc space
• Its main significance lies in the fact that it may result in the wrong spinal level being identified preoperatively – a useful landmark is that the level of the iliac crests usually correlates with the L4/5 disc
• Lumbarization of S1 is less frequently seen

Cervical ribs Additional ribs arising from the 7th cervical vertebra
• *Differentiating feature:* the transverse processes of T1 tend to be directed superiorly (they are directed inferiorly with a cervical rib)

SPINAL INSTABILITY – C2

Os odontoideum Separation of the odontoid process from the body of the axis – this may represent a congenital failure of fusion, or a previous fracture of the odontoid synchondrosis before its closure

True hypoplasia of the dens Associated with more complex fusion anomalies, especially those that restrict rotation at C1/2

SPONDYLOLYSIS

Definition A defect within the pars interarticularis of a vertebral body (not to be confused with spondylosis) ▶ they probably represent stress fractures through the pars interarticularis of the laminae (resulting in a hypertrophic pseudoarthrosis)
• Spondylolytic defects are relatively common at the lumbosacral junction in young athletic adults

Oblique lumbar XR The 'Scottie dog' appearance with the pars defect represented by a dark 'collar' along its 'neck' (the pars intrarticularis)

Congenital type This is uncommon and is associated with absent pedicles, an absent superior articular facet, hypoplastic laminae with deviation of the spinous process and hypertrophy of the contralateral pedicle ▶ it is found within the cervical and lumbar regions

Bilateral spondylolysis This may result in a true spondylolisthesis (i.e. anterior displacement of an affected vertebral body relative to the vertebral body below) ▶ it must be differentiated from a degenerative spondylolisthesis (a pseudospondylolisthesis)
• *Anterolisthesis:* there is anterior displacement
• *Retrolisthesis:* there is posterior displacement with subsequent narrowing of the intervertebral foramina
• It is graded depending upon the degree of anterior displacement: Grade 1 (<25%) ▶ Grade 2 (25–50%) ▶ Grade 3 (50–75%) ▶ Grade 4 (75–100%)

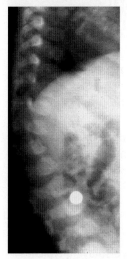

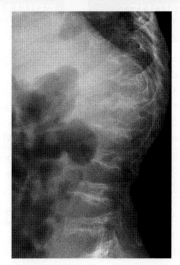

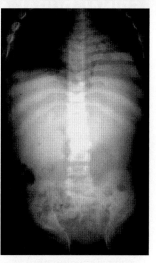

Hurler syndrome. There is hypoplasia of the anterosuperior aspect of the vertebral body at the thoracolumbar junction resulting in an anteroinferior beaking appearance. The other vertebral bodies have a short anteroposterior dimension and are ovoid with concave anterior and posterior margins and convex superior and inferior end plates. Thoracolumbar gibbus deformity is typically present in Hurler syndrome.©35

Morquio syndrome. There is universal vertebra plana, or flattened vertebral bodies. This can be distinguished from the ovoid vertebral bodies of Hurler syndrome and other mucopolysaccharidoses. The central anterior beaking of Morquio syndrome also differs from the anteroinferior beaking of Hurler syndrome and other mucopolysaccharidoses.©35

Hurler syndrome. The ribs are oar-shaped and wider than the intercostal spaces but become narrower in the paravertebral region. The iliac wings of the pelvis are flared, and the iliac body is constricted inferiorly.©35

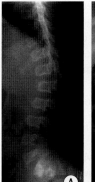
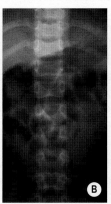
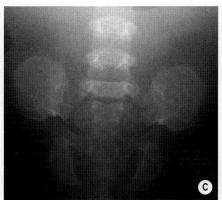
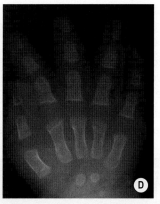

Achondroplasia. (A) Lateral radiograph of spine. Note posterior scalloping, bullet-shaped vertebral bodies, short pedicles and horizontal orientation of the sacrum. (B) Anteroposterior radiograph of the spine. There is abnormal narrowing of the interpedicular distances from L1 to L5 (should get progressively wider). This narrowing is not seen in infants. (C) Anteroposterior radiograph of the pelvis. Typical changes include horizontal acetabular roofs, trident acetabula and square iliac wings. (D) Anteroposterior radiograph shows a trident hand and bullet-shaped phalanges.©35

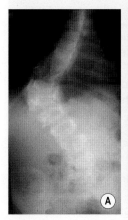
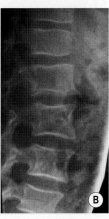
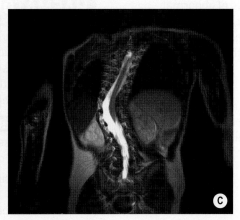

Type 1 neurofibromatosis with a short angular thoracolumbar curve as seen on an anteroposterior radiograph (A), lateral radiograph (B) and coronal T2WI (C). There is scalloping of the posterior vertebral body wall and enlargement of the exit foramen. The MR image demonstrates dural ectasia with a widened spinal canal.©35

SPINAL DURAL ARTERIOVENOUS FISTULA (SDAVF)

Definition These represent >80% of all spinal arteriovenous malformations ▶ middle aged me leading to gait disturbance, paresthesia and incontinence

- *Location:* located within the spinal dura mater close to a root sleeve ▶ they are commonly found within the thoracic region (although within the cervical spine they are only found around the foramen magnum)
- *Anatomy:* usually supplied by 1–2 radiculomeningeal arterial branches with shunting via a single vein into an intradural vein ▶ symptomatic lesions demonstrate slow and anomalous venous drainage which remains intradural through a greater part of the spinal canal than normal (venous stagnation is an important cause of a clinical myelopathy)

Radiological features

MRI

- T2WI: ill defined central intramedullary high SI extending over multiple levels (representing venous hypertensive oedema) ± cord expansion ± low SI rim ▶ engorged perimedullary veins seen as flow voids (dorsal > ventral surface)
- T1WI + Gad: diffuse enhancement of the cord ▶ enhancing perimedullary veins ▶ this may demonstrate the site of the dural fistula

Digital subtraction angiography (DSA) This is the gold standard investigation, also allowing access for interventional therapy (e.g. embolization)

Pearl Embolization of arteries supplying a fistula may be feasible (if they can be shown not to supply the cord)

SPINAL ARTERIOVENOUS MALFORMATIONS (SAVMs)

Definition In contrast to SDAVFs, these are fed by spinal arteries (radiculomedullary/radicullopial) and are more prone to haemorrhage (intramedullary or subarachnoid)

- *Glomerular AVMs (plexiform or nidus type):* the most common, contains a cluster or nidus of abnormal vessels between the feeding artery and draining vein
- *Fistulous AVMs (intradural AV fistula):* direct AV shunts commonly located superficially on the cord

Radiological features

MRI

- T2WI: serpiginous flow voids (dilated veins) ▶ oedema (venous congestion) as ill defined high SI with cord expansion
- T1WI + Gad: enhancement

SPINAL CORD CAVERNOUS MALFORMATION (SCCM)

Definition Rare vascular malformations composed of sinusoidal-type vessels in immediate apposition to each other without normal intervening parenchyma

- Extradural/intradural–extramedullary/intramedullary (commonest)

Clinical presentation Discrete episodes of neurological deterioration separated by variable time intervals ± recovery ▶ slowly progressive myelopathy ▶ acute neurological deficit with either gradual or rapid decline

Radiological features

MRI

- T1WI + T2WI: heterogenous lesions displaying typical 'popcorn' appearances (blood products of differing ages) ▶ low SI T2WI rim and hypointense 'blooming' on GE sequences (haemosiderin deposition)

SPINAL CORD INFARCTION

Definition A rare complication of arteriosclerotic vascular disease (rich anastomotic blood supply) ▶ it may also complicate an aortic dissection or aortic aneurysm surgery

- Thoracolumbar > cervical cord (arterial border zones) ▶ located in the central/anterior territories of the anterior spinal artery – resulting in classical sensory pattern loss of pain and temperature sensation with preservation of touch and proprioception
- A venous infarction (due to extensive thrombosis of the local pial veins) is rare

MRI

- T2WI: high SI within the central cord ('owl's eyes' or 'snake's eyes' appearance) ▶ mild cord swelling
- T1WI + Gad: mild enhancement (breakdown of the blood–brain barrier)
- DWI: very sensitive in the acute phase

SPONTANEOUS EPIDURAL HAEMATOMA

Definition A rare, devastating condition requiring emergency surgical treatment to preserve spinal cord function ▶ a cause is rarely identified

- It presents with acute back pain and a progressive flaccid paraplegia developing over hours

Radiological features

CT A hyperdense epidural mass, which can be broad based, lentiform or biconvex in shape

MRI Variable signal intensities depending upon the haematoma age

- T1WI + Gad: focal enhancement represents active bleeding

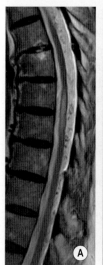
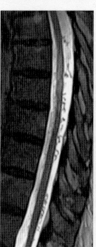
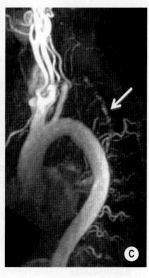
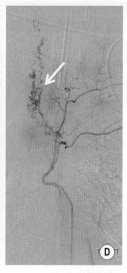

Spinal dural arteriovenous fistula (SDAVF). (A) Sagittal T2 demonstrating intrinsic T2 cord hyperintensity in keeping with spinal cord oedema. Serpiginous flow voids of the dilated perimedullary veins are more prominent on the dorsal surface and appear more conspicuous on (B) the CISS sequence. (C) Sagittal reconstruction of TWIST sequence at the level of the thoracic aorta suggests presence of a fistula in the upper thoracic cord (arrow). A SDAVF was confirmed by DSA (D) following selective catheterization of left supreme intercostal trunk which demonstrated the fistulous point (arrow).**

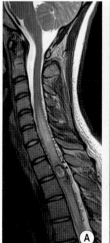
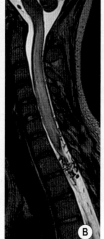
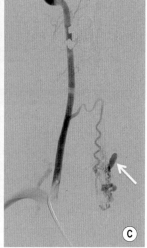

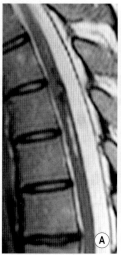
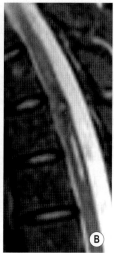

Spinal arteriovenous malformation (SAVM). (A) Sagittal T2 MRI demonstrating an intramedullary lesion at T1/2 with a hypointense rim in keeping with haemosiderosis. Note the cord expansion and associated cord oedema. Note also the serpiginous flow voids, which are more prominent on the dorsal surface of the cord. These are much more conspicuous on heavily weighted T2 sequences such as (B) CISS sequence, right parasagittal slice. (C) Selective catheterization of the right vertebral artery on DSA confirms the presence of an arteriovenous malformation. Note the intranidal aneurysm (arrow).**

Spinal cord cavernous malformation (SCCM). (A) Sagittal T2 and (B) with fat suppression demonstrating intramedullary lesion with heterogeneous signal intensity and T2 hypointense rim in keeping with blood products. Note the associated intrinsic cord T2 hyperintensity, which extends for several segments above and below the lesion.**

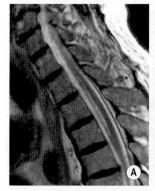
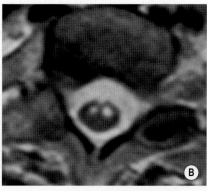
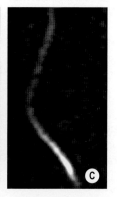

Acute spinal cord ischaemia with acute onset of symptoms in a male patient following aortic repair. (A) On sagittal T2 of the cervicothoracic spine linear hyperintensity is shown in the ventral part of the spinal cord extending over three vertebral segments. (B) Axial T2 demonstrates 'snake's eyes' appearance, indicating involvement of the ventral grey matter of the spinal cord. (C) Sagittal trace DWI demonstrates high signal consistent with restricted diffusion.**

SPINAL TUMOUR CATEGORIES

- *Intramedullary*
  - 10% of all primary spinal tumours ▶ astrocytomas and ependymomas (90%) ▶ 10–15 times less common than primary intracranial tumours
- *Intradural extramedullary*
  - 30% of all primary spinal tumours ▶ results in displacement of the cord to the contralateral side and widening of the ipsilateral CSF space ▶ the majority are extramedullary ▶ meningiomas, nerve sheath tumours (schwannomas and neurofibromas) and drop metastases being the most common ▶ frequently present with progressive myelopathy and weakness
- *Extradural*
  - 60% of all primary spinal tumours ▶ usually arises from the vertebrae ▶ much less frequent than metastatic disease
  - 75% vertebral body lesions are malignant ▶ 70% of benign lesions within posterior elements
  - Adults: 2/3 malignant ▶ children: 2/3 benign

INTRAMEDULLARY TUMOURS

Ependymoma

Definition Arises from the ependymal cells lining the central ependymal canal (therefore frequently centrally located within the cord, explaining the frequent sensory symptoms, with motor deficits only presenting later)
- Well demarcated and compresses rather than invades the adjacent cord

Clinical presentation Most frequent intramedullary tumour in adults ▶ sporadic in children (outside of the setting of NF-2) ▶ low grade (WHO Grade 2) with an indolent course
- Peak incidence: 4th and 5th decades

Radiological features Often found in the cervical cord, less frequently the upper thoracic cord ▶ mean tumour size is usually 3 vertebral body segments ▶ syrinx is a characteristic finding (especially in the cervical region)

CT Canal widening ▶ scoliosis ▶ vertebral body scalloping

MRI Central well circumscribed lesions ▶ T1WI: normal to low SI ▶ T2WI: low to high SI ▶ T1WI + Gad: avid homogenous enhancement
- *'Cap' sign:* T2WI: low SI areas at both sides of the tumour limits (haemosiderin deposits due to chronic haemorrhage)

Astrocytoma

Definition The most common intramedullary tumour in children (30% of intramedullary tumours in adults)
- Usually low grade tumours ▶ infiltrative with poorly defined boundaries

Clinical presentation Peak incidence: 1–5 years ▶ 3rd and 4th decade ▶ slightly more common in males

Radiological features Most common site: thoracic cord (70%) followed by the cervical cord ▶ frequently involve a large proportion of the cord – entire cord involvement ('holocord' tumour) is rare but more common in children

MRI Necrotic-cystic degeneration (60%) with a 'cyst with mural nodule' appearance ▶ solid (40%)
- T1WI: solid component: normal to low SI ▶ necrotic-cystic component: low SI
- T2WI: solid component: high SI ▶ necrotic-cystic component: very high SI
- T1WI + Gad: increasing enhancement with tumour grade

Haemangioblastoma

Definition Rare, benign (low grade) richly vascularized tumours
- Solitary (80%) or multiple (20%) when associated with von Hippel–Lindau syndrome ▶ up to 90% of patients with VHL may have spinal lesions

Clinical presentation More common in adults ▶ peak incidence 4th decade

Radiological features
- *Location:* cervical or thoracic level ▶ multiple sites at all levels in VHL
- *Two presentations:*
  1. Small nodular lesion located in the subpial region and surrounded by extensive intramedullary oedema
  2. Small nodule associated with huge and extensive intramedullary cystic components
- T1WI: solid tumour nodule: normal to low SI
- T2WI: solid tumour nodule: normal to slightly high SI
- T1WI + Gad: intense homogenous enhancement of the subpial nodule

Ganglioglioma

Definition Composed of a combination of neoplastic ganglion cells and glial elements ▶ typically low grade but a propensity for local recurrence (the glial element may progress to high grade)

Radiological features **Location:** cervical and upper thoracic cord – may extend to the medullaoblongata through the foramen magnum ▶ eccentric location within the cord ▶ may extend over >8 vertebral body segments

CT May demonstrate calcification

MRI Non-specific highly variable imaging findings ▶ can be solid or cystic
- Features: long tumour length ▶ tumoral cysts ▶ absence of oedema ▶ T1WI mixed SI ▶ focal or patchy enhancement (rarely involving whole tumour)

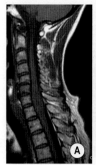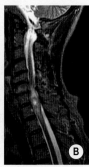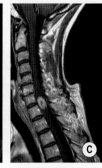

Spinal cord ependymoma. Sagittal T1 (A) and T2 (B) show clearly focal spinal cord enlargement at the cervicothoracic junction. The lesion is iso- to slightly hypointense on T1, and very heterogeneous on T 2 with areas of low signal intensity within the tumour. There is some associated oedema within the cord. Gd-enhanced T 1 (C) shows focal nodular contrast enhancement centrally within the spinal cord. Straightening of the spine and multilevel degenerative changes of the lower C-spine are observed.**

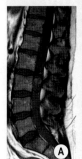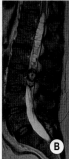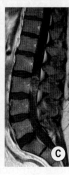

Myxopapillary ependymoma. Sagittal T 1 (A) and T 2 (B) show a well-defined heterogeneous mass at the L3 level. The lesion is slightly hyperintense on T 1, which may be explained by the presence of mucin, but it shows low signal on T2, and has a low signal intensity rim, suggestive for haemorrhage within the tumour. Inferior to the mass, trapped CSF has high T1 and T2 signal, possibly caused by a high protein content. Extensive cyst formation with enlargement of the spinal cord is observed proximal to the tumour with some oedema at the border with the normal cord. Sagittal gadolinium-enhanced T 1 (C) shows enhancement of the tumour mass.**

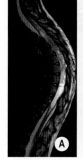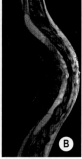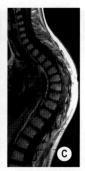

Spinal cord astrocytoma. Follow-up study with sagittal T2 (A, B) in an 11-year-old girl who had partial resection of the tumour 2 and 3 years before, respectively. Final diagnosis at that time was grade 2 fibrillary astrocytoma. Progressive enlargement of the associated polar cysts proximal and distal to the resected tumour is observed. Also the spinal cord oedema has increased. Sagittal contrast-enhanced T1 of the most recent follow-up study (C) shows heterogeneous enhancement, not present on the previous examination, which is indicative of progressive disease. Note the hyperkyphosis and scoliosis in this girl, which are frequently indirect signs of intradural spinal tumours in children.**

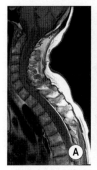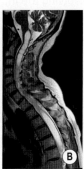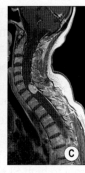

Cervical haemangioblastoma. Sagittal T1 (A) and T2 (B) show a diffuse enlargement of the spinal cord. Extensive oedema and multiple cyst formation can be seen extending up to the level of the obex. Sagittal (C) gadolinium-enhanced T1 show the presence of an intense enhancing tumour at the C7 level. Flow voids can be observed within the enhancing tumour. Enhancement is also visible in dilated veins along the posterior aspect of the spinal cord.** (Case courtesy of M. Voormolen, Antwerp, Belgium.)

Intramedullary tumours			
	Astrocytoma	**Ependymoma**	**Haemangioblastoma**
Definition	A primary intramedullary glioma (most commonly found in the paediatric population)	An ependymal tumour lining the spinal cord central canal (most commonly found in the adult population)	A capillary-rich neoplasm ▶ most are solitary but multiple lesions suggest von Hippel–Lindau syndrome
Predominant location	Thoracic > cervical cord (it is rare within the filum terminale)	It predominantly affects the filum terminale (especially in children where it is usually the myxopapillary type)	Thoracic = cervical cord ▶ it almost always involves the posterior columns of the spinal cord (abutting a pial surface)
Size	Cord expansion: > 4 vertebral segments	Cord expansion: 3–4 vertebral segments	Cord expansion: a few mm up to a few cm
Appearance	A poorly defined infiltrating mass	A well-circumscribed mass	A mass with round and well-defined margins
*T1WI**	Intermediate SI	Intermediate SI	Low-to-intermediate SI (larger lesions can demonstrate flow voids)
*T2WI**	High SI	High SI 'cap' sign: extreme hypointensity (haemosiderin) at its cranial or caudal margin	High SI (± flow voids)
T1WI + Gad	It usually enhances	There is intense enhancement	Intense enhancement (small lesions) ▶ heterogeneous enhancement (large lesions)

*An astrocytoma or ependymoma cannot be distinguished reliably with MRI (or distinguished reliably from many inflammatory processes)

INTRADURAL EXTRAMEDULLARY TUMOURS

Nerve sheath tumours (schwannoma/neurofibroma)

Definition

- **Schwannoma**: benign tumour arising from the dorsal sensory nerve roots ▶ most common intradural extramedullary tumour

Clinical presentation

- **Schwannoma:** more common in adults ▶ far less common in children (can be seen in NF-2)

Radiological features

- **Schwannoma:** usually solitary
  - Location: cervical and lumbar region
    - Intradural extramedullary (70%)
    - Extradural (15%)
    - 'Dumbbell' shape involving the intra- and extradural space (15%)

MRI Well-encapsulated tumours ± cystic components ▶ calcification and haemorrhage are rare

T1WI Isointense to cord ▶ T2WI: high SI ▶ T1WI + Gad: variable enhancement

- **Neurofibroma:** often multiple tumours

MRI Not well encapsulated and ill defined ▶ unable to differentiate between a solitary neurofibroma or schwannoma

T2WI Normal to high SI ▶ 'target' sign: hyperintense rim with a low-to-intermediate SI centre

Meningioma

Definition

- Dural-based intradural tumours ▶ 95% are benign

Clinical presentation

- 2nd most common intraspinal tumour, occurring most frequently in older patients (peak age 5th and 6th decades) ▶ uncommon in children outside of NF-2 ▶ F>M
- Very slow growing and major cord compression can be seen with minor symptoms

Radiological features

- *Location:* thoracic region (80%) with a female preponderance ▶ in men 50% are in the thoracic region and 40% are cervical
- Mostly located posterolaterally in the thoracic region and anteriorly in the cervical region
- Usually solitary tumours (can be multiple in NF-2)

CT Iso- to hyperattenuating ± calcification ▶ hyperostosis is less common than with the intracranial forms

MRI T1WI: normal to low SI ▶ T2WI: slightly high SI ▶ T1WI + Gad: strong and homogenous enhancement ▶ low SI on all sequences if heavily calcified ▶ classical 'dural tail' is less commonly seen than with intracranial lesions

Metastases

Definition

- Leptomeningeal metastases: secondary tumours arising from a primary outside of the CNS (e.g. breast)
  - 'Drop' metastasis: spread of a CNS tumour (e.g. medulloblastoma)
- Leptomeningeal dissemination from CNS neoplasms occurs in younger patients – metastases from lung or breast primaries tends to occur in older patients

Radiological features

CT/MRI 3 patterns of enhancement:
- Diffuse contrast enhancement along the pia of the spinal cord and nerve roots ('sugar coating' pattern)
- Multiple small contrast enhancing nodules in the subarachnoid space
- Single contrast enhancing mass

EXTRADURAL TUMOURS – BENIGN

Vertebral haemangioma

Definition

- Most common benign spinal tumour ▶ can be asymptomatic, or more aggressive with symptoms
- Usually occurs within the vertebral body (10% extend into the pedicles)

Radiological features

CT *'Polka-dot'* pattern: multiple dots seen on axial imaging (reinforced trabeculae) ▶ *'honeycomb'* or *'jail bar'* pattern: parallel linear streaks in a vertebral body of reduced density seen on sagittal imaging

MRI T1WI / T2WI: high SI (fibro-adipose tissue insinuating between the sinusoidal blood channels) ▶ T1WI + Gad: enhancement

- Aggressive lesions characterized by prominent soft tissue that can invade the epidural space and encroach on the spinal canal

EXTRADURAL TUMOURS – MALIGNANT

Metastases

Radiological features

- *Location:* thoracic spine (70%) ▶ lumbar spine (20%) ▶ cervical spine (10%) ▶ multiple levels (30%)

CT Lytic/sclerotic lesions with irregular non-sclerotic margins ± cortical breach/paravertebral or epidural extension
- *Osteolytic:* lung/breast/thyroid/kidney/colon
- *Osteoblastic:* prostate/breast

MRI T1WI: low SI ▶ T2WI: high SI or low SI (if sclerotic)

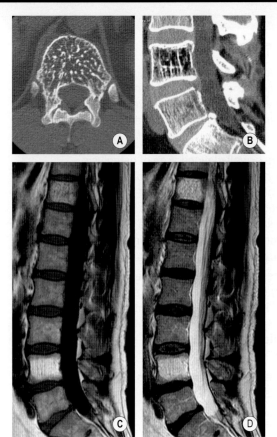

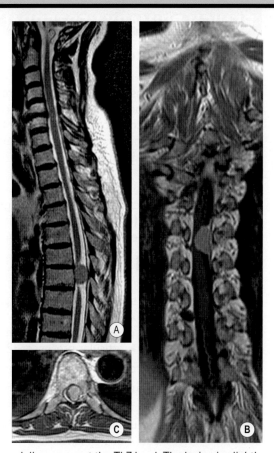

Asymptomatic vertebral haemangioma. Axial CT (A) shows numerous high-attenuation dots within the vertebral bone marrow, simulating the 'polka-dot' pattern on clothing. On a sagittal reformatted image (B) a so-called 'corduroy sign' may be observed: vertically oriented, thickened trabeculations, replacing the normal cancellous bone, surrounded by fatty bone marrow or vascular lacunae. Sagittal T1 (C) and T2 (D) MR images show high (fat) signal intensity throughout the Th11 and L4 vertebral body with linear striations of low signal intensity due to thickened trabeculae.**

Mid-thoracic meningioma. Sagittal T2 (A) demonstrates an ovoid intradural extramedullary mass at the Th7 level. The lesion is slightly hyperintense relative to the spinal cord. Coronal (B) and axial (C) gadolinium-enhanced T1 show avid contrast enhancement. Note the broad attachment to the dura with the presence of a typical dural tail. The tumour causes severe spinal canal narrowing and spinal cord compression and right lateral displacement of the spinal cord.**

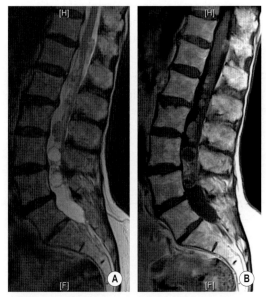

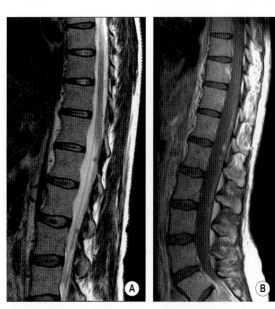

Multiple neurofibromas in a young woman with neurofibromatosis type 1. Sagittal T2 (A) and sagittal gadolinium-enhanced T1 (B) show multiple bulky and nodular tumours arising from spinal nerve roots which are a typical representation of neurofibromatosis type 1. They are iso- to hyperintense on T2 and show strong homogeneous enhancement. MR imaging of the complete neuraxis is mandatory in the work-up of neurofibromatosis patients.**

Intradural extramedullary metastases in a young woman with aggressive cervical cancer. Sagittal T2 (A) and sagittal gadolinium-enhanced T1 (B). Nodular enhancing lesions along the nerve roots of the cauda equina are observed. Without proper clinical information, these lesions are indiscernible from multiple schwannomas as typically encountered in patients with NF-2.**

BENIGN PRIMARY VERTEBRAL TUMOURS

Osteoid osteoma/osteoblastoma
Definition

- Benign tumours consisting of osteoblasts producing osteoid and woven bone ▶ osteoblastomas can undergo malignant transformation and tend to be more aggressive (occasionally requiring surgical excision)
- Osteoid osteoma: <1.5 cm ▶ osteoblastoma: >1.5 cm

Clinical presentation

- *Osteoid osteoma:* localized pain, worse at night and relieved by NSAIDs (can have a painful scoliosis)
  - Peak incidence: second decade ▶ M:F 2-4:1

Radiological features

- *Osteoid osteoma*
  - Location: lumbar spine (60%) ▶ cervical spine (30%) ▶ thoracic spine (10%)
    - A lesion of the posterior elements: lamina or pedicles (50%) ▶ articular processes (20%)

XR Lucent nidus surrounded by variable sclerosis

CT Area of low attenuation with variable surrounding sclerosis

MRI T2WI: low SI nidus surrounded by high SI marrow oedema ▶ T1WI + Gad: nidus enhancement

- *Osteoblastoma*
  - Location: also a tendency to affect the posterior spine

CT Similar appearance to osteoid osteoma, but with less reactive sclerosis ▶ there can be central expansion (similar to an ABC)

Aneurysmal bone cyst (ABC)
Definition

- Aetiology uncertain, may be a non-neoplastic reactive condition, which can be aggressive in its ability to destroy and expand bone

Clinical presentation

- 20–35% of ABC tumours occur in the spine
- Predominantly affects children with a peak incidence in the 2nd decade of life
- Pain, neurological deficit, scoliosis or kyphosis

Radiological features

- Predilection for the lumbar spine, followed by an equal occurrence in the thoracic and cervical spine
  - Can involve all aspects of the vertebral body, but 60% occur in the pedicles, laminae and spinous processes

CT

- *Initial phase:* well-defined area of osteolysis
- *Growth phase:* the lesion has a purely lytic pattern ± ill-defined margins
- *Stabilization phase:* characteristic ballooning multilobulated cystic lesion with a 'soap-bubble' appearance (maturation of the bony shell)

MRI Fluid–fluid levels with variable SI on T1WI and T2WI (different ages of haemorrhage) ▶ low SI rim (intact periosteum) ▶ peritumoral oedema seen on T2 and STIR imaging ▶ T1WI + Gad: enhancement

Eosinophilic granuloma
Definition

- One of the 3 clinical presentations of Langerhans cell histiocytosis (LCH)

Clinical presentation

- Asymptomatic ▶ pain ▶ restricted movement ▶ neurological symptoms

Radiological features

- Classic presentation is with 'vertebra plana', with a predilection for the thoracic spine ▶ vertebral bodies and anterior element more commonly involved than posterior elements ▶ single or multiple lesions ▶ preservation of adjacent discs

XR Lytic lesion with sharp borders

MRI T1WI: isointense SI ▶ T2WI: high SI ▶ T1WI + Gad: avid enhancement

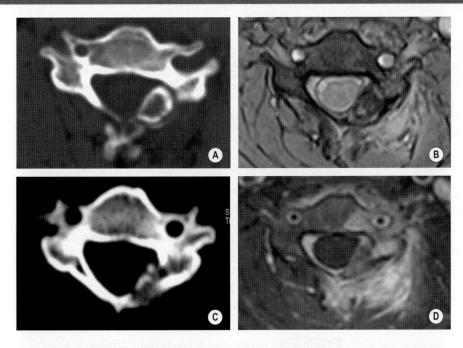

Osteoblastoma of the vertebral arch. Axial CT images (A, B) demonstrate a partially calcified lesion at the left vertebral lamina. On axial T1 (C) merely low signal intensity of the calcified lesion's component. Corresponding T1 after contrast injection (D) shows marked contrast enhancement of the surrounding osseous and soft tissues.**

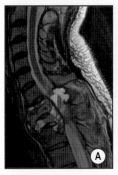
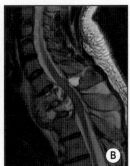
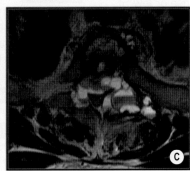

Aneurysmal bone cyst. Sagittal (A, B) and axial (C) T2 show an expansile process involving several segments of two thoracic vertebrae. Extension toward the spinal canal with spinal cord compression is observed. Presence of multiple fluid–fluid levels proves the haemorrhagic content of the lesions.**

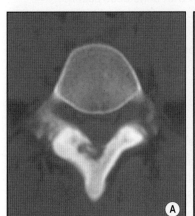
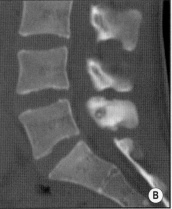
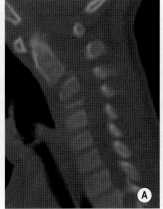
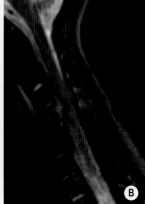

Osteoid osteoma of the posterior elements. Axial CT image (A) and sagittal reformatted image (B) show a sclerotic bone lesion with a small central lucent nidus and dense calcified centre arising at the junction of the laminae of the L5 vertebra.**

Eosinophilic granuloma in a 6-year-old girl with Langerhans cell histiocytosis. Sagittal CT reformat of the C-spine (A) shows marked C4 vertebral compression ('vertebra plana') with kyphosis. Sagittal T2-weighted imaging (B) demonstrates intact vertebral endplates and adjacent disk spaces. A hyperintense soft tissue mass extending in the prevertebral tissues and anterior epidural space is observed.** (Case courtesy of C. Venstermans, Antwerp, Belgium.)

LOCALLY AGGRESSIVE PRIMARY VERTEBRAL TUMOURS

Chordoma

Definition Arise from embryonic remnants of the notochord ▶ most common primary bone tumour of the sacrum and mobile spine ▶ 2 sites of predilection at the sacrum (50%) and skull base (35%)
- Low-grade slow-growing locally aggressive lesions

Clinical presentation Peak incidence between 50–60 years ▶ M>F
- Often quite large at presentation, often resulting in difficulties in surgical resection
- Although not typically metastatic, late presentation makes metastases more likely (5% showing metastases to lungs, bone, skin and brain)

Radiological features Midline lesions, often appearing as destructive bone lesions with an epicentre in the vertebral body and a surrounding soft tissue mass

CT Expansive midline lytic lesion with irregular borders and local tissue infiltration ▶ calcification and sclerosis are frequently present

MRI Heterogenous lesions ▶ T1WI: isointense or low SI relative to muscle with any haemorrhage leading to high SI ▶ T2WI striking high SI (abundant mucin) ▶ T1WI + Gad: homogenous to peripheral septal enhancemnet
- Soft tissue mass spanning several vertebral segments in the mobile spine
- *'Collar button'* appearance on sagittal images
- *Cervical chordomas:* 'dumbbell' morphology or 'mushroom' appearance without bone involvement and enlarging the neuroforamen

Giant cell tumours

Clinical presentation Spinal tumours are rare ▶ occur in skeletally mature patients (2nd to 4th decades) ▶ M>F ▶ 2nd most common primary tumour of the sacrum (after chordoma)

Radiological features *Location:* usually occur in the sacrum, followed by the thoracic, cervical and lumbar segments (decreasing order of frequency) ▶ usually located in the upper part of the sacrum and frequently lateralized in a sacral wing ▶ extraosseous involvement in 79%
- Spine: vertebral body (55%) ▶ involvement of body and posterior elements (30%)

XR Well demarcated lytic and expansile lesion often crossing the midline in the sacrum, and may cross the SI joint ▶ a narrow zone of transition

CT Demonstrates a lack of mineralization and lack of a sclerotic rim at the tumour margin

MRI T1WI: low-to-intermediate SI ▶ T2WI: low-to-intermediate SI ▶ T1WI + Gad: enhancement
- Can see cystic areas, foci of haemorrhage, fluid-fluid levels and a peripheral low SI pseudocapsule

Multiple myeloma/plasmacytoma

Definition Disease of infiltrative plasma B cells

Clinical presentation 5% of patients present with a solitary plasmacytoma ▶ 2M>1F ▶ peak incidence at 35 years old

Radiological features *Location:* vertebral body is the most common site of involvement, but can extend to the pedicles ▶ tends to replace cancellous bone, preserving the cortical bone ▶ preference for the thoracic spine

XR Lytic and usually expansile bone lesion with thickened trabeculae and a multicystic appearance ▶ in one-third of cases, appearances are less characteristic (multicystic 'soap-bubble' appearance simulating a haemangioma)
- Multiple myeloma: diffuse lytic 'punched-out' lesions within single or multiple vertebrae

MRI T1WI: low SI ▶ T2WI: high SI ▶ T1WI + Gad: avid homogenous enhancement

Chondrosarcoma

Definition Usually low-grade lesions arising de novo, or as secondary transformation of an osteochondroma or Paget's disease ▶ the neoplastic tissue is fully developed cartilage without tumour osteoid directly formed by sarcomatous stroma ▶ calcification or ossification may be present

Clinical presentation 2–4M>1F ▶ mean patient age is 45 years

Radiological features *Location:* thoracic and lumbar spine most commonly affected (sacrum only rarely) ▶ vertebral body (15%), posterior elements (40%), both (45%)

CT Large calcified mass with bone destruction ▶ chondroid matrix mineralization (true ossification may be seen)

MRI (Non-mineralized portion): T1WI: low-to-intermediate SI ▶ T2WI: very high SI (water content of hyaline cartilage) ▶ T1WI + Gad: 'rings and arcs' enhancement pattern (reflecting the lobulated growth pattern)

Ewing's sarcoma

Definition Primary vertebral Ewing's sarcoma is rare

Clinical presentation Pain, neurological deficits
- 2nd decade of life ▶ slight male predominance

Radiological features *Location:* can involve all segments of the spine ▶ sacral involvement in 50% – the ala is the commonest sacral site (65%) ▶ 60% of lesions in the mobile spine originate in the posterior elements with vertebral body extension

XR Permeative appearance mimicking osteomyelitis

MRI Variable findings
- *Non-mineralized tumours:* T1WI: low SI ▶ T2WI: high SI
- *Mineralized tumours:* T1WI: low SI ▶ T2WI: high SI
- *T1WI + Gad:* enhancement

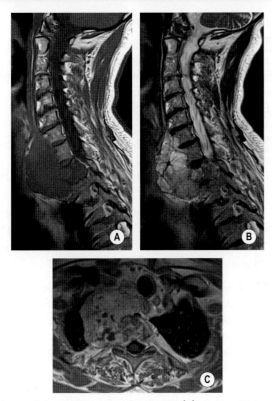

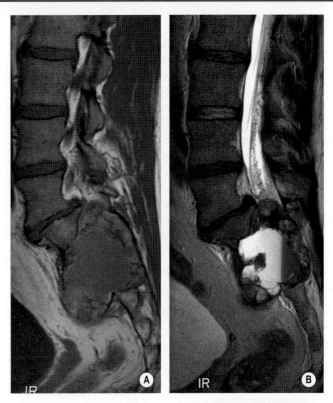

Chordoma of the mobile spine. Sagittal T1 (A), and sagittal T2-weighted images and axial T1 image after Gd injection (C) show a polylobular lesion originating at the body of Th1 and extending anteriorly, invading the anterior aspect of the C6 and C7 vertebral bodies. The lesion is of intermediate signal intensity on T1 (A) and has mixed, intermediate and high signal intensity on T2 (B). There is marked, non-homogeneous contrast enhancement of both the osseous and soft-tissue component of the tumour (C).**

Giant cell tumour from the sacrum. Heterogeneous expansile tumour arising at the S1–S2 level. Low signal intensity components at the periphery of the lesion on both sagittal T1 (A) and T2 (B). Large fluid–fluid level with low signal intensity of the dependent part due to sedimentation of blood components on T2-weighted image.**

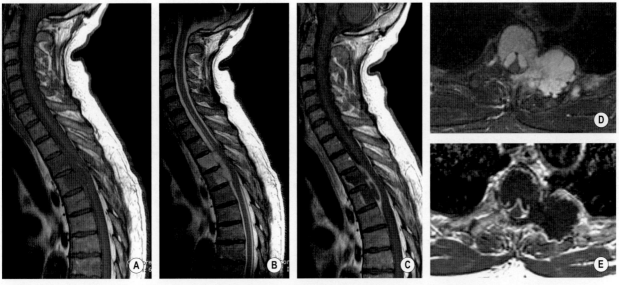

Chondrosarcoma. Sagittal T1 (A), T2 (B) and contrast-enhanced T1 (C) show invasion of the Th3 and Th4 vertebral bodies with low-to-intermediate signal intensity on T1 and very high signal intensity on T2. Extension of the tumour in the anterior epidural space with spinal cord compression is observed. Peripheral irregular enhancement of the tumour. CT-guided percutaneous biopsy of the paravertebral extension of the tumour was performed, and the final diagnosis of low-grade chondrosarcoma was made.**

NON-TUMORAL SPINAL CORD LESIONS

Multiple sclerosis

- *Focal lesions:* oval- or wedge-shaped high T2 signal lesions, located preferentially in the lateral and posterior parts of the spinal cord (which may be swollen) ▶ lesion enhancement is less common than in the brain, and may be subtle ▶ ring- like or intense nodular enhancement can be seen
- *Diffuse involvement:* diffuse signal intensity abnormalities extending over multiple vertebral body segments resembling transverse myelitis
- *Axonal loss/spinal cord atrophy:* more common in the upper cord, and associated with disability
- *Tumefactive lesions:* can mimic tumours ▶ >2 cm circumscribed lesions with little mass effect or oedema ▶ may involve the spinal cord

Acute disseminated encephalomyelitis (ADEM)

- Spinal cord is involved in 30–40% of cases

MRI Non-enhancing high SI lesions in the spinal cord ▶ skip lesions can be seen

Acute transverse myelitis

Definition Aetiology usually unknown, but can be associated with infectious or autoimmune disease

Clinical presentation Weakness, sensory loss and autonomic dysfunction ▶ outcomes can range from complete recovery to death from respiratory failure

MRI Intramedullary high T2 SI with cord swelling ▶ there can be enhancement ▶ lesions tend to involve >⅔ of the cord cross sectional area (cf. MS where lesions do not take up >½ the cross sectional area) ▶ extensive diffuse signal changes diminish over 2–3 months leaving smaller residual lesions (mainly within the cord white matter) ▶ T1WI + Gad: non-persisting enhancement within areas or more extensive signal change

- Longitudinally extensive TM (LETM): abnormalities >2 segments
- Acute partial TM (APTM): abnormalities <2 segments

Neuromyelitis optica

Definition Severe inflammatory disorder affecting the optic nerves and spinal cord ▶ relapsing in 80% ▶ 9F>1M ▶ presents with either optic neuritis or LETM and spinal symptoms

MRI (Spine): T2WI: intramedullary high SI often extending >3 vertebral body segments (LETM) with cavitation's and patchy enhancement ▶ late-stage atrophy and central cavities (predominantly within the posterior fascicle)

Systemic lupus erythematous (SLE)

Definition Relapsing/remitting chronic multisystem autoimmune disease ▶ SLE-related myelitis is rare (1–2%) and usually occurs during an acute exacerbation (occasionally the 1st presentation)

- SLE myelitis manifests mostly as a transverse myelopathy

Clinical presentation Mid-thoracic cord most commonly affected resulting in a sensory level and frequently paraplegia ▶ cauda equine and cervical myelopathy often only causes partial motor and sensory loss

MRI T2WI: high SI and oedema, often with spinal cord expansion ▶ T1WI + Gad: patchy enhancement during the acute phase

Sarcoidosis

Definition Systemic disease of unknown aetiology characterized by non-caseating granulomatosis

- Spinal involvement may be osseous, discal, meningeal or involve the cord itself
- *Leptomeningeal enhancement* (most common spinal cord manifestation)

MRI T1WI + Gad: thin linear or nodular enhancement frequently extending along the surface of the nerve roots ▶ dural involvement is more nodular in appearance

- *Intramedullary spinal lesions:* uncommon and often associated with a neurological deficit

MRI T2WI: high SI with fusiform enlargement of the spinal cord ▶ T1WI + Gad: enhancement

Spinal cord neurological injury

- Mild cord oedema has a good prognosis for neurological improvement ▶ cord haemorrhage is a poor prognostic indicator ▶ cord transection has the worst prognosis
  - Cord haematomas <4 mm in diameter has a better prognosis
- Acute injury:
  - Cord haemorrhage (T2WI): low SI (deoxyhaemoglobin) ▶ variable (up to 10 days) increasing in SI (methaemoglobin) ▶ the zone of high SI begins at the periphery of the lesion ▶ GE sequences will be more sensitive to the presence of haemoglobin
- Delayed worsening of neurology post injury may be due to the development of a spinal cord syrinx ▶ progressive enlargement can cause progressive neurology

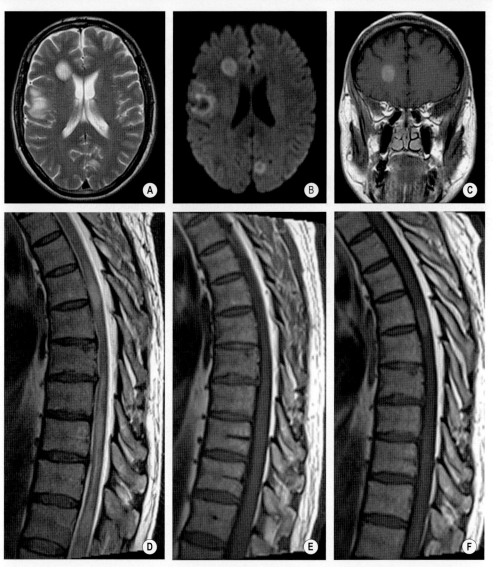

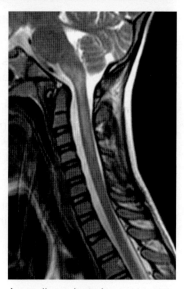

Acute disseminated encephalomyelitis (ADEM) with brain and spinal cord involvement in a child with acute onset of symptoms following viral infection. Sagittal T2 of the cervical spine shows homogeneous high-signal-intensity abnormality in the cervical spinal cord and medulla oblongata. On post-contrast T1 no enhancement is observed (not shown).**

Tumefactive MS. (A) Axial T2 demonstrating multiple hyperintense lesions within the right frontal and left occipital lobes. The lesions are relatively well defined with little mass effect. Other lesions were also present (not shown). (B) DWI shows a rim of restricted diffusion in the larger lesion; the ring is incomplete laterally, which is a typical finding in tumefactive MS lesions. (C) Coronal post-contrast T1 demonstrating enhancement of the right frontal lobe lesion. (D) Sagittal T2 of the thoracic spine demonstrating multiple T 2 hyperintense lesions, the caudal of which extends over several segments. The lesions are not clearly seen on (E) sagittal T1, but demonstrate ring-like enhancement post-contrast administration on (F) sagittal T 1 post contrast.**

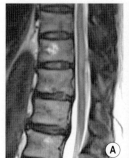
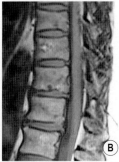
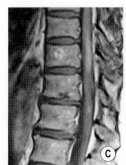
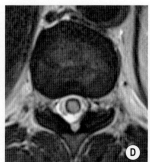
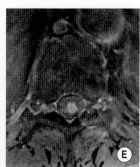

Acute transverse myelitis (ATM). (A) Sagittal T2 showing diffuse hyperintensity extending over several segments. Sagittal T1 pre-four (B) and post-four (C) contrast showing enhancement of the lesion. Axial T2 (D) and axial post-contrast T1 (E) demonstrate that the lesion occupies more than two-thirds of the spinal cord cross-section.**

VERTEBRAL OSTEOMYELITIS

Pyogenic vertebral osteomyelitis

Definition

- Usually from haematogenous seeding – can also be from direct extension ▶ usual organism is *S. aureus*
  - Pyogenic infection almost always begins in the intervertebral disc, spreading to the endplate and along the longitudinal ligaments ▶ contiguous end plate destruction occurs with extension of the abscess into the paravertebral soft tissues

Clinical presentation

- Back pain (sharp pain may indicate an epidural abscess) ▶ fever ▶ motor or sensory involvement

Radiological features

XR Not sensitive

CT Main role for planning any biopsy

MRI Usually 1 disc space and the 2 adjacent vertebral bodies are involved ▶ endplate destruction around the disc ▶ epidural/paraspinal abscesses are seen as high T2WI SI collections (more common in TB infection)
- T1WI: low SI in the disc ▶ bone marrow – low SI (oedema)
- T2WI: high SI in the disc ▶ bone marrow – high SI (oedema)
- T1WI + Gad: homogenous and diffuse enhancement of the vertebral bodies (cf. heterogenous and localized enhancement in TB infection)

Gallium imaging Uptake
- ^{99m}Tc scintigraphy only positive after a few days

Tuberculous vertebral osteomyelitis

Definition

- Usually a secondary infection via haematogenous spread from a primary lung or GU origin ▶ infection usually occurs at the anterior ends of the vertebral bodies, spreading under the longitudinal ligament to involve contiguous vertebrae (posterior element involvement is rare) ▶ skip lesions can occur due to haematogenous spread

Clinical presentation

- Most common at the thoracolumbar junction

Radiological features

XR Tuberculous Vertebral Body Ostemomyelitis Radiological Features

Pearls

- 3 patterns of vertebral body involvement:
  1. *Para-discal lesion* (most common): involvement of subchondral bone adjacent to an intervertebral disc, with reduction in disc height
  2. *Anterior lesions:* loss of blood supply to the vertebral body can lead to necrosis and infection ▶ abscess formation may occur with resultant stripping of the periosteum from the vertebral body, causing scalloping and multiple level involvements
  3. *Central lesions:* these involve the centre of the vertebral body with loss of height resulting in vertebra plana ▶ 'gibbus' deformities can occur due to vertebral body collapse manifesting as acute spine angulation

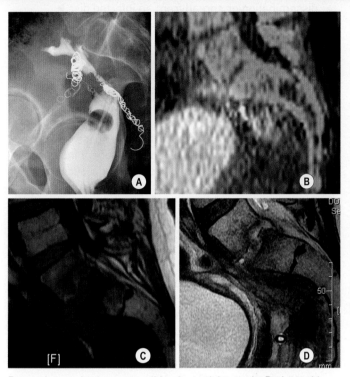

Pyogenic vertebral osteomyelitis after pelvic sepsis. Patient with a presacral abscess following radiotherapy and AP resection for rectal cancer. (A) Contrast enema showing a sinus track to the prevertebral region at L5/S1. (B) Sagittal-fused PET-CT image shows increased uptake of FDG tracer in the presacral region, but not the disc. (C, D) Sagittal T1 and T2 images show the presacral abnormality consistent with granulation tissue extending to the L5/S1 disc, with typical appearances of infective discitis.**

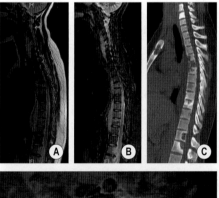

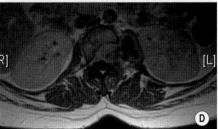

Multilevel involvement in tuberculous spondylitis. Multilevel involvement is a common presentation in tuberculous vertebral osteomyelitis. This may be caused by spread along the anterior longitudinal ligament. Multilevel haematogenous-borne skip lesions also occur. (A,B) Sagittal T2W and STIR images demonstrate multilevel involvement with subligamentous extension at multiple sites. Note the preservation of the intervertebral discs. (C) Sagittal reformatted CT demonstrates lytic lesions at the sites of bone involvement, with surrounding sclerosis. (D) Axial-enhanced MRI of lumbar vertebrae shows chronic bone destruction and a large left paraspinal collection which extends laterally to abut the left kidney.**

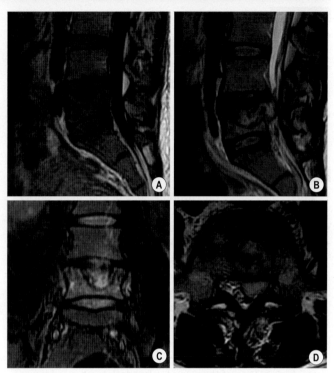

Tuberculous vertebral osteomyelitis. (A, B) Sagittal T1W and T2W images through the spine show discitis of L4/5 vertebra extending to superior end-plate of L5 vertebra, extending to the vertebral body. There is also extension of the abscess into the spinal canal. (C) Axial T2 image at the same level shows the well-defined vertebral body abscess. The abscess component extends into the thecal sac and causes compression of nerve roots on the left. (D) Coronal PD SPIR image shows the well-defined abscess, with relatively little inflammation of surrounding soft tissue, the so-called 'cold abscess'.**

Differentiation between pyogenic and tuberculous vertebral osteomyelitis on imaging	
Pyogenic spinal infection	**Tuberculosis of spine**
1. Lumbar spine involvement common	More common in thoracic spine
2. Commonly single site with disc space infection and involvement of two adjacent vertebra	Multilevel involvement and skip lesions are common, spread may occur along anterior longitudinal ligament
3. Disc abscess with end-plate destruction occurs	Intraosseous and paraspinal abscess occurs more frequently
4. Significant surrounding inflammation with diffuse oedema of vertebral bodies	Inflammation is more localized and formation of cold abscess
5. Enhanced images show diffuse vertebral body enhancement, irregular enhancement of thick-walled abscesses	Enhancement of vertebral bodies more localized and show rim enhancement of thin-walled abscess cavities

DISCITIS

Definition

- This usually follows haematogenous seeding to a degenerative disc ▶ it can also follow spinal surgery
- Infection is usually centred on a disc and involves the two adjacent vertebral bodies (infection confined to 1 vertebral body is rare)
- The likeliest infective location within the spine is the disc space – disease centred on bone is unlikely to be infective in nature

Radiological features

- *Early:* disc space narrowing ▶ loss of end-plate clarity ▶ paravertebral swelling
- *Intermediate:* bone erosion at the disc margins
- *Late:* necrosis ▶ cloacae ▶ sequestra ▶ paraspinal, bone and epidural abscesses ▶ vertebral body collapse (with kyphosis and possible cord compression) ▶ prominent heterotopic new sclerotic bone formation (with peripheral dense spurs bridging the discs) ▶ joint ankylosis

XR/CT Punched-out erosions of bone adjacent to an involved disc ('moth-eaten' appearance) ▶ progressive disc space loss ▶ loss of the vertebral end plates ▶ wedging of adjacent vertebrae ▶ regional subluxation or kyphosis

- There is often prominent sclerosis (which may be associated with small dense sequestra)

MRI This is the imaging modality of choice (allowing a diagnosis to be made at least 2–3 weeks before XR or CT)

- T1WI: low SI throughout the disc and adjacent vertebral bodies
- T2WI: high SI throughout the disc and adjacent vertebral bodies
- T1WI/T2WI: fragmentation and eventual loss of the dark line of the vertebral end plates above and below the affected disc
- T1WI + Gad: diffuse enhancement with active infection

Pearls

- Non-discogenic forms of infective spondylitis present as a localized process, which can be difficult to distinguish from a neoplasia (especially metastases)
- Infection beneath the anterior longitudinal ligament facilitates vertical spread (which is common with indolent infections such as tuberculosis)
- **Vertebral osteomyelitis:** usually based on a destructive discovertebral lesion and rarely affects the neural arches

- **Epidural abscess:** following haematogenous dissemination or spread from an infected disc ▶ commonly extensive

SPINAL MENINGITIS (ARACHNOIDITIS)

Definition

- Inflammation within the subarachnoid space – this may lead to organizing exudates and permanent intradural adhesions ▶ it usually involves the caudal sac (rarely ascending above the L3/4 disc)
- Commonly introgenic ▶ other causes include accidental trauma, spinal subarachnoid haemorrhage, intradural infections

Radiological features

MRI Tapering or obstruction of the lower subarachnoid space ▶ central clumping (± peripheral adhesion of the cauda equina roots) which can appear as an empty thecal sac with thickened walls ▶ loculation and deformity of the subarachnoid spaces (± an irregular spinal cord deformity)

- T1WI + Gad: diffuse intradural enhancement is seen with some infectious agents

SPINAL CORD INFECTION

- **Bacterial spinal cord abscess:** rare (epidural abscesses more common) ▶ ring-like or peripheral enhancement with a high SI centre and marked cord oedema
- **Tuberculous spinal cord abscess:** rare compared with extradural collections ▶ lesions exhibit low SI (T1WI) and high SI (T2WI) with peripheral capsular enhancement
- **Viral myelitis:** non-specific imaging findings with intramedullary high T2WI SI
- **Intramedullary cysticercosis:**
  - *Early vesicular stage:* T2WI: well-defined high SI cyst in the cord ▶ T1WI: the cyst will have low SI with a high SI scolex
  - *Late (colloidal) stage:* thickened cyst capsule with high SI on T2WI and low SI on T1WI ▶ high SI cyst contents (T1WI) ▶ scolex becomes invisible

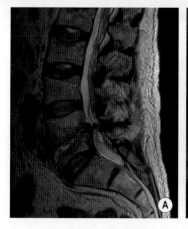
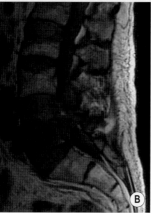
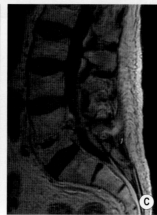

Discovertebral osteomyelitis. The L4/5 disc space is narrowed and on sagittal T2WI there is high SI (pus) within and abnormal SI in the adjacent vertebrae and destruction of the superior surface of L5. On sagittal T1WI (B) it is difficult to distinguish the infected disc from the infected adjacent vertebrae, both of which are of intermediate SI. On sagittal T1WI + Gad (C), there is no enhancement of the pus within the infected disc but the margins of the disc and the infected adjacent vertebrae enhance avidly.*

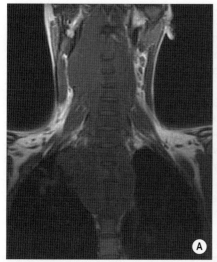
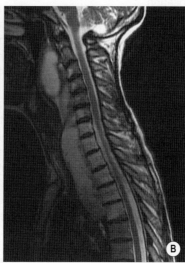

Tuberculosis and osteomyelitis. (A) Coronal T1WI and (B) sagittal T2WI show a huge prevertebral collection and abnormal vertebrae and abnormal material in the epidural space surrounding and narrowing the cord. There is also an extensive retropharyngeal collection.*

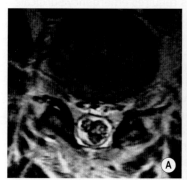
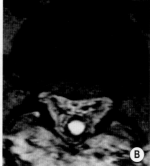
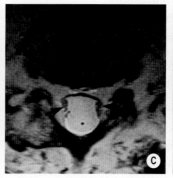
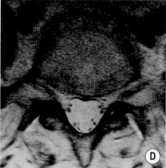

Spinal adhesive arachnoiditis. Axial high-resolution T2WI of the lumbar spine showing the three main diagnostic features of this condition on MRI. (A) Central clumping of nerve roots. (B) Peripheral adhesion of roots, leaving a clear central subarachnoid space. (C) Adhesion of the margins of the thecal sac near the point of exit of the root sheaths (arrows). Compare this with (D), which is normal ▶ here rootlets are clearly seen as they enter the spinal root sheaths on each side.*

SPINAL CORD TRAUMA

DEFINITION

Acute post-traumatic myelopathy

- This usually results from a burst fracture, a fracture–dislocation, an acute disc herniation or rarely an epidural haematoma (the myelopathy is often incomplete with a better prospect for recovery)
- Functional recovery is unlikely if there is complete loss of cord function for >24 h
- Management is conservative

Delayed post-traumatic myelopathy

- This refers to neurological impairment appearing a few hours after injury (often no explanation is found) ▶ if it appears months or years after an injury it may be due to spinal instability (which is often a fracture–dislocation reduced by traction during the early post-injury period) or from a post-traumatic deformity causing progressive cord damage
- Imaging is indicated to exclude any compressive lesion (e.g. an acute disc herniation or an epidural haematoma)

Progressive post-traumatic myelopathy

- This refers to worsening of an existing disability or ascending functional loss
- The spinal cord is usually extensively damaged well beyond the injury site ▶ the damage manifests as diffuse atrophy with necrosis, cell loss and gliosis and extensive cord cavitation

Radiological features

CT Fractures involving only the anterior part of the vertebral body are stable ▶ fractures involving the posterior part of the body and neural arches are potentially unstable

MRI This accurately demonstrates the state of the spinal cord ▶ it is usually abnormal in an acute post-traumatic myelopathy (whether or not a bony injury has occurred) ▶ it will also demonstrate lesions that may acutely compress the spinal cord (e.g. an acute disc herniation, bone fragment or epidural haematoma)

- T1WI: there may be high cord signal, but this is infrequent (although cord contusions are usually haemorrhagic this is only evident in ≤50% of cases)
- T2WI: there is a diffuse increase in cord signal (usually at the injury site or for only 1–2 segments beyond) ▶ cord swelling is usually only slight and not always present ▶ a circumscribed area of low SI within a more extensive area of high SI (and associated with a focal cord swelling) probably represents an intramedullary haematoma
- The extent of signal change within an acutely damaged spinal cord is related to the injury severity
- With paediatric spinal cord injuries extensive cord signal change can occur with a minor spinal injury and is usually followed by persistent functional loss
- Haematomyelia is a poor prognostic indicator
- Progression from an acute injury to a localized cystic myelopathy does not usually lead to further functional loss

THE POSTOPERATIVE SPINE

Perioperative hardware complications

- *Misplaced transpedicular screws:* these should be wholly contained within the pedicles and covered by cortical bone ▶ the screw tip should approach but not breach the anterior vertebral body cortex ▶ misplaced screws may impinge on the spinal canal or neural foramen

Early complications

- *Haemorrhage:* uncommon ▶ airway compression in the cervical spine is a surgical emergency ▶ spinal cord or cauda equine compression is suspicious for epidural haematoma
- *CSF leak:* uncommon ▶ secondary to unrecognized or unrepaired dural breach ▶ extravasation of CSF can lead to a pseudomeningocele or a cutaneous CSF fistula
- *Infection:* wound infection/discitis/vertebral osteomyelitis/epidural abscess/paraspinal abscess ▶

a spinal epidural abscess requires emergency surgical decompression

Late complications

- *Hardware failure:* fractured or extruded screws, plates or rods ▶ misplacement or subsistence of interbody cages ▶ screws: peri-implant lucency may indicate loosening ▶ delayed hardware failure: displacement can lead to pseudoarthrosis and instability
  - Hardware provides only temporary support, and is destined to fail if osseous fusion does not occur with development of a pseudoarthrosis
  - *Pseudoarthrosis:* XR: bone graft resorption ▶ progressive misalignment (>4 mm translation or >10° of angular motion between adjacent vertebrae on flexion/extension views) ▶ CT: a lucent line between bone and graft material ▶ MRI: low T1WI line

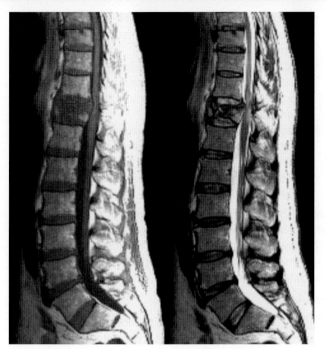

Thoracic burst fracture. Sagittal T1WI (left) and T2WI (right) show retropulsion of the posterior portion of the T11 vertebral body resulting in cord compression. Cord T2 high SI is consistent with oedema. A contusion should be suspected based on the degree of compression ▶ however there is no T2 or gradient-echo low SI to confirm the presence of haemorrhage.⁺⁺

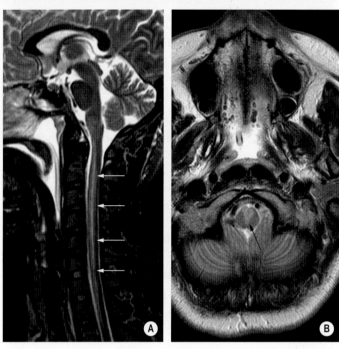

Cord infarct post trauma. (A) Sagittal T2 and FS image following traumatic interruption to the anterior spinal artery. High T2 signal (arrows) corresponds to areas of cord damage. (B) Similar changes can also be seen on axial imaging (arrow).

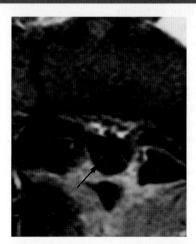

Extraspinal wound abscess and infected pseudo-meningocele. Axial T1W image at L4/5 with fat presaturation and IV gadolinium showing a low signal cavity surrounded by a very thick white wall of granulation tissue. Operation revealed a cavity containing fluid infected by *Staphylococcus aureus*. These appearances can be mimicked by sterile postoperative pseudomeningoceles.*

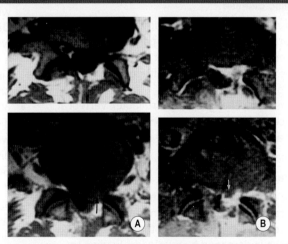

Epidural scar and residual/recurrent disc protrusion. (A) Axial T1W MRI just below (above) and through (below) the L4/5 disc, showing a large epidural mass (black arrow) on the left side. (B) Images at similar levels made after IV gadolinium and using fat presaturation, showing marked enhancement of most of the epidural mass, but also a central non-enhancing region in contact with the discal margin (arrow). At operation, recurrent disc material was found at this site, embedded in dense fibrous tissue.*

DEGENERATIVE SPINAL DISEASE

Spondylosis

Definition Degenerative spinal disease with osteophyte formation ▶ intervertebral disc degeneration is usually related to the mobility of the involved segments (the discs adjacent to any fused spinal segments are especially vulnerable)

- *Involved areas*: multiple levels within the cervical region ▶ L4/5 and L5/S1 ▶ the upper lumbar and lower thoracic spine

Pearl Disc degeneration is closely associated with radial fissuring of the annulus fibrosus (transverse fissures may also develop and can intermittently fill with gaseous nitrogen during movement)

- The central disc ultimately becomes less hydrated and loses volume

Degenerative spondylolisthesis (pseudospondylolisthesis)

Definition Remodelling and fragmentation can result in facet joint instability with vertebral body displacement relative to its inferior vertebra (retrolisthesis is the opposite)

- It can also be caused by trauma, stress fractures and surgical interventions

Schmorl's node

Definition An intraosseus disc herniation through a weakened vertebral end plate (caused by a weak spot generated by regression of nutrient vessels leaving a scar)

Limbus vertebra

Definition Herniation of the nucleus pulposus through the ring apophysis before bony fusion, isolating a segment of vertebral rim

Degenerative disc disease

- Controversial relationship between lumbar spine imaging abnormalities and low-back pain
  - Loss of intervertebral space height is the earliest sign of disc degeneration on XR (although no direct relationship)
  - Late degenerative changes (more reliable): vertebral endplate sclerosis ▶ osteophytes ▶ vacuum phenomena and calcification

MRI T2WI signal loss ('black disc')

Annular disc tears

- Discs become more fibrous and less elastic with age ▶ clinical significance uncertain ▶ degenerative changes are accelerated when the integrity of the posterior annulus fibrosus is damaged by overload – leading to fissures in the annulus fibrosus ('annular tear')

- *Concentric tears*: circumferential lesions found in the outer layers of the annulus fibrosus – post-traumatic from torsion overload injuries
- *Transverse tears* ('rim' lesion): horizontal ruptures of the Sharpey's fibres near the insertion in the bony ring apophysis ▶ post-traumatic ▶ clinical significance unclear
- *Radial tears*: annular tears permeating from the deep central part of the disc extending outward towards the annulus (craniocaudal or transverse plane) ▶ most do not reach the pain-sensitive outer disc margin ▶ associated with disc degeneration

MRI T2WI: high SI ▶ T1WI + Gad: foci of annular enhancement ▶ high intensity zone (HIZ): increased SI with inflammation – a combination of radial and concentric annular tears merging at the disc periphery (hence associated with pain)

Disc bulge

Definition Circumferential disc expansion (>180°) beyond the vertebral margins (this is not a herniation)

- The annulus fibrosis may normally bulge a little beyond the vertebral margins (especially in children) but bulging of >2–3 mm is abnormal

Disc herniation

Definition Displacement of disc material beyond the limits of the intervertebral disc space ▶ these usually extend within the anterior epidural space cranial or caudal to the disc with the migratory fragments usually passing either side of the midline

- **Sequestered fragment:** a free disc fragment that is not in continuity with the parent disc
- **Disc extrusion:** a focal bulge of the annulus fibrosus with its base narrower than its height
- **Disc protrusion:** a focal bulge of the annulus fibrosus with its base wider than its height ▶ it is associated with a radial tear that can occur anywhere along the disc circumference ▶ focal: <25% of the disc circumference ▶ broad based: 25–50% of the disc circumference
- 60–70% of intraspinal fibrocartilaginous masses of discogenic origin resolve spontaneously over a few weeks or months ▶ a relentless progression to a severe disability can occasionally occur
- Severe degenerative change can progress to a destructive discovertebral lesion mimicking an infective spondylitis – however, with infection there will be high SI on T2WI (there is usually low SI with degenerative disease)

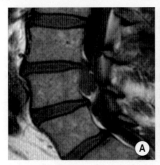
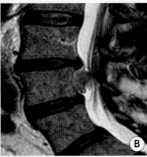
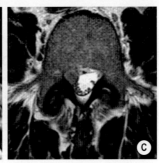

Downward-migrating disc herniation. Sagittal T1 (A), sagittal (B) and axial (C) T2 images of a 59-year-old man show a large disc fragment descending into the right lateral recess behind the L4 vertebral body. The disc is hypointense on T2 imaging, indicating a fibrous nature.**

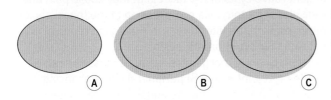

Bulging disc. Symmetrical and asymmetrical bulging disc on transverse CT or MRI images. Normally the intervertebral disc (grey) does not extend beyond the edges of the ring apophyses (black line) (A). In an asymmetrically bulging disc, the disc tissue extends concentrically beyond the edges of the ring apophyses (50–100% of disc circumference) (B). An asymmetrical bulging disc can be associated with scoliosis. Bulging discs are not considered a form of herniation (C).**

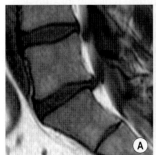
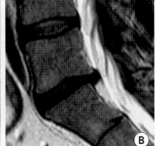
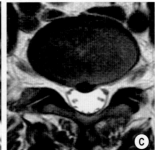

Central disc herniation. Sagittal (A) T1 image; sagittal (B) and axial (C) T2 images. Focal central disc herniation at L5–S1 without compression of the nerve roots. The hypointense signal intensity of the disc indicates a fibrous nature.**

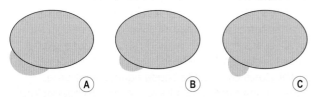

Disc herniations. Types of disc herniations are seen on transverse CT or MRI images. In protrusions: the base of the herniated disc material is broader than the apex. Protrusions can be broad-based (A) or focal (B). In extrusions (C) the base of the herniation is narrower than the apex (toothpaste sign).**

Types of disc protrusion	
Posterolateral	The commonest type
Midline posterior	Previously known as a 'central' protrusion
Lateral	Lateral to the spinal canal and which can involve the dorsal root ganglion
Far lateral	Beyond the foramen and potentially affecting the ventral rami
Broad based	Involvement of 90–180° of the circumference

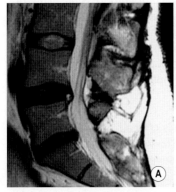
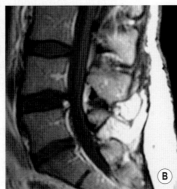
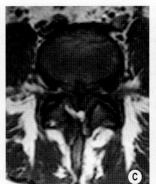
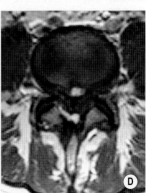

Enhancing annular tear. Pre-contrast sagittal T2 (A) and axial (C) T1 images; post-gadolinium sagittal (B) and axial (D) T1 images. On the T2 sagittal image a posterior annular tear and central disc herniation is seen at the level L4–L5. After gadolinium administration, there is a linear area of enhancement in the posterior annulus, indicating a concentric tear.**

DEGENERATIVE SPINAL DISEASE

Reactive vertebral body changes

- Reactive changes occur within the vertebral bodies, both in the peripheral disc margin (osteophytes) and also within the cancellous bone adjacent to the vertebral end-plates
  - **Cervical spine:** disc margin osteophytes commonly involve the spinal canal and can result in fusion ▶ a reduction in cord cross sectional area by >50–60% (approximately 40 mm³) is associated with a poor operative outcome
  - **Elsewhere within the spine:** disc-related osteophytes do not usually involve the spinal canal (even if large)
- **Modic vertebral body reactive changes:** these occur within the cancellous bone adjacent to the vertebral end-plates:
  - *Type I:* acute inflammatory stage
  - *Type II:* fatty replacement of red marrow
  - *Type III:* bony sclerosis
- **Isolated spondylosis deformans:** degenerative change of the annulus fibrosus associated with anterior or anterolateral disc herniation
- **Uncovertebral joint degeneration:** narrowing of the exiting foramina with compression of the nerve roots at that level

Posterior joints and ligaments

- **Facet joint syndrome:** a range of symptoms resulting in diffuse pain that does not follow a clear nerve root pattern
- **Osteoarthritic changes:** these can develop within the facet joints at all levels (usually in close association with concomitant degeneration within the intervertebral disc) but are most commonly found in the lordotic cervical and lumbar regions ▶ there is resultant articular process hypertrophy with thickening of the capsule, flaval and accessory ligaments ▶ this can lead to encroachment of the posterolateral spinal canal and intervertebral foramina (with canal stenosis) ± pain
- **Ossification of the posterior longitudinal ligament (OPLL):** this involves the mid and lower cervical region in >90% of cases ▶ diffuse, segmental and mixed forms are recognized
- **Ossification of the ligamentum flavum:** small tongues of ossification can extend into the ligaments from the superior borders of the laminae ▶ calcifications of the ligamentum flavum at the insertions are normal variants – at the periarticular level are thought to be degenerative
  - **CT:** bilateral intense radio-dense lines highlighting the lamina, developing from the medial aspect of the pedicle near the insertion of the ligamentum flavum and progressing towards the midline creating a V-shaped ossification
- **Degenerative cysts arising from the facet joints:** periarticular synovial cysts attached to the joint by a membrane ▶ filled with yellow or clear mucinous fluid (haemorrhage or inflammation may vary the fluid consistency) ▶ most commonly seen in the lumbar spine (especially L4–L5) – cervical and thoracic cases are less common ▶ related to adjacent osteoarthritic change ▶ degenerative cysts of the facet joint may cause pain and radicular symptoms via compression of the thecal sac or nerve roots in the lateral recess ▶ surgical removal is indicated for symptomatic cysts
  - **MRI** Sharply marginated epidural masses near the facet joint ▶ low SI peripheral rim (enhancing with Gad) ▶ cyst contents equal SI to CSF (unless haemorrhage)
- **Cysts of the ligamentum flavum:** typically located at L4–L5 with the same imaging characteristics as facet joint cysts (but with no rim calcification) ▶ an extradural intraspinal mass in close relation to the ligamentum flavum

Degenerative spinal canal stenosis

- Acquired spinal canal stenosis is the most common type of stenosis at the cervical and lumbar level (less frequent in the thoracic spine)
- Posterior and central marginal osteophytes can reduce spinal canal diameter with possible cord compression ▶ a bony protrusion at facet level may cause lateral radicular compression by radicular entrapment in the lateral recess ▶ disc herniation can also cause lateral recess narrowing ▶ posterior and central marginal osteophytosis can lead to cauda equine syndrome (cauda equina nerve roots have a higher ischaemic risk if compression is at more than one level) ▶ osteoarthritis of the facet joints may cause stenosis of the central spinal canal and the lateral or foraminal recesses
- Patients often remain asymptomatic until an acute event occurs
  - *Lateral or foraminal radicular compression:* acute or chronic limb pain
  - *Lumbar canal stenosis:* sensory and motor deficits associated with lower limb pain during walking and in an upright position ▶ forward bending and the supine position may relieve symptoms (associated increasing spinal canal diameter)
- Average AP diameter:
  - C4–C7: 17 mm (<14 mm is critical)
  - Lumbar: mild stenosis (12–14 mm) ▶ moderate stenosis (10–12 mm) ▶ severe stenosis (<10 mm)

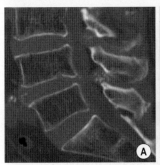
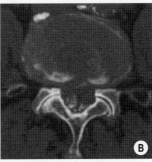

Ligamentum flavum hypertrophy and calcification. Sagittal (A) and axial (B) reformatted CT images. Calcification and hypertrophy of the ligamentum flavum at L4–L5 and in a lesser extend at L3–L4, resulting in a spinal canal stenosis at L4–L5. Calcifications of the ligamentum flavum are also seen in patients with pseudogout. Pseudogout is a crystal-induced arthropathy, which is a debilitating illness in which pain and joint inflammation are caused by the formation of calcium pyrophosphate (CPP) crystals within the joint space. It is sometimes referred to as calcium pyrophosphate disease (CPPD).**

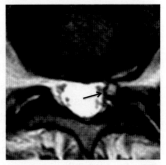

Juxtafacet (ganglion) cyst. Axial T2 image shows a small cystic lesion (arrow) arising from the anteromedial aspect of the left facet joint L5–S1.**

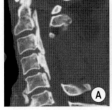
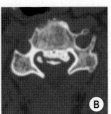

Calcification of posterior longitudinal ligament. Sagittal (A) and axial (B) reformatted CT images show a postoperative condition after posterior laminectomy for a spinal canal stenosis caused by calcifications of the posterior longitudinal ligament from C2 to C5, also known as Japanese disease.**

\multicolumn{2}{l}{Criteria for grading osteoarthritis of the facet joints}
Grade	**Criteria**
0	Normal facet joint space (2–4 mm width)
1	Narrowing of the facet joint space (<2 mm) and/or small osteophytes and/or mild hypertrophy of the articular processes
2	Narrowing of the facet joint space and/or moderate osteophytes and/or moderate hypertrophy of the articular processes and/or mild subarticular bone erosions
3	Narrowing of the facet joint space and/or large osteophytes and/or severe hypertrophy of the articular processes and/or severe subarticular bone erosions and/or subchondral cysts

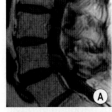
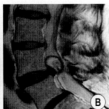
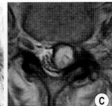

Juxtafacet (ganglion) cyst. Sagittal T1 (A) image; sagittal (B) and axial (C) T2 images. A large cystic lesion arising from the anteromedial aspect of the left facet joint. The content from the cyst appears mildly hyperintense on T2 image (B) and is of intermediate signal intensity on T1 image (A). A low signal intensity rim is observed on the T2 images (B, C). The cyst causes compression of the thecal sac and obliteration of the left lateral recess is seen.**

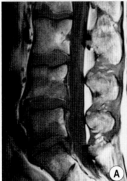
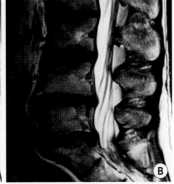

Modic type 1 changes. Sagittal T1 (A) and T2 (B) images. There is a decreased signal intensity on T1 images and increased signal intensity on T2 images in both endplates at level L5–S1 and also in the upper endplate at L4–L5, indicating bone marrow oedema associated with acute or subacute inflammation.**

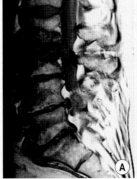
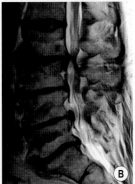

Modic type 2 changes. Sagittal T1 (A) and T2 (B) images. There is an increased signal intensity on T1 and T2 images at L3–L4, L4–L5 and L5–S1, indicating replacement of normal bone marrow by fat. There are also more acute Modic type 1 changes at L2–L3.**

DEGENERATIVE SPINAL DISEASE

Radiological features

- The relation between low-back pain and lumbar abnormalities is controversial, as abnormal findings are often seen in asymptomatic patients

XR Sclerosis ▶ osteophytes ▶ disc space narrowing ▶ calcified or ossified disc material and ligaments ▶ alignment abnormalities ▶ intervertebral space height loss
- A mid-sagittal cervical canal diameter <10 mm suggests the presence of cord compression

CT Annular disc bulges and protrusions ▶ nuclear herniations and migratory fragments ▶ bubbles of nitrogen within a disc ▶ enlarged degenerate ligaments ▶ synovial cysts ▶ spinal canal narrowing (due to osteoarthritis and soft-tissue thickening)
- CT is not usually recommended for the cervical and thoracic regions

MRI This is the optimal investigation
- **Degenerate discs:** these generally return lower SI than healthy discs
  - T1WI: low SI (calcium precipitation may generate high SI)
  - T2WI: low SI (fluid-filled clefts may generate high SI) ▶ annulus fibrosus tears may be visible as high SI foci ▶ migratory fragments can demonstrate higher SI than the nucleus of the disc of origin
- **Modic changes within adjacent vertebral bodies**
  - *Type I:* T1WI: low SI ▶ T2WI: high SI
  - *Type II:* T1WI: high SI ▶ T2WI: normal–high SI
  - *Type III:* T1WI and T2WI: low SI
- **Neural structures:** spinal cord compression is well shown on axial imaging ▶ distortion of the cord shape may be due to compression alone or reflect underlying structural damage
  - *Structural damage:* this is usually reflected by signal change within the cord substance (if it is present it is usually associated with a clinical myelopathy) ▶ it does not always indicate permanent damage as it can often disappear after decompressive surgery
    - T2WI: any high SI is usually focal and occurs at or slightly caudal to the site of compression ▶ it usually involves the central cord areas (often with the appearance of bilateral lesions likened to snakes' or cats' eyes)

- **Spinal nerves:** these are directly shown, and their ganglia can be affected by a far lateral disc protrusion ▶ there is occasionally focal (and mainly extradural) abnormal enhancement of a compressed nerve root which occasionally extends intradurally for several cm

PEARLS

Involvement of neural structures

- Degenerative change, and subsequent mechanical compression, can damage the spinal cord or the nerve roots ▶ the severity of this compression is not linearly related to the degree of damage or its clinical effects
- **Spinal cord**
  - *Cervical region:* compression is usually intermittent or intermittently accentuated by neck movement ▶ damage is sustained only when the sagittal cord diameter is reduced by more than 50%
  - *Thoracic region:* far greater compression is tolerated without any damage (due to the reduced mobility of this part of spine) – calcified fibrocartilagenous masses can occupy up to 60% of the spinal canal without a significant clinical effect
- **Spinal roots**
  - *Cervical region:* the spinal roots are usually compressed by osteophytes and fibrocartilaginous masses located near the entrance of the intervertebral canals
  - *Lumbar region:* the nerve roots are usually compressed by a posterolateral disc protrusion or from migratory fragments within the anterior epidural space ▶ this usually affects the nerve root crossing the abnormal disc to reach the next inferior intervertebral foramen (lying within the lateral extremity of the spinal canal under cover of the articular facet and within the thecal sac)
    - *Far lateral posterior protrusion:* this is much rarer and can compress the dorsal root ganglion ventral ramus (as it exits cranial to the disc and is located within the intervertebral foramen)

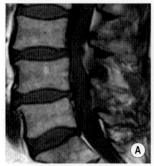
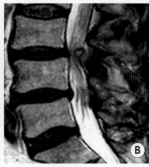
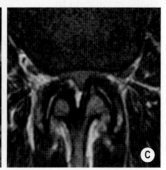

Spinal canal stenosis L3–L4 with synovial facet joint cyst. Sagittal T1 (A) and sagittal (B) and axial (C) T2 images. The axial T2 image shows a hypertrophic facet joint at L3–L4 with a small synovial cyst at the anteromedial aspect of the left facet joint, resulting in a spinal canal stenosis. Also note the discrete anterolisthesis at L3–L4 caused by facet joint osteoarthritis.**

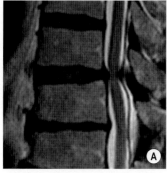
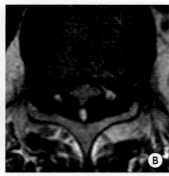
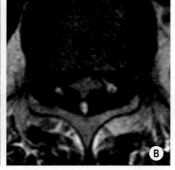

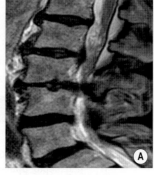
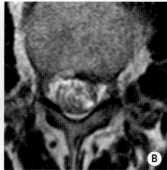

Thoracic spinal canal stenosis. Sagittal (A) and axial (B) T2 images. There is a lateral stenosis of the spinal canal at a low thoracic level due to hypertrophy of the ligamenta flava (B) and a broad-based disc protrusion.**

Spinal canal stenosis with redundant nerve roots. Sagittal (A) and axial (B) T2-weighted images. A case of a spinal canal stenosis at L3–L4 as a result of anterolisthesis caused by facet joint osteoarthritis. As seen on the sagittal image (A), it is a case of a concentric spinal canal stenosis with hypertrophy of the ligamenta flava and disc bulging. Proximal of the stenosis there are redundant nerve roots of the cauda equina, as seen on the sagittal (A) and axial images (B).**

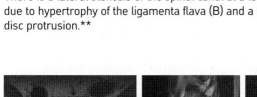
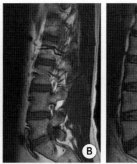
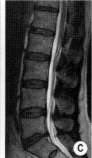

Lateral posterior disc protrusion. (A) On the axial T1WI there is a large lateral L5/S1 protrusion distorting the left dorsal root ganglion and ventral ramus. (B) On the parasagittal T1WI the left L5 foramen is filled with disc material. (C) Note how relatively normal the midline sagittal T2WI appears in this patient. Note also how a lateral disc affects the ventral ramus cranial to the affected disc – unlike the usual disc lesion that affects the root that will emerge at the more caudal level.*

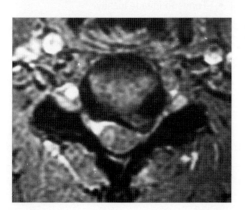

Axial MR image of the cervical spine in a patient with brachalgia at the C4/5 level. There is a left-of-centre posterior disc lesion impinging on the spinal cord and the left C5 roots.*

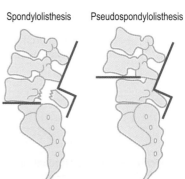

Spondylolisthesis   Pseudospondylolisthesis

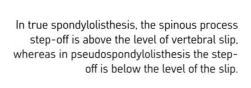

In true spondylolisthesis, the spinous process step-off is above the level of vertebral slip, whereas in pseudospondylolisthesis the step-off is below the level of the slip.

7.7 THE ORBIT

Definition Disease processes can be classified according to the anatomical site involved – this is usually in relation to the rectus muscle pyramid (the 'cone')

Intraconal (within the muscle cone)

- Optic nerve glioma
- Optic nerve meningioma
- Haemangioma
- Inflammatory orbital pseudotumour
- Lymphoma ▶ metastases

Arising from the muscle cone

- Inflammatory orbital pseudotumour
- Dysthyroid ophthalmopathy

- Rhabdomyosarcoma (the commonest cause of a paediatric primary orbital mass)

Extraconal (outside the muscle cone)

- Orbital cellulitis or abscess
- Lymphoma ▶ metastases
- Dermoid ▶ epidermoid ▶ teratoma
- Lymphangioma ▶ lymphohaemangioma

Within or involving the globe

- Retinoblastoma
- Melanoma
- Metastases

	Pathology	**Clinical features**	**Key imaging findings**
Congenital	Optic nerve hypoplasia	• Can be isolated or part of a syndrome (e.g. septo-optic dysplasia)	• Decreased size of the optic nerve
Inflammatory	Optic neuritis	• About 50% of patients with idiopathic optic neuritis develop multiple sclerosis • Other causes include sarcoid, radiation, pseudotumour, toxoplasmosis, TB, syphilis, virus infection	• Best seen on gadolinium-enhanced T1W imaging • If present, look for brain demyelination using T2W imaging
Tumour	Leukaemia	• Reported in 13–16% of cases of leukaemia • More commonly an acute lymphoblastic leukaemia but described in AML and adult leukaemias • Presents with papilloedema and variable loss of acuity	• Diffuse enlargement of the optic nerve with variable enhancement
	Haemangioblastoma	• Associated with von Hippel–Lindau (VHL) disease • Progressive loss of vision • Retinal lesions occur in 60% of patients with VHL	• Rarely affects the orbit or optic nerve • Sharply demarcated from the nerve • Densely enhancing • Usually affects the prechiasmatic nerve
	Haemangiopericytoma	• Mean age 40–60 years • More common in women • Presents with proptosis, optic nerve and extraocular dysfunction	• Superior orbital masses • Tends to invade locally • Marked contrast enhancement • Florid blush on angiography
	Neurofibroma/ schwannoma	• About 1% of orbital tumours • Affects young adults • Usually presents with proptosis • Neurofibromatosis in 2–18%	• Smooth, ovoid, solitary mass • Usually in the superior orbit • May be intraconal, extraconal or intramuscular • Isodense with homogeneous contrast medium enhancement on CT • Isointense on T1 and hyperintense on T2WI
Miscellaneous	Raised intracranial pressure	• Papilloedema, loss of venous pulsation	• Dilatation of the optic nerve sheath

The imaging findings of some less common diseases of the conal and intraconal compartments*

The imaging findings of some less common diseases of the globe*

	Pathology	Clinical features	Key imaging findings
Congenital	PHPV (persistent hyperplastic primary vitreous)	• The primary vitreous normally involutes by the 6th fetal month, but occasionally persists and undergoes hyperplasia • Presents with leucocoria • Affects male infants more than female • Secondary retinal detachment is common (a V-shaped structure within the globe on axial imaging)	• A microphthalmic globe with enhancing and increased density in the vitreous humour on CT • A soft tissue cone or band from the back of the lens to the posterior globe • Can be unilateral or bilateral
	Retinopathy of prematurity	• A history of prolonged ventilation with high O_2 concentration in a premature baby • Pathology shows abnormal and disorganized proliferation of retinal vascular buds ▶ may cause retinal detachment	• Bilateral increased density in the vitreous • Calcification is rare
	Coat's disease	• A congenital vascular malformation of the retina with telangiectasia ▶ usually unilateral ▶ presents in childhood • Exudation from abnormal vessels leads to retinal detachment ▶ disease nature if progressive	• Increased density in all or part of the vitreous • Normal-sized globe • No calcification
	Microphthalmia	• Congenital underdevelopment or acquired diminution in size of the globe • Associated with congenital rubella, PHPV, retinopathy of prematurity and Lowe syndrome	• Congenital = small globe in a small orbit • Acquired = small, calcified globe
	Macrophthalmia	• Enlargement of the globe • The most severe form is called buphthalmos • Associated with juvenile glaucoma	• A large globe in a large orbit • Also seen in Marfan's/Ehlers–Danlos syndrome
	Coloboma	• A defect in the globe, usually near the optic nerve head • It involves the sclera, uvea and retina • It is caused by a defect in fetal optic fissure	• A small globe with cystic outpouching of the vitreous • There may be a retro-ocular cyst
Degenerative	Drusen	• Accretion of hyaline material on the optic disc • It may be asymptomatic or associated with headache or visual field defects	• Discrete, flat calcification of the optic nerve head • Bilateral in 75%
	Phthisis bulbi	• An end-stage injured eye	• A collapsed globe • It may be calcified
Inflammatory	Scleritis	• Anterior scleritis presents with pain, erythema, photophobia and tenderness • Posterior scleritis is painless and may mimic melanoma	• Thickened enhancing sclera • Choroidal detachment may be present
	Sclerosing endophthalmitis	• A 2–8-year-old child exposed to soil contaminated by dog faeces • Ingestion of the ova of *Toxocara canis* results in ophthalmitis	• Dense vitreous without a discrete mass • No calcification
Tumour	Choroidal haemangioma	• Can be isolated or associated with Sturge–Weber syndrome • A benign vascular lesion	• Lenticular or flat densely enhancing eye wall mass
	Medulloepithelioma	• Mean age of onset 4 years • It presents with a ciliary body mass, lens coloboma, lens subluxation, cataract, cyclitic membrane and glaucoma • About 50% are teratoid and 50% non-teratoid	• Involvement of the ciliary body helps differentiate from a retinoblastoma • Only 10–15% are calcified • It rarely may involve the optic nerve and other locations in the CNS

The imaging findings of some less common diseases of the extraconal compartment*			
	Pathology	**Clinical features**	**Key imaging findings**
Congenital	Cephalocele	• Present soon after birth • A soft mass near the medial canthus • It may be pulsatile and increased with Valsalva	• Soft tissue and CSF continuous with the intracranial contents
	Dermoid	• Usually the upper outer quadrant of the orbit • A fullness or small lump	• Usually anterior between the globe and periosteum • A well-defined cystic mass • Epidermoid – fluid density, dermoid – fat density on CT • May be related to sutures
Lacrimal gland inflammatory	Postviral	• The commonest cause of acute inflammatory enlargement in younger patients	• Smooth enlargement of the gland
	Sjögren's syndrome	• Decreased lacrimation and dry mouth • May be primary or secondary to autoimmune connective tissue diseases • Histology = lymphocytic infiltration of the gland	• Non-specific enlargement of the gland in the acute phase • The gland may be small in chronic phase • Enhancement is patchy or absent
	Mikulicz disease/ syndrome	• Mikulicz disease is similar to primary Sjögren's syndrome • Mikulicz syndrome is gland enlargement associated with sarcoid, lymphoma, leukaemia or TB	• As for Sjögren's syndrome
Tumour	Benign mixed tumour	• Same as a pleomorphic adenoma • Benign • Represents about 50% of primary lacrimal gland neoplasms (the rest are malignant) • It can undergo malignant change	• Well-defined, smooth enlargement of gland • Long-standing so there may be bone remodelling • May not enhance
	Adenoid cystic carcinoma	• The most common malignant primary tumour (followed by malignant mixed tumour, adenocarcinoma and mucoepidermoid carcinoma)	• Tumour is hard enough to indent the globe • The gland may have a serrated edge • A tendency for perineural spread • Enhances well
	Lymphoma (NHL)	• The lacrimal gland is a common site for NHL in the orbit	• Infiltrating mass • Enhances well

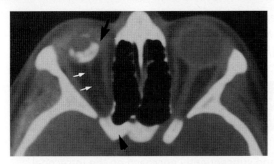

Congenital microphthalmos. Axial CT image. There is choroidal calcification (large black arrow) with a small globe, a thinned optic nerve (small white arrows) and a small orbit. Note the hypoplastic optic canal (black arrowhead).*

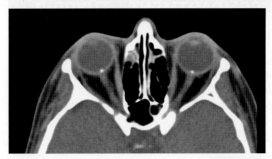

Drusen. Axial CT. There are small foci of calcification at both optic nerve heads.*

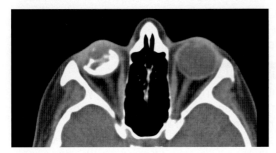

Phthisis bulbi. Axial CT. The patient had been stabbed in the right eye 2 years previously. The globe is small and densely calcified.*

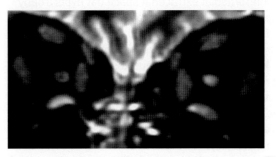

Optic neuritis. Coronal T2WI with inversion recovery. There is high signal in the left optic nerve, indicating optic neuritis. The patient was symptomatic and had multiple demyelinating lesions in the cerebral white matter.*

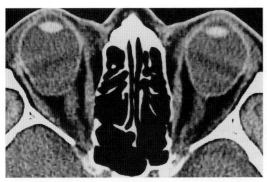

Coloboma. Axial CT image demonstrates bilateral retinal defects with outpouching in the region of the optic nerve head.†

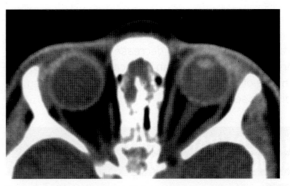

Persistent hypertrophic primary vitreous. Axial CT of the orbits demonstrates a small left globe with a V-shaped retrolental density (A).**

CONAL COMPARTMENT – THYROID OPHTHALMOPATHY

Definition This results from deposits of hygroscopic mucopolysaccharides and infiltration of the lymphocytes, mast and plasma cells

- It is the commonest cause of an adult unilateral or bilateral exophthalmos
- 85% are bilateral (but are often asymmetrical)

Clinical presentation An insidious and painless exophthalmos (± lid lag) ▶ only 10% of patients are euthyroid ▶ 4th–5th decade ▶ F:M – 4:1

Radiological features

CT/MRI An increased intraorbital fat volume – especially within the anteromedial extraconal space (fat hypertrophy may also be seen with steroid therapy and Cushing's disease) ▶ fusiform enlargement and enhancement of the extraocular muscle bellies (with sparing of the tendinous insertions) ▶ the hypertrophied muscles and increased fat content may lead to crowding of the orbital apex (with possible optic nerve compression and decreased vision)

- All of the intraocular muscles are usually involved ▶ if there is isolated enlargement of the lateral rectus muscle belly, then causes other than a thyroid ophthalmopathy should be sought (e.g. a pseudotumour)
  - *The order of muscular involvement:* **i**nferior rectus ▶ **m**edial rectus ▶ **s**uperior rectus ▶ **l**ateral rectus ▶ the **o**blique muscles ('**I'M SLOW**')
- With advanced disease the lamina papyracea may demonstrate a concavity due to the raised intraorbital pressure
- *Dynamic contrast-enhanced MRI:* the mean of peak enhancement ratio values for the extraocular muscles in Graves' disease tends to decrease according to the severity of the clinical and anatomical changes ▶ the mean rate of enhancement also decreases according to the disease severity

CONAL COMPARTMENT – RHABDOMYOSARCOMA

Definition A highly malignant primary orbital tumour originating from the extraocular muscles, nasopharynx and paranasal sinuses (this is the most common site for a head and neck rhabdomyosarcoma)

Clinical presentation It is seen in children aged 2–5 years and presents with a rapidly progressive exopthalmos ▶ metastases are typically haematogeneous (lung/bone the most common)

Radiological features

CT A bulky aggressive-looking isodense or slightly hyperdense mass usually located within the superomedial orbit ▶ it demonstrates uniform enhancement and is associated with bone destruction ▶ no calcification

MRI T1WI/T2WI: intermediate SI

EXTRACONAL COMPARTMENT – RETROBULBAR METASTASES

Definition Most retrobulbar metastases are extraconal in location and subsequently encroach on the intraconal compartment as they increase in size ▶ they usually produce an infiltrating poorly marginated mass ▶ they usually originate from the greater sphenoid wing with associated bone destruction

- *Adults:* an infiltrative retrobulbar mass (+ enophthalmos) is characteristic of a scirrhous carcinoma of the breast
- *Children:* smooth extraconal masses related to the posterior lateral orbital wall is seen with metastases from a neuroblastoma or Ewing's sarcoma

Radiological features

CT An infiltrating poorly marginated mass which is isodense or hyperdense ▶ there is enhancement following IV contrast medium administration

- Their baseline hyperdensity and lack of invasion of the preseptal compartment differentiates them from a rhabdomyosarcoma

EXTRACONAL COMPARTMENT – DERMOID/EPIDERMOID

Definition A cystic lesion resulting from a congenital epithelial inclusion ▶ it is classified as a true choristoma (i.e. a tumour composed of tissue not normally found at the site of occurrence) ▶ it is the commonest periorbital mass lesion found in infants and children

- *Dermoid:* composed of epithelial and dermal elements
- *Epidermoid:* composed of epithelial elements only

Radiological features

CT An ovoid, well-demarcated cystic mass lesion ▶ there may be fat (50%) or calcification (15%) present ▶ there can be bone remodelling and rim enhancement ▶ the lesion may rupture

- The majority are found within an extraconal location, occupying the superolateral aspect of the anterior orbit (and related to the frontozygomatic suture)

MRI T1WI: high SI (if fatty) or intermediate SI ▶ T2WI: low-to-intermediate SI ▶ T1WI + Gad: thin rim enhancement unless rupture has occurred

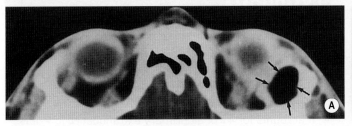 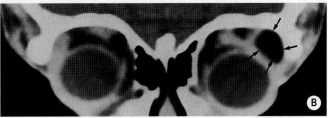

Dermoid. (A) Axial and (B) coronal CECT. There is a fat density mass in the superolateral left orbit with a thick enhancing capsule (arrows). Subtle deformity of the adjacent bone is noted.*

Differentiation between a pseudotumour and thyroid ophthalmopathy		
	Pseudotumour	**Thyroid ophthalmopathy**
Involvement	Usually unilateral	Usually bilateral
Tendon involvement	Yes	No
Orbital fat	Hyperdense (inflammation)	Increased amounts
Effect of steroids	Marked	Minor

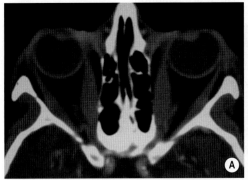 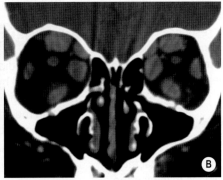 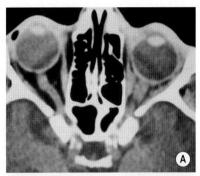

Thyroid ophthalmopathy. (A) Axial and (B) coronal CT imaging. There is generalized enlargement of the bellies of all the extraocular muscles, proptosis and increased intraorbital fat.*

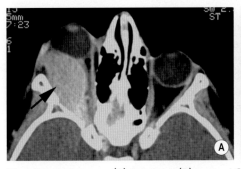 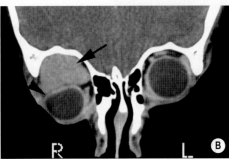 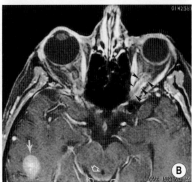

Rhabdomyosarcoma. (A) Axial and (B) coronal CECT. There is a large uniformly enhancing mass in the superior right orbit which is difficult to separate from the extraocular muscles.*

Breast metastasis to the left orbit. (A) Breast carcinoma with enophthalmos of the left globe secondary to the tumour desmoplastic reaction. (B) T1WI + Gad FS: there is subarachnoid seeding along the optic nerve (arrowheads) and in the posterior midbrain (open arrow). Also note the large mass in the right temporal region (arrow).+

IDIOPATHIC ORBITAL PSEUDOTUMOUR

DEFINITION

- An autoimmune idiopathic inflammatory condition affecting the orbital soft tissues ▶ it is the commonest cause of an adult intraorbital mass
- Affects any age ▶ M=F
- Any orbital structure can be affected, in the following order of frequency: the retrobulbar fat ▶ the extraocular muscles ▶ lacrimal gland ▶ the optic nerve ▶ the globe (the uveal-scleral area)
  - *Tumefactive type:* there is diffuse involvement of the conal and intraconal structures
  - *Myositic type:* this involves the extraocular muscles
  - *Tolosa–Hunt syndrome:* an idiopathic inflammatory condition similar to a pseudotumour and affecting the cavernous sinus and orbital apex (it can also present with a painful ophthalmoplegia)

CLINICAL PRESENTATION

- There is a rapid onset in middle age with a unilateral painful ophthalmoplegia, proptosis and chemosis
  - *Acute:* there is a rapid and lasting response to steroids ▶ this is the more common presentation
  - *Chronic:* there is a poor response to steroids with subsequent fibrosis (requiring chemotherapy and radiotherapy)

RADIOLOGICAL FEATURES

`CT` 'Dirty fat': subtle hyperdensity of the intraorbital fat ▶ there is enhancement of the affected regions following the administration of IV contrast medium

`MRI` T2WI: low SI (true tumours generate high SI)

PEARLS

- *10% are associated with other systemic autoimmune conditions:* Wegener's granulomatosis ▶ fibrosing mediastinitis ▶ Riedel's thyroiditis ▶ sclerosing cholangitis ▶ retroperitoneal fibrosis ▶ polyarteritis nodosa ▶ dermatomyositis ▶ rheumatoid arthritis
- Involvement of a unilateral single extraocular muscle (*including the tendinous insertion*) is highly suggestive of a pseudotumour rather than thyroid ophthalmopathy ▶ the tendon is spared in thyroid disease ▶ frequency of muscular involvement: medial rectus > superior rectus > lateral rectus > inferior rectus

LYMPHOMA

DEFINITION

- This is usually a non-Hodgkin's lymphoma (NHL) of the B-cell variety – Hodgkin's disease of the orbit is rarely seen
- It accounts for 4% of all primary extranodal NHL ▶ it is the commonest primary orbital malignancy in adults (accounting for 10–15% of orbital masses)
- Secondary orbital involvement occurs in 3.5–5% of both Hodgkin's disease and non-Hodgkin's lymphoma
- Any orbital structure may be affected but it usually affects the lacrimal gland followed by the conal and intraconal compartments (the commonest involved extraocular muscle is superior rectus) ▶ the optic nerve and sheath complex can also be affected (where it may mimic an optic nerve meningioma or neuritis)

CLINICAL PRESENTATION

- It presents during middle age with a painless orbital swelling and proptosis (there is usually no evidence of systemic disease at presentation)

RADIOLOGICAL FEATURES

`CT` The radiological findings can vary between a well-defined hyperdense enhancing mass, or diffuse infiltration with destruction of the normal anatomy
- It will mould to the orbital contour without any associated bone destruction (unless very aggressive)

`MRI` T1WI: low SI ▶ T2WI: high SI ▶ T1WI + Gad: enhancement

`CT-PET` Positive

PEARLS

- Bilateral orbital masses suggest the diagnosis of lymphoma
- Lymphoma tends to be more superiorly placed within the orbit than a pseudotumour
- Orbital involvement in leukaemia is rare ▶ any orbital structure can be involved – infiltration of the optic nerve is an oncological emergency due to the threat to vision ▶ can present as a mass or diffuse infiltration

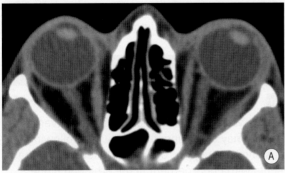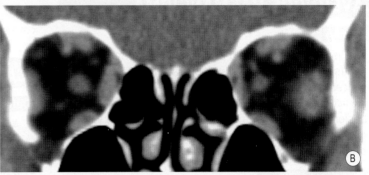

Idiopathic orbital inflammation (orbital pseudotumour). Axial (A) and coronal (B) CT reconstructions of the orbits demonstrating asymmetrical swelling of the left lateral rectus muscle and tendon. Note the stranding of the adjacent orbital fat indicative of an active inflammatory process.**

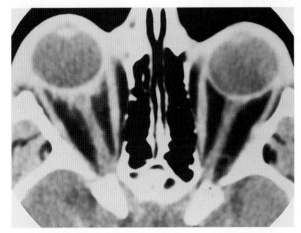

Scleral pseudotumour. Marked thickening and irregularity of the sclera of the right globe involves the adjacent retro-orbital fat.†

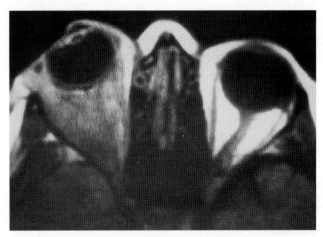

Diffuse pseudotumour. Axial MR T1-weighted image showing a diffuse mass in the right orbit due to pseudotumour.†

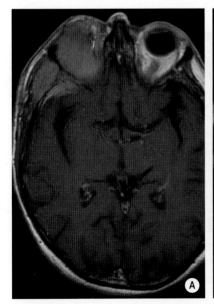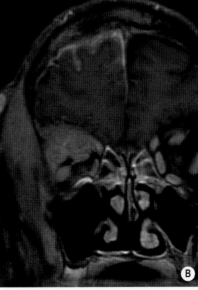

Lymphoma. (A) Axial T1WI + Gad. (B) Coronal T1WI + Gad FS. There is a homogeneously enhancing mass in the superior right orbit that extends outside the orbit to involve the temporal fossa. On coronal imaging, there is thick meningeal enhancement indicating intracranial spread of lymphoma.*

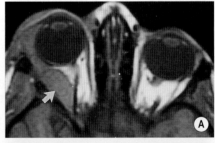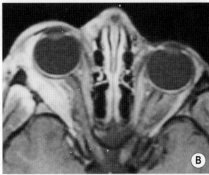

Lymphoma. T1-weighted MR image (A) demonstrates proptosis of right globe due to a large intermediate signal intensity lesion that involves the lacrimal fossa and the right lateral rectus muscle (arrow), with extension posteriorly in the extraconal compartment. Postcontrast image (B) demonstrates homogeneous enhancement.†

849

CAVERNOUS HAEMANGIOMA

Definition

- This is the most common primary orbital tumour in adults consisting of large endothelial-lined vascular spaces with a fibrous pseudocapsule ▶ they are usually intraconal in location
- Lesions occur in adults aged between 20 and 40 years old (M>F) ▶ patents present with a painless slow proptosis but their vision is usually unaffected

Radiological features

CT A sharply demarcated, rounded or oval hyperdense enhancing mass that spares the orbital apex ▶ bone deformities following erosion may occur (but there is no bone destruction)

MRI This is better at demonstrating the relationship of the optic nerve and extraocular muscles

- T1WI: normal or low SI ▶ T2WI: high SI ▶ T1WI + Gad: enhancement (progressive on delayed imaging)
- There are no recognizable arterial feeders or draining veins ▶ there may be associated phleboliths and surrounding haemosiderin or ferritin deposition ▶ intralesional haemorrhage is rare

CAPILLARY HAEMANGIOMA

Definition

- A mass resulting from the proliferation of endothelial cells with multiple capillaries present
- It presents with proptosis in infants who are <1 year old ▶ it spontaneously regresses during the first few years of life

Radiological features

CT/MRI An ill-defined irregular enhancing mass spanning the intraconal and extraconal compartments ▶ MRI can demonstrate the multiple punctuate low SI flow voids present within a mass

LYMPHANGIOMA

Definition

- A harmatoma arising embryologically from the primitive vascular tree ▶ it is composed of varying amounts of solid and cystic material with haemorrhagic products of differing ages ▶ it is largely extraconal but can commonly cross boundaries
- It presents with a slowly progressive exophthalmos in childhood or with sudden proptosis due to intratumoural haemorrhage ▶ does not enlarge with Valsalva stress

Radiological features

CT A poorly defined lobulated mass of mixed attenuation demonstrating variable enhancement

MRI T2WI: heterogeneous cystic and haemorrhagic components ▶ T1WI + Gad: minimal enhancement

CAROTID-CAVERNOUS FISTULAE

Definition

- A fistula between the carotid siphon and the cavernous sinus which may occur spontaneously (e.g. following a carotid siphon aneurysm rupture) or following trauma
- It presents with engorgement of the orbit and globe, a pulsating exophthalmos and bruit with, eventually, glaucoma and visual loss

Radiological features

MRI Signs of orbital venous hypertension (e.g. an enlarged and engorged superior ophthalmic vein and extraocular muscles) ▶ signal voids within the cavernous sinus and superior ophthalmic vein (due to the presence of fast-flowing arterial blood)

- The enlarged cavernous sinus may be bowed (convex to the middle cranial fossa)

MRA There is filling of the cavernous sinus and superior ophthalmic vein in conjunction with the arterial anterior intracranial circulation

Conventional angiography There is filling of the ipsilateral or contralateral cavernous sinus via the intercavernous sinuses ▶ drainage is into the ipsilateral or bilateral superior ophthalmic veins, inferior petrosal sinuses, or even the cortical veins or sphenoparietal sinuses (when severe)

VASCULAR LESIONS – VENOUS VARIX

Definition

- A massively dilated intraconal vein representing a congenital or acquired (e.g. post-traumatic) venous malformation ▶ it may be associated with an intra-orbital or intracranial arteriovenous malformation
- It presents with intermittent proptosis (upon straining and coughing) and retrobulbar pain

Radiological Features

CT An intraconal hyperdense lobulated mass demonstrating strong enhancement ▶ phleboliths and thrombus may be present ▶ it may require the Valsalva manoeuvre for demonstration (if small)

MRI This may reveal slow-flow phenomena ▶ clot following a spontaneous thrombosis is common (generating variable signal intensities)

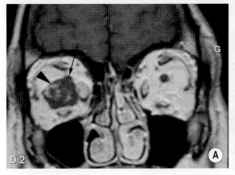
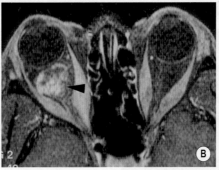
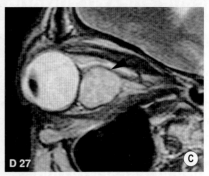

Cavernous haemangioma. (A) Coronal T1WI + Gad. The heterogeneous mass (black arrowhead) lies inferolateral to the optic nerve (arrow). (B) Axial T1WI + Gad FS. The heterogeneous enhancement of the mass (black arrowhead) corresponds to pooling of contrast medium within intratumoural vascular spaces. (C) Sagittal T2WI. The lesion (black arrowhead) is high SI and has a low-intensity rim, probably because of a combination of fibrous tissue and haemosiderin/ferritin in the capsule.*

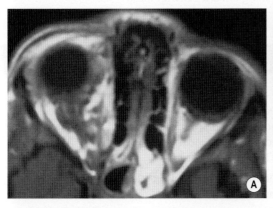
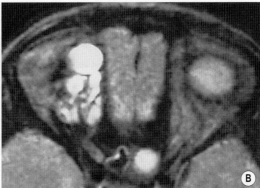

Lymphangioma. Axial T1WI (A) and T2WI (B) demonstrate mild right proptosis due to a complex, multiloculated, cystic, extra-axial lesion in the superomedial aspect of the right orbit.*

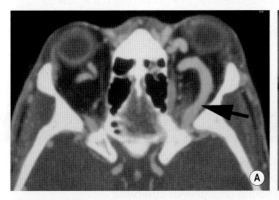
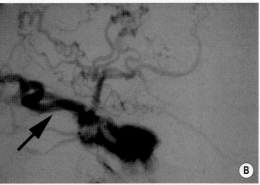

Post-traumatic high-flow carotid-cavernous fistula. (A) Axial CECT shows marked dilatation of the left superior ophthalmic vein (arrow) and moderate dilatation of the right superior ophthalmic vein. (B) Carotid angiography shows early filling of the cavernous sinus and left superior ophthalmic vein (arrow).*

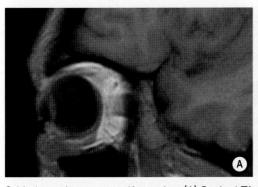
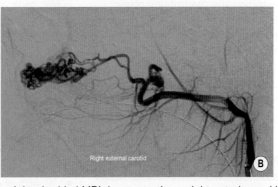

Orbital arteriovenous malformation. (A) Sagittal T1-weighted orbital MRI demonstrating a right anterior and inferior subtle orbital mass. Selective digital subtraction angiography (DSA) of the right internal maxillary artery (B) demonstrates arteriovenous shunting through the mass through a tangle of abnormal vessels representing the nidus of an AVM.**

NERVE SHEATH TUMOUR

DEFINITION

Schwannoma is the commonest orbital nerve sheath tumour ▶ a slow-growing benign peripheral nerve sheath tumour ▶ usually seen in adults ▶ frequently arise from sensory branches of the ophthalmic nerve (V1), explaining the sometimes extraconal location

CLINICAL PRESENTATION

Painless progressive proptosis

RADIOLOGICAL FEATURES

MRI T1WI: low SI ▶ T2WI: high SI ▶ T1WI + Gad: enhancement

PEARLS

- Neurofibroma can also develop in the orbit with similar imaging features to schwannoma ▶ it can arise in isolation or as part of NF-1
- Plexiform neurofibroma is associated with hypoplasia of the greater wing of the sphenoid
- Calcification can be present in some neurofibromata, distinguishing it from schwannoma

OPTIC NERVE GLIOMA

DEFINITION

- A slow-growing low-grade pilocytic astrocytoma seen during childhood (75% of cases are less than 10 years old)
- It is the commonest primary optic nerve tumour
- 15% of patients with neurofibromatosis type 1 have an optic nerve or chiasmatic glioma – if this is bilateral it is then pathognomonic for neurofibromatosis
- It presents with decreased vision with minimal proptosis

RADIOLOGICAL FEATURES

- Tortuous optic or nerve sheath complex thickening that is commonly tubular (but may be fusiform or excrescent)

- ▶ unlike an optic nerve meningioma, a glioma cannot be separated from the optic nerve
- It does not tend to spread from the optic nerve to the intracranial compartment (although only 25% are confined to the optic nerve)

CT An isodense mass ▶ calcification is rare (except following radiotherapy)

MRI T1WI: intermediate SI ▶ T2WI: high SI ▶ due to arachnoidal gliomatosis there may be low SI with a high SI rim in neurofibromatosis ▶ there may be a cystic component ▶ T1WI + Gad: 50% enhance

RETINOBLASTOMA

DEFINITION

- A tumour derived from primitive photoreceptors or neuronal retinal cells (histologically resembling other primitive neuroectodermal tumours)
- It is a highly malignant tumour that may spread haematogenously, via the lymphatics, or along the optic nerve to the intracranial compartment (giving drop metastases within the subarachnoid space)
- It is the commonest paediatric tumour of the globe
  - It occurs in children <3 years old (presenting with leucocoria)

RADIOLOGICAL FEATURES

CT 95% of cases demonstrate clumped or punctate calcification within the posterior globe which extends into the vitreous (it may fill the globe if it is advanced)

- Calcification within an intraocular mass in a child who is less than 3 years old should be considered a retinoblastoma until proven otherwise

MRI This is better for the detection of any tumour extension intracranially or along the optic nerve

- T1WI: high SI ▶ T2WI: low SI ▶ T1WI + Gad: minimal enhancement

PEARLS

- 75% are unilateral and unifocal ▶ 25% are bilateral or unilateral and multifocal
  - *Trilateral retinoblastoma*: bilateral retinoblastomas in conjunction with a pineoblastoma
- 10–40% of cases are familial (autosomal dominant) – these tend to be bilateral and associated with other non-ocular tumours (e.g. an osteosarcoma)

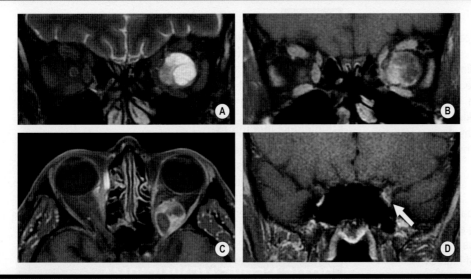

Nerve sheath tumour. Coronal STIR (A), coronal (B, D) and axial (C) T1-weighted post-gadolinium fat-suppressed MRI of the orbits demonstrating a well-circumscribed heterogeneous signalled and heterogeneously enhancing left orbital apex mass, extending through the superior orbital fissure (white arrow). Mass reveals avid and homogeneous enhancement.**

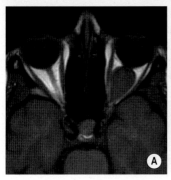
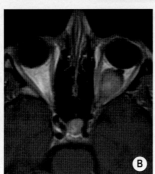
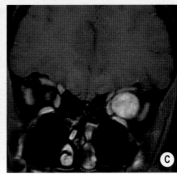

Optic nerve glioma. (A) Axial T1WI, (B) axial T1WI + Gad, (C) coronal T1WI + Gad FS. There is smooth expansion of the left optic nerve extending to the orbital apex. On contrast-enhanced imaging, there is homogeneous enhancement of the mass, and the nerve cannot be distinguished from it.*

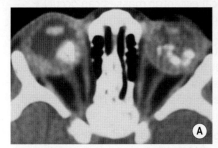
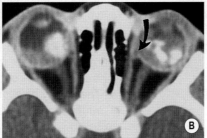

Retinoblastoma. NECT (A) demonstrates bilateral partially calcified intraocular masses. CECT (B) demonstrates spread through sclera and into intraconal compartment (arrow), predicting a poor prognosis.†

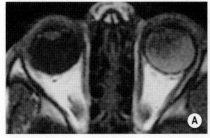
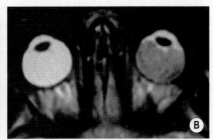

Axial T1-weighted (A) and T2-weighted (B) MR images demonstrate the full extent of a large lesion within the left globe. High signal intensity on T1WIs, and low signal intensity on T2WIs, is consistent with the dense cellular nature of this tumour.†

ORBITAL INFECTION

Definition

- The orbital septum acts as a mechanical barrier to the spread of infection into the orbit
- *Preseptal cellulitis:* this is usually confined to the eyelids
- *Postseptal infection:* this is much more serious ▶ it can arise from sinus disease, bacteraemia, trauma and the spread of serious infection from the skin
- Intraorbital infection spread via paranasal sinus infection can lead to superior ophthalmic vein thrombosis ± cavernous sinus thrombosis

Radiological features

CT/MRI There are ill-defined retrobulbar tissue planes
- There may be a soft tissue mass (ring enhancement ± pockets of gas is suggestive of abscess formation)
- T1WI/T2WI: there is loss of the normal high SI
- *Subperiosteal abscess:* this can develop in association with an ethmoid sinusitis ▶ it can be identified as a soft tissue mass (± central fluid) that is centred on the bony (and usually medial) orbital wall ▶ there is displacement of the adjacent extraocular muscles ▶ a thin layer of extraconal fat is preserved and the lamina papyracea may or may not be destroyed
- The CT and MRI appearances are non-specific for any particular ocular infection

Pearls

- Endophthalmitis can be nematodal (*Toxocara*), fungal (*Candida*), or bacterial (*Staphylococcus/Streptococcus*)
- Infectious uveitis can be bacterial, viral, fungal or parasitic

UVEAL MELANOMA

Definition

- This is the most common adult primary intraocular malignancy ▶ it is usually found unilaterally within the choroid and metastasizes to the liver and lungs ▶ extensive spread beyond the globe is common ('collar button' lesion)
- Progressive visual loss

Radiological features

CT A hyperdense soft tissue mass centred on the outer layers of the globe ▶ the mass bulges inward into the vitreous ▶ it may be small and flat, crescentic, or large and sharply demarcated with a 'mushroom cloud' appearance ▶ tumour morphology can vary from nodular, to plaque-like lesions and diffuse infiltration ▶ it enhances after contrast medium administration

MRI T1WI: high SI ▶ T2WI: low SI (both are due to the presence of paramagnetic melanin ± haemorrhage) ▶ T1WI + Gad: enhancement
- *Amelanotic melanomas:* T1WI: low SI ▶ T2WI: high SI

OCULAR METASTASES

Definition

- Only 50% of patients with an ocular metastasis have a known primary (they occur most commonly to the uveal tract)
  - *Male:* GI tract
  - *Female:* lung or breast

Radiological features

CT Small multiple areas of hyperdense thickening (occasionally with subretinal fluid)
- Lesions found bilaterally and within the posterior temporal regions near each macula suggest a metastatic diagnosis (rather than choroidal haemangiomas in association with Sturge–Weber syndrome)

OPTIC NERVE MENINGIOMA

Definition

- These tumours arise from the arachnoid layer of the leptomeninges that surround the optic nerve (without infiltrating it) ▶ this leads to tubular thickening of the optic nerve and sheath complex (rather than fusiform or excrescent thickening) ▶ there may be intracranial spread – but this is only to the prechiasmatic optic nerve sheath
  - It is the 2nd commonest primary optic nerve tumour after a glioma
  - It may be bilateral when seen in association with neurofibromatosis type 2
  - It presents with a progressive loss of vision and commonly affects middle-aged women (rarely children with neurofibromatosis type 2)

Radiological features

CT Circumferential or fusiform enlargement of the optic nerve sheath (focal eccentric masses can occur) ▶ a hyperdense enhancing optic nerve meningioma is seen separate from the optic nerve – intense enhancement leads to a 'tram-track' sign (axial images) or a 'doughnut sign' (coronal images) ▶ calcification (due to psammoma bodies) is seen in 20–50% of cases
- There may be hyperostosis affecting a remodelled and widened optic canal

MRI This is better for assessing orbital apex or intracanalicular lesions (the surrounding bone makes this area difficult to outline accurately on CT)
- T1WI: low SI ▶ T2WI: high SI ▶ T1WI + Gad: there is strong enhancement

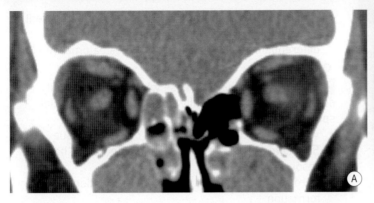 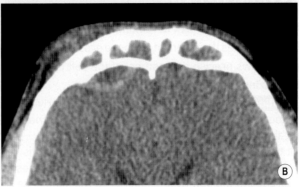

Orbital infection. Coronal CT of the orbits (A) in a patient with right orbital cellulitis, demonstrating subtle stranding of the intraorbital fat on the right with asymmetric swelling of the superior-rectus levator complex and a soft-tissue inflammatory mass superior to it. Note the extensive opacification of the maxillary antra and right ethmoidal air cells. Axial CT of the brain in this patient (B) revealed an empyema subjacent to opacified frontal sinuses and right forehead cellulitis.**

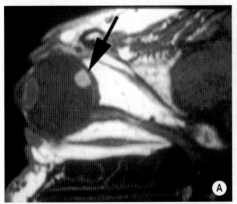 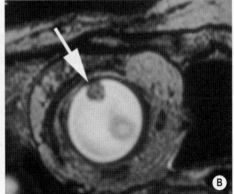

Malignant melanoma of the choroid. (A) Oblique sagittal T1WI. (B) Oblique coronal T2WI. There is a nodule applied to the wall of the globe that is high SI on unenhanced T1- (black arrow) and low SI on T2-weighted (white arrow) images. These signal intensities are in keeping with melanin.*

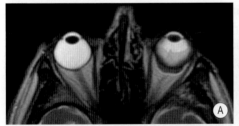 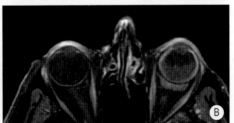

Ocular metastasis from systemic lymphoma. (A) Axial T2WI and (B) axial T1WI + Gad FS. There is thickening of the wall of the globe with soft tissue and enhancement extending into the vitreous and retrobulbar space.*

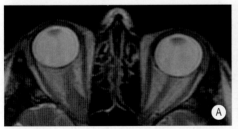 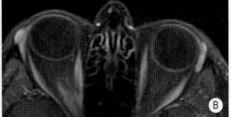

Optic nerve meningioma. (A) Axial T2WI, (B) axial T1WI + Gad FS. There is a mass at the right orbital apex, closely applied to the optic nerve but seen separate to it. On the contrast-enhanced image, 'tram-track' enhancement along the nerve can be seen.*

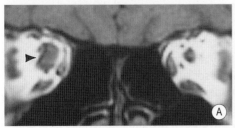 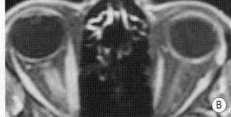

Optic nerve meningioma. Coronal T1-weighted MR image (A) demonstrates marked thickening of right optic nerve sheath (arrowhead). Axial T1-weighted postcontrast fat-saturated image (B) demonstrates peripheral enhancement of the thickened right optic nerve sheath. Non-enhancing soft tissue within represents the encased optic nerve.[†]

7.8 EAR, NOSE AND THROAT RADIOLOGY

EXTERNAL EAR

Squamous or basal cell carcinoma

HRCT Defines the extent of any bone erosion or destruction

MRI Allows precise assessment of the soft tissue mass

Necrotizing otitis externa

Definition An osteomyelitis/necrosis particularly affecting the floor of the external auditory canal ▶ *Pseudomonas* is a typical initiating organism

- It typically affects an elderly diabetic patient and is associated with a facial nerve palsy as the diseases spreads to the soft tissues inferior to the skull base

Osteoma of the external ear

Definition A benign tumour that can arise spontaneously but usually occurs in individuals fond of swimming in cold water ('surfer's ear')

- They enlarge slowly and present with late conductive deafness (as the tumour fills the external meatus)

CT A well-defined homogeneous dense tumour ▶ pedunculated, unilateral and lateral to the bone

MIDDLE EAR

Chronic suppurative otitis media and acquired cholesteatoma (keratoma)

Definition Eustachian tube dysfunction generates a negative pressure within the middle ear (drawing the tympanic membrane inwards) ▶ if any desquamating epithelium from the tympanic membrane cannot be cleared by the natural processes of ear toilet, the desquamated skin accumulates and forms a ball of skin which is known as a keratoma (cholesteatoma) ▶ this can subsequently enlarge and cause bone destruction

- *If the superior tympanic membrane (the pars flaccida) is involved, skin accumulation occurs within the superior Prussak's space (the attic)*

CT A soft tissue mass within Prussak's space with erosion of the scutum ▶ ossicular erosion (commonly affecting the long process of the incus) with *medial* displacement of the ossicles

MRI T1WI: low SI ▶ T2WI: high SI ▶ T1WI + Gad: there is little enhancement

- *If the inferior tympanic membrane (the pars tensa) is involved, skin accumulation occurs within the inferior sinus tympani*

CT A sinus tympani-based mass that can fill the middle ear cavity and invade the mastoid bone ▶ it commonly erodes the ossicles with *lateral* displacement of the ossicles

MRI T1WI: low SI ▶ T2WI: high SI ▶ T1WI + Gad: there is little enhancement

Congenital cholesteatoma (epidermoid)

Definition This originates from ectodermal cell rests which may arise within any cranial bone (the petrous temporal bone is the most common)

- It is usually found within the petrous apex, producing a clearly defined 'punched-out' area of bone destruction

- **Cholesterol granuloma:** this is an important differential and is a form of granulation tissue ▶ it can be differentiated from a congenital cholesteatoma with MRI

Otosclerosis

Definition A localized disease whereby the normally dense otic capsule is initially replaced by new vascular spongy bone (with later sclerosis)

- *Acute phase:* deposition of islets of osteoid tissue
- *Subacute phase:* remodelling and osteoclastic bone resorption
- *Chronic phase:* new osteoblast-induced sclerotic bone formation
- **Fenestral:** initially starts at the anterior margin of the oval window ▶ it can lead to fusion of the stapes foot plate to the oval window (causing a conductive hearing loss)
- **Retrofenestral (cochlear):** this initially starts within the pericochlear bony labyrinth ▶ it can lead to a sensorineural hearing loss

INNER EAR

Glomus tumours

Definition These are usually benign tumours arising from chemoreceptor cells ▶ glomus jugular tumours arise in the jugular foramen extending into the middle ear cleft ▶ globus tympanicum tumours arise on the medial wall of the middle ear cavity on the cochlear promontory

- Both present clinically with pulsatile tinnitus and as a mass within the inferior aspect of the tympanic membrane
- **Glomus jugulare (glomus jugulotympanicum) tumour:**

CT A jugular foraminal mass with adjacent destructive and permeative bone changes ▶ it rarely extends below the level of the hyoid bone

MRI T1WI/T2WI: high SI (due to haemorrhage and slow vascular flow) ▶ T1WI + Gad: there is intense enhancement

- *'Salt and pepper' appearance:* this is due to multiple low SI flow voids + subacute haemorrhage
- **Glomus tympanicum tumour:**

CT / MRI An enhancing mass with a flat base located on the cochlear promontory

- T1WI + Gad: there is intense enhancement

Bell's (facial nerve) palsy

Definition Typically this describes a sudden facial paralysis which recovers fully or incompletely after 2–3 months

MRI T2WI: nerve swelling and high SI ▶ T1WI + Gad: pathological nerve enhancement is well described

Trauma

Definition Skull base fractures involving the petrous bone are uncommon ▶ they are important to identify because (1) there may be an associated CSF leak, (2) the facial nerve may be damaged and (3) the ossicular chain may be disrupted.

- Classically they have been divided into longitudinal and transverse subtypes (although most take a complex course through a complex bone)

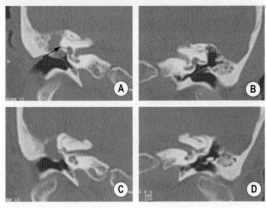

Chronic suppurative otitis media. (A) Coronal CT showing erosion of horizontal semicircular canal (HSCC, arrow), with normal (B) for comparison. A large mass can be seen filling the attic. It has eroded into the HSCC, destroyed the ossicles and partially covers the oval window. (C) Coronal CT of erosion of the lateral wall. By comparing this with the normal side (D) the destruction of the lateral attic wall can be appreciated.*

Temporal bone fractures[ʃʃ]		
Parameter	**Longitudinal fractures (middle ear fracture)**	**Transverse fractures (inner ear fracture)**
Frequency	80%	20%
Fracture line	Parallel to long axis	Perpendicular to long axis
Labyrinth	Spared	Involved: vertigo, sensorineural hearing loss
Ossicles	Involved: conductive hearing loss	
Tympanic membrane	Involved	Spared
Facial paralysis	20%	50%

	Congenital cholesteatoma	**Cholesterol granuloma**
T1WI	Low SI	High SI (cholesterol content)
T2WI	High SI	High SI

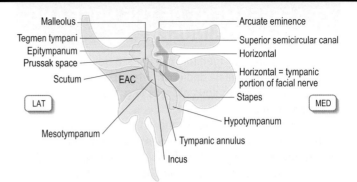

Schematic diagram showing the anatomy of the middle ear.

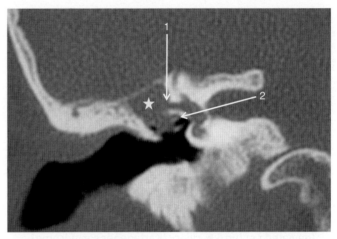

Coronal CT of right petrous temporal bone. Star = cholesteatoma in attic; 1 = eroded otic capsule over lateral SCC; 2 = facial nerve (tympanic segment).**

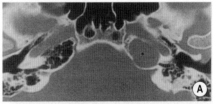

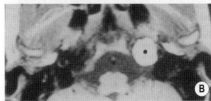

(A) Axial CT section showing an expansile lesion in the petrous apex (asterisk). (B) High signal on both T1W and T2W images confirmed that this was a cholesterol granuloma.[†]

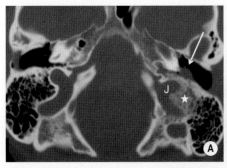

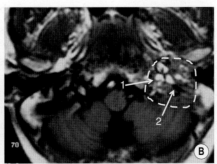

(A) Axial CT of petrous temporal bone. Star = classic permeative appearance of a glomus tumour. Note also the loss of the dense cortical line of the jugular foramen (J). The tumour extends into the middle ear (white arrow), which is the tip of the iceberg of a large glomus jugulotympanicum (GJT). (B) Axial T1W MR image of the same patient. Interrupted white line outlines the GJT. The 'salt and pepper' appearance of the tumour is shown. 1 = T1W high signal of foci of haemorrhage; 2 = signal void of large feeding vessel.**

CT ASSESSMENT OF THE NOSE AND PARANASAL SINUSES

- *Identification of congenital variations:* a deviated nasal septum ▶ hypoplasia and enlargement of the normal structures ▶ anomalous air cells (e.g. Haller and Agger nasi air cells)
- *Identification of disease extent:* which sinuses are involved or spared ▶ if there is involvement of the osteomeatal complex or sphenoethmoidal recess ▶ if there is disease extension into the orbit or cranium
- *Identification of bone destruction:* this may indicate malignancy
- *Identification of complications:* e.g. an orbital or intracranial abscess

Osteomeatal complex

- This is the drainage point for the frontal, anterior ethmoidal and maxillary sinuses ▶ its infundibulum leads to its opening (the hiatus semilunaris)
  - *Medial wall:* the uncinate process
  - *Superolateral wall:* the inferior orbital wall

RHINOSINUSITIS

Definition An extremely common condition that does not usually require radiological investigation
- *Causes:* allergic ▶ vasomotor ▶ infective ▶ mechanical (deviated septum) ▶ ciliary (Kartagener's syndrome)

CT/MRI A thickened and enhancing sinonasal mucosa

NASAL POLYPOSIS

Definition

- Non-neoplastic inflammatory swelling of the sinonasal mucosa
- This is common in adults, but in children cystic fibrosis or a midline congenital anomaly (e.g. a meningocele or encephalocele) needs to be excluded
- The aetiology is uncertain (although allergies are important)
- It can be controlled by steroids, but surgery is frequently required (with resection via an endoscope)

CT/MRI Polypoid soft tissue masses with enhancement of the peripheral surrounding mucosa

Antrochoanal polyp

- A special unilateral polyp arising within the maxillary antrum, passing out through the ostium (which it has enlarged) and then projecting backwards into the postnasal space ▶ it causes unilateral nasal obstruction and the radiological hallmark is the enlarged ostium

MUCOCELES

Definition A blocked sinus ostium generates a mucus-filled ostium (which is not usually infected) ▶ this acts as a slow-growing mass lesion and thins the bony sinus wall ▶ it is commonly located within the frontal and ethmoid sinuses ▶ usually sterile

Clinical presentation It is usually painless and asymptomatic
- *Posterior ethmoid mucocele:* this may encroach upon the optic nerve leading to visual failure
- *Frontal or anterior ethmoid mucocele:* this may extend into the orbit (causing proptosis)

CT Characteristic sinus expansion with a very thin membrane of surrounding bone ▶ there is only peripheral enhancement if it is secondarily infected

MRI T1WI: low SI (due to its mucus water content) ▶ T2WI: high SI

NASAL/PARANASAL TUMOURS

Osteoma

- A common slow growing benign tumour which is usually found within the frontal sinus ▶ it is frequently an isolated incidental finding (but can also be part of a genetic disorder such as Gardner's syndrome) ▶ a large frontal sinus osteoma may sinus obstruct drainage with secondary infection

CT A well-defined sessile or pedunculated bone density lesion ▶ there is no enhancement

MRI T1WI/T2WI: low SI (bone content) ▶ it may have internal marrow signal

Inverting papilloma

- This frequently presents as a unilateral nasal polyp causing obstruction and epistaxis ▶ locally invasive tumours require full surgical excision ▶ calcification (10%) ▶ lobulated outline

Juvenile angiofibroma

- A benign lesion characteristically presenting in adolescent boys with heavy epistaxis ▶ it originates within the sphenopalatine foramen and widens the pterygopalatine fissure (a nasal mass with a widened fissure is therefore pathognomonic) ▶ angiography has a valuable preoperative role (and also permits therapeutic embolization)

CT/MRI A soft tissue mass with associated bone destruction (it may spread across the skull base) ▶ it will demonstrate intense enhancement (± multiple flow voids on MRI)

Malignant tumours

- These are commonly a squamous carcinoma (followed by adenocarcinoma, adenoid cystic carcinoma and melanoma) ▶ a lymphoma can be primary or secondary

CT This assesses any bone destruction

MRI This assesses any soft tissue component

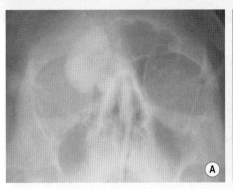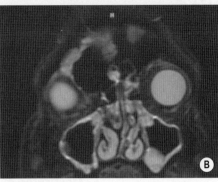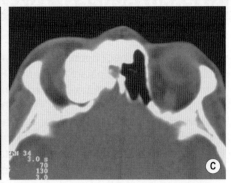

Osteoma. (A) A rare use for a plain radiograph. The osteoma can be clearly appreciated, but the image gives no details of its involvement with the intracranial space or orbit. (B) The coronal STIR images underestimate the lesion since bone and air are both black on T2WI. (C) The axial CT shows extension into the orbit.*

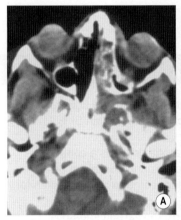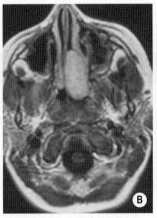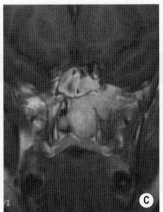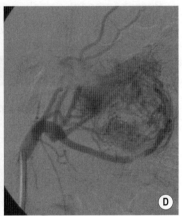

Juvenile angiofibroma in a teenager with epistaxis. (A) This axial CT shows widening of the pterygopalatine fissure on the left side. This is virtually diagnostic of an angiofibroma. (B) T1WI + Gad image reveals an enhancing, well-defined mass in the nose. (C) Coronal image revealing the mass at the level of the posterior choana with lateral extension towards the infratemporal fossa. (D) Angiography. Lateral superselective injection into the maxillary artery shows the highly vascular nature of the tumour.*

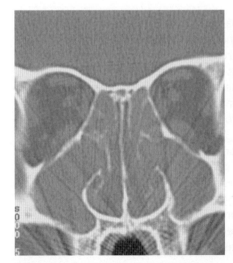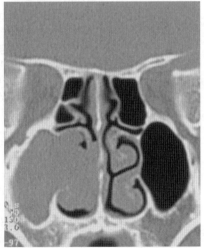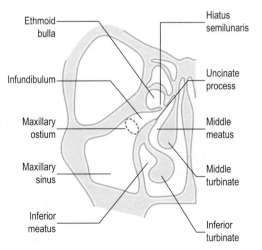

Severe nasal polyposis and airway obstruction. CT at the level of the ostia of the maxillary antra. Note the complete opacity of the nasal airway. The ostia are widened by benign polyps and the nasal turbinates are partially eroded.*

Antrochoanal polyp. CT showing polyp in the maxillary antrum, widening the osteum, lying between middle and inferior turbinates.

Schematic diagram showing the anatomy of the paranasal sinuses.

NASOPHARYNGEAL ANATOMY

The nasopharynx

- The area of the neck bounded by the skull base (superiorly) and the palate (inferiorly) ▶ it is divided into a number of complex compartments – some of these (e.g. the parapharyngeal, retropharyngeal and prevertebral compartments) can serve as a major potential vertical transmission route for disease
  - Each compartment will initially contain any pathological process but there will eventually be spread beyond the fascial planes

The compartments and their contents

- *Pharyngeal mucosal:* stratified squamous epithelium ▶ small salivary glands ▶ adenoids ▶ pharyngeal constrictor muscles ▶ levator palatini muscle
- *Parapharyngeal:* parapharyngeal fat ▶ rare for pathology to develop here

- The direction of effacement of the parapharyngeal fat can point to the site of original disease:
  - *Anteriorly:* masticator space
  - *Posteriorly:* carotid space
  - *Medially:* pharyngeal mucosal space
  - *Laterally:* parotid space
- *Retropharyngeal:* fat (route for infection spread into the mediastinum)
- *Prevertebral:* prevertebral muscles
- *Masticator:* muscles of mastication ▶ mandible ▶ teeth
- *Carotid:* carotid artery ▶ jugular vein ▶ vagus and glossopharyngeal nerves ▶ sympathetic trunk
- *Parotid:* parotid gland ▶ retromandibular vein ▶ facial nerve

PATHOLOGY

Mucosal and parapharyngeal spaces

- **Nasopharyngeal carcinoma:** this is a squamous cell carcinoma usually arising from the lateral pharyngeal recess ▶ it is usually advanced at diagnosis (it can infiltrate the parapharyngeal fat 'silently') with 90% of patients demonstrating positive nodes at presentation ▶ skull base invasion and intracranial extension seen ▶ it is associated with the Epstein–Barr virus and is common in the Chinese population

  CT/MRI These demonstrate the lesion well (the tumour demonstrates mild enhancement)
- Surgery is not usually an option – the treatment is radiotherapy (requiring radiological planning)

Masticator space

- **Tumour** (of the muscles of mastication): this is rare and usually a rhabdomyosarcoma
- **Sepsis:** this usually arises around the teeth ▶ it can occasionally present with trismus
- **Atrophy:** atrophy of the muscles of mastication can be caused by trigeminal nerve dysfunction (occasionally atrophy of one side is misinterpreted as overgrowth of the other)

Carotid space

- **Vagal neuroma:** this is usually a benign schwannoma originating within the carotid sheath (spreading the carotid and jugular vessels apart) ▶ it may reach a large size due to its very slow rate of growth

  MRI T1WI: variable SI ▶ T2WI: characteristically high SI ▶ T1WI + Gad: avid enhancement
- **Paraganglionoma:** carotid bulb tumours are tumours of the chemoreceptor cells arising within the carotid body (and are similar to a glomus jugulare tumour) ▶ as 10% are multiple, both sites should always be examined

  MRI T1WI: a 'salt and pepper' appearance if a lesion is >1.5 cm (this is due to a combination of high SI

due to subacute haemorrhage and low SI flow voids, respectively) ▶ T2WI: intermediate or high SI ▶ T1WI + Gad: avid enhancement

- **Vascular anomaly:** the carotid artery is a common site for atheroma ▶ less commonly there can be an aneurysm (which can appear complex and mistaken for tumour)
- **Lymph node enlargement:** the carotid sheath is invested with a double layer of fascia and is resistant to invasion by local disease – however, lymph nodes within the carotid sheath can enlarge as part of a systemic disease (e.g. lymphoma) or if the sheath is directly invaded by tumour

Parotid space

- The majority of parotid tumours are benign and are pleomorphic adenomas ▶ 20% are malignant and a heterogeneous group of carcinomas, lymphomas and adenolymphomas (Warthin's tumour)
  - Tumours of the deep lobe can spread medially into the parapharyngeal fat and are sometimes difficult to differentiate from laterally spreading parapharyngeal tumours
  - Although the precise location of the intraparotid facial nerve is surgically important, it is currently impossible to identify it radiologically
- Malignancy is suggested by heterogeneity, irregular margins (± local invasion) and lymphadenopathy
- **Pleomorphic adenoma:** a well-demarcated slow-growing mass (malignant transformation is seen in 5%)

  US A hypoechoic mass

  CT Calcification is suggestive of the diagnosis

  MRI T1WI: low SI ▶ T2WI: high SI

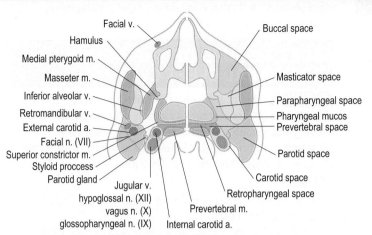

Anatomy of the parotid and parapharyngeal spaces.

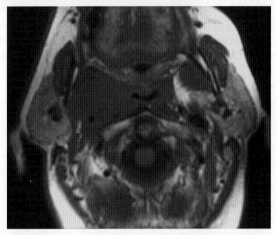

Nasopharyngeal carcinoma. Axial T1WI shows a large parapharyngeal mass in contact with the deep lobe of the parotid laterally and partially encasing the carotid.*

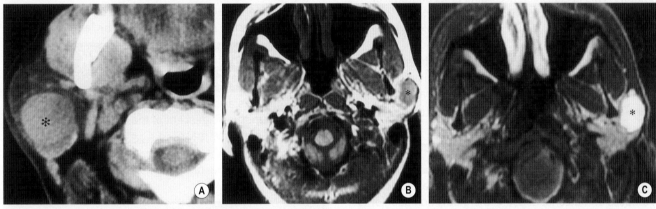

Pleomorphic adenoma. (A) CT demonstrating a well-defined mass (*) within the superficial right parotid gland. (B) T1WI demonstrating a pleomorphic adenoma within the left parotid gland. (C) The high SI on T2WI (in the face of a T1WI that does not look like a cyst) suggests a pleomorphic adenoma.+

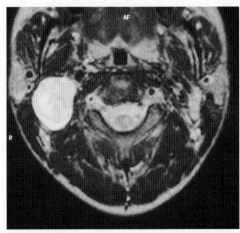

Vagal neuroma. Axial T2WI shows a well-defined mass of high SI on the right side just posterior and lateral to the flow void of the carotid artery.*

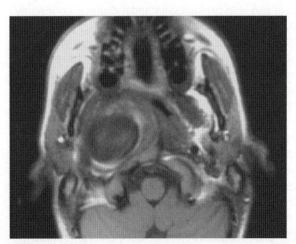

Carotid aneurysm. Axial T1WI MRI at nasopharynx level shows a low SI aneurysm in the lumen and organized thrombus in the wall.*

OROPHARYNX – CARCINOMA OF THE TONGUE

Definition This is usually a squamous carcinoma and can range between a small lesion (representing an aphthous ulcer) to a large lesion (demonstrating widespread tongue infiltration)

- *Small lesions:* these are resected or ablated
- *Large lesions:* a full glossectomy or hemiglossectomy is performed (the tongue can function well from the muscular action on one side against a myocutaneous flap replacement)

CT/MRI The following features will require radical surgery or radiotherapy:

- Crossing of the midline
- Erosion or infiltration of the mandible
- Involvement of the epiglottic root (and impaired function) by the posterior aspect of the tumour

OROPHARYNX – CARCINOMA OF THE PHARYNX

Definition This is classified according to its anatomical origin (e.g. a pyriform fossa carcinoma or supraglottic carcinoma) ▶ faucial tonsil and anterior tonsillar pillar are commonest sites

- Surgical resection and reconstruction may be impossible ▶ the integrity of the epiglottic mechanism is of paramount importance (as it prevents aspiration)

CT/MRI All tumours infiltrate adjacent structures and along epithelial surfaces

CARCINOMA OF THE LARYNX

Definition This is a squamous cell carcinoma, associated with tobacco and alcohol abuse ▶ the glottis and subglottis (which has few vascular and lymphatic channels) is embryologically distinct from the supraglottic region (which has many vascular and lymphatic channels)

- *Supraglottic tumour:* this can present late with a large mass (it can also present with nodal disease, commonly involving the deep cervical lymph nodes)
- *Glottic tumour:* this is the most common type and is usually small at presentation (as it tends to have an immediate effect on the voice) – it can therefore usually be completely removed with a good prognosis
  - It can spread locally to the contralateral cord (via the anterior commissure) with an adverse effect on the prognosis ▶ nodes at presentation rare
- *Subglottic:* the least common type ▶ the undersurface of the cord is the usual site (which is difficult to assess endoscopically) ▶ can present late with a large mass (as this is a clinically silent area) ▶ there are early nodal metastases and poor prognosis

CT/MRI *Critical observations:* Is there anterior spread through the thyroid notch? ▶ Has the tumour crossed the midline? ▶ Is there spread into the supraglottis or upper oesophagus? ▶ Is there invasion of the cartilaginous structures of the larynx?

SOFT TISSUES OF THE NECK – BRANCHIAL CLEFT CYST

Definition This is a developmental cyst of water attenuation or signal intensity which occurs due to incomplete involution of the branchial apparatus ▶ although it is congenital, it is usually identified during the 2nd to 4th decades and may become infected

CT/MRI

- *1st branchial cyst:* this is found within the parotid or preauricular region
- *2nd branchial cyst:* this can appear as a fistula, sinus or cyst ▶ it is commonly located posterolateral to the submandibular gland and anteromedial to the sternocleidomastoid muscle ▶ it accounts for 95% of branchial anomalies
- *3rd branchial cyst:* this is located within the posterior triangle of the neck
- *4th branchial cyst:* located anywhere from the left pyriform sinus to the superior aspect of the left thyroid lobe

SOFT TISSUES OF THE NECK – THYROGLOSSAL CYST

Definition This arises from epithelial tissue trapped during the embryonic descent of the thyroid gland ▶ it presents as a midline mass

Location Between the tongue base (the foramen caecum) and thyroid gland ▶ usually located anterior to the hyoid bone

SOFT TISSUES OF THE NECK – LYMPHANGIOMA/CYSTIC HYGROMA

Definition This follows abnormal lymphatic development

CT/MRI It appears as a uni- or multiloculated mass that is not confined to any one neck compartment (insinuating itself between structures) ▶ demonstrates fluid imaging characteristics with little enhancement (unless it is infected)

SOFT TISSUES OF THE NECK – VENOUS VASCULAR MALFORMATION (CAVERNOUS HAEMANGIOMA)

Definition A vascular malformation consisting of multiple venous channels

CT A lobulated soft tissue mass with multiple phleboliths present

MRI Variable SI and enhancement ▶ flow voids are uncommon

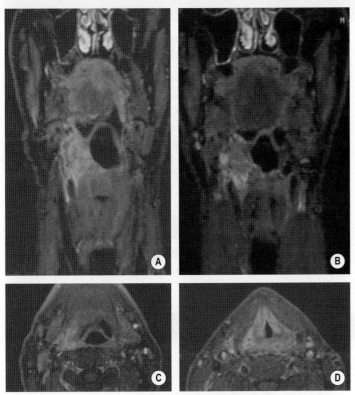

Carcinoma of the larynx. (A,B) Coronal STIR and (C,D) axial T1WI + Gad FS. The coronal images demonstrate the superior and inferior extents while the axial images define the extent more accurately.

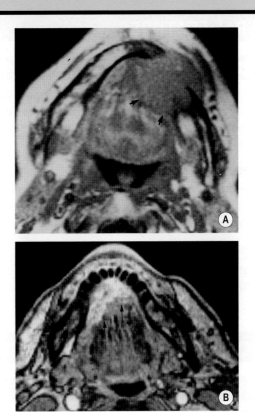

Carcinoma of the floor of the mouth. (A) Axial T1WI showing the lesion as an area of low SI (arrows) extending through the mandible into the buccal sulcus. (B) T1WI + Gad of another case showing enhancing tumour (arrows).[†]

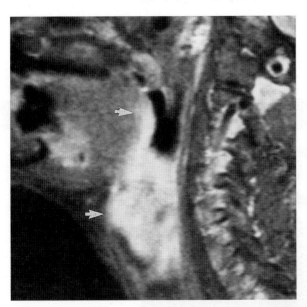

Sagittal STIR showing a hypopharyngeal carcinoma extending into the base of the tongue (arrows).[†]

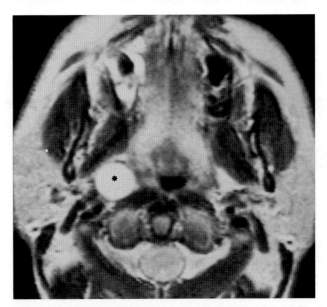

Branchial cyst. Axial T2WI of the neck shows a small fluid-filled high SI branchial cyst (asterisk).[†]

7.9 DENTAL RADIOLOGY

GENERAL FEATURES

DEFINITION

- Cysts occur more frequently within the jaw than in any other bone due to the numerous epithelial cell residues left after tooth formation ▶ these cysts are slow growing and painless (unless they become infected)

Odontogenic cysts

- These arise from epithelial residues of tooth-forming tissues and include: radicular (dental) and residual cysts ▶ dentigerous cysts ▶ odontogenic keratocysts

Non-odontogenic cysts (uncommon)

- These are mainly developmental and arise from epithelium that is not involved in tooth formation

RADIOLOGICAL FEATURES

XR The features are characteristic of slow-growing lesions (i.e. a radiolucent lesion with well-defined cortical margins) ▶ raised intracystic pressures and expansion by tissue fluid transudation results in its circular or oval shape (except for an odontogenic keratocyst) ▶ if the lesion is sufficiently large, then the cortex may become thinned, expanded and then perforated ▶ there is displacement of any adjacent structures (e.g. the tooth roots)

PEARL

- Solitary and aneurysmal bone cysts resemble jaw cysts but have no epithelial lining

RADICULAR CYST ('RESIDUAL CYST')

DEFINITION

- This is the most common odontogenic cyst (>50%) and is derived from epithelial remnants of root formation
- It develops at the apex of a non-vital tooth with the majority found on the permanent anterior teeth or 1st molars

PEARL

- Extraction of the causative tooth brings about resolution (if this does not occur it is termed a 'residual cyst') ▶ however, many regress without treatment

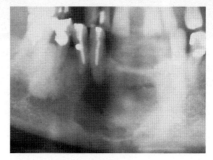

A well-defined radicular cyst is related to the right lower canine.[†]

DENTIGEROUS CYST (FOLLICULAR CYST)

DEFINITION

- This arises from reduced enamel epithelium surrounding the crown of an unerupted tooth (therefore it is only found on buried teeth)

PEARL

- Cystic enlargement of the tooth follicle produces a pericoronal radiolucency (attached to the tooth at its neck) with the crown appearing to lie within the cyst lumen

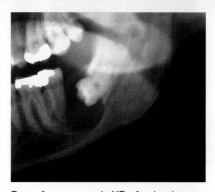

Part of a panoramic XR of a dentigerous cyst arising on a lower left wisdom tooth, which is unerupted and lying horizontally. It appears as a well-defined, circular radiolucency attached to the tooth at its neck. The inferior alveolar canal has been displaced inferiorly.[*]

ODONTOGENIC KERATOCYST (KERATOCYSTIC ODONTOGENIC TUMOUR)

DEFINITION

- This arises from remnants of the dental lamina ▶ it demonstrates a higher mitotic activity than the oral mucosa and so behaves more like a benign neoplasm ▶ recurrences are common (5–20%)

RADIOLOGICAL FEATURES

XR It appears as a unilocular or multiloculated, elongated, irregularly shaped radiolucency with a scalloped, well-defined margin ▶ it lacks the more ballooning characteristics of other odontogenic cysts (which is an important diagnostic feature) ▶ it frequently occurs within the lower 3rd molar or ramus region (and may displace an unerupted wisdom tooth where it can resemble a dentigerous cyst)

CT It demonstrates higher attenuation values of its cyst fluid than other jaw cysts (due to its high protein or keratin content) ▶ NECT: 30–200HU

MRI T1WI: low/intermediate SI ▶ T2WI: high SI

PEARL

- Gorlin–Goltz syndrome: multiple keratocysts and multiple basal cell naevi

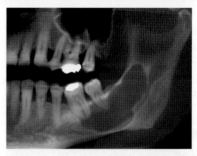

Part of a panoramic-style MPR on CBCT of an odontogenic keratocyst which appears as an elongated, loculated radiolucency extending from the mandibular foramen to the lower first molar region. There is thinning of the bony cortices but no jaw expansion, a feature associated with odontogenic keratocysts.**

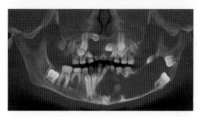

Panoramic-style MPR on CBCT showing odontogenic keratocysts in the left mandible and anterior maxilla consistent with Gorlin–Goltz syndrome. There is marked displacement of teeth by the cysts, which show minimal expansion.**

SOLITARY BONE CYST

DEFINITION

- This occurs during the 1st two decades of life (mainly in the premolar or molar regions of the mandible)

RADIOLOGICAL FEATURES

XR It has a less well-defined margin than that of an odontogenic cyst and its superior border arches up between the roots of the adjacent teeth ▶ tooth displacement and root resorption is uncommon

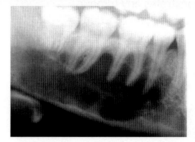

Part of a panoramic XR showing a partially corticated radiolucency in the right mandible involving the apices of the 2nd premolar and 1st and 2nd molars diagnosed as a solitary bone cyst. Note the characteristic scalloping between the roots of the molars.*

ANEURYSMAL BONE CYST

DEFINITION

- This is considered a reactive lesion of bone (characterized by a fibrous connective tissue stroma containing many cavernous blood-filled spaces) ▶ it is rare and occurs mainly in the young (<30 years old)

RADIOLOGICAL FEATURES

XR It is typically found within the posterior mandible and appears as a well-defined, multilocular, often septated, circular radiolucency ▶ there is often marked cortical expansion

CT/MRI Multiple fluid levels can be seen ▶ T1WI/T2WI: low to intermediate SI

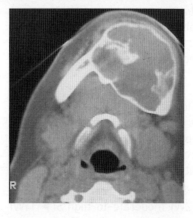

Fibrous dysplasia and resulting degeneration into aneurysmal bone cyst. CT shows the expanded mandible and the now essentially cystic nature of the lesion.†

JAW OSTEOMA

Definition A benign bone-forming tumour ▶ usually slow growing and painless ▶ affects the mandible more commonly than the maxilla (usually located posteromedially)

- *Gardner's syndrome:* multiple osteomas + familial adenomatous polyposis
  - Osteoma development precedes any intestinal colonic polyposis

OSTEOSARCOMA

Definition A malignant osteoid-producing bone tumour ▶ it is uncommon in the jaw and tends to be slower growing and occurs about 10 years later than seen with a long bone osteosarcoma ▶ the mandible is more commonly affected than the maxilla

- Maxillary lesions tend to arise from the alveolar ridge ▶ mandibular lesions tend to arise from the body

Radiological features

XR A destructive appearance ▶ the tumour can be radiolucent, patchily radio-opaque or sclerotic ▶ a 'hair-on-end', 'sunray' or 'onion skin' appearance (due to an elevated periosteum)

- *A widened periodontal ligament space:* this is an important early sign due to tumour spread along the periodontal ligament ▶ it is also seen with other sarcomas (e.g. fibrosarcoma and Ewing's sarcoma)

CT This accurately demonstrates any tumour calcification, bone destruction or bone reaction

MRI This assesses any intramedullary or extraosseous tumour component ▶ heterogeneous SI

- T1WI: intermediate SI ▶ T2WI: high SI ▶ there may be areas of low SI due to mineralization

AMELOBLASTOMA

Definition A locally invasive benign tumour arising from the odontogenic epithelium ▶ the commonest odontogenic tumour (11%) ▶ 30–50 years of age

- Usually found within the molar or ramus mandibular region (commonly centred on the 3rd molar)
- It is locally aggressive (requiring a wide excision margin) and can potentially involve the infratemporal fossa, orbit or skull base ▶ it can rarely undergo malignant transformation with lung metastases

Radiological features

XR A unilocular or multilocular radiolucency ▶ it typically contains septa and locules of variable size producing a honeycombed 'bubbly' appearance ▶ a well-defined margin and often corticated ▶ a large mass will cause jaw expansion with cortical perforation ▶ there can be knife-edge resorption of tooth roots by the tumour

MRI T1WI: mixed SI ▶ T2WI: moderate-to-high SI ▶ T1WI + Gad: enhancement of the septae and solid regions

ODONTOME

- A developmental malformation or hamartoma consisting of dental hard tissues or tooth-like structures
- *Compound odontome:* a collection of small discrete teeth (denticles) ▶ typically found in the anterior region of maxilla
- *Complex odontome:* randomly arranged mass of enamel, dentine and cementum ▶ found mostly in the lower premolar/molar region

OTHER ODONTOGENIC TUMOURS

Definition Mostly benign, these arise from either the odontogenic epithelium or the ectomesenchyme

Odontogenic myxoma A benign, locally aggressive tumour of the odontogenic mesenchyme affecting patients <45 years old ▶ usually located within the mandible (premolar or molar region) ▶ a well-defined, unilocular mass with coarse internal trabeculations

Calcifying epithelial odontogenic tumour Premolar or molar regions of the mandible ▶ middle-aged patients (M>F) ▶ a well-defined mass with variable amounts of focal mineral deposits

Adenomatoid odontogenic tumour This arises anteriorly (especially within the maxilla) ▶ females during the 2nd decade of life ▶ associated with an unerupted tooth ▶ a well-defined mass with variable amounts of focal mineral deposits

Cementoblastoma A neoplasm of the cementum ▶ rare (affecting young males) ▶ an encapsulated radio-opaque mass attached to a root (usually of a lower posterior tooth)

JAW METASTASES

Definition These are uncommon and occur predominantly within the posterior mandible

- Common primary sites: breast, kidney, lung, colon or prostate

XR/CT A lesion with ill-defined destructive margins (without new bone formation) ▶ metastases are usually lytic (although prostate metastases can appear sclerotic)

OTHER JAW TUMOURS

Extranodal lymphoma This can affect the maxilla or posterior aspect of the mandible ▶ an ill-defined non-corticated radiolucency

Myeloma This is uncommon ▶ it affects the mandible more commonly than the maxilla (with a predilection for the posterior body and angle) ▶ it is typically well defined but lacks a cortical margin (giving a 'punched-out' appearance)

Ewing's tumour This affects the same age group within the jaw as elsewhere ▶ lesions are predominantly lytic and it is associated with a poor prognosis

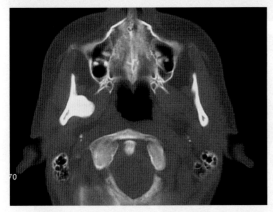

Bone window setting of an axial CT showing a dense (compact) osteoma arising from the medial aspect of the ramus of the right mandible.*

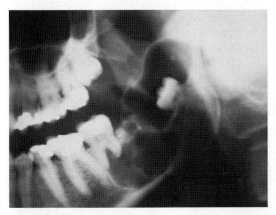

Ameloblastoma. A multilocular cystic lesion erodes the root of a molar but also prevents eruption of a wisdom tooth. The ameloblastoma may be secondary to a dentigerous cyst.*

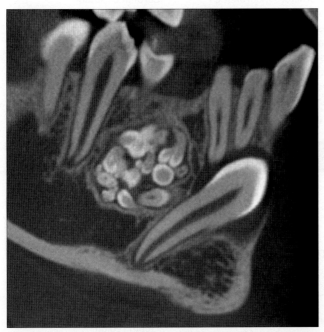

CBCT parasagittal slice showing a compound odontome consisting of numerous small teeth (denticles). The odontome has displaced and prevented the lower right canine from erupting.**

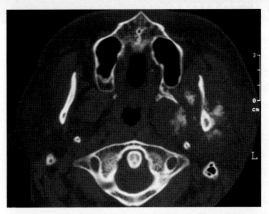

Bone window setting of an axial CT of osteogenic sarcoma of the left mandibular ramus. There is bone destruction in the region of the sigmoid notch. The lesion contains areas of neoplastic bone formation and extends medially towards the lateral pterygoid plate, posteriorly to the styloid process and laterally resulting in facial swelling.*

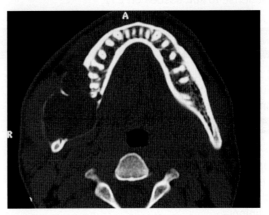

An axial CT on bone window setting of a large cystic ameloblastoma of the right side of the mandible showing marked thinning and expansion of the bone and the presence of root resorption.*

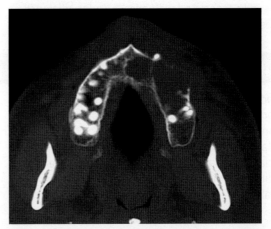

Extranodal lymphoma of the maxilla shown on a bone window setting axial CT at the level of the alveolus. Although a few areas of the lesion are well defined, the overall appearance is destructive with loss of much of the buccal alveolar plate.*

ORBITAL TRAUMA

Blunt trauma
- Can result in:
  - *Retinal detachment:* this results in a V-shaped membrane with the apex of the V at the optic disc ▶ the associated subretinal fluid may be hyperintense (T1WI) due to proteinaceous fluid or haematoma
  - *Choroidal detachment:* this is distinguished by the fact that it does not extend to the optic nerve head (because of the tethering effect of the vortex veins)
  - *Globe rupture or laceration* (uncommon): there will be loss of the normal globe contour on CT and MRI
  - *Lens dislocation:* this is uncommon

Penetrating intraocular foreign bodies

CT This is helpful to demonstrate glass, metal or bone fragments

MRI This is contraindicated for a metallic intraocular body ▶ it is better for assessing wood splinters and thorns (these are isodense to soft tissues on CT)

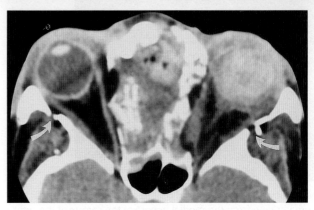

Ruptured globe. Opacification of ethmoids with blood and fluid secondary to extensive comminuted nasal and ethmoid fractures. Bilateral fractures of lateral orbital wall (arrows). Hyperdense blood fills ruptured and misshapen left globe. There is contusion of retro-orbital fat as well as preseptal soft tissue swelling.[†]

BLOW-OUT FRACTURE

Definition A sudden increase in intraocular pressure (e.g. following blunt trauma to the head) leads to fracturing of the thin orbital floor – the orbital rim remains intact

Clinical presentation Enophthalmos ▶ diplopia

XR/CT

- *'Tear drop' sign:* orbital fat, and the inferior oblique and inferior rectus muscles may prolapse into the maxillary sinus ▶ this may lead to entrapped tissues, fibrosis and possible diplopia
- *'Eyebrow' sign:* emphysema (following fracture of the adjacent sinuses) rising superiorly within the intraorbital cavity
  - There may also be associated fluid within the maxillary sinus
  - It is usually associated with a fractured medial wall (representing the lamina papyracea of the orbit)

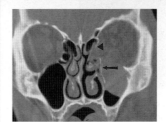

Inferior and medial blow-out fractures. Coronal CT demonstrating inferomedial displacement of bony fragments of the left orbital floor (arrow) as well as an accompanying fracture of the left lamina papyracea (arrowhead).[†]

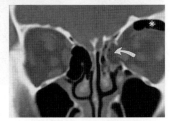

Medial blow-out fracture. Coronal CT image demonstrates partial herniation of medial rectus muscle and orbital fat into the left ethmoid air cells through a fractured lamina papyracea (arrow). 'Eyebrow' sign: there is associated intraorbital emphysema (asterisk).[†]

MANDIBULAR FRACTURE

- *The common fracture sites:* the parasymphyseal region ▶ the body of the mandible ▶ the angle of the mandible ▶ the condylar neck or coronoid process
  - A unilateral mandibular fracture is frequently associated with a contralateral fracture (as the mandible is a 'ring' structure) – this is commonly the contralateral condylar neck

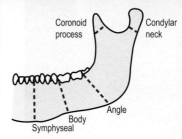

Line diagram showing common sites of fracture of the mandible.[**]

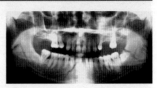

Panoramic radiograph showing bilateral fractures of the mandible in the right canine region and left wisdom tooth region.[*]

FRACTURES OF THE ZYGOMATIC COMPLEX

Definition The zygomatic bone contributes to the lateral and inferior orbital margins, the lateral wall of the maxillary sinus and the anterior end of the zygomatic arch

- Usually fractures in the region of the zygomatico-frontal suture, zygomatico-temporal suture, infra-orbital rim and lateral wall of the antrum
- It is the 2nd most common facial fracture (after a nasal bone fracture) following a direct blow to the side of the face
- The presence of one fracture should raise the suspicion that others are present

XR/CT

- It may be an isolated fracture but is more often a 'tripod' fracture involving:
  - Diastasis of the zygomaticofrontal suture
  - A fracture of the inferior orbital rim and lateral maxillary wall
  - A fracture of the posterior zygomatic arch

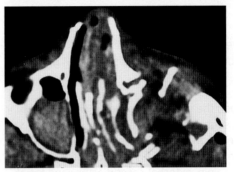

Comminuted fracture of the left zygoma on axial CT. There are multiple fractures of the anterior, posterolateral and medial walls of the maxillary sinus. There is air in the soft tissues of the cheek and infratemporal fossa.*

Diagram of the usual sites of fracture of the zygoma and of the zygomatic arch: o, orbit ▶ a, antrum.

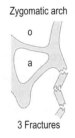

Zygomatic arch

o

a

3 Fractures

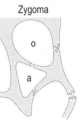

Zygoma

o

a

4 Fractures

LE FORT FRACTURES

DEFINITION

This describes maxillary fractures following blunt trauma

Le Fort I fracture

- Trauma to the lower face results in a transverse fracture across the entire lower maxilla (separating the tooth-bearing part of the maxilla from the remaining midface)
- The fracture line runs from the piriform fossa posteriorly to the pterygoid plates and involves the lower part of nasal septum

Le Fort II fracture

- The fracture line runs along the nasal bridge, through the lacrimal bones across the medial orbital walls and orbital rims, to involve the anterior and posterolateral walls of the maxillary sinuses and pterygoid plates
- The nasal septum is fractured at a variable level

Le Fort III fracture

- This results in craniofacial dysjunction (with complete separation of the midface from the cranial base, resulting in clinical lengthening of the face)
- The fracture line runs through the nasal bones, the frontal maxillary processes, posterolaterally through the medial and lateral orbital walls and finally through the zygomatic arches
- The nasal septum is fractured superiorly

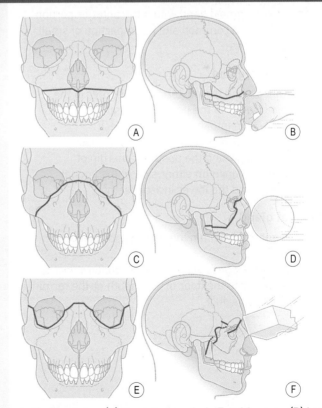

LeFort fractures. (A) Frontal view of a LeFort I fracture. (B) Lateral view of a LeFort I fracture. (C) Frontal view of a LeFort II fracture. (D) Lateral view of a LeFort II fracture. (E) Frontal view of a LeFort III fracture. (F) Lateral view of a LeFort III fracture.

SALIVARY GLAND IMAGING TECHNIQUES

ANATOMY

- There are three paired major salivary glands: the parotid, the submandibular and the sublingual glands

Parotid gland

- This lies between the posterior border of the mandibular ramus and the segment of the sternocleidomastoid muscle attaching to the mastoid process
- It is enclosed in deep cervical fascia and traversed by the retromandibular vein, external carotid artery and facial nerve
- The plane of the dividing facial nerve plexus lies just lateral to the retromandibular vein (dividing the gland into a larger superficial and smaller deep portion)
- Whereas tumours are more common in the superficial lobe, the surgical approach to the deep lobe involves dissection of the nerve branches with the associated risk of nerve damage
- *Parotid drainage is via Stensen's duct:*
  - This runs horizontally (1 cm below the zygomatic arch) on the surface of the masseter muscle ▶ it then perforates the buccinator muscle and emerges on the buccal mucosa opposite the 1st maxillary molar tooth
  - The sharp sigmoid bend within the anterior portion of the duct is a common site for impaction of small salivary stones

Submandibular gland

- This wraps around the posterior free border of the mylohyoid (medial to the posterior mandible) and descends 2–3 cm into the suprahyoid neck
- *Submandibular drainage is via Wharton's duct:*
  - This passes around the posterior margin of mylohyoid to open on either side of the lingual frenum behind the lower incisor teeth

Sublingual gland

- This lies anteriorly within the mouth floor (above mylohyoid)
- *Sublingual drainage is via a single Bartholin's duct or multiple ducts* into the floor of the mouth or the terminal part of Wharton's duct

RADIOLOGICAL TECHNIQUES

XR This is of limited value

Sialography This is highly sensitive for ductal abnormalities but limited for parenchymal disease
- Cannulation of the parotid duct is usually straightforward but cannulation of the submandibular duct can be difficult ▶ the sublingual anatomy is usually only incidentally demonstrated
- Small mobile stones may be extracted by Dormia basket or balloon catheter ▶ duct strictures may be dilated by angioplasty balloon

US This is the first-line investigation for salivary gland masses (it is highly sensitive for 70–80% of superficial parotid tumours) ▶ it can also detect calculi or resultant duct dilatation

CT This is sensitive for calculi detection ▶ it has been superseded by MRI for tumour assessment

MRI MR sialography (using heavily T2WI) allows noninvasive assessment of obstructive disease ▶ T1WI + Gad is not usually required for uncomplicated cases

Radionuclide radiology This assesses glandular function in obstruction and inflammatory conditions ▶ it has limited value in tumour imaging (due to its low resolution and lack of uptake in Warthin's tumours)

99mTc-pertechnetate time activity curves This can quantify salivary gland function ▶ it may distinguish between a functioning, obstructed or non-functional gland

FDG PET Whilst actively taken up by growing neoplasms, it is also concentrated within lymphoid tissue and salivary glands ▶ it has a higher uptake in malignant tumours and benign Warthin's tumour
- It is used for assessing the post-treatment neck but may not distinguish tumour from acute infection or early wound healing

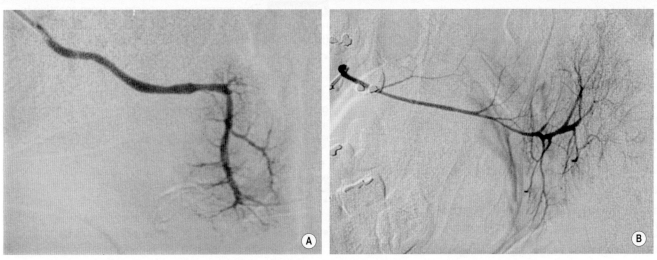

Digital subtracted images showing (A) a normal submandibular sialogram and (B) a normal parotid sialogram.†

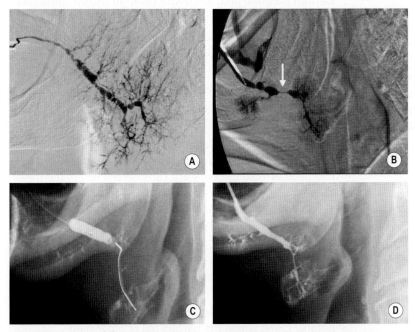

Parotid sialogram. (A) Multiple strictures in the main and in some of the branch ducts. Digital subtraction image. (B) Parotid sialogram shows an inflammatory parotid duct stricture (arrow) secondary to stone disease. Digital subtracted image. (C) Balloon dilatation of the stricture. (D) Postprocedure sialogram.†

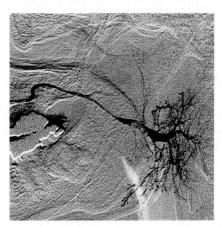

Collection of calculi at hilum of parotid gland. There is minor sialectasis (irregularity of calibre of some intraglandular ducts).*

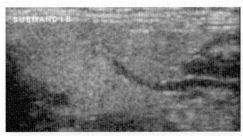

Longitudinal oblique US of a submandibular gland showing the main (Wharton's) duct.†

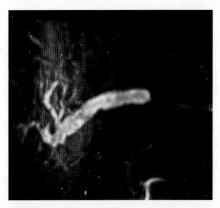

MR sialography image showing gross dilatation of the main duct and some of the secondary ducts. Areas of low SI in the main duct are due to the presence of several large stones. The distal part of the duct is normal.*

Calculi and strictures

- **Calculi:** Salivary gland obstruction results in mealtime-related swelling of the affected gland ▶ obstruction predisposes to infection, sialectasis, strictures and eventual gland atrophy
- **Strictures:** These result from inflammation caused by infection or calculi ▶ they account for 25% of salivary obstruction
- There can be focal or diffuse forms (with proximal dilatation of the duct system)
- *'Sialodochitis':* a combination of duct dilatation and stenosis following obstruction complicated by infection

Inflammatory conditions

Infective sialadenitis (viral and bacterial)

`Definition` This leads to generalized glandular enlargement

`US` Heterogeneous reduced salivary gland echogenicity

`CT` Increased salivary gland attenuation

`MRI` T2WI: high SI ▶ there can be inflammatory stranding involving the overlying tissues

- *Kuttner tumour:* a focal chronic inflammatory sialadenitis that may be mistaken for tumour

Sjögren's syndrome

`Definition` This autoimmune disease can damage the intercalated salivary ducts with leak of contrast media during sialography (giving a characteristic fine punctate sialectasis evenly distributed throughout the salivary tissue)

- There is an increased risk of developing a mucosa-associated lymphoid tissue (MALT) lymphoma

`US` A heterogeneous reticular pattern of small low reflective foci

`MRI` T1WI/T2WI: a specific speckled honeycomb appearance

- MR sialography has an improved sensitivity and specificity over conventional sialography

Sarcoid

`Definition` There is generalized glandular enlargement with multiple small granulomatous areas

`US` Low echoreflectivity

`CT` Glandular enlargement with multiple small hypodense granulomatous areas

`MRI` Diffuse high SI

`67Ga scintigraphy` Increased activity

Human immunodeficiency virus (HIV)-associated salivary gland disease

`Definition` This covers a spectrum of disorders including lymphoepithelial infiltration, which may progress to lymphoma ▶ it can occur at any stage of HIV disease

`CT/MRI` A combination of multiple intraparotid cysts (which are otherwise rare) and cervical lymphadenopathy raises this possibility

Benign lymphoepithelial infiltration

`Definition` This represents a spectrum from reactive to neoplastic change ▶ it can occur as an isolated abnormality (but is more commonly a feature of Sjögren's syndrome)

- It can be complicated by malignant lymphoma (5%) and anaplastic carcinoma (1%)

`CT` With advanced disease there are grossly enlarged glands containing multiple well-defined round areas of low attenuation

`67Ga scintigraphy` This can assess disease progression

Salivary gland tumours

`Definition` Usually benign and can develop at any age

- *Location:* parotid gland (80%) ▶ submandibular gland (5%) ▶ sublingual gland (1%) ▶ minor salivary glands (15%)
- *Benign features:* the presence of a capsule or well-defined outline ▶ a homogeneous, hypoechoic appearance without regional lymphadenopathy
- *Malignant features:* neoangiogenesis

Benign pleomorphic adenoma (benign mixed tumours) (80%)

`Definition` These usually arise within the superficial portion of the parotid gland and are commonly seen in middle-aged women

`US` A uni- or mildly loculated hypoechoic lesion

`MRI` T1WI: characteristic low SI ▶ T2WI: high SI

Adenocarcinoma

`Definition` These are commonly an adenoid cystic carcinoma or mucoepidermoid carcinoma ▶ mucoepidermoid tumours are commonest within the minor salivary glands of the palate

- They are slow growing and difficult to eradicate (the adenoid cystic type has a propensity for insidious perineural spread)

`MRI` This can usually identify the presence (but can underestimate the extent) of any perineural spread

Warthin's tumour

`Definition` This is a benign adenolymphoma ▶ it is notably found within the parotid tail of older men

- Multiple (20%) ▶ occasionally bilateral (6.5%)

Lipoma

`US` This has a characteristic hypoechoic appearance with numerous layered highly reflective internal strands

`CT` There is markedly low fat attenuation

Lymphoma

`Definition` All the salivary glands may be involved (the parotid gland is the most frequently affected) ▶ many of the patients are middle-aged women and a history of Sjögren's disease is common

`US` Hypoechoic masses

`CT` Single or multiple well-defined masses are seen (which are of higher density than the surrounding gland)

`MRI` T1WI/T2WI: intermediate SI

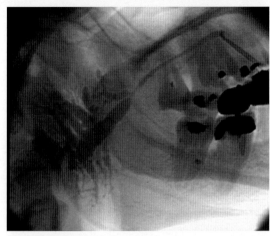

Sialogram showing a diffuse stricture at the entrance to the hilum of the parotid gland.*

Salivary gland calculi		
	Submandibular gland	**Parotid gland**
Incidence of calculi	85%	15%
Radio-opaque calculi	60–80%	20–40%
Common location of calculi	At the duct genu (where it makes an acute bend over the posterior free border of the mylohyoid muscle)	The parotid hilum or the main duct overlying the masseter muscle

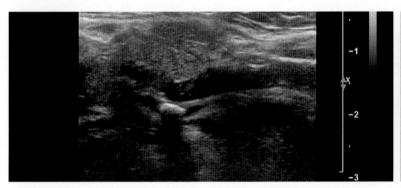

US of a salivary stone in the proximal portion of the submandibular duct.*

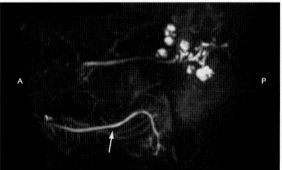

MR sialography image showing chronic sialadenitis of the parotid gland with focal globular high signal areas of sialectasis within the parenchyma of the gland. The main duct appears normal. The submandibular duct and gland (arrow) appear normal.*

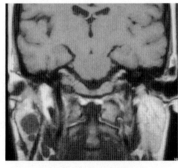

Unenhanced coronal T1WI through the parotid glands showing a well-circumscribed bilobed mass in the right superficial lobe. Diagnosis: pleomorphic adenoma.†

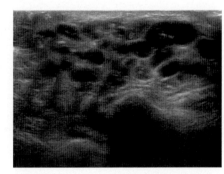

Ultrasound image of the parotid gland showing the honeycomb pattern of hypoechogenic change in Sjögren's syndrome.**

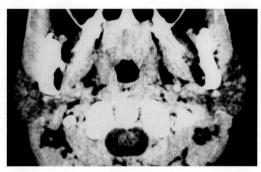

Sarcoid of the parotid glands. There is generalized glandular enlargement and multiple small areas of decreased attenuation.**

ENDOCRINE SYSTEM

8.1 THYROID DISORDERS

THYROID CANCER

DEFINITION

- A malignant tumour arising from the thyroid or parafollicular C cells ▶ it is an uncommon tumour (accounting for 0.5% of all cancer deaths)
- *Risk factors:* previous radiation exposure ▶ iodine excess ▶ a genetic predisposition ▶ alcohol excess

CLINICAL PRESENTATION

- It presents with a painless solitary thyroid nodule ▶ there can be hoarseness (due to recurrent laryngeal nerve involvement), dysphagia or hyperthyroidism
- There is a peak incidence at 25–35 years (M>F)

RADIOLOGICAL FEATURES

US A hypoechoic nodule ± an irregular ill-defined border ± cervical adenopathy ± destruction of any adjacent structures

US-guided FNAC This is less sensitive for a cystic papillary carcinoma ▶ it cannot differentiate between a follicular adenoma or adenocarcinoma (histologically the distinction relies on documenting capsular or venous invasion and this requires a core biopsy)

99mTc-pertechnetate scintigraphy The pertechnetate anion is actively transported against a concentration gradient into the thyroid gland (via the same channel as the iodide anion) ▶ once in the thyroid gland it is not incorporated into thyroglobulin

- ^{99m}Tc-pertechnetate is not used for detecting metastatic disease
- *Other sites demonstrating similar uptake:* salivary glands ▶ gastric mucosa ▶ choroid plexus

- *More than 80% of solitary nodules are hypofunctioning 'cold' nodules:* up to 20% of these are tumours
- *Approximately 10% of solitary nodules are hyperfunctioning 'warm' nodules (on a background of normal thyroid activity):* up to 10% of these will be tumours ▶ if one of these lesions is malignant it will usually be cold with ^{123}I imaging
- *Up to 5% of solitary nodules are hyperfunctioning 'hot' nodules (on a background of suppressed remaining thyroid activity):* these are very rarely malignant
- *There is a reduced incidence of malignancy with an increasing number of nodules detected:* whilst less likely than with a solitary nodule, a cold nodule within a multinodular goitre can still represent a malignancy

^{123}I scintigraphy As the iodide anion is incorporated into thyroglobulin, this represents a more physiological representation than seen with ^{99m}Tc-pertechnetate ▶ it can be used for detecting metastatic disease

- ^{123}I decays with a 159 keV photon but requires cyclotron production
- ^{131}I decays with a 364 keV photon and can be used for therapeutic ablation

PET This is used for detecting recurrent or metastatic disease ▶ there is increasing uptake with less differentiated tumour types ▶ it can also be used in medullary cancer

CT This is not routinely used – it can assess metastatic nodal involvement, the presence of distant metastases (e.g. miliary lung nodules) or demonstrate any retrosternal or tracheal spread

- Thyroid nodules appear as low attenuation lesions (particularly after IV contrast medium)
- US features of benign and malignant thyroid nodules (FNAC is still required for suspicious lesions)

US features of benign and malignant thyroid nodules (FNAC is still required for suspicious lesions)		
	Benign	**Malignant**
Nodule characteristics	• A cystic nodule ± debris ± septations ▶ a sponge-like nodule • Posterior acoustic shadowing • A hyperechoic nodule • 'Comet tail' artefact (colloid nodule) • Multiple isoechoic nodules (multinodular goitre) • Multiple hypoechoic nodules (Hashimoto's thyroiditis) • Indeterminate: a solid well-defined nodule ± cystic components	• Solid nodules protruding into the cystic space • No posterior acoustic shadowing
Peripheral halo	• A thin uniform halo	• An incomplete, irregular or thickened halo
Nodule margin	• Smooth regular margins	• An irregular, lobulated or poorly defined margin
Calcification	• This is generally absent (eggshell calcification may be present)	• Microcalcification ▶ fine or coarse calcification (commonly papillary or medullary carcinomas)
Metastatic spread		• Invasion of the adjacent tissues ± enlarged ipsilateral or bilateral cervical lymph nodes

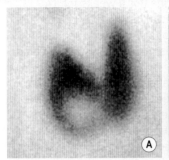
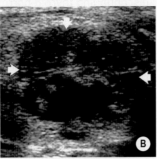

Thyroid carcinoma presenting as a cold nodule. (A) ^{99m}Tc-pertechnetate scintigram shows a 'cold' nodule in the lower pole of the right lobe of the thyroid gland. (B) Transverse US corresponding to the lesion in (A) shows an inhomogeneous nodule (arrows).*

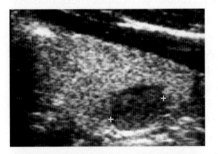

Medullary carcinoma. The appearance of this solid hypoechoic nodule (cursors) is very similar to that of papillary carcinoma.¶

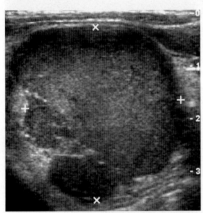

Anaplastic carcinoma. Transverse view shows a large lobulated solid hypoechoic mass (cursors) replacing the entire thyroid.¶

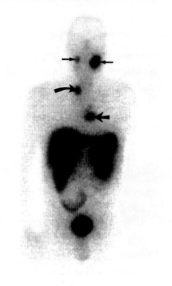

MEN type IIB. ^{111}In-pentetreotide image shows a patient with medullary carcinoma of the thyroid (curved arrow) and bilateral glomus tumours (small arrows) and a paraganglioma (large arrow) in the lower mediastinum.*

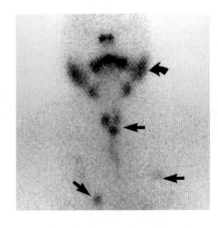

Well-differentiated thyroid carcinoma imaged 3 days after ^{131}iodine. Imaging shows increased uptake in thyroid bed, right hilar region and left upper chest (arrows). Salivary activity, which is a normal feature (curved arrow), is also noted.*

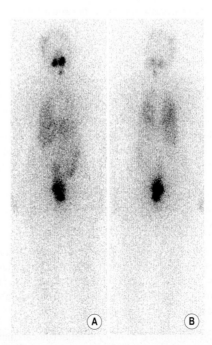

^{131}I scintigraphy. (A) anterior view and (B) posterior view. Follicular thyroid carcinoma treated with a total thyroidectomy and ^{131}I ablation now demonstrates diffuse uptake throughout both lungs consistent with miliary lung metastases.§§

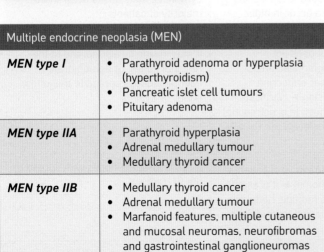

Multiple endocrine neoplasia (MEN)	
MEN type I	• Parathyroid adenoma or hyperplasia (hyperthyroidism) • Pancreatic islet cell tumours • Pituitary adenoma
MEN type IIA	• Parathyroid hyperplasia • Adrenal medullary tumour • Medullary thyroid cancer
MEN type IIB	• Medullary thyroid cancer • Adrenal medullary tumour • Marfanoid features, multiple cutaneous and mucosal neuromas, neurofibromas and gastrointestinal ganglioneuromas

PEARLS

Diagnosis Cytology or histology (FNAC) from a thyroid nodule or after the removal of a cervical lymph node

Prognostic factors The patient's age ▶ the size of the tumour ▶ the degree of differentiation ▶ the presence of invasion, nodal or distant metastases

Treatment

- *Papillary/follicular tumours:* thyroidectomy ± lymph node dissection ± postoperative ^{131}I-ablation therapy ▶ thyroglobulin can be used as a postoperative tumour marker if there has been complete resection ▶ radical radiotherapy and chemotherapy can be used for locally advanced or metastatic disease
- *Anaplastic tumours:* radical or palliative radiotherapy ± chemotherapy
- *Medullary carcinoma:* thyroidectomy ± radiotherapy (with chemotherapy for advanced disease)

Subsequent follow-up ^{131}I-scintigraphy and serum thyroglobulin measurement is performed 6–12 months later to assess the adequacy of ablation and to detect and treat any metastatic disease (under an elevated TSH drive) ▶ anaplastic and medullary cancers do not concentrate ^{131}I and are thus not detectable by iodine scanning

- Whole-body iodine imaging is performed after discontinuing thyroid hormone (for 4 weeks for T4 or for 2 weeks for T3) and establishing that TSH concentrations are >30 µmol/L ▶ one can then identify most functioning metastases, which are usually located in the neck, lungs or bone
- In patients following removal of a medullary carcinoma, serum calcitonin concentrations are used to diagnose recurrence ▶ if they become elevated, pentavalent ^{99m}Tc-DMSA, ^{111}In-DTPA-octreotide, or ^{123}I-MIBG can be used for the detection of recurrent or residual disease ▶ in cases of ^{123}I-MIBG-positive disease, therapy with ^{131}I-MIBG can be instituted

MRI This can be used for the detection of recurrent disease ▶ like CT, false-positive results can be caused by inflammatory lymphatic hyperplasia and granulation tissue

US This is useful during follow-up to detect neck masses or lymph nodes

Multinodular goitre

- Generally (but not always) this is a benign disorder
- Dominant cold nodules (especially enlarging ones) require further evaluation by aspiration biopsy
- Autonomous foci are common and if extensive will ultimately result in hyperthyroidism (a toxic multinodular goitre or Plummer's disease)

Thyroid malignancies – key features

	Description	Pattern of spread
Papillary carcinoma (70–80%)	Low-grade tumours with a good prognosis (histologically multicentric) ▶ tumours concentrate radio-iodine	Early lymph node spread (metastatic lymph nodes may be normal in size, cystic, calcified, haemorrhagic or contain colloid) ▶ distant metastases are rare (and usually to the lungs)
Follicular carcinoma (10–20%)	Slow growing ▶ tumours concentrate radio-iodine	It rarely metastasizes to the regional lymph nodes ▶ the tendency is to spread via the bloodstream and disseminate to the lungs, bones or liver
Anaplastic carcinoma (1–2%)	Undifferentiated malignant tumours (which do not concentrate radio-iodine) ▶ there is a poor prognosis ▶ they tend to occur in older patients ▶ punctate calcification and necrosis is frequently present	Lymphatic metastases occur in the majority of patients
Medullary carcinoma (5–10%)	This originates from the parafollicular C cells ▶ it does not concentrate radio-iodine ▶ it may be sporadic or familial (and associated with the MEN type II syndrome or other endocrine neoplasms) ▶ it is usually a unilateral solitary lesion ▶ calcification is seen in 10% ▶ ^{123}I-MIBG and somatostatin analogues (e.g. octreotide) can be used for evaluation ▶ circulating calcitonin levels are usually elevated	It may invade locally, spread to the regional nodes, or demonstrate haematogenous spread to the lungs, bones or liver
Lymphoma (10%)	It is usually a non-Hodgkin's lymphoma ▶ it occurs in $\frac{1}{3}$ of patients with Hashimoto's thyroiditis (a MALT-type lymphoma) ▶ it presents as a rapidly enlarging solitary nodule (80%) or as multiple nodules (imaging cannot distinguish between a lymphoma and thyroiditis) ▶ necrosis and calcification is uncommon	It can involve the nodes with spread to the GI tract
Metastases (<1%)	The commonest primary is renal cell carcinoma	

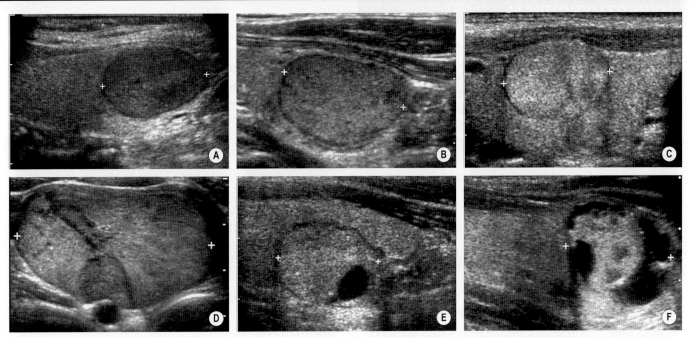

Follicular adenomas in different patients. (A) Solid hypoechoic nodule (cursors) with a thin peripheral hypoechoic halo. (B) Solid isoechoic nodule (cursors) with a peripheral halo. (C) Solid hyperechoic nodule (cursors) with a peripheral halo. (D) Large solid hyperechoic nodule (cursors) with scattered internal regions of decreased echogenicity. (E) Predominantly solid isoechoic nodule (cursors) with a peripheral halo and a well-defined internal cyst. (F) Complex cystic and solid nodule (cursors) that simulates nodular hyperplasia.¶

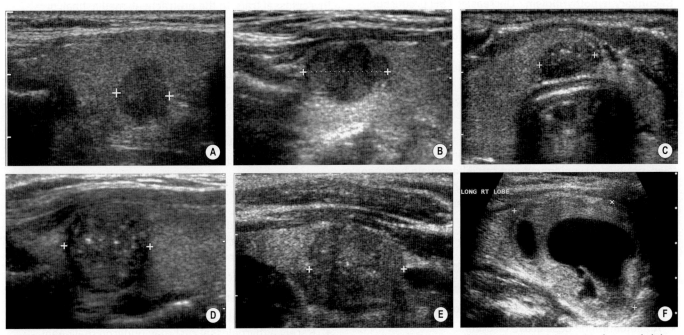

Papillary thyroid cancer in different patients. (A) Longitudinal view shows a hypoechoic homogeneous entirely solid lesion (cursors). (B) Longitudinal view shows a homogeneous hypoechoic slightly lobulated solid lesion (cursors). (C) Transverse view shows a hypoechoic solid lesion (cursors) that contains a few microcalcifications. (D) Longitudinal view shows an entirely solid hypoechoic lesion with scattered microcalcifications and an irregular halo. (E) Longitudinal view shows a solid slightly heterogeneous nodule (cursors) containing a few microcalcifications. (F) Longitudinal view shows a large complex lesion (cursors) that is solid but contains large internal cystic components. This is a follicular variant of papillary carcinoma.¶

HYPERTHYROIDISM

Graves' disease This is an autoimmune disorder in which a circulating immunoglobulin (produced largely by intrathyroidal lymphocytes) stimulates the thyroid gland by binding to TSH receptors ▶ with a pre-existing normal thyroid this will result in a diffuse toxic goitre ▶ there may underlying thyroid disease in 5–10% of patients (e.g. solitary thyroid nodules, a multinodular goitre, or Hashimoto's thyroiditis)

US A diffusely hyperechoic gland without any discrete nodules

- *Colour Doppler:* increased vascularity

^{99m}Tc-pertechnetate/^{123}I scintigraphy Diffuse increased uptake

Toxic multinodular goitre (Plummer's disease) This may present either as a toxic goitre with hyperfunctioning nodules and a suppressed stroma, or as diffuse toxicity of the thyroid stroma with intervening nodules

Scintigraphy A single toxic nodule shows high uptake of tracer with the remaining normal thyroid tissue showing poor or virtually no activity

HYPOTHYROIDISM

Primary hypothyroidism This is due to an endogenous thyroid disorder

Secondary hypothyroidism Decreased TSH production secondary to pituitary disease

- *Causes:* surgery ▶ radiation ablation for Graves' disease or thyroid cancer ▶ primary idiopathic hypothyroidism ▶ Hashimoto's thyroiditis ▶ iodine deficiency ▶ congenital hypothyroidism

Tertiary hypothyroidism Decreased TRH secretion secondary to a hypothalamic disorder

^{99m}Tc-pertechnetate scintigraphy This will help to confirm the presence of a normal gland in patients with a false-positive screening test and can differentiate between the subgroups of primary congenital hypothyroidism:
- Non-visualization of functioning thyroid tissue
- Hypoplastic and ectopic glands
- Dyshormonogenesis

THYROIDITIS

Hashimoto's thyroiditis (chronic lymphocytic thyroiditis)

- An autoimmune destructive disorder

US This can demonstrate variable appearances:
- A normal or enlarged thyroid with a diffuse heterogeneous echo texture
- There may be numerous poorly defined hypoechoic regions separated by fibrous strands ▶ less commonly there may be discrete nodules and adjacent adenopathy

- *End-stage appearance:* a small fibrotic gland that is ill defined and heterogeneous
- *US follow-up:* this is required due to the risk of developing a non-Hodgkin's lymphoma

Scintigraphy There is no typical pattern ▶ uptake is most commonly heterogeneous and patchy, but may be uniformly increased or decreased

Silent or painless thyroiditis An autoimmune disorder in which radio-iodine uptake is initially very low, but in the recovery (hypothyroid) phase it may be normal to elevated

Scintigraphy

- *Mild subacute (viral) thyroiditis:* patchy uptake within an enlarged and tender thyroid gland
- *Extensive disease:* uptake is markedly suppressed by both the disruptive effect of inflammation and the ensuing hyperthyroidism

Riedel's thyroiditis A fibrosing reaction that destroys the thyroid

US A hypoechoic thyroid

CT A hypodense thyroid

MRI T1WI and T2WI: low SI

CONGENITAL DISORDERS

Ectopic thyroid This may occur anywhere from the foramen caecum (the base of the tongue), and via the thyroglossal tract, to the pretracheal, mediastinal, or pericardiac areas

- *'Lingual thyroid':* residual thyroid tissue at the foramen caecum

Hypoplasia or agenesis of a thyroid lobe This always involves the left side ▶ conversely, a small right lobe is usually the result of disease rather than an anatomical variation

Thyroglossal cysts

- Over 50% of cysts have normal thyroid tissue within their walls
  - *Location:* infrahyoid (65%) ▶ suprahyoid (20%) ▶ hyoid (15%)
- They normally demonstrate imaging features of cyst ▶ however if the cyst is infected, haemorrhagic, or has a high protein content, the following will be seen:

  US Internal echoes

  CT A hyperdense cyst

  MRI T1WI and T2WI: high SI

- Rarely a thyroglossal cyst may undergo malignant change into a papillary carcinoma (with a soft tissue component existing within or around the cyst)

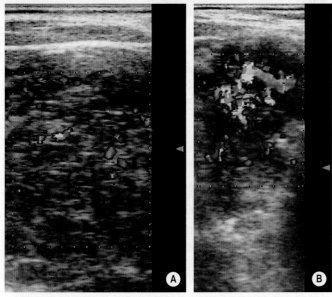

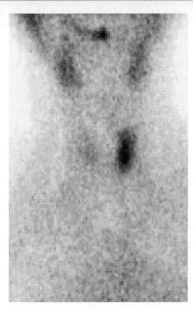

(A) Longitudinal US through the left lobe of the thyroid in a patient known to have Hashimoto's thyroiditis reveals a loose heterogeneous echotexture with abnormal colour flow. There are enlarged neck nodes (B), again with abnormal colour flow in this patient who has developed lymphoma.

Thyroid scintigraphy demonstrating chronic thyroiditis affecting only the right lobe.[†]

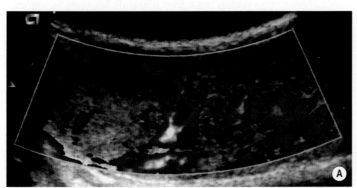

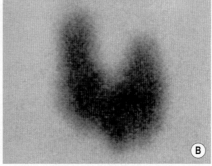

Graves' disease. (A) Longitudinal US with colour Doppler shows diffusely increased vascularity of the thyroid gland. (B) ^{99m}Tc-pertechnetate imaging shows diffusely increased tracer uptake.*

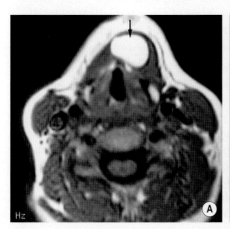

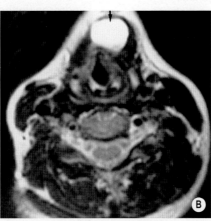

Thyroglossal duct cyst. (A) Axial T1WI and (B) T2WI demonstrating a well-defined high SI thyroglossal duct cyst just anterior to the hyoid bone.*

8.2 ADRENAL DISORDERS

NON-HYPERFUNCTIONING ADRENAL ADENOMA

Definition This is due to non-neoplastic overgrowth of the adrenocortical cells of the zona fasciculate

- More common in some inherited diseases (e.g. MEN 1/Beckwith–Weidman syndrome/Carney complex)
- It is detected incidentally in up to 5% of CT examinations ▶ the number and size of any nodules increases with age (but generally they are <6 cm in diameter)
- Most commonly seen in obese diabetics/elderly women
- 6% of 60 year olds have an adrenal adenoma (80% of these are benign non-functioning adenomas) ▶ in patients with a known malignancy, only 25–35% of adrenal masses are malignant

Investigation of incidental adrenal mass

- *Biochemical evaluation:* hyperfunctioning or non-hyperfunctioning status dictates further management
- If there is no history of malignancy, a unilateral non-hyperfunctioning adrenal mass rarely, if ever, represents a metastasis (adenoma or carcinoma)
- Smaller adrenal masses (<4 cm) are more likely to be benign (this is not a reliable indicator)
  - Adenomas have an increased intracellular lipid content ▶ if an adrenal mass measures ≤10 HU on a NECT, it is an adenoma (contrast imaging is not required) ▶ if NECT attenuation is >10 HU, it may be a lipid-poor adenoma-further imaging is required
  - Even lipid-poor tumours demonstrate a rapid washout of IV contrast medium
  - $$\%\text{ absolute contrast enhancement washout} = \frac{\text{CECT attenuation @ 60 s} - \text{CECT attenuation @ 15 min}}{\text{CECT attenuation @ 60 s} - \text{NECT attenuation}} \times 100$$

    Washout ≥60% = adrenal adenoma
- **Histogram analysis method:** ROI drawn over at least $\frac{2}{3}$ of the adrenal mass (excluding necrosis); pixel attenuation values are plotted against their frequency ▶ 97% of adenomas have negative pixels (metastases have no negative pixels)

MRI 90% of adenomas demonstrate homogenous or ring enhancement (60% of malignant masses have heterogeneous enhancement) ▶ adenomas show early peak enhancement (the value of peak enhancement does not distinguish between adenomas and metastases) ▶ fat-rich adenomas will lose signal on out-of-phase imaging – quantitative analysis can be made using the adrenal – splenic ratio (the liver can be unreliable due to either fatty or iron deposition, and skeletal muscle can undergo fatty infiltration in the elderly)

FDG-PET Maximum SUV uptake is lower for adenomas than metastases; however 48% of adenomas demonstrate moderate and high FDG uptake and can mimic malignant masses (limiting its role) ▶ quantitative evaluation using a SUV cutoff of 2.68–3.0 has a high sensitivity and specificity for separating benign from malignant masses

- *False positive:* adrenal adenoma/phaeochromocytoma/inflammatory lesions
- *False negative:* adrenal metastases with haemorrhage or necrosis/small metastatic nodules/metastases from bronchioloalveolar carcinoma or carcinoid tumours
- Phaeochromocytomas can have similar attenuation and washout characteristics as an adenoma; if concerned biochemical and clinical evaluation is required

INFECTION

- **Granulomatous infections (tuberculosis, histoplasmosis, or blastomycosis)**

CT There is bilateral but asymmetric involvement of the adrenal glands ▶ with active infection the adrenal glands are enlarged and heterogeneous (particularly after contrast administration) ▶ they may demonstrate small non-enhancing areas of caseous necrosis (± calcification) during the acute phase or with healing ▶ long-standing infection can result in atrophy of the adrenal glands

- **AIDS patients with extrapulmonary *Pneumocystis carinii* infection:** there may be punctuate or coarse calcification within the adrenal glands (as well as within the spleen, liver, kidney and lymph nodes)
- **Adrenal abscesses:** these are rare, with most found in neonates with pre-existing adrenal haemorrhage ▶ an abscess will appear as a thick-walled cystic lesion

ADRENAL HYPOFUNCTION (ADDISON'S DISEASE)

Definition Results from primary adrenal insufficiency or secondary to hypothalamic-pituitary ACTH deficiency ▶ manifests when >90% of the gland destroyed ▶ acute (rare, and usually due to haemorrhage) or chronic

- *Primary insufficiency causes:* autoimmune (commonest western cause)/TB (commonest worldwide cause)/AIDS/drugs/adrenal haemorrhage/Waterhouse–Friderichsen syndrome (in the context of septicaemia)/sarcoidosis/amyloidosis/haemochromatosis /congenital

CT/MRI

- *Haemorrhage/haematoma:* T1WI and T2WI signal evolves over time ▶ need to exclude an underlying mass lesion (e.g. metastases or melanoma) ▶ an underlying mass may demonstrate enhancement ▶ acute haemorrhage can precipitate an Addisonian crisis, chronic haemorrhage chronically calcify or turn cystic
- *Subacute Addison's disease:* hypofunction <2 yrs ▶ usually secondary to adrenalitis – with adrenal hypertrophy ± central necrosis and rim enhancement
- *Calcification:* usually seen in granulomatous disease (e.g. TB/sarcoidosis)
- *Chronic changes:* the adrenal glands can be extremely small and may be difficult to identify

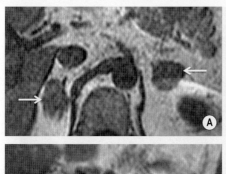
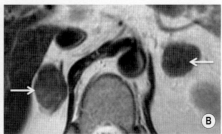
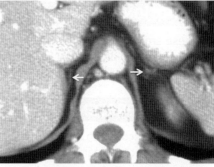

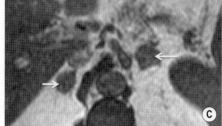
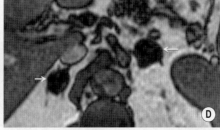

Contrast-enhanced CT 60 s after contrast medium administration. Both adrenal glands are very small, irregular and difficult to detect. The appearances are typical for autoimmune adrenal atrophy.**

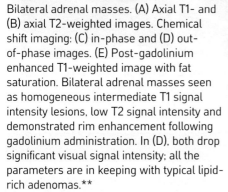
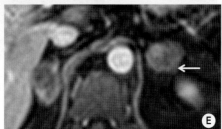

Bilateral adrenal masses. (A) Axial T1- and (B) axial T2-weighted images. Chemical shift imaging: (C) in-phase and (D) out-of-phase images. (E) Post-gadolinium enhanced T1-weighted image with fat saturation. Bilateral adrenal masses seen as homogeneous intermediate T1 signal intensity lesions, low T2 signal intensity and demonstrated rim enhancement following gadolinium administration. In (D), both drop significant visual signal intensity; all the parameters are in keeping with typical lipid-rich adenomas.**

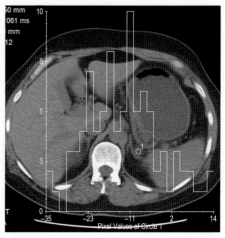

Histogram analysis of adenoma. A small left-sided adrenal lesion is seen on the unenhanced CT. The attenuation value is 14 HU and therefore indeterminate on unenhanced CT alone. On histogram analysis, obtained by drawing a region of interest over the mass, there are pixels ranging between −35 HU and +14 HU (x-axis). The presence of more than 5% negative pixels indicates an adenoma. This was confirmed on washout criteria.**

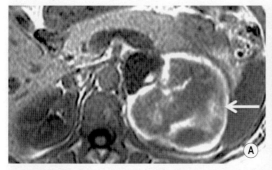
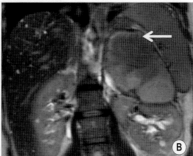
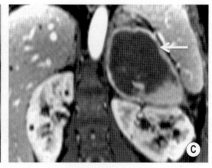

(A) Axial T1-, (B) coronal T2- and (C) coronal T1-weighted image with fat saturation and gadolinium enhancement of a sporadic large left adrenal haemorrhage in a 43-year-old man. There is a high T1 signal intensity rim, low T2 signal intensity foci within the lesion and no internal contrast enhancement. The lack of internal architecture and enhancement excludes an underlying lesion.**

ADRENAL CYSTS

DEFINITION

- These are usually endothelial or epithelial in origin (they may also be parasitic) ▶ pseudocysts (following haemorrhage or necrosis) are more common

CLINICAL PRESENTATION

- They are uncommon and usually unilateral (F>M)
- If large can cause pain

RADIOLOGICAL FEATURES

CT/MRI Thin-walled cysts with fluid attenuation and signal characteristics ▶ they are non-enhancing ▶ there can be peripheral and curvilinear calcification (15% of cases)

- T1WI: increased SI can be seen with the presence of proteinaceous material, infectious debris or haemorrhage
- Solid components/thickened walls/septae suggest possible necrotic mass or infective cyst

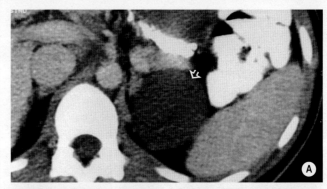
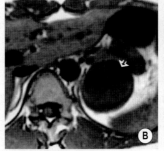
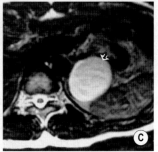

Adrenal cyst. (A) CECT showing the typical appearance of a cyst (arrow) within the left adrenal gland. (B) T1WI shows the low signal intensity of a simple cyst (arrow). (C) T2WI shows the uniformly high SI of a fluid-filled lesion (arrow).*

ADRENAL METASTASES

DEFINITION

- These most commonly follow tumours of the lung, kidney, breast, GI tract and ovary (and also with melanoma) ▶ they very rarely result in hypoadrenalism

RADIOLOGICAL FEATURES

CT A metastasis tends to be larger than an adenoma ▶ they are also heterogeneous, less well-defined and have a thick, irregular enhancing rim ▶ they are more commonly unilateral

MRI T1WI: low SI (compared to liver) ▶ T2WI: high SI (compared to liver)

PEARLS

- The presence of an adrenal mass in a patient with a known malignancy does not necessarily indicate the presence of metastatic disease: 40–50% of lesions are non-metastatic and represent adenomas (even bilateral adrenal masses are more likely to be adenomas rather than metastatic deposits)
- It may require percutaneous biopsy if the primary is unknown
- Increased likelihood of malignancy: size >4 cm ▶ rapid size increase

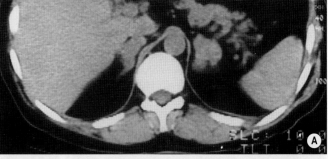
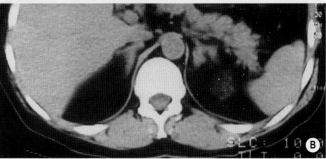

Adrenal metastases. (A) NECT demonstrates bilateral nodular adrenal masses. (B) After chemotherapy, the adrenal masses are smaller.ſ

ADRENAL HAEMORRHAGE

Traumatic

- This is seen on CT in 2% of patients who sustain severe trauma

CT A round or oval well-defined adrenal haematoma (seen in the majority) is more common than uniform adrenal enlargement or diffuse irregular haemorrhage obliterating the gland

Non-traumatic

- *This is usually associated with:* anticoagulants (or other bleeding disorders) ▶ recent surgery or severe burns ▶ sepsis (in particular meningococcal) leading to the Waterhouse–Friderichsen syndrome ▶ hypotension ▶ tumour (particularly a melanoma)

CT Haemorrhage is unilateral in the majority (R>L) ▶ calcification may develop after a few months ▶ occasionally a haematoma will liquefy and persists as a pseudocyst

- *Acute or subacute phase:* the enlarged adrenals are of increased density (50–70 HU)
- *Later stages:* there is reduced density and size of the lesion (which usually resolves)

Adrenal apoplexy

- Bilateral adrenal haemorrhage may result in acute adrenal insufficiency

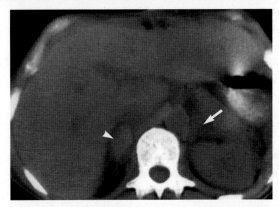

Adrenal haemorrhage. NECT showing bilateral enlargement due to adrenal haemorrhage (arrow). An area of high attenuation due to bleeding is demonstrated within the right adrenal gland (arrowhead).*

MRI appearances of adrenal haemorrhage		
Acute	T1WI/T2WI: low SI	Intracellular deoxyhaemoglobin
Subacute	T1WI: high SI	Methaemoglobin
Chronic	T1WI/T2WI: low peripheral SI rim	Haemosiderin/calcification

PRIMARY ADRENAL LYMPHOMA

DEFINITION

- The adrenal glands are more commonly involved with widespread lymphoma (and seen in 4% of non-Hodgkin's lymphoma (NHL) but in up to 25% at autopsy)
- Primary lymphoma is very rare, and tends to be extranodal

RADIOLOGICAL FEATURES

CT Solid homogeneous masses of soft tissue density (the adrenal glands enlarge but retain their adreniform shape) ▶ there is mild enhancement ▶ calcification is unusual without previous radiotherapy

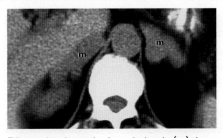

Bilateral enlarged adrenal glands (m) due to lymphomatous infiltration.†

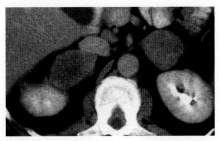

Adrenal lymphoma. CECT showing bilateral large inhomogeneous soft tissue masses. No other evidence of disease could be detected elsewhere and a core biopsy showed the presence of NHL.

PRIMARY ADRENOCORTICAL CARCINOMA

DEFINITION

- This is a rare and highly malignant tumour ▶ 90% produce steroids but only 50% cause symptoms related to excess hormone production
- Functioning carcinomas most commonly result in Cushing's syndrome, but virilization, feminization and hyperaldosteronism (Conn's syndrome) may also occur

CLINICAL PRESENTATION

- It is common in adults (with a peak incidence at 45–55 years) but is also occasionally seen in children (<5 years) ▶ F>M

RADIOLOGICAL FEATURES

CT They are usually large (85% are >6 cm in diameter) at the time of diagnosis (tumours <6 cm are usually functional and therefore present earlier)
- They are more commonly found on the left (10% are bilateral)
- There is patchy, irregular or nodular calcification

- Internal haemorrhage and necrosis is common
- There can be heterogeneous enhancement or a thick nodular rim
- Local invasion into the adjacent organs and extension into the IVC may be demonstrated

MRI T1WI: it is isointense to liver ▶ T2WI: it is hyperintense to liver

Scintigraphy NP-59 (^{131}I-6-iodomethyl-19-norcholesterol): reduced uptake

PEARLS

Metastases These occur to the liver, lungs and bones
- Metastases are common at presentation and contribute to the poor prognosis

Associations Li–Fraumeni and Beckwith–Wiedemann syndromes

Treatment Surgical resection (even with associated IVC involvement)
- Chemotherapy (mitotane)
- Tumours are radiotherapy resistant

ADRENAL MYELOLIPOMAS

DEFINITION

- A rare, benign neoplasm composed of fat and hematopoietic bone marrow tissue in varying proportions; hormonally inactive

CLINICAL PRESENTATION

- Most are asymptomatic and nonfunctioning, but larger lesions can present with pain or retroperitoneal haemorrhage ▶ they are usually small (<5 cm) and solitary
- It is usually an incidental finding on imaging
- Haemorrhage or necrosis within the tumour may cause pain

RADIOLOGICAL FEATURES

- **CT**
  - Can be predominantly soft tissue with small regions of fatty tissue, or almost completely composed of fat ▶ recognizable capsule ▶ may contain calcification ▶ the soft tissue component usually enhances ▶ in nearly all lesions some area of fat (<30 HU) can be identified on NECT ▶ the amount of fat in an adenoma is not usually less than –20 HU
- **MRI**
  - Fat is of high signal on T1WI and T2WI ▶ hematopoietic marrow elements are low signal on T1WI and intermediate signal on T2WI ▶ the signal intensity of any haemorrhage depends upon the age of the blood ▶ areas of fat will lose high T1WI signal on fat saturated and out-of-phase sequences

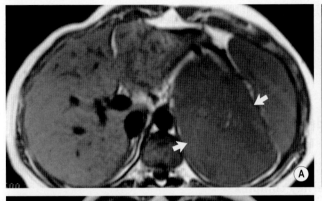

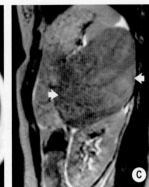

Adrenal carcinoma on MRI. (A) Axial T1WI, (B) axial T2WI and (C) sagittal T2WI show a large left adrenal cancer (arrows). The size of the lesion and the high SI on the T2WI are typical of an adrenal carcinoma.*

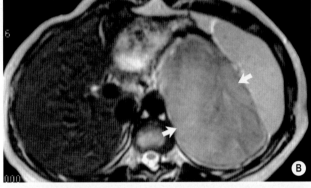

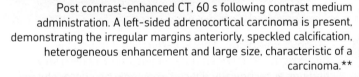

Post contrast-enhanced CT, 60 s following contrast medium administration. A left-sided adrenocortical carcinoma is present, demonstrating the irregular margins anteriorly, speckled calcification, heterogeneous enhancement and large size, characteristic of a carcinoma.**

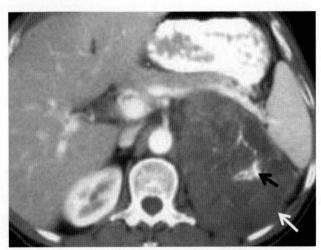

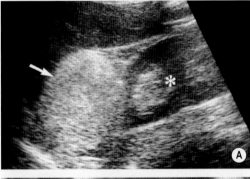

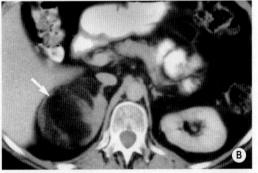

Myelolipoma. (A) A longitudinal US showing a hyperechoic mass (arrow) lying above the right kidney (*) and behind the liver. (B) CECT showing large right adrenal mass (arrow) consisting predominantly of fat. (C) Corresponding T1WI showing a mass (arrow) consisting predominantly of fat of similar SI to the surrounding perirenal fat. (D) STIR sequence showing suppression of the signal from fat within the mass (arrow).*

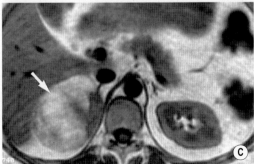

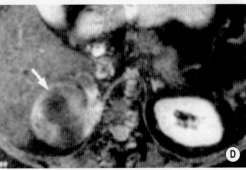

ENDOGENOUS CUSHING'S SYNDROME

- Cushing's syndrome is made up of symptoms and signs resulting from long-term elevated glucocorticoid levels
- ACTH Dependent (80%): secondary to a pituitary ACTH secreting tumour (Cushing's Disease)
- ACTH Independent (20%): due to primary adrenal disease

ACTH-dependent Cushing's disease

- This will result in bilateral adrenal hyperplasia ▶ it is due to a pituitary cause (i.e. Cushing's disease) in 85%, with the remaining 15% due to ectopic ACTH secretion, which can be either overt or occult:
  - *Overt:* this is usually clinically apparent, presenting with a short history and lacking the clinical features of Cushing's syndrome ▶ it is most commonly from a small cell lung cancer
  - *Occult:* this presents with a more chronic clinical picture and is often indistinguishable from Cushing's syndrome due to either a pituitary or adrenal adenoma ▶ it usually results from a bronchial carcinoid tumour (less frequently an islet cell tumour of the pancreas, phaeochromocytoma, medullary thyroid carcinoma, or thymic carcinoid tumour)

Adrenocortical adenoma

- This accounts for 10–20% of cases of Cushing's syndrome ▶ such adenomas are usually >2 cm in diameter and the contralateral gland is usually normal (but may be atrophic due to reduced ACTH secretion) ▶ necrosis or haemorrhage can be seen with larger lesions

Adrenal carcinoma

- This accounts for 10–15% of cases of Cushing's syndrome (see Section 5 Chapter 7)

Carney complex

- An autosomal dominant syndrome characterized by:
  - Myxoma's (of the heart, skin and breast)
  - Abnormal skin pigmentation
  - Endocrine abnormalities (commonly primary pigmented nodular adrenocortical disease leading to ACTH-independent Cushing's syndrome)

PRIMARY HYPERALDOSTERONISM (CONN'S SYNDROME)

DEFINITION

Primary hyperaldosteronism is due to excess aldosterone production ▶ severe hypertension, biochemical alkalosis, hypokalaemia and hypernatraemia ▶ the distinction between an aldosteronoma and bilateral adrenal hyperplasia is crucial, as surgery can treat adrenal masses, and medical treatment is used for adrenal hyperplasia

Causes

- A benign cortical adenoma (80%)
- Bilateral adrenal hyperplasia (20%)
- An adrenocortical carcinoma (rare)

Adrenocortical adenoma (Conn's tumour)

- These are usually <2 cm ▶ can be difficult to detect

CT The lesion is low density (<10 HU) because of its high cytoplasmic lipid content ▶ there is no significant enhancement ▶ it rarely calcifies

MRI T1WI: low-to-intermediate SI ▶ T2WI: intermediate-to-high SI ▶ signal loss on out-of-phase imaging

Venous sampling This is performed if there is a disagreement between the imaging and biochemistry findings ▶ technically difficult, may only be successful in 50% of patients

- It is the most accurate means of localizing an aldosteronoma
- Its sensitivity approaches 100% (with a positive predictive value of 90%)

Adrenal scintigraphy This is performed with a cholesterol-based radiopharmaceutical such as NP-59 (^{131}I-6-iodomethyl-19-norcholesterol, which localizes masses arising from the adrenal cortex) and dexamethasone suppression

- It is able to distinguish between a unilateral adenoma and a bilateral hyperplasia
- It is seldom used, as its sensitivity is dependent on the size of the adenoma (and is less accurate than CT)

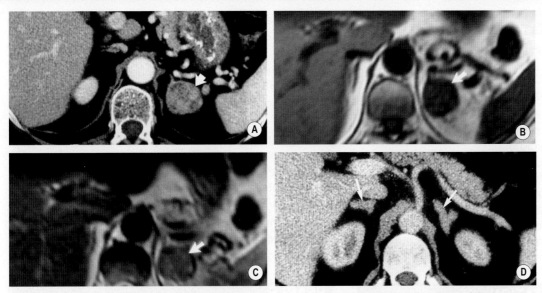

Cushing's syndrome due to adrenocortical adenoma. (A) Contrast-enhanced CT, (B) T1WI and (C) T2WI all show a 3 cm adenoma (arrows) in the left adrenal gland. (D) CECT of bilateral adrenal hyperplasia (arrows) in a different patient with Cushing's disease.*

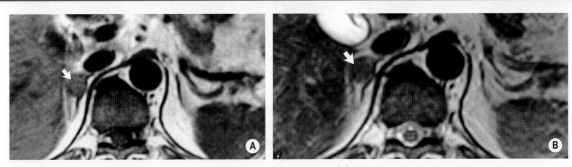

Conn's syndrome due to an adrenocortical adenoma. (A) T1WI and (B) T2WI images showing the typical appearance of a small aldosterone-producing adenoma (arrow) in the right adrenal gland.*

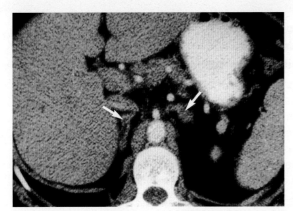

Conn's syndrome due to bilateral nodular adrenal hyperplasia. Contrast-enhanced CT shows small nodules in the adrenal glands (arrows).*

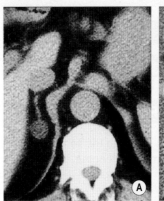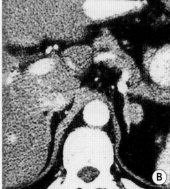

Conn's syndrome. CT appearances of (A) a right adrenal nodule and (B) a left adrenal nodule in a different patient.†

PHAEOCHROMOCYTOMAS

DEFINITION

- Catecholamine-producing tumours that arise from the paraganglion cells anywhere within the autonomic nervous system
- *Phaeochromocytoma* (90%): tumours arising from the chromaffin cells of the adrenal medulla ▶ these are more commonly endocrinologically active (90%) than extra-adrenal tumours (50%)
- *Paraganglioma* (10%): tumours arising from the extra-adrenal chromaffin tissue:
  - Paravertebral sympathetic ganglia > the organ of Zuckerkandl (at the aortic bifurcation) > within the head and neck (e.g. carotid body tumours or glomus tympanicum, jugulare or vagale tumours) > the bladder

CLINICAL PRESENTATION

- Symptoms are attributable to excess catecholamine secretion (e.g. tachycardia, headache, hypertension) ▶ it can present at any age (M = F)

RADIOLOGICAL FEATURES

USS Well defined, ovoid or round suprarenal mass ▶ can be heterogeneous (haemorrhage/necrosis)

NECT Round masses (which are isodense to surrounding soft tissue structures) ▶ they may demonstrate a fluid-filled centre (as haemorrhage and necrosis is frequent) ▶ there can be speckled calcification ▶ the average size at presentation is 5 cm, with a smaller size seen in cases of MEN II ▶ preservation of the periadrenal fat planes indicates that no invasion is present

CECT Intense enhancement ▶ use a non-ionic contrast medium to avoid a hypertensive crisis

MRI T1WI: low SI (high SI in areas of haemorrhage) ▶ T2WI: extremely high SI (and may give rise to a 'light bulb' appearance) ▶ T1WI + Gad: intense enhancement ▶ there is no significant SI loss with in-phase and out-of-phase imaging

MIBG scintigraphy MIBG is a guanethidine analogue that concentrates within the medullary tissue – increased uptake is seen with a phaeochromocytoma ▶ it can also be used for detecting metastatic or locally recurrent disease

FDG-PET Abnormally increased uptake (which is greater in malignant tumours) ▶ it allows assessment of any metastatic disease ▶ relatively low sensitivity and not recommended for initial diagnostic evaluation

PEARLS

10% rule 10% are extra-adrenal ▶ 10% are bilateral ▶ 10% are malignant ▶ 10% are calcified ▶ 10% are inherited ▶ 10% are non-functioning ▶ 10% invade the IVC or renal vein

Malignant lesions These can demonstrate local invasion, IVC and renal vein invasion and local lymph node spread ▶ there is haematogenous spread to the bones (most common), liver and lungs

Associations (and the phaeochromocytoma prevalence) Multiple endocrine neoplasia type II (50%) ▶ neurofibromatosis type I (10%) ▶ Von Hippel–Lindau syndrome (10%)

Treatment Surgical resection (with ^{131}I-MIBG for incomplete resection or metastatic spread) or chemotherapy ▶ medical management with α and β blockade can control any symptoms
- Urinary free catecholamine measurement aids diagnosis

ADRENOGENITAL SYNDROME

DEFINITION

- Androgen-producing adrenal tumours are usually carcinomas (less commonly an adenoma)

RADIOLOGICAL FEATURES

CT They are usually >2 cm in size with the same imaging characteristics as for a carcinoma or adenoma

PEARLS

Congenital adrenocortical hyperplasia

- This is the commonest adrenal cause of androgen excess in childhood and due to an inborn 21-hydroxylase enzyme deficiency (which causes a partial block in the synthesis of adrenocortical steroids and a resultant increase in the production of androgens) ▶ the compensatory elevation of ACTH production results in gross adrenal enlargement ▶ long-term stimulation can result in transformation of a hyperplastic nodule into an adenoma or even a carcinoma
- In virilism, imaging is used to detect a tumour within the adrenals, ovaries or testes ▶ can also lead to ambiguous genitalia

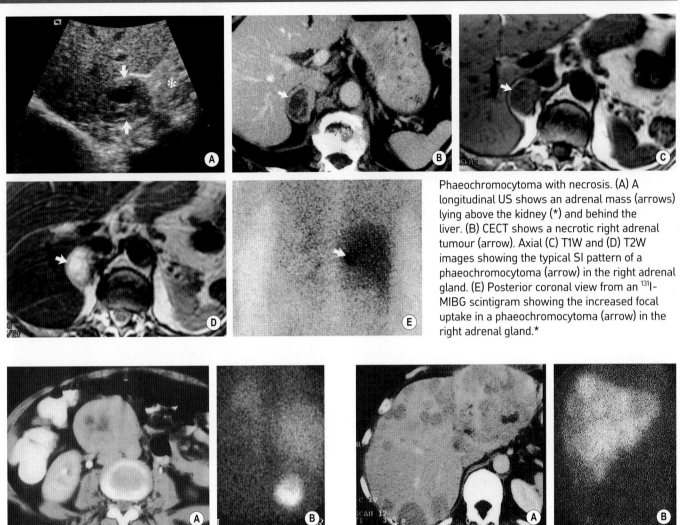

Phaeochromocytoma with necrosis. (A) A longitudinal US shows an adrenal mass (arrows) lying above the kidney (*) and behind the liver. (B) CECT shows a necrotic right adrenal tumour (arrow). Axial (C) T1W and (D) T2W images showing the typical SI pattern of a phaeochromocytoma (arrow) in the right adrenal gland. (E) Posterior coronal view from an ^{131}I-MIBG scintigram showing the increased focal uptake in a phaeochromocytoma (arrow) in the right adrenal gland.*

Paraganglioma. (A) CT demonstrating a non-specific tumour anterior to the aorta which was intensely active on (B) MIBG scintigraphy.[†]

Malignant phaeochromocytoma. (A) Non-specific liver metastases. (B) MIBG scintigraphy shows these to be functioning adrenal metastases.[†]

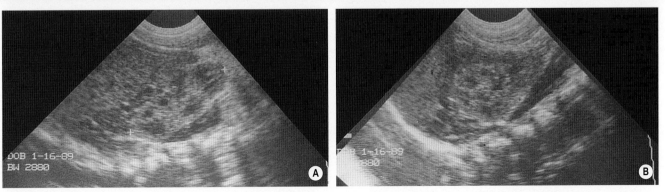

Congenital adrenal hyperplasia in a patient with male pseudohermaphroditism. Sagittal US of the (A) right and (B) left adrenal glands demonstrates mass-like enlargement.[ʃ]

LYMPHOMA

INTRODUCTION

DEFINITION

- The lymphomas are caused by the malignant clonal expansion of either T or B lymphocytes – these can accumulate within lymph nodes (causing lymphadenopathy) or infiltrate solid organs
- NB: if malignant lymphocytic change predominantly involves the lymph nodes (± extranodal sites) this is described as a lymphoma ▶ if bone marrow or peripheral blood involvement predominates it is then known as a leukaemia

Hodgkin's disease (HD)

- The defining cell is the Reed–Sternberg cell (usually derived from germinal centre B cells or, rarely, peripheral T cells) ▶ it is subclassified into four histological types:
  - *Lymphocyte-rich classical HD (5%):* an often indolent disease occurring within peripheral lymph nodes
  - *Mixed cellularity (MC) classical HD (20–25%):* this is more commonly seen in males and is associated with B symptoms
  - *Nodular sclerosing (NS) classical HD (70%):* many fibrotic bands are present ▶ it typically presents in young females as a bulky mediastinal or neck mass
  - *Lymphocyte-depleted (LD) classical HD (< 5%):* this is seen with HIV-associated disease

Non-Hodgkin's lymphoma (NHL)

- Most NHLs arise from the cells of the lymph node germinal follicle and are classified according to the WHO classification ▶ the majority (> 90%) are B-cell lymphomas

CLINICAL PRESENTATION

Painless superficial lymph node enlargement

- Cervical (up to 80%) ▶ axillary (up to 20%) ▶ inguinal (up to 15%) ▶ hepatosplenomegaly (30%)

Systemic 'B' symptoms (up to 40%)

- These are more commonly seen with HD and include: fever ▶ drenching night sweats ▶ weight loss (>10% of the patients body weight)
  - *Other constitutional symptoms:* pruritus ▶ fatigue ▶ anorexia ▶ rarely alcohol-induced pain at the site of any enlarged lymph nodes

HD This tends to spread in a contiguous fashion from one lymph node group to the next – primary extranodal HD is rare ▶ lymph node involvement is usually the only manifestation of disease ▶ lymph nodes tend to be smaller in HL than NHL

- HD demonstrates a bimodal age distribution (with a peak incidence at 20–30 years and a second smaller peak within the elderly population)

NHL Although the majority present with painless nodal disease, extranodal disease is a lot more commonly seen than in HD ▶ B symptoms are less frequent than in HD (20%)

- This is mainly a disease of the elderly, with a median age at diagnosis of 65 years (the incidence increases exponentially with age after 20 years) ▶ immunosuppression is an important aetiological factor, with a high incidence in AIDS patients and those on long-term immunosuprression
- HD is less common than NHL (3.7 vs 15.1/100 000/year, respectively) ▶ whilst the incidence of HD has remained stable, that of NHL has risen significantly (which is explained in part by the use of new classification techniques and also as a consequence of the increased incidence of NHL associated with immune deficiencies)

AETIOLOGY

Infectious agents

- *Epstein–Barr virus (EBV):* this is present in > 90% of cases of Burkitt's lymphoma ▶ it is also an important trigger for lymphomas occurring in congenital immunodeficiencies, immunosuppressed organ transplant patients and patients receiving chemotherapy ▶ also found in HL (mixed cellularity type)
- *Retrovirus human lymphotropic virus type 1 (HTLV-1):* this has been implicated in the causation of adult T-cell lymphomas
- *Human herpes virus 8:* implicated as a cause of primary effusion large cell lymphoma
- *Helicobacter pylori:* this is necessary for developing a gastric lymphoma of the mucosa-associated lymphoid tissue (MALT) type

Pre-existing immunosuppression

- MALT-type lymphomas can arise in organ specific autoimmune disease (e.g. Hashimoto's thyroiditis and Sjögren's syndrome) ▶ in severe immunodeficiency states (e.g. AIDS and with organ transplantation) lymphomas are often EBV-driven large B-cell lymphomas

Genetic factors

- There is an increased risk with a family history of lymphoma (this does not extend to the histological type)

Gender and race

- There is a higher frequency in whites than blacks or Asians ▶ there is also a slight male preponderance for HD and NHL
  - *HD:* M:F 1.4:1
  - *NHL:* M:F 1.1:1

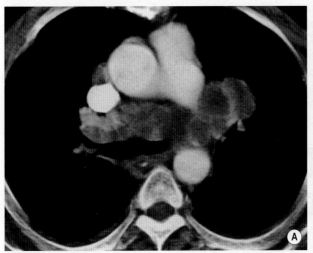 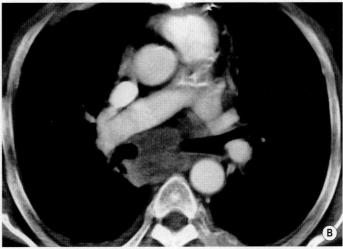

Middle mediastinal nodal disease. (A) CECT showing marked enlargement of the paratracheal and precarinal group of nodes, extending laterally into the left aortopulmonary nodes and continuing inferiorly into the subcarinal group (B) in the same patient.*

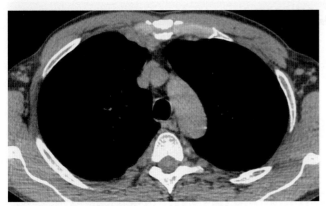

Internal mammary lymphadenopathy. Axial CT showing marked enlargement of the right internal mammary lymph nodes. Note the minimal bilateral axillary lymph node enlargement and paravertebral extrapleural disease bilaterally.**

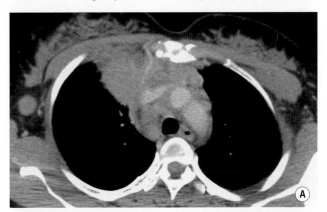

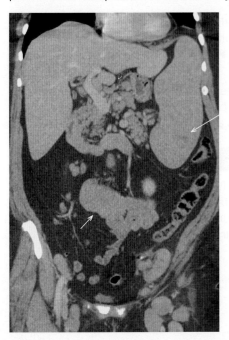

Upper abdominal lymph node enlargement. Coronal reformatted contrast-enhanced CT showing lymph node enlargement around the coeliac axis and porta hepatis (arrowhead), the splenic hilum, the mesentery (short arrow), the left external iliac chain and both inguinal regions. There is splenomegaly and a focal splenic lesion (long arrow).**

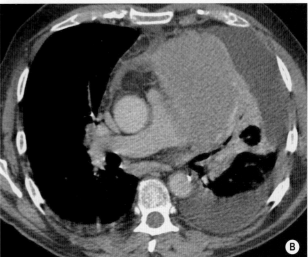

Mediastinal masses in lymphoma. (A) Contrast enhanced CT showing a large anterior mass involving the chest wall in a young patient with Hodgkin's lymphoma. Note the right axillary nodal disease. (B) Contrast-enhanced CT in a patient with primary mediastinal large B-cell lymphoma (PMBL) in the anterior and middle mediastinum. Note the pericardial involvement, compressive atelectasis of the left upper lobe and large left pleural effusion.**

STAGING

- HD and NHL both use the Cotswold's modification of the Ann Arbor staging system

PROGNOSIS

HD

- Failure to achieve an initial complete, or almost complete, response to first-line treatment (or recurrence within the first year) are both associated with a very poor prognosis
- The following are also thought to have a prognostic significance:
  - The patient's age (with a poorer prognosis in older patients)
  - The tumour subtype (mixed cellularity and lymphocyte-depleted types have a worse prognosis)
  - A raised ESR
  - Mutiple sites of disease
  - Bulky mediastinal disease
  - B symptoms

NHL

- Low-grade tumours, although incurable, have an indolent course ▶ high-grade tumours carry a worse prognosis but are potentially curable
- Factors with a prognostic significance:
  - Age > 60 years
  - An elevated serum lactate dehydrogenase (LDH)
  - A performance status > 1 (i.e. non-ambulatory)
  - Advanced stage III or IV
  - The presence of > 1 extranodal sites of disease

TREATMENT

HD

- *Localized disease* (stages 1A and 11A): early stage non-bulky disease: combination chemotherapy ▶ radiotherapy to involved nodes is an option
  - Radiotherapy is avoided in young patients where possible ▶ although HD is highly radiosensitive there is risk of secondary cancers (e.g. thyroid and breast) within the area of the mantle radiotherapy field
- *Advanced disease* (stages 11B, IIIA/B and IVA/B): extensive combination chemotherapy is used in the first instance (± subsequent consolidatory radiotherapy to any sites of 'bulky' disease to reduce risk of local recurrence)
  - A large mediastinal mass (i.e. > $\frac{1}{3}$ of the intrathoracic diameter at the level of T5) is generally treated with a moderate amount of initial chemotherapy in order to shrink the mass prior to any subsequent radiotherapy – this aims to avoid any excessive irradiation of the lung parenchyma and subsequent radiation fibrosis

NHL

- Unlike HD, the histological subtype is the major determinant of treatment
- This is usually combination chemotherapy, since around 80% of patients will have advanced disease at presentation ▶ radiotherapy alone is considered for the small proportion of patients with stage I disease and no adverse factors (in whom surgical excision alone is considered inappropriate)

BURKITT'S LYMPHOMA

DEFINITION

- A highly aggressive B-cell variant of NHL which is associated with the Epstein–Barr virus (EBV) ▶ it is associated with immunodeficiency (usually HIV)

CLINICAL PRESENTATION

- 2M:1F ▶ mean age 7 years (2–16 years)
- Endemic (mainly African children) or non-endemic (mainly white children)
- Extranodal disease is common and there is a risk of CNS disease (leptomeningeal disease can be seen at presentation and is a site of relapse)
- Retroperitoneal and paraspinal disease can cause paraplegia (a presenting feature in up to 15%)
- Thoracic disease is rare

RADIOLOGICAL FEATURES

Endemic form The jaw and orbit are involved in 50% of cases ▶ the ovaries, kidneys and breast may also be affected

XR A 'floating' teeth appearance: a destructive jaw lesion starting in the medulla and later affecting the cortex (± periosteal reaction) ▶ there is a similar appearance in other bones

Sporadic form There is a predilection for the ileocaecal region and patients can present with an intussusception ▶ the ovaries, kidneys and breasts are commonly involved

PEARLS

- It accounts for only 2–3% of NHL in immunocompetent adults (but 30–50% of all childhood lymphomas)
- Although these tumours are extremely aggressive, they are potentially curable (chemotherapy)

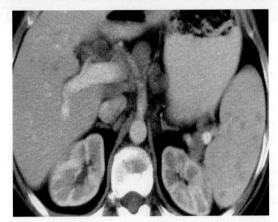

CECT showing lymph node enlargement in the region of the splenic hilum around the coeliac axis and in the porta hepatis. Multiple small, non-enhancing foci are demonstrated within the spleen, typical of splenic involvement.

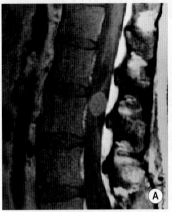
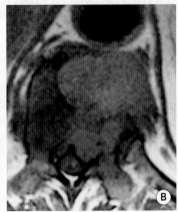

(A) Sagittal T1WI showing a well-defined lesion within the dura due to a lymphomatous deposit within the meninges. (B) Lymphomatous infiltration of the spinal canal. T1WI showing a mass of intermediate-to-high SI in the paravertebral soft tissues, extending into the vertebral body and into the spinal canal.

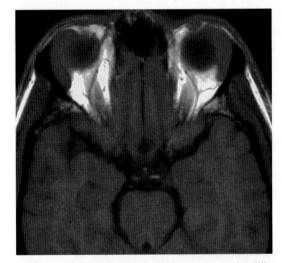

Bilateral orbital lymphoma. T1WI demonstrating bilateral orbital masses arising in the region of the lacrimal glands.*

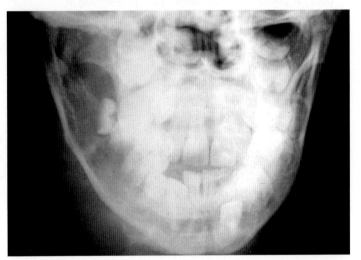

Burkitt's lymphoma. Destruction of the right side of the mandible has resulted in 'floating teeth' and an associated large soft tissue mass.*

Cotswold's modification of the Ann Arbor staging classification of Hodgkin's disease*	
Stage	**Classification**
I	Involvement of a single lymph node region (I) or a single extralymphatic organ or site (IE)
II	Involvement of two or more lymph node regions on the same side of the diaphragm (II) or one or more lymph node regions plus an extralymphatic site (IIE)
III	Involvement of lymph node regions on both sides of the diaphragm (III) (the spleen is included in stage III) ▶ subdivided into: 　III(1): involvement of the spleen and/or splenic hilar, coeliac and portal nodes 　III(2): with para-aortic, iliac, or mesenteric nodes
IV	Involvement of one or more extralymphatic organs (e.g. lung, liver, bone, bone marrow) with or without lymph node involvement
Additional qualifiers denote the following:	A: asymptomatic B: fever, night sweats and weight loss of >10% body weight X: bulky disease (defined as a lymph node mass >10 cm in diameter or, if involving the mediastinum, a mass greater than $\frac{1}{3}$ of the intrathoracic diameter at the level of T5) E: involvement of a single extranodal site, contiguous with a known nodal site

SPECIFIC FORMS OF LYMPHOMA

MUCOSA-ASSOCIATED LYMPHOID TISSUE (MALT) LYMPHOMAS

- These arise from mucosal sites that normally have no organized lymphoid tissue, but within which acquired lymphoid tissue has arisen as a result of chronic inflammation or autoimmunity:
  - *Hashimoto's thyroiditis:* a 70× increased risk of thyroid lymphoma
  - *Sjögren's syndrome:* a 44× risk of lymphoma
  - *Helicobacter-induced chronic follicular gastritis*
- There is a median age of 60 years (F>M) ▶ most patients present with stage IE or IIE disease, which tends to be indolent
- **Sites:** the GI tract is the commonest site (50%), and within the GI tract the stomach is the most often affected (85%) ▶ the small bowel and colon are involved in immunoproliferative small intestinal disease (IPSID), which was previously known as alpha-chain disease ▶ bone marrow involvement is seen in 10% ▶ other sites of involvement include the lungs, head, neck, ocular adnexae, skin, thyroid and breast
  - Multiple extranodal sites are involved in up to 25% but this does not appear to have the same poor prognostic import as other forms of NHL
  - Up to 20% of lymphomas involving Waldeyer's ring are of the MALT type with the tonsils the most commonly affected ▶ the commonest pattern is asymmetrical thickening of the pharyngeal mucosa

LYMPHOMA IN THE IMMUNOCOMPROMISED

- There are four broad groupings associated with an increased incidence of lymphoma and lymphoproliferative disorders:
  - Primary immunodeficiency syndromes
  - Infection with the human immunodeficiency virus (HIV)
  - Iatrogenic immunosuppression after solid organ or bone marrow allografts
  - Iatrogenic immunosuppression from methotrexate (usually for autoimmune disorders)

Lymphomas associated with HIV

- Lymphoma is the first AIDS-defining illness in up to 5% of HIV patients (the incidence of all subtypes of NHL is increased 60–200-fold and the incidence of HD is increased up to 8-fold) ▶ EBV positivity occurs in up to 70% of patients
  - Various types are seen, including those in immunocompetent patients such as BL and DLBCL, but some occur more frequently in HIV patients (e.g. primary effusion lymphoma and plasmablastic

lymphoma of the oral cavity) ▶ DLBCL tends to occur later, whereas BL occurs in less immunodeficient patients
- Most tumours are aggressive, with advanced stage, bulky disease and a high serum LDH at presentation ▶ there is a marked propensity to involve extranodal sites (especially the GI tract, CNS, liver and bone marrow) ▶ multiple sites of extranodal involvement are common (> 75%) ▶ peripheral lymph node enlargement is relatively uncommon
- **Chest:** NHL is usually extranodal ▶ pleural effusions, nodules, acinar and interstitial opacities are common ▶ hilar and mediastinal nodal enlargement is generally mild
- **Abdomen:** the GI tract, liver, kidneys, adrenal glands and lower GU tract are commonly involved ▶ imaging appearances are similar to those seen in immunocompetent patients (although mesenteric and retroperitoneal nodal enlargement is less common)
- **PCNSL:** deep white matter lesions ▶ rim enhancement and multifocality are seen more often than in the immunocompetent population (causing confusion with cerebral toxoplasmosis although the location of PCNSL within the deep white matter is suggestive)

Post-transplant lymphoproliferative disorders (PTLD)

- This occurs in 2–4% of solid organ transplant recipient patients ▶ marrow allograft recipients in general have a low risk (1%)
  - The lowest frequency is seen in renal transplant recipients (1%) ▶ the highest frequency is seen in heart–lung or liver–bowel allografts (5%)
- Most are associated with EBV infection and appear to represent EBV-induced monoclonal or, more rarely, polyclonal B-cell or T-cell proliferation as a consequence of immune suppression
  - EBV-positive cases occur earlier than EBV-negative cases (the latter occurring 4–5 years after transplantation)
- PTLD develops earlier in patients receiving ciclosporin rather than azathioprine (with a mean interval of 48 months)
  - In patients receiving azathioprine, the allograft itself and the CNS are often involved (in patients who have received ciclosporin the GI tract is affected more than the CNS)
- In all cases extranodal disease is disproportionately commoner (CNS disease is rare)
- The bone marrow, liver and lung are often affected ▶ multiple intrapulmonary masses, pleural effusions, and involvement of multiple segments of bowel and the transplanted organ have all been reported

Differentiating between Hodgkin's disease and Non-Hodgkin's lymphoma		
	Hodgkin's disease (HD)	**Non-Hodgkin's lymphoma (NHL)**
General features	• Lymph node involvement is usually the only manifestation of disease	• Nodal disease is frequently associated with extranodal sites of tumour ▶ involved nodes tend to be larger than in HD
	• Nodes tend to displace adjacent structures rather than invade them	
Short-axis diameter criteria for size enlargement (mm)	• Usually a short-axis diameter > 10 mm is considered pathological ▶ clustering of small nodes can be abnormal • **Exceptions:** jugulodigastric nodes > 13 mm ▶ gastrohepatic ligament/porta hepatis nodes > 8 mm ▶ retrocrural nodes > 6 mm ▶ supraclavicular nodes > 5 mm ▶ pelvic nodes > 8 mm ▶ any nodes seen at the splenic hilum, or presacral and perirectal areas are considered unusual	
CT	• Homogeneous, soft tissue density nodal masses demonstrating mild-to-moderate uniform enhancement • Calcification is uncommon – but can be seen post treatment • Necrosis is rarely seen within large nodal masses – but again is more frequently seen post treatment	
PET-CT	Superior diagnostic accuracy than CT alone ▶ can get false negative studies with low grade lymphomas ▶ certain organ involvement (e.g. stomach and CNS) can be difficult to recognize due to high physiological uptake	
MRI	• T1WI: low-to-intermediate SI ▶ T2WI: intermediate-to-high SI ▶ STIR: very high SI	
Neck	• Affecting 60–80% of patients at presentation • Spread is usually to contiguous nodal groups • The internal jugular chain is usually involved first with subsequent spread to the deep lymphatic chains ▶ supraclaviclar or bilateral neck adenopathy is not associated with an increased risk of infradiaphragmatic disease	• Cervical adenopathy is less common • There is usually non-contiguous involvement • Waldeyer's ring is the most frequently affected region ▶ 40–60% of patients presenting with head and neck involvement will have disseminated NHL
Thorax	• 60–85% of patients at presentation • Prevascular and paratracheal (85%) > hilar (28%) and subcarinal (22%) > other sites • Usually affects > 2 nodal groups ▶ the paracardiac nodes are an important site of recurrence as they are not included in the classical 'mantle' radiation field	• 25–40% of patients at presentation • Superior mediastinal nodes (35%) > hilar and subcarinal nodes (9%) • Usually affects only one nodal group in 50% of patients
	• Involved nodes are usually bilateral but *asymmetrical* (cf. sarcoidosis) ▶ they can be discrete or matted together with cystic changes seen within large anterior mediastinal masses • Hilar enlargement is rare without mediastinal involvement (particularly in HD) • The posterior mediastinum is infrequently involved, however lower mediastinal disease is associated with retrocrural disease • All the mediastial sites (other than the paracardiac and posterior mediastinal nodes) are more frequently involved in HD than NHL • Nodal calcification is commonly seen post therapy • Large anterior mediastinal masses usually represent thymic infiltration as well as nodal disease	
Abdomen and pelvis	• Retroperitoneal nodes are involved in 25–35% of patients at presentation • Mesenteric nodes are involved in < 5% • Coeliac axis, splenic hilar and porta hepatis nodes are involved in 30% ▶ splenic hilar involvement is almost always associated with diffuse splenic infiltration • Nodal spread is contiguous from one lymph node group to another • Notes are often normal in size or minimally enlarged	• Retroperitoneal nodes are involved in 45–55% of patients at presentation • Mesenteric nodes are involved in > 50% • 'Hamburger' sign: nodal mesenteric and retro-peritoneal involvement compressing a loop of bowel between the two large nodal masses • Additional sites (such as the porta hepatis or around the splenic hilum) are more frequently involved than in HD ▶ regional nodal involvement is frequently seen with primary extranodal lymphoma involving an abdominal viscus • Nodal spread is non-contiguous, bulky and more frequently associated with extranodal disease
	• Involved nodes tend to enhance uniformly ▶ the presence of central necrosis or multilocular enhancement suggests an alternative diagnosis (e.g. tuberculosis or atypical infection)	
Pelvis	• All nodal groups may be involved in both HD and NHL ▶ inguinal or femoral adenopathy is seen in < 20% of HD patients at presentation	

CNS LYMPHOMA

Definition This is usually a primary high-grade B-cell lymphoma (secondary lymphoma is rare) ▶ there is an increasing incidence (3% of all primary brain tumours) – partly due to an increasing association with transplant-related immunosuppressive therapy and an increasing AIDS population

- Secondary lymphoma: this occurs during the course of NHL in 15% ▶ it is very rare in HD
- *Risk factors:* stage IV disease ▶ a testicular or ovarian presentation ▶ a high-grade histology Burkitt's lymphoma
- *Affected patients:* those with AIDS or immunocompromised for other reasons (peak incidence 4th decade) ▶ immunocompetent patients (peak incidence 6th and 7th decades)

Radiological features

Primary lymphoma More than 50% of tumours occur within the cerebral white matter, close to or within the corpus callosum and often abutting the ependyma ▶ most touch the ependymal lining of the ventricles or the leptomeningeal surfaces

- *'Butterfly' distribution:* tumour crossing the corpus callosum is a typical finding (but can also be seen with a glioblastoma multiforme)
- The majority (90%) are supratentorial with 15% of cases affecting the deep grey matter of the thalamus and basal ganglia ▶ 10% arise within the posterior fossa ▶ 15% of cases are multifocal

CT A well-defined hyperdense mass (NECT) due to its high cellular density ▶ it is virtually never calcified ▶ there is little surrounding vasogenic oedema or mass effect ▶ there is uniform enhancement in immunocompetent

patients ▶ ring-like enhancement in immunocompromised patients (central necrosis)

MRI T1WI: low-to-intermediate SI ▶ T2WI: low SI (may be heterogeneous due to haemorrhage or necrosis) ▶ T1WI + Gad: avid homogeneous enhancement ▶ DWI: restricted diffusion with a lower ADC than seen with a glioma or toxoplasmosis

Secondary lymphoma

CT/MRI Extra-axial disease (epidural, subdural and subarachnoid) and disease within the spinal epidural and subarachnoid spaces is more commonly seen than an intra-axial mass

- Enhancing plaques over the cerebral convexities and around the basal meninges ▶ diffuse meningeal involvement is more common with secondary lymphoma (but relatively rare with primary disease)
- Spinal epidural disease can result in cord compression or a cauda equina syndrome ▶ *'dumb-bell' tumour:* epidural extension of tumour into the spinal canal from a paravertebral mass is the commonest cause
- Vertebral involvement can lead to epidural spread and extrinsic thecal compression (less common)

Pearls Rapid tumour resolution can follow steroid administration ± radiotherapy

HIV-infected population Tumour tends to be multifocal with periventricular spread ▶ necrosis and haemorrhage is common ▶ the main differential is toxoplasmosis infection

- Differentiation from toxoplasmosis:
  - *Lymphoma:* hyperdense (NECT) ▶ callosal involvement and ependymal spread ▶ positive thallium imaging
  - *Toxoplasmosis:* more commonly presents with multiple lesions

HEAD AND NECK LYMPHOMA

- True extranodal involvement is rare in HD ▶ conversely, 10% of patients with NHL present with extranodal head and neck involvement, accounting for 5% of all head and neck cancers (50% will have disseminated lymphoma)

Waldeyer's ring

- This comprises lymphoid tissue in the nasopharynx, oropharynx, the faucial and palatine tonsil and the lingual tonsil
- The commonest site of head and neck lymphoma with circumferential or multifocal involvement ▶ tonsils most commonly affected (with asymmetrical thickening of the pharyngeal mucosa)
- Associated with synchronous or metachronous involvement of the GI tract (probably as many are of the MALT type)

- Secondary invasion from adjacent nodal masses is also a common occurrence

Paranasal sinuses

- NHL comprises 8% of paranasal sinus tumours ▶ disease often spreads from one sinus to another in a contiguous fashion ▶ bony destruction is considerably less marked than with a squamous cell carcinoma ▶ locally aggressive (spread through the skull base into the cranium in 40%)
  - **Western population:** the disease affects middle-aged men and commonly the maxillary sinus (commonly DLBCL)
  - **Asian population:** commonly the aggressive diffuse T-cell type and linked with EBV (diffuse T-cell type)

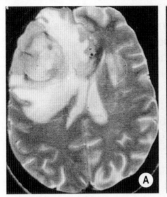
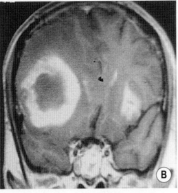

Primary CNS lymphoma in an AIDS patient. (A) T2WI demonstrating a large amount of vasogenic oedema associated with the mass and extension across the corpus callosum. (B) Coronal T1WI + Gad demonstrating thick irregular ring enhancement. Subependymal enhancement around the anterior aspect of the frontal horns is also evident, a characteristic feature of cerebral lymphoma.[†]

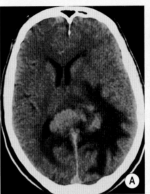
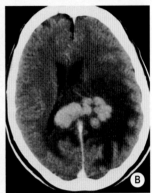

Primary cerebral lymphoma. NECT (A) and CECT (B). An irregular mass that is hyperdense to grey matter expands the splenium of the corpus callosum and extends into the left hemisphere. It is surrounded by extensive white matter oedema and enhances avidly with contrast.[*]

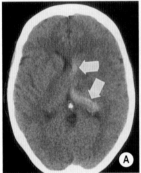
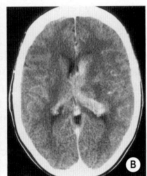

Periventricular lymphoma. (A) Pre- and (B) post-contrast CT images demonstrate a hyperdense mass (arrows) that intensely enhances and infiltrates the ventricular ependymal surface.[+]

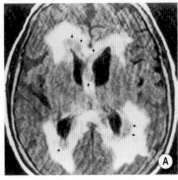
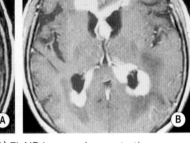

Ependymal lymphoma spread. (A) FLAIR images demonstrating periventricular low SI (arrows) and (B) T1WI + Gad demonstrating ependymal enhancement.[+]

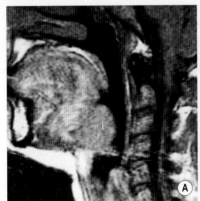
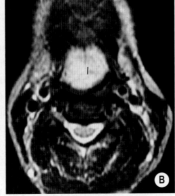

Oropharyngeal lymphoma. (A) Sagittal T1WI reveals a round exophytic mass within the tongue base (l) secondary to lymphoma. (B) T2WI demonstrating that the SI of the lesion is markedly hyperintense, which would be unusual for a squamous cell carcinoma.[+]

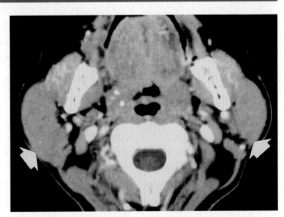

CECT of the parotid glands showing diffuse enlargement of both glands, which are of increased attenuation (arrows). This was infiltration by NHL.[†]

PULMONARY LYMPHOMA

Definition

- Pulmonary parenchymal involvement can be broadly divided into:
  - *That occurring in association with existing or previously treated nodal disease* ▶ as it is usually due to the direct extension of nodal disease, it will demonstrate a paramediastinal location
  - *That due to primary lymphoma of the lung* ▶ this is rare, accounting for < 1% of all lymphomas

Radiological features

- Parenchymal involvement increases with disease progression (and is seen particularly in relapsed patients) ▶ the general radiographic appearance can vary:
  - *Multiple pulmonary nodules* (common) ▶ these are less well defined and dense than metastases ▶ they tend to spread out from the hila along lymphatic channels ▶ cavitation can be seen
  - *One or more areas of pulmonary consolidation resembling a pneumonia* (less common): due to lymphoma filling the pulmonary acini
  - *Miliary nodulation or reticulonodular shadowing* (rare): this can resemble lymphangitis carcinomatosis

Hodgkin's disease

- *Nodal involvement* (60–85%): the anterior mediastinum is the most often involved and may cause SVC obstruction or tracheal compression ▶ it is frequently bilateral but often asymmetrical (unlike sarcoidosis)
- *Lung involvement* (12%): this is three times as frequent compared with NHL ▶ it is usually secondary to widespread disease and therefore accompanied by visible intrathoracic adenopathy ▶ primary pulmonary HD is extremely rare (patients with an intrapulmonary lesion and no mediastinal disease are unlikely to have lymphomatous disease of the lung unless there has been previous mediastinal irradiation)
  - *Segmental or lobar areas of consolidation which may contain bronchograms:* these often radiate from the hila without conforming to any segmental anatomy in keeping with direct invasion from the involved mediastinal nodes

Non-Hodgkin's lymphoma

- *Nodal involvement* (25–40%)
- *Lung involvement* (4%): isolated lung involvement without intrathoracic adenopathy is common and seen in 50% of patients (cf. HD)
  - Radiographic features are similar to Hodgkin's disease
- *Chest wall involvement:* this is more commonly seen than in HD ▶ it is usually secondary to direct infiltration by an anterior mediastinal mass or spread from axillary or supraclavicular nodes ▶ bone destruction is rare and should suggest a diagnosis of carcinoma or infection

- Pleural involvement may also occur – either from direct extension from a chest wall mass or parenchymal lung disease, or from direct seeding (giving plaque-like opacities)
- *Primary pulmonary NHL:* this is very uncommon (it is almost never seen in HD) ▶ it is usually a low-grade B-cell MALT lymphoma – a high-grade lymphoid granulomatosis is the 2nd most common type
  - *MALT lymphoma:* a low-grade indolent disease tending to occur in the 5th and 6th decades ▶ many patients have a prior history of inflammatory or autoimmune disease ▶ it appears as solitary or multifocal, round or segmental areas of consolidation with no lobar predilection ▶ it can be centrally or peripherally located ▶ air bronchograms may be a striking feature ▶ cavitation and pleural effusions are rare ▶ calcification does not occur
  - *High-grade lymphoid granulomatosis:* solitary or multiple pulmonary nodules (characteristically growing very rapidly)

Pearls

- **Patterns of intrathoracic nodal involvement:** large anterior masses usually indicate thymic involvement as well as a nodal mass ▶ the posterior mediastinum is infrequently involved (it may represent contiguous retrocrural involvement) ▶ all the mediastinal nodes other than the paracardiac and posterior mediastinal nodes are more frequently involved in HD than NHL ▶ hilar adenopathy is rare in the absence of mediastinal adenopathy
  - *HD nodes:* often enlargement of ≥ 2 nodal groups ▶ prevascular and paratracheal > hilar > subcarinal nodes
  - *NHL nodes:* often only 1 nodal group is involved ▶ hilar and subcarinal involvement is rarer than with HD
- **Eggshell calcification:** this may occur in mediastinal lymph nodes following radio- or chemotherapy
- **Atelectasis due to extrinsic lymph node compression:** this is rare and is usually due to endobronchial lymphoma
- **Pleural effusions:** these are common except with a MALT lymphoma usually exudates secondary to central lymphatic or venous obstruction ▶ they are usually unilateral and accompanied by intrathoracic adenopathy ▶ they usually disappear once the mediastinal nodes have been irradiated (as they were probable due to venous or lymphatic obstruction rather than neoplastic pleural involvement)
- **Following previous mediastinal or hilar node irradiation:** isolated pulmonary recurrence may be seen in both HD and NHL ▶ paracardiac nodes are important potential sites as they are not within the classical 'mantle' filed of irradiation

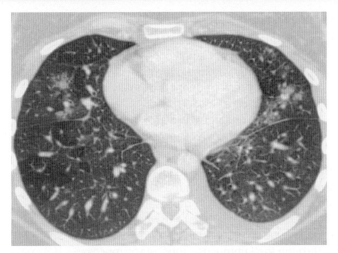

Pulmonary involvement in a patient with Hodgkin's lymphoma. CT performed at the time of presentation, showing widespread ill-defined intrapulmonary nodular shadowing scattered throughout both lungs with a bronchocentric distribution. Note also the abnormal thickened interlobular septae and patchy ground-glass opacity.**

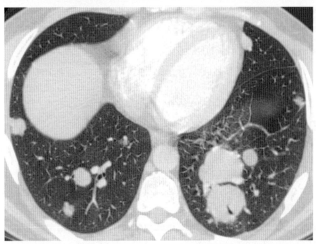

Lung involvement in recurrent Hodgkin's lymphoma. CT showing multiple rounded nodules: the left lower lobe nodule is beginning to cavitate.**

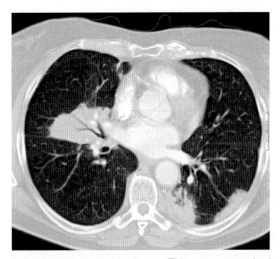

Primary pulmonary lymphoma. This appearance had been very slowly progressive over several years.*

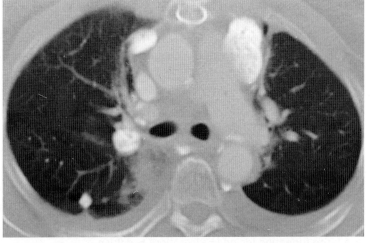

Hodgkin's disease. CT demonstrating extensive calcification within the mediastinal nodes following previous treatment.†

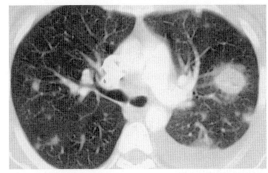

Lymphomatoid granulomatosis. CT demonstrating multiple pulmonary nodules and a larger mass in the left upper lobe with an air bronchogram. Subcarinal lymph node enlargement and a left pleural effusion are also present.†

Differentiating between Hodgkin's disease and Non-Hodgkin's lymphoma		
	Hodgkin's disease	**Non-Hodgkin's lymphoma**
Nodal involvement	60–85%	25–40%
Lung involvement	12%	4%
Lung involvement (without adenopathy)	Rare	Common (50%)
Chest wall involvement	Less common	Common
Pleural effusions	7% at presentation	10% at presentation

LYMPHOMA OF THE GI TRACT

DEFINITION

Primary extranodal NHL

- The GI tract is the commonest site of disease ▶ usually a non-Hodgkin's B-cell lymphoma (T-cell lymphoma in coeliac disease)

Primary HD of the GI tract

- Rare ▶ usually unifocal ▶ it arises from the lymphoid tissue of the lamina propria submucosa ▶ it usually occurs in patients < 10 years old (Burkitt's lymphoma) or during the 6th decade (MALT type and enteropathy associated T-cell type)

Secondary lymphomatous involvement of the GI tract

- Extremely common ▶ usually follows direct extension from involved lymph nodes

RADIOLOGICAL FEATURES

Oesophagus (very rare)

- Usually NHL ▶ associated with disease elsewhere
  - It begins as a submucosal lesion (distal $\frac{1}{3}$ of the oesophagus) resulting in a smooth luminal narrowing with an intact overlying mucosa (± later ulceration)
  - Secondary involvement by contiguous spread from adjacent nodal disease is more common but rarely results in dysphagia

Stomach (50%)

- Primary lymphoma originates within the submucosa (2–5% of gastric tumours) ▶ antrum > body or cardia (the duodenum is often involved if the antrum is affected)
  - *MALT lymphoma:* the commonest site is the stomach (and usually arises within mucosa-associated lymphoid tissue in response to *H. pylori* infection)

Barium meal Multiple nodules (± central ulceration) ▶ a large fungating lesion (± ulceration) ▶ diffuse infiltration with marked wall thickening and luminal narrowing (mimicking linitis plastica) ▶ diffuse gastric fold enlargement (10%)

- *Low-grade MALT lymphoma:* shallow ulceration and nodulation

CT Lymphoma may mimic a gastric carcinoma but the wall thickening (4–5 cm) is much greater (except with a MALT lymphoma where there is minimal thickening) ▶ infiltration of adjacent organs is unusual (unlike a gastric carcinoma) ▶ antral extension into the proximal duodenum is more characteristic of a lymphoma

Small intestine (35%)

- Lymphoma (usually of B-cell lineage) accounts for up to 50% of all primary small bowel tumours ▶ it occurs most frequently within the terminal ileum, becoming progressively less frequent proximally ▶ duodenal lymphoma is rare
  - Disease is multifocal in 50% ▶ mural thickening with constriction of bowel segments is typical – (often obstructive symptoms)

Barium follow-through Irregular thickened valvulae conniventes ▶ extraluminal mass ▶ strictures ▶ broad-based ulceration ▶ mucosal destruction (± shouldering of the margins) ▶ cavitation ▶ ileo-ileal fistula

- *Long 'tube-like' segments:* progressive tumour spread through the submucosa/muscularis mucosa
- *Aneurysmal dilatation of long segments:* infiltration of the autonomic plexus
  - Such alternating areas of dilatation and constriction are a common feature of small bowel involvement
- Infiltration can be predominantly submucosal, resulting in multiple nodules or polyps (predominantly within the terminal ileum) ▶ this often results in an intussusception (particularly in children > 6 years old)

CT/MRI Wall thickening ▶ secondary small bowel invasion

- *'Sandwich'/'hamburger' complex:* small bowel encasement by large ill-defined confluent mesenteric lymph nodes
- *Peritoneal disease* (similar to ovarian carcinoma): this occurs late with advanced disease

Large bowel (15%)

- Usually a Burkitt's or MALT lymphoma ▶ usually arises within the caecum or rectum

Barium enema/CT

- **Generalized pattern (common)**
  - Diffuse or segmental small nodules (0.2–2.0 cm) typically with an intact mucosa
  - Ulceration simulates aphthoid ulcers
  - *Advanced disease:* marked colonic or rectal fold thickening ▶ focal strictures ▶ fissures or ulcerative masses with fistula formation
    - A lymphoma stricture > carcinoma stricture
    - Irregular excavation mass suggests lymphoma
- **Localized pattern (less common)**
  - *Solitary polypoid mass:* usually caecal ▶ infiltrating (± a large pericolic mass) ▶ indistinguishable from a carcinoma (terminal ileal involvement is more suggestive of lymphoma)
  - *Annular mass:* smooth and non-obstructing (± aneurysmal dilatation)

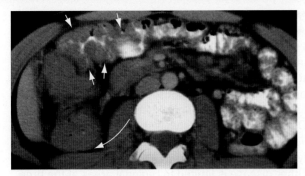

Involvement of large bowel in NHL. CT showing marked and extensive diffuse, uniform thickening of the wall of the transverse colon (arrows). Mesenteric nodes can also be identified. There is also very marked thickening of the wall of the ascending colon (curved arrow) and caecum.*

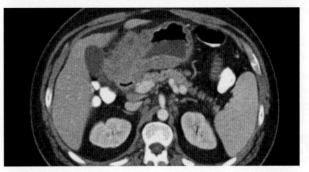

CT of a large non-obstructing gastric lymphoma involving the distal stomach.••

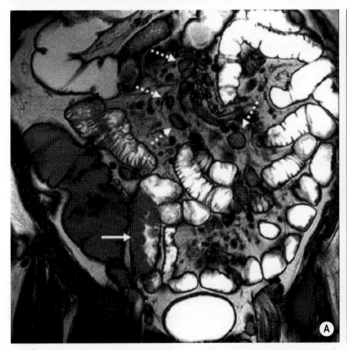

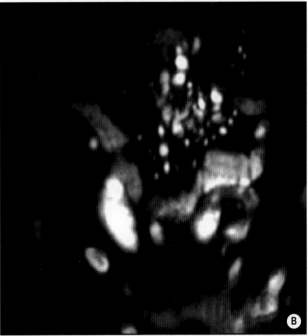

Patient with small intestinal lymphoma. The coronal true FISP image (A) shows significant mural thickening of the terminal ileum (arrow) and multiple, small and large, in size, mesenteric lymph nodes (dotted arrows). (B) DWI with a b-value of 1000 s/mm² renders the lesions with high SI compatible with the presence of a restricted water diffusion pattern due to hypercellularity.*

Staging of GI lymphoma	
CT staging	
Stage I	Tumour confined to bowel wall
Stage II	Regional lymphadenopathy
Stage III	Widespread lymphadenopathy
Stage IV	Spread to bone marrow, liver and other organs

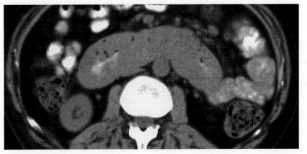

NHL involving the duodenum. Diffuse concentric duodenal wall thickening due to lymphomatous infiltration with prominent lymph nodes in the mesentery and retroperitoneum.*

MUSCULOSKELETAL SYSTEM

- Involvement of the bone, bone marrow and skeletal muscles can occur in both HD and NHL ▶ bone and bone marrow are important sites of disease relapse
- Involvement of osseous bone does not necessarily imply bone marrow involvement (unless it is particularly widespread) ▶ bone scintigraphy has no predictive value in determining marrow involvement

BONE MARROW LYMPHOMA

DEFINITION

- As the bone marrow is an integral part of the reticuloendothelial system, lymphoma may arise within the marrow as a true primary disease (stage IE disease) ▶ more often the marrow is involved as part of a disseminated process (stage IV disease)

NHL

- Marrow involvement is present in 20–40% of patients at presentation and is associated with a poorer prognosis than either liver or lung involvement (bone marrow biopsy is included in the staging of NHL)
- *Low-grade NHL:* there is usually diffuse involvement
- *High-grade NHL:* there is usually focal involvement

HD

- Marrow involvement is rare at presentation but will develop during the course of the disease in 5–15% (thus bone marrow biopsy is not routinely included in the staging of clinical early-stage HD)

RADIOLOGICAL FEATURES

MRI This is very sensitive in detecting bone marrow involvement (upstaging as many as 30% of patients with negative iliac crest biopsies) ▶ a positive study appears to confer a poorer prognosis, regardless of bone marrow biopsy status
- T1WI: low SI ▶ STIR: high SI

FDG-PET This is moderately sensitive for bone marrow involvement at presentation (upstaging a similar proportion of patients as MRI when compared to bone marrow biopsy)

PEARL

MRI/FDG-PET False-negative studies can occur with microscopic infiltration as well as a low-grade lymphoma ▶ diffuse or heterogeneous increased uptake in a pretreatment image may indicate reactive marrow hyperplasia rather than infiltration ▶ both techniques can be used to monitor the effects of treatment (especially where other imaging modalities have failed to demonstrate disease)

PRIMARY BONE LYMPHOMA

DEFINITION

- It is nearly always a non-Hodgkin's B-cell lymphoma (primary Hodgkin's disease is extremely rare) ▶ infiltration of bone can also occur secondary to direct invasion from adjacent soft tissues
- A diagnosis of a primary bone lymphoma requires that:
  - Only a single bone is involved
  - There is unequivocal histological evidence of lymphoma
  - Other disease is limited to regional areas at the time of presentation
  - The primary tumour precedes metastases by at least 6 months

CLINICAL PRESENTATION

- Chronic pain and a palpable mass (33%) ▶ pathological fractures are common (25%)
- The mean age at presentation is 50 years (50% of cases occur between the ages of 10 and 30 years) ▶ there is a slightly biphasic distribution, with peaks at 20 and 50 years ▶ M:F 1.6:1
- Secondary bone involvement affects the axial skeleton more than the appendicular skeleton (affecting 20% of patients with HD and up to 6% of patients with NHL)

Location Lymphoma usually occurs within the appendicular skeleton, affecting the metadiaphyses of the long bones (femur > tibia > humerus) ▶ it can also affect the flat bones (ilium/scapula) and spine

RADIOLOGICAL FEATURES

XR Primary and secondary NHL, HD and other bone tumours (e.g. Ewing's sarcoma) may be indistinguishable ▶ a relative absence of cortical destruction is characteristic
- Other features: transarticular extension, periosteal reaction, reactive sclerosis, sequestra formation
- *NHL:* bone lesions are permeative and osteolytic in 80% of cases (and sclerotic in 4% and mixed in 16% of cases)
- *HD:* this typically gives sclerotic or mixed sclerotic and lytic lesions (86%) ▶ primarily lytic lesions are far less common (14%) ▶ most lesions are found within the skull, spine and femora ▶ ribs: multiple lytic lesions associated with soft tissue masses
  - The classic finding of the sclerotic 'ivory' vertebra

MRI A soft tissue mass is demonstrated with all imaged cases ▶ there is often extensive involvement of the medullary canal ▶ the combination of a large soft tissue mass and relative preservation of the cortex is a well-recognized feature of lymphoma

PEARL

- Anterior mediastinal and paravertebral masses involve the sternum and vertebra, respectively, resulting in scalloping or destruction

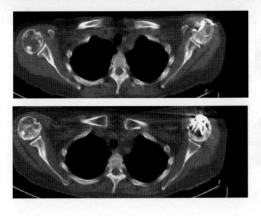

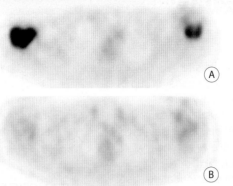

Non-Hodgkin's lymphoma of bone. (A) Axial CT on bone settings at the level of the humeri with corresponding axial PET image. Lymphomatous deposits in both humeral heads are intensely metabolically active. Note the pathological fracture on the right. (B) After successful treatment, there has been complete metabolic resolution.*

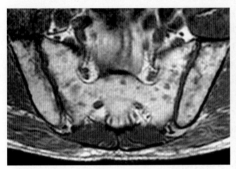

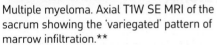

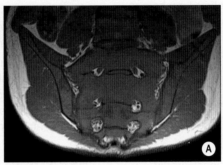

Multiple myeloma. Axial T1W SE MRI of the sacrum showing the 'variegated' pattern of marrow infiltration.**

Primary multifocal osseous lymphoma. (A) Coronal T1W SE and (B) STIR MRI showing diffuse reduction of T1W and increased STIR marrow SI.**

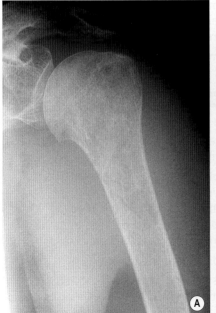

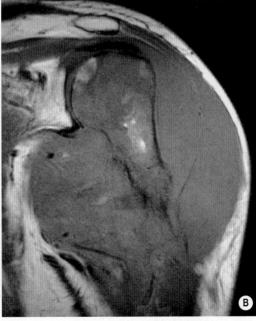

Primary lymphoma of bone. (A) AP XR of the proximal humerus shows a permeative destructive lesion in the metadiaphysis. (B) Coronal T1WI of the proximal humerus shows a large soft tissue extension.*

EXTRANODAL MANIFESTATIONS

GENERAL

- Primary involvement of an extranodal site in 30–40% of NHL cases (involvement limited to a regional group of nodes) ▶ primary extranodal HD is very rare
- Secondary extranodal involvement usually occurs in the presence of widespread advanced disease elsewhere and is an adverse prognostic feature ▶ secondary involvement is more common with NHL
- There is an increased incidence of extranodal disease in children (especially in the GI tract, major abdominal viscera, and extranodal locations within the head and neck) as well as within the immunocompromised
  - Extranodal involvement usually involves lymphomas of a more aggressive histological type
  - *Lymphomas with a propensity to arise within extranodal sites:* mantle cell (a diffuse low-grade B-cell lymphoma) ▶ lymphoblastic lymphomas (80% of which are T-cell) ▶ Burkitt's (small cell non-cleaved) lymphoma ▶ MALT lymphoma

THYMUS

- Primary thymic HD is rare, but thymic involvement is seen with mediastinal adenopathy in 30–50% at presentation
- Mediastinal large B-cell lymphoma characteristically involves the thymus (typically young women between the ages of 25 and 40 years) ▶ rapidly growing bulky disease is typical (up to 40% have SVC obstruction)
- Benign thymic rebound hyperplasia can develop after completion of chemotherapy ▶ this can be difficult to differentiate from recurrent disease with functional imaging - (gallium-67 or FDG-PET) is unable to differentiate

CT Differentiation from enlarged mediastinal lymph nodes can be difficult as the thymus involved by lymphoma usually has a homogeneous soft tissue density or a heterogeneous nodular appearance ▶ thymic involvement usually retains the shape of the normal thymus and has a smooth contour (nodal masses are usually lobulated)

MRI Mixed SI similar to involved nodes ▶ there may occasionally be cysts measuring up to 3 cm in diameter

SPLEEN

HD The spleen is involved in 30–40% at presentation and is usually associated with stage III disease

NHL The spleen is involved in up to 40% at some stage
- Primary splenic NHL is rare (1% of all patients with NHL) ▶ patients present with splenomegaly (which is often marked) ▶ focal masses are usual

CT *Secondary HD:* splenomegaly ▶ focal lesions (10–25%) can be seen if > 1 cm in size
  - ⅓ of patients have splenomegaly without infiltration ▶ ⅓ of normal-sized spleens are found to contain tumour following splenectomy
- *Secondary NHL:* a solitary mass ▶ miliary nodules ▶ multiple masses

FDG-PET This is more accurate than CT

PANCREAS

- *Primary involvement:* pancreatic lymphoma accounts for only 1.3% of all pancreatic malignancies (2% of patients with NHL) ▶ NHL ≫ HD
- *Secondary involvement:* this usually results from direct infiltration from an adjacent nodal mass

CT A solitary mass lesion, usually within the head of the pancreas ± biliary or pancreatic ductal obstruction (mimicking a pancreatic adenocarcinoma) ▶ calcification and necrosis is rare ▶ there is less commonly diffuse uniform enlargement

HEPATIC LYMPHOMA

Definition

- Primary lymphoma of the liver is a rare entity (although the liver is a common secondary site of lymphomatous involvement)

NHL Liver involvement is seen in 15% of adults at presentation (a higher incidence is seen in the paediatric population and with recurrent disease)

HLD Liver involvement is seen in 5% of patients at presentation (almost invariably with splenic involvement)

Radiological features

Primary lymphoma A large multilobulated mass that enhances poorly ▶ central necrosis is frequent ▶ up to 25% of patients are hepatitis B or C positive

Secondary lymphoma Diffusely infiltrative or micronodular involvement (hepatomegaly strongly suggests diffuse infiltration) ▶ larger focal areas of infiltration may demonstrate miliary nodules or larger solitary or multiple masses (resembling metastases)

US hypoechoic and well-defined lesions

CT hypodense masses (pre- and post-contrast administration) ▶ periportal infiltration manifests as periportal low attenuation

MRI T2WI: lesions demonstrate higher SI than surrounding parenchyma

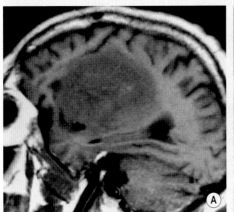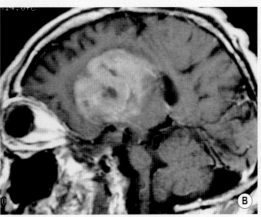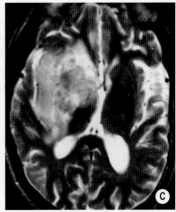

Cerebral non-Hodgkin's lymphoma. (A) T1-weighted sagittal MRI showing a mass of low signal intensity within the right parietal lobe. (B) This enhances intensely following intravenous administration of gadolinium-DTPA and can be seen to be causing marked mass effect with compression of the right lateral ventricle on (C), an axial T2-weighted image.*

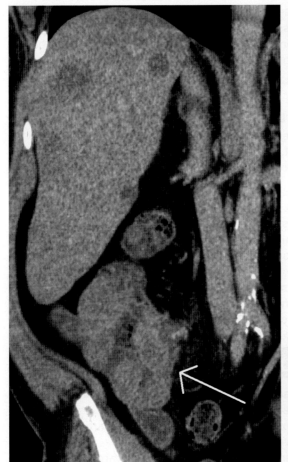

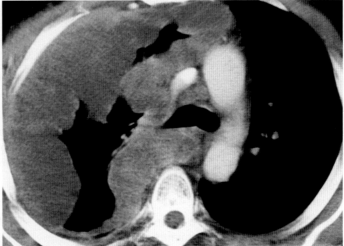

Pleural disease in lymphoma. CT showing a typical appearance of pleural involvement in a patient with NHL. There is a lobulated mass encasing the right hemithorax involving all the pleural surfaces, encasing and narrowing the superior vena cava.*

Lymphomatous infiltration of the liver. There are multiple poorly defined low-density lesions in the liver in this patient with T-cell NHL of the small bowel (arrowed).**

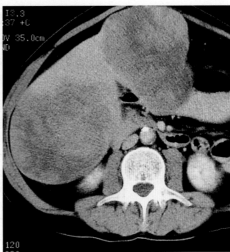

Lymphomatous infiltration of the liver. Transverse US of the liver, showing multiple large hypoechoic lesions corresponding to the large focal masses demonstrated on CECT.*

909

GENITOURINARY TRACT

- A true primary GU lymphoma is rare as there is very little lymphoid tissue present within the GU tract
  - Although the GU is not commonly involved at presentation (<5%), more than half of patients will have involvement at autopsy
  - Testis > kidney and perirenal space > bladder, prostate, uterus, vagina, or ovaries (rare involvement)

Kidney

- Primary lymphoma of the kidney is very rare (as no lymphatic tissue is present within the kidneys) ▶ secondary lymphoma is due to haematogenous spread or contiguous invasion from adjacent retroperitoneal lymphadenopathy ▶ close to 90% of cases are associated with a high-grade NHL
- The commonest pattern is the presence of multiple masses (a solitary renal mass is only seen in 15% and may be indistinguishable from a RCC) ▶ 2nd commonest presentation is direct infiltration of the kidney by contig-uous retroperitoneal nodal masses ▶ in 10% soft tissue masses are seen in the perirenal space (occasionally encasing the kidney without evidence of parenchymal invasion) ▶ diffuse renal infiltration (resulting in global enlargement) is the least common presentation – renal vessel and hilar encasement can mimic TCC
- No retroperitoneal lymph node involvement in >50% of renal masses

US Hypoechoic renal deposits without posterior acoustic enhancement

NECT Well-defined homogeneous iso- or hypo-attentuating masses

CECT A 'density reversal pattern': a lesion is more dense than surrounding renal parenchyma before contrast medium administration and less dense after

MRI T1WI: intermediate SI ▶ T2WI: intermediate-to-low SI ▶ STIR: high SI
- Direct infiltration of the kidney by contiguous retroperitoneal nodal masses is the 2nd commonest presentation ▶ diffuse renal infiltration (resulting in global enlargement) is the least common presentation

Bladder

Primary extranodal involvement
- The bladder is a rare site (< 1% of all bladder tumours), occurring more frequently in women in the 6th decade who often have a history of recurrent cystitis ▶ small cell and MALT lymphomas are seen with a generally good prognosis

IVU/CT Large multilobular submucosal masses with minimal or no mucosal ulceration ▶ transmural spread into adjacent pelvic organs can occur

Secondary lymphoma
- This is seen in 10–15% of patients with lymphoma at autopsy ▶ it is manifest as intrinsic bladder disease or as contiguous spread from adjacent involved nodes ▶ microscopic infiltration more common than gross disease

CT Non-specific appearances indistinguishable from a TCC (diffuse widespread thickening of the bladder wall or a large nodular mass)

Prostate

- Primary lymphoma is extremely rare, with a very poor prognosis (cf. bladder NHL)
- Usually prostatic involvement is secondary to spread from adjacent nodes in the setting of advanced disease
- There is diffuse infiltration with periprostatic spread (solitary nodules are uncommon)

Testis

- This accounts for 5% of primary testicular tumours overall (but 25–50% in patients > 50 years and is the commonest primary tumour in patients > 60 years)
- It is very rare in HD but seen in 1% of NHL patients at presentation ▶ up to 25% of cases are bilateral and relapse can occur within the contralateral testis
- It is associated with lymphoma of Waldeyer's ring, the skin and CNS (staging therefore requires a whole body CT + brain imaging)

US Focal hypoechoic areas or a more diffuse decrease in testicular reflectivity

Female genital tract

- Isolated involvement is rare (1% of extranodal NHL) ▶ 75% of patients are postmenopausal
- Cervix > uterus and vagina > ovary

MRI

- *Cervix / vagina:* a large soft tissue mass ▶ T2WI: high SI
- *Uterus:* diffuse enlargement (often with a lobulated contour mimicking a fibroid) ▶ the mucosa and junctional zone are intact ▶ there is a good prognosis
- *Ovary:* this has a very poor prognosis as it often presents late and disease is frequently bilateral ▶ imaging is similar to an ovarian carcinoma (although haemorrhage, necrosis and calcification is rare)

CARDIAC

- Cardiac involvement may be present with little evidence of disease elsewhere – characteristically it takes the form of diffuse myocardial infiltration (particularly the right ventricular outflow tract)
- Primary and secondary (metastatic) cardiac lymphoma occurs more commonly in immunocompromised patients – patients with HIV typically have an aggressive B-cell lymphoma
  - Primary cardiac lymphoma typically involves the right atrium with pericardial extension (the valves are rarely involved)
- Pericardial effusions are evidence of pericardial involvement

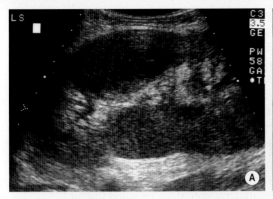

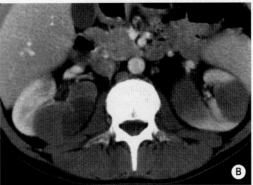

Multiple lymphomatous renal masses. (A) Longitudinal US of the left kidney showing multiple hypoechoic masses. (B) CT in the same patient showing multiple masses, well defined from the normally enhancing adjacent renal parenchyma. Note the absence of retroperitoneal lymph node enlargement.*

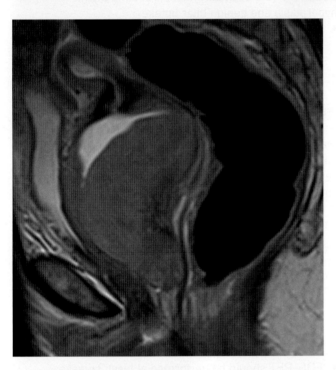

Lymphoma involving the vagina. Sagittal T2-weighted MRI of the patient described in the adjacent figure demonstrates a large intermediate-to-high signal intensity mass, substantially larger than seen usually in a squamous carcinoma of the cervix. Biopsy showed an aggressive B-cell lymphoma.**

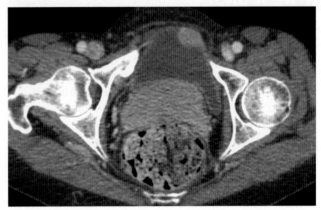

Bladder lymphoma. Contrast-enhanced CT of the pelvis in a female patient showing a polypoid soft-tissue mass arising from the wall of the bladder. There is involvement of the vagina.**

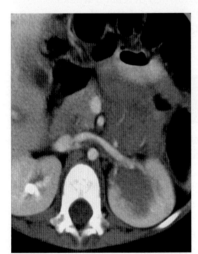

Renal lymphomatous mass (NHL). A left renal mass is seen within the renal pelvis (CECT). The inferior aspect of a large pancreatic mass is also seen.*

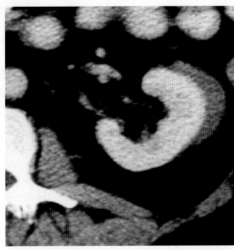

Perirenal lymphoma. CECT showing a mass in the perirenal space.*

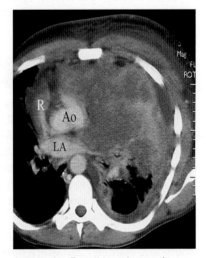

Aggressive B-cell lymphoma. A large heterogeneous soft tissue mass is invading the mediastinum, pericardium, heart, and left pleural space. Ao, aortic root ▶ LA, left atrium ▶ R, right atrial appendage.

MONITORING THE RESPONSE TO THERAPY

DEFINITION

- Achievement of a complete response after treatment is the most important factor for predicting prolonged survival in both HD and NHL
- CT is conventionally used for evaluating treatment response within the neck, chest, abdomen and pelvis
  - The optimal timing of any reassessment varies across centres, with some favouring assessment 1 month after therapy completion, and others favouring an interim reassessment after two cycles of chemotherapy

FDG-PET IN THE MONITORING OF RESPONSE

- FDG-PET gives more prognostic information than CT alone (detecting changes in functional/metabolic activity long before structural changes have occurred)
- FDG-PET performed after one-to-three cycles of chemotherapy predicts the eventual outcome in NHL more accurately than PET at the end of treatment and more accurately than conventional imaging ▶ early FDG-PET may allow a change in therapy
- Recommended that the time from chemotherapy to imaging should be as close as possible to the next cycle to reduce the risk of false-negative results due to 'tumour stunning' ▶ various response criteria have been proposed for interim PET images (including a category of 'minimal residual uptake' – 'MRU', lower or equal to that in the liver)
- Gallium imaging is limited by its lower sensitivity, and that there is a significant proportion of non-gallium-avid tumours

RESIDUAL MASSES

- Successfully treated, enlarged nodes often return to a normal size in both HD and NHL
- However, a 'sterilized' mass of fibrous tissue occurs in up to 85% of patients treated for HD (usually within the mediastinum) and 40% of patients with NHL ▶ this is more frequent in patients with bulky disease and it is uncertain as to whether such residual masses predispose to relapse

CT Residual masses are those that are > 1.5 cm in short-axis diameter, but which have reduced by > 75% of the sum of the products of the greatest diameters of the pre-treatment mass ▶ it cannot distinguish between fibrotic tissue and residual active disease on the basis of density alone ▶ if masses remain static after 1 year they are considered inactive – any increase in size suggests relapse

MRI This may help to differentiate between active tumour and necrosis but may not detect small foci of tumour ▶ false positives occur (especially early after treatment) because of non-specific inflammation and necrosis

- Most tumours have high T2WI SI and this decreases with a response ▶ persistent heterogeneous high SI or recurrent high SI in a residual mass suggests residual or recurrent disease, respectively

Gallium-67 This is a better predictor of disease relapse than CT in both HD and NHL but is difficult to use ▶ false-positive studies can occur with non-specific treatment-related inflammation, rebound thymic hyperplasia and benign hilar uptake

- If no uptake is shown in a residual mass that was previously gallium-avid, this suggests that the mass is fibrotic
- Persistent uptake of gallium-67 in a residual mass (after treatment) is a bad prognostic sign

FDG-PET Gallium-67 has been superseded by FDG-PET ▶ can detect and quantify changes in functional and metabolic activity long before any structural changes have taken place ▶ at the end of treatment, FDG-PET has a very high positive predictive value for early relapse ▶ its specificity, overall accuracy and positive predictive value is much higher than that of CT (and is more sensitive than gallium imaging)

- Its greater sensitivity means that false positives (e.g. due to a pneumonitis or thymic hyperplasia) can be a problem
- FDG-PET predicts for early relapse and false-negative studies do occur with late relapse
- FDG-PET suggested for end of therapy response assessment in DLBCL and HL, but not for other NHL (unless the CR rate is a primary endpoint of a clinical trial)
- FDG-PET should be performed at least 3 weeks (preferably 6–8 weeks) after completion of chemotherapy, and 8–12 weeks after radiation or chemoradiotherapy

SURVEILLANCE AND DETECTION OF RELAPSE

- Relapse after a satisfactory response to initial treatment occurs in 10–40% of patients with HD and > 50% of patients with NHL
  - *HD:* relapse usually occurs within the first 2 years after treatment and patients are followed up closely during this period
  - *Residual masses in HD and NHL:* follow-up depends on the size of the mass, the site of involvement and the extent of disease ▶ a residual mass of fibrous tissue can persist in up to 80% of HL patients (usually within the mediastinum) and 20–60% of NHL patients who are in clinical CR
- Functional imaging can identify early relapse before CT and development of clinical signs

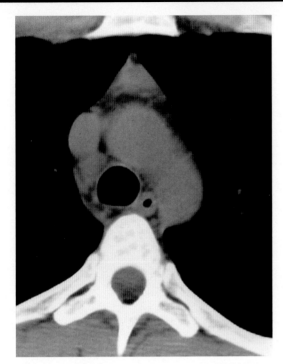

Thoracic residual mass in a patient with HD. After treatment, follow-up CT at 6 months shows a residual right paratracheal mass. Surveillance CTs done several years later have demonstrated the stability of this small mass, consistent with inactive residual disease.*

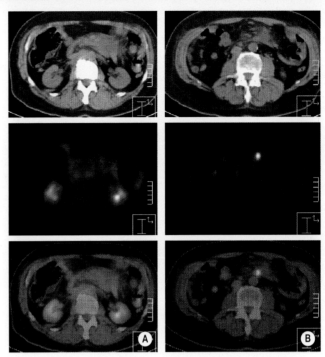

PET in monitoring disease progress. (A) CT, PET and fused PET-CT images demonstrating a large residual mass that is PET negative. (B) At a lower level, there is a small nodule in the inferior part of the mass that is metabolically active, indicating residual disease.*

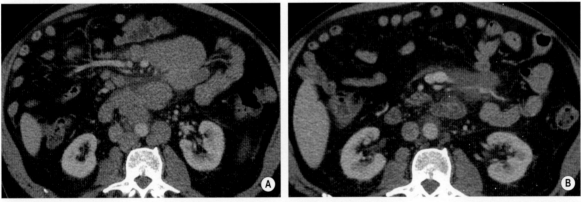

Mesenteric residual mass. (A) Contrast-enhanced CT in a patient with NHL presenting with a large mesenteric nodal mass and bilateral para-aortic nodal disease. (B) Follow-up CT performed 1 year after treatment shows a persistent low-density soft-tissue mass within the mesentery encasing the mesenteric vessels, whilst the retroperitoneal nodal enlargement has resolved.**

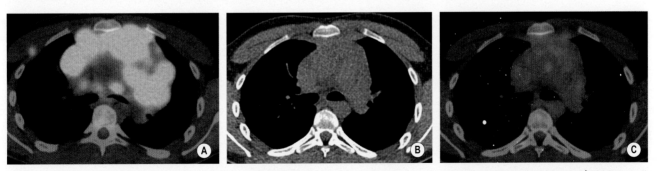

PET in assessment of the residual mass. (A) Fused PET/CT image demonstrating a large metabolically active anterior/middle mediastinal mass and metabolically active but normal-sized right subpectoral lymph node. (B) Post-treatment CT shows a residual anterior mediastinal mass. (C) The mass has normal levels of FDG uptake, identical to that of the remainder of the mediastinum (a metabolic CR by the IHP criteria).**

FUNCTIONAL IMAGING

10.1 FUNCTIONAL IMAGING

POSITRON EMISSION TOMOGRAPHY - CT (PET-CT)

General principles PET imaging is based on the detection of an injected positron-emitting radioactive tracer – PET relies on the co-incidence detection of the annihilation photons (γ) released when a positron combines with an electron; it cannot differentiate individual species that are radiolabelled

- PET has a high sensitivity but low spatial resolution – PET-CT combines cross sectional anatomic information (CT) with metabolic information (PET)
  - FDG (2-[fluorine-18]fluoro-2-deoxy-d-glucose) is a glucose analogue used in oncology imaging which is taken up by metabolically active cells; it undergoes phosphorylation to form FDG-6-phosphate, which unlike glucose, cannot undergo further metabolism and becomes trapped within the cell
  - Malignant cells demonstrate increased glucose metabolism relative to normal tissues

Indications for PET-CT in oncology imaging

- Differentiation of a malignant from a benign lesion (e.g. evaluation of a solitary pulmonary nodule)
- Tumour staging; evaluation of any tumour recurrence:
  - Non-small cell lung carcinoma; lymphoma; melanoma; head and neck cancers; breast cancer; colorectal cancer

Technique Imaging is started 60 minutes following FDG injection; an enhanced whole-body CT study (scan time 60-70 seconds) is followed by whole-body PET imaging (scan time 30-45 minutes)

- A hybrid PET-CT scanner provides co-registered functional (PET) and anatomic (CT) images on the same scanner and without moving the patient

Fasting A patient must be fasted for 4-6 hrs prior to imaging – the resultant low background glucose levels will enhance FDG tumour uptake and also minimize cardiac uptake

- Before injecting FDG, the blood glucose level is measured (it should be < 150 mg/dL); good blood glucose control is essential as FDG uptake is competitively inhibited by glucose (they share a common transport mechanism)

Strenuous activity This must be avoided prior to imaging (and following radioisotope injection) to avoid physiological muscle FDG uptake

- Patient activity and speech is limited for 20 minutes prior to radioisotope injection

Optional Bladder catheterization (or voiding prior to imaging); bowel opacification; IV contrast medium

Image interpretation PET-CT relies on CT transmission data to correct for any inherent attenuation differences

- As PET imaging relies on the emission of photons, the proportion of photons naturally absorbed by different parts of the body needs to be taken into account when assessing the activity from a given source
- PET and CT studies are compared by visual inspection (as well as using fused images); PET is generally not sensitive for lesions <1 cm in size (e.g. a pulmonary nodule)
- *Standardized uptake value (SUV)*: this is a semi-quantitative assessment of the radiotracer uptake from a static PET image; malignant tumours typically have a SUV > 2.5-3

$$SUV = \frac{\text{Activity per unit mass of tissue}}{\text{Injected activity per unit body mass}}$$

Limitations and artifacts of PET-CT

Motion artefact This will affect the co-registration of the CT and PET studies; it can be due to patient motion, respiration, cardiac or bowel motion

Attenuation (transmission) correction artifacts These may occur where there are highly attenuating objects within the path of the CT beam

- Correction software normally corrects for photon absorption by using the CT transmission data and adjusting accordingly; it may 'overcorrect' a photopaenic area next to a high attenuating structure giving it a falsely elevated SUV on the corrected images (unlike a true lesion, this will remain photopaenic on the uncorrected image)

Physiological muscle uptake No corresponding mass lesion will be seen on CT; this uptake also usually appears symmetric and diffuse on PET imaging

Differentiating physiological from pathological uptake

As well as identifying areas of neoplasia, FDG will accumulate within various normal organs

Sites of physiological FDG uptake

- *Brain* (it is exclusively dependent on glucose metabolism): cerebral cortex; basal ganglia; thalamus; cerebellum
- *Myocardium:* this relies on a mixture of glucose and free fatty acid metabolism
- *Skeletal muscle:* particularly following exercise and hyperventilation; with tension (cervical muscle contraction); with speaking (affecting the laryngeal muscles)
- *GI tract:* stomach; small intestine; colon; distal oesophagus (particularly with reflux)
- *GU tract:* FDG is not reabsorbed by the renal tubules and therefore collects within the renal collecting system
- *Brown adipose tissue:* symmetric uptake is seen within the brown adipose tissues of the supraclavicular, mid-axillary, and paraspinal regions; this can mimic pathological uptake
  - The normal function of brown fat is to generate heat (rather than ATP)
  - Precise correlation with the CT images will identify normal anatomical structures
  - Beta blockers or diazepam may be helpful in reducing erroneous uptake
- *Salivary glands:* low to moderate uptake; uptake can also be seen within the parotid gland and the lymphatic tissues of Waldeyer's ring

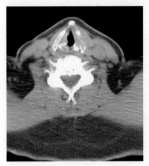 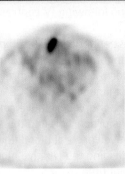 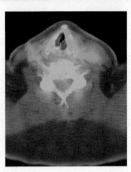

Paralysed vocal cord artefact on PET imaging. CT, PET and PET–CT images reveal unilateral uptake within the neck, localizing to the right vocal cord. The left vocal cord was found to be paralysed. This uptake could be confused with a lymph node metastasis or a head and neck carcinoma if CT correlation is not used.[§§]

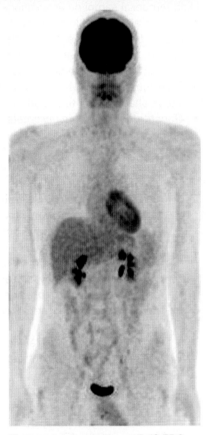

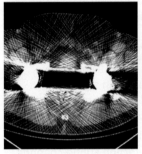 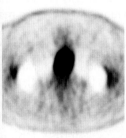 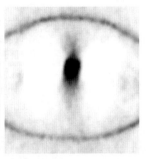

Metal artefact. Axial CT and PET images show beam-hardening artefact on CT (left) from bilateral hip prostheses. The attenuation corrected PET image (middle) shows artifactually increased uptake along the lateral margins of the prostheses, which is significantly decreased on non-attenuation corrected images (right).[§§]

The normal distribution of F-18 FDG: uptake is normally intense within the brain and urinary tract, moderately intense within the liver, and variable within the muscles, heart and bowel.[§§]

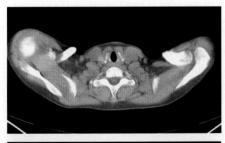 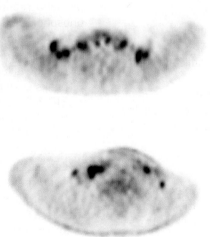 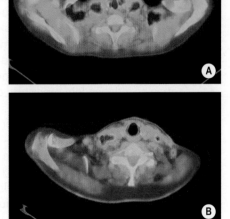

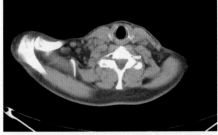

FDG PET appearance of 'brown fat' activity. (A) Abnormal supraclavicular uptake localizes to the fat on fused images. (B) Lymphoma involvement within the supraclavicular region can appear similar to brown fat uptake, but fused images localize the activity to involved lymph nodes.[§§]

Dynamic contrast enhanced CT (DCE-CT) *Perfusion CT:*
High temporal sampling acquisitions over a large volume

- Temporal changes in attenuation can be modelled to assess tissue vascularity; the situation is more complex for MRI (complex relationship between MR signal intensity and local tissue contrast concentration)
- *Semi-quantitative functional parameters:* describing the 'curve shape' of the tissue attenuation time graph
- *Quantitative functional parameters:* derived from kinetic modelling
- **Parameters:**
  - *Regional tumour blood flow:* blood flow per unit volume or unit mass of tissue
  - *Regional tumour blood volume:* proportion of tissue that compromises flowing blood
  - *Mean transit time:* average time for contrast to traverse the tissue vasculature
  - *Extraction fraction:* rate of transfer of contrast material from the intravascular space to the EES
  - *Permeability – surface area product:* characterises the rate of diffusion from the intravascular compartment to the EES
  - K^{trans}: Baseline volume transfer constant – the volume transfer coefficient of contrast between the blood plasma and the EES
    - Elevation is controversial in terms of prognosis; may be used to demonstrate which tumours are responding to therapy (e.g. anti-angiogenic drugs)
  - Changes in DCE-CT parameters reflect microvascular changes during angiogenesis; DCE-CT may distinguish between benign and malignant lesions (although there is some overlap between malignant and inflammatory lesions); higher perfusion parameters are reported in malignant lesions (although there can be variability between different tumours and within the same tumour type); DCE-CT can be used in the assessment of anti-vascular effects of chemotherapy and interventional procedures targeting the vasculature
  - DCE-CT can also have a role in risk stratification and as a predictive biomarker of treatment:
    - *Squamous cell carcinoma of the head:* pre-treatment primary blood flow and permeability may be independent predictors of disease recurrence
    - *Pancreatic cancer:* a low K^{trans} predicts a poorer response to treatment
    - *Colorectal cancer:* tumours with a low blood flow at staging are more likely to have nodal metastases
    - *Rectal tumours:* a lower blood flow are likely to respond poorly to chemoradiation

Dynamic contrast enhanced MRI (DCE-MRI) Serial MRI acquisitions following IV contrast agent in a similar manner to DCE-CT

- Contrast enhanced MRI can provide a qualitative snapshot of tissue enhancement, or more quantitatively in the form of DCE-MRI (providing a fuller description of contrast kinetics as for DCE-CT
  - *Neuroimaging:* relative cerebral blood volume (rCBV): this is proportional to the area under the curve; relative cerebral blood flow (rCBF) can be estimated by dividing the relative blood volume by the mean transit time
  - *Other measurements:* arrival time (T_0); time to peak (Tp); mean transit time (MTT); the rCBF can be estimated by dividing the relative blood volume by the mean transit time
- DCE-MRI reproducibility may be less between centres (differences in hardware and scanning protocols); MR signal is not directly proportional to contrast agent concentration and therefore more complex quantitative date analysis is required

Dynamic susceptibility contrast MRI (DSC-MRI) DSC-MRI measures induced alterations in the transverse relaxation times (T2 and T2*), resulting in signal loss (acting as a negative contrast); its application for extracerebral tumours is under investigation

MR spectroscopy (MRS) MRS allows the measurement of several tissue metabolites by detecting subtle changes in the nuclear resonance frequently exerted by the atomic structure of the constituent molecule (for example hydrogen nuclei in water have a different resonant frequency than in fat); multiple metabolites can be simultaneously assessed

- Common metabolites that can be assessed: choline containing molecules (Cho) / creatine (Cr) / phosphocreatine (PCr) / N-acetylaspartate (NAA) / phosphorus-31 (^{31}P) / lactate
  - NAA predominantly found in neurones (loss can be seen in stroke or tumour)
  - Choline is found in cell membranes, with increased peaks seen in tumours
  - 31P-MRS can detect cellular ATP levels – tumours tend to demonstrate elevated levels (this can be used as a marker for tumour aggressiveness and assess response to therapy)
  - Lactate can be found in areas of abnormality
- Measurement of the frequency shift of a peak relative to a standard (e.g. water) allows a molecule to be identified
- The area under the curve of the peak gives an indication of the molecule concentration
- An example of a high grade neurological malignancy:
  - A high Cho/Cr ration of 2:1 (normal ratio is 1)
  - Decreased NAA (neuronal loss)
  - High lactate (necrosis)

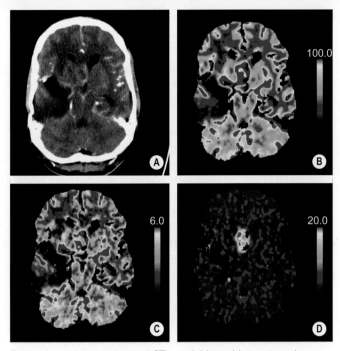

Dynamic contrast-enhanced CT acquisition with parametric maps from a glioblastoma multiforme tumour. (A) Contrast-enhanced CT, (B) regional blood flow, (C) blood volume and (D) permeability–surface area product. The images demonstrate a vascular solid component with disruption of the blood–brain barrier best seen on the permeability–surface area product map.**

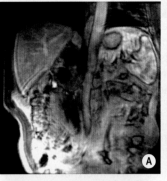
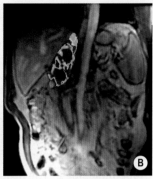
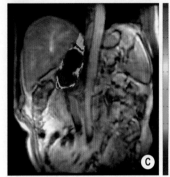

Example parameter maps for a renal cell carcinoma metastasis. (A) Image from a dynamic contrast-enhanced acquisition, (B) initial area under the gadolinium curve (over 90 s; IAUGC90) map before treatment, (C) IAUGC90 map 48 h after treatment with an anti-angiogenic agent (bevacizumab), showing decrease in the tumour perfusion with colour scale.** (Images courtesy of Andrew Gill, Dr Andrew Priest, Professor Duncan Jodrell and Professor Tim Eisen, Addenbrooke's Hospital, Cambridge.)

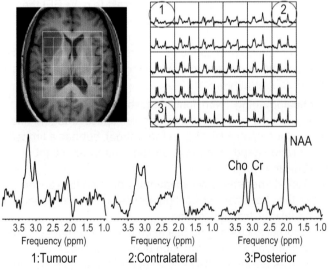

1:Tumour   2:Contralateral   3:Posterior

Example of magnetic resonance spectroscopy (MRS) in a patient with a brain tumour. Localised spectroscopy has been acquired from a patient with a low-grade glioma. Three voxels have been enlarged to include: (1) tumour; (2) normal contralateral brain; and (3) normal ipsilateral brain. Common metabolites identified are: choline-containing molecules (Cho); creatine (Cr); and N-acetylaspartate (NAA). NAA is present predominately in neurons and loss of NAA is associated with neuronal damage. The glioma demonstrates low levels of NAA and a Cho peak which is larger relative to the Cr peak.** (Images courtesy of Dr Mary McLean, Cancer Research UK, Cambridge Institute.)

Most common pharmacokinetic parameters used in DCE-MRI analysis[32,40]		
Parameter (units)	**Alternative nomenclature**	**Definition**
K^{trans} (min^{-1})	EF, K^{PS}	Volume transfer constant between blood plasma and EES
v_e (a.u.)	Interstitial space	EES volume per unit tissue volume
v_p (a.u.)		Blood plasma volume per unit tissue volume
k_{ep} (min^{-1})	k_{21}	Rate constant from EES to blood plasma $k_{ep} = K^{trans} / v_e$
k_{pe} (min^{-1})	k_{12}	Rate constant from blood plasma to EES
k_{el} (min^{-1})		Elimination rate constant
Amp (a.u.)	A	Amplitude of the normalised dynamic curve

Adapted from Yang et al.[40] and Tofts et al.[32]; a.u., arbitrary units.
[32] Tofts PS, Brix G, Buckley DL, et al. Estimating kinetic parameters from dynamic contrast-enhanced T(1)-weighted MRI of a diffusable tracer: standardized quantities and symbols. J Magn Reson Imaging 1999;10(3):223–32.
[40] Yang X, Knopp MV. Quantifying tumor vascular heterogeneity with dynamic contrast-enhanced magnetic resonance imaging: a review. J Biomed Biotechnol 2011;2011:732848.

Diffusion weighted imaging (DWI) This exploits the presence of random (Brownian) motion of water molecules in order to generate image contrast

- DWI can detect, characterise and stage tumours, predict and monitor response to therapy, and evaluate for tumour recurrence; whole body DWI is a future application
- It relies on modification of a standard T2WI sequence: a pair of diffusion sensitizing gradients are applied symmetrically around a 180° refocusing RF pulse

Static molecules The acquired phase information after the 1st pulse is completely reversed by a 2nd pulse with no change in measured signal intensity

Mobile molecules Movement results in the acquisition of phase shifts between molecules after the 1st pulse which will not be completely rephrased by the 2nd pulse – this results in signal loss (with signal loss proportional to the degree of microscopic motion that occurs during the pulse sequence)

- DWI: stationary water molecules appear much brighter than areas with higher molecular diffusion
- **'b-value':** the degree of phase shift or signal loss depends upon the strength and duration of the diffusion sensitizing gradient – this is expressed by the 'b-value'; molecules that do not easily diffuse will only demonstrate signal loss with high b-values
- Quantitative analysis of the apparent diffusion coefficient (ADC) requires sequences with at least two different b-values; there is increased signal loss within the more cystic components with higher b-values (relative to the more cellular components that demonstrate reduced diffusion)
  - For an individual pixel, the slope of the line plotted for the logarithm of the relative signal intensity of the tissue (y-axis) vs. the b-values applied (x-axis) describes the ADC
  - All the pixel data can be combined to visually produce an **'ADC map'**
  - Areas with a decreased ADC appear dark on ADC maps (this is converse to DWI where areas of decreased diffusion appear bright)
- *Qualitative assessment:* relative DWI changes compared with surrounding tissue
- *Quantitative assessment:* by calculation of the apparent diffusion coefficient (ADC) – this is calculated from the slope of the relative SI (on a log scale) against a series of *b*-values
- **'T2-shine through':** areas with a naturally high background T2WI signal intensity may retain high signal on DWI and be mistaken for restricted diffusion (this can be reduced to some extent by using a high b-value)

Diffusion tension imaging (DTI) This characterizes the anisotropy that is seen within the brain on a pixel-by-pixel basis; it allows for the mapping of the white matter tracts

- Diffusion in the brain is directionally dependent (or anisotropic) – this is particularly prominent in compacted white matter tracts and least evident within grey matter

Functional magnetic resonance imaging (fMRI) This measures the tiny increase in signal intensity on T2*WI during neuronal activation and is used to study cortical activation

- During cortical activation there is an increased rCBF and increased oxygen delivery to the activated brain (with a net increase in oxyhaemoglobin concentration); as oxyhaemoglobin is diamagnetic whilst deoxyhaemoglobin is paramagnetic this results in a tiny increase in MR signal (the so called blood oxygenation level dependent or BOLD effect)
- **Major advantages of fMRI over PET:** there is a lack of ionizing radiation and higher temporal resolution
- **fMRI disadvantages:** there is inferior time resolution compared with EEG (due to the haemodynamic response time); the magnitude of the MR signal change is not directly proportional to the rCBF change (therefore absolute quantification is not possible - although relative changes may be more important during activation tasks)

Emerging techniques

Ultrasound Microbubbles with a gaseous central core are injected IV; local application of a resonant frequency ultrasound pulse causes the bubbles to burst significantly enhancing the ultrasound signal giving an enhanced image of the vascular space; if these bubbles are conjugated to a targeted probe for a protein of interest (e.g. VEGF) the subsequent burst gives an idea of the distribution of the protein of interest; a developing technique is the use of drug containing microbubbles, where the microbubbles are burst within an area of interest giving high concentrations where it is required

Optical imaging Non-ionising technology using light to probe cellular and molecular function; optical imaging has a very high spatial resolution (nm range), but has a limited penetration depth due to the strong scattering of light in biological tissues

- Optical spectroscopy can identify and monitor cancer as the characteristics of light emission change during neoplastic transformation
- Fluorescence imaging has been used for tumour margin delineation and identification of involved nodes, as well as during Gl / GU endoscopic screening for occult dysplastic lesions
- Raman spectroscopy: if monochromatic laser light is directed at a molecule, some of the photons will scatter and lose energy (Raman effect) – the molecular structure and composition of any material is encoded as a set of frequency shifts in the Raman scattered light (giving it a spectral unique signature)

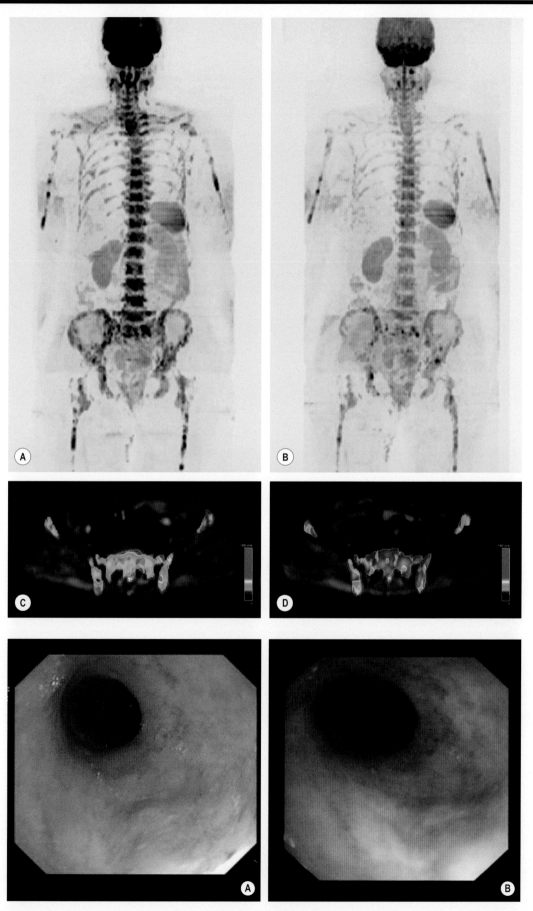

Example of whole-body diffusion-weighted imaging. Serial changes in a 64-year-old woman with metastatic breast cancer treated with chemotherapy and bisphosphonates. (A) Inverted 3D maximum intensity projection (MIP) diffusion-weighted images showing widespread metastatic bone disease; (B) there is a subsequent decrease in the restricted diffusion and disease extent following treatment. (C) Colour ADC map of the pelvis in the same patient before treatment; (D) after treatment there is an increase in ADC, demonstrated by the colour change, indicating a response to treatment.** (Images courtesy of Professor Anwar Padhani, Mount Vernon Cancer Centre, Northwood, Middlesex.)

Example of a clinical application of optical imaging: the detection of Barrett's oesophagus on endoscopy. (A) The Barrett's lesion is inconspicuous on standard white-light imaging; (B) autofluorescent imaging shows an abnormal purple area with normal surrounding green tissue; the abnormal area was confirmed histologically as low-grade dysplasia. Autofluorescence imaging is based on the detection of fluorescence emitted by endogenous molecules within tissue; changes in these molecules between normal and abnormal tissue can be exploited for the detection of dysplastic tissue that would otherwise be difficult to detect.** (Images courtesy of Dr Rebecca Fitzgerald, Addenbrooke's Hospital, Cambridge.)

INTERVENTIONAL RADIOLOGY

CATHETER ANGIOGRAPHY

VASCULAR ACCESS

Contraindications Very few absolute contra-indications – caution with patients on anticoagulants / systemic hypertension / prolonged steroid treatment / connective tissue disorders

The right common femoral arterial approach is preferred (other sites include the axillary, brachial or radial artery) this allows good access with well defined puncture landmarks and a low complication rate

- *Arterial puncture technique:* can use a single (anterior artery wall) or double puncture (anterior and posterior arterial walls) technique, followed by guidewire insertion and then exchange with dilators / catheters, and a heparinized saline flush injection ▶ the most common problem with antegrade femoral artery puncture is catheterisation of the profunda femoris
- *Landmarks for a fluoroscopic guided puncture:* the skin entry point is at the inferior margin of the femoral head ▶ the arterial entry point is at the mid-femoral head level ▶ puncture is usually achieved under direct US guidance
  - *Puncturing too high (above the inguinal ligament):* this increases the risk of bleeding and also means that direct pressure to maintain haemostasis is difficult
  - *Puncturing too low (e.g. into the superficial femoral artery):* this increases the risk of false aneurysm and arteriovenous fistula formation
- The guidewire should never be advanced without fluoroscopic guidance and never against resistance

Potential complications

- *Haemorrhage:* retroperitoneal bleeding may occur if the puncture site is above the inguinal ligament – it can also occur if a normal puncture penetrates the femoral sheath (downward extension of pelvic fascia around the femoral vessels, allowing bleeding to enter the retroperitoneum / abdominal wall) ▶ peritoneal bleeding occasionally with punctures above the inguinal ligament
- *Local vascular complications:* late stenosis or occlusion ▶ local sepsis / local nerve damage
  - *False aneurysm formation:* this occurs where there has been inadequate haemostasis and is more likely to occur with a low CFA puncture where the artery cannot be compressed against the femoral head ▶ the treatment options include US guided compression, thrombin injection and surgical repair
  - *Arteriovenous fistula formation:* this is uncommon with a CFA puncture but is more likely with a SFA puncture (as the femoral vein lies deep to it)

- *Thrombosis:* due to severe vessel trauma during puncture or thrombus wiped off the outside of the arterial catheter during extraction acts as a nidus ▶ this is more likely if the artery is severely diseased at the puncture site
- *Arterial dissection following angioplasty:* this usually occurs with an antegrade approach ▶ retrograde dissections are usually self limiting
- *Distal microembolization:* this follows thrombus or atheroma breaking off from the vessel wall
- *Perivascular contrast injection:* pain ▶ possible to dissect and occlude a vessel with a subintimal injection
- *Catheter complications:* thrombi in or on a catheter and entering the vascular system ▶ vascular injuries (commonly dissection of the tunica intima forming a flap that can occlude a vessel) ▶ organ injuries (following ischaemia during arteriographic procedures) ▶ guidewire fracture

Vascular sheath

- This provides an atraumatic access route (e.g. preventing the wings of a deflated angioplasty balloon creating an arteriotomy as it is removed)
  - It consists of a hollow tube connected to a haemostatic valve (through which catheters are inserted) and a side arm for flushing

Haemostasis As well as direct pressure applied to the puncture site, other alternatives are available:

- **Suture mediated closure devices** (e.g. Perclose): the technique relies on a complex mechanism whereby 2 needles pass through the vessel wall adjacent to the puncture site and then retrieve a suture loop ▶ the suture loop is then pulled through and out of the skin (it closes the puncture site as it is tightened and a slipknot is formed)
  - It allows immediate haemostasis and repuncture (if required)
- **Collagen plug and anchor** (e.g. Angioseal): a collagen footplate is deployed within the arterial lumen ▶ this is attached to an anchor on the external side of the arterial lumen (this has collagen wadding which forms a plug at the puncture site) ▶ the collagen footplate dissolves after approximately 10 weeks
  - Unlike the suture mediated method a repuncture should not happen within 3 months as there is a risk of dislodging the anchor plate

CATHETERS

- High flow catheters with end and side holes are used for central vessels (e.g. the aorta) ▶ low flow catheters with end holes only are used for selective arterial catheterization

Catheter outer diameter This determines the catheter size
- *'French' (Fr) size:* the outer circumference in millimeters (the French size divided by 3 gives the approximate outer diameter)

Catheter inner diameter this is measured in 1/1000 of an inch

Catheter length This is commonly 65 cm (abdominal work) or 100 cm (aortic arch and carotid work)

Non selective catheters
- *Pigtail catheter:* this is used within the aorta ▶ it has a large endhole and smaller sideholes with a pigtail loop and measures approximately 15 mm in diameter

Selective catheters
- *Cobra:* visceral and peripheral angiography
- *Sidewinder:* visceral and aortic arch angiography
- *Berenstein:* this has an endhole only and an angled tip ▶ it is useful for anterior aortic arch vessels
- *Headhunter:* this has a forward facing primary curve (± sideholes) ▶ it is used for head and neck vessels

Microcatheters Coaxial catheters (2-3Fr) that can catheterize small vessels

Guide catheters large caliber (7-9Fr) catheters providing a safe conduit from the arterial puncture site to the target vessel ostium

	Endhole catheters	Sidehole catheters
Advantages	These can be used for embolization	These can be used for pump injection runs (the multiple sideholes can deliver a fast flow rate)
Disadvantages	Pump injections can be hazardous (as the high pressures generated through a single endhole can displace the catheter)	These cannot be used for embolization (due to an unpredictable flow of embolic material through the sideholes)

GUIDEWIRES

Steerable
- **Hydrophilic guidewires** (Terumo, Road-runner): these have a hydrophilic coating and must be kept wet – their frictionless nature allows them to cross narrow stenoses

Non steerable
- **3 mm J guidewire:** this has a 3 mm radius to its distal curve – 5, 10 and 15 mm curves are also available
- **Bentson wire:** this has a very floppy atraumatic tip
- **Amplatz super stiff:** this is a very strong wire (again with a floppy tip) that is strong enough to provide support for introducing stents

Outer diameter This is measured in 1/1000 of an inch (0.018 to 0.038)

Length 140 cm (standard length), but can be up to 260 cm (e.g. if working in the upper limb from the groin)

ANGIOPLASTY

Definition
- a balloon catheter can be used for the treatment of a vascular stenosis or occlusion ▶ the inflated balloon fractures the wall intima and any atherosclerotic plaque as well as stretching the muscular media ▶ healing is by intimal hyperplasia over a period of weeks (which restores the smooth intimal surface)

Technique
- The balloon catheter is advanced to the site of the lesion and then inflated for a short period of time (a wire must always remain across the lesion) ▶ an inflation handle with a pressure gauge ensures that the balloon is used at the correct pressure ▶ a post deflation angiogram is required
  - A residual stenosis of < 30% is the aim and there must also be adequate run off ▶ most angioplasty sites will demonstrate a minor dissection flap that is only significant if it impedes distal flow
  - *Good prognostic indicators:* proximal lesions within large vessels ▶ stenoses (vs. occlusions) ▶ short lesions ▶ focal disease ▶ a good inflow and outflow
- The diameter of the arterial segment immediately adjacent to the lesion should guide the balloon size:

Aorta	10–15 mm
Common iliac	8 mm
External iliac	7 mm
CFA and proximal SFA	6 mm
Distal SFA	5 mm
Popliteal	4 mm

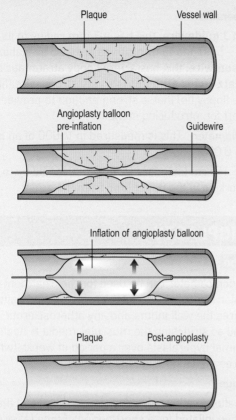

- Angioplasty catheters can range between 2 and 25 mm in diameter (with lengths between 60 and 120 cm) ▶ some even have razor blades within their walls
- If a balloon ruptures they are designed to tear longitudinally (a circumferential tear makes extraction through the sheath difficult)

Specific vessels

- **Aorta:** angioplasty is ideal for focal infrarenal stenoses ▶ stents are reserved for recurrent stenoses and heavily calcified vessels
- **Iliac arteries:** there are reduced angioplasty patency rates for occlusions, heavily calcified lesions and stenotic disease that is > 10 cm in length (stenting should then be considered) ▶ complications are more frequent with occlusions than stenoses and for lesions affecting the external iliac vessels
- **CFA:** lesions are often treated by surgical endarterectomy (due to their superficial location)
- **SFA:** poorer angioplasty results are obtained for stenoses or occlusions > 10 cm in length ▶ stents are reserved for 'bail out' procedures
- **Popliteal artery:** stents are to be avoided (due to repeated flexion)
- **Renal artery:** the majority of stenoses are due to atherosclerosis affecting the proximal or ostial arterial segments (with the poorest angioplasty success rates) ▶ fibromuscular dysplasia can affect any renal arterial segment (with a characteristic 'beaded' appearance) and has the highest angioplasty success rates
  - Ostial lesions can also be treated with primary stenting

STENTING

Definition

- a metallic mesh tube placed cross a vascular stenosis or occlusion
  - *Primary stenting*: iliac arterial occlusions are often treated in this way to reduce any distal embolization
  - *Secondary stenting*: this is used for salvage of an unsuccessful procedure (e.g. a failed angioplasty)

Balloon expandable endoprostheses

- These are usually made of stainless steel and are mounted on a balloon catheter and deployed by inflating the balloon ▶ they allow precise placement but are less flexible ▶ they have a high radial strength (which is advantageous in calcified lesions) ▶ there is usually some minor shortening during deployment ▶ stents are often oversized by 1 mm to ensure secure fixation

Self-expanding stents (e.g. Wallstent)

- These are compressed on a delivery catheter and released by withdrawing an outer sheath (they expand by their own radial force) ▶ placement is less precise but their flexible nature allows placement within tortuous vessels (they are better at conforming to the vessel wall)

Stent grafts

- covered stents reline a vessel and can treat a rupture, exclude an aneurysm, or treat a rupture occurring during angioplasty ▶ the stent covering can be either Dacron (polyester) or PTFE (polytetrafluorethylene)

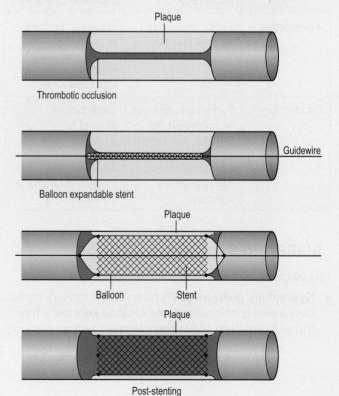

Post-stenting

EMBOLIZATION

Definition Occlusion of a blood vessel by injection of embolic material through a percutaneously passed catheter ▶ it will cause infarction if it involves a distal vessel (proximal occlusion may not compromise any collateral flow)

- It may be a definitive treatment (for non-malignant lesions) or may be used pre-operatively to reduce blood loss and alleviate symptoms
- *Common indications:* visceral haemorrhage from the GI tract or kidneys ▶ arteriovenous malformations ▶ preoperative devascularization ▶ as an adjunct to another interventional procedure (e.g. internal iliac artery embolization prior to an aortic stent graft insertion)

Embolic agents The choice of embolic agent depends on the anatomical site, nature of the lesion, and operator preference.

Temporary particulate emboli

- These can be used to control haemorrhage when recanalization of the parent vessel may be desirable once the 'acute' lesion has healed
- *Autologous blood clot:* this is rarely used as it only induces a temporary occlusion
- *Gelofoam:* this dissolves after a few weeks ▶ it is formed from a sheet which is cut into pledgets 1–2 mm in size and injected via a catheter

Permanent particulate emboli (e.g. for benign or malignant tumours)

- Used for benign and malignant tumours ▶ may be used in combination with chemotherapeutic agents (drug eluting beads) in hepatic chemoembolisation
- *Coils:* these cause blockage via intimal damage (generating thrombogenic agents), by providing a large thrombogenic surface, and by direct physical blockage ▶ most are made of stainless steel or platinum with fibres attached to promote thrombosis
  - Coils are used in situations analogous to the surgical tying of a vessel ▶ a knowledge of the vascular anatomy is important to avoid retrograde filling from any collateral vessels (it is therefore best used for end arteries) ▶ it is useful for packing a pseudoaneurysm lumen and can also be placed across a pseudoaneurysm neck to prevent 'front and back door' blood entry
  - *Technique:* a coil is pushed through a catheter (using a 'pusher' device) and when extruded at the distal catheter end will coil into its predetermined shape ▶ coils should be packed tightly together (requiring correct sizing) and the catheter should be slightly withdrawn with each coil placement
- **Polyvinyl alcohol:** particles (150-1500 μm) are suspended in contrast medium (as they themselves are not radio-opaque) and injected through a catheter to the site of the lesion where it will silt up the blood supply and cause an occlusion
- **Liquid embolic agents:** these include sclerosants such as absolute alcohol, sodium tetradecyl sulphate (STD), glue (e.g. n-butyl-2-cyanoacylate) and newer agents such as Onyx ▶ they can be particularly difficult to control ▶ not uncommon for the agent to be infused over 24–48h ▶ they are useful for venous embolization (e.g. varicoceles) ▶ glue-like materials are useful for arteriovenous malformations

THROMBOLYSIS

DEFINITION

- Blood clot dissolution within an artery or vein by injection or infusion of a thrombolytic drug directly into a thrombus (via a percutaneous catheter) ▶ it can also be used to treat graft thromboses
  - Infusion usually occurs over 24–48h with a periodic check angiogram to assess progress
- Urokinase and r-tPA (expensive) can be used as thrombolytic agents (requiring close monitoring) – revascularization of a non viable limb may cause renal failure or cardiovascular collapse due to release of toxic metabolites
- Usually a successful thrombus clearance reveals an underlying causative lesion (which should be treated by angioplasty or stenting during the same procedure)

MULTIDETECTOR CT ANGIOGRAPHY (MDCTA)

- Rapid IV injection of contrast (3-5 mL/s) ▶ automated contrast bolus detection techniques: the 'arrival of contrast medium is measured within a vessel at a single level, and data acquisition initiated when a certain density threshold is reached
  - *Multiplanar reconstruction (MPR):* useful for the rapid review of blood vessels in any plane (and assessment of vessel walls that might be obscured in MIP and VR techniques ▶ curved MPR allows tortuous vessels to be 'straightened'
  - *Maximum Intensity Projection (MIP):* produces a planar image from a volume of data within which the pixel values are determined by the highest voxel value in a ray projected along the data set in a specified direction ▶ mimics a conventional arteriogram ▶ however tissue of high density (e.g. bone) will be reprojected in the final image and may misrepresent a blood vessel
  - *Volume Rendering Techniques (VR):* assesses the entire volume of data with an attenuation threshold for display producing a 3D image (final images can be rotated) ▶ vascular stenosis can be overestimated
- Preferred for vascular aneurysm assessment over MRA as more sensitive for detecting wall calcification

MAGNETIC RESONANCE ANGIOGRAPHY (MRA)

Unenhanced time-of-flight (TOF) MRA

- This utilizes differences in magnetization with a very short time to repetition (TR) – contrast is provided between stationary background spins and inflowing, fresh blood ▶ gradient-echo sequences (with high T1 weighting) are often used ▶ it can be acquired at a very short TR (maximizing the TOF contrast)
  - *Stationary spins:* these are repeatedly exposed to the excitation pulse ▶ due to the short TR there is not enough time for their longitudinal magnetization to return to equilibrium ▶ they therefore become saturated, with a lack of magnetization with which to form a signal
  - *Inflowing blood:* as flowing blood enters the area being imaged it has undergone a limited number of excitation pulses so it is not saturated, giving it a much higher signal than saturated stationary tissue – therefore areas with slow flow (such as large aneurysms) may not be well visualized ▶ an oblique course of a blood vessel being imaged in relation to the slice orientation may also result in poor visualization
- Data is acquired perpendicular to the expected flow direction ▶ the TR must be sufficiently long to allow an adequate 'inflow' of fully relaxed protons into the imaging slice (the TR is therefore dictated by the expected flow rates)
  - *Selective arteriogram:* this employs a saturation pulse placed downstream of the imaging slice (eliminating venous return from the opposite direction)
  - *Selective venogram:* the saturation pulse is upstream of the imaging slice (eliminating arterial signal)
- Severity and length of stenosis may be overestimated due to intravoxel dephasing secondary to turbulent or slow flow (unlike CEMRA) – as a result has not had a major impact on clinical practice outside of the brain (TOF MRA remains the technique of choice for depicting intracranial arteries)
- *Carotid artery stenosis:* intramural calcification does not interfere with stenosis grading (unlike in CTA)

Contrast enhanced MRA (CEMRA)

- Intravascular signal depends on T1 shortening induced by injection of a paramagnetic contrast agent leading to increased signal on T1WI ▶ ultrafast 3D acquisitions are available (using the shortest TRs possible)
  - The unique nature of k-space (where the central lines determine image contrast and the peripheral lines image resolution) can be uniquely exploited – acquisition of the contrast-defining central lines of k-space during the arterial peak and collection of resolution defining peripheral lines during venous enhancement reduces venous contamination
- High contrast-to-noise ratio ▶ high spatial resolution ▶ rapid acquisition ▶ relatively artefact free
- Intravascular signal is not dependent on any inherent flow properties (unlike non-contrast techniques) ▶ images can be acquired in any plane
- *Post processing techniques:* maximum intensity projection (MIP) ▶ multiplanar reformatting ▶ volume rendering ▶ surface-shade displays

Unenhanced phase contrast techniques

- Now almost universally replaced by contrast enhanced techniques
- This utilizes the basic phenomenon that phase changes are introduced to the transverse magnetization when spins are exposed to a magnetic field gradient
  - *Stationary spins:* if the phase-encode gradient is reversed after a time delay, then any spin phase differences introduced by the initial gradient will be completely reversed by the second gradient
  - *Moving spins:* if a spin has moved in the direction of the gradient between its initial application and reversal, then the second gradient will not be able to perfectly return any spin phase differences to their initial state – an overall phase change will have developed
- The magnitude, duration and time interval between these additional 'bipolar gradients' will determine any experienced phase changes ▶ this can be used to quantitate the velocity of any moving spins (as any phase shift is proportional to the blood velocity)

11.3 SPECIFIC DRAINAGE TECHNIQUES

CHEST

- Pleural drainage catheters are smaller than surgical drains (up to 16Fr) – haemothorax is better treated with surgical drains (36–38Fr)
- USS is adequate for uncomplicated collections, but CT is usually needed for drainage of multiloculated pleural collections
- It is recommended that the dependent portion of the collection is accessed just above the adjacent rib (away from the neurovascular bundle) and avoiding insertion close to the scapula
  - *'Vacuthorax'* phenomenon: a pneumothorax following pleural drainage (due to inadequate surfactant or the presence of restrictive pleural disease precipitating an asymptomatic hydropneumothorax)
- A chest drain placed for a pneumothorax can be removed 24 hours after the pneumothorax has resolved
- *Options for a partially treated pleural collection:* catheter repositioning / exchange for a larger catheter / instillation of a fibrinolytic agent for an inadequately draining complex collection
- *Pleurodesis:* this is used to prevent recurrence of effusion or pneumothorax by generating pleural inflammation and fibrosis causing obliteration of the plural space (e.g. with the installation of a chemical agent such as Bleomycin)

LIVER

- Catheter directed drainage is favoured for pyogenic collections, but for an amoebic collection only if it has failed medical management, is > 6-8 cm in size, or rupture is imminent
- Catheter drainage of an infected tumour in a non-surgical candidate is likely to remain permanently
- Ideally normal hepatic parenchyma should be traversed prior to entering the collection
- Pleural transgression should be avoided if possible

PANCREAS

- Access to the head of pancreas is often obtained using an anterior approach through the gastrocolic ligament – access to the tail of pancreas generally through the anterior pararenal space ▶ the liver and stomach can be transgressed (but not the small or large bowel)
- Pseudocysts can be drained if infected, intractable pain, or GI / biliary obstruction
- Drainage of an infected acute necrotic collection is often a bridge to surgery (high surgical morbidity in the first 4 weeks) ▶ the merits of drainage of non-infected acute necrotic collections is debatable
- If pancreatic ductal communication is demonstrated (e.g. catheter injection under fluoroscopy) endoscopic pancreatic duct stent placement is an option (transcather embolization if leakage persists)

DEEP PELVIC COLLECTIONS

- Transrectal drainage is favoured over transvaginal drainage where possible
- Prone positioning is favoured for transgluteal drainage of deep pelvic collections, often via CT guidance
  - Optimal transgluteal drain insertion is at the level of the sacrospinous ligament inferior to the piriformis muscle and close to the sacrum in order to reduce pain and the risk of blood vessel and nerve injury

RADIOFREQUENCY ABLATION (RFA)

- Monopolar RFA involves the application of high frequency (460-500 kHz) alternating current to the target tissue using a needle like applicator (dispersive grounding pads are attached to the patient's trunk / thigh) ▸ the resultant alternating electric field around the uninsulated probe tip causes 'radiofrequency' agitation of water molecules (inherently polarized) and local frictional heating within a few mm of the probe tip
- Coagulative necrosis results if the target tissue is maintained at temperatures > 45°C (RFA can induce temperatures of 100–110°C within a few millimetres of the probe) – beyond this it relies on conductive heating
- Reproducible 3-5 cm spheres of tissue destruction can be achieved within 15-20 minutes ▸ larger ablation volumes can be achieved by 'clustering' needles on a single-hand piece, expandable multi-tined devices or via multipolar arrays ▸ rapidly switching multiple electrode solutions simultaneous ablation zones
  - The temperature of the tissue at the lesion edge needs to be high enough to avoid marginal recurrences – the aim is to ablate an adequate margin of adjacent normal tissue
  - The heating effect on a tumour can be inadvertently reduced by the 'heat-sink' effect of blood flow in adjacent vessels >3 mm in diameter ▸ adjacent temporary vessel occlusion or embolization may help
  - Over aggressive RFA can lead to dessication and charring which increases tissue impedance, and prevents the application of additional current and temperature ▸ internal electrode cooling to limit charring may help
  - RFA ablation zones can vary according to the local tissue environment (e.g. aerated lung tissue is associated with high impedance and therefore poor heat transfer)

MICROWAVE ABLATION (MWA)

- Needle like probes harbouring a microwave broadcast antenna towards the needle tip (900-2400 MHz) ▸ antenna design will affect the size and shape of the ablation zone (e.g. elongated or rounded) ▸ multiple antennae can create zones of constructive or destructive wave interaction
- Water molecules oscillate when subjected to microwave radiation with significant local tissue heating ▸ in contrast to electric currents with RFA, microwaves radiate through all tissues including those with high electrical impedance – MWA can produce faster (approx. 5 mins) and larger ablation zones in multiple tissue types compared with RFA
  - *Advantages over RFA:* faster ablations ▸ higher temperatures without tissue impedance limitations ▸ reduced sensitivity to tissue types and more consistent results ▸ relative insensitivity to 'heat-sinks' ▸ the ability to create larger ablation zones

  - *Disadvantages over RFA:* potential for increased normal tissue damage due to potentially larger ablation zones generated

Cryoablation

- Uses narrow gauge (17G) argon cryoprobes – the phase change of liquid to gaseous argon can induce temperatures as low as -150°C to -170°C within the immediate vicinity
  - Faster freezing leads to intracellular ice formation which disrupts cellular organelles ▸ slower freezing leads to extracellular ice formation and osmotic dehydration which causes cellular disruption, also compounded by microvascular endothelial injury
  - The cell lethal isotherm lies at -20°C to -30°C and is ensured by the use of a double freeze-thaw cycle
  - Cell death may only occur 8 mm deep to the edge of the visualized ice ball
- In practice several probes (3-4) are placed into the tumour (approx. 10 mm from the edge and 15-20 mm apart)
  - *Advantage:* the main advantage is the production of a predictable physical iceball that can be monitored with USS, CT or MRI (cf. RFA)
  - *Disadvantages:* as the ablation zone is reperfused after the ice ball melts, the rapid release of cellular debris may explain the increased systemic complications (cryoshock) that can be seen compared with coagulative techniques ▸ as there is no diathermy effect, bleeding complications are more common ▸ longer ablation times required (25-30mins than with RFA or MWA)

FOCUSED ULTRASOUND

- Small focal areas of tissue destruction are achieved by focusing sound energy in the 1 MHz range using an extracoporeal acoustic lens – although avoiding breaching the body wall sound energy can be severely attenuated by intervening tissues
- The focused energy results in small ovoids of tissue destruction usually of rice grain size – these areas are stacked together to create larger ablation zones

IRREVERSIBLE ELECTROPORATION (IRE)

- A non-thermal ablative technique that acts by the application of millisecond pulses of direct current between monopolar probes or a single bipolar probe
- Sufficient bursts of current can disrupt the electrical potential of the cell membrane and perforate (or 'porate') the cell membrane leading to controlled cell death
- The major disadvantage is the accompanying severe muscle contractions when the current is applied require the use of general anaesthesia and muscle relaxants

CHEMICAL ABLATION

- Chemical agents that denature tissue (e.g. absolute alcohol and acetic acid) are instilled into a lesion

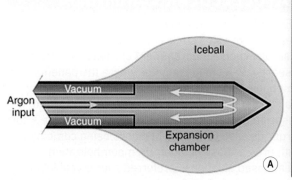

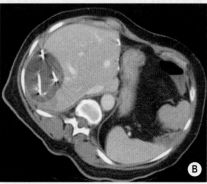

Cryoablation. **A,** Schematic illustration of tip of a cryoprobe with surrounding iceball formation. **B,** Axial contrast-enhanced computed tomography image demonstrates multiple cryoprobes placed and iceball formation during cryoablation of tumor in right lobe of liver. (From Ahmed M, Brace CL, Lee FT Jr, Goldberg SN. Principles of and advances in percutaneous ablation. Radiology 2011;258:351–69.)

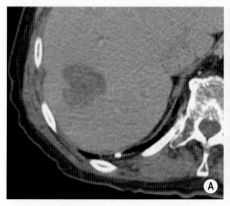

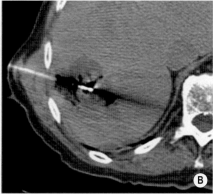

Example demonstrating the problem of outgassing following RFA or MWA. (A) Colorectal metastases in segment 7 for microwave ablation. (B) At initial probe placement and treatment there is considerable 'outgassing' obscuring the target tumour and rendering probe repositioning and treatment dosimetry difficult.**

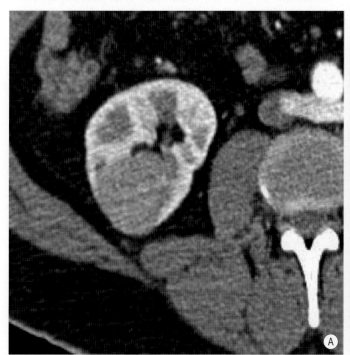

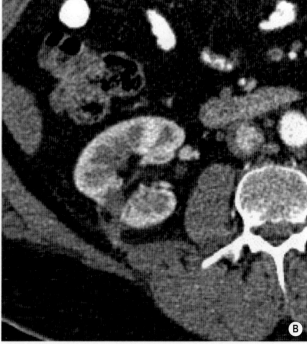

Sequential images showing involution of a successfully cryoablated 44-mm renal cell carcinoma on late arterial phase CT. (A) Pre-treatment. (B) Sixteen months post-treatment.**

PRE-PROCEDURAL PLANNING

- Ablative techniques are generally aimed at smaller tumours (<5 cm) with the best results seen in tumours <3 cm
- Injury to structures (e.g. bowel) can be avoided by physical displacement ('hydrodissection') through the use of injected 5% dextrose (± dilute contrast for visualization) ▶ carbon dioxide gas insufflation can also be used within the retroperitoneum to displace adjacent bowel in renal ablation

POST PROCEDURE IMAGING

- Non enhancement is a surrogate marker for tumour ablation ▶ other surrogates:
  - ▪ *Kidney:* 'post-treatment' halo artifact within the perirenal fat
  - ▪ *Lung:* contiguous circumferential ground glass opacification around completely denatured lung tumours
- Follow up imaging can be delayed for 1-2 weeks to allow ablation zone maturation and resolution of penumbral arterialization (which can take up to 3 months) ▶ degraded blood products should not be mistaken for viable enhancing residual tissue
- Over time the ablation zone should slowly involute, becoming darker on CT with an increasingly well defined and sharp margin without residual enhancing (irregular or nodular) residual tissue
- *Suggested follow up imaging protocol:* 3 monthly for the 1st year ▶ 6 monthly for the next 2 years ▶ annually out to 5 years

RENAL CANCER

- Ablation is effective for tumours <5 cm – increasing size increases the risk of an incomplete ablation and recurrence
- Cryoablation may be more effective than RFA with lower rates of local recurrence, achieving similar results to surgical resection with lower morbidity
- Hydrodissection plays a greater role than with hepatic ablations (proximity of bowel, pancreas and ureter)
- Central tumours and those adjacent to vulnerable structures may benefit from the precision offered by cryoablation ▶ IRE may also have a role for tumours near the renal pelvis / ureter (as this does not damage these structures)
- Treatment of tumours near the ureter may benefit from placement of a ureteral stent and pyeloperfusion

HEPATOCELLULAR CARCINOMA

- ▪ RFA and MWA plays an increasing role in the treatment of sub 5 cm lesions with a lower morbidity than resection – the treatment of choice in nodular disease < 2-3 cm in diameter where the patient is not amenable to transplantation or if on the transplant waiting list ▶ treatment of larger tumours (>3 cm) is associated with higher rates of local recurrence ▶ for larger disease (4-6 cm) ablation is being combined with pre- or post-ablation chemoembolization
- ▪ Heat based ablation is preferred over cryoablation (providing improved haemostasis and reduced risk of cryoshock)

COLORECTAL LIVER METASTASES

- Increasing interest in whether ablation can replace surgery for small isolated metastases (or extend the scope of surgery when combined with resection)
- Data suggests that metastases are more difficult to ablate than HCC of a similar size with higher local recurrence rates – ablation tends to be confined to lesions <3 cm in size

LUNG TUMOUR ABLATION

- Surgical resection is the preferred treatment but may be limited by poor lung function
- Metastases suitable for ablation are usually < 3 per hemithorax, < 3.5 cm in diameter and located in well aerated lung, and usually at least 2-3 cm from hilar structures
- RFA may give mixed results (air has a high electric impedance that limits current flow and tissue heating)
- Cryoablation is relatively resistant to the cold sink effect of ventilation (cf. RFA) ▶ also useful for those tumours close to the mediastinum or chest wall (visible iceball) ▶ associated with minimal postprocedural pain
- Microwave ablation can generate large and predictable ablation zones even in the presence of aerated lung

BONE TUMOUR ABLATION

- RFA and cryoablation are used for the treatment of small osteoid osteomas, osteoblastomas and chondroblastomas ▶ also used in the palliation of larger malignant tumours (e.g. renal cell carcinoma metastases)

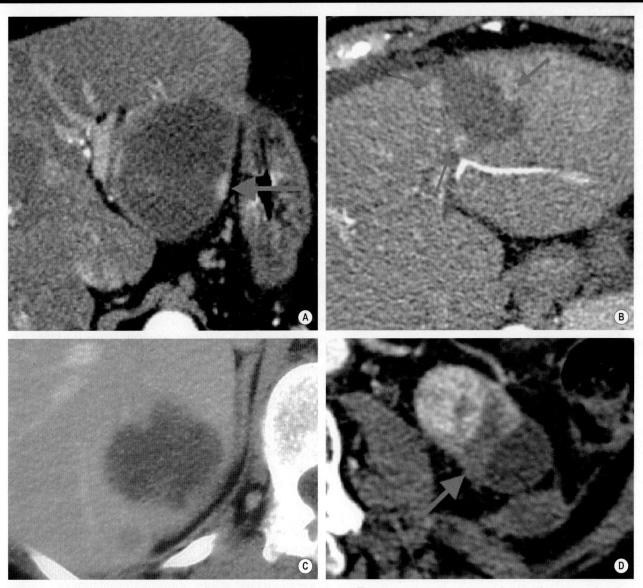

Patterns of local recurrence can vary according mainly to tumour type. Examples of local recurrence in hepatic tumours but the patterns can apply to all tumour locations. (A) Peripheral nodular recurrence on late arterial phase CT, seen in the subtotal treatment of hepatocellular carcinoma. (B) A patchy peripheral recurrence on late arterial phase CT, sometimes referred to as a 'halo' recurrence. (C) An enlarging (with reference to the ablation zone) low density lesion with increasing ill-defined treatment margin. This form of 'expanding' recurrence is seen with inadequate treatment of a colorectal metastasis. (D) Crescenteric peripheral enhancement on late arterial phase CT indicative of a subtotal treatment.**

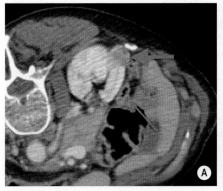 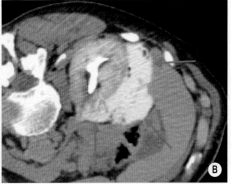

Sequence demonstrating the need for hydrodissection during cryoablation of a renal tumour (thick arrow). (A) Portal venous phase CT; directly adjacent loops of small bowel (thin arrow) that would be at risk if incorporated in the ablation zone. (B) A hydrodissection needle is placed to the interposed retroperitoneum and contrast-tinted saline injected (arrowed), displacing adjacent at risk structures.**

11.5 HEPATOBILIARY INTERVENTION

LIVER BIOPSY

- Spring-powered cutting sheath biopsy devices collect more consistent core biopsies with less crush artefact than a manually operated system
- The traditional route for liver intervention uses a horizontal right lateral intercostal approach ▶ an anterior subcostal approach (that does not traverse the pleura) is less likely to cause pulmonary complications
- It is preferable to biopsy lesions using a route through intervening normal liver as this probably reduces the risk of haemorrhage ▶ the presence of ascites is not by itself a contraindication to biopsy
- US is usually used as the real-time capability allows faster positioning of the needle or catheter and allows selection of an oblique approach (CT is limited to axial imaging)
- *Complications:* haemorrhage ▶ pneumothorax ▶ biliary peritonitis ▶ perforation of the bowel or gallbladder ▶ haemobilia ▶ arterioportal shunt formation

BILIARY SYSTEM

- MRCP and ERCP have replaced many previous roles served by biliary intervention / diagnosis
- Mid to lower biliary obstruction is treated endoscopically in the first instance – lesions at the liver hilum are challenging to treat at ERCP and best dealt with percutaneous biliary drainage ▶ with biliary-enteric anastomoses an ERCP approach is unlikely to be possible (e.g. Roux loop or Billroth II gastric anastomosis)

Indications Obstructive jaundice / cholangitis / evaluation and treatment of a biliary-enteric anastomosis / access for stone disease treatment/ evaluation of bile duct injuries

- Biliary drainage often performed for patients who have failed endoscopic treatment or have altered anatomy

Technique Supine position – right arm resting above the head ▶ conscious sedation or GA + local anaesthesia ▶ antibiotic prophylaxis ▶ lower edge of the right liver lobe is normally accessed in the mid-axillary line just above the 10th rib, and the needle directed towards the opposite shoulder under fluoroscopic guidance ▶ stylet is removed and contrast gently injected as the needle is incrementally withdrawn ▶ bile duct access is indicated by the 'dripping wax' appearance (contrast dissipating into the bile ducts) ▶ biliary access on the right is preferably through an inferior duct with a straight course to the hepatic hilum (better future catheter or stent placement) ▶ proximity of left lobe ducts to the anterior abdominal wall is conducive to USS guided placement and subsequent injection under fluroscopy

- *One-stick technique:* employs a small needle (e.g. 22G Chiba needle), microwire and dilator system to access the biliary tree

- *Two-stick technique:* begins with biliary access and opacification using a small needle, followed by separate biliary access with a larger needle and conventional wire

Biliary drainage An external drain left above the level of obstruction is a temporary measure ▶ an internal – external drain (percutaneous biliary transhepatic drainage – PTBD) from the duodenum through the biliary system to the skin is preferred ▶ it can be used after biliary stenting to preserve access to the biliary tree for a few days (e.g. if there is blood in the biliary tree)

- If a biliary stricture cannot be crossed at a first attempt, a stent can be left in situ until a repeat attempt ▶ once a stent is placed balloon dilatation can be used to bring the stent up to its nominal diameter ▶ a combined percutaneous and ERCP rendezvous approach can be considered

Complications Pain ▶ bile leak ▶ haemobilia ▶ septicaemia

Plastic stents These offer a lower patency rate due to encrustation of bile and often require a larger tract through the liver (10–12Fr) ▶ they are easily removed and can be used preoperatively in patients who require drainage prior to surgery

Metallic stents These offer better patency rates than plastic stents (larger lumen reduces effects of bile encrustation) ▶ as they self expand to a predefined diameter they can be placed through smaller tracts (6-8Fr) ▶ as they elicit a marked fibrotic reaction they should not be used in benign disease or preoperatively ▶ occlusion can occur from tumour overgrowth through the stent interstices or overgrowth at the end of the stent ▶ stenting through the sphincter of Oddi may give better drainage at the risk of increased infection (enteric reflux) ▶ 10–30% will require re-intervention following blockage

Covered metallic stents Aims to prevent tumour ingrowth ▶ drawbacks include increased migration and side branch coverage (cholecystitis and pancreatitis)

BENIGN DISEASE

- Transhepatic drainage can be performed to:
  - Drain an obstructed infected system (not amenable to endoscopic drainage)
  - Dilate benign strictures (ductal injury secondary to laparoscopic cholecystectomy / biliary-enteric anastomotic strictures / post hepatic transplantation ischaemic strictures / sclerosing cholangitis)
  - Treat intrahepatic or ductal calculi
- *Benign strictures:* balloon dilatation with an 8-10 mm balloon, with at least 2 weeks of biliary drainage with the catheter across the stricture ▶ useful to leave an access catheter in place for 6 weeks to facilitate redilatation if early restenosis occurs
- *Distal CBD calculi:* usually managed by ERCP ▶ after passage of a guidewire past the calculus, a balloon

catheter dilates the sphincter of Oddi, it is then deflated, placed above the calculus, reinflated and pushed forward to move the calculus into the duodenum

GALLBLADDER

- Used for patients with acute cholecystitis who are poor surgical candidates
- Preference is to traverse hepatic parenchyma prior to entering the gallbladder to help secure

catheter placement and reduce the risk of peritoneal contamination
- Catheters placed for calculous cholecystitis remain in place until surgery
- Catheters placed for acalculous cholecystitis are removed after 6 weeks if: well patient / no gallstones / patent cystic duct / established tract from gallbladder to skin

LIVER VASCULAR INTERVENTIONAL TECHNIQUES

TRANSARTERIAL CHEMOEMBOLISATION (TACE)

- Malignant tumours usually derive most of their blood supply from the hepatic arterial branches (the portal vein provides > 70% of the parenchymal blood supply) – a tumour can therefore be rendered ischaemic by occluding its arterial supply (whilst preserving parenchymal blood flow)
- Local delivery of chemotherapy directly to the tumour reduces systemic effects – embolization should be performed as super-selectively as possible using slow controlled injections ▶ the end point is elimination of the tumour blush but not complete arterial stasis

Indications *HCC:* to reduce tumour bulk to allow an unresectable tumour to become resectable ▶ to control or reduce tumour bulk in HCC until a transplant becomes available
- Requirements: preserved liver function ▶ ECOG performance status 0–1 without extrahepatic disease
  - *Metastases:* disease confined to the liver or stable extra hepatic disease

Contraindications *>50-75%* of liver parenchyma replaced by tumour ▶ advanced cirrhosis ▶ advanced or progressive extrahepatic disease
- *Relative contra-indications*: portal vein thrombosis ▶ Chlid Pugh Class C ▶ hepatic encephalopathy ▶ active GI bleeding ▶ refractory ascites ▶ serum bilirubin > 5 mg/dL ▶ TIPS stent
- Prior sphincterotomy / CBD stents are at higher risk of reflux and liver abscess formation – prophylactic antibiotics required

Complications Hepatic failure due to infarction ▶ abscess ▶ biliary necrosis ± stricture ▶ tumour rupture ▶ non target embolization (e.g. gallbladder)
- *Post Embolisation Syndrome (PES):* occurs following cytokine release ▶ develops within 12 hours, lasting for 2-7 days ▶ nausea, vomiting, pain, fever ▶ supportive treatment

Treatment response CT / MRI tumour response assessed after 6 weeks (further imaging follow up at 3-6 monthly intervals) ▶ mRECIST response criteria (assessing viable enhancing tumour) may be more appropriate than standard RECIST criteria

RADIOEMBOLISATION – SELECTIVE INTRA-ARTERIAL RADIOTHERAPY

- Micron sized particles containing radioisotope are delivered directly to the tumour via its feeding arteries (minimising dose to surrounding tissues)
- Spheres impregnated with yttrium-90 (^{90}Y) emitting β particles
  - *TheraSpheres:* glass spheres
  - *SIR-Sphere:* resin spheres

Indications Unresectable lesion ▶ lack of fitness for transplantation ▶ unsuitable for thermal ablation ▶ failed chemotherapy ▶ life expectancy > 12 weeks
- Detailed pre-treatment angiography is required to:
  - Identify variant arterial anatomy
  - Tumour arterial supply (e.g. if there is dual tumour supply – for example parasitized flow from phrenic vessels in liver dome lesions)
  - Determine any arterio-portal shunting
- Non target embolization is a greater problem than with chemoembolization, as ^{90}Y also causes radiation damage in addition to ischaemia ▶ planning angiography allows identification of GI branches that could cause significant issues – these can be embolised pre SIRT (e.g. GDA, gastric arteries) although there is a risk of GI haemorrhage or pancreatitis ▶ proximal coils do not usually cause bowel ischaemia (rich collateral supply)
- HCC is characterised by significant shunting – planning angiography allows determination of lung shunt fraction (LSF) with a technetium ^{99m}Tc albumin aggregated shunt study (^{99m}Tc-MAA) – the MAA particle size is the same as ^{90}Y ▶ if LSF >20%, radioembolisation is not safe

- One liver lobe is treated at any one time (with 4 weeks between lobar treatments) ▶ repeat angiography is required before treatment repeat
- ^{90}Y *complications:* post-radioembolisation syndrome (similar to post-embolization syndrome) ▶ hepatic dysfunction ▶ biliary strictures ▶ radiation pneumonitis
- Response assessment is similar to that following TACE

HEPATIC ARTERIAL EMBOLIZATION

Control of haemorrhage   Arterial bleeding may occur into the biliary tree, hepatic parenchyma, or peritoneal space

- *Causes:* accidental or iatrogenic trauma ▶ neoplastic disease ▶ arteritides (e.g. polyarteritis nodosa)
- Surgical ligation of the main hepatic artery may be insufficient (there may be an extensive collateral arterial supply)
- It requires the selective catheterization and occlusion of the abnormal vessel ▶ embolization can be performed with coils, particles or liquid embolic agents such as glue

PORTAL VEIN EMBOLIZATION (PVE)

Used in cases where the future liver remnant (FLR) will not provide sufficient function post tumour resection, exploiting the ability of the liver to regenerate ▶ embolization with glue, coils, plugs or a combination ▶ usually performed 4–6 weeks prior to surgical resection

  ▪ PVE considered if: FLR < 25% (normal liver) ▶ FLR < 40% (cirrhotic liver)

TRANSJUGULAR INTRAHEPATIC PORTOSYSTEMIC SHUNT (TIPSS) INSERTION

This involves the creation of a track between the portal vein (usually right branch) and one of the hepatic veins, followed by insertion of a metallic covered stent to maintain its patency

- Its major indication is in patients with acute variceal haemorrhage which is resistant to emergency endoscopic sclerotherapy

Other indications   Refractory ascites ▶ Budd Chiari syndrome ▶ hepatorenal syndrome

- After stent insertion pressure measurements are performed to ensure adequate shunting has occurred (pressure <12 mmHg or halving the portosystemic gradient) ▶ residual opacifying varices should be embolised if a significant variceal bleed has occurred
- Resultant haemodynamic changes can lead to cardiac failure with a risk of encephalopathy
- Complications: hepatic arterial injury ▶ capsular perforation ▶ intraperitoneal haemorrhage (extrahepatic portal vein puncture) ▶ bile duct injury ▶ right atrial perforation

HEPATIC VENOUS INTERVENTION

Its major indication is to investigate and treat Budd Chiari syndrome (obstruction of the hepatic venous outflow may occur at any level from the hepatic venules to the suprahepatic IVC) ▶ the options available are:

- Surgical fashioning of a portosystemic shunt (if the liver function is stable)
- Angioplasty ± stent insertion (in patients with a short segment hepatic vein or an IVC occlusion)
- TIPSS insertion (this is an alternative to surgical shunting if there are impassable intrahepatic occlusions or extensive venous thrombosis) ▶ its advantages to a surgical shunt include:
  ▪ It does not compromise any subsequent hepatic transplantation
  ▪ It bypasses any caval stenosis that is commonly present in patients with Budd Chiari syndrome

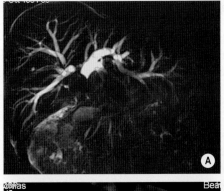

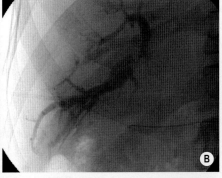

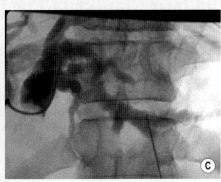

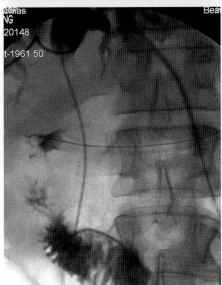

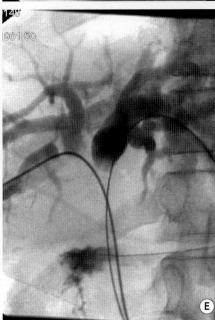

A 50-year-old male with metastatic colorectal cancer to liver causing a hilar obstruction resulting in marked jaundice and pruritus. MRCP demonstrates that the right and left main hepatic ducts do not communicate (A). A PTC was performed via the right side (B) confirming no communication between the ducts. The left side was then punctured (C) and the long stricture within the hilum and common duct was elicited (D). Therefore it was elected to place metallic biliary stents from both the right and left sides in a Y configuration. Guidewires were placed through the stricture via both sides (E).**

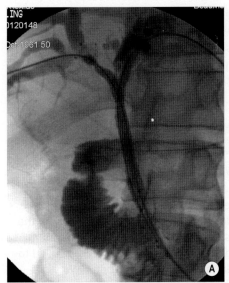

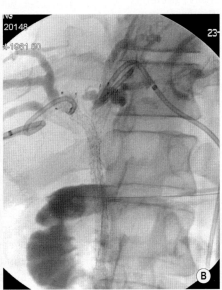

Ten-millimetre metallic self-expanding stents were deployed simultaneously across the stricture; note the tight stricture proximally within the right-sided stent which required balloon dilatation with an 8-mm balloon (A). Following balloon dilatation, the stents are widely patent, with safety external biliary drains placed for 24 hours (B).**

PERCUTANEOUS RENAL ACCESS

- The safest point for calyceal puncture is the centre of the calyx, approached through the relatively avascular plane (Brödel's line) between the branches of the anterior and posterior divisions of the renal artery
- Puncturing the centre of the calyx avoids injury to the arcuate divisions that course around the infundibulum – puncture into the infundibulum or renal pelvis may lacerate larger arterial branches
- A further potential hazard is the posterior renal artery division (the only major division lying posterior to the collecting system) ▶ typically it lies behind the upper renal pelvis but is occasionally behind the upper pole infundibulum (where it can be injured by an infundibular puncture)
- Typically the upper and lower pole calyces are fused (therefore larger and easier to access
- The posterior calyx is ideal for access (closer to the skin surface) and also allow better intrarenal navigation (access to the PUJ is easier from an interpolar or upper pole calyx)
- Upper pole access may require an intercostal entry

Access needle

- *Two-part 21G needle system* (micropuncture access system): puncture with a 21G needle through which a 0.018 inch platinum tipped wire is inserted, followed by a 4Fr dilator and finally a 0.035 inch working guidewire ▶ smaller puncture site
- *One-part 18G 4Fr sheath system:* 18G diamond point needle, over which a 4Fr sheath and the whole is inserted as a single unit

Guidewires

- A soft flexible with good torque to navigate out of the calyx (rigidity less vital) – e.g. a straight tipped Bentson wire
- Once out of the calyx and into the renal pelvis / ureter, rigidity becomes more important (e.g. stiffer Amplatz type wire) ▶ a stiff shaft hydrophilic wire is less prone to kinking than other wires

Catheters

- *Navigation:* a short angled-tip (e.g. Kumpe) or Cobra shape high torque catheter is best ▶ hydrophilic catheters are useful for bypassing tight ureteric strictures
- *Drainage:* a pigtail catheter with large side holes ▶ a pigtail may not easily form in a small renal pelvis

PERCUTANEOUS NEPHROSTOMY (PCN)

- *Indications:* urinary tract obstruction ▶ pyonephrosis ▶ urinary leakage / fistula / access for interventional or endoscopic procedures

- Data suggest that PCN and ureteric stents are equally effective
- No absolute contraindications (severe coagulopathy is a relative contraindication) ▶ in patients with a limited life expectancy a nephrostomy should only be inserted only if it leads to improved quality of life and survival
- INR < 1.3 ▶ platelets >80,000/dL ▶ antibiotic prophylaxis
- *Technique*
  - Prone / prone oblique position ▶ performed under monitored sedo-analgesia + local anaesthetic infiltration down to the renal capsule
  - Following appropriate puncture of an appropriate calyx, urine is aspirated to confirm position ▶ contrast medium (10 ml) injected to confirm puncture site if there are no signs of sepsis ▶ overdistension should be avoided to avoid bacteraemia ▶ if the puncture site is suitable, a wire is inserted and the tract dilated for catheter insertion
- Nephrostomy removal should be performed under fluoroscopic guidance using a guidewire

Single puncture USS guided PCN

- posterior calyces are the most superficial and medial with the patient lying prone

Single puncture fluoroscopically guided PCN

- IV contrast medium can be used to identify a suitable calyx ▶ on fluoroscopy of an opacified system calyces demonstrating the largest range of movement on screening are the most posterior calyces and also the least densely opacified in a prone position (as they are non-dependent) ▶ once identified, the needle is inserted under fluoroscopy

Double puncture combined USS and fluoroscopy guided PCN

- if definitive calyceal entry is not possible under fluoroscopy, the any access point identified under USS is punctured with a 22G needle, a contrast pyelogram performed and used to select a target calyx which is then punctured under fluoroscopy

CT guided PCN

safer technique when variant anatomy suspected, using a planning pyelographic phase CT ▶ then performed under CT or combined CT / fluoroscopic guidance

COMPLICATED NEPHROSTOMIES

Non dilated kidneys

- the double contrast technique can be used – if the renal pelvis can be seen on US then this can be punctured with a 22G needle and a pyelogram used to identify the posterior calyces ▶ if no part of the collecting system is seen on US, then IV contrast medium can be used to opacify the system and select a posterior calyx

Horseshoe kidney

- a medial upper pole calyx should be chosen for PCN (a lower pole lateral entry may damage large anterior division arteries or accessory branches from the iliac artery)

Transplant kidney

- a lateral, upper pole entry is preferred to avoid puncturing the peritoneum ▶ often marked capsular fibrosis can make dilatation and catheter insertion difficult

Paediatric PCN

- Performed under GA ▶ the collecting system can rapidly decompress on needle entry and access may be lost (the catheter must be inserted as quickly as possible) ▶ special neonatal nephrostomy catheters are available

Complications

- *Sepsis:* pre-procedural antibiotics ▶ over-distension and manipulation should be avoided
- *Haematuria:* not uncommon ▶ usually resolves spontaneously but may require bladder washout ▶ venous bleeding usually resolves with continued nephrostomy drainage and catheter tamponade ▶ arterial bleeding may require more prolonged catheter tamponade or embolization
- *Renal / pelvic injury:* usually due to poor technique ▶ usually treated with prolonged internal or external drainage
- *Rare:* bowel injury ▶ pneumothorax ▶ empyema ▶ haemothorax

PERCUTANEOUS NEPHROLITHOTOMY (PCNL)

- **Indications:** renal pelvic stones >2 cm ▶ staghorn calculi ▶ lower pole stones >1 cm ▶ stones in kidneys with poor drainage
  - *Less common indications:* resection of TCC of the renal pelvis ▶ balloon dilatation / incision of PUJ obstruction
  - *Relative indications:* stones >1000 HU ▶ cysteine stones
- Key steps are tract dilatation and sheath insertion
- **Tract Planning:** if complete stone clearance is not possible, the renal pelvis should be cleared to de obstruct the kidney ▶ lower pole calyces should be cleared as residual fragments may not drain naturally
- **Tract Dilatation:** 30 Fr is usual ▶ 2 guidewires - a stiff wire for dilatation and a safety wire
  - *Systems available for dilatation:* balloon mounted sheath system ▶ serial plastic dilators ▶ concentric telescopic metal dilators

- **Complications:** bleeding (7.8%) ▶ renal pelvic injury (3.4%) ▶ pleural effusion (1.8%) ▶ bowel and visceral injury (rare)
  - *Delayed complications:* late pseudoaneurysm ▶ haemorrhage ▶ ischaemic stricture of the collecting system

Antegrade ureteric stents

- Stents function both as a splint and drainage tube ▶ stents can irritate the urothelium and become infected ▶ all will eventually occlude either due to malignant overgrowth or encrustation
  - All stents lead to reactive urothelial hyperplasia, thickened mucosa and peri-ureteral inflammation, together with reduced ureteric peristalsis
  - long term stents should be exchanged every 3–6 months using an antegrade or retrograde approach
- **Indications:** relief of ureteric obstruction ▶ ureteric splinting after stricture balloon dilatation ▶ prior to stone therapy (relative indication)
  - Primary stenting is contraindicated with infected obstructed systems
- **Plastic stents:** double pigtail (double J) along the full ureter ▶ require regular exchange
- **Metal stents:** these become permanently incorporated into the wall by epithelialization ▶ only the Memokath 051 is specifically designed for the urinary tract (it does not epithelialize and can be removed)
- **Technique of Antegrade Stenting:** interpolar or upper pole renal access is preferred ▶ a stricture can be negotiated with a curved tip hydrophilic wire combined with an angled tip, high torque catheter for stricture cannulation (or with a straight tip guidewire combined with a Cobra shape catheter ▶ once the stricture is crossed, the catheter is advanced into the bladder and the wire exchanged for a stiff guidewire to support stent insertion ▶ the tract is dilated to 1–2 Fr larger than the stent
- **Stent lumen size:** 8 Fr (malignant or ischaemic/post-surgical strictures ▶ 6 Fr (bypass ureteric calculi or inflammatory strictures) ▶ 6–8 mm diameter (metal stents)
  - *Peri-stent drainage:* benign strictures allow drainage around the stent
  - as the ureter dilates (not seen in malignant lesions)
- **Stent length:** <175 cm height: 22 cm long stent ▶ 175–195 cm: 24 cm stent ▶ >195 cm: 26 cm stent ▶ urostomy: 22 cm or shorter
- **Additional Issues:**
  - *Retroperitoneal looping of the stent / wire:* secondary to a long retroperitoneal tract or extrarenal cavity (e.g. urinoma) - the tract can be supported using a stiff wire and peel-away sheath
  - *False passage creation during stricture cannulation:* stop, start antibiotics and insert nephrostomy ▶ reattempt stenting after 3–7 days of external drainage

- *Tortuous ureter:* use a high-torque, angled tip catheter
- *Tight /rigid stricture:* the stiff end of a hydrophilic wire can be placed forcefully across such a stricture ▶ if a subintimal passage is made, stenting is still possible once the true lumen has been re-entered ▶ a long dilator or balloon may help ▶ reattempting after 1week of nephrostomy drainage is often successful
- *Stent cannot be advanced across a stricture after dilatation:* the distal tip of a hydrophilic wire can be snared in the bladder and externalized out of the urethra, allowing a push-pull maneouvre with a stent forced across the stricture
- *Extra anatomical stenting (if a stricture cannot be bypassed with a guidewire):* rendezvous technique for bladder level strictures - a combined antegrade and retrograde approach with a curved tip catheter wedged in the stricture and directed towards the bladder with the stiff end of a hydrophilic wire used to puncture through the tumour / bladder wall

Balloon dilatation of ureteric strictures

- High recurrence rate ▶ a failed balloon dilatation does not prevent surgical repair
- *Technique:* an interpolar calyx is ideal for access ▶ an angled tip catheter and hydrophilic guidewire to cross the stenosis (a hydrophilic catheter may be required if the stricture is very tight) ▶ a peel-away sheath helps support the catheter and wire during exchange ▶ the hydrophilic guidewire is then exchanged for a stiff guidewire and the stricture dilated using a 6–8 mm balloon (high dilatation pressures may be needed) ▶ ideally looking for abolition of the 'waist' of the stricture with minimal contained extravasation ▶ a stent is then placed as a splint for 4–6 weeks ▶ if perforation occurs up to 1 week should be allowed for the perforation to heal before a repeat attempt

INTERVENTIONAL PROCEDURES IN THE PROSTATE

- *Transrectal approach:* performed in the left lateral position under local anaesthesia ▶ a risk of haemorrhage and infection which can be severe
- *Transperineal route:* negligible risk of major complications ▶ painful requiring a GA or generous sedation
- *Drainage of Prostatic Abscesses:* transrectal route is technically easier but may not be tolerated due to pain ▶ using a prostate biopsy needle guide attached to the transrectal probe and directing an 18G needle into the abscess

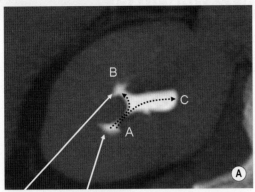

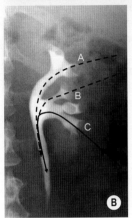

Calyceal selection for renal access. These two images illustrate the importance of choosing the right calyx for renal access. (A) Axial CT image showing entry into a posterior-facing calyx A allows easy navigation into the anterior calyx B as well as towards the infundibulum and the renal pelvis C. Entry into an anterior calyx B would be poor for intrarenal navigation. (B) Coronal fluoroscopic image demonstrating that upper pole A or interpolar entry B is better for ureteric access. Lower pole entry C is less favourable.**

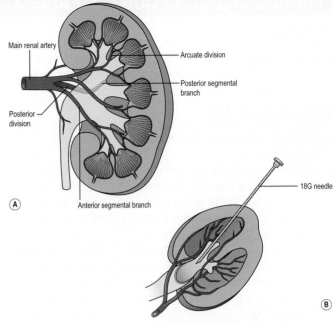

(A) Normal renal arterial anatomy as seen from the front. Note that the posterior division of the main renal artery lies behind the collecting system, and is vulnerable during percutaneous renal access in the prone position, especially if a more medial puncture is made. (B) The safest place to puncture a calyx is its middle, (see text).**

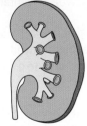

Principles of PCNL access
Aims
1. Aim for complete stone clearance
2. If complete clearance is not possible:
   • Clear renal pelvis to improve renal drainage.
   • Clear lower pole calyces as these may not respond to ESWL.
   • Residual stones in the upper/interpolar calyces can later be treated with ESWL.

Renal access
1. Posterior calyces allow access to anterior calyces.
2. Anterior calyceal entry poorer for intrarenal navigation.
3. Upper pole entry allows deep access of the PUJ/upper ureter:
   • May puncture posterior division artery.
   • May puncture pleura
4. Some interpolar calyces may be difficult with either lower or upper entry.

(A)

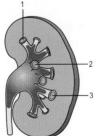

Complete staghorn
Stone clearance may be impossible with a single puncture.

1. Route 1 or 2 may be preferred—with Route 3 PUJ/ureteric clearance may be difficult.
2. With either routes some interpolar calyces may be difficult.

(B)

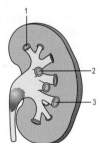

Stone in renal pelvis
Stone removed with minimal fragmentation. Ureteric fragments may be difficult to chase. Access planned according to PUJ anatomy.

1. Routes 1 and 2 are preferred with straight navigation to PUJ.
2. Route 3 may be difficult if the infundibulo-pelvic angle is acute and distal stone may be beyond reach.

(C)

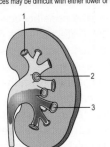

Stone in pelvis and lower calyces
Complete clearance is important (see under Principles/Aims).

1. Route 1 is often best.
2. Poor views of the interpolar calyx.
3. Poor views of upper ureter

(D)

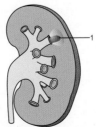

Stone in calyceal diverticulum with tight neck
Complete clearance is ideal. To decrease chances of recurrence, the neck should be dilated (thereby improving drainage) or the diverticulum should be obliterated.Direct puncture onto stone (1). Hydrophilic wire and good distension (with air/CO_2) help in searching for neck.

(E)

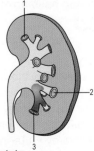

Lower-pole branched calculus
Stones in anterior and posterior parallel calyces. Complete clearance as ESWL may not work.
1. Route 1 preferred as both parallel calyces can be seen.
2. Route 2 (posterior calyx) better than 3 (anterior calyx) as navigation easier.

(F)

(A–F) The principles of tract planning for PCNL. A well-planned tract should allow for maximal/all stone removal and easy intrarenal navigation, such that most/all calyces should be endoscopically accessible.**

11.7 WOMAN'S IMAGING – INTERVENTIONAL RADIOLOGY

FIBROID EMBOLIZATION – UTERINE ARTERY EMBOLIZATION (UAE)

Definition

- Uterine fibroids are the commonest tumour found in reproductive women – the prevalence increases up to the menopause (up to 80% in Afrocarribean women)

Radiological features

- **USS:** operator dependent ▶ poor assessment of vascularity
- **MRI:** contrast enhancement should be used routinely (occasionally a non enhancing fibroid unsuitable for embolization can be demonstrated) ▶ adenomyosisis not a contra-indication to embolization but outcomes are less robust than with fibroids
  - Surgery may be more effective than UAE where there is a submucosal fibroid on a stalk where surgery is simple and effective ▶ controversy surrounds pedunculated subserosal fibroids and very large lesions

UAE technique

- Overnight stay to manage the post embolization pain which can be severe (analgesia administered prior, during and after UAE)
- Prophylactic antibiotics
- Access from the right common femoral artery (4–5F cobra catheter), crossing the aortic bifurcation and the contralateral anterior division of the internal iliac artery selected (the use of a coaxial catheter at this stage to select the uterine artery minimizes the risk of spasm allowing free flow embolization) ▶ catheter is withdrawn and then the ipsilateral internal iliac and uterine artery is selected and embolised
- Choice of embolic agent is operator dependent ▶ more expensive options are no more effective than standard non-spherical PVA ▶ embolic end point is complete stasis in the uterine artery
- Complications: post embolization syndrome (pain, fever, raised inflammatory markers) ▶ vaginal discharge and infection ▶ severe complications include fibroid expulsion and premature ovarian failure

Post partum haemorrhage (PPH)

Definition

- *Primary PPH:* blood loss >500 ml within 24 hours of delivery
- *Secondary PPH:* blood loss >24 hours after delivery, linked to either retained products ± infection
- *Causes:* uterine atony ▶ genital tract lacerations ▶ abnormal placentation ▶ post caesarean section or hysterectomy ▶ uterine AVM (rare)

Management

- Embolization is never the first line treatment, but should also not be used as the last resort

- *Initial options:* uterotonics ▶ removal of retained products ▶ intrauterine balloon ▶ uterine compression suture (if abdomen already opened)

Technique

- Similar to that for fibroids
- Access is best from a bilateral common femoral artery approach with catheterization of the anterior divisions of the internal iliacs and embolization of the bleeding point (usually the uterine artery) with Gelofoam v ▶ bilateral embolization is usually required as there is good cross flow collateralisation
- A negative angiogram is not uncommon with uterine atony
- Continued bleeding may require a hysterectomy
- Major complications: buttock and lower limb ischaemia ▶ small bowel, uterine, vaginal, cervical and bladder wall necrosis ▶ sciatic nerve damage

Abnormal placentation

Definition

- Abnormal placentation occurs when a defect within the decidua basilis allows invasion of the chorionic villi into the myometrium
  - *Placenta accreta* (least invasive): placental tissue invading the myometrium
  - *Placenta increta:* placental tissue reaching the serosa
  - *Placenta percreta:* placental tissue invading beyond the serosa into adjacent structures (e.g. bladder)

Management

- If identified pre-natally a pre-delivery strategy should be formed involving an interventional radiologist ▶ options include trying to preserve the uterus (possibly leaving the placenta in situ) or a planned caesarean hysterectomy
- Bilateral common femoral artery access should be established ▶ options include:
- Waiting to see how the caesarean section progresses (if bleeding can be controlled surgically no embolization is required) ▶ Gelfoam is the usual embolic agent
- Placing at least guidewires and possibly occlusion balloons in the common iliac, internal iliacs or uterine arteries and inflating these just prior to incising the uterus or placenta ▶ there are reports of parasitic supply to the uterus form branches from the common femoral artery (therefore a balloon placement in the common iliac arteries will cater for most extra uterine supply) ▶ if balloon inflation controls the haemorrhage, embolization may not be required (embolization may be required if bleeding occurs after balloon deflation) ▶ there have been reports of child anoxia where the balloons have been inflated within the uterine arteries which are sensitive to spasm

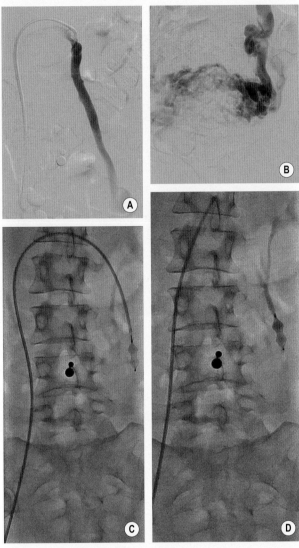

Ovarian vein embolisation. (A) Left renal venogram shows reflux into the left ovarian vein. (B) Venogram shows enlarged left ovarian vein and tortuous pelvic veins crossing midline. (C, D) Deployment of Amplatzer vascular plug in the left ovarian vein from right femoral vein approach.**

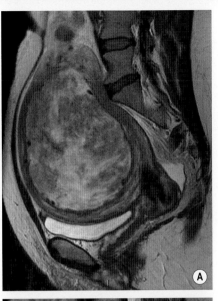

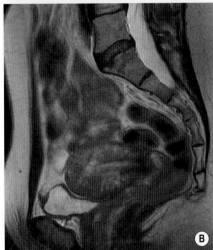

Fibroid uterus. (A) Sagittal T2-weighted image showing a large intramural fibroid. (B) Sagittal T2-weighted image following uterine artery embolisation shows complete resolution of fibroid.**

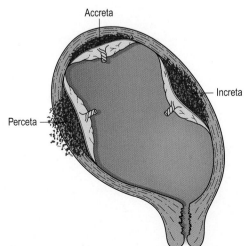

Classification of invasive placenta. Image showing different degrees of placental invasion into the uterine wall.**

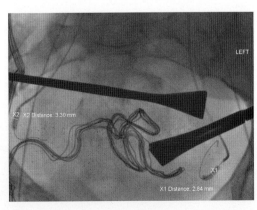

Uterine artery balloon occlusion. Patient with an invasive placenta undergoing prophylactic balloon occlusion of both uterine arteries to minimise blood loss during caesarean section.**

943

APPENDICES

12.1 GENERAL PEARLS

INTRAVASCULAR CONTRAST MEDIA

Barium based contrast agents

- For assessment of the GI tract
- Based on very poorly soluble barium sulphate ($BaSo_4$) ▶ administered PO or PR
- Can lead to barium peritonitis if leaks into the peritoneal cavity

Iodine based contrast media

- For general use in angiography and CT
- No marked pharmacological actions – can interfere with clotting times (avoid clotting tests for 6 hours after administration)
- Excreted unchanged via the kidneys ▶ >80% excreted after 4 hours with a normal GFR (>60 mL/min/1.73 m^2)
- Iodine provides the radio opacity – the other elements of the molecule act as carriers of iodine
- Low osmolar non-ionic contrast media
  - *iohexol/iopamidol/iomeron/iopromide/ioversol/ ioxilan/iobitridol/ iopentol/iobiditrol*
- Iso osmolar non-ionic contrast media
  - *isomenol/iotrolan/iodixanol*
  - High viscosity makes injection through thin IV lines difficult – requires preheating

MR contrast agents

- Gadolinium (Gd) has 7 unpaired electrons and therefore demonstrates a very large magnetic dipole moment
- Paramagnetic ions (Gd) reduce the T1 and T2 relaxation times
  - *omniscan/optimark/magnevist/gadovist/prohance/ dotarem*
- Gadolinium (Gd) is very toxic – it requires encapsulation with a chelate (linear or cyclic/cyclic or macrocyclic/ionic or non ionic)
  - *Cyclic:* Gd caged in a molecular ring
  - *Acyclic:* Gd held less tightly
- Excreted by passive glomerular filtration (95% by 24 hours)
  - Can cause spurious hypocalcaemia (interferes with assay method)
  - Gd chelates do not cross the blood brain barrier
- Gd itself does not change the signal intensity – the surroundings change signal when the agent is there
  - *T1 images:* increased signal intensity
  - *T2 images:* no effect

- Supraparamagnetic ions (Fe^{2+})
  - *T1 images:* increased signal intensity (low concentration) ▶ minimal effect (high concentrations)
  - *T2 images:* reduced signal intensity (high concentrations)
- Hepatobiliary Agents (Gadolinium disodium – Primovist)
  - Excreted 50% biliary tree / 50% kidneys
  1. Rapidly distribute into the vascular/interstitial space, allowing acquisition of dynamic images
     a. As only ¼ of the dose of extracellular agents s required, this may be suboptimal
  2. Then enter *functioning* hepatocytes via OATP8 receptors – these can be imaged after 20 minutes (hepatobiliary phase T1 images)

USS contrast agents

- Gas filled microbubbles (2-6 μm) that enhance US signals and which are small enough to cross the lung capillary bed so that systemic US enhancement can follow venous injection
- A shell that can be either stiff (e.g. denatured albumin) or flexible (e.g. phospholipids) surrounding low solubility gases (e.g. perfluorocarbon) – this shell prevents bubble collapse due to the high surface tension
  - Confined to the intravascular space
- As they contain gas, they change size in response to alternating pressures in the US filed (in contrast to tissue which is virtually incompressible) – they therefore resonate if there is a match between their diameter and ultrasonic wavelength
  - As the response is asymmetrical (they resist compression more than expansion) this results in higher frequencies (harmonics) present in the echoes they generate
- Microbubble specific methods have been developed to select for these harmonics to produce real time images solely of the microbubbles (usually displayed adjacent to a B-mode image for anatomical localisation
  - Based on the cancellation and/or separation of linear USS signals from tissue and utilization of the non-linear response from microbubbles
  - *Low acoustic pressure imaging:* non linear response from non disrupted microbubbles
  - *High acoustic pressure imaging:* non linear response secondary to microbubble disruption

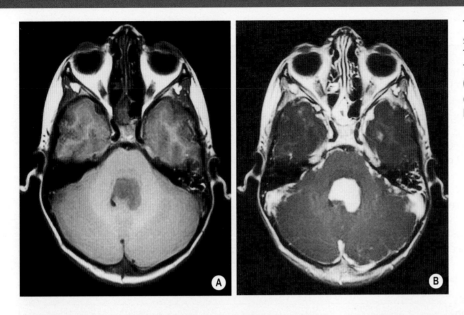

Typical appearance of a brain tumour, specifically a cerebellar medulloblastoma. (A) The tumour has a low signal on spin-echo T1-weighted image owing to a prolonged T1. (B) After the injection of Gd-DTPA, the tumour enhances avidly, depicting breakdown of the blood–brain barrier.**

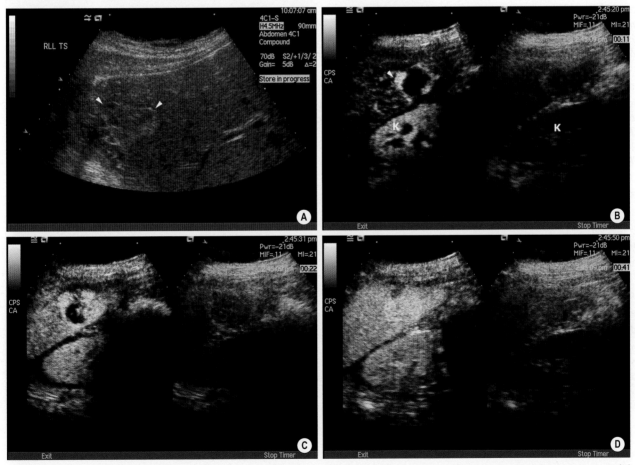

Contrast-enhanced ultrasound (CEUS) of a haemangioma. The baseline transverse section through the right lobe of the liver (A) shows a subtle lesion (arrowheads). The system was then reset to display the contrast image on the left (using contrast pulse sequences) and the B-mode image on the right, both with low mechanical indices. SonoVue (2.4 mL) was given IV and the haemodynamics of the flow through the lesion observed in real time. At 11 s after injection (B), the lesion showed peripheral nodular enhancement (arrowhead). By 22 s (C), the lesion shows centripetal filling and by 41 s (D) it had almost completely filled, a pattern characteristic of a haemangioma. The liver and the kidney also show enhancement. The ability to provide a firm diagnosis of a benign mass as soon as it was detected is a benefit of CEUS. K = kidney.**

947

INTRAVENOUS CONTRAST AGENT ADMINISTRATION IN ADULTS

CT

Renal impairment

- Renal impairment combined with diabetes mellitus carries significant risk
- Congestive heart failure, old age (> 70 years), and concurrent nephrotoxic drugs are also risk factors for contrast nephrotoxicity
- Insufficient evidence supporting the use of pharmacological means to reduce the incidence of contrast nephrotoxicity
- Serum creatinine is a poor indicator of renal function, and eGFR should be used where possible
  - All elective patients with renal disease or diabetes should have a recent eGFR (within 3 months)
  - All angiographic procedures require an eGFR (higher doses used)
- Renal impairment = eGFR < 60 ml/min/1.73 m – determine eGFR within 7 days of contrast administration
- *eGFR 30-60 ml/min/1.73 m*
  - Check scan indication
  - Ensure the patient is well hydrated before and after the procedure (PO or IV) (e.g. IV saline 1–1.5 mL/kg/h for 6 hours before and after contrast medium)
  - Use the smallest amount of contrast possible
  - Consider an iso-osmolar non-ionic dimeric contrast agent (e.g. Visipaque), although their exact preventative role is unclear
- *eGFR < 30 ml/min/1.73 m*
  - Use contrast only if essential and after discussion with referring clinicians

Previous allergies

- Review the need for contrast administration
- No conclusive evidence that prophylactic steroids are of benefit
- *If contrast is required:*
  - Use a non-ionic low or iso-osmolar agent
  - Maintain close medical supervision, leaving a cannula in place with 30 min of observation post investigation
  - Ensure adequate resuscitation facilities are in place

Metformin

- Metformin accumulation in renal impairment may result in lactic acidosis, although there is no convincing evidence that lactic acidosis is an issue after iodinated contrast medium in patients taking metformin
- *eGFR > 60 ml/min/1.73 m*
  - No need to stop metformin
- *eGFR < 60 ml/min/1.73 m*
  - Consult with referring clinician regarding stopping metformin for 48 h after contrast administration + hydration

Asthma

- No precautions necessary
- If uncontrolled asthma, defer imaging

Pregnancy

- Administer iodinated contrast medium only in exceptional cases
- Thyroid function should be measured in the fetus in the 1st week after birth

Lactation

- No special precautions or cessation of breastfeeding required

Thyroid

- Iodinated contrast should not be given if the patient is hyperthyroid
- Iodinated contrast will preclude therapeutic radio-iodine therapy for 2 months – MRI is the preferred staging method
- Isotope thyroid imaging should be avoided for 2 months after iodinated contrast

©33

MRI

Gadolinium Agents and NSF	
HIGHEST RISK OF NSF	Gadodiamide (Omniscan); Gadopentetate dimeglumaine (Magnevist); Gadoversetamide (Optimark)
Contraindicated: CKD 4 and 5 (GFR < 30 mL/min) – including if on dialysis; acute renal insufficiency; pregnancy; neonates	
Used with caution: CKD 3 (GFR = 30-60 mL/min) – at least 7 days between injections; children < 1 yr	
Lactating women: stop breastfeeding for 24 hrs and discard milk	
eGFR and clinical assessment mandatory before administration; never given in doses > 0.1 mmol/kg	
INTERMEDIATE RISK OF NSF	Gadobenate dimeglumine (Multihance); Gadofosveset trisodium (Vasovist); Gadoxetate disodium (Primovist)
LOWEST RISK OF NSF	Gadobutrol (Gadovist); Gadoterate meglumine (Dotarem); Gadoteridol (Prohance)
Used with caution: CKD 4 and 5 (GFR <30 mL/min) – at least 7 days between injections	
Pregnant women: can be used to give essential information	
Lactating women: discussion required whether to discard breast milk for 24 hours after injection	
eGFR testing not manadatory	

SEDATION AND PAIN RELIEF IN INTERVENTIONAL RADIOLOGY

Agent	Effects	Dosing	Onset of action	Duration of action
Sedation				
Benzodiazepines: facilitate the action of γ-aminobutyric acid (main CNS inhibitory neurotransmitter) ► benzodiazepines act synergistically with opiods • *Overdose:* flumazenil (0.2 mg IV every 60s, up to 1 mg)				
Diazepam	Sedation ► anxiolytic effects	2–10 mg IM/IV every 3–4 hours PRN (max 30 mg)	2–3 min	6 hours
Midazolam	Sedation ► anxiolytic effects ► amnesia	1-2.5 mg IV over 2 mins PRN – titrate to effect every 2 mins (max 5 mg)	2 min	45–60 min
Pain relief				
Opiods: shorter acting narcotics (e.g. fentanyl) are used for most interventional procedures • *Overdose:* naloxone (0.1-0.3 mg IV every 30–60s – no max dose)				
Morphine	Analgesia	2–10 mg/70 kg IV – titrate to effect	3–10 min	3–4 hours
Pethidine	Analgesia		15 mins	2–4 hours
Fentanyl	Analgesia	50–100 µg IV titrate to effect ► repeat every 1–2 hrs PRN (max 2 µg/kg)	2–3 min	30–60 min
Non opiods				
Voltarol	Analgesia	PO: 75–150 mg daily in 2–3 divided doses ► PR: 75–150 mg daily in divided doses	30 mins	6–8 hours
Local anaesthetics				
• *Short Acting:* Lidocaine • *Longer Acting:* Bupivicaine • *Local Anaesthetic Systemic Toxicity (LAST):* early signs: lightheadedness / mouth numbness / ringing in the ears / metallic taste sensation ► late signs: blurred vision / tremors / seizures / cardiovascular collapse ▪ Rapid anaesthetic review required if suspected				
Lidocaine (plain)	Analgesia	Max dose: 3–5 mg/kg ► <300 mg	2–5 mins	Up to 2 hours
Lidocaine (with adrenaline)	Analgesia	Max dose: 5–7 mg/kg ► <500 mg	2–5 mins	Up to 3 hours
Bupivicaine	Analgesia	Max dose: 2.5 mg/kg ► <175 mg	5–10 mins	4–8 hours

CONTRAST MEDIUM REACTION TREATMENT

Nausea/vomiting

- *Transient:* supportive treatment
- *Severe, protracted:* appropriate antiemetic drugs should be considered

Urticaria

- *Scattered, transient:* supportive treatment, including observation
- *Scattered, protracted:* appropriate H_1-antihistamine IM, PO, or IV should be considered
- *Profound:* consider adrenaline 1:1000, 0.1–0.3 ml (0.1–0.3 mg) IM. Repeat as needed

Bronchospasm

- O_2 by mask (6–10 L/min)
- β_2 agonist metered dose inhaler (2–3 deep inhalations)
- *Adrenaline:*
  - *Normal blood pressure:* adrenaline 1:1000, 0.1–0.3 ml (0.1–0.3 mg) IM. Use a smaller dose in a patient with coronary artery disease or in an elderly patient
  - *Decreased blood pressure:* adrenaline 1:1000, 0.5 ml (0.5 mg) IM

Laryngeal oedema

- O_2 by mask (6–10 L/min)
- Adrenaline 1:1000, 0.5 ml (0.5 mg) IM. Repeat as needed

Hypotension

- *Isolated hypotension:*
  - Elevate patients legs
  - O_2 by mask (6–10 L/min)
  - Rapid IV fluids: normal saline or lactated Ringer's solution
  - If unresponsive: adrenaline 1:1000, 0.5 ml (0.5 mg) IM. Repeat as needed
- *Vagal reaction (hypotension and bradycardia):*
  - Elevate patients legs
  - O_2 by mask (6-10 L/min)
  - Atropine 0.6-1.0 mg IV. Repeat if necessary after 3 min, to a total of 3 mg (0.04 mg/kg)
  - Rapid IV fluids: normal saline or lactated Ringer's solution

Generalized anaphylactoid reaction

- Call for the resuscitation team
- Suction airway, if needed
- Elevate the patient's legs, if hypotensive
- O_2 by mask (6–10 L/min)
- Adrenaline 1:1000, 0.5 ml (0.5 mg) IM
- H_1 blocker (e.g. diphenhydramine 25–50 mg IV)

Contrast medium extravasation

- Elevate the affected limb
- Apply ice packs to the affected area
- If symptoms do not resolve quickly, consider admitting the patient for monitoring
  - Skin blistering, paraesthesia, altered tissue perfusion and increasing or persistent pain (> 4 h) suggests severe injury
- More aggressive therapy with surgical suction or topical aspiration of the extravasated contrast media is controversial
- Record the event in the radiology report and patient notes

Adapted from: RCR Standards for IV Contrast Agent Administration to Adult Patients, 2nd edition (February 2010).

ANTI-COAGULATION AGENTS AND INTERVENTIONAL RADIOLOGY

		Low risk	Moderate risk	High risk
		Thoracentesis ▶ paracentesis ▶ superficial aspiration or drainage ▶ superficial biopsy	Intra-abdominal and chest biopsy or drainage (excluding high risk) ▶ cholecystotomy ▶ simple RFA	Renal, hepatic or splenic biopsy ▶ biliary intervention ▶ complex RFA ▶ nephrostomy
Unfractionated Heparin	Interval between last dose and procedure	1 hour	4 hours	4–6 hours
Unfractionated Heparin	Resumption after procedure	1 hour	1 hour	1 hour
Warfarin	Interval between last dose and procedure	5 days	5 days	5 days
Warfarin	Resumption after procedure	12 hours	12 hours	12–24 hours
LMWH	Interval between last dose and procedure	12 hours	12 hours	24 hours
LMWH	Resumption after procedure	6 hours	6 hours	6 hours
Clopidogrel	Interval between last dose and procedure	5 days	5 days	5 days
Clopigogrel	Resumption after procedure	Immediate	Immediate	Immediate
Aspirin (low dose)	Interval between last dose and procedure	Do not withhold	Do not withhold	Do not withhold
Aspirin (high dose)	Interval between last dose and procedure	Do not withhold	5 days	5 days (Heparin 'bridge' may be required)
Aspirin	Resumption after procedure	Immediate	Immediate	Immediate
NSAIDs	Interval between last dose and procedure	None	None	5 days
NSAIDs	Resumption after procedure	Immediate	Immediate	Immediate

Warfarin

- Withhold warfarin therapy for 5 days pre procedure; goal of INR < 1.5 ▶ heparin bridge may be required for those who need continuing anticoagulation ▶ restart warfarin within 12 hours (low/moderate risk procedure) and 24 hours (high risk procedure)
  - Reversal with administered fresh frozen plasma (FFP) and vitamin K

Heparin

- Heparin effect monitored via APTT measurement (target window of 1.5 to 2.5 times the normal value) ▶ platelets should be monitored to evaluate for heparin induced thrombocytopaenia
  - Reversal with protamine – 1 mg of protamine reverses 100 IU of unfractionated heparin

SUMMARY OF THE RESPONSE EVALUATION CRITERIA IN SOLID TUMOURS (RECIST 1.1)

- This provides a standard approach for the objective assessment of change in the *overall* tumour burden for use in cancer clinical trials. It is not applicable when studying malignant lymphoma (separate guidelines exist). The following criteria are based on CT assessment and require a CT scan slice thickness no greater than 5 mm:

Measurability of lesions at baseline	
Tumour	A minimum longest diameter within the plane of measurement of 10 mm ▶ only the *long*-axis measurement is used for follow-up
Malignant lymph node	A short-axis measurement ≥ 15 mm ▶ only the *short*-axis measurement is used for follow-up
Non-measurable	Small lesions (with a longest diameter < 10 mm) ▶ pathological lymph nodes with a short axis of ≥ 10 mm and < 15 mm ▶ leptomeningeal disease ▶ ascites ▶ pleural or pericardial effusions ▶ inflammatory breast disease ▶ lymphangitic skin or lung involvement

Baseline documentation of 'target' and 'non-target' lesions	
Target lesions	There should be a maximum of 5 lesions in total (with a maximum of 2 lesions per organ) ▶ the lesions should be representative of all the involved organs and have the longest diameters
Lymph nodes	A short-axis measurement ≥ 15 mm
Non-target lesions	This includes all other sites of disease or pathological lymph nodes with a short-axis measurement of ≥ 10 mm but < 15 mm ▶ these should be recorded but their measurements are not required and should be followed as 'present' or 'absent'
A sum of the diameters (the long axis for non-nodal and the short axis for nodal lesions) for all target lesions will be reported as the baseline sum diameters.	

Response criteria for target lesions	
Complete response (CR)	Disappearance of all target lesions* ▶ any pathological lymph nodes (target or non-target) must have had their short-axis dimension reduced to < 10 mm
Partial response (PR)	There is at least a 30% decrease in the sum of the target lesion diameters (taking the baseline sum diameter as the reference measurement)
Progressive disease (PD)	There has been at least a 20% increase in the sum of the target lesion diameters, taking as a reference the smallest sum on the study (including the baseline sum if this is the smallest) ▶ in addition, the sum must also demonstrate an absolute increase of ≥ 5 mm ▶ 1 or more new lesions is also considered progression
Stable disease (SD)	There has been neither a PR or PD (with the smallest sum diameter during the study taken as a reference)
*If a target lesion becomes too small to measure accurately it should be assigned a default value of 5 mm (or 0 mm if it has disappeared) ▶ if a target lesion splits, the longest diameter of the fragmented portions should be added together ▶ if target lesions coalesce, then the longest diameter of the coalesced lesion should be measured.	

Response criteria for non-target lesions	
Complete response (CR)	There has been disappearance of all non-target lesions and normalization of tumour marker levels ▶ all lymph nodes must be non-pathological in size (< 10 mm short-axis diameter)
Non-CR/non-PD	There is persistence of ≥ 1 non-target lesions (± maintenance of tumour marker levels)
Progressive disease (PD)	There has been unequivocal progression of existing non-target lesions ▶ 1 or more new lesions is also considered progression

Reference: new response evaluation criteria in solid tumours: revised RECIST guideline (version 1.1).©32

CERVICAL LYMPH NODE LEVELS

SOFT TISSUES OF THE NECK – LYMPH NODES

- Patterns suggestive of malignant involvement:
  - A round lobular shape (a short axis measurement > 1 cm is significant)
  - Absence of a fatty hilum ▶ an irregular outline ▶ a heterogeneous internal pattern
  - A disorganized peripheral colour flow pattern (Doppler US)
  - Nodal clusters or fusion of nodes

Level	Nodal group	Space occupied
Level I	*Submental/ submandibular nodes*	Above the hyoid bone, below the mylohyoid muscle and anterior to the posterior aspect of the submandibular gland
Level IA	*Submental nodes*	Between the medial margins of the anterior bellies of the digastric muscles
Level IB	*Submandibular nodes*	Lateral to the level IA nodes and anterior to the posterior aspect of the submandibular gland
Level II	*Upper internal jugular nodes*	Anterior to the posterior aspect of the sternocleidomastoid muscle, posterior to the back of the submandibular gland, and above the base of the hyoid bone
Level IIA		A node that does not lie posterior to the internal jugular vein, or if it does is not separable from the vein
Level IIB		A node that lies posterior to the internal jugular vein with a fat plane separating it and the vein
Level III	*Middle internal jugular nodes*	Anterior to the posterior aspect of the sternocleidomastoid muscle, and between the base of the hyoid bone and the base of the cricoid arch
Level IV	*Low internal jugular (Virchow) nodes*	Anterior to a line connecting the posterior aspect of the sternocleidomastoid muscle and the posterolateral margin of the anterior scalene muscle, and between the base of the cricoid arch and the level of the clavicles
Level V	*Posterior triangle nodes*	From the skull base to the level of the clavicle, anterior to the anterior margin of the trapezius muscle, and posterior to the posterior aspect of the sternocleidomastoid muscle
Level VA		Above the level of the base of the cricoid arch
Level VB		Below the level of the base of the cricoid arch and above the clavicle ▶ nodes lie posterolateral to the posterior aspect of the sternocleidomastoid muscle and the posterolateral margin of the anterior scalene muscle
Level VI	*Upper visceral nodes*	Between the base of the hyoid bone and manubrium ▶ between the carotid arteries ▶ this includes the paratracheal, pretracheal, parathyroid and precricoid nodes
Level VII	*Superior mediastinal nodes*	Below the manubrium but above the innominate vein ▶ between the carotid arteries

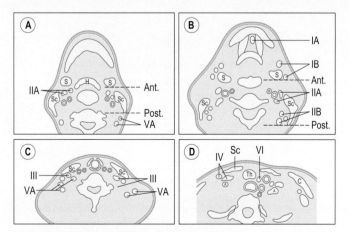

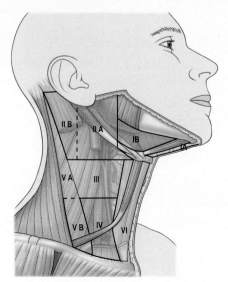

Drawing of the right side of the neck with the sternocleidomastoid muscle and right submandibular salivary gland removed and the IJV tied off, demonstrating the nodal levels (1–6). Level 7 (superior mediastinum) has not been covered.**

Transaxial diagram of cervical lymph node stations at the level of the floor of the mouth and submandibular gland (s) ▶ (A) the hyoid bone (h) ▶ (B) thyroid cartilage and cricoid cartilage (C) and just above the clavicles (c) (D) with a portion of the thyroid gland (Th) in view. Note the appearance of the sternocleidomastoid muscle (Sc), which is a key landmark.

LIVER SEGMENT ANATOMY

Couinaud classification

- The liver is subdivided anatomically into 8 segments in an anticlockwise fashion:
  - The horizontal left and right portal veins separate the superior segments (II, IVa, VIII, VII) from the inferior segments (III, IVb, V, VI)
  - The three vertical hepatic vein branches further subdivide the segments:
    - *Right branch:* this separates segments VII, VI from VIII, V
    - *Middle branch:* this separates segments VIII, V from IVa, IVb
    - *Left branch:* this separates segments IVa, IVb from II, III
  - *The caudate lobe (segment I):* this is autonomous, receiving vessels from both the left and right portal vein branches and the hepatic artery ▶ it has an independent venous drainage directly into the IVC

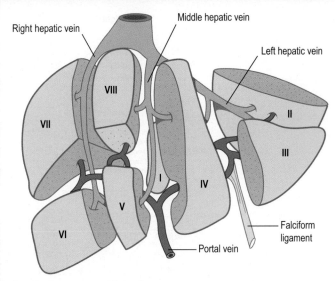

Surgical segments of the liver.

MIDDLE EAR ANATOMY

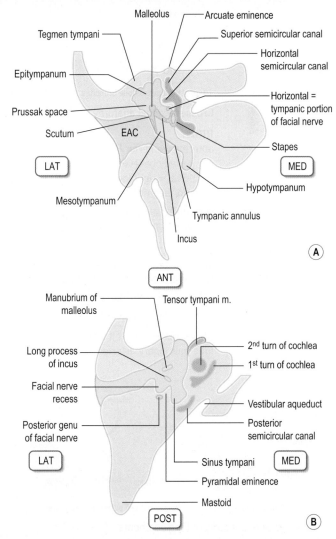

(A) Coronal tomogram of temporal bone. (B) Axial tomogram of temporal bone.

LUNG SEGMENT ANATOMY

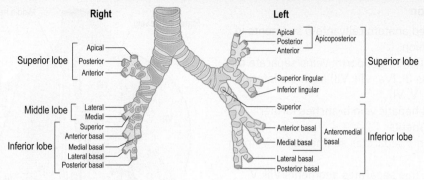

Anatomy of the bronchial tree.

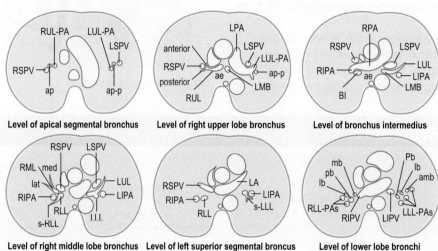

Level of apical segmental bronchus — Level of right upper lobe bronchus — Level of bronchus intermedius

Level of right middle lobe bronchus — Level of left superior segmental broncus — Level of lower lobe bronchi

Cross-sectional anatomy of bronchovascular divisions.

RIGHT

anterior = anterior RUL, ap = apical RUL, BI = bronchus intermedius, lat = lateral RML, mb = mediobasal RLL, med = medial RML, pb = posterobasal RLL, post = posterior RUL, RLL = right lower lobe, RML = right middle lobe, RUL = right upper lobe, s-RLL = superior segment.

RIPV/LIPV = right/left inferior pulmonary vein, RPA/LPA = right/left pulmonary artery, RUL-PA/LUL-PA = right/left upper lobe pulmonary artery.

LEFT

amb = anteromediobasal LLL, ap-p = apicoposterior LUL, lb = laterobasal LLL, LLL = left lower lobe, LMB = left main bronchus, LUL = left upper lobe, pb = posterobasal LLL, s-LLL = superior segment.

ae = azygoesophageal recess.

RIPA/LIPA = right/left inferior pulmonary artery, RLL-PAs/LLL-PAs = right/left lower lobe pulmonary arteries, RSPV/LSPV = right/left superior pulmonary vein.

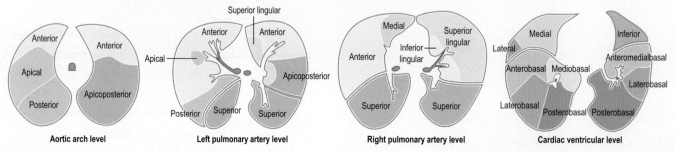

Aortic arch level — Left pulmonary artery level — Right pulmonary artery level — Cardiac ventricular level

Cross-sectional anatomy of lung segments.

INTRAABDOMINAL PERITONEAL COMPARTMENTS

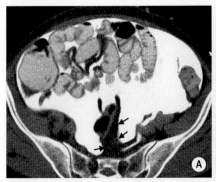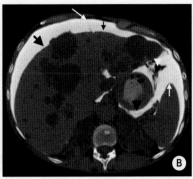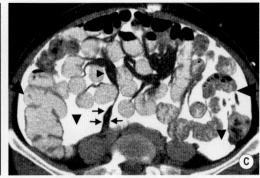

Peritoneal spaces of a woman suffering chronic renal failure, after intraperitoneal injection of water-soluble contrast material on CT. (A) The opacified fluid in the left inframesocolic space is partly bounded by the sigmoid mesocolon seen as the fatty plane extending from the sigmoid colon to the sacrum (arrows). (B) Contrast medium opacifies the right subphrenic (large black arrow) and the left posterior subphrenic (small white arrow) space. The left anterior perihepatic space (small black arrow) is bounded on the right by the falciform ligament (large white arrow). The lesser sac (black arrowhead) is delineated behind the stomach and its superior extension around the caudate lobe of the liver is demonstrated. The gastrosplenic ligament (white arrowhead) is demonstrated as the fatty space between the lesser sac and the splachnic splenic surface. The bare area of the liver at the reflection of the right coronary ligament is uncovered by contrast material. (C) Inframesocolic compartment. The opacified fluid delineates the right (large black arrow) and the left paracolic gutters. The right and the left inframesocolic spaces are also opacified (large arrowheads). A triangle-shaped opacified area (small arrowhead) intervenes between folds of small-bowel mesentery that are seen as lucent bands. The fat within the root of the small-bowel mesentery (small arrows) is outlined by fluid.

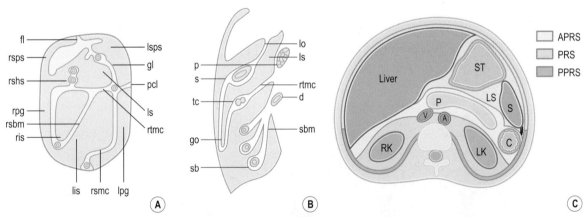

(A) Coronal diagram showing the division of the peritoneal cavity according to its peritoneal attachments to the posterior abdominal wall. (B) Midsagittal diagram of the upper abdomen. d, duodenum; fl, falciform ligament; gl, gastrosplenic ligament; go, greater omentum; lis, left infracolic space; lo, lesser omentum; lpg, left paracolic gutter; ls, lesser sac; lsps, left subphrenic space; p, pancreas; pcl, phrenicocolic ligament; ris, right infracolic space; rpg, right paracolic gutter; rsbm, root of small-bowel mesentery; rshs, right subhepatic space; rsps, right subdiaphragmatic space; rtmc, root of transverse mesocolon; s, stomach; sb, small bowel; sbm, small-bowel mesentery; tc, transverse colon. (C) Retroperitoneal compartments. The pancreas (P) lies in the anterior pararenal space (APRS) together with the ascending and descending colon (C) and duodenum. A, aorta; LK, left kidney; LS, lesser sac; PPRS, posterior pararenal space; PRS, pararenal space; RK, right kidney; S, spleen; ST, stomach; V, inferior vena cava.

STROKE VASCULAR TERRITORIES

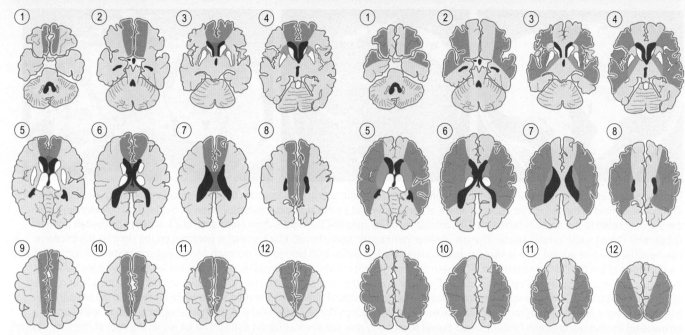

ACA distribution. Shaded areas of these axial diagrams, arranged in sequence from base to vertex outline the territory of ACA including the medial lenticulostriate (medium shading), callosal (dark shading) and hemispheric branches (light shading).

MCA distribrtion. This diagram of the axial sections, arranged in sequence from base to vertex, outlines the MCA distribution with the lateral lenticulostriate (medium shading) and hemisphenric branches (light shading).

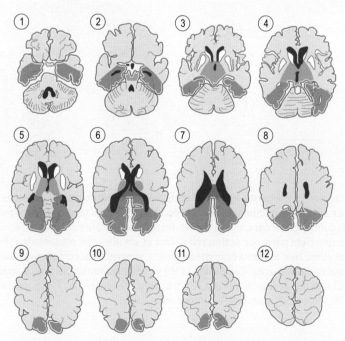

PCA distribution. Axial diagrams arranged in sequence from base to vertex outline supply from the PCA, the thalami and midbrain perforators (medium shading), callosal (dark shading) and hemispheric branches (light shading).

RADIOLOGICAL FEATURES OF COMMON ENDOCRINOLOGICAL CONDITIONS

Radiological features of acromegaly

Skull	Vault thickened Paranasal and mastoid air cells enlarged Pituitary fossa enlarged Floor of the fossa asymmetrical or ballooned
Mandible	Prognathism with increased angle
Spine	Kyphosis Enlarged vertebral bodies Posterior scalloping of vertebral bodies
Chest	Increased anteroposterior diameter Ribs increased in calibre and length
Hands	General enlargement Enlarged bases of phalanges and terminal tufts, spade-like Enlarged muscle attachments
Feet	Thickening of 'heel pad': M > 23 mm, F > 21.5 mm
Long bones	Thickened by periosteal new bone formation
Joints	Widening of joint spaces due to thickened cartilage Premature degeneration (OA) changes (shoulders, hips, knees) Chondrocalcinosis
Soft tissues	Enlarged heart, kidneys, liver Calcification of pinna of ears

Radiological features of Cushing's syndrome

Skull	Pituitary fossa usually normal
Skeleton	Osteoporosis Vertebral collapse Kyphosis Concave vertebral margins Wedged vertebral bodies Rib fractures – multiple, painless with excess callus Necrosis of femoral heads Secondary osteoarthritis

Radiological features of hypopituitarism

Skull	Unfused sutures
Skeleton	Small but normal proportions (Lorain dwarf) Slender bones Small pituitary fossa Unfused epiphyses

Radiological features of hyperthyroidism (thyrotoxicosis)

Skull	Exophthalmos
Skeleton	Osteopenia Cortical striation – acropachy In childhood, early appearance and accelerated growth of ossification centres
Heart	Cardiac enlargement Cardiac failure
Thymus	Enlargement

Radiological features of hypothyroidism (cretinism and juvenile myxoedema)

Skull	Delayed closure of fontanelles Relatively large sella Poorly developed paranasal sinus Usually brachycephalic Dentition delayed: dental caries Wormian bones
Skeleton	Dwarfism Increased density
Ossification centres	Retarded growth Multicentric and irregular Bilateral and symmetrical
Epiphyses	Delayed fusion and appearance Inhomogeneous epiphyses Fine or coarse stippling Fragmentation
Spine	Kyphosis Flattening of bodies Increase in width of intervertebral space Bullet-shaped vertebral bodies, usually L1 and L2
Long bones	Short Dense transverse bands at metaphyseal ends
Pelvis	Narrow with coxa vara

Radiological features of myxoedema

Heart	Enlargement
Body cavities	Pleural effusion Ascites
Gastrointestinal tract	Abnormalities of oesophageal peristalsis Decreased incidence of peristalsis Constipation 'Pseudo-obstruction'

HISTOLOGICAL TYPING: BONE TUMOURS

Histological typing of primary bone tumours (modified from WHO classification)

	Benign	Malignant
I. Bone-forming tumours	Osteoma Osteoid osteoma Osteoblastoma	Osteosarcoma Parosteal osteosarcoma Periosteal osteosarcoma Telangiectatic osteosarcoma and many other types
II. Cartilage-forming tumours	Chondroma Osteochondroma (cartilage capped exostosis) Chondroblastoma Chondromyxoid fibroma	Chondrosarcoma Mesenchymal chondrosarcoma Clear-cell chondrosarcoma
III. Giant cell tumour		Malignant giant cell tumour
IV. Marrow tumours a. Round cell tumours b. Lymphoma c. Plasma cell tumours d. Leukaemia		{ Ewing's sarcoma Atypical Ewing's sarcoma Primitive neuroectodermal tumours { Hodgkin's disease Non-Hodgkin's lymphoma Solitary myeloma (plasmacytoma) Granulocytic sarcoma (chloroma)

V. Vascular tumours	Haemangioma
	Lymphangioma
	Glomus tumour
	    Intermediate
	    Haemangiopericytoma
	    Massive osteolysis	

VI. Other connective tissue tumours	Non-ossifying fibroma Benign fibrous histiocytoma Desmoplastic fibroma Lipoma Fibromatoses	Fibrosarcoma Malignant fibrous histiocytoma Liposarcoma Malignant mesenchymoma
VII. Other miscellaneous disorders	Neurilemmoma Neurofibroma	Neurosarcoma Chordoma Adamantinoma of long bones
VIII. Unclassified tumours		Undifferentiated primary sarcoma
IX. Tumour-like lesions	Solitary bone cyst Aneurysmal bone cyst Langerhans' cell histiocytosis (eosinophilic granuloma) Fibrous dysplasia Implantation epidermoid Reparative giant cell granuloma	

SUMMARY OF RADIOLOGICAL FEATURES IN JOINT DISEASE

Inflammatory	Chondropathic	Depositional
Periarticular (synovial) erosions *Osteoporosis* *Tendon-related erosions* *Periosteal reaction* *Syndesmophytes* *Malalignment*	*Subchondral erosions* *Subchondral sclerosis* *Osteophytes* *Chondrocalcinosis* *Normal bone density*	*Soft tissue masses* *Extra-articular* *erosions* *Normal bone* *density*

Rheumatoid and its variants	**Seronegative**	**Degenerative**	**Metabolic**	
Symmetrical Small joints (e.g. MCPJ/PIPJ) Osteoporosis	Asymmetrical Large joints (e.g. SIJ/spine/DIPJ) Osteoporosis less marked Periosteal reaction Syndesmophytes	Weight-bearing joints (e.g. DIPJ/1st CMCJ) Localized cartilage loss Marginal calcification	Atypical distribution Uniform cartilage loss Diffuse chondrocalcinosis Large subchondral cysts Greater destruction	
Rheumatoid arthritis *SLE* *Scleroderma* *Dermatomyositis*	*Ankylosing spondylitis* *Reiter's syndrome* *Psoriatic arthropathy* *Enteropathic arthritis* *Juvenile idiopathic arthritis*	*Osteoarthritis* *Neuropathic* *Haemophilic*	*Calcium pyrophosphate* *Haemochromatosis* *Alkaptonuria* *Hyperparathyroidism* *Wilson's disease*	*Gout* *Reticulohistiocytosis* *Amyloidosis*

©12

HAEMATOMA MR APPEARANCES

	Hyperacute (< 12 h)	Acute (hours to days)	Early subacute (few days)	Late subacute (up to 1 month)	Chronic (1 month +)
Underlying pathology	Extravasation	Deoxygenation	Clot retraction + deoxy-Hb is oxidized to met-Hb	Cell lysis	Clot digestion (macrophages)
Erythrocyte status	Intact	Intact – hypoxic	Intact – severely hypoxic	Lysis	Absent
Haemoglobin status	Intracellular oxy-Hb	Intracellular deoxy-Hb	Intracellular met-Hb	Extracellular met-Hb	Haemosiderin ferritin
T1WI	↔ or ↓	↔ or ↓	↑↑	↑↑	↔ or ↓
T2WI	↑	↓	↓↓	↑↑	↓↓

deoxy-Hb, deoxyhaemoglobin ▶ met-Hb, methaemoglobin ▶ oxy-Hb, oxyhaemoglobin

EPONYMS FOR COMMON FRACTURES

Fracture	Description
Face	
Le Fort I	Detachment of the upper jaw from the maxillofacial skeleton – a 'floating palate'
Le Fort II	A pyramidal fracture of the midfacial skeleton – a 'floating maxilla'
Le Fort III	A transverse craniofacial dissociation involving the zygomatic arch – a 'floating face'
Spine	
Jefferson	A burst fracture of the atlas (C1 vertebra)
Hangman	A fracture of the neural arch of C2 vertebra (bilateral pars fractures)
Teardrop	An avulsion fracture of the anterior/inferior margin of a cervical vertebral body (that looks like a teardrop) ▶ this is an unstable injury
Clay-shoveler's	An avulsion fracture of a spinous process (usually C7/T1 vertebra)
Chance	A horizontal fracture through a spinous process, pedicles and vertebral body (this is usually a flexion injury of the thoracolumbar spine)
Upper extremity	
Hill-Sachs	An impaction fracture of the posterolateral humeral head
Bankart	A fracture of the anterior glenoid rim
Reverse Bankart	A fracture of the posterior glenoid rim
Monteggia	A fracture of the ulna with dislocation of the proximal radius
Galeazzi	A fracture of the radius with dislocation of the distal radioulnar joint
Colles's	A fracture of the distal radius with dorsal angulation
Smith's	A fracture of the distal radius with volar angulation
Barton's	An intra-articular fracture/dislocation of the distal radius
Bennett's	A fracture of the base of the first metacarpal with dislocation of the MCP joint
Rolando	A comminuted fracture of the base of the first metacarpal with dorsal subluxation of the metacarpal
Boxer's	A fracture of the neck/shaft of the 4th or 5th metacarpal
Gamekeeper's	An injury to the ulnar collateral ligament of the 1st MCP joint
Chauffer's	An intra-articular fracture of the radial styloid

Table continued

Table continued

Fracture	Description
Lower extremity	
Segond	An avulsion fracture of the lateral tibia at the attachment of the lateral capsular ligament ▶ this is associated with an ACL injury
Pilon	An intra-articular comminuted compression injury of the distal tibia
Tillaux	A Salter–Harris III injury of the lateral distal tibia
Maisonneuve	Disruption of the distal tibiofibular syndesmosis with an associated fracture of the proximal fibula (± a fracture of the medial malleolus)
Jones	A transverse fracture located 1.5–2 cm distal from the proximal tip of the 5th metatarsal
Lisfranc	A fracture dislocation of the tarsometatarsal joints
March	A stress fracture of the metatarsal neck
Nutcracker	A cuboid fracture following an indirect compressive force
Pelvis	
Duverney	An isolated fracture of the iliac wing
Malgaigne	Double vertical fractures of the pelvis ▶ the anterior fracture is usually through both pubic rami but there may be disruption of the symphysis pubis ▶ the posterior fracture is usually through the sacrum but there may be dislocation of the sacroiliac joint
Bucket handle	A fracture through the sacrum or disruption of the sacroiliac joint with a fracture of the contralateral pubic rami
Straddle	A fracture of all 4 pubic rami

12.4 PATTERNS OF TUMOUR SPREAD

INITIAL COMMON PATTERNS OF TUMOUR SPREAD

Lung (NSCLC)

Local spread	• Mediastinal invasion ▶ chest wall invasion ▶ brachial plexus invasion (Pancoast's tumour)
Lymph node spread	• Hilar and mediastinal nodes are often present at diagnosis • ***Spread is usually sequential:*** ipsilateral peribronchial (± ipsilateral) hilar and intrapulmonary nodes (N1) > ipsilateral mediastinal (± subcarinal) nodes (N2) > ipsilateral mediastinal (± subcarinal) nodes (N3)

Haematogenous spread	• Liver > adrenal > brain > bone > kidney
	  ▪ Adrenal mass < 2 cm: likely adenoma
	  ▪ Adrenal mass > 2 cm: likely metastasis

PEARL	• Squamous cell tumours are the least likely type to metastasize ▶ SCLCs have usually metastasized at presentation

Oesophagus

Local spread	• Early local invasion of adjacent structures due to lack of a serosal barrier – therefore usually at an advanced stage at diagnosis

Lymph node spread	• Involved nodes are usually at the same level as the tumour
	• Oesophageal lymphatics tend to course longitudinally, however 'skip' nodal involvement can occur
	  ▪ *Cervical oesophagus:* cervical and supraclavicular nodes
	  ▪ *Upper and middle third:* mediastinal nodes
	  ▪ *Lower third:* lower medistinal, left gastric, coeliac, and para-aortic nodes

Haematogenous spread	• Common (tumour has easy access to lymphatics and blood vessels) • Liver > lungs > bone > kidney > brain

Stomach

Local spread	• Local spread into adjacent structures (e.g. pancreas, colon, spleen)
Lymph node spread	• ***Perigastric:*** pericardial ▶ lesser curvature ▶ greater curvature ▶ suprapyloric • ***Extraperigastric:*** left gastric ▶ common hepatic ▶ coeliac ▶ splenic hilum and artery ▶ hepatic pedicle ▶ retropancreatic ▶ mesenteric root ▶ middle colic ▶ para-aortic • NB: retropancreatic, para-aortic and mesenteric nodes are classified as M1 metastatic disease
Haematogenous spread	• Via the portal vein to the liver (25% at presentation) ▶ a similar number will have peritoneal metastases
PEARL	• Transcoelomic spread can occur through the peritoneum (e.g. Kruckenberg tumours)

Rectum

Local spread	• Invasion through the bowel wall into the perirectal fat – an important predictor of local recurrence and survival • Extramural venous invasion is an adverse prognostic factor
Lymph node spread	• From the level of the tumour cranially within the mesorectum – proximal blockage (e.g. extensive adenopathy) may cause retrograde spread with lower rectal tumours rarely spreading to the inguinal nodes • Pelvic side wall spread is unusual
Haematogenous spread	• Liver (via the portal vein)
PEARLS	• Involvement of the circumferential resection margin (CRM) is an adverse prognostic feature (including disruption during surgery) • Perforation of the peritoneal membrane can result in transcoelomic spread as well as an increased risk of recurrence • Transcoelomic spread favours the lower right small bowel mesentery and the pouch of Douglas

Hepatocellular carcinoma (HCC)

Local spread	• Vascular invasion of the portal or hepatic veins
Lymph node spread	• Spread to lymph nodes along the hepatoduodenal ligament
Haematogenous spread	• Lung = bone > adrenals > peritoneum
PEARL	• Abdominal lymph nodes are often enlarged with cirrhosis

Cholangiocarcinoma

Local spread	• Vascular invasion of the portal or hepatic veins
Lymph node spread	• Spread to lymph nodes along the hepatoduodenal ligament – with a propensity to spread to the portocaval lymph node chain as well as the anterior and posterior pancreaticoduodenal chain
Haematogenous spread	• Less common than with HCC – remote metastases are usually to the lung (less commonly to bone, the adrenals and peritoneum)

Renal cell carcinoma

Local spread	• Perinephric fat ▶ ipsilateral adrenal ▶ adjacent viscera (including muscles) • Renal vein invasion (± IVC)
Lymph node spread	• Via lymphatics following the renal vessels to the ipsilateral para-aortic nodes ▶ direct connections with the thoracic duct and mediastinum also exist
Haematogenous spread	• Common sites: lungs > bones, CNS, adrenals
PEARL	• IVC tumour thrombus extending above the hepatic veins requires a transthoracic surgical approach – right atrial involvement requires cardiopulmonary bypass

Pancreas

Local spread	• 70% of tumours arise within the pancreatic head • Tumour spreads by direct perivascular and perineural invasion • ***Head/uncinate process tumours:*** these usually extend along the SMA and mesenteric root • ***Body/tail tumours:*** these usually infiltrate the coeliac, hepatic or splenic arteries • Local invasion can involve the stomach, duodenum and retroperitoneum
Lymph node spread	• Early micrometastases at presentation are common • ***Primary drainage:*** superior, inferior, anterior, posterior and splenic lymph nodes • ***Secondary drainage:*** porta hepatis, common hepatic, coeliac, mesenteric root lymph nodes • ***Tertiary drainage:*** peri-aortic and distal superior mesenteric lymph nodes
Haematogenous spread	• Early micrometastases at presentation are common • These usually involve the liver and peritoneal surfaces
PEARL	• Usually only tumours of the head and uncinate process are surgically resectable (tumours of the body and tail usually have perivascular or perineural metastases at presentation)

Bladder

Local spread	• Initially perivesical fat infiltration ▶ subsequent invasion of adjacent pelvic organs and the pelvic side wall by direct invasion
Lymph node spread	• Rare for superficial (<T2b) tumours • Increasing incidence with deep muscle invasion, and then extravesical spread • Initial nodal involvement: anterior and lateral perivesical nodes ▶ presacral nodes ▶ hypogastric, obturator and external iliac nodes • Late nodal involvement: common iliac and para-aortic nodes • Nodal involvement above the diaphragm is rare
Haematogenous spread	• A late presentation • Sites: bone, lungs, brain, liver

Prostate

Local spread	• Direct extension through the prostate capsule into the seminal vesicles and bladder base
Lymph node spread	• Order of nodal involvement: obturator ▶ presacral ▶ internal iliac ▶ common iliac
Haematogenous spread	• Bone > lung and liver ▶ rarely intracranial or adrenal involvement • Spinal bone metasases are the commonest site (due to the direct communication between the presacral and periprostatic veins)
PEARLS	• Apical tumours are more likely to demonstrate extracapsular extension due to relatively little capsule at this level • Denonvilliers' fascia forms a relative natural barrier to rectal spread

Testis

Lymph node spread	• Lymphatics drain the testis via the spermatic cord to drain into the retroperitoneal lymph nodes
	  ▪ Iliac or inguinal nodes are usually only involved if there is associated cryptorchidism or a history of scrotal surgery
	• **Right-sided tumours:** right paracaval ▶ pre- and retrocaval nodes ▶ aortocaval nodes
	  ▪ A common site for initial presentation is an aortocaval or right paracaval node below the right renal hilum
	• **Left-sided tumours:** left para-aortic nodes ▶ preaortic nodes
	  ▪ A common site for initial presentation is a para-aortic node just below the left renal vein
	• More advanced disease can involve nodes above the level of the renal vessels ▶ retrocrural adenopathy can be followed by posterior mediastinal and subcarinal adenopathy
	• Tumour spread via the thoracic duct can lead to supraclavicular adenopathy

Haematogenous spread	• Usually to the lungs • Rare sites: brain, bone and liver
PEARLS	• Right-sided tumours tend to spread to right-sided retroperitoneal nodes (and vice versa) – contralateral nodal involvement in the absence of ipsilateral nodal involvement is rare • Contralateral nodal involvement is more common when the ipsialteral nodes are larger than 2 cm in size • **'Echelon' node:** a right-sided node lateral to the paracaval group (between the 1st and 3rd lumbar vertebrae) can also be involved

Breast

Local spread	• Chest wall

Lymph node spread	• The axillary nodes are the principal site of metastases, and the likelihood of involvement is related to the size of the primary tumour
	• Nodal involvement is usually sequential, with level 3 involvement carrying a poor prognosis:
	  ▪ **Proximal (level 1):** medial to pectoralis minor
	  ▪ **Middle (level 2):** beneath pectoralis minor
	  ▪ **Distal (level 3):** lateral to pectoralis minor
	• The internal mammary lymph node chain is another potential metastatic site, and most often seen with inner quadrant or central tumours (although these will still most commonly involve the axillary nodes)
	• Supraclavicular lymph node involvement is a late stage of axillary disease with a corresponding poor prognosis

Haematogenous spread	• Although metastatic disease can involve any organ ▶ radiologically demonstrable metastatic disease at presentation is unusual ▪ Bone > lung > liver > pleura > adrenals > skin > brain • Chest involvement can take the form of mediastinal adenopathy, infiltrative mediastinal disease, pulmonary metastases, lymphangitis, or pleural effusions
PEARLS	• The internal mammary lymph node chain is a common site of relapse (as it is not routinely treated with surgery or radiotherapy) • **Sentinel node:** the first lymph node draining a tumour will show metastatic disease if this is present – a sentinel node can be identified by injection of the primary tumour with blue dye or radiopharmaceuticals

Ovary

Local spread	• Uterus and broad ligament (via the fallopian tube) • Direct invasion of the rectum, colon, bladder and pelvic side wall
Lymph node spread	• **Via lymphatics** travelling along with the ovarian vessels to terminate in retroperitoneal nodes • **Via the broad ligament** to terminate in the internal iliac and obturator nodes • **Via the round ligament** to terminate in the external iliac and inguinal nodes
Transcoelomic spread	• This occurs due to the shedding of tumour cells into the peritoneal cavity following disruption of the ovarian serosal epithelial lining ▶ intra-abdominal peritoneal flow dynamics tends to draw the fluid to the undersurface of the diaphragm (having been drawn along the para-aortic gutters and over the omentum) ▪ *Common sites*: undersurface of the diaphragm ▶ liver surface ▶ pouch of Douglas ▶ omentum ▶ serosal bowel surfaces
Haematogenous spread	• This occurs late during the disease • Liver > lungs, kidney, bone
PEARLS	• Occlusion of retroperitoneal lymph nodes can lead to an obstructive ascites • Communication between abdominal and pleural lymphatic vessels can lead to a pleural effusion

Endometrium

Local spread	• Superficial and then deep myometrial invasion • Invasion of adjacent organs once the serosa has been breached
Lymph node spread	• **Tumours within the upper uterus:** common iliac and para-aortic nodes • **Tumours within the lower uterus:** initially to the parametrial, paracervical and obturator nodes ▶ subsequently to iliac and retroperitoneal nodes • Inguinal nodes can be involved via the round ligament
Transcoelomic spread	• Peritoneal spread can occur once the serosa has been breached
Haematogenous spread	• Lungs ▶ liver ▶ bone ▶ brain

Cervix

Local spread	• *Superior:* uterine body • *Inferior:* proximal vagina • *Anterior:* bladder • *Posterior:* rectum • *Pelvic side wall:* via the uterine ligaments
Lymph node spread	• *Initial nodal involvement:* paracervical ▶ parametrial ▶ presacral • *Subsequent nodal involvement:* external iliac ▶ internal iliac, common iliac
Haematogenous spread	• Spread to the lungs, bone and liver is unusual
PEARL	• Hydronephrosis is a common finding secondary to ureteric involvement by parametrial spread

Thyroid

Local spread	• *Papillary thyroid carcinoma* ▪ Thyroid capsule ± surrounding neck structures • *Follicular thyroid carcinoma* ▪ Thyroid capsule ± surrounding neck structures • *Anaplastic thyroid carcinoma* ▪ Local invasion (e.g. trachea or oesophagus) is common • *Medullary thyroid carcinoma* ▪ Thyroid capsule ± surrounding neck structures
Lymph node spread	• *Papillary thyroid carcinoma* ▪ Propensity to spread to regional lymph nodes (≥ 75%) • *Follicular thyroid carcinoma* ▪ Rarely spreads to regional lymph nodes • *Anaplastic thyroid carcinoma* ▪ Uni- or bilateral lymph node involvement is almost universal • *Medullary thyroid carcinoma* ▪ Early spread to regional lymph nodes is common
Haematogenous spread	• *Papillary thyroid carcinoma* ▪ Uncommon (5%) ▶ usually to the lungs • *Follicular thyroid carcinoma* ▪ Tendency for haematogenous spread to bone, liver or lungs • *Anaplastic thyroid carcinoma* ▪ Early haematogenous spread (50% at presentation) ▶ lung > bone > brain • *Medullary thyroid carcinoma* ▪ Distant metastases are seen within the liver, lungs, bone and brain
PEARL	• Papillary thyroid carcinoma lymph node metastases have no bearing on the prognosis

Paranasal sinus neoplasms (squamous)

Local spread	• By direct extension into adjacent structures or via perineural spread
	  ▪ ***Superior maxillary antral tumours:*** ethmoid and orbital spread
	  ▪ ***Posterior maxillary antral tumours:*** initially direct spread into pterygo-palatine fossa and pterygoid plates ▶ later perineural spread into the masticator space
	  ▪ ***Inferomedial maxillary antral tumours:*** alveolus and nasal cavity involvement
	  ▪ ***Ethmoid tumours:*** cribriform plate (± intracranial extension) ▶ lateral orbital spread

Lymph node spread	• Uncommon (retropharyngeal > level I and II nodes) • Indicates tumour spread outside of the nasal cavity (e.g. skin extension)
Haematogenous spread	• Uncommon (10% at presentation)
PEARLS	• Central necrosis is a good indicator of malignant nodal involvement • Orbital involvement carries a poor prognosis ▶ periosteal involvement requires orbital exenteration

Nasopharyngeal carcinoma

Local spread	• Tumours often arise within Rosenmüller's fossa
	  ▪ ***Lateral spread:*** parapharyngeal space
	  ▪ ***Posterolateral spread:*** carotid space ± jugular foramen
	  ▪ ***Superior spread:*** skull base ± intracranial extension
	  ▪ ***Anterior spread:*** nasal cavity ± pterygopalatine fossa
	  ▪ ***Posterior spread:*** prevertebral muscles ± vertebral bodies

Lymph node spread	• Common • Retropharyngeal nodes are the primary draining nodes
Haematogenous spread	• Relatively rare, although higher than with other head and neck tumours

CT CHARACTERIZATION OF ADRENAL MASS LESIONS

- Adenomas contain lipid and will be of low attenuation at unenhanced CT
- Adenomas rapidly washout contrast material (> 60%)

Technique	
Injection	150 ml contrast at 2 ml/s
Initial enhanced attenuation	Measured at 60 s
Delayed attenuation	Measured at 15 min
Measurement area	ROI at least 50% of the adrenal lesion

Size of lesion	Follow-up
< 1 cm	No endocrinology referral or further imaging required

1-4 cm	**HU < 10 = adenoma**
	Suggested wording in report:
	    ■ *'CT findings in keeping with an adrenal adenoma. Consider endocrinology referral if the patient is hypertensive or hypokalaemic.'*
	HU > 10
	Arrange a dedicated CT adrenal:
	  ● Adenoma (i.e. unenhanced HU < 10 or washout characteristics in keeping with adenoma)
	    ■ *'CT findings in keeping with an adrenal adenoma. Consider endocrinology referral if the patient is hypertensive or hypokalaemic.'*
	  ● Washout characteristics not in keeping with an adenoma
	    ■ *'Endocrinology referral is required'*

> 4 cm	*'Urgent endocrinology referral is advised'* (Unless typical features of a myelolipoma, i.e. a very low HU – where no referral and no further imaging is required)

Contrast washout

Absolute wash out

$$\frac{\text{Enhanced CT (HU)} - \text{Delayed CT (HU)}}{\text{Enhanced CT (HU)} - \text{Unenhanced CT (HU)}} \times 100\%$$

Relative wash out

$$\frac{\text{Enhanced CT (HU)} - \text{Delayed CT (HU)}}{\text{Enhanced CT (HU)}} \times 100\%$$

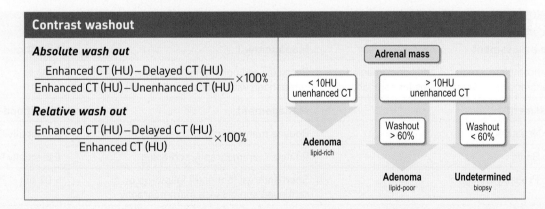

FOLLOW-UP IMAGING

- Follow-up ALL incidental adrenal lesions > 1 cm
  (*whether adenoma or not*)
  - *Single* follow-up un-enhanced CT (adrenals only) at 6 months
    - If > 5 mm increase alert referring clinician
    - If no change in size or increase < 5 mm no further imaging is required

12.5 TNM STAGING OF COMMON CANCERS

BREAST CANCER

T stage

Tx	The primary tumour is not assessable	
T0	There is no evidence of primary tumour	
Tis	Carcinoma in situ (DCIS, LCIS, or Paget's disease without a tumour mass)	
T1	The tumour measures ≤ 2 cm*	
	T1mic	Micro-invasion ≤ 0.1 cm*
	T1a	> 0.1 cm but ≤ 0.5 cm*
	T1b	> 0.5 cm but ≤ 1 cm*
	T1c	> 1 cm but ≤ 2 cm*
T2	The tumour measures > 2 cm but ≤ 5 cm*	
T3	The tumour measures > 5 cm*	
T4	A tumour of any size involving the chest wall or skin (including inflammatory breast cancer)	
	T4a	Chest wall extension
	T4b	Oedema ▶ breast skin ulceration ▶ satellite skin nodules to the same breast
	T4c	Combined T4a and T4b features
	T4d	An inflammatory carcinoma

*Greatest dimension

N stage

Nx	The nearby lymph nodes are not assessable	
N0	There is no spread	
N1	There is spread to movable ipsilateral level I and II axillary nodes	
N2	There is spread to fixed ipsilateral level I and II axillary nodes, or ipsilateral internal mammary nodes *without* axillary involvement	
	N2a	There is spread to fixed level I and II ipsilateral axillary nodes
	N2b	There is spread to ipsilateral internal mammary nodes without axillary node involvement
N3	Metastases in ipsilateral infraclavicular (level III axillary) lymph node(s) with or without level I, II axillary lymph node involvement	
	N3a	Metastases in ipsilateral infraclavicular lymph node(s).
	N3b	Metastases in ipsilateral internal mammary lymph node(s) and axillary lymph node(s)
	N3c	Metastases in ipsilateral supraclavicular lymph node(s)

M stage

M0	There is no distant spread
M1	There is distant spread

AMERICAN COLLEGE OF RADIOLOGY BI-RADS

Assessment categories

Incomplete assessment	Management	Likelihood of cancer
Category 0: incomplete – requires additional imaging evaluation and/or prior mammograms for comparison	Recall for additional imaging and/or comparison with prior examination(s)	N/A
Final assessment	**Management**	**Likelihood of cancer**
Category 1: Negative	Routine mammography screening	Essentially 0%
Category 2: Benign	Routine mammography screening	Essentially 0%
Category 3: Probably Benign	Short-interval (6 month) follow-up or continued surveillance mammography	> 0% but ≤ 2%
Category 4: Suspicious	Tissue diagnosis	> 2% but < 95%
• Category 4A: Low suspicion for malignancy		> 2% to ≤ 10%
• Category 4B: Moderate suspicion for malignancy		> 10% to ≤ 50%
• Category 4C: High suspicion for malignancy		≥ 50% to < 95%
Category 5: Highly suggestive of malignancy	Tissue diagnosis	≥ 95%
Category 6: Known biopsy-proven malignancy	Surgical excision when clinically appropriate	N/A

NB: a similar scoring table is used for USS or MRI assessment with the appropriate designation, for example U3 / M3 rather than B3
Taken from ACR BI-RADS ATLAS (5th Edition) 2013

LUNG CANCER

T stage

TX	Tumour cannot be assessed (or is not visualized)
T0	There is no evidence of a primary tumour
Tis	Carcinoma in situ
T1	A tumour measuring < 3 cm (greatest dimension) ▶ it is surrounded by lung or visceral pleura ▶ there is no bronchoscopic evidence of invasion within the main bronchus

	T1(mi) *T1a*	*Minimally invasive adenocarcinoma* *Tumour measuring ≤1 cm (greatest dimension)*
	T1b *T1c*	*Tumour measuring >1 cm but ≤2 cm (greatest dimension)* *Tumour measuring >2 cm but ≤3 cm*

T2	Tumour measuring >3 cm but ≤ 5 cm, or tumour with any of the following features: • Tumour involving the main bronchus regardless of distance from carina, but without involvement of the carina • Invades the visceral pleura • Associated with atelectasis or obstructive pneumonitis that extends to the hilar region, involving part or all of the lung

	T2a	*Tumour measuring > 3 cm but ≤4 cm (greatest dimension) ▶ invasion across a fissure*
	T2b	*Tumour measuring > 4 cm but ≤5 cm (greatest dimension)*

T3	Tumour measuring > 5 cm but not more than 7 cm (greatest dimension) or directly invades any of the following structures: • Chest wall (including parietal pleura and superior sulcus tumours), phrenic nerve, parietal pericardium • Or associated with separate tumour nodule (s) in the same lobe as the primary
T4	Tumour measuring > 7 cm (greatest dimension) or of any size that invades any of the following structures: • Diaphragm, mediastinum heart, great vessels, trachea, recurrent laryngeal nerve, oesophagus, vertebral body, carina Or associated with separate tumour nodule(s) in a different ipsilateral lobe to that of the primary.

N stage

Nx	The lymph nodes are not assessable
N0	There is no regional nodal involvement
N1	There are involved ipsilateral peribronchial (± ipsilateral) hilar and intrapulmonary lymph nodes
N2	There are involved ipsilateral mediastinal (± subcarinal) lymph nodes
N3	There are involved contralateral mediastinal or hilar nodes, ipsilateral or contralateral scalene nodes, or supraclavicular nodes

M stage

M0	There are no distant metastases
M1	There are distant metastases

	M1a	*Separate tumour nodule(s) in a contralateral lobe ▶ tumour with pleural or pericardial nodule(s) or a malignant pleural or pericardial effusion*
	M1b *M1c*	*Single extrathoracic metastasis in a single organ* *Multiple extrathoracic metastases in one or several organs*

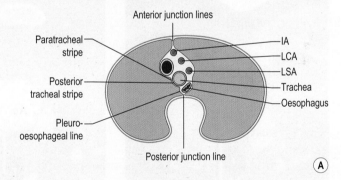

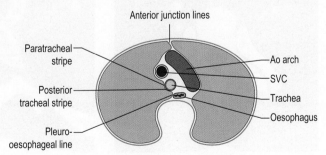

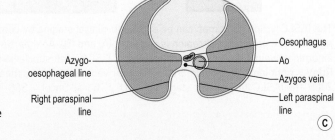

Diagrams illustrating the mediastinal boundaries and junction lines. The visualisation of the junction lines on a plain chest radiograph is variable, depending on how much fat is present in the mediastinum and on how closely the two lungs approximate to one another. (A) Section just above the level of the aortic arch. (B) Section through the aortic arch. (C) Section through the heart.**

IASLC LYMPH NODE MAP

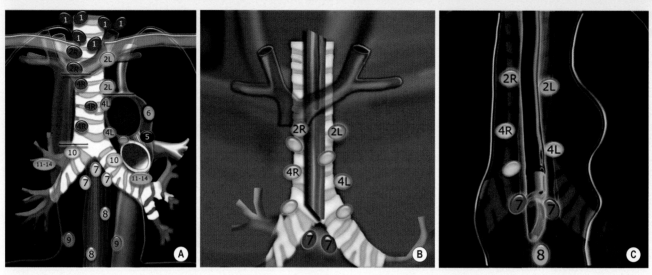

The International Association for the Study of Lung Cancer (IASLC) lymph node map grouping the lymph node stations into 'zones' for purpose of prognostic analysis (from: <http://www.radiologyassistant.nl/en/4646f1278c26f>). Please see explanations in table below.**

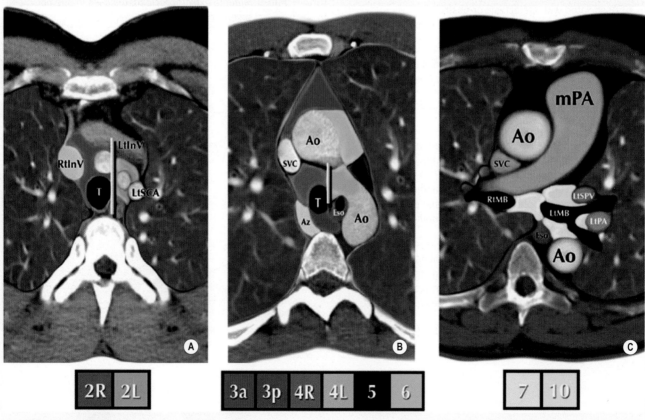

The IASLC lymph node map can be applied to clinical staging by computed tomography in axial (A–C) views. The border between the right and left paratracheal region is shown in (A) and (B). Ao = aorta; Az = azygos vein; MB = main bronchus; Eso = oesophagus; IV = innominate vein; LtInV = left innominate vein; LtSCA = left subclavian artery; PA = pulmonary artery; SPV = superior pulmonary vein; RtInV = right innominate vein; SVC = superior vena cava; T = trachea.** (With permission from Rusch VW, Asamura H, Watanabe H et al 2009 The IASLC lung cancer staging project. J Thorac Oncol 4: 568–577.)

IASLC map for regional lymph nodes*

Zone	Side	Border	Anatomical structure
1		Upper	Lower margin of cricoid cartilage
1		Lower	Clavicles/manubrium
1		Left/right	Midline of trachea
2R	Right	Upper	Apex of right lung/upper border of manubrium
2R	Right	Lower	Intersection of caudal margin of innominate vein with trachea/ nodes to left lateral border of trachea
2L	Left	Upper	Apex of left lung/upper border of manubrium
2L	Left	Lower	Superior border of aortic arch
3a	Anterior	Upper	Apex of chest
3a	Anterior	Lower	Level of carina
3a	Anterior	Anterior	Posterior aspect of sternum
3a	Anterior	Posterior	Anterior border of superior vena cava
3a	Anterior	Upper	Apex of chest
3a	Anterior	Lower	Level of carina
3a	Anterior	Anterior	Posterior aspect of sternum
3a	Anterior	Posterior	Left carotid artery
3p	Posterior	Upper	Apex of chest
3p	Posterior	Lower	Carina
4R	Right	Para-/pretracheal—upper	Intersection of caudal margin of innominate vein with trachea
4R	Right	Right para-/pretracheal—lower	Lower border of azygos vein
4L	Left	Left paratracheal to lig. art.—upper	Upper margin of aortic arch
4L	Left	Left paratracheal to lig. art.—lower	Upper rim of left main pulmonary artery
5		Subaortic lateral to lig. art.—upper	Lower border of aortic arch
5		Subaortic lateral to lig. art.—lower	Upper rim of left main pulmonary artery
6		Anterior and lateral to ascending aorta and aortic—upper	Line tangential to upper border of aortic arch
6		Anterior and lateral to ascending aorta and aortic—lower	Lower border of aortic arch
7		Mediastinal subcarinal—upper	Carina of trachea
7	Right	Mediastinal subcarinal—lower	Lower border of bronchus intermedius
7	Left	Mediastinal subcarinal—lower	Upper border of lower lobe bronchus
8	Right	Paraoesophageal excluding subcarinal—upper	Lower border of bronchus intermedius
8	Left	Paraoesophageal excluding subcarinal—upper	Upper border of lower lobe bronchus
8		Paraoesophageal excluding subcarinal—lower	Diaphragm
9		Within pulmonary ligament incl. inf. pulm. vein—upper	Inferior pulmonary vein
9		Within pulmonary ligament incl. inf. pulm. vein—lower	Diaphragm
10	Right	Hilar—adjacent to mainstem bronchi and hilar vessels—upper	Lower rim of azygos vein
10	Left	Hilar—adjacent to mainstem bronchi and hilar vessels—lower	Upper rim of pulmonary artery
10		Hilar—adjacent to mainstem bronchi and hilar vessels	Interlobar region bilaterally
11	Right	Interlobar—superior subgroup	a#11s: between upper lobe bronchus and bronchus intermedius
11	Right	Interlobar—inferior subgroup	a#11i: between middle and lower lobe bronchi
11	Left	Interlobar	Between upper lobe bronchus and lower lobe bronchi
12		Lobar	Adjacent to lobar bronchi
13		Segmental	Adjacent to segmental bronchi
14		Subsegmental	Adjacent to subsegmental bronchi

*International lymph node map in the seventh edition of the TNM classification for lung cancer.

OESOPHAGEAL CANCER

T stage		
Tx	Tumour is not assessable	
T0	No primary tumour	
Tis	Carcinoma in situ; high grade dysplasia	
T1	Tumour invades the lamina propria, muscularis mucosae, or submucosa	
	T1a	Lamina propria or muscularis mucosae
	T1b	Submucosa
T2	Tumour invades the muscularis propria	
T3	Tumour invades the adventitia	
T4	Tumour invades adjacent structures	
	T4a	Involvement of the pleura, pericardium, diaphragm, or adjacent peritoneum
	T4b	Unresectable tumour involving other adjacent structures (e.g. aorta, vertebral body, or trachea)

N stage		
NX	Regional lymph nodes cannot be assessed	
N0	There is no regional nodal disease	
N1	There are regional nodal metastases	
	N1	1 to 2 regional lymph nodes
	N2	3 to 6 regional lymph nodes
	N3	>6 regional lymph nodes

M stage	
M0	There are no tumour metastases
M1	There are distant metastases

Oesophagogastric junction
- Cancers involving the esophagogastric junction (OGJ) that have their epicenter within the proximal 2 cm of the cardia (Siewert types I/II) are to be staged as esophageal cancers.
- Cancers whose epicenter is more than 2 cm distal from the OGJ, even if the OGJ is involved, will be staged using the stomach cancer TNM

STOMACH CANCER

T stage		
Tx	Primary tumour is not assessable	
T0	There is no evidence of primary tumour	
Tis	Carcinoma in situ	
T1	Tumour invades the lamina propria or submucosa	
	T1a	Invasion of the lamina propria or muscularis mucosae
	T1b	Invasion of the submucosa
T2	Tumour invades the muscularis propria	
T3	Tumour invades the subserosa without invading any adjacent structures	
T4	Tumour perforates the serosa or invades adjacent structures	
	T4a	Perforation of the serosa (visceral peritoneum)
	T4b	Invades adjacent structures

N stage		
Nx	The lymph nodes are not assessable	
N0	There is no regional nodal involvement	
N1	Tumour spread to 1–2 regional nodes	
N2	Tumour spread to 3–6 regional nodes	
N3	Tumour spread to ≥ 7 regional nodes	
	N3a	7–15 nodes
	N3b	≥ 16 nodes

M stage	
M0	There is no distant spread
M1	There is distant spread

RECTAL CANCER

T stage

Tx	Primary tumour is not assessable
T0	There is no evidence of a primary tumour
T1	Tumour invades the submucosa
T2	Tumour invades, but does not penetrate, the muscularis propria
T3	Tumour invades the subserosa (through the muscularis propria) ▶ there is no involvement of the neighbouring tissues or organs

	T3a	The tumour extends < 1 mm beyond the muscularis propria
	T3b	The tumour extends 1–5 mm beyond the muscularis propria
	T3c	The tumour extends > 5–15 mm beyond the muscularis propria
	T3d	The tumour extends > 15 mm beyond the muscularis propria

T4	Tumour invades the neighbouring tissues or organs ± perforates the visceral peritoneum
	T4a	Perforates the visceral peritoneum
	T4b	Directly invades neighbouring tissues or organs

N stage

Nx	Lymph nodes are not assessable
N0	There is no regional nodal involvement
N1	Involvement of 1–3 regional nodes

	N1a	1 regional node
	N1b	2–3 regional nodes
	N1c	Tumour within the subserosa, mesentery, or non-perionealized pericolic or perirectal tissues without regional nodal metastasis

N2	There are > 4 regional involved nodes
	N2a	4–6 regional nodes
	N2b	≥7 regional nodes

M stage

M0	There is no distant tumour spread
M1	There is distant tumour spread

	M1a	Metastasis confined to 1 organ
	M1b	Metastasis in more than one organ
	M1c	Metastasis to the peritoneum with or without other organ involvement

Definition of tumour deposit

Tumour deposits (satellites) are discrete macroscopic or microscopic nodules of cancer in the pericolorectal adipose tissue's lymph drainage area of a primary carcinoma that are discontinuous from the primary and without histological evidence of residual lymph node or identifiable vascular or neural structures. If a vessel wall is identifiable on H&E, elastic or other stains, it should be classified as venous invasion (V1/2) or lymphatic invasion (L1). Similarly, if neural structures are identifiable, the lesion should be classified as perineural invasion (Pn1). The presence of tumour deposits does not change the primary tumour T category, but changes the node status (N) to N1c if all regional lymph nodes are negative on pathological examination

ANAL CANCER

T stage

Tx	The primary tumour is not assessable
T0	No primary tumour
Tis	Carcinoma in situ
T1	Tumour ≤ 2 cm (greatest dimension)
T2	Tumour >2 cm but ≤ 5 cm (greatest dimension)
T3	Tumour > 5 cm (greatest dimension)
T4	Tumour of any size invades the adjacent organs (eg, vagina, urethra, bladder) • Direct invasion of the rectal wall, perirectal skin, subcutaneous tissue or sphincter muscle is NOT classified as T4

N stage

Nx	The lymph nodes are not assessable
N0	There is no regional nodal involvement
N1	Metastasis in regional lymph node (s)

	N1a	Metastases in inguinal, mesorectal, and/or internal iliac nodes
	N1b	Metastases in external iliac nodes
	N1c	Metastases in external iliac and inguinal, mesorectal and/or internal iliac nodes

M stage

M0	There is no distant metastasis
M1	Distant metastasis

COLON CANCER

T stage	
Tx	The primary tumour is not assessable
T0	No primary tumour
Tis	Carcinoma in situ
T1	Tumour invades the submucosa
T2	Tumour invades (but does not penetrate) the muscularis propria
T3	Tumour invades the subserosa (through the muscularis propria) ▶ there is no involvement of the neighbouring tissues or organs
T4	Tumour invades the neighbouring tissues or organs ± perforates the visceral peritoneum
	T4a	Tumour penetrates the visceral peritoneum
	T4b	Directly invades neighbouring tissues or organs

N stage	
Nx	The lymph nodes are not assessable
N0	There is no regional nodal involvement
N1	Involvement of 1–3 regional nodes
	N1a	1 regional node
	N1b	2–3 regional nodes
	N1c	Tumour within the subserosa, mesentery, or non-perionealized pericolic or perirectal tissues (without regional nodal metastasis)
N2	Involvement of ≥4 regional nodes
	N2a	4–6 regional nodes
	N2b	≥7 regional nodes

M stage	
M0	There is no distant metastasis
M1	Distant metastasis
	M1a	Metastasis confined to 1 organ
	M1b	Metastasis in more than one organ
	M1c	Metastasis to the peritoneum with or without other organ involvement

PANCREATIC CANCER

T stage	
Tx	Primary tumour cannot be assessed
T0	No evidence of tumour
Tis	Carcinoma in situ (a non-invasive flat carcinoma)
T1	Tumour confined to the pancreas (≤ 2 cm)
	T1a	Tumour < 0.5 cm
	T1b	Tumour > 0.5 cm and < 1 cm
	T1c	Tumour > 1 cm but < 2 cm
T2	Tumour confined to the pancreas (> 2 cm but < 4 cm)
T3	Tumour > 4 cm in greatest dimension
T4	Tumour involves the celiac axis, the superior mesenteric artery and/or common hepatic artery (unresectable)

N stage	
Nx	The lymph nodes are not assessable
N0	There is no regional nodal involvement
N1	Metastases in 1 to 3 nodes
N2	Metastases in 4 or more nodes

M stage	
M0	There is no distant spread
M1	There is distant spread

HEPATOCELLULAR CARCINOMA

T stage

Tx	The primary tumour is not assessable
T0	No tumour is present
T1	A single tumour (of any size) *without* blood vessel invasion
	T1a: Solitary tumour < 2 cm (greatest dimension) without vascular invasion
	T1b: Solitary tumour > 2 cm (greatest dimension) without vascular invasion
T2	A single tumour > 2 cm *with* vascular invasion or multiple tumours (none > 5 cm)
T3	Multiple tumours, any more > 5 cm
T4	Tumour(s) invading a major branch of the portal or hepatic vein with direct invasion of adjacent organs including the diaphragm (other than gallbladder) or with perforation of the visceral liver peritoneum

N stage

Nx	The lymph nodes are not assessable
N0	There is no regional nodal involvement
N1	There is regional nodal involvement

M stage

M0	There is no distant tumour spread
M1	There is distant tumour spread

Milan criteria for liver transplantation

1 tumour ≤ 5 cm in diameter, or
Up to 3 tumours ≤ 3 cm in diameter
+ No vascular invasion
+ No extrahepatic disease

Note

The TNM staging classification does not take into account the background liver function, which is often impaired in cirrhosis and will affect treatment options and prognosis. Other staging systems take into account both disease extent and liver function, but have not been compared accurately against one another:
- Barcelona Clinic Liver Cancer (BCLC) system
- Cancer of the Liver Italian Program (CLIP) system
- Okuda system

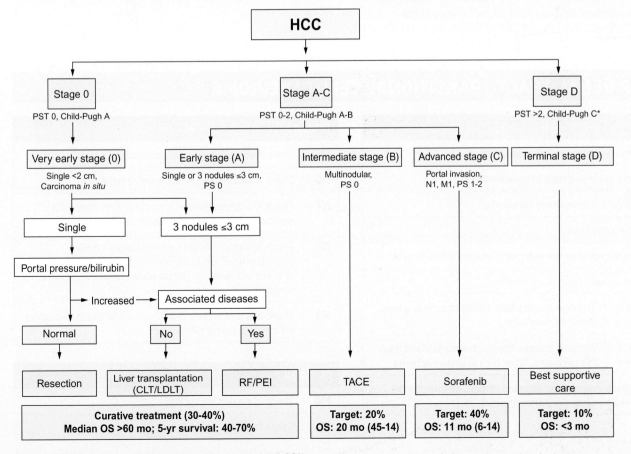

Updated BCLC staging system and treatment strategy, 2011.

RENAL CELL CARCINOMA

T stage		
Tx	The primary tumour is not assessable	
T0	There is no evidence of primary tumour	
T1	Tumour is limited to the kidney and ≤ 7 cm in size	
	T1a	*Tumour measuring ≤ 4 cm**
	T1b	*Tumour measuring > 4 cm but ≤ 7 cm**
T2	Tumour is limited to the kidney but measures > 7 cm*	
	T2a	*Tumour > 7 cm but ≤ 10 cm in greatest dimension, limited to the kidney*
	T2b	*Tumour > 10 cm, limited to the kidney*
T3	Tumour extends into the major veins or perinephric tissues (but not the ipsilateral adrenal gland or beyond Gerota's fascia)	
	T3a	*Tumour grossly extends into the renal vein, or invades the peri-renal fat and/or renal sinus fat (but not beyond Gerota's fascia)*
	T3b	*Tumour grossly extends into the infra-diaphragmatic IVC*
	T3c	*Tumour extends into the supradiaphragmatic IVC or invades the IVC wall*
T4	There is tumour extension beyond Gerota's fascia	

*Greatest dimension

N stage	
Nx	The lymph nodes are not assessable
N0	There is no regional nodal involvement
N1	Regional node metastasis

M stage	
M0	There is no distant spread
M1	There is distant spread

UPPER RENAL TRACT TRANSITIONAL CELL CARCINOMA

T stage		
Tx	Primary tumour is not assessable	
T0	There is no evidence of primary tumour	
Ta	Papillary non-invasive carcinoma	
Tis	Carcinoma in situ	
T1	Tumour invades the subepithelial connective tissues	
T2	Tumour invades the muscularis	
T3	Ureter	Tumour invades beyond the muscularis into the periureteric fat
	Renal pelvis	Tumour invades beyond the muscularis into the peripelvic fat or the renal parenchyma
T4	Tumour invades any adjacent organs, or through the kidney and into the perinephric fat	

N stage	
Nx	The lymph nodes are not assessable
N0	There is no regional nodal involvement
N1	There is a metastasis in a single lymph node which measures ≤ 2 cm in greatest dimension
N2	There is a metastasis in a single lymph node (measuring > 2 cm but ≤ 5 cm in greatest dimension) ▶ or there are multiple lymph nodes (measuring ≤ 5 cm in greatest dimension)
N3	There is a metastasis in a lymph node which measures > 5 cm in greatest dimension

M stage	
M0	There is no distant spread
M1	There is distant spread

BLADDER CANCER

T stage

Tx	Primary tumour cannot be assessed	
T0	No evidence of primary tumour	
Ta	Non-invasive papillary carcinoma	
Tis	Carcinoma in situ (non-invasive flat carcinoma)	
T1	Tumour invasion into the subepithelial connective tissue	
T2	Tumour invasion into the muscle	
	T2a	The inner half of the muscle layer is involved
	T2b	The outer half of muscle layer is involved
T3	Tumour invades the extravesical fat	
	T3a	Microscopic extravesical fat invasion
	T3b	Macroscopic extravesical fat invasion
T4	Involvement of adjacent structures	
	T4a	Tumour invades the prostate, uterus or vagina
	T4b	Tumour invades the pelvic or abdominal wall$^{\alpha}$

$^{\alpha}$including tumour extension to within 3 mm of the abdominal wall muscles (± obturator internus involvement)

N stage

Nx	The lymph nodes are not assessable
N0	No regional nodal involvement
N1	A single regiona l lymph node metastasis within the true pelvis*
N2	Multiple regiona l lymph node metastases within the true pelvis*
N3	Common iliac lymph node metastases

*Hypogastric, obturator, external iliac, or presacral lymph nodes

M stage

M0	No distant spread	
M1	Distant spread	
	M1a	Non regional lymph nodes
	M1b	Other distant metastasis

PROSTATE CANCER

T stage

Tx	Primary tumour is not assessable	
T0	There is no evidence of primary tumour	
T1	Tumour is not clinically palpable or detected with imaging	
	T1a	An incidental histological finding in ≤ 5% of resected tissue (e.g. TURP)
	T1b	An incidental histological finding in > 5% of resected tissue (e.g. TURP)
	T1c	Tumour is identified by needle biopsy
T2	Prostate-confined tumour which is clinically palpable or detected with imaging	
	T2a	Tumour involves ≤ ½ of one prostate lobe
	T2b	Tumour involves > ½ of one prostate lobe (but not both lobes)
	T2c	Tumour involves both lobes
T3	There is tumour extension through the prostate capsule	
	T3a	Unilateral or bilateral tumour extension through the prostate capsule
	T3b	Seminal vesical involvement
T4	Tumour invades structures other than the seminal vesicles (e.g. the bladder neck, rectum, or pelvic wall)	

N stage

Nx	The lymph nodes are not assessable
N0	There is no tumour spread
N1	There is tumour spread to one or more regional pelvic nodes

M stage

M0	There is no tumour spread beyond the regional pelvic nodes	
M1	There is tumour spread beyond the regional pelvic nodes	
	M1a	Tumour spread to nodes outside of the pelvis
	M1b	Tumour spread to bones
	M1c	Tumour spread to other organs (e.g. lung, liver and brain) ± bone involvement

AMERICAN COLLEGE OF RADIOLOGY PI-RADS

Scoring systems

Score criteria

T2WI for peripheral zone

1   Uniform high signal intensity
2   Linear, wedge-shaped, or geographic areas of lower SI, usually not well demarcated
3   Heterogeneous signal intensity or non-circumscribed, rounded, moderate hypointensity. Or other not in categories 1/2 or 4/5
4   Circumscribed, homogeneous moderate hypointense focus/mass confined to prostate and <1.5 cm in greatest dimension
5   Same as 4 but ≥1.5 cm in greatest dimension or definite ECE/invasive behaviour

T2WI for transition zone

1   Heterogeneous intermediate SI
2   Circumscribed hypointense or heterogeneous encapsulated nodule(s) (BPH)
3   Heterogeneous signal intensity with obscured margins. Or other not in categories 1/2 or 4/5
4   Lenticular or non-circumscribed, homogeneous, moderately hypointense, and <1.5 cm in greatest dimension
5   Same as 4, but ≥1.5 cm in greatest dimension or definite ECE/invasive behaviour

DWI

1   No abnormality (i.e. normal) on ADC and high b-value DWI
2   Indistinct hypointense on ADC
3   Focal mildly/moderately hypointense on ADC and isointense/mildly hyperintense on high b-value DWI
4   Focal markedly hypointense on ADC and markedly hyperintense on high b-value DWI; <1.5 cm in greatest dimension
5   Same as 4 but ≥1.5 cm in greatest dimension or definite ECE/invasive behaviour

Dynamic contrast-enhanced MRI

- No early enhancement **OR**
   Diffuse enhancement not corresponding to a focal fingding on T2 and/or DWI **OR**
   Focal enhancement corresponding to a lesion demonstrating features of BPH on T2WI
+ Focal **AND**
   Earlier than or contemporaneously with enhancement of adjacent normal prostatic tissues **AND** Corresponds to suspicious finding on T2 and/or DWI

PI-RADS v2, Prostate Imaging—Reporting and Data System version 2; T2WI, T2-weighted imaging; SI, signal intensity; ECE, extra-capsular extension; BPH, benign prostatic hypertrophy; ADC, apparent diffusion coefficient; DWI, diffusion-weighted imaging; MRI, magnetic resonance imaging.

Guidance for overall score

Peripheral zone				Transition zone			
DWI score (dominant sequence)	DCE score (secondary sequence)	T2WI score	Overall PI-RADS v2 score	DWI score (dominant sequence)	DCE score (secondary sequence)	DCE score	Overall PI-RADS v2 score
1	Any	Any	1	1	Any	Any	1
2	Any	Any	2	2	Any	Any	2
3	-	Any	3	3	≤4	Any	3
3	+	Any	4	3	5	Any	4
4	Any	Any	4	4	Any	Any	4
5	Any	Any	5	5	Any	Any	5

PI-RADS v2, Prostate imaging—Reporting and Data System version 2; T2WI, T2-weighted imaging; DWI, diffusion-weighted imaging; DCE dynamic contrast-enhanced.

NEUROBLASTOMA

International neuroblastoma staging system

Stage 1	Localized tumour confined to the area of origin ▶ complete gross resection, with or without microscopic residual disease ▶ identifiable ipsilateral and contralateral lymph nodes which are negative microscopically
Stage 2A	Localized tumour with an incomplete gross excision ▶ identifiable ipsilateral and contralateral lymph nodes which are negative microscopically
Stage 2B	Unilateral tumour with complete or incomplete gross resection with positive ipsilateral regional lymph nodes ▶ the contralateral lymph nodes are negative microscopically
Stage 3	Unresectable tumour infiltrating across the midline with or without regional lymph node involvement ▶ a unilateral tumour with contralateral regional lymph node involvement, or a midline tumour with bilateral regional lymph node involvement
Stage 4	Dissemination of tumour to distant lymph nodes, bones, bone marrow, liver, skin or other organs (except as defined in Stage 4S)
Stage 4S	Localized primary tumour (as defined for Stages 1, 2A or 2B) with dissemination limited to the skin, liver, or bone marrow (< 10% tumour cells, and a negative marrow meta-iodobenzylguanidine scintigram). This is limited to infants younger than 1 year old

ENDOMETRIAL CARCINOMA

FIGO staging of endometrial carcinoma with corresponding MR findings

FIGO stage	Description of stage	MRI findings
Stage I	Tumour confined to the corpus uteri	
Ia	Tumour extending to <50% of myometrial depth	Abnormal signal intensity extends into <50% of the myometrium
Ib	Tumour extending to ≥50% of myometrial depth	Abnormal signal intensity extends into ≥50% of the myometrium
Stage II	Tumour invades cervical stroma, but does not extend beyond the uterus	Disruption of low signal intensity cervical stroma by tumour. A widened internal os with tumour protruding into the endocervical canal does not represent stromal invasion
Stage III	Local and/or regional spread of the tumour	
IIIa*	Tumour invades the serosa of the corpus uteri and/or adnexa	Disruption of continuity of outer myometrium. Irregular uterine configuration
IIIb	Vaginal and/or parametrial involvement	Segmental loss of hypointense vaginal wall
IIIc	Metastases to pelvic and/or para-aortic lymph nodes	Regional or para-aortic nodes >1 cm in short-axis diameter. Additional suspicious features include multiple small rounded lymph nodes, irregular lymph node contour, abnormal signal intensity similar to that of the primary tumour, presence of necrosis
IIIc1	Positive pelvic nodes	
IIIc2	Positive para-aortic lymph nodes ± positive pelvic lymph nodes	
Stage IV	Tumour invades bladder and/or bowel mucosa, and/or distant metastases	
IVa	Tumour invades bladder and/or bowel mucosa (biopsy proven)	Abnormal signal intensity disrupts normal low signal intensity bladder/rectal mucosa. Note that bullous oedema does not indicate stage IVa
IVb	Distant metastases, including intra-abdominal metastases and/or inguinal lymph nodes	Tumour in distant sites or organs

*Positive cytology obtained at peritoneal washings should be recorded but does not alter any stage.

CERVICAL CANCER

Stage 1	*Tumour confined to the cervix (extension into the uterine body is disregarded)*		
	Stage IA	*This is a microscopic diagnosis*	
		Stage IAI	*Area of invasion: ≤ 3 mm deep ▶ ≤ 7 mm wide*
		Stage IA2	*Area of invasion: > 3 mm but not > 5 mm deep ▶ ≤ 7 mm wide*
	Stage IB	*Macroscopically visible or a microscopic lesion*	
		Stage IB1	*Macroscopically visible: ≤ 4 cm (greatest dimension)*
		Stage IB2	*Macroscopically visible: > 4 cm (greatest dimension)*
Stage II	*Tumour extension beyond the uterus, but not to the pelvic wall or lower ⅓ of the vagina*		
	Stage IIA	*No parametrial invasion*	
		Stage IIA1	*Macroscopically: ≤ 4 cm (greatest dimension)*
		Stage IIA2	*Macroscopically visible: > 4 cm (greatest dimension)*
	Stage IIB	*Parametrial tumour invasion*	
Stage III	*Tumour extension to the lower ⅓ of the vagina or pelvic wall, or tumour that causes hydronephrosis (or a non-functioning kidney)*		
	Stage IIIA	*Involvement of the lower ⅓ of the vagina*	
	Stage IIIB	*Pelvic wall invasion (± hydronephrosis or a non-functioning kidney)*	
Stage IV	*Spread to the adjacent organs or distant tumour spread*		
	Stage IVA	*Spread to the adjacent organs (e.g. the bladder or rectum)*	
	Stage IVB	*Distant tumour spread*	
Classified according to the FIGO classification (clinical not surgical staging)			

FIGO staging of cervical carcinoma with corresponding MR findings		
FIGO stage	**Description of stage**	**MRI findings**
Stage I	The carcinoma is strictly confined to the cervix	
Ia	Invasive carcinoma which can be diagnosed only by microscopy, with deepest invasion <5 mm and largest extension >7 mm	MRI is not indicated in stage Ia as tumour is not seen (except in cases considered for fertility sparing surgery such as trachelectomy)
Ia1	Measured stromal invasion of <3 mm in depth and extension <7 mm	
Ia2	Measured stromal invasion of >3 mm and not >5 mm with an extension of not >7 mm	
Ib	Clinically visible lesions limited to the cervix uteri or preclinical cancers greater than stage Ia	Intermediate signal intensity mass on T2WI. MRI can accurately delineate the tumour and its location and provide accurate size measurement (including distance from the internal os and cervical length in cases considered for trachelectomy)
Ib1	Clinically visible lesions <4 cm in greatest dimension	
Ib2	Clinically visible lesions >4 cm in greatest dimension	
Stage II	Cervical carcinoma invades beyond the uterus, but not to the pelvic wall or to the lower third of the vagina	Accurate evaluation of tumour location and tumour size. Invasion of the upper two-thirds of vagina is indicated by disruption of the low signal intensity vaginal wall by high signal intensity tumour on T2WI
IIa	Without parametrial invasion	
IIa1	Clinically visible lesion <4 cm in greatest dimension	
IIa2	Clinically visible lesion >4 cm in greatest dimension	
IIb	With obvious parametrial invasion	Parametrial invasion is indicated by disruption of the low signal intensity stromal ring, presence of a spiculated tumour/parametrium interface, gross nodular tumour extension into the parametrium or encasement of the uterine vessels by tumour
Stage III	The tumour extends to the pelvic wall and/or involves the lower third of the vagina and/or causes hydronephrosis or non-functioning kidney	
IIIa	Tumour involves lower third vagina, no extension to pelvic wall	Invasion of the lower third of vagina is indicated by disruption of the low signal intensity vaginal wall by high signal intensity tumour on T2WI
IIIb	Extension to the pelvic wall and/or hydronephrosis/non-functioning kidney	Pelvic side-wall invasion is indicated by tumour extension within 3 mm of pelvic side wall. Hydronephrosis is an indication of ureteral and/or bladder invasion
Stage IV	The carcinoma has extended beyond the true pelvis or has involved (biopsy proven) the mucosa of the bladder or rectum	Bladder or rectal invasion is indicated by loss of perivesical/perirectal fat planes and disruption of the normal low signal intensity bladder/rectal mucosa. Note that bullous oedema does not indicate stage IVa
IVa	Spread to adjacent organs	
IVb	Distant metastases (including intra-abdominal metastases) and/or inguinal lymph nodes	Tumour in distant sites or organs

T2WI, T2-weighted image.

OVARIAN CARCINOMA

Stage I (T1N0M0)	Tumour is limited to the ovaries (one or both)	
	Stage IA (T1a)	**Tumour limited to 1 ovary or fallopian tube** *Intact capsule; tumour is not present on the outer ovarian surface; there are no tumour cells seen within either ascites or peritoneal washings*
	Stage IB (T1b)	**Tumour present within both ovaries** *Intact capsule; tumour is not present on the outer ovarian surface; there are no tumour cells seen within either ascites or peritoneal washings*
	Stage IC1 (T1c1)	**Surgical spill**
	Stage iC2 (T1c2)	**Capsule ruptured before surgery or tumour on surface of ovary or tube**
	Stage IC3 (T1c3)	**Malignant cells in ascites or peritoneal washings**
Stage II (T2N0M0)	Pelvic extension below pelvic brim or primary peritoneal cancer	
	Stage IIA (T2a)	**Tumour invades (± implants on) the uterus, fallopian tubes or ovary(ies)**
	Stage IIB (T2b)	**Spread to other pelvic organs**
Stage III (T3M0 ± N1)	Peritoneal metastasis beyond pelvis and/or regional lymph node metastasis	
	Stage IIIA1 (T1/2N1)	**Retroperitoneal lymph nodes only**
	Stage IIIA2 (T3a)	**Microscopic peritoneal metastasis**
	Stage IIIB (T3b)	**Macroscopic peritoneal metastasis (≤ 2 cm)**
	Stage IIIC (T3c)	**Peritoneal metastasis > 2 cm**
Stage IV (Any T, Any N, M1)	Distant metastases (excluding peritoneal metastases)	
	Stage IVA	Pleural effusion positive cytology
	Stage IVB	Parenchymal metastases
Classified according to the FIGO classification (TNM staging in brackets)		

FIGO staging of ovarian carcinoma with corresponding CT findings

FIGO stage	Description of stage	CT findings
Stage I	Tumour limited to ovaries (one/both)	
Ia	Tumour limited to one ovary, capsule intact, no tumour on ovarian surface, no malignant cells in ascites or peritoneal washings[a]	Enlarged or normal ovary and ascites may be present
Ib	Tumour limited to both ovaries, capsule intact, no tumour on ovarian surface, no malignant cells in ascites or peritoneal washings[a]	Enlarged or normal ovaries and ascites may be present
Ic	Tumour limited to one or both ovaries with any of the following: capsular rupture, tumour on ovarian surface, malignant cells in ascites or peritoneal washings[a]	Unilateral or bilateral mixed cystic/solid or solid adnexal mass with irregular contour, heterogeneous enhancement of solid components and thick septa. Ascites
Stage II	Tumour involves one or both ovaries with pelvic extensions or implants	
IIa	Tumour extension and/or implants on uterus/fallopian tube(s), no malignant cells in ascites or peritoneal washings[a]	Irregularity or obliteration of the fat plane between the uterus and the adnexal mass. Dilated fallopian tubes which may contain enhancing soft-tissue nodules. Ascites
IIb	Tumour extension and/or implants on other pelvic tissue, no malignant cells in ascites or peritoneal washings	Loss of the normal fat plane around the rectum or bladder, less than 3 mm between the tumour and the pelvic side wall, and/or displacement or encasement of the iliac vessels. Ascites
Stage III	Tumour involves one or both ovaries with microscopically confirmed peritoneal metastasis outside the pelvis	
IIIa	Microscopically confirmed peritoneal metastasis[b] outside the pelvis (no macroscopic tumour)	Microscopic extra-pelvic peritoneal implants are not detectable with CT
IIIb	Macroscopically peritoneal metastasis outside the pelvis is 2 cm or less in dimension	Peritoneal/serosal deposits <2 cm outside the pelvis
IIIc	Macroscopically peritoneal metastasis outside the pelvis is >2 cm and/or involved regional lymph nodes	Peritoneal implants of >2 cm. Omental cake. Note that subcapsular liver implants and those along the diaphragm, lesser sac, porta hepatis, intersegmental fissure, gall bladder fossa; gastrosplenic, gastrohepatic ligament and small bowel mesentery are 'difficult to resect'. Enlarged inguinal and retroperitoneal lymph nodes
Stage IV	Distant metastasis beyond the peritoneal cavity. Enlarged lymph nodes above the level of the renal hilum	Liver parenchymal metastases, pleural effusion.[c] Enlarged lymph nodes above the level of the renal hilum

[a] The presence of ascites does not affect staging unless malignant cells are present.
[b] Liver capsule metastasis is stage III; liver parenchymal metastasis is stage IV.
[c] Stage IV: pleural effusion must have positive cytology.

INDEX

Page numbers followed by '*f*' indicate figures, '*t*' indicate tables, and '*b*' indicate boxes.

D